369 0077133

KU-279-091

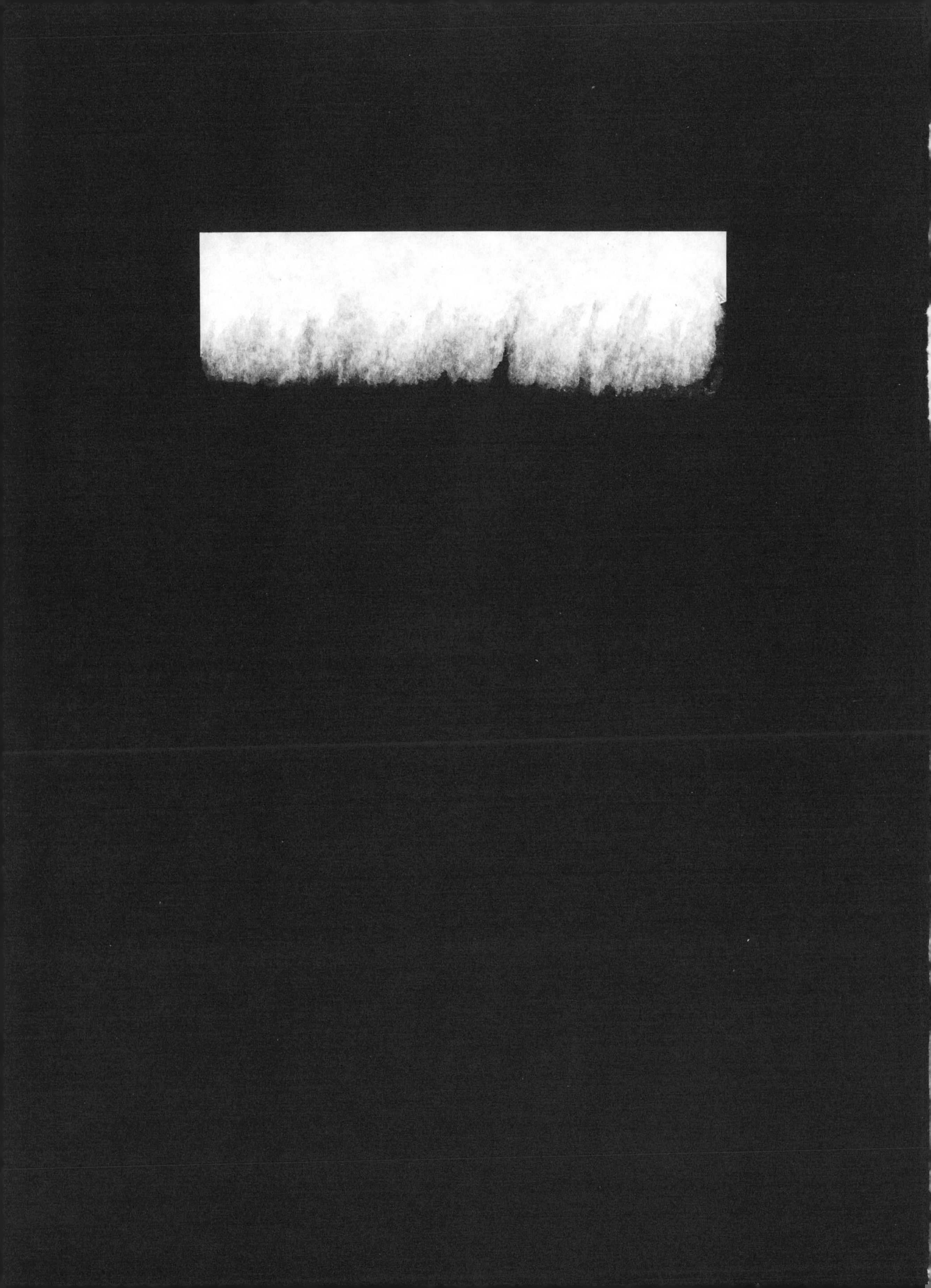

Estrogens and Progestogens in Clinical Practice

DEDICATIONS

'In general, Estrogen is the hormone of the woman, it assures the development of the genital and mammary apparatus; progesterone is the hormone of the mother, it is indispensable for reproduction.'

Robert Courrier; *Biologie Des Hormones Sexuelles Femelles*, 1937 (translation)

To Dorothy, Lindsay, Gael and Rowan
Ian S Fraser

To Diana, Wendy, Alice, Peter and Christopher
Robert P S Jansen

To Jessie, Maggie and Ross
Rogerio A Lobo

To Oliver and Barnaby for painting and crayoning the proofs so beautifully
Malcolm I Whitehead

Estrogens and Progestogens in Clinical Practice

Edited by

Ian S Fraser MD BSc(Hons) FRACOG FRCOG CREI
Professor in Reproductive Medicine, Department of Obstetrics and Gynaecology, Sydney Centre for Reproductive Health Research, Queen Elizabeth II Research Institute for Mothers and Infants, University of Sydney, Sydney, Australia

Associate Editors

Robert P S Jansen MD (Syd) BS Bsc(Med) FRACP FRACOG CREI
Medical Director Sydney IVF, Professor Department of Reproductive Endocrinology and Infertility, University of Sydney, Sydney, Australia

Rogerio A Lobo MD
Professor and Chairman, Department of Obstetrics and Gynecology, Sloane Hospital for Women, Columbia University, New York, USA

Malcolm I Whitehead MD FRCOG
Consultant Gynaecologist, The Menopause Clinic, King's College Hospital, Denmark Hill, London, UK

Foreword by

Daniel R Mishell Jr
Lyle G McNeil Professor of Obstetrics and Gynecology, University of Southern California School of Medicine, Women's and Childrens Hospital, Los Angeles, California, USA

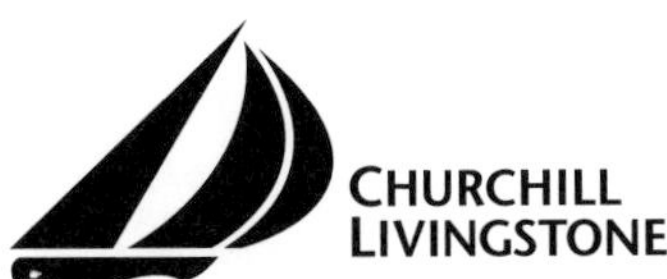

LONDON EDINBURGH NEW YORK PHILADELPHIA SAN FRANCISCO SYDNEY 1998

CHURCHILL LIVINGSTONE
A division of Harcourt Brace & Co Limited

ISBN 0 443 04706 5

British Library Cataloguing in Publication Data
A catalogue record for this book is available from the British Library.

Library of Congress Cataloging in Publication Data
A catalog record for this book is available from the Library of Congress.

Printed in China
NPCC/01

Contents

Color plates follow prelims

Hormonal contraception

Menopause

Cancer of reproductive organs

Metabolic actions and long term side-effects of therapeutic steroids used for contraception, hormone replacement and gynecologic disease

Contributors

Mats Åkerlund MD
Professor of Obstetrics and Gynaecology
Department of Obstetrics and Gynaecology
University Hospital, Lund, Sweden

R A Atkinson MBBS MRCS LRCP FRCA
Consultant Pain Clinician, Director of Pain Services, Royal Hallamshire Hospital, Sheffield, UK

David T Baird DSc FRCOG FRCP
Professor of Reproductive Biology, MRC Clinical Research Centre for Reproductive Biology, University of Edinburgh, Edinburgh, UK

Robert L Barbieri MD
Department of Obstetrics and Gynecology
Brigham and Women's Hospital, Boston, Massachusetts, USA

Patrick L Blohm MD
Associate Professor, Department of Obstetrics and Gynecology, Duke University Medical Center, Durham, North Carolina, USA

Phillipe Bouchard MD
Professor and Chairman of Endocrinology, Hôpital Saint Antoine and University Pierre and Marie Curie, Paris, France

Mark P Brincat MRCS LRCP PhD (Lon) MRCOG
Dean, Faculty of Medicine and Surgery, Department of Obstetrics and Gynaecology, University of Malta Medical School, Gwardamangia, Malta

Charles G D Brook MA MD FRCP FRCPCH
Professor of Paediatric Endocrinology, Director of London Centre for Paediatric Endocrinology, Department of Endocrinology, University College London, London, UK

P R Brzechffa MD
Center for Health Sciences, University of California, Los Angeles, California, USA

Henry G Burger MD FRACP FRACOG FRCP(Lon) FCP(SA) AO FAA
Director, Prince Henry's Institute of Medical Research, Monash Medical Centre, Monash University, Clayton, Victoria, Australia

Iain T Cameron BSc MD MRCOG MRACOG
Regius Professor of Obstetrics and Gynaecology, University of Glasgow, The Queen Mother's Hospital, Yorkhill, Glasgow, UK

Bruce R Carr BS MD
Paul C MacDonald Professor of Obstetrics and Gynecology, Division of Reproductive Endocrinology, The University of Texas, Southwestern Medical Center, Dallas, Texas, USA

David S Celemajer MBBS PhD FRACP
Associate Professor of Medicine, Consultant Cardiologist, University of Sydney, Royal Prince Alfred Hospital, Camperdown, New South Wales, Australia

Nathalie Chabbert-Buffet MD
Chef de Clinique-Assistante, Department of Endocrinology, Hôpital Saint Antoine and University Pierre and Marie Curie, Paris, France

John R G Challis MD
Chairman, Department of Physiology, Faculty of Medicine, University of Toronto, Toronto, Canada

Claus Christiansen MD
Centre of Clinical and Basic Research, Ballerup, Denmark

John A Collins MD
Department of Obstetrics and Gynecology, Department of Epidemiology and Biostatistics, Faculty of Health Sciences, McMaster University, Hamilton, Ontario, Canada

William P Collins DSc FRCOG
Professor of Reproductive Biochemistry, Department of Steroid Biochemistry, King's College Hospital, Denmark Hill, London, UK

Elizabeth B Connell MD
Department of Obstetrics and Gynecology, Emory University School of Medicine, Atlanta, Georgia, USA

Ian D Cooke MD FRCOG
Professor and Head, Department of Obstetrics and Gynaecology, Jessop Hospital for Women, Sheffield, UK

Sybil L Crawford PhD
Senior Research Scientist, New England Research Institute, Watertown, Massachusetts, USA

Hilary O D Critchley BSc MBChB MD MRCOG FRACOG
Senior Lecturer in Obstetrics and Gynaecology, Centre for Reproductive Biology, University of Edinburgh, Edinburgh, UK

David Crook PhD
Senior Research Fellow, Department of Cardiovascular Biochemistry, St Bartholomew's Hospital, Medical College London, London, UK

Phillip D Darney MD MSc
Professor in Residence and Attending Gynecologist, Department of Obstetrics, Gynecology and Reproductive Sciences, University of California, San Francisco, California, USA

M Dattani MBBS MRCP
London Centre for Paediatric Endocrinology, Department of Endocrinology, University College London, London, UK

Graham C Davies MBBS MDMRCOG
Clinical Research Physician, Eli Lilly and Co Ltd, Basingstoke, UK

Lorraine Dennerstein MBBS PhD DPM FRANZCP
Director, Office for Gender and Health, Department of Psychiatry, University of Melbourne, Victoria, Australia

Egon Diczfalusy MD PhD FRCOG FACOG(Hons)
Professor Emeritus, Karolinska Institutet, Stockholm, Sweden

John A Eden MD FRACOG CREI
Associate Professor, University of New South Wales, Frank Rundle House, Royal Hospital for Women, Paddington, New South Wales, Australia

Richard A Edgren BS MS PhD
Consultant, 50 Oakhaven Way, Woodside, California, USA

John A Edwards PhD
Vice-President and Director Emeritus, Institute of Organic Chemistry, Syntex Research, Palo Alto, California, USA

Johann W Faigle
Emeritus Senior Research Associate, Department of Research and Development, Pharmaceuticals Division, Ciba-Geigy Ltd, Basel, Switzerland

Juan C Felix MD
Associate Professor of Pathology, Obstetrics and Gynecology, Department of Pathology, University of Southern California Medical Center, Los Angeles, California, USA

Ian S Fentiman MD FRCS
Professor of Surgical Oncology Unit, Hedley Atkins Breast Unit, Guy's Hospital, London, UK

L A Fitzpatrick MD
Professor of Medicine, Division of Endocrinology and Internal Medicine, Mayo Clinic and Mayo Foundation, Rochester, Minnesota, USA

M Formosa
Faculty of Medicine and Surgery, Department of Obstetrics and Gynaecology, University of Malta Medical School, Gwardamangia, Malta

Ian S Fraser MD BSc(Hons) FRACOG FRCOG CREI
Department of Obstetrics and Gynaecology, Professor in Reproductive Medicine, Sydney Centre for Reproductive Health Research, Queen Elizabeth II Research Institute for Mothers and Infants, University of Sydney, Sydney, Australia

Mark A Fritz MD
Professor, School of Medicine, University of North Carolina, Chapel Hill, North Carolina, USA

Ian F Godsland BA PhD
Senior Lecturer, Department of Metabolic Medicine, Division of Medicine, Imperial College School of Medicine, National Heart and Lung Institute, London, UK

Joseph W Goldzieher MD FACE FACOG
Distinguished Professor, Department of Obstetrics and Gynecology, Texas Tech University, Health Sciences Center, Amarillo, Texas, USA

Charles B Hammond MD FACOG
EC Hamblen Professor and Chairman Department of Obstetrics and Gynecology, Duke University Medical Center, Durham, North Carolina, USA

Susan E Hankinson MD
Department of Epidemiology and Nutrition, Harvard School of Public Health, Harvard Medical School and Brigham's Women's Hospital, Boston, Massachusetts, USA

David L Healy FRACOG PhD
Chairman of Monash University Department of Obstetrics and Gynaecology, Monash Medical Centre, Clayton, Victoria, Australia

Milan Henzl MD PhD
Clinical Professor, Department of Obstetrics and Gynecology, Stanford University School of Medicine, Stanford, California, USA

Martha Hickey MD BA(Hons) MBChB MRCOG
Clinical Lecturer, Department of Obstetrics and Gynaecology, Imperial College of Science Technology and Medicine, St Mary's Hospital, Paddington, London, UK

Stephen G Hillier PhD DSc FRCPath
Professor of Reproductive Medicine, Centre for Reproductive Biology, University of Edinburgh, Edinburgh, UK

William H Hindle MD
Professor of Clinical Obstetrics and Gynecology, University of Southern California Medical School, Director, Breast Diagnostic Center, Women's and Children's Hospital, Los Angeles, California, USA

Tamas Horvath DVM
Assistant Professor, Department of Obstetrics and Gynecology, Yale University School of Medicine, New Haven, Connecticut, USA

Myra Hunter BA(Hons) DipClinPsy PhD AFBP(S)
Clinical Psychologist/Senior Lecturer, Sub-Department of Clinical Health Psychology, University College London, London, UK

Peter J Illingworth MBChB MD(Hon) MRCOG FRACOG
Director of Reproductive Endocrinology and Infertility, Westmead Fertility Centre, Westmead Hospital, Westmead, New South Wales, Australia

Robert P S Jansen MD (Syd) BS BSc(Med) FRACP FRACOG CREI
Medical Director Sydney IVF, Professor, Department of Reproductive Endocrinology, and Infertility, University of Sydney, Sydney, Australia

Shawna Johnston MD FRCSC
Assistant Professor of Urogynaecology, Queen's University, Kingston, Ontario, Canada

Warren R Jones AO MD PhD FRACOG FRCOG
Emeritus Professor and Senior Visiting Specialist, Department of Obstetrics and Gynaecology, Flinders Medical Centre, Bedford Park, South Australia, Australia

Henrik L Jørgensen MD
Senior Physician, Centre for Clinical and Basic Research, Ballerup, Denmark

Howard L Judd MD
Center for Health Sciences, University of California, Los Angeles, California, USA

Raymond H Kaufman MD
Department of Obstetrics and Gynaecology, Baylor College of Medicine, Houston, Texas, USA

William R Keye Jr MD
Division of Reproductive Endocrinology and Infertility, William Beaumont Hospital, Royal Oak, Michigan, USA

Sundeep Khosla MD
Associate Professor, Division of Endocrinology, Metabolism, Nutrition, and Internal Medicine, Mayo Clinic and Foundation, Rochester, Minnesota, USA

Gabor T Kovacs MD FRCOG FRACOG CREI
Professor of Obstetrics and Gynaecology, Monash Medical School, Monash University, Clayton, Victoria, Australia

Robert J Kurman MD
Professor of Pathology, Department of Pathology, USC Medical Center, Los Angeles, California, USA

Bruce A Lessey PhD MD
Associate Professor, School of Medicine, University of North Carolina, Chapel Hill, North Carolina, USA

Lih-Mei Liao BSc(Hon) MSc PhD AFB(S)
Clinical Psychologist, Sub-Department of Clinical Health Psychology, University College London, London, UK

Christopher Longcope MD
Professor of Medicine and Obstetrics and Gynecology, University of Massachusetts Medical School, Worcester, Massachusetts, USA

Rogerio A Lobo
Professor and Chairman, Department of Obstetrics and Gynecology, Sloane Hospital for Women, Columbia University, New York, USA

S J Lye MD
Department of Physiology, Faculty of Medicine, University of Toronto, Toronto, Canada

Mary Ann Lumsden MD MRCOG
Senior Lecturer in Obstetrics and Gynaecology, University of Glasgow, Queen Mother's Hospital, Glasgow, UK

Jane R McCrohon MBBS FRACP
Department of Cardiology, Royal Prince Alfred Hospital, Camperdown, New South Wales, Australia

Donald P McDonnell PhD
Associate Professor, Director of Graduate Studies, Department of Pharmacology and Cancer Biology, Duke University Medical Center, Durham, North Carolina, USA

Sonja M McKinlay PhD
President, New England Research Institutes Inc, New England Research Institute, Watertown, Massachusetts, USA

Alan S McNeilly BSc PhD DSc FRSE
MRC Reproductive Biology Unit, University of Edinburgh, Edinburgh, UK

Sophie Christin-Maître MD
Department of Endocrinology, Hôpital Saint Antoine and University Pierre and Marie Curie, Paris, France

Phillip L Matson BSc(Hons) PhD
Scientific Director, Concept Fertility Centre, King Edward Memorial Hospital, Subiaco, Westmead, Australia

L Joseph Melton III MD
Michael Eisenberg Professor, Mayo Clinic and Mayo Foundation, Rochester, Minnesota, USA

Virginia M Miller PhD
Professor of Surgery and Physiology, Department of Surgery, Mayo Clinic, Rochester, Minnesota, USA

Frederic Naftolin MD DPhil FACOG FRCOG
Professor and Chairman/Professor of Biology, Department of Obstetrics and Gynecology, Center for Research in Reproductive Biology, Yale University, New Haven, Connecticut, USA

Jane E Norman MD MRCOG
Senior Lecturer, Department of Obstetrics and Gynaecology, Glasgow Royal Infirmary, Glasgow, UK

Robert Norman MBChB(Hons) MD FRACOG FRCPA CREI
Associate Professor, Department of Obstetrics and Gynaecology, University of Adelaide, Queen Elizabeth Hospital, Woodville, Adelaide, Australia

Olusegun A Odukoya MBBS FMCOG(Nig) MRCOG FWACS MD
Clinical Lecturer, Department of Obstetrics and Gynaecology, Jessop Hospital for Women, University of Sheffield, Sheffield, UK

Nicholas Panay BSc MRCOG MFFP
Specialist Registrar, Department of Obstetrics and Gynaecology, Chelsea and Westminster Hospital, London, UK

Greg Phillipson MBChB FRNZCOG FRACOG CREI
Specialist in Reproductive Endocrinology and Infertility, Deputy Director, New Zealand Centre for Reproductive Medicine, Christchurch Women's Hospital, Christchurch, New Zealand

Tibor Polcz MD
Department of Obstetrics and Gynecology, Center for Research in Reproductive Biology, Yale University, New Haven, Connecticut, USA

Y S Prakash PhD
Research Associate, Department of Anesthesia, Mayo Clinic and Mayo Foundation, Rochester, Minnesota, USA

Phillipa A Ramsay MBBS FRACOG COGU
Department of Foetal Medicine and Ultrasound, King George V Memorial Hospital, Camperdown, New South Wales, Australia

Peter A Rogers PhD
Principal Research Fellow, Department of Obstetrics and Gynaecology, Monash Medical Centre, Clayton, Victoria, Australia

Robert H Sands MRCOG
Medical Adviser, Organon Laboratories Ltd, Cambridge, UK

G C Sieck PhD
Professor of Anesthesia, Department of Anesthesia, Mayo Clinic and Mayo Foundation, Rochester, Minnesota, USA

Lotte Schenkel MD (deceased)
Formerly Emeritus Senior Research Associate, Research and Development Department, Pharmaceuticals Division, CIBA-GEIGY, Basel, Switzerland

James J Schlesselman PhD
Department of Epidemiology and Public Health, Sylvester Comprehensive Cancer Center, University of Miami, Florida, USA

Joe Leigh Simpson MD
Chairman, Professor of Molecular and Human Genetics, Department of Obstetrics and Gynaecology, Baylor College of Medicine, Houston, Texas, USA

Frank Z Stanczyk MD
Professor of Research, Department of Obstetrics and Gynecology, University of Southern California Women's and Children's Hospital, Los Angeles, California, USA

Stuart Stanton FRCS FRCOG
Professor of Urogynaecology and Pelvic Floor Reconstruction, Urogynaecology Unit, Department of Obstetrics and Gynaecology, St George's Hospital Medical School, London, UK

Meir Stampfer MD PhD
Professor of Epidemiology and Nutrition, Harvard School of Public Health, Harvard Medical School and Brigham's Women's Hospital, Boston, Massachusetts, USA

John W W Studd DSc MD FRCOG
Consultant Gynaecologist, Department of Obstetrics and Gynaecology, Chelsea and Westminster Hospital, London, UK

Beverley J Vollenhoven PhD FRACOG CREI
Senior Lecturer, Department of Obstetrics and Gynaecology, Monash Medical Center, Monash University, Clayton, Victoria, Australia

Brandee L Wagner PhD
Research Associate, Joslin Diabetes Center, Boston, Massachusetts, USA

Edith Weisberg MMed MBBS FACSHP
Director of Research, Sydney Centre for Reproductive Health Research, Family Planning NSW, Ashfield, New South Wales, Australia

Malcolm I Whitehead MD FRCOG
Consultant Gynaecologist, The Menopause Clinic, King's College Hospital, Denmark Hill, London, UK

Bent Winding MD
Project Leader, Cancer and Bone Group, Center for Clinical and Basic Research, Ballerup, Denmark

John L Yovich MBBS MD FRCOG FACOG
Medical Director, PIVET Medical Centre, Perth, Western Australia, Australia

Foreword

During the past century, both estrogens and progestogens have been chemically characterized and synthesized. Thereafter, physiologic effects of these steroids upon organs of the reproductive tract and other organ systems, have been extensively studied at the molecular, cellular and tissue level. In addition to the naturally occurring steroids, a great number of pharmacologic agents with both estrogenic and progestogenic actions have been synthesized and administered to animals and humans.

Techniques have been developed to assay natural and synthetic reproductive steroid hormones in tissue, blood, urine and saliva which has made it possible to understand their pharmacokinetic properties. Exogenous administration of both estrogens and progestogens has been used to treat many pathologic conditions, as well as to provide effective contraception, treat the problems caused by postmenopausal estrogen deficiency and assist in the treatment of the infertile couple. The beneficial, as well as the adverse effects of therapeutic use of these steroids, has been widely studied.

This volume, Estrogens and Progestogens in Clinical Practice, provides an extremely comprehensive and current summary of each of these aspects of steroid reproductive hormones. Each author contributing to the chapters in this volume is a recognized expert in the subject area about which they have written. They have utilized their expertise to provide the reader with an excellent analysis of existing data. This book will be of great use to both research and clinical scientists whose areas of investigation involve these steroids. In addition, clinicians who utilize these hormones for therapy of various pathologic entities, as contraceptive agents, for hormone replacement or to treat the infertile couple will enhance their knowledge by reading this volume. The clear figures, concise tables and comprehensive bibliography provided in each chapter help make this book an excellent resource for all individuals interested in obtaining additional current information about the subject matter. The completeness of the subject material and the expertise of the individual authors and editors make this volume the definitive text of reproductive steroid hormones.

Daniel R Mishell Jr
Lyle G McNeil Professor of
Obstetrics and Gynecology,
University of Southern California
School of Medicine,
Women's and Childrens Hospital,
Los Angeles,
California, USA

Preface

At all ages estrogens and progesterone are the key hormones in the coordination of reproductive processes, and function and malfunction of the reproductive tract. They are also major therapeutic agents for a range of gynecological and other conditions. They have such a central role in physiology, pathophysiology, pharmacology and therapy for the reproductive tract, that we saw a real need for a detailed publication aimed at linking each of these areas together in a coherent manner. We have also tried to ensure that the roles, functions and effects of estrogens and progestogens have been placed in perspective with other relevant molecules, mechanisms and therapies.

Readers will become aware that we have encouraged a degree of overlap between certain chapters. This has been deliberate in certain fields where there can be differences of opinion or a particular degree of complexity that can be viewed from different perspectives. It has been our intention that each chapter should be able to stand on its own, but liberal cross-referencing has been used. We have aimed to provide a broad balance of views over the whole book. Authors have also been encouraged to consider and emphasise the strength of available published evidence in line with current medical thought on the concept of 'evidence-based medicine', although it has become clear that much of our 'knowledge' is not yet based on the highest quality of evidence.

Throughout this book we have utilised the term 'progestogen' rather than enter the confused debate on alternative terminologies such as 'progestin' and 'gestagen'.

We have been able to assemble a broad international array of acknowledged expert clinicians and scientists in every field, and we are especially grateful to all of them for the time, effort, expertise and cooperation they have invested in the preparation of their chapters. They have provided us with a superb basis of sound and intelligible science and medicine.

This book has been developed on the basis that it will act as a valuable digest of current thought and recommendations on all aspects of estrogens and progestogens. Essentially, its major use will be as a ready reference source for physicians and scientists working in relevant fields, but we also see this volume as an important tool for those training in the reproductive sciences and medicine. Fields of medicine where this book will have direct relevance particularly include gynecology, obstetrics, endocrinology, reproductive medicine, family planning, women's health, menopausal medicine and reproductive epidemiology.

We are indebted to the many people at Churchill Livingstone in London who have shepherded the editors and authors through the gestation process, from Tim Horne, Lucy Gardner, who stimulated and facilitated the initial conception, through Antonia Seymour, Prudence Daniels, Miranda Bromage and Nora Naughton, who ensured expert ongoing care and ultimate delivery in conjunction with the copy editing and production teams.

Ian S Fraser
Robert P S Jansen
Rogerio A Lobo
Malcolm I Whitehead

Glossary

AR	Androgen receptor
Analyte	The substance to be quantified in a test specimen
Anti-allotypic antibody	An antibody raised against any part of another antibody other than the antigen binding site
Antigen	A substance that binds reversibly and noncovalently to a specific site on the Fab fragment of an antibody
Anti-idiopathic antibody	An antibody raised against the antigen binding site of another antibody
Binding protein	A protein used to quantify or detect an analyte (e.g. antibodies, receptor proteins)
Bias profile	A graphical representation of the numerical difference between the average of a series of estimates and the true or accepted value of the concentrations of analyte being measured
Binding site	That part of a molecule (antibody, analyte or antigen) which takes part in a specified binding reaction
Bispecific antibody	A single antibody with binding sites for two different antigens, one of which might function as a label
C21	carbon atom 21
Ca	Calcium
Capture antibodies	Nonlabeled antibodies which are immobilized and used in excess in a non-competitive assay to bind to a selected epitope of the analyte
Cross-reaction	The ability of substances other than the analyte to bind to antibodies, and the ability of substances other than the antibodies to bind to the analyte
CBG	Corticosteroid-binding globulin
CI	Confidence interval
COC	Combined oral contraceptive
CNS	Central nervous system
CVD	Cardiovascular disease
Detection limit	The smallest amount or concentration which can be distinguished from zero dose with stated confidence (commonly two standard derivations).
Dipstick	A solid phase in the form of a stick coated with a reagent
DMPA	Depot medroxyprogesterone acetate
Dose–response curve	The graphical relationship between the amount of reference material and the response of the detector
DNA	Deoxyribonucleic acid
E_2	Estradiol
EGF	Epidermal growth factor
Epitope	A binding site on an antigen
ER	Estrogen receptor
FSH	Follicle stimulating hormone
GnSAF	Gonadotropin surge-attenuating factor
GnRH	Gonadotropin-releasing hormone

GR	Glucocorticoid receptor
Hapten	A substance that is an antigen, but which is not by itself immunogenic (i.e. will not stimulate the production of an antibody
HRT	Hormone replacement therapy (menopausal)
Hybridoma	A fusion product of two cells – one immortalized and one producing a desired antibody
ICAM	Intracellular adhesion molecule
Immunochromatography	The chromatographic separation (usually on a strip) of immunologically active reagents and analyte
IL	Interleukin
i.m.	Intramuscular
i.v.	Intravenous
Label	A particle or substance attached to one of the assay reagents in order to monitor and quantify the immunological reaction
Ligand	A substance that is reversibly and noncovalently bound by a binding agent
LH	Luteinizing hormone
LNG	Levonorgestrel
Matrix	The solution containing the reference standard or the biological fluid containing the analyte
MI	Mitotic index
Monoclonal antibodies	Antibodies derived from a single clone of lymphocytes
NET	Norethindrone (Norethisterone)
NO	Nitric oxide
Nonspecific binding	The fraction of the label that is present in the end-point signal due to components in the assay system other than the desired agent
OC	Oral contraceptive
OR	Odds ratio
OVX	Ovariectomy; oophorectomy
Polyclonal antibodies	Antibodies derived from many clones of lymphocytes
PCNA	Proliferating cell nuclear antigen
$PGF_{2\alpha}$	Prostaglandin F2 alpha
PMS	Premenstrual syndrome
PR	Progesterone receptor
Precision profile	The agreement between replicate measurements represented as a curve or set of values relating the statistics for variability (usually coefficient of variation) of the responses to the concentration of analyte measured
PRL	Prolactin
P_4	Progesterone
Reference preparation	An identified preparation of reference material of attested suitabiity containing a specific analyte and intended for assessment of quality or quantitation in an assay system
RNA	Ribonucleic acid
RR	Relative risk
s.c.	Subcutaneous
SHBG	Sex hormone-binding globulin
Specificity	The specificity of an assay is the degree to which it is not influenced by cross-reacting substances or other factors
TNF	Tumor necrosis factor
TGF	Transforming growth factor
TR	Thyrotropin receptor
VEGF	Vascular endothelial growth factor
Within assay	Occurring within a batch of standards and test samples
Working range	The range of analyte concentration in test specimens for which an assay (or test) gives results with acceptable precision (usually with a coefficient of variation <10%)
17OH	17 hydroxy (as in 17 hydroxyprogesterone)
β-hCG	β-subunit of human chorionic gonadotropin

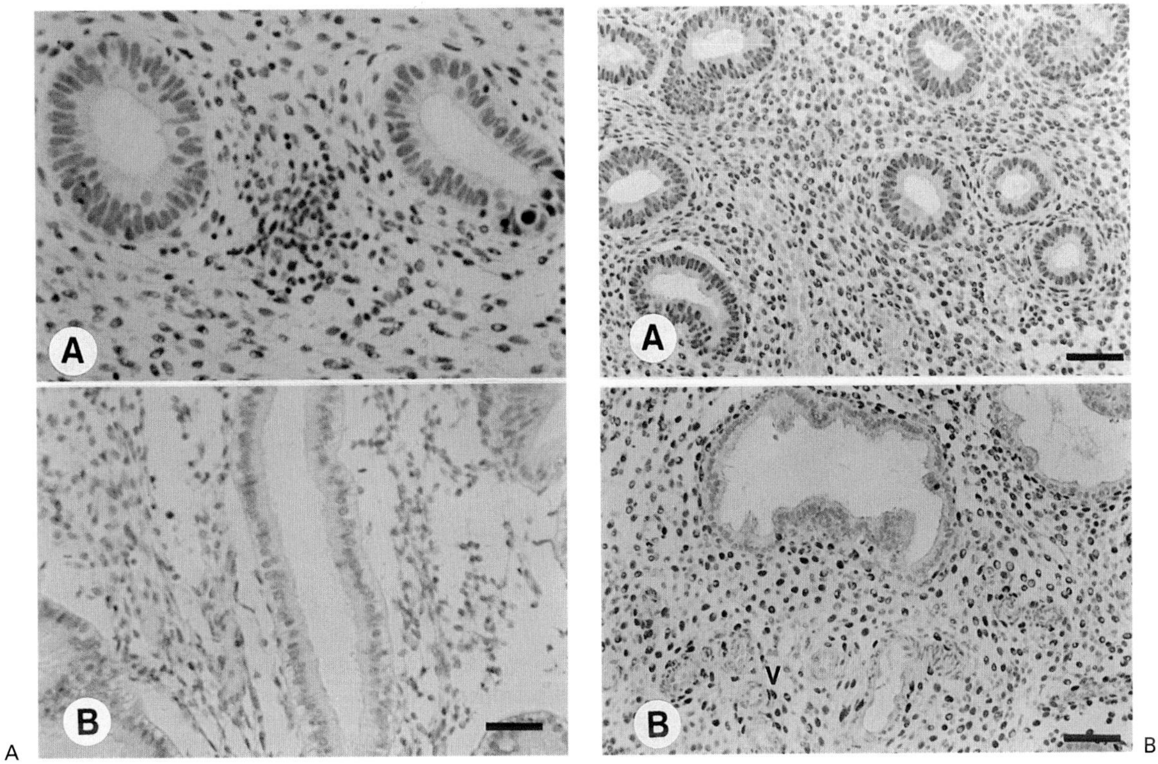

Fig. 13.11 Photomicrographs: **A** estrogen receptor immunoreactivity; **B** progesterone receptor immunoreactivity across the phases of the normal menstrual cycle. A: proliferative phase; B: secretory phase; V: vessel. (see p154)

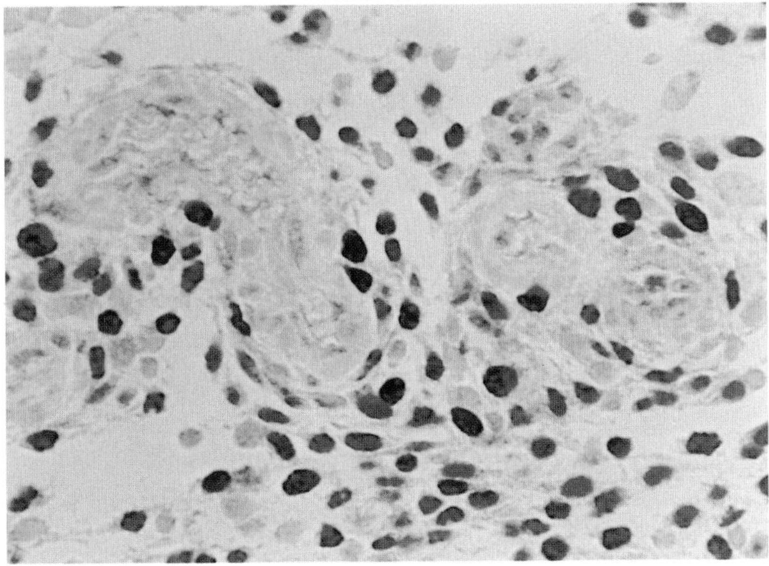

Fig. 13.12 Photomicrograph of late secretory phase endometrium demonstrating perivascular localisation of progesterone receptor immunoreactivity. (see p154)

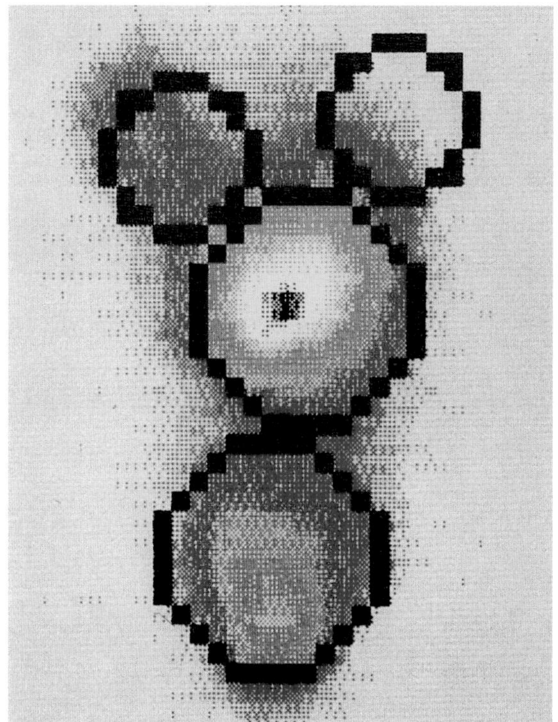

Fig. 15.3 Radioscintographic image of the distribution of technicium-labeled microspheres 16 minutes after placement in the cervix in the late follicular phase. Note that myosalpingeal contractions have resulted in preferential passage of spheres into the right fallopian tube (the left side of the figure), ipsilateral to the side of ovulation.[21] (see p175)

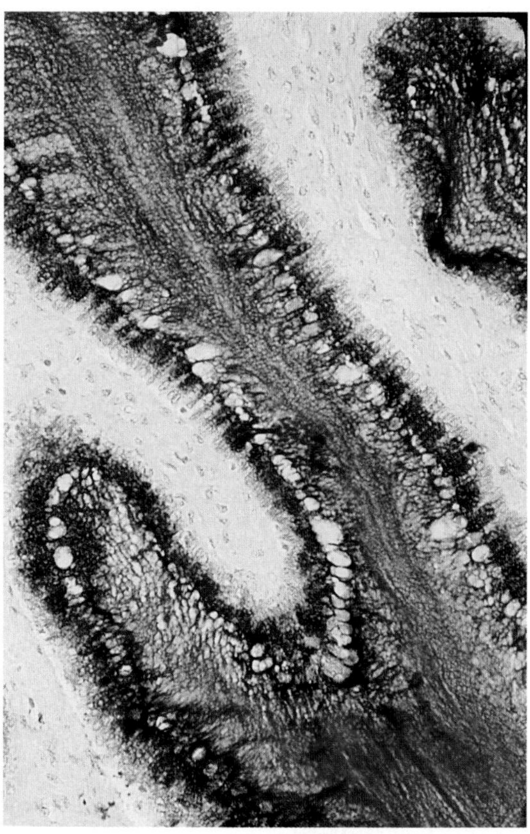

Fig. 15.6 Longitudinal section through the endocervical canal, showing the highly acidic mucus glycoproteins that result from the action of estradiol. Alcian blue. (see p180)

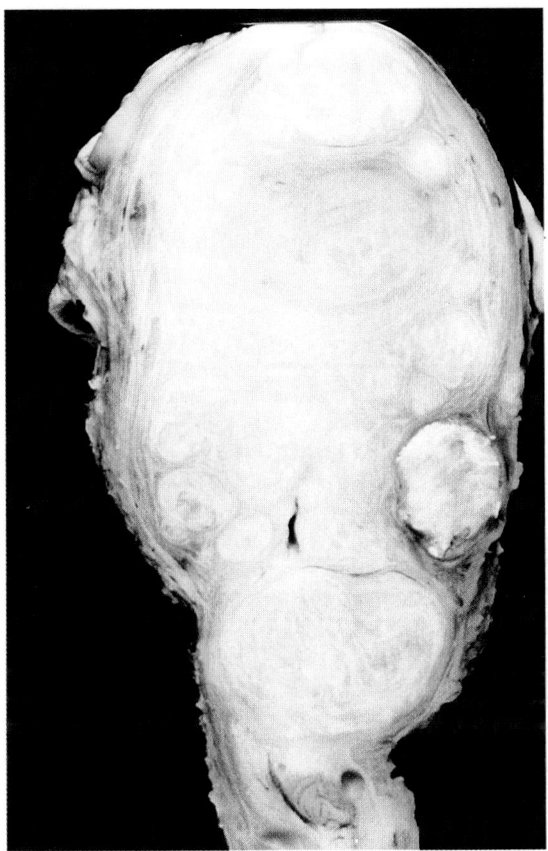

Fig. 38.1 An enlarged uterus showing multiple fibroids. The fibroids are submucosal (causing cavity distortion), intramural and subserosal. The subserosal fibroid has undergone degeneration. (see p471)

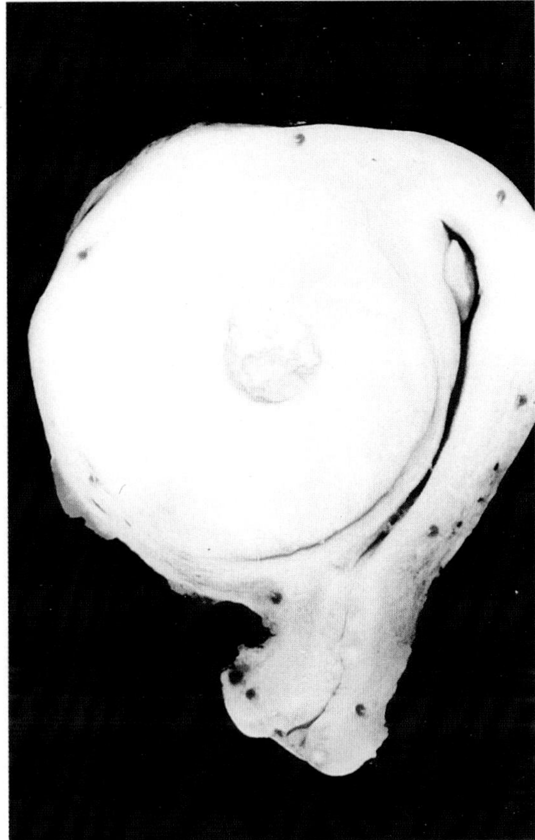

Fig. 38.2 A large intramural fibroid with central degeneration and a single polypoid submucous fibroid. (see p472)

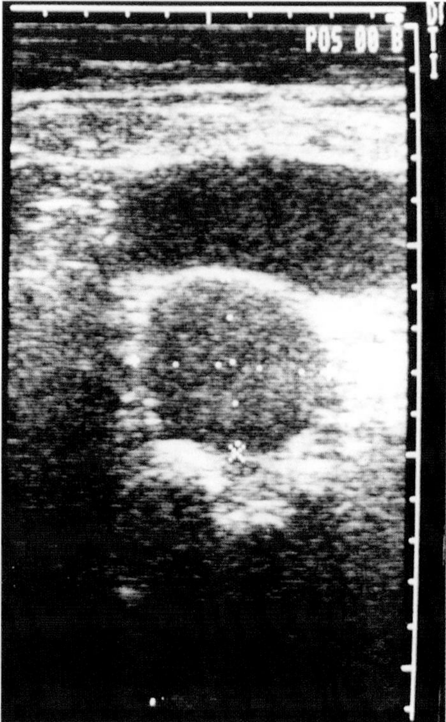

Fig. 38.3 The typical appearance of a fibroid on transabdominal ultrasound. (see p476)

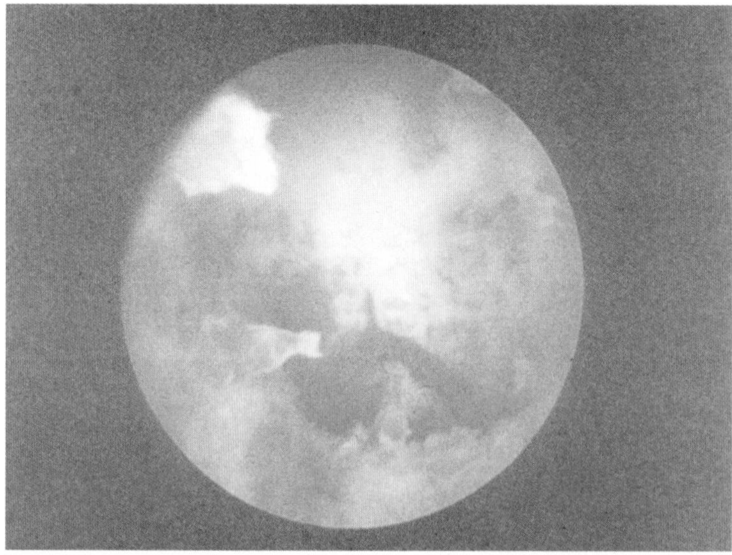

Fig. 38.4 The typical appearance of a fibroid on diagnostic hysteroscopy. (see p476)

SECTION 1

Historical overview

CONTENTS

1. The discovery of reproductive steroid hormones and recognition of their physiological roles

Egon Diczfalusy Ian S. Fraser

Introduction

The scientific elucidation of the physiological roles of estrogens and progestogens has been a long and complex path, which is still far from reaching its ultimate destination. Progress in the understanding of reproduction made little headway in the early millenia of human existence, and it is only within the past century that we have seen a rapidly accelerating and focused scientific enquiry into the understanding of reproductive processes and the hormones which control them. This has been a field in which progress has been especially erratic and notoriously influenced by prevailing political and religious ideologies. Through a major part of recorded human history, the origins of human life have been regarded as sacrosanct by those in positions of power, and meaningful study, or even speculation, has usually been proscribed, often on pain of death! Nevertheless, some innovative and lateral thinkers were able to contribute to true advances in understanding, even in ancient times.

The general principles of logical scientific inquiry have been demonstrated by a small number of astute observers at all ages: over the centuries they have been applied to the solving of a variety of 'scientific' problems facing societies (especially in the disciplines of mathematics, physics and chemistry), or in the elucidation of various natural phenomena. However, the definition and the popularization of a systematic approach to understanding the biological and reproductive sciences has really had to wait until the present century. In addition to effective inhibitory religious and political influences, the rate of progress was inevitably influenced by prevailing education, ideas, availability of investigative tools and benevolent patronage (sponsorship).

The origins of the knowledge that vaginal penetration and male ejaculation during sexual intercourse were necessary for fertility, and that removal of the testes (castration) led to infertility, reach back into antiquity and are now lost in the mists of time. The ancients were apparently aware that orchidectomy led to loss of the ability of the male animal or human to procreate, and that this operation was also followed by behavioral and sexual changes amounting to loss of virility. The name of Herophilus is linked with the discovery in the 4th century BC of the ovaries, when they appear to have been recognized as 'female testicles'. It took a further 600 years before Soranus of Ephesus described their size, shape and position in detail in the 2nd century AD. At about the same time, Galen was carrying out animal dissections, and issuing a number of influential writings on anatomy that included descriptions of the relationships of the reproductive tract. This became the prevailing teaching until the 16th century.

The overt physical and behavioral markers of animal cycles have been recognized for thousands of years, and the times of maximum fertility appear to have been precisely determined for many domesticated species. During their reproductive cycles, many of these animals exhibit one prominent behavioral event associated with vaginal bleeding, around the time of maximal fertility, the phenomenon called estrus. The nature of the relationship between estrus in lower orders of animals and periodic menstruation in primates has confused scientists, physicians and naturalists since antiquity. The completely different nature of menstruation and the timing of ovulation and maximal fertility in women has only been clarified in the 20th century.

Meanwhile, the egg of birds was recognized as a reproductive unit produced within the uterus, and Aristotle believed that the human egg was also produced in the uterus. This belief persisted well into the 17th century. The uterus was also recognized as the origin of the blood-stained flow in women, called menstruation, and the estrus discharge of lower animals. The menstruating woman has been regarded as 'unclean' by most cultures and even dangerous to male health by some. Most of the ancient writers such as Hippocrates, Aristotle, Galen and Pliny have assumed that menstruation was a cleansing process.

True scientific inquiry into the biology of the reproductive organs began in the 15th and 16th centuries, and these ideas and observations are described in more detail below. The complicated and erroneous medieval views were mainly based on speculation and prevailing social views on gender, and are well described by Audrey Eccles[1] and Clara Pinto-Correia.[2]

The brevity of the present chapter has prevented listing of all original sources, but the location of the original references to most of these reports is elaborated in the very detailed publications by Pinto-Correia,[2] O'Dowd and Philipp,[3] and Corner.[4]

RECOGNITION OF THE ROLES OF THE UTERUS, OVARIES, PITUITARY AND PLACENTA IN REPRODUCTION

Understanding of the specific roles of the major players in the small reproductive endocrine orchestra has come slowly and erratically through a number of lines of enquiry. Anatomical dissection and behavioral observations gave the earliest opportunities for scientific enlightenment, and gradually led to specifically designed experiments to answer major questions.

Microanatomical recognition and description of reproductive structures

The main reproductive organs such as ovary, testis, uterus, cervix and vagina were recognized and described in antiquity, but the pituitary gland was not described until 1543, when Andreas Vesalius published the first edition of his book *De Humani Corporis Fabrica*. In addition to his description of the 'glandula pituitam cerebri excipiens' this father of modern anatomy also gives the first thorough description of the ovaries, its follicles and what appears to be a corpus luteum. In 1621 Fabricius de Aquapendente recognized the hen's ovary as the organ of egg formation and was the first to use the term 'ovarium'. Gian Matteo de Gradi had already speculated in the early 1500s that the mammalian female 'testicles' were the site of egg formation, but it was not until the mid-1600s that Dutch and Danish anatomists convincingly demonstrated this concept in mammals. Regnier de Graaf is credited with the first clear description of the development of the large follicles that bear his name, although he thought that the entire follicle was the ovum.

The pioneer microscopist Marcello Malpighi provided a detailed description of the corpus luteum and first used this term in 1681 at about the same time that Anton van Leeuwenhoek was gaining recognition for his discovery of spermatozoa. In the early 1700s Hermann Boerhaave speculated that the egg left the corpus luteum behind as it left the ovary, and also that sperm fertilized the egg before entry to the uterus. Karl von Baer in 1827 was the first to recognize and describe the mammalian ovum inside the ovarian follicles of a dog. He observed a tiny yellowish white point inside each large ovarian follicle, opened one of the follicles, and examined the white speck:

> When I placed it under the microscope I was utterly astonished, I saw an ovule ... and so clearly that a blind man could hardly deny it. It is truly wonderful and surprising to be able to demonstrate to the eye, by so simple a procedure, a thing that has been sought so persistently and discussed *ad nauseam* in every textbook of physiology as insoluble.

Other important anatomical observations from this time were the description of the anterior pituitary portal vessel system by Liutand in 1742. Leonardo da Vinci (1452–1519) was the first to represent the human uterus as having a single cavity, and William Hunter (1718–1783) produced a series of very detailed illustrations of gravid human uteri and their contents. Hunter also described the presence of two corpora lutea in a case of twins. Somewhat later, Edward Pflüger (1863) deduced that the corpus luteum developed from the Graafian follicle.

Surgical removal and transplantation experiments

It was known from ancient times that castration of males led to infertility, behavioral effects and sometimes impotence, and castration of female animals led to uterine shrinkage and infertility. Percival Pott (1775) was one of the first to link removal of human ovaries to amenorrhea and decrease in breast size when he removed both ovaries in a hernia in a young woman. Carl Ludwig (1858) was able to extend and define these observations ('castrate atrophy') more precisely once the operation of oophorectomy became more frequent. Many theorized that this castrate atrophy was due to interference with the blood or nerve supply to the genital tract during the surgery.

The next step was taken by Emil Knauer (1896), who was able to prevent uterine atrophy after oophorectomy in rabbits by grafting small pieces of ovary back into various new sites. A few years later (1900) he was able to postulate ovarian 'secretions' as an explanation for this phenomenon. Josef Halban (1900) extended these observations by grafting bits of adult ovary under the skin of infantile guinea pigs and discovering that the uterus grew to adult size. He then clearly expounded the theory of an ovarian secretion that was 'absolutely' necessary for the maintenance of the genital organs and the mammary glands.

Surgical procedures were also crucial to an understanding of the corpus luteum. Ludwig Fraenkel (1901, 1910) carried out a series of experiments to destroy the corpora lutea of rabbits prior to embryo implantation in order to test the theory of Gustav Born that secretions of the corpus luteum were concerned with protection of the early embryo. After various types of destructive interventions, Fraenkel was able to present completely convincing data to demonstrate the effects of removal of the corpora lutea on loss of the embryos. At the same time (1901) Vilhelm Magnus was carrying out similar experiments which allowed him to make the important observation that although removal of the corpora lutea alone caused abortion, it did not lead to uterine atrophy. He speculated that the ovary must produce more than one secretion.

Also, at around the same time (1910) the French histologists Paul Bouin and Ancel were describing the remarkable microscopic changes which occur in the endometrium of early pregnancy in the rabbit, and demonstrating that these were caused by the corpora lutea. They were able to prove this by a series of experiments where they mated fertile female rabbits to males who had undergone vasectomy and then studied the endometrium when the corpora lutea were left intact, were destroyed or when the ovaries were removed. George Corner refined these experiments in 1928 to demonstrate that destruction of the corpora lutea leads to early embryonic death because the uterine lining has not been appropriately prepared to receive them.

Surgical procedures have also been important in understanding the roles of the pituitary and the hypothalamus in the control of reproduction. It was recognized early in the 20th century that destructive pathological lesions of the anterior pituitary caused genital atrophy, and this began to be defined much more clearly following the first experimental hypophysectomy procedures carried out in 1910 in dogs in Harvey Cushing's laboratory. Complex and precise surgical procedures were also utilized by several groups of investigators (including Flerko, Wislocki, Harris and Naftolin) in the 1930s, 40s and 50s to demonstrate the importance of the pituitary stalk, the pituitary portal vessels and various centers in the hypothalamus in the control of reproduction.

RECOGNITION OF THE CONCEPT OF REPRODUCTIVE HORMONES

The discipline of reproductive endocrinology belongs entirely to the 20th century, but speculation that organs such as the thyroid gland released substances into the bloodstream dates back to Ruysch at the end of the 17th century. The term 'endocrine' means inwardly secreting and derives from the Greek *endon* (within) and *krinein* (to separate). The word 'hormone' means to excite or arouse, and comes from the Greek *hormao*. The word was apparently first suggested by Sir William B. Hardy and W. T. Vesey of Cambridge and was first used in a public lecture by Professor Ernst Henry Starling in his 1905 Croonian Lecture on 'The Chemical Correlation of the Functions of the Body'.

Claude Bernard, of 'milieu interieur' fame, was the first to introduce the concept of internal secretions in 1855, but in 1890 Charles Eduoard Brown-Sequard, the French physiologist born in Mauritius, was the first to use gonadal extracts for behavioral or therapeutic effect. He found a substantial effect on sexual function and 'vigor' with self-injection of aqueous extracts of animal testes, but his aqueous ovarian extracts had no obvious effect in women. Brown-Sequard also postulated that the adrenals, thyroid, pancreas, liver, spleen and kidneys were organs producing secretions which entered the bloodstream, and had the potential to be used in treatment. Louis Auguste Prenant was the first to postulate in 1898 that the corpus luteum was a gland of internal secretion.

Numerous attempts were made by many investigators to prepare extracts from ovary, corpus luteum and placenta, but failed to define the proper chemical steps until two groups prepared active extracts of ovary using lipid solvents (alcohol, ether, acetone and chloroform). The first effective extracts were prepared by Henri Iscovesco in Paris and Ottfried Fellner in Vienna in 1912–13, and these were refined and extended to include corpus luteum and placenta extracts over the next two years by Robert Frank (New York) and Edmond Herrmann (Vienna).

The next step was the requirement for a precise test to demonstrate the presence of this 'secretion'. F. Lataste had made the first observations of a correlation between the cyclical ovarian changes and those in vaginal epithelial cytology (1886), but Charles Stockard and George Papanicolaou were able to describe these changes in vaginal cytology in rodents very precisely (1917). This became a simple, cheap and accurate method to determine the stage of the estrus cycle. It also provided a precise bioassay to act as the basis for testing extracts for the isolation of estrogens and progesterone. Unfortunately, the changes in vaginal cytology in women were less precise, albeit still useful.

The changes in the endometrium during the menstrual cycle in women could also be used as a 'bioassay' and were correlated with the corpus luteum by the German gynecologists Robert Schröder (in 1909), Robert Meyer (in 1911) and Carl Ruge (in 1913). Schröder was the first to use the terms 'proliferative' and 'secretory' endometrium. George Corner extended these endocrine studies further in the 1920s and 30s by the use of progestin and estrin extracts in rhesus monkeys and clearly defined the roles of each hormone on the endometrium and menstruation. He also found that menstruation could be inhibited by 'progestin' if given in sufficient quantities and continuously, while 'estrin' prevented bleeding only if the endometrium was in the proliferative phase. At this time (1931) George Bartelmez was studying the spiral arterioles of the endometrium and demonstrating their remarkable changes in structure during the secretory phase and menstruation.

These investigations were the background for a series of beautifully descriptive and meticulous observational studies by John Markee (1932, 1940, 1948), who transplanted fragments of endometrium to the anterior chamber of the eye in rhesus monkeys. Markee's descriptions of the microscopic vascular and tissue changes in these endometrial transplants during the process of menstruation still form the basis of our present day understanding of menstruation in women.

Josef Halban was the first to suggest (in 1905) an endocrine secretory function for the placenta, but it was many years (1927) before Sellman Aschheim and Bernhard Zondek were able to identify a gonadotropin and an ovarian hormone (an estrogen) in human pregnancy urine. J. B. Collip from Canada (in 1930) was able to report that the placenta secreted an 'ovarian-stimulating hormone'. This was finally defined when Ernst Philipp and coworkers (in 1930 and 1936) demonstrated the virtual absence of gonadotropin from the pituitaries of more than 100 pregnant women and G. Gey, Georgeanna Seegar Jones and Lou Hellman (in 1938) reported the production of a gonadotropic substance from placental chorionic cells in culture. Histochemical techniques were used to demonstrate that steroids (Wislocki and Bennett in 1943) and gonadotropin (Pierce and Midgley in 1963) were both elaborated by the chorionic syncitium.

ISOLATION, CHARACTERIZATION AND SYNTHESIS OF ESTROGENS AND PROGESTERONE

The landmarks of the estrogen and progesterone stories are highlighted in Tables 1.1 and 1.2. The gradual unfolding of the numerous individual steps in these stories has been memorably recorded by George Corner in his *The Hormones in Human Reproduction*.[4] O'Dowd and Philipp[3] have also faithfully summarized the key events and references in this fascinating story. Diczfalusy and Lauritzen[5] have authored the most extensive review about estrogens in women in 1961 (with 2207 references).

The characterization of estrogens and progesterone really began in the mid 1920s with the identification of rich sources of estrogens, such as follicular fluid (by Edgar Allen and Edward Doisy in 1923) and pregnancy urine (Aschheim in 1927), and rich sources of progesterone (corpus luteum and placenta).

The chemical characterization began with the preparation of concentrated, purified and even crystalline extracts. Edgar Allen and Edward Doisy were the first group to achieve in 1923 a satisfactory extraction, partial purification and biological testing of an estrogenic ovarian hormone from follicular fluid. The extraction of 'estrogen' from ovarian tissue proved surprisingly difficult because of all the tissue fats and oils, so that the detection of an estrogenic substance in urine by Loewe and Lange in 1926, and the extraction of large amounts of the hormone from pregnancy urine by Sellman Aschheim in 1927, was of great assistance to the chemists. A pure crystalline estrogen was isolated from urine by several groups of investigators during 1928 and 1930 (including Doisy, Allen and Butenandt), and Butenandt in Germany was able to propose the chemical formula for this estrogen, which was later called estrone. Browne isolated estriol from placenta in 1930 and found it to be a much less potent estrogen than estrone, but it was several years (1936) before MacCorquodale, Thayer and Doisy were able to crystallize a few mg of estradiol from two tons of ovaries!

The structures of all these estrogens were rapidly determined in the early to mid 1930s once they were obtained in pure form, and following on from the demonstration of the structure of the common sterol, cholesterol, by the German chemist Heinrich Wieland in 1932. It was soon confirmed that the structures of the sex hormones estrone, estriol, estradiol and indeed progesterone and testosterone were all based on the four-ring steroid nucleus.

Progesterone turned out to be equally difficult to isolate in pure form. George Corner[4] gives a colorful

Table 1.1 Landmarks in the estrogen story.

Antiquity		Castration of female animals prevents breeding and leads to uterine shrinkage
1760	De Haen	Amenorrhea in a woman with a pituitary tumor
1775	Percival Pott	Linked destruction of ovaries to shrinkage of breast and cessation of menstruation
1809	Ephraim McDowell	First oophorectomy; allowed observation of effects of ovarian removal
1858	Carl Ludwig	Loss of human ovaries caused uterine shrinkage and amenorrhea ('castrate atrophy')
1886	F. Lataste	First correlated cyclical ovarian changes with cytological vaginal epithelial changes
1890	Charles Brown-Sequard	Aqueous ovarian extracts ineffective as therapy, although extracts of testis had beneficial sexual effects in males
1896	Emil Knauer	Prevention of uterine atrophy by oophorectomy and grafting the ovary at new sites (guinea pigs)
1900	Josef Halban	Graft of adult ovaries in infantile guinea pigs caused normal uterine growth and development
1912–14	Henri Iscovesco (Paris); Ottfried Fellner (Vienna); Robert Frank (New York); Edmond Herrman (Vienna)	Lipid extracts (in alcohol, ether, acetone, chloroform) of ovary, corpus luteum and placenta caused growth and development of uterus and mammary glands
1917	Charles Stockard & George Papanicolaou	Precise bioassay of vaginal cytology changes with stages of estrus cycle in guinea pig
1918	Arthur Robinson	Estrus is due to a product of ovarian follicles
1923	Edward Doisy & Edgar Allen	Injection of follicle fluid under skin of castrate rats and mice; potent lipid extract of follicular fluid, but still very impure
1929	Doisy; Adolf Butenandt	Synthesis of active hormonal principle (estrone) in crystalline form extracted from pregnancy urine or stallion's urine (called 'theelin' by Doisy, 'progynon' by Butenandt, 'oestrin' by Parkes).
1935	D. MacCorquodale; Thayer & Doisy	Extracted two tons of swine ovaries to obtain a few mg of estradiol
1936	E.C. Dodds	Synthesis of 'synthetic' estrogens including diethyl stilbestrol
1936	League of Nations Commission on Biological Standardization	International standard unit of estrone and pure supply of standard hormone
1939	George Corner	Proposed his theory of the existence of a pituitary-ovarian-endometrial axis

and humble account of the extraction of minced corpora lutea in hot alcohol, from which was obtained a 'crude oily extract looking like a poor grade of automobile grease' but which contained the long-sought hormone in ample quantity. This material was able to fully substitute for the removed corpora lutea in early rabbit pregnancy. Corner and Allen were able to maintain rabbit pregnancy from 18 hours following mating all the way to normal birth in seven out of their first 14 attempts (in spite of paying no attention to the possible estrogen content of the extract or its requirement for the pregnancy maintenance process). Elucidation of the progesterone story was far from straightforward and Corner recollects memories of bafflement, comedy, hard work and modest success. He goes on to say: Can I forget the time I went racing up the steps of the laboratory in Rochester carrying a glass syringe containing the world's entire supply of crude progesterone, stumbled, fell and lost it all? Or the day Willard Allen showed me his first glittering crystals of the hormone, chemically pure at last?'.

Final chemical purification of progesterone required numerous chemical steps to remove various other lipids and related sterols without destroying progesterone itself. Four groups isolated the

Table 1.2 Landmarks in the progesterone story.

1555	Andreas Vesalius	First illustration of corpus luteum in *De Humani Corporis Fabrica*
1681	Marcello Malpighi	Term 'corpus luteum' first used
c. 1720	Hermann Boerhaave	Speculation on corpus luteum formation after the egg leaves the ovary
c. 1750	William Hunter	Detailed description of corpus luteum and two corpora lutea with twins
1863	Edward Pflüger	Deduced that corpus luteum developed from Graafian follicle
1898	Louis-Auguste Prenant	Corpus luteum postulated to be an organ of internal secretion
1900	Gustav Born	Postulated that an internal secretion of the corpus luteum is concerned with protection of the embryo
1901	Ludwig Fraenkel & F. Cohn	Destruction of corpora lutea in pregnant rabbits caused abortion or failure of implantation
1901	Vilhelm Magnus	Postulation of two hormones coming from ovary
1910	Paul Bouin & P. Ancel	Demonstrated that the corpus luteum is essential for the dramatic histological changes in endometrium during early pregnancy
1911	Robert Meyer	Stages of development of corpus luteum were related to changes in the endometrium
1928	George Corner	Corpora lutea necessary for nutrition and protection of the embryo and for implantation
1929	George Corner, Willard Allen & Walter Bloor	Discovery of gestational hormonal effects of an oily extract of corpora lutea called 'progestin'
1934	Allen & Wintersteiner; Butenandt, Westphal & Hohlweg; Slotta, Ruschig & Fels; Haustmann & Wettstein	Purification and structure of 'progesterone'
1934	Butenandt & Schmidt	Synthesis of 'luteosterone' (progesterone)
1935	Second International Conference on the Standardization of Sex Hormones, London	The active hormone named as progesterone
1936	League of Nations Commission on Biological Standardization	International standard of potency for progesterone

compound at virtually the same time in 1934: W.M. Allen and O. Wintersteiner; A. Butenandt, U. Westphal and W. Hohlweg; K.H. Slotta, H. Ruschig and E. Fels; and M. Hartmann and A. Wettstein. Its structure was elucidated by Butenandt and Schmidt in the same year.

All of these chemical processes gave meagre yields of pure hormone, and most of the initial structural analyses were achieved with amounts varying between 20–75 mg. The need to extract gallons of pregnancy urine or many kilograms of ovary meant that extracts used for therapeutic purposes in the late 1930s were very expensive. All of this suddenly changed in the 1940s, called by Carl Djerassi 'the decade of Mexican jungle chemistry', when the brilliant and unorthodox chemical maverick, Russell Marker, developed a spectacularly simple process for chemically transforming a sapogenin called diosgenin into progesterone.[6] He then discovered that diosgenin was particularly abundant in certain yams which grow profusely in Mexico. When pharmaceutical companies showed little interest, he went to Mexico on his own and collected ten tons of yams which he extracted in a rented laboratory. He took the syrupy extract back to the USA where he isolated pure diosgenin in the industrial laboratory of a friend and converted it into 3000 g of pure progesterone (worth, at that time, US $80 per gram). This success encouraged him to set up in 1944 a primitive production facility in Mexico City, a precursor to the Syntex Company that was later responsible for many major breakthroughs in steroid synthesis, resulting in the large-scale manufacture of testosterone, cortisone, highly potent synthetic corticosteroids and orally active progestogens, such as norethindrone and chlormadinone acetate.

The obvious clinical need for therapeutic steroids for men and women with androgen or estrogen deficiencies and for other therapeutic purposes rapidly led to an urgent chemical search for synthetic estrogens and progestogens that were straightforward to synthesize and active orally (which the natural estrogens and progesterone were not). Ethinyl estradiol was synthesized by Inhoffen and coworkers of Schering-Berlin already in 1938, and a series of inexpensive nonsteroidal estrogens were synthesized the same year by Dodds and his group at the Middlesex Hospital in London. The development of a brilliant method for the removal of the angular methyl group of testosterone by Birch (in 1950) then opened the way to the synthesis of the first orally active progestogenic 19-norsteroids: norethindrone by Djerassi and colleagues in 1951 and norethynodrel by Colton in 1953.

E.C. Dodds and his group at the Middlesex Hospital synthesized a series of nonsteroidal substances with estrogenic activity, including diethyl stilbestrol in 1938. Orally active progesterones were more difficult, and it took until November 1951 before the Syntex group filed its patent for norethindrone, followed in 1953 by Frank Colton of Searle with norethynodrel. It is of interest that the highly active synthetic steroidal estrogens, mestranol and ethinyl estradiol, were not specifically designed and 'hunted', but were discovered and identified as by-products and contaminants of the original oral progestogen formulations!

Nomenclature of steroids was initially confusing, but a series of international conferences on nomenclature and biological standardization in the mid 1930s allowed agreement on structures, international units of potency, and standardized preparations.

The availability of pure estrogens and progesterone allowed physiological studies to begin in earnest on secretion and its control, transport, metabolism, and end-organ effect. It also became necessary to develop sensitive methods to measure the tiny concentrations of the natural hormones circulating in the bloodstream. Much of the information arising from these studies is elaborated in other chapters of this book, but some of the major early landmarks are highlighted in the next section.

EARLY STUDIES OF THE PHYSIOLOGY OF ESTROGENS AND PROGESTERONE

The earliest physiological observations have been recorded earlier in this chapter. After the isolation of relatively pure extracts of estrogens and progesterone it became relatively straightforward to explore the effects of these hormones on the endometrium, cervix and vaginal cytology of women. It even became possible to demonstrate the concept of 'negative feedback' as early as 1932 (Karl Moore and Dorothy Price) and the first evidence in 1934 of a positive feedback effect (Walter Hohlweg). George Corner was responsible for a comprehensive series of studies on endometrial and menstrual effects in rhesus monkeys and this led to his theory of a pituitary-ovarian-endometrial axis in 1939. The precise histological changes in the endometrium during the secretory phase were most accurately defined by Noyes, Hertig and Rock in 1950.

It gradually became clear that estrogens and progesterone had to gain access to the cell in order to exert their actions and that they needed to exhibit specific actions only in the cells of certain organs. The concept of specific hormone binding in particular cells that was born, and thus developed the need for receptive cells to express molecules (receptors) would precisely recognize the particular hormone. Early estrogen receptor studies were described in detail by Jensen and Jacobsen in 1962.

There was an early interest in the ability of the corpus luteum and the follicle to actively synthesize steroids, and much effort was invested into defining the biosynthetic pathways, mainly through the use of radioactively labelled precursor molecules. By the early 1960s a clear picture of ovarian follicular (granulosa and theca) and luteal steroid biosynthesis was beginning to emerge, partly through the monumental contribution of Elwood Jensen but also through the work of investigators like Savard, Marsh, Ryan and James. This led directly to a focused interest in the mechanisms by which FSH and LH activated their receptors in ovarian target cells through the cyclic AMP and other pathways by several groups including those of McKerns, Channing, Niswender and Jaffe. The field of molecular mechanisms in reproductive hormone synthesis, secretion and action has become almost unbelievably complex since these early days!

The end-result of hormone synthesis is release of the hormone from the cell surface and passage of the free hormone into the bloodstream and other body fluids. Detailed study of hormone secretion, changes in serum levels, transport in the circulation, metabolism and excretion all required the development of sensitive and specific assays. The first substance for which an assay was developed in 1938 was the main human urinary metabolite of progesterone, pregnanediol glucuronide (Venning). The early chemical assays were colorimetric or fluorimetric, were relatively insensitive, and could not be used on serum because of extraction difficulties and low hormone concentrations. Hence, most of the early work on changes in secretion was based on extrapolation from measurements in urine. The first assay for urinary estrone, estradiol and estriol that fulfilled the recognized criteria of reliability was developed by Jim Brown in 1955, while working in Edinburgh. A similarly reliable and robust method for the measurement of urinary pregnanediol was also developed in Edinburgh by Klopper, Michie and Brown, in the same year. These assays permitted a wide range of *in vivo* and *in vitro* studies of secretion and metabolism in animals and in women under different circumstances, and laid very sound foundations for our present understanding of ovarian function.

Measurement of estrogens in blood was altogether a more complex challenge. The first (in 1968) specific and accurate, but laborious, chemical assay for estradiol and estrone in serum was that of David Baird and permitted eight samples to be processed over a three day period. Introduction of the concept of radioimmunoassay (for insulin) by Berson and Yalow in 1956 led to a revolution in the field of serum protein hormone assay, and after a further development phase, was followed in the 1970s by the appearance of a range of sensitive, precise and reliable radioimmunoassays and protein-binding assays for steroids.[7] Application of these was soon followed by an explosion of information on short-term, long-term and cyclical changes in circulating ovarian steroids and pituitary gonadotropins, and a definition of their interrelationships. The endocrinology of the specific phases of puberty, perimenopause and postmenopause began to be realistically explored in the 1970s.

A combination of these tools with specific surgical techniques to access the placenta, amniotic fluid and the fetal circulation began to reveal some of the endocrine mysteries of the unique state of pregnancy. One of us (ed) established a group in Stockholm very active in the early 1960s which was responsible for elaborating much of the knowledge we have today on the individual endocrine synthetic capabilities of the fetus and placenta in early pregnancy and of the complex interactions between the two. They also proposed the concept of the feto-placental unit.[8] Others have explored the numerous endocrine functions of the placenta in late pregnancy, and much attention has been directed to the investigation of endocrine changes responsible for the onset of parturition. Among these earlier investigators, Sir Graham 'Mont' Liggins of Auckland stands out for demonstrating that parturition in sheep is initiated by a rise in fetal cortisol, which induces 17-hydroxylase activity in the placenta, resulting in a fall in progesterone and a rise in estradiol, which lead to increased uterine prostaglandins and uterine contractions — a unique demonstration of the importance of both components of the feto-placental unit.

Conclusion

This overview of the discovery of estrogenic and progestogenic hormones and their physiological roles has been heavily reliant on a number of much more detailed publications,[1–12] in addition to the personal experience and involvement of one of us (ED). The reader is referred especially to the beautifully written historical and first hand 1942 account of the discovery of estrogens and progesterone by George Corner — a true classic.[4] This volume has been reprinted and republished in a number of different editions. A reader with an interest in the history of the scientific foundations of reproduction and reproductive hormones is recommended to consult all of these texts, but will find particular enjoyment in the Sir Henry Dale Lectures of the Society for Endocrinology and published in the *Journal of Endocrinology* (Diczfalusy 1978,[8] Corner 1964,[9] Parkes 1966,[10] Marrian 1966,[11] Greep 1967[12]).

The studies of these pioneers and their myriad predecessors, collaborators and successors were able to establish a sound basis for an unprecedented assault on the manipulation of these processes for purposes of therapy, contraception and postmenopausal hormone replacement therapy (see chapter 2 and other relevant sections of this book).

REFERENCES

1. Eccles A 1982 Obstetrics and gynaecology in Tudor and Stuart England. Croom Helm, London, pp 26–32
2. Pinto-Correia C 1997 The ovary of Eve. University of Chicago Press, Chicago
3. O'Dowd MJ, Philipp EE 1994 The history of obstetrics and gynaecology. Parthenon Publishing Group, London, pp 255–289
4. Corner GW 1942 The hormones in human reproduction. Princeton University Press, Princeton
5. Diczfalusy E, Lauritzen Ch 1961 Oestrogene beim Menschen. Springer-Verlag, Berlin
6. Djerassi C 1979 The chemical history of the pill. The Politics of Contraception. W.W. Norton, New York, pp 227–255
7. Diczfalusy E, Diczfalusy A (eds) 1970 Steroid assay by protein binding. Second Karolinska Symposium on Research Methods in Reproductive Endocrinology. Acta Endocrinologica Suppl. 147
8. Diczfalusy E 1978 Reproductive endocrinology and the merry post-war period. Journal of Endocrinology 79: i–xvii
9. Corner GW 1964 The early history of the oestrogenic hormone. Journal of Endocrinology 31: iii–xvii
10. Parkes AS 1966 The rise of reproductive endocrinology, 1926–1940. Journal of Endocrinology 34: xix–xxxii
11. Marrian GF 1966 Early work on the chemistry of pregnanediol and the oestrogenic hormones. Journal of Endocrinology 35: vi–xvi
12. Greep RO 1967 The saga and the science of the gonadotrophins. Journal of Endocrinology 39: i–ix

2. Historical overview of estrogens and progestogens as therapeutic agents

Joseph W. Goldzieher

Introduction

Although physiologists had explored for decades the endocrinology of the reproductive system in minute detail and in many species, including nonhuman primates and man,[1] this was of little clinical utility until the chemical structure of the hormones involved became known. No sooner had the steroid nature of progesterone[2] and the estrogens[3] been elucidated than the chemists set to work to synthesize these and related, clinically useful substances. The natural estrogens and progestogens are highly insoluble in water and therefore not orally active (micronization was not perfected at the time); moreover their half-life is very short. Crystalline suspensions in aqueous media for injection turned out to be painful and unacceptable. Therefore, lipid-soluble esters with a prolonged half-life (estradiol benzoate, cypionate; 17-hydroxyprogesterone caproate, etc.) to be administered intramuscularly in oil vehicles were among the first preparations suitable for clinical use. However, these agents were still short-lived and inconvenient, and progesterone in oil, for example, was far too expensive for use at the dosages now known to be required. Another option for estrogen administration was to use the orally effective water-soluble sulfoconjugates, which can be extracted commercially from the urine of pregnant mares. This mix ('conjugated equine estrogens') of nearly a dozen human and equine estrogens of varying potencies has been in clinical use for half a century.[4] Synthetic conjugates such as estrone sulfate itself also became available. Eventually, in the 1930s the chemists prepared ethinyl estradiol, which proved to be orally active and extremely potent. Several decades later, the methyl ether of this compound fortuitously turned up as a contaminant of certain synthetic progestogens, but more of that later. In 1938, Dodds and his associates[5] in England synthesized a large series of nonsteroidal estrogens which included diethylstilbestrol, a highly potent, orally active, inexpensive compound that was made available to the medical profession without patent restrictions.

Although estrogens can be absorbed in effective amounts through the skin or vaginal wall from appropriate vehicles, clinical usage by these routes came only much later. Basically, the oral approach served clinical purposes very well, although the injectables, despite their poor pharmacokinetic profile, continue to be used to this day.

Schering's *de facto* monopoly of progesterone, produced by a lengthy process,[6] was broken in 1943 by the American chemist, Russell Marker, who devised a synthesis starting with a steroid found in a common, large Mexican yam;[7] in 1943 this brought the price of progesterone down from $1000 a gram to $80. Nevertheless, better agents than progesterone itself were needed. 17-hydroxyprogesterone caproate dissolved in an oily base served as a moderately long-lived injectable, but all other efforts to modify the progesterone molecule failed until the synthesis of the C_{21}-steroid medroxyprogesterone acetate in the mid-1950s[8] (and eventually, related compounds such as megestrol and chlormadinone) yielded highly potent, orally active agents. An injectable microcrystalline suspension of medroxyprogesterone acetate also found an important therapeutic niche. The final step in the development of progestational agents took place in 1952 when chemists at Syntex SA in Mexico and G.D. Searle Co. in the USA independently discovered that certain derivatives of 17-ethynyl 19-nortestosterone were powerful, orally active progestogens.[7] A later modification, the substitution of an 18-ethyl for an 18-methyl group as part of the total synthesis of 19-norsteroids, accomplished in 1963 by Herchel Smith, created the class of gonanes (levonorgestrel, gestodene, desogestrel), which are among the most widely used progestogens (especially in oral contraceptives) today.

GYNECOLOGICAL APPLICATIONS

Clinical use of the estrogens and progestogens centered on several major areas: replacement therapy in case of endogenous deficiency (e.g. primary ovarian failure, menopause, senile vaginitis); corrective therapy (as in the management of dysfunctional uterine bleeding, hormonal deficiencies during pregnancy or endocrine infertility); therapy of prostate cancer; and contraception. Enthusiasm for the use of estrogens, especially for menopausal problems, was tempered by concern over tumorigenicity, which had been observed in rodent experiments. A 1938a report of breast tumors developing in mice treated with estrogen was the beginning of the clinical nightmare of 'hormones cause [breast] cancer' which is with us to this day. The fact that these mice had to be of a special strain, had to be infected with MMT virus and had to have intact pituitaries (prolactin was essential for tumor development) did not lessen clinical fearfulness. In fact, it was not until 1994 that authoritative groups[9] at last formally questioned the dogma that giving estrogen to breast cancer survivors would accelerate recurrences. Chiefly because of the fear of promoting breast cancer, the Council on Pharmacy of the American Medical Association maintained into the 1990s that estrogens should be used for menopause management in minimal doses to alleviate symptoms and for the shortest time possible. What warning symptoms of an impending osteoporotic hip fracture or myocardial infarction were to be looked for was not specified.

Another discouragement of menopausal estrogen therapy eventually appeared: an increased frequency of a relatively benign, well-differentiated endometrial carcinoma in long-term estrogen-only users.[10] It was soon determined that this hazard could be avoided by concomitant exposure of the endometrium to progestogens, but this overemphasized, easily preventable consequence of long-term estrogen-only use augmented the hesitancy to use estrogen replacement therapy. When in 1966 a New York City gynecologist, Robert Wilson, published a bestseller entitled *Feminine Forever*,[11] in which he advocated lifelong estrogen use for most women, he was expelled from his specialty society for unprofessionalism.

Just as with the introduction of birth control pills, when the medical profession had to be dragged reluctantly into the oral contraceptive era, we are now seeing the medical profession, equally reluctantly, come to the realization (just as Wilson perceived) that the era of hormone replacement therapy for ovarian failure is an imperative for the proper care of the peri- and postmenopausal woman.

In the late 1930s and on into the 1940s, menstrual dysfunctions (delayed menarche, irregular menstrual bleeding, secondary amenorrhea, dysmenorrhea) were treated by superimposing a therapeutic estrogen-progestogen cyclic regimen on the presumed disordered ovarian activity, largely on an empirical basis, since assays for ovarian and pituitary hormones, if available at all, were not often of practical utility.[4,12] Oral estrogens (stilbestrol in particular) were used to treat dysmenorrhea by inhibiting ovulation and therefore progesterone production. Application of this treatment in the context of contraception apparently never occurred to anyone.

Use in pregnancy

It was evident from studies in animals that endocrinological normalcy is necessary for initiation and maintenance of pregnancy (although the fundamental differences between rodent and primate gestation were not yet appreciated).[18] As assays for urinary pregnandiol glucuronide became available, Smith and Smith[13] in Boston hypothesized that some cases of repeated abortion (and threatened abortion as well) were due to insufficient production of placental progesterone and that this, in turn, was due to insufficient estrogen production. At the same time Priscilla White,[14] also of Boston and a collaborator of Smith and Smith, believed that similar endocrinopathy was at the root of the late pregnancy wastage in diabetics. With the availability of an inexpensive estrogen like stilbestrol, they developed an incremental estrogen regimen ending with 125 mg daily in the 35th week of gestation. White and the Smiths reported live-birth salvage rates in both observational and controlled studies that were far better than with any other therapy that had been tried, and this form of therapy came into wide use, especially since giving estrogen in a state already characterized by high estrogen levels (the estrogen output in a normal pregnancy is approximately equal to the annual estrogen output of 150 cycling women) seemed a reasonable and 'obviously harmless' intervention. Others failed to confirm these results, disagreed with the pregnandiol findings of Smith and Smith, and felt that the treatment was no better than placebo.[15] Actually, it was not until 1986 that Castracane et al[16] proved the Smith and Smith mechanism of an estrogen-dependency of placental progesterone production to be correct. Unfortunately, during these years the rules of clinical experimental design, the control of biases, the statistical evaluation of data and other aspects of good investigational technique were not as well understood as at present, and much flawed work was published, leading to controversy that remained unsettled.[17]

One aspect of this gestational therapy that concerned many obstetricians was the tumorigenicity and teratogenicity of stilbestrol (and other estrogens) in pregnant rodents. Experimental tumor formation in a wide variety of tissues, major alterations of both male and female genital tracts, abnormalities of hair growth and dentition, etc. were reported. These effects varied from species to species. Reproductive biologists[18] emphasized that estrogens were toxic to rodent pregnancy to begin with, that the experimental doses used were out of proportion to human therapy, and that extrapolation to human use was thus unwarranted. One must record in passing, however, that one Texas obstetrician gave women with threatened or recurrent abortion total dosages that exceeded 180 000 mg with no sign of ill effects to mother or fetus.[19]

In 1971 Herbst[20] in Boston reported a cluster of seven young women with a rare malignancy — clear cell carcinoma of the vagina — and noted that six of their mothers had been given stilbestrol during gestation of these children. This was not a proper case/control study, but enormous publicity resulted. A registry was set up by Herbst (it should be noted that such registries are of no value for most epidemiological calculations) and major retrospective studies were undertaken throughout the United States. Subsequently it was reported that T-shaped uteri, salpingeal atresia and a variety of other reproductive tract disorders (in both male and female offspring) were present in larger numbers in stilbestrol-exposed offspring than expected from control populations.[17] It is now generally believed that stilbestrol exposure is causally related to some cases of clear-cell carcinoma of the vagina (although at least a fourth of the cases in the Herbst registry have no evidence of such exposure). The inadequacy of the epidemiological studies of this issue was meticulously documented by McFarlane et al[21] in 1986, but without much effect on the beliefs of the obstetrical and oncological establishments. This piece of history gave stilbestrol such a bad name that it is now virtually never used in the USA. The fundamental biologic question remains: if all estrogens act through the same receptor mechanism, why and how should (nonsteroidal) stilbestrol alone cause this unique malignancy at this particular site? DES exposure in pregnancy is considered further in chapter 43.

CONTRACEPTIVE APPLICATIONS

Another major clinical role of estrogens and progestogens lies in the field of contraception. Most people believe that this application began with the development of 'the pill' in the late 1950s.[22] In fact, the idea of contraception with an ovarian (progestational) hormone is explicit in the studies of Haberlandt in Austria in the 1920s and 1930s.[23] Since pure compounds were unavailable, he did not achieve his goal, although he tried to market an oral preparation called 'Infecundin'. As early as 1912 others noted the ovulation-inhibiting effect of estrogenic extracts.[7] In their paper describing the synthesis of stilbestrol Dodds et al[5] specifically mentioned the possibility of using estrogen to inhibit ovulation or to prevent pregnancy in the manner we now describe as the 'morning-after-pill'. Their ideas were advanced for their time, and it was not until 1960 that clinical research into 'sequential' oral contraceptives using mestranol or ethinyl estradiol for ovulation inhibition and cycle-end progestogen simply for its endometrial effect began.

The specific search for a steroid contraceptive[7,22] re-emerged when Pincus and Chang repeated the 1937 studies of Makepeace et al,[24] confirming the antiovulatory effect of progesterone in rabbits. Pincus was a consultant to the GD Searle Co. in the USA, and they sent him selected newly-synthesized steroids for his studies; these compounds eventually included the 19-norsteroids norethynodrel and norethisterone. These agents provided orally active progestogens potent enough to do in humans what progesterone did in rabbits. Clinical studies in Puerto Rico and eventually by Syntex in Mexico and the USA by several investigators[7] confirmed the efficacy of 'the pill'. What Pincus and his colleagues at first ignored was a contamination of their norethynodrel with mestranol, yet we know today that the 150 μg of this estrogen present in their original clinical formulation was by itself sufficient to account for the contraceptive effect. Eventually the individual and combined effects of ethynyl estrogens and 19-norprogestogens were worked out and the synergistic effect on the hypothalamopituitary system identified,[25] thus making possible the very low dose oral contraceptive formulations in use today.

Large doses of stilbestrol or other estrogens for 'interception' were presently supplanted by less unpleasant but equally brief exposure to high dose ethinyl estradiol/levonorgestrel oral contraceptives; these regimens will no doubt be replaced by the timely use of oral antiprogestational compounds such as mifepristone.

The ethynyl estrogens mestranol and ethinyl estradiol have a gonadotropin-inhibiting potency disproportionate to their other estrogenic effects,[25] but even with these estrogens 60–75 μg per day are required for consistent ovulation inhibition; thus the 'sequential' type of oral contraceptive fell into disuse as lowering of the contraceptive dosage was pursued. By contrast, the 19-norprogestogens have several contraceptive actions (q.v.), making possible the progestogen-only minipill.[26] Further, micronized medroxyprogesterone acetate, a compound currently not used in oral contraceptive formulations, was shown in 1966 to be a highly effective injectable contraceptive, with a three month duration of action.[27] More recently, the World Health Organization Human Reproduction Programme has sponsored the development of several monthly injectable estrogen/progestogen formulations.[28] Much research has been done over the past 30 years with implantable devices delivering various progestogens and having effectiveness for up to five years or more. Norplant, containing levonorgestrel, is the only system marketed worldwide at the present time.

Special considerations

The idea of providing contraception with a drug differs profoundly from the idea of using a drug to treat an ailment, and raises some highly charged religious and sociocultural issues that do not occur in the course of ordinary therapeutics. It is therefore not surprising that even anecdotal reports of adverse effects attributed to hormonal contraceptives gained (and still gain) immediate and worldwide attention. These adverse effect reports not only alerted the medical professional to problems that had to be addressed, but were — and still are — invoked through the media by religious or 'moral' opponents of contraception, and others with special agendas of their own.

Over the last 30 years, this attention has resulted in the most intensive scrutiny accorded to any pharmacological agent in history. The unfortunate result of a sometimes unbalanced assessment of benefits v. risks has been to frighten large numbers of women away from this most effective form of contraception. In the USA it was estimated that over a million unintended pregnancies occurred per year because of oral contraceptive failure, misuse or discontinuation, and that misperceptions about oral contraceptive efficacy and safety account for up to 60% of this total.[29] It is education, not intrinsic efficacy or safety, that is currently the limiting factor in this form of contraception.

REFERENCES

1. Medvei VC 1992 The history of clinical endocrinology. Parthenon Publishing Group, New York
2. Allen WM 1974 Recollections of my life with progesterone. Gynecological Investigation 5: 142–182
3. Allen E, Doisy A 1923 An ovarian hormone: preliminary report on its localization, extraction, partial purification and action in test animals. Journal of the American Medical Association 81: 819–821
4. Haus LW, Goldzieher JW, Hamblen EC 1947 Dysmenorrhea and ovulation: correlation of the effect of estrogen therapy on pain, the endometrium, and the basal body temperature. American Journal of Obstetrics and Gynecology 54: 820–828
5. Dodds EC, Golberg L, Lawson W, Robinson R 1939 Synthetic oestrogenic compounds related to stilbene and diphenylethane. Part I. Proceedings of the Royal Society of London 127: 140–152
6. Butenandt A, Westphal U 1974 Isolation of progesterone — 40 years ago. American Journal of Obstetrics and Gynecology 120: 137–141
7. Perone N, Goldzieher JW 1995 Historical perspective. In: Goldzieher JW, Fotherby K (eds) Pharmacology of the contraceptive steroids. Raven Press, New York, pp 5–26
8. Vecchio TJ 1993 Birth control by injection. The story of depo-provera. Vantage Press, New York

8a. Lacassagne AL 1932 Apparition des cancers de la mamelle chez la souris malè soumis a des injections de folliculine. Compt Rend Seances Soc Biol Filiales 195: 632–638

9. Cobleigh MA, Berris RF, Bush T et al 1994 Estrogen replacement therapy in breast cancer survivors. Journal of the American Medical Association 272: 540–545
10. Ziel HK, Finkle WD 1975 Increasd risk to endometrial cancer among users of conjugated estrogens. New England Journal of Medicine 293: 1167–1170
11. Wilson RB 1966 Feminine forever M. Evans & Co., New York
12. Goldzieher JW, Haus LW, Hamblem EC 1947 The characteristics of uterine bleeding following cyclic oral therapy with estrogen and progesterone. American Journal of Obstetrics and Gynecology 54: 636–642
13. Smith OW, Smith GVS 1949 The influence of diethylstilbestrol on the progress and outcome of pregnancy as based on a comparison of treated with untreated primigravidas. American Journal of Obstetrics and Gynecology 58: 994–1003
14. White P 1945 Pregnancy complicating diabetes. Journal of the American Medical Association 128: 181–193
15. Ferguson JH 1953 Effect of stilbestrol on pregnancy compared to the effect of a placebo. American Journal of Obstetrics and Gynecology 65: 592–595
16. Castracane VD, Goldzieher JW 1986 The relationship of estrogen to placental steroidogenesis in the baboon. Journal of Clinical Endocrinology and Metabolism 62: 1163–1166
17. Edelman DA 1986 DES/diethylstilbestrol — new perspectives. MTP Press, Lancaster
18. Greene RR, Burrill MW, Ivy AC 1940 Experimental intersexuality. The effects of estrogens on the antenatal sexual development of the rat. American Journal of Anatomy 67: 305–323

19. Karnaky KJ 1947 Estrogenic tolerance in pregnant women. American Journal of Obstetrics and Gynecology 53: 312–315
20. Herbst AL, Scully RE 1970 Adenocarcinoma of the vagina in adolescence. A report of 7 cases including 6 clear-cell carcinomas (so-called mesonephromas. Cancer 25: 745–757
21. McFarlane MJ, Feinstein AR, Horwitz RI 1986 Diethylstilbestrol and clear-cell vaginal carcinoma. Reappraisal of the epidemiologic evidence. American Journal of Medicine 81: 855–863
22. Sawin C 1995 Gregory Pincus and the 'Pill'. Endocrine Practice 1: 216–218
23. Haberlandt L 1921 Hormonal sterilisation of female animals. Münchner Med Wochenschr 68: 1577–1578
24. Makepeace SW, Winstein GL, Friedman NW 1937 The effect of progestin and progesterone on ovulation in the rabbit. American Journal of Physiology 119: 512–519
25. Goldzieher JW, De la Pena A, Chenault CB, Cervantes A 1975 Comparative studies of ethynyl estrogens used in oral contraceptives. II. Effect on plasma gonadotropins. American Journal of Obstetrics and Gynecology 122: 619–624
26. McCann MF, Potter LS 1994 Progestin-only contraception; a comprehensive review. Contraception 50: S1–S198
27. Zanartu J, Rice-Wray E, Goldzieher JW 1966 Fertility control with long-acting injectable steroids. A preliminary report. Obstetrics and Gynecology 17: 676–683
28. Sang GW, Shao QX, Ge RS et al 1995 A multicentered phase III comparative clinical trial of Mesigyna, Cyclofem and Injectable No. 1 given monthly by intramuscular injection to Chinese women. Contraception 51: 167–192
29. Rosenberg MJ, Waugh MS, Long S 1995 Unintended pregnancies and use, misuse and discontinuation of oral contraceptives. Journal of Reproductive Medicine 40: 355–360

3. Drug regulatory testing

Richard A. Edgren

Introduction

The twin objectives of premarketing studies on drugs is to provide convincing evidence of efficacy and to assure safety. Regulatory agencies establish requirements for development that must be met prior to marketing. These regulations vary from country to country, partly because of variations in medical requirements but also because of variable attitudes toward health needs and political pressures controlling the regulatory agencies.

This chapter discusses what may generally be considered basic scientific needs and considers the published requirements of the US Food and Drug Administration (FDA), which are in many respects the world's most restrictive and most comprehensive. The FDA dominated early regulatory activity with regard to the oral contraceptives and provided unofficial standards for many other countries.[1] The World Health Organization has since focused on certain of these regulations and has provided a degree of relaxation without compromising safety.[2] More recently, the impact of general safety information, particularly on the oral contraceptives, has resulted in some relaxation of some of the more restrictive demands by the FDA.[3] Nonetheless, over the past 40 years or so requirements have become progressively more stringent as the drugs themselves have become more potent and effective. It is remarkable how modifications of steroidal sex hormones, particularly those employed as oral contraceptives, have dominated the thinking of regulatory agencies, in spite of the fact that these products have always been among the safest and most effective of drug classes.

PRECLINICAL STUDIES

Endocrine pharmacology

New steroidal entities or hormone-like agents that mimic the effects of the natural hormones must be subjected to a range of biological testing procedures. These are well-defined and have been basic to new-drug filings for many years. Estrogenic substances have a relatively restricted range of pharmacological activities, whereas the progestogens have a broad range; the use of combined estrogen and progestogen therapy in contraceptive formulations (and more recently in hormone replacement regimens) requires special considerations. The overlap in activities, particularly among the progestogens, means that much the same testing is required for all classes of sex hormone-like drugs.

I have recently reviewed my experience with drug regulatory testing of steroids that are components of oral contraceptives[4] and have provided protocols in papers referred to in that review. More detailed discussions have also been published elsewhere.[5]

Receptor binding

The primary actions of steroid hormones are mediated by binding to cellular receptors. Receptors for all five classes of steroid hormones: estrogens, progestogens, androgens, glucocorticoids and mineralocorticoids can be extracted in sufficiently pure form to permit precise qualitative assessment of binding and quantitative estimates of binding affinity. Most steroids currently employed in therapy were, however, developed and marketed prior to development of these assays. Binding information is now available on these drugs and such information is a prerequisite for the development of new drugs.

Although biochemically specific, binding data have limitations and must be supplemented with other pharmacological approaches. For example, mestranol, the 3-methyl ether of ethinyl estradiol used in many early oral contraceptives, must be demethylated before it binds to the estrogen receptor. Progestogens such as ethynodiol diacetate, norethindrone acetate and desogestrel, and perhaps norgestimate, require metabolic alteration before binding to the progesterone receptor. Thus these substances will fail to bind to their appropriate receptors *in vitro*, but will have measurable biological activity in bioassays. Furthermore there is some association of specific steroids with receptors for other classes, i.e. progestogens related to acetoxyprogesterone will bind to corticoid receptors as well as to the progesterone receptor, and those related to 19-nortestosterone bind to the androgen receptor. Such binding was often apparent from classical endocrine biaoassays before *in vitro* receptor binding methods became available.

Bioassays

The main purpose of bioassays today is to better characterize new compounds prior to their clinical use. Because the assays are based on common mammalian physiological mechanisms and employ natural steroidal substances as standards, the classical assays for steroidal sex hormone-like activity project well to human situations qualitatively. In contrast, quantitative bioassay data are much less predictive: in a very general sense, highly potent compounds tend to be so both in laboratory animals and in the clinic; weak substances tend to be weak in the laboratory and the clinic. In my opinion precise quantification will not project to humans.

Estrogenic activity

The natural estrogenic hormones are active in a broad range of laboratory animal systems. The induction of vaginal cornification, i.e. keratinization of the vaginal epithelium in spayed female rats or mice (the Allen-Doisy test), and growth of the rodent uterus in spayed or prepubertal animals are the most common approaches employed. These assays have been used for decades and their strengths and limitations are well understood.[6] The vaginal smear assays appear to be more *specific* than the uterine growth assays, because androgens and progestogens also are effective in stimulating uterine growth, particularly in the rat. Uterine growth assays, in contrast, are more *precise*, i.e. the results are less variable.

In vitro bioassays, employing cell lines often derived from human breast cancer cells, have achieved a degree of popularity with many cancer researchers. The correspondence of these assays with *in vivo* systems and particularly their clinical correlations remain to be established.

Progestational activity

Most bioassays, both qualitative and quantitative, depend upon secretory transformation of the uterine epithelium. Rabbits have been used extensively for this purpose. McPhail provided a grading system that depends upon the degree of glandular proliferation of the epithelium in estrogen-primed animals.[7] Two assays employ the McPhail system: the Clauberg assay employs systemic administration, either oral or parenteral, to immature estrogen-treated rabbits;[8] the McGinty assay involves direct injection into an isolated segment of the uterus of spayed, adult estrogen-primed animals.[9]

Rats have been extensively employed in pregnancy maintenance tests. When pregnant rats are spayed during gestation the embryos are resorbed. Administration of progesterone and various synthetic progestogens maintain normal embryonic and fetal development through to the expected time of parturition.

Certain qualitative problems arise in interpretation of data from these assays. Such extensively employed human progestogens as norethynodrel and norethisterone produce a minimal degree of glandular proliferation in the Clauberg test, but they fail to produce development comparable to that of progesterone itself; they have little or no effect in the McGinty test, and they do not maintain pregnancy in spayed, pregnant rats.[10] In addition, norgestrel, which has characteristic progesterone-like activities in most assay systems, maintains pregnancy in rats only at low doses, and is ineffective at higher levels.

Androgenic activity

Classically, testing for male-hormone-like activity depends upon growth of the prostate or seminal vesicles of castrated rats, either immature[11] or adult.[12] Prostate growth is the more specific, because estrogens as well as androgens stimulate seminal vesicle growth. Correspondence with human activity is generally good, although classic end-points for assessment of androgenic activity in humans (e.g. acne, hirsutes, vocal changes) remain variable and subjective. Suppression of levels of HDL-cholesterol might provide a precise, specific parameter for screening for androgenic activity but has not been employed for comparative purposes.

Corticoid activity

Glucocorticoid assessment can be based upon a broad series of assays, including anti-inflammatory tests such as the Selye pouch test and the cotton wad granuloma test; liver glycogen content of adrenalectomized rats and thymolymphatic involution are also satisfactory bioassays. Estrogens tend to be ineffective in such tests, although a degree of thymic involution can be produced in intact animals. Progestogens, at least the C21-acetoxyprogesterone derivatives, display a significant degree of glucocorticoid activity, which corresponds to binding to the glucocorticoid receptor; the 19-nortestosterone derivatives appear to have little effect in these assays.

Mineralcorticoid effects may be demonstrated by evaluation of sodium retention in adrenalectomized rats,[13] and the potent anti-aldosterone compounds often show a degree of progestational activity.[14]

Hormone antagonist activity

Most of the assays cited above, if performed precisely enough, can be adapted to measure antagonistic effects. Progestogens and androgens tend to have anti-estrogenic effects. The estrogens will inhibit the effects of progesterone. Androgenic activities are often reversed by simultaneous administration of progestogens. The anti-estrogenic effects of progestogens can be of crucial importance in assessing potential progestogen-only contraceptives, which act by reversing estrogen-induced changes in cervical mucus at mid-cycle in women.

Other activities

Estrogens and progestogens often have effects on pharmacological activities far removed from their primary sex hormone activities. For example, high-dose estrogens often produce gastric ulcers in rats, presumably as a result of activation of endogenous glucocorticoids, i.e. they act as stressors. Progestational agents have anaesthetic effects, particularly when administered intravenously. In the initial testing of estrogens and progestogens it is mandatory to subject a new agent to an extended range of pharmacological assays — most will produce negative results, but some might identify unexpected but clinically important activities.

Toxicology and carcinogenicity

Standard toxicological studies are probably the most straightforward and least disputed area for consideration here. Acute toxicity usually involves a single administration of a high dose of a compound followed by observation of the animals for a week or more, followed finally by sacrifice and detailed autopsy. If deaths occur or other untoward observations are made, examinations are required to determine cause. Fortunately, estrogens and progestogens and their combinations in oral contraceptives have little acute toxicity — as a result such studies with these drugs are of limited significance.

Subchronic and chronic studies require relatively long-term administration of test compound. Currently, for a New Drug Application for oral contraceptives, the FDA requires a six month toxicology test in rats and a 12 month test in monkeys. Subchronic tests are variable, but the duration of the animal studies must equal the proposed duration of the clinical trial, up to the maxima indicated for the NDA. A two year carcinogenicity study is also required in rats or mice. These requirements seem neither onerous nor excessive, and are a welcome simplification from earlier requirements, which included two year studies in rats, dogs and monkeys as well as seven year carcinogenic studies in dogs and ten year studies in monkeys. Doses to be employed are based upon blood levels determined from human studies, and are proposed to produce a ten fold higher blood level in the laboratory animals than are found in women.

One must question the use of circulating levels of drugs as a basis for setting a standard for testing. It has been known for decades that steroids are sequestered and retained in target organs long after they are cleared from the blood. Thus one might expect that activity, including toxicity, be more likely related to tissue levels than to blood levels. Unfortunately, determining tissue levels on a routine basis is beyond current technical capabilities. Arbitrary multiples of clinical dose levels would seem appropriate, provided these are within biologically meaningful limits. The FDA-required 25-fold multiples of the clinical doses of norgestrel (racemate) and ethinyl estradiol on a mg/kg basis were practically ineffective in standard assays, i.e. these doses were of questionable toxicological significance. Multiples based upon biologically meaningful levels for the species employed in the toxicity study would seem adequate.

Carcinogenic studies on the sex steroids in rats and mice have been carried out for decades without producing clinically relevant results. In both species, estrogens tend to increase the incidence of mammary tumors, especially in sensitive strains of rodents, but specific studies with the high-dose oral contraceptive formulations available at the time showed little effect.[15] Meaningful projection of these findings to women has proved elusive, and one cannot help but wonder in retrospect whether the continued effort and expense of such studies is warranted.

In the wake of recriminations following the discovery of mammary carcinoma in dogs treated with a chloroethynyl derivative of 19-nortestosterone, and the establishment of the fact that C21-acetoxyprogesterone derivatives were associated with a very high incidence of benign mammary nodules in beagle bitches, the FDA mandated that seven-year dog and 10-year monkey carcinogenic studies be initiated prior to filing of an NDA; NDA approval was granted before the studies were completed. The expense and problems associated with such studies drove many potential developers out of the field of reproduction — a problem that still exists, and limits development of new estrogens, progestogens and oral contraceptives. That these tests were controversial from the beginning was obvious to researchers active in this area at the time, and many of us believed that we were simply working with a specific problem restricted to dogs, and perhaps even to beagle bitches! These early doubts have since been borne out and the dog testing requirements have been rescinded.[16] Similarly, the monkey data generated showed little beyond exaggerated pharmacological effects of the drugs,[17] and testing has now been abandoned.[3]

Reproductive toxicology

A specialized area of concern for drugs active on the reproductive system involves their potential for untoward effects on the reproductive system of treated subjects and on their offspring if treated when pregnant. Such concerns have not been restricted to natural and synthetic sex steroids, but have also been exended to other classes of therapeutic agents and recently to environmental pollutants.

Various special testing procedures have been required by the FDA for the evaluation of contraceptives:

Genotoxicity

The FDA recommends an *in vitro* mammalian cell gene mutation assay with and without metabolic activation, an *in vitro* chromosome aberration test in mammalian cells with and without metabolic activation, and the mouse micronucleus test for chromosome damage.[3] The relevance of these tests to human genetic problems remains to be demonstrated; there is no available evidence to suggest that the use of hormonal contraceptives is followed by genetic abnormalities.

Teratology

Teratological studies are warranted since, for example, androgenic progestogens in the past have been associated with masculinization of the human female fetus,[18] and estrogens,[19] particularly the nonsteroidal estrogen diethylstilbestrol, are associated with developmental anomalies of the genital tract (in both male and female fetuses). In each case these abnormalities occurred when the drug was employed, often at massive doses, in what at the time was considered a high risk of threatened pregnancy. Exposure of the fetus to oral contraceptives in the event of an unrecognized pregnancy has not been associated with anomalies of the neonate. Use during pregnancy is nonetheless warned against in current labeling requirements for oral contraceptives.

Perinatal and postnatal exposure

Administration of progestogens in late pregnancy prevents parturition and produces dystocia and fetal and maternal death in rats;[20] but the same is not true in humans. Both estrogens and progestogens inhibit lactation and are secreted in the milk. The use of estrogens or progestogens and the administration of hormonal contraceptives during lactation remains controversial. For many years estrogens were employed to inhibit lactation, but this use has fallen into disfavor in recent times.

Return to fertility

Evidence both in women and in laboratory animals supports the concept that fertility returns normally in women treated with estrogens and progestogens orally, although occasional delays are reported; whether such delays are drug related remains conjectural. Long-acting injectable agents have been associated with protracted delays in occasional women, usually interpreted as resulting from idiosyncratic clearance of drug from certain subjects.

CLINICAL STUDIES

Clinical evaluation of all drugs, including hormonal contraceptives, estrogens and progestogens is characteristically carried out in three stages.

Human safety (phase I trials)

Phase I studies are generally short-term, high-dose studies. Doses are chosen on the basis of pharmacological and toxicological assessment and given to volunteer subjects; classically these subjects have been young, healthy males, in order to assure that new, untried drugs are not inadvertently given to women in early pregnancy. Current pregnancy diagnosis techniques have largely obviated this concern, and clearly this is not a problem with drugs designed for menopausal women. Fortunately, estrogens and progestogens demonstrate little in the way of acute toxicity, so such studies are of limited significance.

Dose finding (phase II trials) and clinical use anticipation (phase III trials)

The purpose of phase II studies is to determine the effective dose or doses of the compound under consideration. This has from the beginning raised major problems — especially with regard to the oral contraceptives — problems that have been inseparable from those encountered in mimicking eventual clinical use (phase III studies).

Initially, both Enovid and Ortho-Novum were marketed with steroid doses that were early recognized as excessive, but decreasing the doses, particularly in the United States, required caution. Prior to liberalization of abortion laws, pregnant women had no recourse to termination of pregancy so sponsors of contraceptive efficiency studies were reticent to move from known effective levels to doses with unknown efficacy. The first dose decrease with Enovid, a halving of the levels of both the estrogen and the progestogen, was satisfactory, but the second halving of the doses was followed by an increase in pregnancies, which was reversed by an increase in the estrogen level.

The first round of dose decreases was directed toward decreasing the progestational component. Reports associating the use of oral contraceptives with thrombotic episodes began to appear early in the 1960s and for reasons that were never substantiated these problems were attributed immediately to the estrogen. This resulted in the major reductions in estrogen content we have seen over the past 40 years. Subsequent epidemiological studies have been interpreted as demonstrating decreased incidence of thrombotic episodes with the lower estrogen products, and regulatory agencies have been active in forcing older higher-dose preparations off the market. Two reviews fail to support a dose–response relationship between thrombotic experiences and estrogen doses.[22] Recent European concerns with venous thromboses and oral contraceptives involved an association with the progestogens gestodene and desogestrel rather than with the estrogens.[23] Peculiarly, in contrast to results with earlier preparations, these same studies appear to suggest a protective effect of the new progestogens on myocardial infarction.[24]

Currently, the FDA requires that a new oral contraceptive be supported by studies based upon 1000–2000 subjects treated for two years with an accumulation of 10 000 or more cycles of exposure. No explanation for this requirement has been made: I presented estimates many years ago that showed that little was gained in precision of estimated pregnancy rates if studies were extended beyond one year and included more than 100 or so patients. I recommended about 100–200 subjects for 12–18 months. Such numbers will not reveal rates of rare untoward events such as thrombotic episodes or breast cancer, but the rates of such complications are too low to be captured by the FDA-recommended studies.

During the 1960s and 1970s, drug testing guidelines for ovarian steroids included extensive studies of blood clotting factors, despite the low incidence of thrombotic episodes, which suggested that such information could not define meaningful risks. There have been no data to suggest that thrombotic episodes occurred in women with predisposing blood clotting problems. Closer attention to basic problems could perhaps have uncovered the factor V Leiden mutation at an earlier date; this is associated with the putative increased tendency to thrombosis both in pregnancy and in oral contraceptive users.[25] The FDA also required extensive studies of glucose metabolism, despite a lack of evidence that oral contraceptive-induced changes in glucose tolerance were diabetic in nature.

In the event a pharmaceutical company now wishes to alter dose without changing the chemical nature of the components, substantially lower numbers of subjects are required (500–600 subjects for six months) *provided the ratio of estrogen to progestogen remains constant.* No biological response to steroid hormone combinations is known that is dependent upon this ratio.

Recently, an FDA working group provided a series of recommendations regarding evaluation of combinations of estrogens and progestogens for menopausal therapy[26] that might arouse ethical concerns. Placebo groups are to be included, even though it is ethically difficult to justify administration of unopposed estrogen to women with intact uteri for a one year period, as is suggested in the guidelines. Similarly, with the anti-osteoporotic effect of estrogen as well established as it is currently, can one justify treating a group of menopausal women with placebo for a two year period? These FDA requirements appear to need reconsideration.

Conclusion

Many oral contraceptives and ovarian steroid preparations have been marketed that are safe and efficacious. However, the process has not been without cost. Onerous regulatory demands have contributed to withdrawal of much of the pharmaceutical industry from reproductive research and have caused significant delays in the development of potentially new therapeutic agents.

REFERENCES

1. Edgren RA 1972 A viewpoint of industry. In: Clinical Proceedings, International Planned Parenthood Federation, Sydney, 14–18 August, pp 144–154
2. Special Programme of Research, Development and Research Training in Human Reproduction. World Health Organization Guidelines for the toxicological and clinical assessment and post-registration surveillance of steroidal contraceptive drugs. In: Michal F (ed) 1989 Safety requirements for contraceptive steroids. Cambridge University Press, Cambridge, pp 416–454
3. Jordan A 1992 FDA requirements for nonclinical testing of contraceptive steroids. Contraception 46: 499–509
4. Edgren RA 1994 Issues in animal pharmacology. In: Goldzieher JW, Fotherby K (eds) Pharmacology of the contraceptive steroids. Raven Press, New York, pp 81–97
5. Dorfman R (ed) 1962–1966 Methods in hormone research, volumes II–V. Academic Press, New York
6. Reel JR, Lamb JC, Neal B (1996) Mammalian estrogen bioassays: current state of the art. Fundamental and Applied Toxicology 34: 288–305
7. McPhail MK 1934 The assay of progestin. Journal of Physiology 83: 145–156
8. Elton RL, Edgren RA 1958 Biological actions of 17α-(2-methallyl)-19-nortestosterone, an orally active progestational agent. Endocrinology 63: 464–472
9. McGinty DA, Anderson CP, McCullough NB 1939 Effect of local application of progesterone on the rabbit uterus. Endocrinology 24: 829–832
10. Edgren RA, Jones RC, Peterson DL 1967 A biological classification of progestational agents. Fertility and Sterility 18: 238–256
11. Hershberger LG, Shipley EG, Meyer RK 1953 Myotrophic activity of 19-nortestosterone and other steroids determined by modified levator ani muscle method. Proceedings of the Society of Experimental Biology and Medicine 83: 175–180
12. Eisenberg E, Gordan GS 1950 The levator ani muscle of the rat as an index of myotrophic activity of steroidal hormones. Journal of Pharmacology and Experimental Therapeutics 99: 38–44
13. Kagawa CM 1964 Anti-aldosterones. In: Dorfman RI (ed) Methods in hormone research, vol III. Academic Press, New York, pp 351–414
14. Edgren RA, Elton RL 1960 Estrogen antagonisms: effects of steroidal spirolactones on estrogen-induced uterine growth in mice. Proceedings of the Society of Experimental Biology and Medicine 104: 664–665
15. Carcinogenicity tests of oral contraceptives. A report by the Committee on Safety of Medicines, 1972. Her Majesty's Stationery Office, London
16. Larsson KS, Machin D 1989 Predictability of the safety of hormonal contraceptives from canine toxicological studies. In: Michel F (ed) Safety requirements for contraceptive steroids. Cambridge University Press, Cambridge, pp 230–269
17. Valerio MG 1989 Sub-human primate studies. In: Michel D (ed) Safety requirements for contraceptive steroids. Cambridge University Press, Cambridge, pp 270–288
18. Wilkins L 1960 Masculinization of female fetus due to use of orally given progestins. Journal of the American Medical Association 172: 1028–1032
19. Herbst AL, Bern HA 1981 Developmental effects of diethyl-stilbestrol (DES) in pregnancy. Thieme Stratton, New York, pp 141–203
20. Edgren RA, Peterson DL 1966 Delay of parturition in rats by various progestational steroids. Proceedings of the Society of Experimental Biology and Medicine 123: 867–869
21. Sturtevant FM 1989 Safety of oral contraceptives related to steroid content: a critical review. International Journal of Fertility 34: 323–332
22. Russell M, Ramcharan S 1987 Oral contraceptive estrogen content and adverse effects: has a dose–response relationship been established? Canadian Family Physician 33: 445–460
23. Spitzer WO, Lewis MA, Heinemann LAJ, Thorogood M, MacRae K 1996 Transnational Research Group on Oral Contraceptives and the Health of Young Women. Third generation oral contraceptives and risk of venous thromboembolic disorders: an international case-control study. British Medical Journal 312: 83–88
24. Lewis MA, Spitzer WO, Heinemann LAJ, MacRae KD, Bruppacher R, Thorogood M 1996 Transnational Research Group on Oral Contraceptives and the Health of Young Women. Third generation oral contraceptives and risk of myocardial infarction: an international case-control study. British Medical Journal 312: 88–90
25. Bloemenkamp KWM, Rosendaal FR, Helmerhorst FM, Buller HR, Vanderbroucke JP 1995 Enhancement by factor V Leiden mutation of risk of deep vein thrombosis associated with oral contraceptives containing a third generation progestogen. Lancet 346: 1593–1596
26. FDA working group 1995 Guidance for clinical evaluation of combination estrogen/progestin products for hormone replacement therapy of postmenopausal women. Menopause 2: 131–136

SECTION 2

Chemistry

CONTENTS

4. Structure-function relationships and metabolism of estrogens and progestogens

Frank Z. Stanczyk

Introduction

A variety of natural or synthetic estrogens and progestogens are available to women for contraception or hormone replacement therapy (HRT). However, most clinical practitioners know very little about the chemical nature of these steroids and how they are transformed in the body. This information forms the foundation for understanding the pharmacokinetics of estrogens and progestogens utilized therapeutically, which will be discussed in subsequent chapters. All of this knowledge is vital in order to prescribe estrogens and progestogens appropriately, to understand particular as well as individual problems that may emerge with a given prescription, and to determine the need for a specific estrogen or progestogen. The objective of the present chapter is to compare the various estrogens and progestogens used therapeutically for contraception or HRT, with respect to their chemical structure, structure-function relationships and biochemical transformation in the body. This chapter will begin with a discussion of structure-function relationships of natural and synthetic estrogens and progestogens, and will follow with a discussion of their metabolism. The endogenous steroids will be discussed in relation to the menstrual cycle, pregnancy and the postmenopausal stage.

STRUCTURE-FUNCTION RELATIONSHIPS OF NATURAL AND SYNTHETIC ESTROGENS

Classification

Estrogens can be divided into two different types: steroidal and nonsteroidal, and each of these categories can be subdivided into natural and synthetic estrogens (Table 4.1).[1]

Table 4.1 Classification of estrogens and examples of each type

	Steroidal	Nonsteroidal
Natural	Estradiol Estrone Estriol	Phytoestrogens Cardiac glycosides
Synthetic	Ethinylestradiol Mestranol	Diethylstilbestrol Chlorotrianisene Clomiphene

Steroidal estrogens

Both natural and synthetic steroidal estrogens are related to the 18 carbon parent structure, estrane, possess an aromatic A ring, and contain oxygenated substituents at carbon number 3 (C-3) and C-17 of the molecule.

Natural estrogens

The three classic estrogens are estrone, estradiol and estriol (Fig. 4.1). They are referred to as classic because they were the first estrogens to be isolated. Of these estrogens, estradiol has the highest biologic activity. Oxidation of the hydroxyl group at C-17 of estradiol gives rise to estrone, which is 50%–70% less active than estradiol. Addition of a hydroxyl group at C-16 of estradiol yields estriol, which is only about one tenth as active as estradiol. When the hydroxyl group at C-17 of estradiol or estriol is transformed from β-orientation to α-orientation, the estrogens (17α-estradiol and epiestriol) lose their biologic activity.

Formation of a double bond between C-7 and C-8 of estrone gives rise to equilin, whereas double bond formation between carbons C-6 and C-7 and between C-8 and C-9 yields equilenin. The sulfated forms of these two estrogens as well as their reduced C-17 ketone metabolites are found in pregnant mare urine, which is used in the preparation of a widely used drug for estrogen replacement therapy, namely Premarin. Premarin is a mixture of at least 10 different conjugated estrogens, of which estrone sulfate

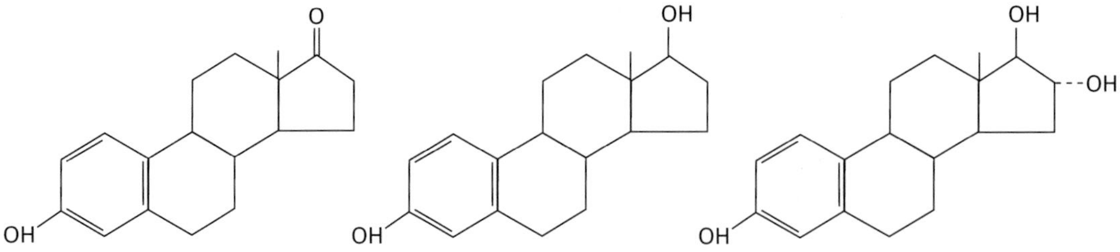

Estrone (E_1) Estradiol (E_2) Estriol (E_3)

Fig. 4.1 Chemical structures of estrone, estradiol and estriol.

comprises approximately 50% of the total. Other major constituents of Premarin include equilin sulfate and 17α-dihydroequilin sulfate; they represent about 25% and 15% of the total, respectively. The remaining 10% of the total consists of 17β-dihydroequilin sulfate, 17α-estradiol sulfate, 17β-estradiol sulfate, equilenin sulfate, 17α-dihydroequilenin sulfate, 17β-dihydroequilinin sulfate, $\Delta^{8,9}$-estrone sulfate.

Synthetic estrogens

A number of potent estrogens have been synthesized and are used orally or parenterally. Structural modification of the estradiol molecule by insertion of an ethinyl group (–C≡CH) at C-17 gives rise to ethinylestradiol, which is a very potent estrogen with high oral activity (Fig. 4.2). This compound is widely used as the estrogenic component of oral contraceptive steroids.

Modification of ethinylestradiol by formation of a methyl ether at C-3 yields mestranol (Fig. 4.2). This estrogen has been widely used as a component of oral contraceptive preparations, but is now used less frequently. The estrogenic effect of mestranol is due to its rapid demethylation in the liver, which results in the formation of ethinylestradiol.

Long-acting, oil soluble, estrogenic preparations used therapeutically are synthesized by esterification of estradiol at C-3 or C-17 with fatty acids. In general, the higher the molecular weight of the estradiol derivative, the more pronounced is the biologic activity of the compound. These products are usually administered intramuscularly. They can be administered orally, but are usually not as potent by this route. For example, estradiol benzoate, which is formed by esterification of estradiol with benzoic acid, is only half as potent when given orally, as compared with its administration intramuscularly.

Nonsteroidal estrogens

Many nonsteroidal estrogens have been isolated from natural sources or have been synthesized. These compounds have estrogenic activity but are different in chemical structure as compared with steroidal estrogens.

Natural estrogens

Numerous nonsteroidal compounds (called phyto-estrogens) that are weakly estrogenic have been isolated from plants. Although some of these compounds are important therapeutic agents (e.g.

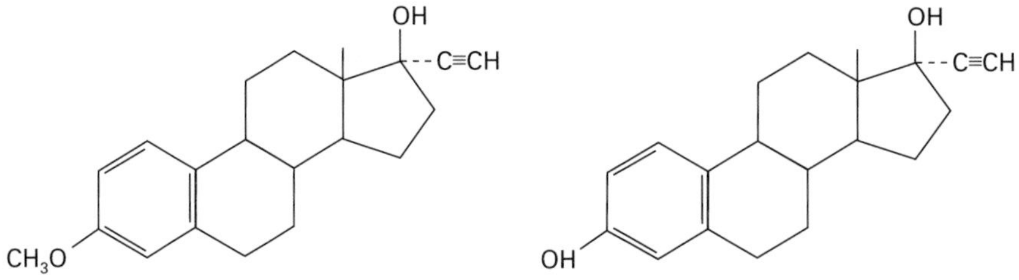

Mestranol Ethinylestradiol

Fig. 4.2 Chemical structures of ethinylestradiol and mestranol.

the cardiac glycosides), none is used for estrogen therapy.

Synthetic estrogens

The most important nonsteroidal estrogens are the stilbesterols, which are derivatives of stilbene (1,2-diphenylethene). Diethylstilbestrol is the best known of these derivatives because it was widely used therapeutically in the 1940s and 1950s. It is synthesized from estrone and is a highly potent, orally active estrogen. In comparison, estrone is orally inactive and not as estrogenic as diethylstilbestrol. However, published reports about potential oncogenic effects of diethylstilbestrol have drastically limited its use as a therapeutic agent.

Modification of the chemical structure of the diethylstilbestrol molecule can result in products with greatly reduced estrogenicity (Fig. 4.3). Examples of two of these products that are widely used therapeutically are chlorotrianisene (TACE) and clomiphene. TACE is a weak estrogen that is used clinically for suppression of postpartum lactation, whereas clomiphene is an antiestrogen that is used to treat anovulation. The latter compound is marketed as clomiphene citrate (Clomid and Serophene). Substitution of an ethyl group for the chloral group in the clomiphene molecule gives rise to tamoxifen which is widely used in the treatment of breast cancer.

STRUCTURE-FUNCTION RELATIONSHIPS OF NATURAL AND SYNTHETIC PROGESTOGENS

Classification

Progestogens can be divided into natural and synthetic compounds (Fig. 4.4).[2–4] There is really only one natural progestogen, and that is progesterone. Synthetic progestogens can be subdivided into those structurally related to progesterone and those structurally related to testosterone. Progestogens structurally related to progesterone can be subdivided further into pregnane and norpregnane derivatives. The pregnane derivatives consist of acetylated and non-acetylated compounds. Similarly, progestogens structurally related to testosterone can be subdivided further into compounds with and without ethinyl groups. The ethinylated derivatives can be subdivided into estrane and gonane derivatives.

Progestogens structurally related to progesterone

Clinical manipulation of the progesterone molecule has led to the development of potent progestogens (Fig. 4.5). Addition of a hydroxyl group at C-17 of progesterone results in loss of progestational activity. However, acetylation of the hydroxyl group gives rise

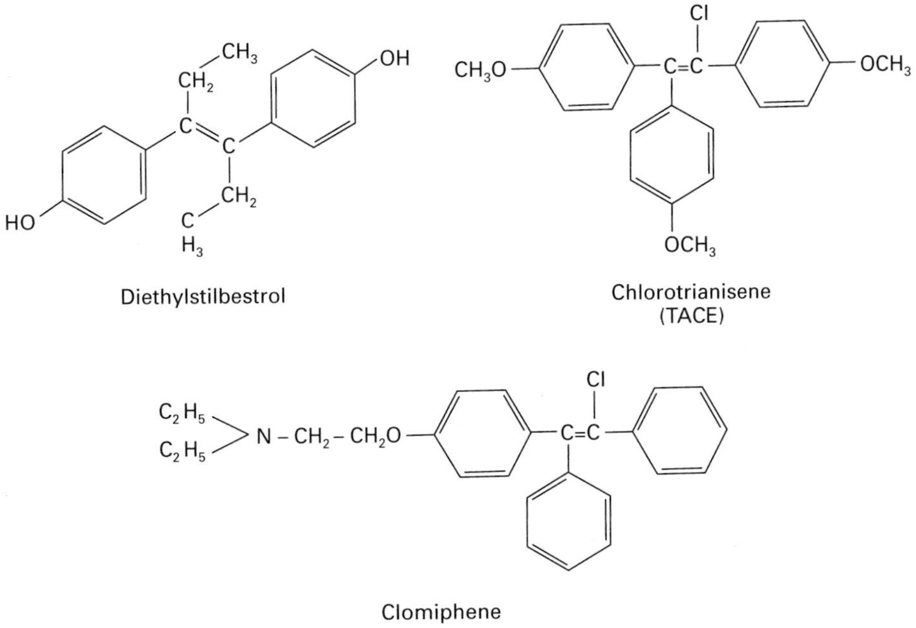

Diethylstilbestrol

Chlorotrianisene (TACE)

Clomiphene

Fig. 4.3 Chemical structures of diethylstilbestrol and its derivatives.

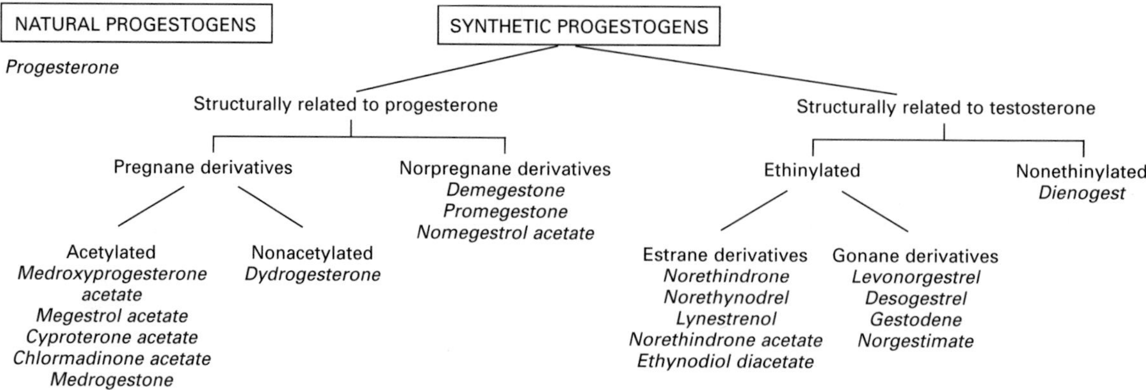

Fig. 4.4 Classification of progestogens and examples of each type.

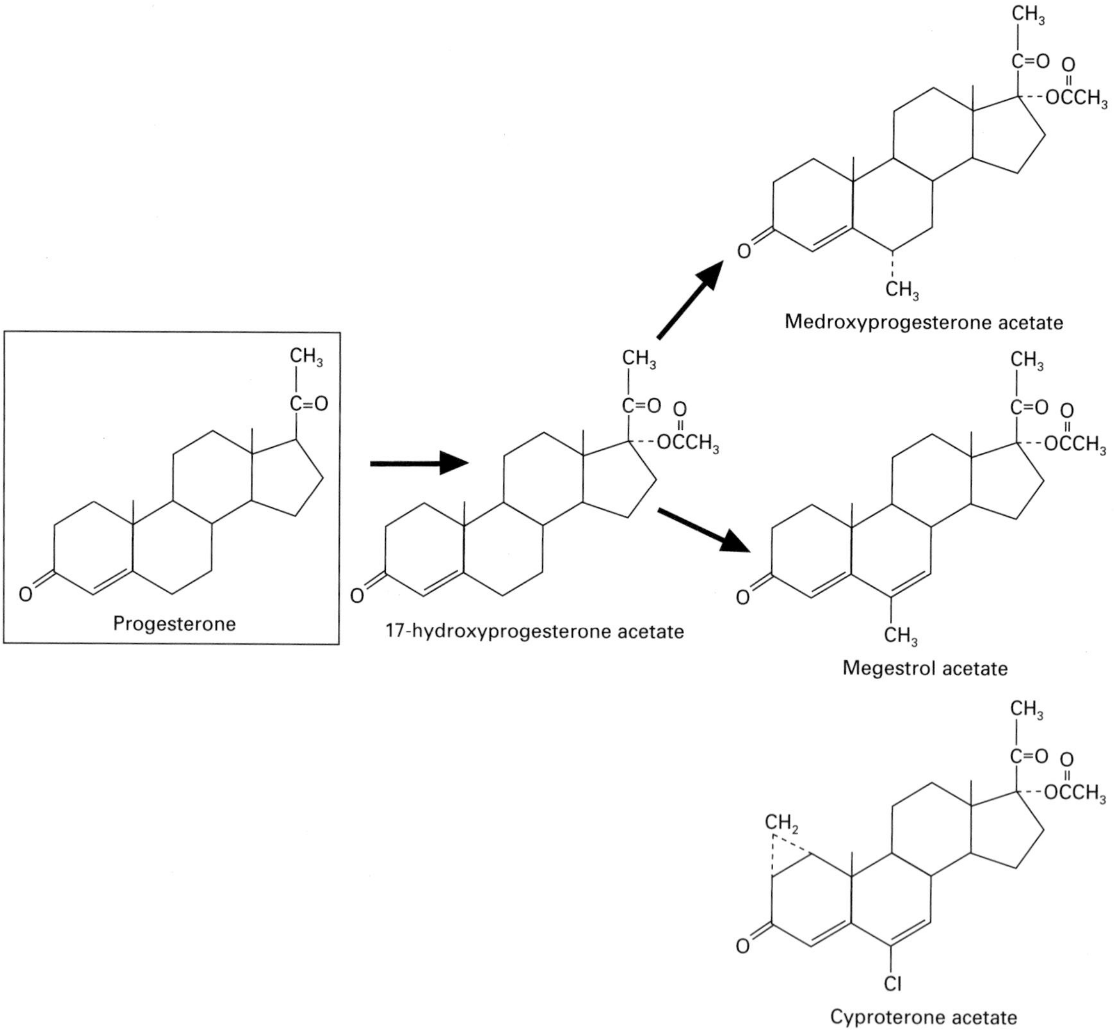

Progesterone

17-hydroxyprogesterone acetate

Medroxyprogesterone acetate

Megestrol acetate

Cyproterone acetate

Fig. 4.5 Chemical structures of progestogens structurally related to progesterone.

to 17-hydroxyprogesterone acetate, which has some progestational activity. Manipulations of the 17-hydroxyprogesterone acetate molecule, primarily at C-6, have produced potent oral as well as parenteral progestogens. These include medroxyprogesterone acetate, megestrol acetate, cyproterone acetate, chlormadinone acetate and medrogestone.

A different manipulation of the progesterone molecule has led to the formation of dydrogesterone. In this molecule, the methyl group at C-10 is in the α-orientation, and the hydrogen at C-9 is in the β-orientation. These two orientations are opposite to those present in progesterone. Also, the molecule has a double bond between C-6 and C-7.

Another group of progestogens structurally related to progesterone lack the methyl group at C-10. The 19-norprogestogens include demogestone, promegestone and nomegestrol acetate.

Progestogens structurally related to testosterone

Chemical alteration of the testosterone molecule has produced potent ethinylated and non-ethinylated oral progestogens, which are related to either the estrane or gonane parent structure. Addition of an ethinyl group at C-17 of testosterone causes the steroid to lose androgenicity substantially and to acquire progestational properties and oral activity. Removal of the methyl group at C-10 further increases oral progestational activity of the molecule and virtually eliminates its androgenicity. The resulting estrane derivative is called norethindrone or norethisterone (European name) (Fig. 4.6).

Four important derivatives of norethindrone are used orally (Fig. 4.7). Norethynodrel differs structurally from norethindrone only in the position of the double bond, which is between C-5 and C-6 in the norethynodrel molecule instead of between C-4 and C-5. Lynestrenol has no oxygenated functional group at C-3. Norethindrone acetate has an acetate group on C-3, whereas ethynodiol diacetate has acetate groups on both C-3 and C-17.

Substitution of an ethyl group in place of the methyl group at C-13 of norethindrone gives rise to an even more potent oral progestogen. This gonane derivative is called norgestrel and is synthesized as a racemic mixture, of which levonorgestrel is the biologically active form (Fig. 4.6).

Potent progestogens have also been synthesized by manipulation of the levonorgestrel molecule (Fig. 4.8). Removal of the ketone group at C-3 and addition of a methylene group at C-11 gives rise to desogestrel. Introduction of a double bond between C-15 and C-16 yields gestodene, and formation of an oxime

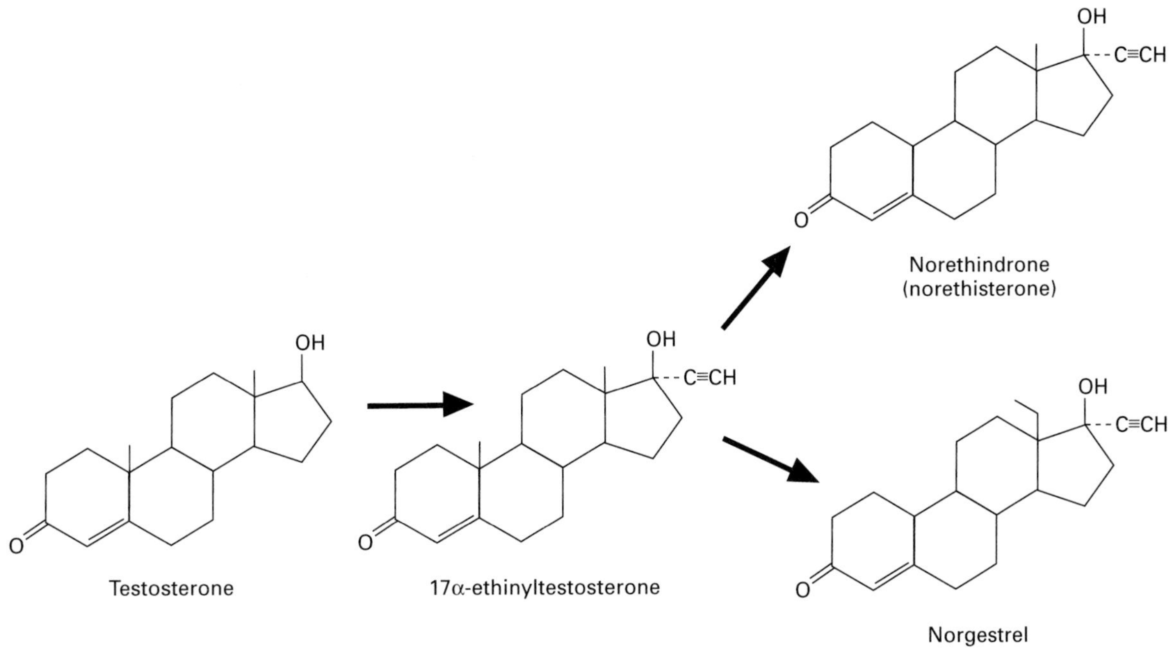

Testosterone

17α-ethinyltestosterone

Norethindrone (norethisterone)

Norgestrel

Fig. 4.6 Chemical structures of progestogens structurally related to testosterone.

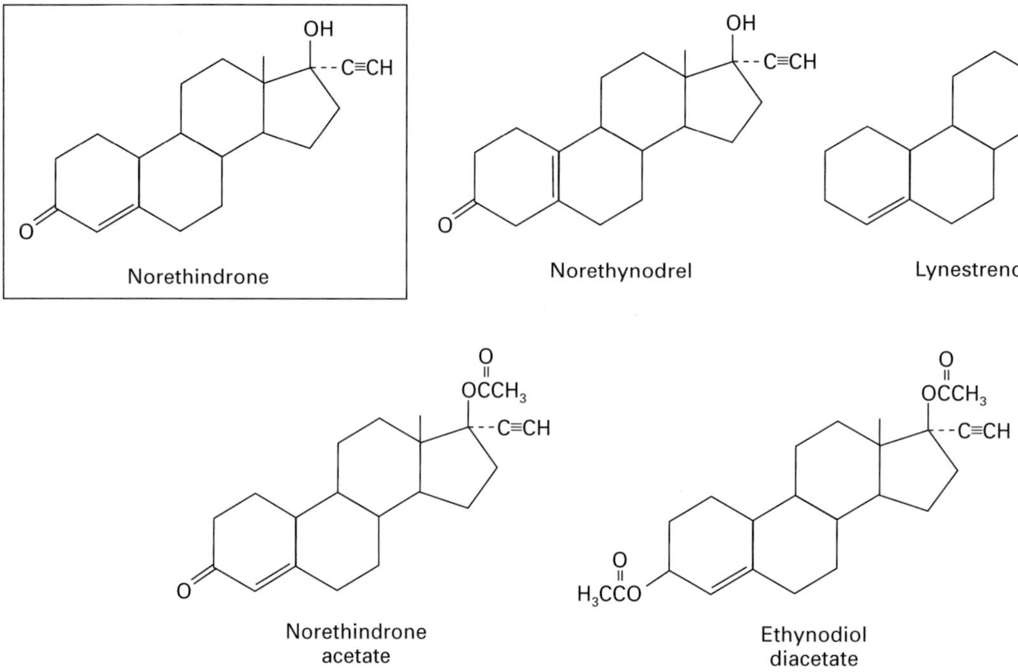

OH C≡CH O Norethindrone

OH C≡CH O Norethynodrel

OH C≡CH Lynestrenol

O OCCH3 C≡CH O Norethindrone acetate

O OCCH3 C≡CH O H3CCO Ethynodiol diacetate

Fig. 4.7 Chemical structures of progestogens structurally related to norethindrone.

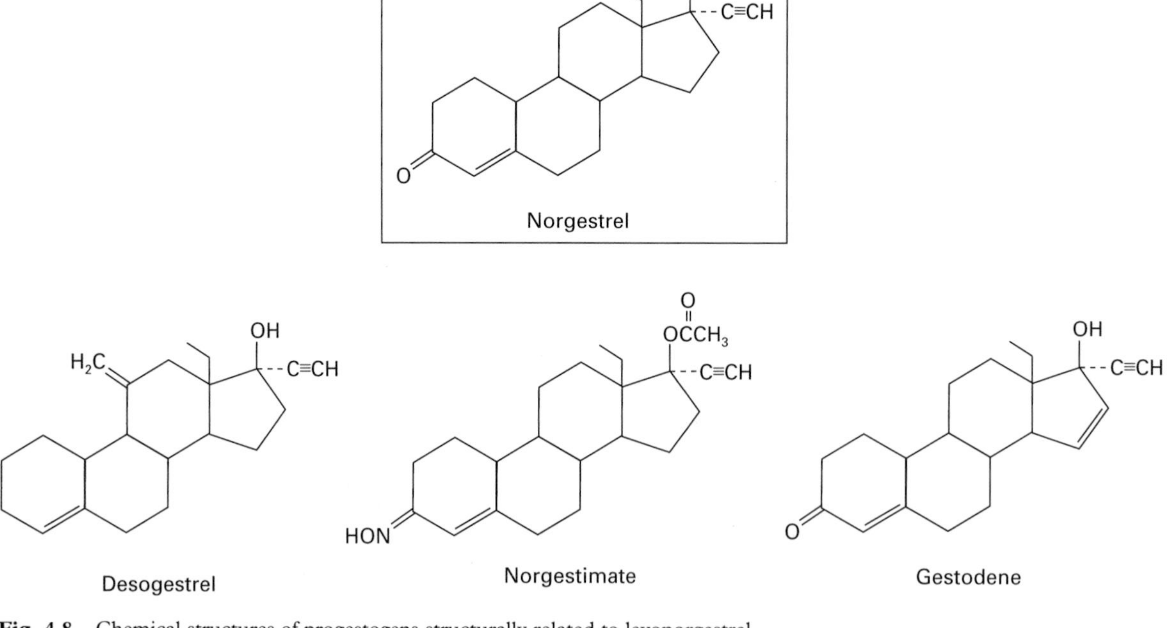

Fig. 4.8 Chemical structures of progestogens structurally related to levonorgestrel.

group at C-3 and an acetate group at C-17 produces norgestimate.

METABOLISM OF ESTROGENS

Natural estrogens

Premenopause

The major estrogens produced in non-pregnant women are estradiol and estrone. In the circulation, about 60% and 40% of the total estradiol is bound to albumin and sex hormone binding globulin (SHBG) respectively; about 2% is unbound (free).[5] In contrast, there is insignificant binding of estrone to SHBG. The lower affinity of SHBG for estrone compared to estradiol accounts for the fact that the metabolic clearance rate (MCR) of estrone (approximately 2200 liters per day) is considerably higher than that of estradiol (approximately 1300 liters per day).

Estradiol is readily converted to the less potent estrogen, estrone, through the action of the enzyme, 17β-hydroxysteroid oxidoreductase (dehydrogenase). This reaction is reversible, however the formation of estrone is favored.

Circulating estrogen metabolites. Major reactions involved in the metabolism of estradiol and estrone include hydroxylation or ketone formation at C-2, C-4, C-6α, C-6β, C-7α, C-14α, C-15α, C-16α, C-16β and C-18, as well as methylation of the hydroxyl group at C-2. Hydroxylation of estradiol or estrone at C-2 or C-4 gives rise to catechol estrogens, which are characterized by the presence of a catechol group (Fig. 4.9). Metabolites of estradiol and estrone circulate as sulfates, glucuronides, or mixed conjugates. Both the unconjugated and conjugated hydroxylated metabolites are present in very low concentrations in blood. For example, during the menstrual cycle circulating levels of 2-hydroxyestrone and estriol are only about 10 pg/ml.

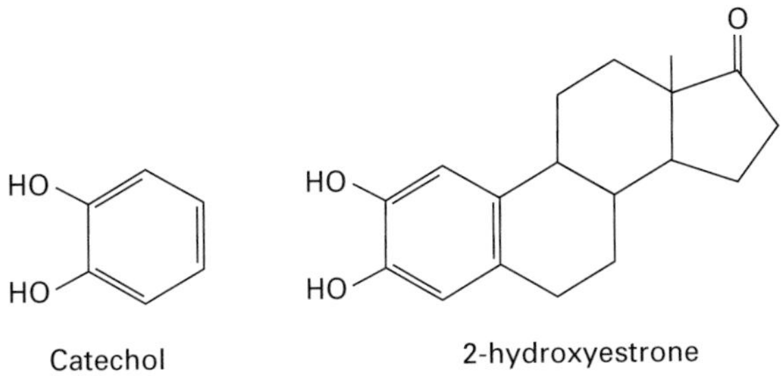

HO HO Catechol

HO HO O 2-hydroxyestrone

Fig. 4.9 Chemical structure of catechol group.

Until recent years, catechol estrogens such as 2-hydroxyestrone and 2-hydroxyestradiol were thought to be merely inactivation products resulting from the metabolism of estrone and estradiol, respectively. There is evidence, however, that catechol estrogens may have a role in the regulation of catecholamines. One proposed mechanism by which this regulation may occur involves competitive inhibition.[8] Catechol estrogens compete strongly for the enzyme catechol O-methyltransferase which inactivates the catecholamines, dopamine and norepinephrine. The affinity of 2-hydroxyestrone and 2-hydroxyestradiol for catechol O-methyltransferase is 10- to 18-fold higher than that of dopamine and norepinephrine. Thus, catechol estrogens may control hormonal actions of catecholamines by inhibiting enzymatic methylation and causing catecholamine inactivation.

Quantitatively the most important circulating estrogen in the premenopausal woman is estrone sulfate (Fig. 4.10).[6] In the follicular phase, it is present in amounts as high as 1000 pg/ml, and in the luteal phase the levels are even higher (approximately 1800 pg/ml). The production rate of estrone sulfate fluctuates during the menstrual cycle, similar to that observed for E_2 and E_1. During the follicular and luteal phases, the estrone sulfate production rates are approximately 100 and 300 μg/day, respectively. Estrone sulfate is not secreted by any endocrine tissue, since essentially all of its blood production can be accounted for by peripheral formation from estradiol and estrone. More than 90% of estrone sulfate is bound to albumin, which accounts for its low MCR (100–180 L/day). The importance of estrone sulfate is evident from studies in which transfer constants were determined for interconversions among estradiol, estrone and estrone sulfate (Fig. 4.11).[7] The data show that 65% and 54% of the estradiol and estrone, respectively, entering the circulation in women with normal menstrual cycles are converted to estrone sulfate, whereas the conversions of the reverse reactions are only 1.4% and 21%, respectively. The large pool of estrone sulfate may be conceptualized as a slowly metabolized estrogen reservoir.

In contrast to estrone sulfate, circulating levels of estrone glucuronide are approximately three- to five-fold lower. This finding is consistent with the fact that the renal clearance rate of steroid sulfates is approximately 10-fold lower than the steroid glucuronide renal clearance rate, and in blood the affinity of albumin for steroid sulfates is greater than for steroid glucuronides.

Urinary estrogen metabolites. In urine, the most abundant metabolites of estrone and estradiol are

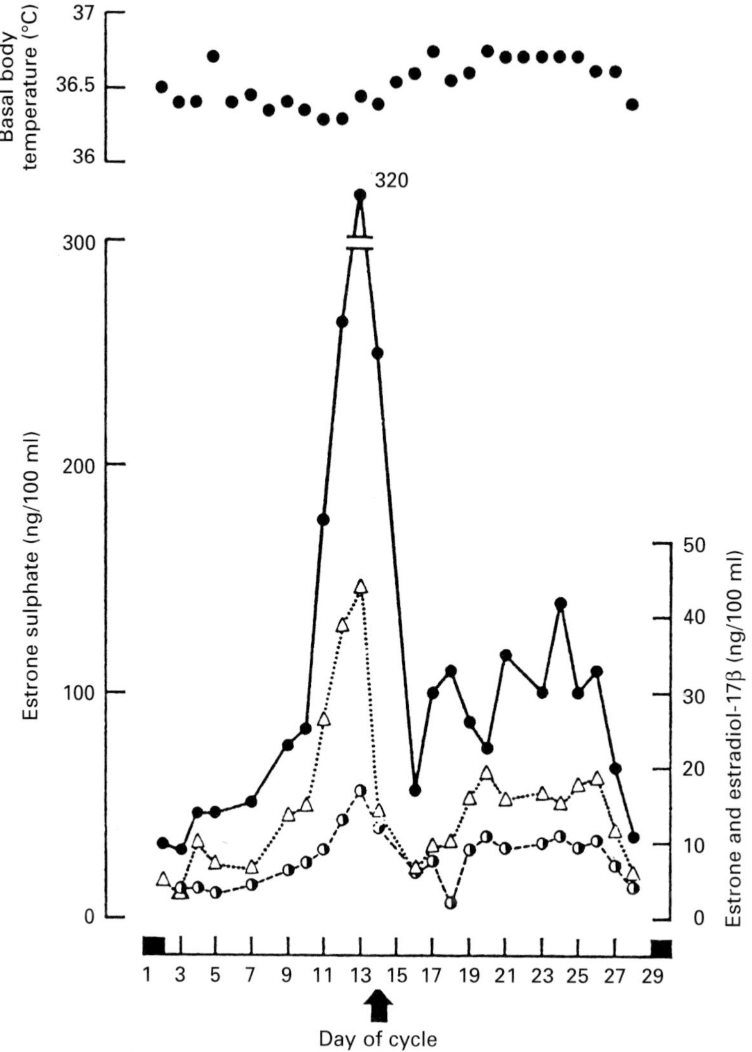

Fig. 4.10 Circulating levels of estrone, estradiol and estrone sulfate during the menstrual cycle.

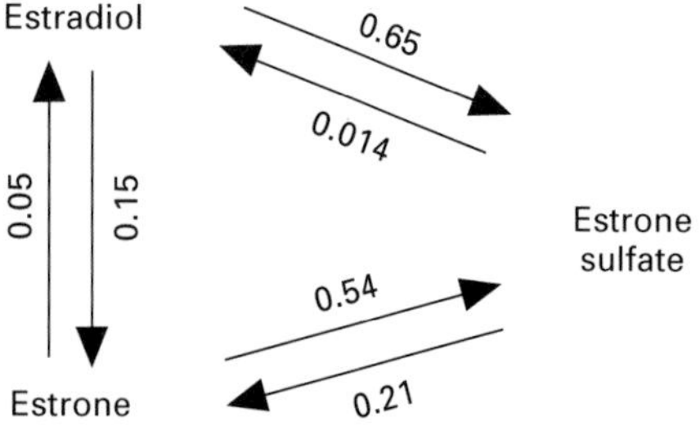

Fig. 4.11 Interconversions among estradiol, estrone and estrone sulfate.

conjugates of 2-hydroxylated and 16α-hydroxylated estrogens. In recent years, these estrogens have been the subject of studies involving breast cancer. It has been proposed that 16α-hydroxylation of estradiol is associated with increased risk of breast cancer, whereas the competing 2-hydroxylation pathway is either neutral or is associated with decreased risk.

Quantitatively, the most important 16α-hydroxylated estrogens in urine are conjugates of estriol, which include sulfates and glucuronides conjugated at C-3, C-16 or C-17, or a combination of these carbons. Mean estriol excretion rates measured following hydrolysis of the estriol conjugates are approximately 10, 25 and 20 μg/24 hr during the follicular, preovulatory and luteal phases, respectively. These values are 1–2 and 3–4 times greater than the corresponding excretion rates reported for estrone and estradiol, respectively.

Individual urinary estrogen conjugates have been tested for predicting ovulation, and determining the beginning and end of the fertile period. Initial studies showed that urinary levels of estrone glucuronide, estradiol-3-glucuronide, estriol-17-glucuronide and estriol-16-glucuronide rise early and steeply prior to ovulation.[9] In 1975, the World Health Organization set up a task force with the objective of developing a noninvasive immunochemical test (e.g. urinary dipstick assay) for determining the fertile period, and they selected estrone glucuronide for further studies. Although a test for predicting ovulation would be of great value for the treatment of infertility and for natural birth control, studies to develop a reliable and practical estrone glucuronide assay kit, which could be used in a physician's office or at home, have not been successful. Major obstacles limiting the availability of such an assay include large intra- and intersubject variability in excretion of urinary estrogens.

Pregnancy

In the pregnant woman, the placenta forms large amounts of estrone, estradiol and estriol which are secreted into the fetal and maternal compartments.[10] These estrogens are formed from androgenic precursors. The placenta cannot form estriol from estrone or estradiol because it lacks 16α-hydroxylase activity.

In the fetal compartment, the three classical estrogens are metabolized extensively. A large proportion of estrone and estradiol undergoes hydroxylation at different carbons of the steroid nucleus. In addition, estrone and estradiol as well as their hydroxylated metabolites are conjugated, forming primarily sulfates and to a lesser extent, glucuronides. Estriol, on the other hand, is hydroxylated only to a minor extent but undergoes extensive conjugation, forming mainly the sulfated metabolites.

The unconjugated estrogens cross the placenta readily and enter the maternal compartment, where they undergo transformations to a variety of unconjugated and conjugated metabolites similar to the metabolic conversions described for estrogens in non-pregnant women. Circulating levels of both unconjugated and conjugated estriol have been used clinically as diagnostic markers of fetal well-being. In the mother, estriol is metabolized almost entirely to four major estrogens: estriol-3-glucuronide, estriol-16-glucuronide, estriol-3-sulfate, estriol-3-sulfate-16-glucuronide. The conjugated forms of estriol represent approximately 90% of the total maternal circulating estriol, whereas unconjugated estriol comprises only about 10% of the total. Total plasma estriol levels at term are about 220 ng/ml.

Menopause

In postmenopausal women, both endogenous and exogenous estrogens are metabolized in the same manner as in premenopausal women. Since many postmenopausal women ingest estrogenic preparations, it is important to understand how these estrogens are transformed during intestinal absorption and the first pass through the liver. Three of the most common oral preparations utilized by postmenopausal women for estrogen replacement therapy are Premarin, Estrace and Ogen. Premarin contains 10 different conjugated equine estrogens, of which estrone sulfate comprises 50%, whereas Ogen consists of the piperazine salt of estrone sulfate. The estrone sulfate in both preparations undergoes hydrolysis in the intestinal mucosa yielding estrone, which is absorbed into the circulation and which can be converted to estradiol by a variety of tissues. In contrast, Estrace consists of micronized estradiol and undergoes oxidation via the enzyme 17β-hydroxysteroid oxidoreductase, to form estrone and estrone sulfate during the first hepatic pass. Thus, all three estrogen preparations give rise to increased circulating levels of estradiol, estrone and estrone sulfate, which are dose dependent. Following a 0.625 mg dose of Premarin, 1 mg of Estrace or 0.625 mg of Ogen, approximate ranges of estradiol and estrone levels found in postmenopausal women are 30–70 pg/ml and 120–200 pg/ml, respectively.

Equine estrogens

Knowledge of equine estrogen metabolism is important because these estrogens comprise approximately 50% of the total composition of Premarin. All of the sulfated equine estrogens can be hydrolyzed to form the corresponding unconjugated compounds. In postmenopausal women, equilin sulfate is converted to equilin, 17β-dihydroequilin, equilenin and 17β-dihydroequilenin.[11] No 17α-reduced metabolites are formed. Thus, the transformation of equilin sulfate to equilin and 17βdihydroequilin is similar to the conversion of estrone sulfate to estrone and estradiol.

Synthetic estrogens

Ethinylestradiol

The metabolism of ethinylestradiol is similar to that of the natural estrogens.[12] Thus, ethinylestradiol undergoes extensive hydroxylation at the C-2 and C-16 positions of the molecule. The 2- and 3-methyl ethers of ethinylestradiol have also been identified as major metabolites. Both ethinylestradiol and its metabolites undergo extensive conjugation. The principal circulating form of ethinlyestradiol appears to be ethinylestradiol sulfate; the ratio of these compounds in plasma was found to be 1:6.5 following the administration of ^{3}H-ethinylestradiol in women.

The presence of significant amounts of de-ethinylated urinary metabolites of ethinylestradiol, such as estrone and estradiol, has been found after oral and intravenous administration of ^{3}H-ethinylestradiol. However, quantification is difficult from the reported data. In a similar study neither ^{3}H-estrone nor ^{3}H-estradiol was found in blood. This finding does not rule out the possibility that other de-ethinylated metabolites of ethinylestradiol, e.g. estrone sulfate, were present in the circulation.

Mestranol

It has been shown that the estrogenic effect of mestranol is due to its rapid demethylation in the liver, forming ethinylestradiol.[12] Other metabolites of mestranol are similar to those described for ethinylestradiol. Like ethinylestradiol, mestranol also undergoes de-ethinylation *in vivo*. The extent of the de-ethinylation has been estimated to be 1–2% of the administered dose of mestranol, based on measurement of derived urinary estrone, estradiol, estriol and 2-hydroxyestrone. This conversion appears to be considerably less than that observed for ethinylestradiol, indicating that there is at least one major difference between the metabolism of mestranol and ethinylestradiol.

Tamoxifen

Following oral administration to humans, tamoxifen is converted to several metabolites. The principal metabolite of tamoxifen is N-desmethyltamoxifen, which is formed by removal of a methyl group from the parent compound. This metabolite is an antiandrogen and is similar in potency and efficacy to tamoxifen. Another important metabolite is 4-hydroxytamoxifen, formed by hydroxylation of tamoxifen at C-4. It is present in serum at approximately one-fiftieth the concentration of the parent compound and has an affinity for the estradiol receptors which is similar to that of estradiol. In serum, steady-state levels of tamoxifen usually range from 50–200 ng/ml, whereas the levels of N-desmethyltamoxifen and 4-hydroxy-tamoxifen range from 75–400 ng/ml and 2–5 ng/ml, respectively.[12]

METABOLISM OF PROGESTOGENS

Progesterone

Most of the progesterone in blood is weakly bound to protein and is metabolized extensively. About 20% of the progesterone is bound with high affinity to corticosteroid-binding globulin (CBG) and most of the remainder is bound to albumin.[5] Progesterone undergoes extensive metabolism, primarily in the liver, by reduction of its double bond (between C-4 and C-5) and ketone groups (at C-3 and C-20). These reactions result in formation of two pregnanedione isomers, four isomers of pregnanolone, as well as eight pregnanediol isomers. In addition, progesterone undergoes some hydroxylation, e.g. at C-21 to form deoxycorticosterone. Metabolites of progesterone are conjugated, forming a variety of sulfate and glucuronide derivatives which are excreted mostly in urine but also in feces. Quantitatively, the most important urinary metabolite of progesterone is 5β-pregnane-3α,20α-diol-3-glucuronide (pregnanediol glucuronide). The quantitative or qualitative determination of midluteal urinary pregnanediol glucuronide is useful for detecting ovulation. Measurement of this metabolite is carried out by immunoassay. A commercial kit for qualitative estimation of pregnanediol glucuronide has been marketed. It is based on a rapid enzyme immunoassay that measures the conjugate in first morning void urine specimens. Studies show that this test can be used at home to confirm whether ovulation has occurred, and provides a practical alternative to other diagnostic tests such as ultrasound and serum progesterone measurements.

During pregnancy, the metabolism of progesterone in the maternal compartment is similar to that in nonpregnant women but differs in both the fetus and placenta. Only a small amount of progesterone is metabolized in the placenta, whereas in the fetus there is extensive conversion of progesterone to a variety of hydroxylated products and their sulfated conjugates, e.g. corticosterone sulfate. Also, the fetal liver is a major site of progesterone reduction and conjugation, similar to the maternal liver.

Because the placenta secretes progesterone primarily into the maternal compartment, large amounts of pregnanediol glucuronide are excreted into the urine. Urinary pregnanediol glucuronide concentrations increase progressively until approximately 32 weeks of pregnancy, at which time the concentrations level off and are maintained until term.

There is evidence for interconversion of progesterone and 20α-dihydroprogesterone in the fetus and placenta. Fetal tissues, but not the placenta, readily transform progesterone to 20α-dihydroprogesterone, whereas in the placenta there is extensive metabolism of 20α-dihydroprogesterone to progesterone.

The clearance of progesterone from blood is rapid. Its MCR during both phases of the menstrual cycle and during pregnancy ranges from 2000–2300 liters per day. In postmenopausal women, progesterone metabolism appears to be the same as in premenopausal women.

Medroxyprogesterone acetate

Considering its wide use for many years throughout the world, little is known about the metabolism of medroxyprogesterone acetate. Following its oral administration, medroxyprogesterone acetate is found in the circulation weakly bound to albumin. The limited data on the metabolism of this progestogen shows that it undergoes reduction of the Δ^4-3-ketone group, hydroxylation (primarily at C-6 and C-21) and formation of glucuronides. It appears that the acetate group of the molecule remains intact during metabolism.

Levonorgestrel and norethindrone

In general, the metabolism of norethindrone and levonorgestrel is similar to that of endogenous steroid hormones and includes reduction, hydroxylation and conjugation.[13] The sulfates and glucuronides of levonorgestrel, norethindrone and their metabolites are excreted primarily in urine, and also in feces. Studies show that following oral administration of levonorgestrel labelled with carbon-14 (^{14}C), plasma levels of unconjugated levonorgestrel are highest, followed by tetrahydrolevonorgestrel sulfate.[14] However, in urine the pattern of levonorgestrel metabolites was opposite to that found in plasma. Tetrahydrolevonorgestrel glucuronide and 16α-hydroxylated tetrahydrolevonorgestrel glucuronide were the most abundant urinary metabolites, followed by tetrahydrolevonorgestrel sulfate. Only minute amounts of unconjugated levonorgestrel were found.

Although there are limited data on the metabolism of norethindrone, it appears that the pattern of its metabolites in plasma and urine is similar to that of levonorgestrel. When ^{14}C-norethindrone was administered orally to a woman in two different doses (25 and 2 mg), it was found that, in plasma, sulfated metabolites of norethindrone were most abundant, followed by unconjugated norethindrone and its metabolites; only minute amounts of the glucuronide metabolites were isolated.[15] In contrast, the glucuronide metabolites of norethindrone were present in highest concentrations in urine.

The higher levels of sulfated metabolites of levonorgestrel and norethindrone in plasma compared to the corresponding glucuronide metabolites is consistent with the distribution of endogenous plasma conjugated steroid hormones. Mechanisms by which elevated levels of sulfated steroids are maintained in blood include a higher affinity of albumin for steroid sulfates than for steroid glucuronides and a higher glomerular filtration rate of the steroid glucuronides compared to the sulfates.

Among the conjugated metabolites isolated in plasma following oral administration of ^{14}C-labelled levonorgestrel and norethindrone were the corresponding sulfated metabolites, i.e. levonorgestrel sulfate and norethindrone sulfate, respectively. The presence of significant plasma levels of these compounds is important because they may contribute to the progestational activity in a woman. Although conjugated steroids are not active, the sulfate moiety in compounds such as levonorgestrel sulfate and norethindrone sulfate can be cleaved off these molecules by sulfatases, present in a number of tissues, thereby yielding the progestationally active parent steroids. This is analogous to the present view that total estrogenicity in a woman is determined not only by circulating levels of estradiol and estrone but also by estrone sulfate.

Derivatives of norethindrone

Four progestogens are generally considered to be prodrugs of norethindrone.[13] Both norethindrone acetate and ethynodiol diacetate undergo rapid hydrolysis to form the parent compound, and it appears that lynestrenol may undergo hydroxylation and subsequent oxidation at C-3, thereby also forming the parent compound. In addition, there is some evidence, but not convincing, that norethynodrel is converted to norethindrone.

Derivatives of levonorgestrel

Desogestrel

It is generally accepted that desogestrel is a prodrug of 3-ketodesogestrel. Evidence to support this view initially came from a study in which a large dose of desogestrel was administered to a woman, and circulating levels of desogestrel and 3-ketodesogestrel were measured.[16] High levels of 3-ketodesogestrel were found. This finding was supported by data showing that ^{3}H-ketodesogestrel was a major metabolite when ^{3}H-desogestrel was incubated with liver homogenate.[17] Additional evidence demonstrating that desogestrel is a prodrug of 3-ketodesogestrel came from a study in which 10 women received a single oral dose of 150 μg of desogestrel in combination with 30 μg of ethinylestradiol, and another group of 10 women received a single oral dose of 150 μg of 3-ketodesogestrel, also combined with 30 μg of ethinylestradiol.[18] After measuring levels of 3-ketodesogestrel in serum obtained from both groups of subjects, it was shown that there was no significant difference in the levels of this metabolite between the two groups.

3-ketodesogestrel is bound mostly to albumin in blood and is metabolized further. Approximately 32% of the total circulating 3-ketodesogestrel is bound to SHBG and 66% is bound to albumin, whereas only 2–3% is unbound.[19] *In vivo* studies of 3-ketodesogestrel metabolism have not been performed. However, on the basis of the data from the *in vitro* study in which radiolabeled desogestrel was incubated with liver homogenate, it appears that 3-ketodesogestrel undergoes further reduction of its Δ^{4}-3-ketone.

Gestodene

There has been only a single study on the *in vivo* metabolism of gestodene.[20] Following oral administration of ^{14}C-labeled gestodene to a group of three women, it was shown that gestodene is transformed to reduced and hydroxylated metabolites, which are conjugated and then excreted in urine. A number of urinary metabolites of gestodene were not identified. No levonorgestrel was identified in either urine or blood, and therefore it is generally accepted that gestodene is not a prodrug. In the circulation, approximately 75% of the total gestodene is bound to SHBG, 24% is bound to albumin and less than 1% is unbound.[19]

Norgestimate

Norgestimate appears to be partly a prodrug for levonorgestrel. In the only *in vivo* study of norgestimate metabolism, it was shown that following oral administration of ^{14}C-norgestimate to a group of five women, levonorgestrel and four of its metabolites were identified in urine.[21] Other metabolites were also isolated but were not characterized. In a subsequent study, it was shown that following oral administration of 350 μg of norgestimate in combination with 70 μg of ethinylestradiol to 10 women, either as a single dose or daily for one week, peak serum levels of norgestimate were only 100 pg/ml, in contrast to peak levels of deacetylated norgestimate (levonorgestrel-3-oxime) which were 4 ng/ml.[22] More recently, a crossover study was carried out in 10 women, who received 250 μg of norgestimate in combination with 35 μg of ethinylestradiol or 250 μg of levonorgestrel combined with 30 μg of ethinylestradiol as a single oral dose.[23] Serum levonorgestrel levels were measured after both doses, and the results show that the levonorgestrel levels measured after the norgestimate dose were about one tenth of those obtained following the levonorgestrel dose. From the ratio of area under the curve (AUC) values obtained after both dosings, the bioavailability of norgestimate-derived levonor gestrel was calculated to be about 22%. These studies support the view that norgestimate is at least partly a prodrug of levonorgestrel.

Conclusion

In this chapter a variety of natural and synthetic estrogens and progestogens were presented with respect to their structure-function relationships and metabolism. It was shown that a practical approach in classifying estrogens and progestogens was to divide estrogens into steroidal and nonsteroidal types, and then to subdivide each group into natural and synthetic types. In contrast, progestogens were first divided into natural and synthetic types, and then the latter group was subdivided in relationship to the parent steroid, progesterone or testosterone. Knowledge of structure-function relationships of steroids used therapeutically is important for understanding their potency, and oral or parenteral activities. Furthermore, knowledge of chemical structures of steroids is the foundation for understanding steroid metabolism and pharmacokinetics.

The present chapter shows that the metabolism of progestogens and steroidal estrogens differs. Progestogens are transformed to a variety of metabolites primarily by reduction of the double bond between C-4 and C-5 and the ketone groups at C-3 and C-20. In contrast, steroidal estrogens are metabolized primarily by hydroxylation of the steroid nucleus. However, both estrogen and progestogen metabolites are conjugated by sulfation or glucuronidation of hydroxyl groups.

It is important to know which progestogens or estrogens act as prodrugs. This knowledge allows us to measure the appropriate circulating metabolite of the prodrug, so that the pharmacokinetics and potency of the drug can be studied.

All of this information will help the physician to choose the optimum estrogen and/or progestogen, as well as the appropriate dosage, when prescribing drugs for oral contraception and hormone replacement therapy.

REFERENCES

1. Stanczyk FZ 1997 Steroid hormones. In: Mishell DR, Jr, Paulson RJ, Shoupe D (eds) Mishell's textbook of infertility, contraception and reproductive endorinology 4th edn, Blackwell Science, Malden, Massachusetts, pp 46–66
2. Stanczyk FZ 1989 Pharmacokinetics of progestogens. Int Proc J 1: 11–20
3. Stanczyk FZ 1994 Structure-function relationships, potency and pharmacokinetics of progestogens. In: Lobo RA (ed) Treatment of the postmenopausal woman. Raven Press, New York, pp 68–69
4. Stanczyk FZ 1996 Structure-function relationships, metabolism, pharmacokinetics and potency of progestins. Med Actual/Drugs of Today (32 Suppl H: 1–14)
5. Westphal V 1986 Steroid-protein interactions. Springer-Verlag, Berlin, pp 192–264
6. Hawkins RA, Oakey RE 1974 Estimation of oestrone sulfate, oestradiol-17β and estrone in peripheral plasma: concentrations during the menstrual cycle and in men. Journal of Endocrinology 60: 3–17
7. Buster JE 1987 Estrogen metabolism. In: Sciara JJ (ed) Endocrinology, infertility, genetics, vol. 5. Harper & Row, Philadelphia, pp 1–11
8. Breuer H 1977 Metabolic pathways of steroid contraceptive drugs. In: Garattini S, Berendes HW (eds) Pharmacology of steroid contraceptive drugs. Raven Press, New York
9. Stanczyk FZ, Miyakawa I, Goebelsmann U 1980 Direct radioimmunoassay of urinary estrogen and pregnanediol glucuronide during the menstrual cycle. American Journal of Obstetrics and Gynecology 137: 443–450
10. Dizfalusy E 1969 Steroid metabolism in the feto-placental unit. In: Pencile A, Finzi C (eds) The feto-placental unit. Excerpta Medica, Amsterdam, p 65
11. Bhavnani BR 1988 The saga of the ring B unsaturated equine estrogens. Endocrinology Reviews 9: 396–416
12. Roy S, Bernstein L, Stanczyk FZ 1988 Analysis of oral contraceptive risks. In: Runnebaum B, Rabe T, Kiesel L (eds) Female contraception. Springer-Verlag, Berlin, pp 21–55
13. Stanczyk FZ, Roy S 1990 Metabolism of levonorgestrel, norethindrone and structurally related contraceptive steroids. Contraception 42: 67–96
14. Sisenwine SF, Kimmel HB, Liu AL, Ruelius HW 1975 The presence of DL-, D-, and L-norgestrel and their metabolites in the plasma of women. Contraception 12: 339–353
15. Braselton WE, Lin TJ, Mills TM, Ellegood JO, Mahesh VG 1977 Identification and measurement by gas chromotography–mass spectrometry of norethindrone and metabolites in human urine and blood. Journal of Steroid Biochemistry 8: 9–18
16. Vinikka L 1979 Radioimmunoassay of a new progestogen, ORG 2969, and its metabolite. Journal of Steroid Biochemistry 9: 979–982
17. Vinikka L 1979 Metabolism of a new synthetic progestogen, ORG 2969, and its metabolite. Journal of Steroid Biochemistry 10: 353–357
18. Hasenack HG, Bosch AMG, Kaar K 1986 Serum levels of 3-ketodesogestrel after oral administration of desogestrel and 3-ketodesogestrel. Contraception 33: 591–596
19. Kuhnz W, Pfeffer M, Al-Yacomb G 1990 Protein binding of the contraceptive steroids gestodene, 3-keto-desogestrel and ethinylestradiol in human serum. Journal of Steroid Biochemistry 35: 313–318
20. Dusterberg B, Tack J-W, Krause W, Humpel M 1987 Pharmacokinetics and biotransformation of gestodene in man. In: Elstein M (ed) Gestodene: development of a new gestodene-containing low-dose oral contraceptive. Parthenon Publishers, London, p 35
21. Alton KB, Hetyel NS, Shaw C, Patrick JE 1984 Biotransformation of norgestimate in women. Contraception 29: 19–29
22. McGuire JL, Phillips A, Hahn DW, Tolman EL, Flor S, Kafrissen ME 1990 Pharmacologic and pharmacokinetic characteristics of norgestimate. American Journal of Obstetrics and Gynecology 163: 2127–2131
23. Kunhz W, Blode H, Mahler M 1994 Systemic availability of levonorgestrel after single oral administration of a norgestimate-containing oral contraceptive to 12 women. Contraception 49: 255–263

5. Chemistry of antihormones

G.C. Davies

Introduction

The term antihormone encompasses a range of molecules with a spectrum of estrogenic/progestogenic activity. These agents may be subdivided into antiestrogens with varying degrees of agonistic activity, molecules with mixed antiestrogenic/antiprogestogenic properties and antiprogestogens. Steroid molecules play a key role in this group.

THE STRUCTURE OF STEROIDS

A steroid (cyclopentanoperhydrophenanthrene) is a hydrocarbon consisting of four rings (A, B, C, D). Rings A, B and C — perhydrophenanthrene — is the saturated derivative of phenanthrene. The five-membered D ring is a cyclopentane. The stereochemistry of the rings markedly affects biological activity. The orientation of the bonds of the steroid ring determine whether the steroid is either a trans (sagittal or coronal) or cis (sagicoronal) isomer.

The biologically active compounds progesterone, testosterone and estrogen are analogues of the 5α-pregnane, 5α-androstane and 5α-estrane steroid classes respectively. The pregnanes contain 21 carbon atoms (C-21), the androstanes C-19 and the estranes C-18. The 5α annotation denotes a hydrogen atom at position 5 on the opposite side to the methyl groups at position 18 and 19, which are assigned to the β side of the molecule. In drawing steroid compounds functional groups on the α side are joined by dotted lines whereas those on the β side are joined by solid lines. The symbol Δ is used to designate a C=C in a steroid. If the carbon double bond is located between positions 4 and 5, as is the case in progesterone, this is described as Δ^4.

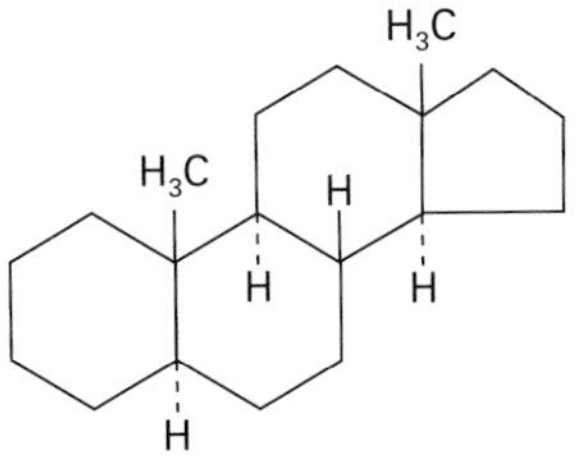

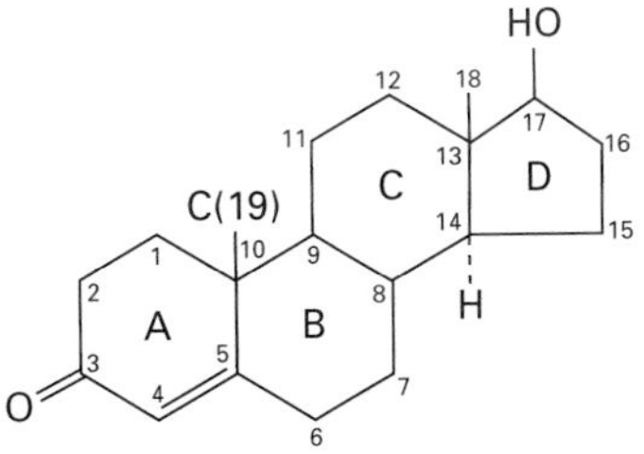

Testosterone (Fig. 5.1)

Testosterone (17β-hydroxyl-4-androsten-3-one) in many target tissues is reduced at the 5α position to dihydrotestosterone which serves as the intracellular mediator of most actions of the steroid.

Fig. 5.1 The chemical structure of the 5α androstane and testosterone.

Estrogen (Fig. 5.2)

The estrane class is typified by 17β estradiol (estra-1, 3,5,(10)-triene-3,17β-diol). It contains a phenolic A ring and a β hydroxyl group at position 17 of ring D. The high selectivity in binding to the estrogen receptor (ER) is dependent on the phenolic A ring, the C-3 hydroxyl substitution, the 17β hydroxyl group, the distance between the two hydroxyl groups and the planar, hydrophobic nature of the molecule.[1] Many compounds possess estrogenic activity; in contrast to

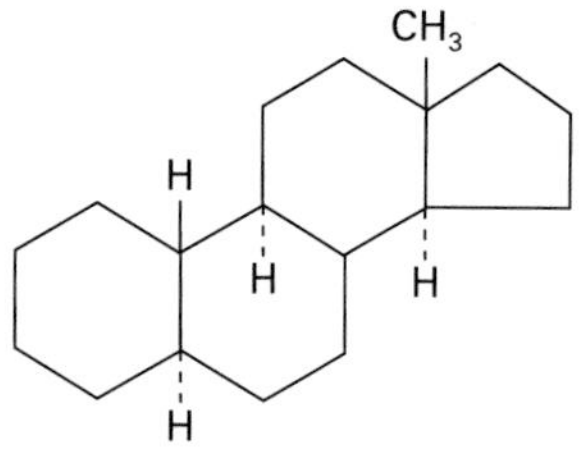

Fig. 5.2 The chemical structure of the 5α-estrane and 17β-estradiol.

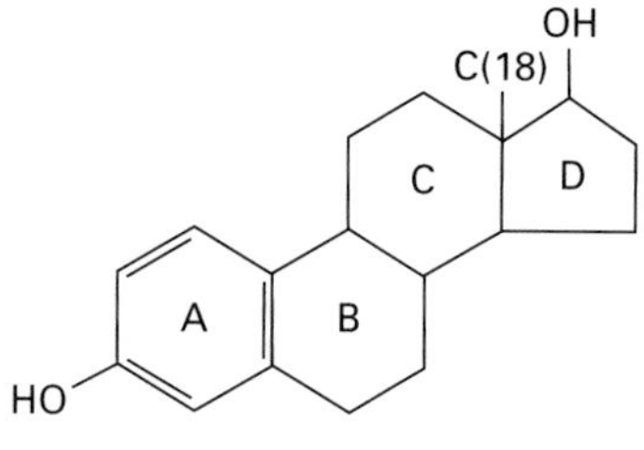

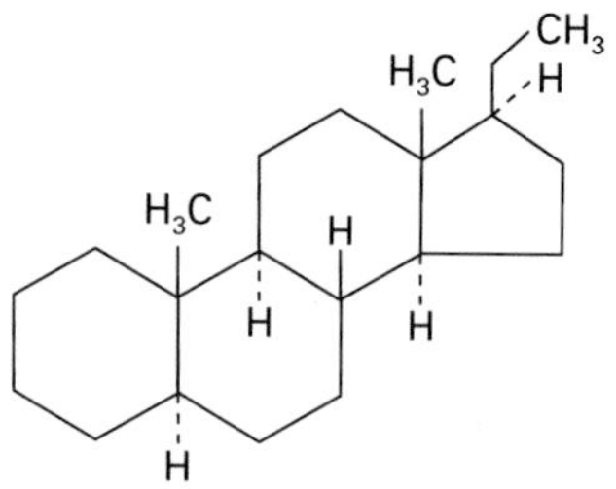

Fig. 5.3 The chemical structure of the 5α-pregnane and progesterone.

other sex hormones, estrogenic activity is not dependent on strict steroidal configurations.

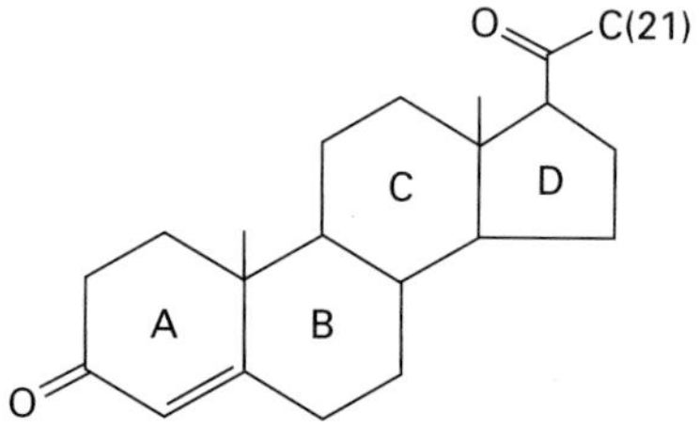

Progesterone (Fig. 5.3)

The progesterone (preg-4-ene-3,20-dione) receptor relies on Δ^4-3-one A ring in an inverted 1β, 2α conformation for receptor specificity.[1] Other steroid receptors also bind with this ring, thus synthetic progestogens frequently possess glucocorticoid, mineralocorticoid and androgenic effects.

Mixed estrogen agonists/antagonists

This group may be subdivided into natural (phytoestrogens) and synthetic agents.

Phytoestrogens (Fig. 5.4)

It has long been recognized that the differing incidence of estrogen and nonestrogen dependent tumours vary amongst cultural groups and this may be due to dietary differences. The presence of dietary phytoestrogens, a group of polycyclic molecules with mixed estrogen agonist/antagonist properties, may be responsible for this demographic variation.

The phytoestrogens demonstrate diversification of structure, origin (Table 5.1) and properties and this is reflected in the increasing number of targets apart from the estrogen receptor which are being discovered. The actions of phytoestrogens are also species specific, the antifertility effects seen in sheep are not seen in cattle but have been described in predatory cats following isoflavinoid ingestion.[2]

Flavonoids are a group of phytoestrogens biosynthetically derived from chalcones. There are at least 12 structurally related flavonoids with the ability to stimulate the transcriptional activity of the estrogen receptor. Phytoestrogens have demonstrated estrogenic properties over a range of 0.1–10 μM concentrations. The activity is thought to be mediated through the estrogen receptor. This has been demonstrated by the ability of the more potent flavonoids to compete with 17β estradiol in cell culture, in contrast to the nonestrogenic flavonoids.[3]

The chalcones, flavones, flavanones and isoflavones all possess phenolic A and B rings. In relationship to estrogenic activity, modifications to the central bridge structure and the hydroxylation pattern of ring A are tolerated in contrast to variations in the hydroxylation pattern of ring B.[3] The 4 hydroxylated isoflavones (genistein and daidzein) demonstrate greater stimulation of transcriptional activity of the estrogen receptor *in vitro* than the 4 methoxylated isoflavones (biochanin A and formononetin).[3]

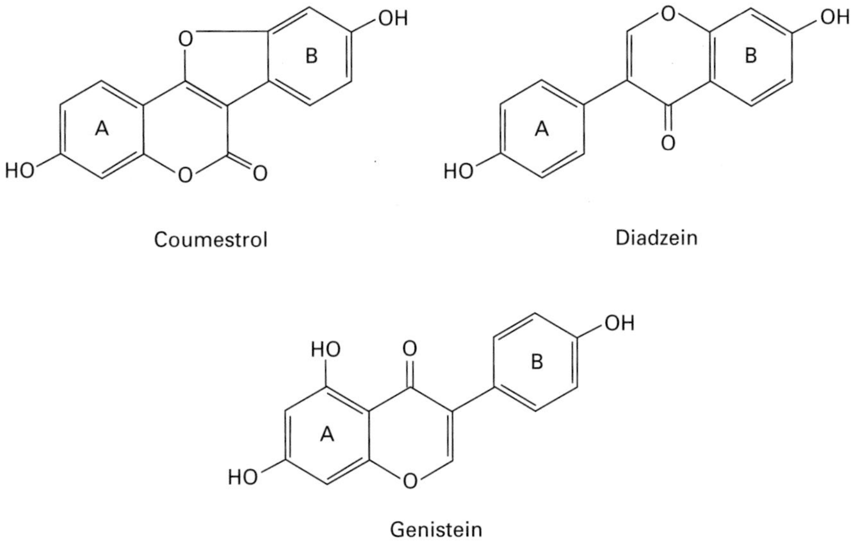

Coumestrol

Diadzein

Genistein

Fig. 5.4 Chemical structures of phytoestrogens coumestrol, daidzein and genistein.

Table 5.1 The source and structure of phytoestrogens.[5]

Structure		Trivial name	Source
Flavonoids	Isoflavone	Genistein	Soy
	Isoflavone	Daidzein	Soy
	Isoflavone	Biochanin A	Clover
	Isoflavone	Formononetin	
	Flavone	Apigenin	
	Flavonol	Kaempferol	
	Chalcone	Phloretin	
	Chalcone	Isoliquiritigenin	
Coumestans		Coumestrol	Clover
Stilbenes		4,4-dihydroxystilbene 3,5-dihydroxystilbene	Wood
Coumarins		Coumarin	Beans
Plant sterols		α-sitosterol β-sitosterol β-sitostanol	Plantoils, leguminous plants, wood
Saponins		α-glycyrrhetinic acid β-glycyrrhetinic acid	
Resorcyclic acid lactones		Zearalenone	Mould (*Fusarium*) infected grain

Coumestrol, which appears in high concentrations in the legume alfalfa, is 30 times more estrogenic than genistein in the mouse uterus and may cause estrogen related disorders in other species.[4]

Soy contains the highest concentrations of phytoestrogens, of which the isoflavinoids, genistein and diadzein predominate.[5]

Synthetic agents (Fig. 5.5)

In the search for enhanced treatments for breast cancer, research in structure-activity relationships has led to the discovery of an increasing number of molecules with improved estrogen antagonistic profiles.

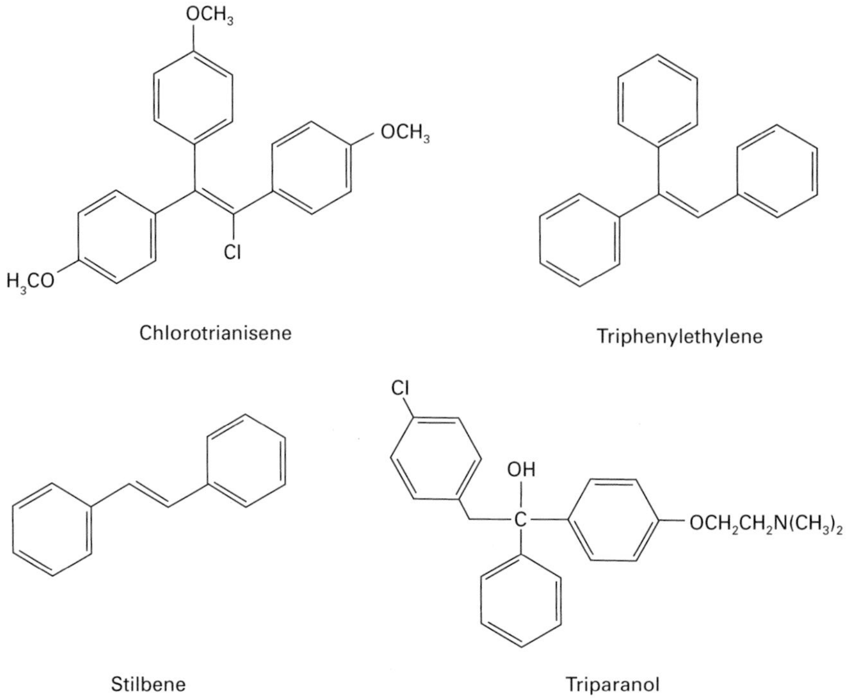

Chlorotrianisene

Triphenylethylene

Stilbene

Triparanol

Fig. 5.5 The structure of chlorotrianisene, triphenylethylene, stilbene and triparanol.

Apart from the development of these molecules in the field of oncology, investigators are looking to this group for agents with beneficial selective profiles. The profile of these agents would be antagonistic or neutral at sites where estrogen may promote carcinogenesis, i.e. breast and uterus, but agonistic at sites where estrogen has potential beneficial activity, i.e. the cardiovascular system, bone and the central nervous system. Some foodstuffs containing phytoestrogens have demonstrated such an effect albeit at a less than optimal degree. This unique group of molecules has been termed selective estrogen receptor modulators (SERM).[6] The degree of selectivity and efficacy varies within the group.

The development of this group of agents followed the discovery that the triarylethylene derivative chlorotrianisene reduced the enlargement of the pituitary in estradiol stimulated rats.[7] The culmination of further research led to the synthesis of the more potent triphenylethylene derivatives, clomiphene, nafoxidine and tamoxifen in the late 1950s. These triphenylethylene derivatives are structurally related to the nonsteroidal estrogen stilbene and antilipidemic agent triparanol.

The fertility agent clomiphene is a mixture of the cis isomer, zuclomiphene, and the trans isomer, enclomiphene. The cis isomer is estrogenic and the trans isomer has mixed activity. Tamoxifen was the first agent with antiestrogenic/estrogenic properties to demonstrate efficacy in breast carcinoma. The stereo isomers of tamoxifen are relatively stable compared to its biologically active metabolites, which undergo enzymatic isomerization.[8]

Agonist or antagonistic properties of tamoxifen and its metabolite 4-hydroxytamoxifen are dependent on the orientation of the alkylaminoethoxy side chain. As the trans isomer, the compound and its metabolite are antagonist; in the cis orientation tamoxifen is oestrogenic and 4-hydroxytamoxifen demonstrates weak agonistic/antagonistic properties.[9] Tamoxifen has approximately 2% the binding capacity of estradiol, the introduction of a hydroxyl group at C-4 imparts a 100-fold increase in antagonistic activity.[10] Tamoxifen is marketed as the trans isomer. Both isomers of 4-hydroxytamoxifen have been found in the breast tumors of women treated with tamoxifen.[10] Recent studies with nonisomerizable analogues of tamoxifen have questioned whether the presence of an estrogenic isomer is the underlying metabolic mechanism in tamoxifen resistance following prolonged use.[11]

With tamoxifen as the current bench mark, triphenylethylene molecules with increased antiestrogenic activity and improved antiestrogenic to estrogenic ratios of activity are under development. These agents include droloxifene,[12] nitromifene,[13] toremifene,[14] and idoxifene[15] (Fig. 5.6).

Groups of compounds with fixed rings are being investigated in an attempt to overcome the potential problem of isomerization. One of the earliest groups to be developed were the naphthylenes (Fig. 5.7) from which the agents nafoxidine and trioxifene were synthesized.[16]

A group of indolic derivatives has been developed (Fig. 5.8). Zindoxifene, 5-acetoxy-2-(4-acetoxyphenyl)-1-ethyl-3-methylindole demonstrates mixed estrogenic activity and antiandrogenic properties. Zindoxifene is currently being developed as an antineoplastic antiestrogen.[17] Another member of this group

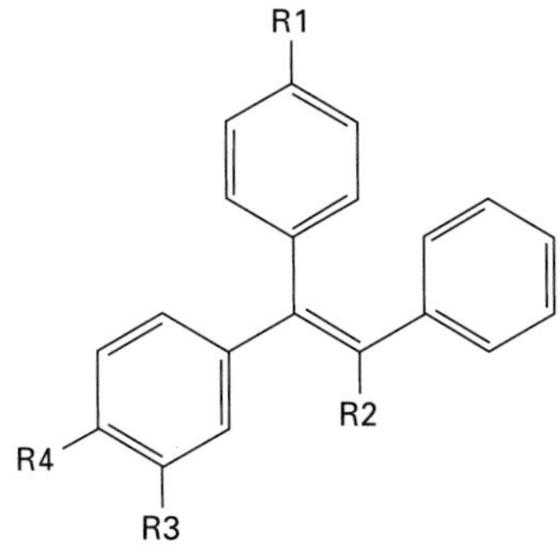

	R1	R2	R3	R4
Clomiphene	OCH2CH2N(C2H5)2	Cl	H	H
Tamoxifen	OCH2CH2N(CH3)2	CH2CH3	H	H
4-hydroxytamoxifen	OCH2CH2N(CH3)2	CH2CH3	H	OH
Droloxifene	OCH2CH2N(CH3)2	CH2CH3	OH	H
Nitromifene	OCH2CH2NC4H8	NO2	H	OCH3
Toremifene	OCH2CH2N(CH3)2	CH2CH2CL	H	H
Idoxifene	OCH2CH2NC4H8	CH2CH3	H	I

Fig. 5.6 The structure of the triphenylethylene derivatives.

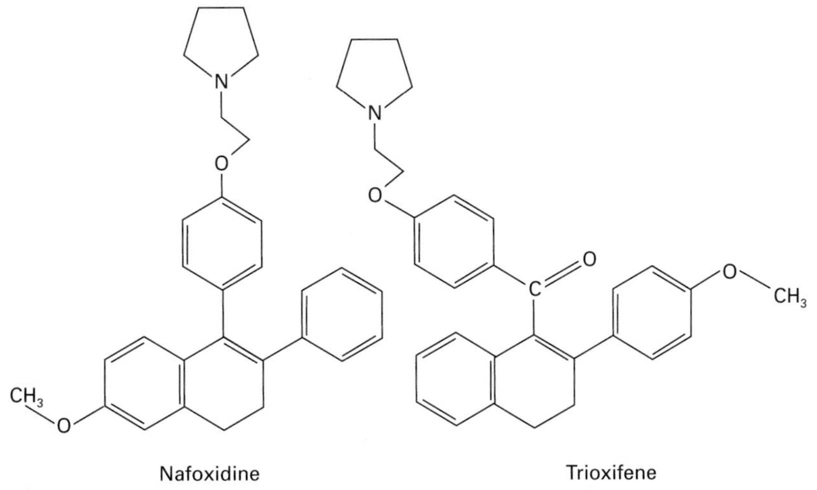

Fig. 5.7 The structure of the naphthylenes, nafoxidine and trioxifene.

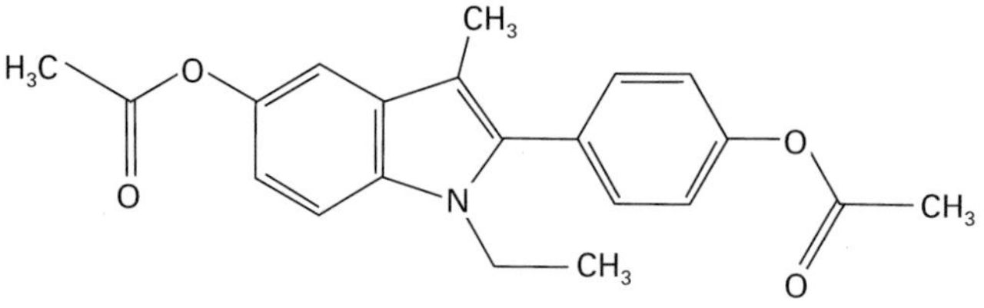

Zindoxifene

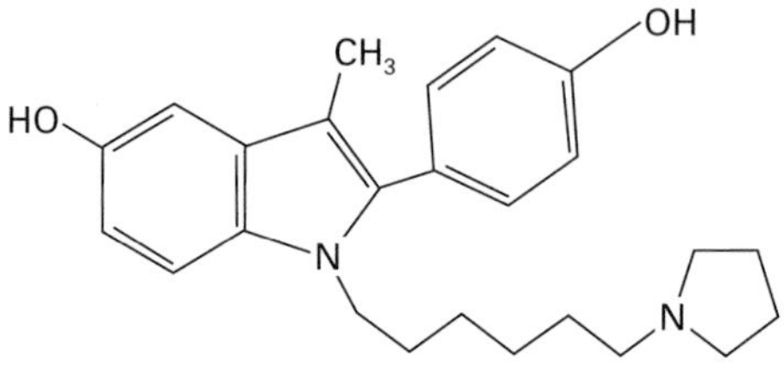

ZK-119010

Fig. 5.8 The indoles, zindoxifene and ZK 119010.

ZK119010 is less estrogenic and more antiestrogenic in rats than zindoxifene. This beneficial ratio is thought to be due to the introduction of the N-pyrrodinyl group to the indole molecule.[18]

The benzothiaphene based agents deviate from the triphenylethylene structure by the incorporation of a ketone or carbonyl bridge linking the phenyl ring containing the piperidinyl or pyrrolidinyl basic side chain with the remainder of the molecule. The benzothiaphene nucleus assures that the stilbene moiety remains in the transmolecular arrangement, thereby precluding the possibility of estrogenic 'cis'-triphenylethylene structures. Raloxifene (Fig. 5.9), previously referred to by the name keoxifene, and its analogues and bioisosteres form the structural basis for a group of molecules with SERM characteristics.

The benzopyrans are another group of agents whose SERM profile is being investigated. The balance of estrogen agonist/antagonist activity of the 2,3-diaryl-2H-1-benzopyrans (DABP) is dependent on substitutions. The DABP phenols have potent antagonist activity and improved affinity for the receptor compared to nonphenolic derivatives. A further hydroxyl substitution at position 7 increases antagonistic activity.[19] The hydroxyl substitutions and the requirement of a side chain is similar to other groups with SERM properties.

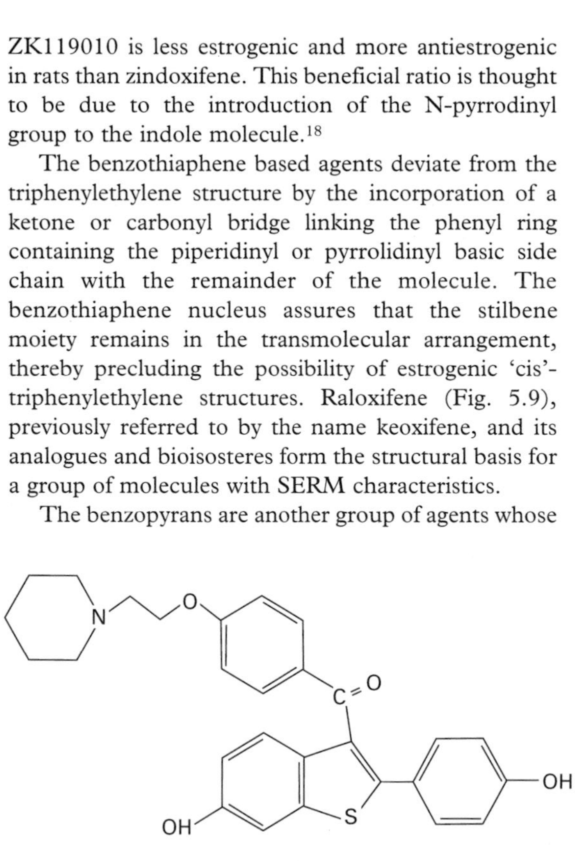

Raloxifene

Fig. 5.9 The structure of the benzothiaphene, raloxifene.

Centchroman (trans-1-[2-[4-(7-methoxy-2,2-dimethyl-3-phenyl-3,4-dihydro-2H-1-benzopyran-4yl)-phenoxy]ethyl]-pyrrolidine hydrochloride) was originally developed as a postcoital contraceptive. It is an estrogenic antagonist with weak estrogenic activity and little effect on the hypothalamic-pituitary-ovarian axis.[20] Recently the SERM properties have been investigated. Centchroman (Fig. 5.10) is a potent inhibitor *in vitro* of osteoclastic bone resorption.[21]

The benzofuroquinoline derivative, KCA 098 (Fig. 5.11) is structurally related to the phytoestrogen, coumestrol and demonstrates both bone resorption inhibitory activity and bone formation enhancing activity *in vitro*.[22] It is devoid of uterine stimulatory activity in the rat.[23]

Antiestrogens

This group may exert their activity by competitive antagonism at the ER, by altering ER dynamics or by inhibition of estrogen synthesis.

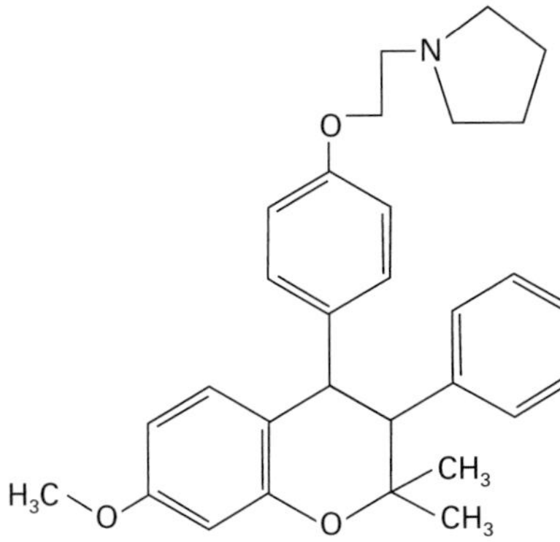

Fig. 5.10 The structure of the benzopyran, centchroman.

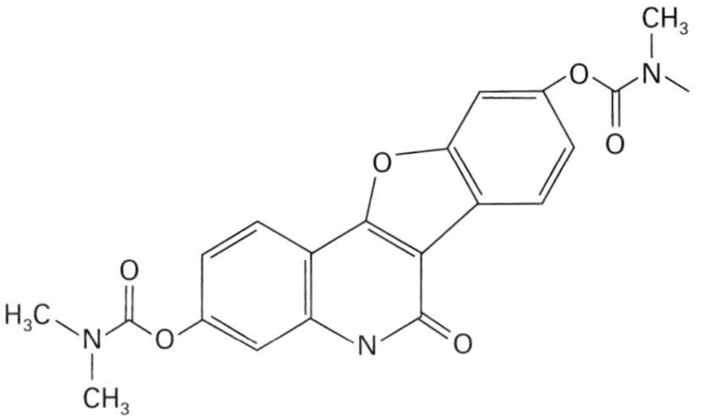

Fig. 5.11 The structure of the benzofuroquinolone, KCA 098.

Steroid antiestrogens

High dose estrogen (diethylstilbestrol), progestogen (megestrol) and androgen (fluoxymestrone) have all demonstrated 'antiestrogenic' effects in hormone dependent breast carcinoma in postmenopausal women.

Pure antiestrogens (Fig. 5.12) are derivatives of 17β estradiol and demonstrate no intrinsic estrogenic properties.[24] The unique action of these agents may be explained by the substitution of long alkanamide or alkanesulfoxide chains to the estradiol molecule. ICI 164384 and RU 58668 are characterized by alkanamide substitutions at the 7α and 11β positions respectively. ICI 182780 is characterized by an alkanesulfoxide chain at the 7α position and has 10 times the potency of ICI 164384.[25] The improved binding affinity of the halo-steroid EM 139 to the estrogen receptor appears to be due to the substitution of a chlorine atom to the 16α position.[26]

Inhibitors of steroid biosynthesis (Fig. 5.13)

Postmenopausal women with breast cancer are susceptible to estrogen produced by peripheral aromatization of adrenal derived androstenedione. The aromatase enzyme complex is responsible for the conversion of androstenedione or testosterone to estrone or estradiol respectively. The enzyme is located in the endoplasmic reticulum of the cell and consists of the cytochrome $P450_{arom}$ protein and NADPH-cytochrome P450 reductase.

The aromatase inhibitors are either competitive or mechanism based. The latter group, termed suicide inhibitors, compete with androstenedione and testosterone for the active site of the enzyme and are converted to reactive alkylating agents by aromatase. These alkylating agents then form covalent bonds close to the active site rendering the enzyme irreversibly

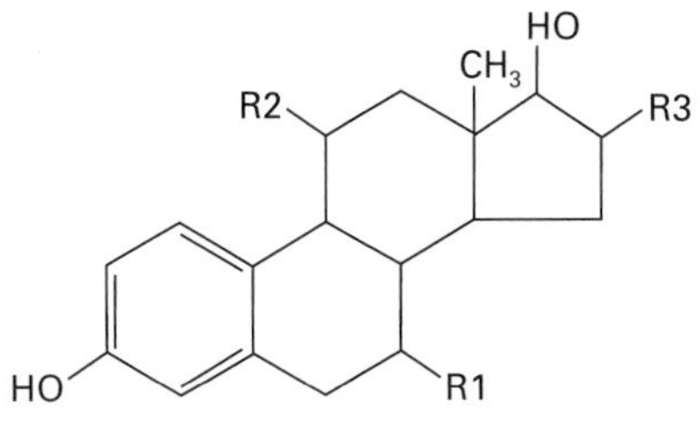

	R1	R2	R3
ICI 164384	$(CH_2)_{10}$CON-n-Bu Me	H	H
ICI 182780	$(CH_2)_9SO(CH_2)_3CF_2CF_3$	H	H
RU 58668	H	β-[4-$(CF_3CF_2(CH_2)_3SO_2(CH_2)_5O)C_6H_4$]-	H
EMI 139	$(CH_2)_{10}$CON Bu Me	H	Cl

Fig. 5.12 The structure of 'pure' antiestrogens.

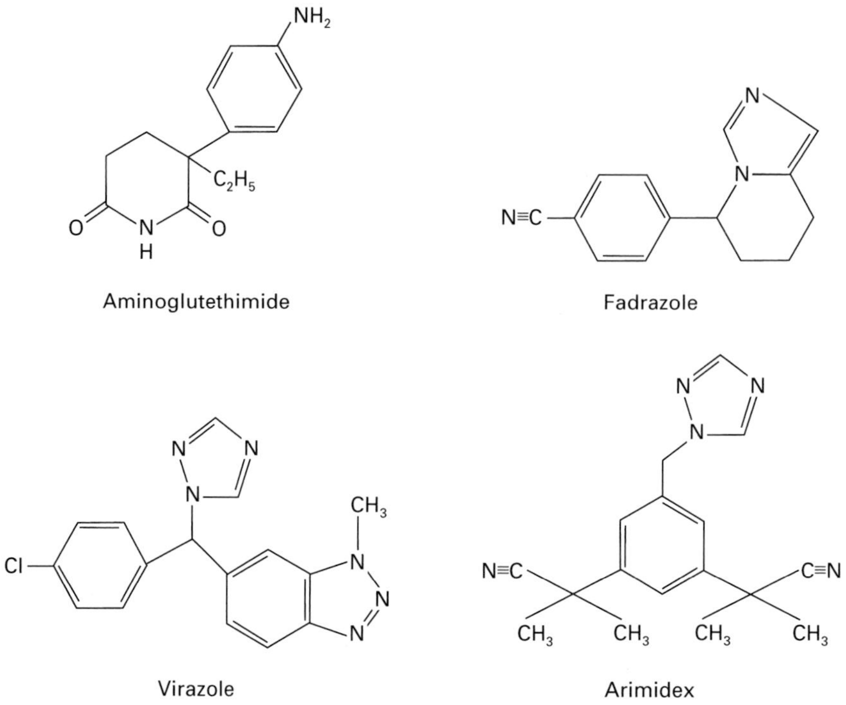

Aminoglutethimide

Fadrazole

Virazole

Arimidex

Fig. 5.13 Structure of selected nonsteroidal aromatase inhibitors.

inactive.[27] Competitive agents may be either nonsteroidal or steroidal in structure.

Aminoglutethimide was the first aromatase inhibitor to be developed; it belongs to the nonsteroidal competitive antagonist group and inhibits both peripheral aromatization and the action of desmolase in the production of pregnenolone from cholesterol. This latter effect necessitates the coadministration of hydrocortisone to prevent ACTH production overriding the blockade. The drug is a mixture of two optical isomers. The D isomer is 5–25 times more potent than the L isomer. Analogues have been developed to maximize the aromatase effect and minimize the desmolase effect and CNS sedative properties of aminoglutethemide. The 4-pyridyl analog, rogletimide (3-ethyl-3-(4-pyridyl)piperidine-2,6-dione) is a less potent aromatase inhibitor than aminoglutethimide *in vitro* but lacks the desmolase inhibitory activity of aminoglutethemide.[28]

A new generation of selective nonsteroidal aromatase inhibitors are under development. Fadrazole ({4 - (5,6,7,8 - tetrahydro - imidazo - [1, 5a] - pyridin-5-yl) benzonitrile monohydrochloride}), a second generation aromatase inhibitor and letrozole ({4,4′-(1H-1,2,4-triazol-1-yl-methylene)-bis-benzonitrile]), a third generation aromatase inhibitor, are imidazole (two nitrogen atoms in a five membered ring) derivatives. Fadrazole has 180–500 times the potency for aromatase inhibition than aminogluthimide *in vitro* but lacks specificity. Letrozole has approximately 1 000–10 000 times the potency of aminoglutethimide and eight times the potency of fadrazole.[29]

The triazole derivatives (three nitrogen atoms in a five membered ring), arimidex (2,2′-[5 - (1H -1,2,4 - triazol-1-yl methyl)-1,3 -phenylene] bis (2-methyl-propiononitrile) and virazole (6- [(4 - chlorophenyl) (1H-1,2,4-triazol-1-yl)-methyl]-1-methyl-1H-benzotriazole) are potent selective aromatase inhibitors that are active orally.[30] A nitrogen atom on the heterocyclic ring is thought to bind with the heme-iron of the cytochrome P450 protein.[31]

Effective steroidal inhibitors are analogs of androstenedione (Fig. 5.14). Those with minimal structural deviation of the A ring and C19 position appear to be the best inhibitors. Steroidal aromatase competitive inhibitors include testolactone, D-homo-17α-oxandrosta-1, 4-diene-3, 17-dione, 7α-amino-phenylthio-4-androstene-3, 17-dione and 6α-bromo-androstene-dione.

The suicide inhibitor group (Fig. 5.15) includes formestane (4-hydroxyandrostenedione), a potent inhibitor but only active parenterally, exemestane

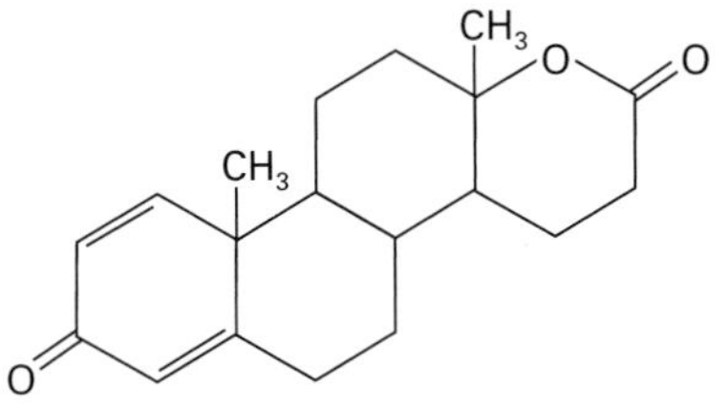

Testolactone

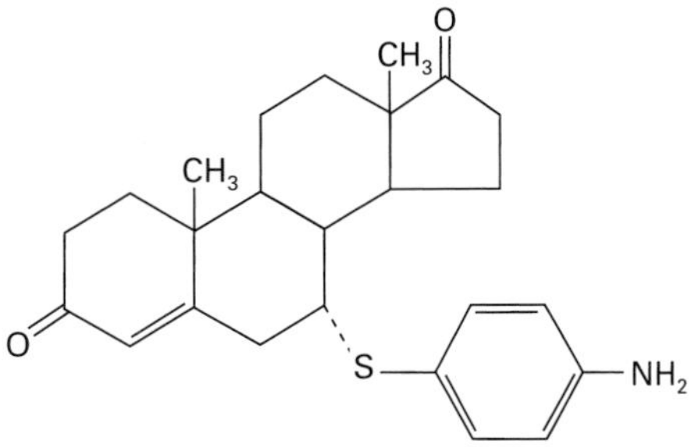

7α-aminophenylthioandrost-1,4-diene-3,17-dione

Fig. 5.14 Structure of selected competitive steroidal aromatase inhibitors.

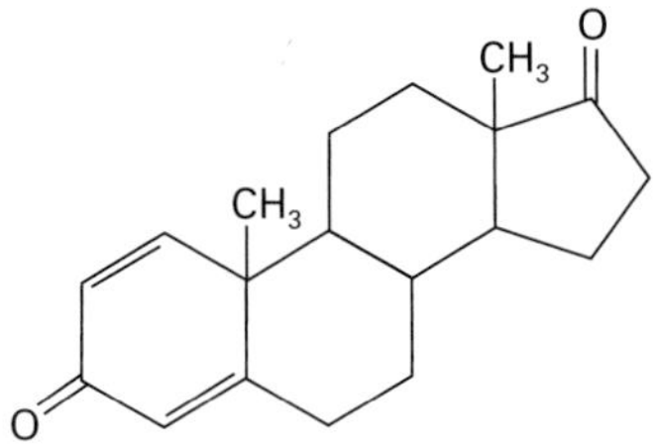

Atamastane

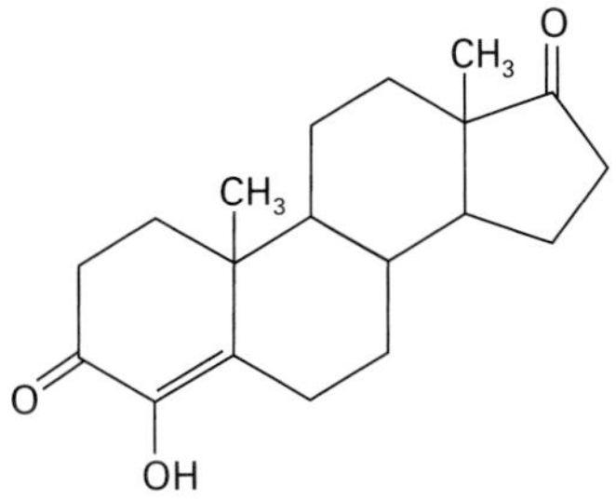

Formestane

Fig. 5.15 Structure of selected suicide aromatase inhibitors.

([4,4′ -(1H-1,2,4-triazol-1-yl-methylene)-bis-benzonitrile]), a selective, potent oral agent under development,[32] and atamestane (1-methyl-1, 4 androstadiene-3,17-dione).[33]

Mixed antiestrogens/antiprogestogens

Steroid derivatives

The androgens danazol (17α-pregna-2,4-diene-20-yn [2,3-d]isoxazol-17-ol) and gestrinone (13-ethyl-17α-ethinyl-17-hydroxy-gona-4,9,11-trien-3-one) are efficacious in the estrogen dependent disorders endometriosis, fibroids and dysfunctional uterine bleeding. Competitive binding to the ER, progesterone receptor (PR) and androgen receptor (AR) with a corresponding reduction in ER and PR concentration *in vitro* appears to be the basis of action of danazol[34] (Fig. 5.16) and gestrinone.[35,36]

Peptides (Fig. 5.17)

The group contains analogues of the decapeptide, gonadotropin releasing hormone (GnRH). Agonists were initially developed as fertility agents. Prolonged treatment leads to 'down regulation' of GnRH receptors in the pituitary gland resulting in 'chemical gonadectomy'; this is also achieved by the utilization of GnRH antagonists. This action may be applied in the control of estrogen dependent gynecological conditions such as endometriosis, fibroids and dysfunctional uterine bleeding and in the treatment of sex hormone dependent tumors such as

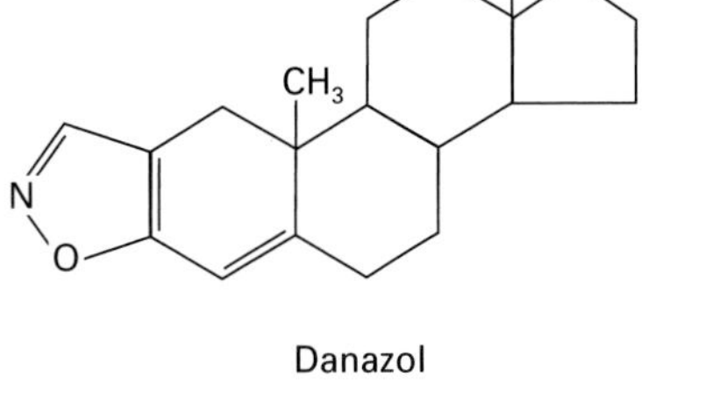

Danazol

Fig. 5.16 Structure of danazol.

	1	2	3	4	5	6	7	8	9	10
GnRH	Pyro Glu	His	Trp	Ser	Tyr	Gly	Leu	Arg	Pro	Gly NH_2
Superagonists										
Buserelin	Pyro Glu	His	Trp	Ser	Tyr	DSer (But)	Leu	Arg	Pro NHET	
Leuprorelin	Pyro Glu	His	Trp	Ser	Tyr	D Leu	Leu	Arg	Pro NHET	
Goserelin	Pyro Glu	His	Trp	Ser	Tyr	DSer (But)	Leu	Arg	Pro Az	Gly NH_2
Antagonists										
Cetrorelix	Ac-D-Nal	D-(pCl) Phe	D-Pal	Ser	Tyr	D Cit	Leu	Arg	Pro	D-Ala NH_2

Fig. 5.17 Structures of GnRH analogues.

premenopausal breast carcinoma and prostatic carcinoma.

The chemistry of the decapeptide GnRH was elucidated in 1971.[37] Since then over 3000 synthetic analogues have been investigated with the aim of increasing potency and duration of action through substitutions within the decapeptide. The first three amino acids, pyro-Glu (5-oxoproline), His and Trp are intrinsic to the activity of GnRH — substitutions in these positions lead to decreases in activity unless the substituents are structurally similar. Increases in potency may be produced by 6 and 10 position substitutions.[38] The hydrophobic nature, size and aromaticity of the substituent may be determinants of potency and duration of action.[38] The superagonist group include buserelin (D-Ser (But) desglycine $NH_2{}^{10}$-GnRH ethylamide), leuprorelin (D-Leu^6-GnRH ethylamide), goserelin (D-Ser (But)^6 Az-Gly^{10}-GnRH), triptorelin (D-Trp^6-GnRH) and nafarelin (D-Nal^6-GnRH). Buserelin is 100 times and goserelin and leuprorelin are 50 times more potent than GnRH.[39,40]

The antagonists of GnRH appear to work through competitive inhibition at the pituitary. Early analogues were complicated by anaphylactic reactions associated with D-arginine or other basic residues at position 6.[41] Highly active antagonists have been developed devoid of anaphylactoid reactions. These agents incorporate neutral hydrophilic D-ureidoalkyl amino acids at position 6. Among this group cetrorelix appears to be the most powerful,[41] its potency and resistance to degradation appears to be due to its five non-natural D-amino acids.[42]

Antiprogestogens (Fig. 5.18)

The antiprogestogens were initially developed as abortifacients but also have demonstrated therapeutic potential for the treatment of breast cancer. The first marketed antiprogestogen was mifepristone, 17β-hydroxy-11β-[4-(dimethylamino)phenyl]-17β-hydroxy-17α-(1-propynl) estra-4,9-dien-3-one. Mifepristone has twice the binding affinity for the PR as progesterone and also demonstrates antiglucocorticoid activity. The mifepristone analogue onapristone, a 13α configured (retro) steroid has reduced glucocorticoid but also reduced progesterone receptor binding affinity.[43] Agents with improved profiles are being developed.

The compounds Org 31710 and Org 31806 (Fig. 5.19) share a spiroether group at C-17 in addition to a β methyl group in the B ring at position 6 and 7 respectively. The antiprogestational activities of these agents are greater than mifepristone and onapristone; they have weak androgenic and antiandrogenic activity with little antiglucocortocoid activity.[44] At present there appears to be no clear cut structure-activity relationship. The most important modifications to the steroid skeleton as far as selectivity is concerned are substitutions to the B ring, changes in the stereochemical structure of the D ring through 13α configuration and the nature of the substituent at the C-17 position.[45] The potent and selective agent, Org 33628 (Fig. 5.19), has the C-11 group occupied by an acetophenone group and the C-17 by a methylene-furan substituent. This molecule demonstrates twice the binding affinity of mifepristone for the PR and 25 fold less the binding affinity for the glucocorticoid

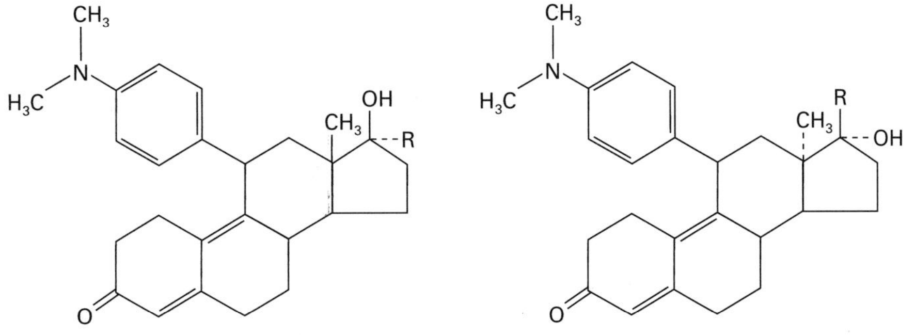

Mifepristone (RU 38,486): R=-C≡C-CH_3 Onapristone (ZK 98,299): R=-CH_2CH_2 CH_2OH

Fig. 5.18 Structure of the antiprogestogens, mifepristone and onapristone.

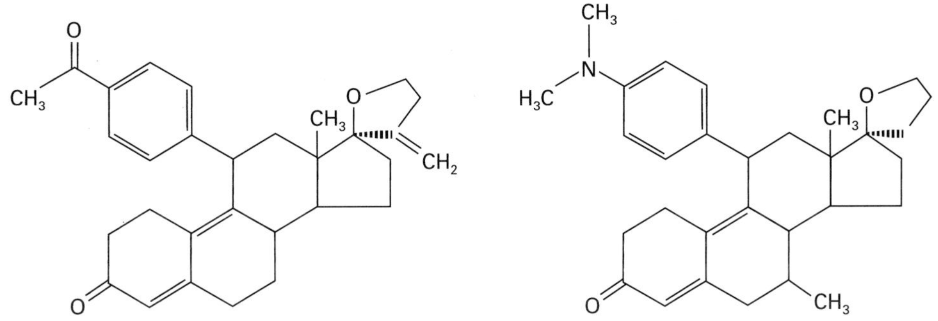

Org 33628 Org 31806

Fig. 5.19 Structure of Org 33628 and Org 31806.

receptor. An improved potency in pregnancy interruption and ovulation inhibition in rats was also demonstrable.[45]

Conclusion

The agents summarized in this chapter represent the 'tip of the antihormone iceberg.' Many will fail the stringent requirements necessary for the development of safe, efficacious medicines. The importance of this group in a wide range of conditions is reflected in a growing number of new chemical entities under development.

REFERENCES

1. Duax WL, Griffin JF, Weeks CM, 1988 The mechanism of action of steroid antagonists: insights from crystalographic studies. Journal of Steroid Biochemistry 31: 481–492
2. Barnes S, Peterson TG 1995 Biochemical targets of the isoflavone Genistein in tumour cell lines. Proceedings of the Society for Experimental Biology and Medicine 208: 103–108
3. Miksicek RJ 1995 Estrogenic flavonoids: structural requirements for biological activity. Proceedings of the Society for Experimental Biology and Medicine 208: 44–50
4. Saloniemi H, Wahala K, Nykanen-Kurki P, Kallela K, Saastamoinen I 1995 Phytoestrogen content and estrogen effect of legume fodder. Proceedings of the Society for Experimental Biology and Medicine 208: 13–17
5. Makela TS, Poutanen J, Lehtimaki M, Kostian ML, Santti R, Vihko R 1995 Estrogen specific 17β-hydroxysteroid oxidoreductase type 1 as a possible target for the action of phytoestrogens. Proceedings of the Society for Experimental Biology and Medicine 208: 51–59
6. Bryant HU, Glasebrook AL, Yang NN, Sato M 1995 A pharmacological review of raloxifene. Journal of Bone Mineral Metabolism 13: 75–83

7. Segal SJ, Thompson CR 1956 Inhibition of estradiol induced pituitary hypertrophy in rats. Proceedings of the Society for Experimental Biology and Medicine 91: 623–625
8. Katznellenbogen JA, Carlson KE, Katznellenbogen BS 1988 Facile geometric isomerization of phenolic non-steroidal estrogens and antiestrogens: limitations to the interpretation of experiments characterizing the activity of individual isomers. Journal of Steroid Biochemistry 22: 589–596
9. Jordan VC, Mittal S, Goden B, Koch R, Lieberman ME 1985 Structure activity relationships of estrogens. Environmental Health Perspectives 61: 97–110
10. Williams ML, Lennard MS, Martin IJ, Tucker GT 1994 Interindividual variation in the isomerization of 4-hydroxytamoxifen by human liver microsomes: involvement of cytochrome P450. Carcinogenesis 15(12): 2733–2738
11. Osborne CK, Jarmen M, McCague R, Coronado EB, Hilsenbeck SG, Wakeling AE 1994 The importance of tamoxifen metabolism in tamoxifen stimulated breast tumour growth. Cancer Chemotherapy and Pharmacology 34: 89–95
12. Rauschning W, Pritchard KI 1994 Droloxifene, a new antiestrogen: its role in metastatic breast cancer. Breast Cancer Research and Treatment 31: 83–94
13. Ruenitz PC, Thompson CB, Srivatsan V 1989 Characterization of MCF 7 breast cancer cell growth inhibition by the antiestrogen nitromifene (CI 628) and selected metabolites. Journal of Steroid Biochemistry 33: 365–369
14. Kangas L 1990 Review of the pharmacological properties of toremifene. Journal of Steroid Biochemistry 36: 191–195
15. Coombes RC, Haynes BP, Dowsett M et al 1995 Idoxifene: report of a phase 1 study in patients with metastatic breast cancer. Cancer Research 55: 1070–1074
16. Lednicer D, Leyster SC, Duncan GW 1967 Mammalian antifertility agents. Basic 3,4-dihydronaphthalenones. Journal of Medical Chemistry 10: 78–84
17. Stein RC, Dowsett M, Cunningham DC et al 1990 Phase I/II study of the anti-oestrogen zindoxifene (D16726) in the treatment of advanced breast cancer. A cancer research campaign phase I/II clinical trials committee study. British Journal of Cancer 61: 451–453
18. Nishino Y, Schneider MR, Michna H, Von Angerer E 1991 Pharmacological characterization of a novel oestrogen antagonist, ZK 119010, in rats and mice. Journal of Endocrinology 130: 409–414
19. Sharma AP, Saeed A, Durani S, Kapil RS 1990 Structure-activity relationships of antiestrogens. Phenolic analogues of 2,3-diaryl-2H-1-benzopyrans. Journal of Medical Chemistry 33: 3222–3229
20. Kamboj VP, Ray S, Dhawan BN 1992 Centchroman, Drugs of Today 28: 227–232
21. Hall TJ, Nyugen M, Schaueblin M, Fournier B 1995 The bone specific estrogen cenchroman inhibits osteoclastic bone resorption in vitro. Biochemical and Biophysical Research Communications 216: 662–668
22. Kojima M, Tsutsumi N, Nagata H et al 1994 Effect of KCA-098, a new benzofuroquinolone derivative, on bone mineral metabolism. Biological Pharmacology Bulletin 17: 504–508
23. Tsutsumi N, Kawashima K, Arai N, Nagata H, Kojima M, Ujiie A, Endo H 1994 In vitro effect of KCA-098, a derivative of coumestrol, on bone resorption of fetal rat femurs. Bone Minerals 24: 201–209
24. Wade GN, Blaustein JD, Gray JM, Meredith JM 1993 ICI 182780: a pure antiestrogen that affects behaviors and energy balance in rats without acting in the brain. American Journal of Physiology 265: 1392–1398
25. Wakeling AE, Dukes M, Bowler J 1991 A potent specific pure antiestrogen with clinical potential. Cancer Research 51: 3867–3873
26. Levesque C, Merand Y, Dufour JM, Labrie C, Labrie F 1991 Synthesis and biological activity of new halo-steroidal antiestrogens. Journal of Medical Chemistry 34: 1624–1630
27. Santen RJ 1990 Clinical use of aromatase inhibitors: current data and therapeutic perspectives. Journal of Enzyme Inhibition 4: 79–99
28. Foster AB, Jarman M, Leung CS 1985 Analogues of aminogluthemide: selective inhibition of aromatase. Journal of Medical Chemistry 28: 200–204
29. Masamura S, Adlercreutz H, Harvey H, Lipton A, Demers L, Santen RJ, Santner SJ 1994 Aromatase inhibitor development for treatment of breast cancer. Breast Cancer Research and Treatment 33: 19–26
30. Goss PE, Gwyn KMEH 1994 Current perspectives on aromatase inhibitors in breast cancer. Journal of Clinical Oncology 12: 2460–2470
31. Brueggemeier RW 1990 Biochemical and molecular aspects of aromatase. Journal of Enzyme Inhibition 4: 101–111
32. Di Salle E, Ornati G, Giudici D, Lassus M, Evans TRJ, Coombes RC 1992 Exemestane (FCE 24304), a new steroidal aromatase inhibitor. Journal of Steroid Biochemistry and Molecular Biology 43: 137–143
33. El Etreby FM 1993 Atamestane: an aromatase inhibitor for the treatment of benign prostatic hyperplasia. A short review. Journal of Steroid Biochemistry and Molecular Biology 44: 565–572
34. Yamashita S, Ohno Y, Watanabe Y et al 1994 Antiestrogenic effects of danazol on rabbit uterus. Gynecologial and Obstetric Investigation 38: 245–248
35. Tamaya T, Fujimoto J, Watanabe Y, Arahori K, Okada H 1986 Gestrinone binding to steroid receptors in human uterine endometrial cytosol. Acta Obstetrica Gynecologica Scandinavica 65: 439–441
36. Tamaya T, Wada K, Imai A, Mori H, Ban H 1991 Rationale for frequency and dose of administration in gestrinone therapy for pelvic endometriosis in the experimental model of rabbit uterus. General Pharmacology 22: 505–510
37. Schally AV, Nair RM, Redding TW, Arimura A 1971 Isolation of the luteinizing hormone and follicle stimulating hormone releasing hormone from porcine hypothalami. Journal of Biological Chemistry 246: 7230–7236
38. Fujino M, Fukuda T, Shinagawa S et al 1974 Synthetic analogs of luteinizing hormone releasing hormone (LH-RH) substituted in position 6 and 10. Biochemical and Biophysical Research Communications 82: 406–413
39. Dutta AS, Furr BJ, Giles MB, Valcaccia B 1978 Synthesis and biological activity of highly active alpha-aza analogues of luliberin. Journal of Medical Chemistry 21: 1018–1024

40. Maynard PV, Nicholson RI 1979 Effects of high doses of a series of new luteinizing hormone releasing hormone analogues in intact female rats. British Journal of Cancer 39: 274–279
41. Gonzalez-Barcena D, Vadillo-Buenfil M, Gomez-Orta F 1994 Responses to the antagonistic analog of LH-RH (SB-75, Cetrorelix) in patients with benign prostatic hyperplasia and prostatic cancer. The Prostate 24: 84–92
42. Muller A, Busker E, Engel J, Kutscher B, Bernd M, Schally AV 1994 Structural investigation of Cetrorelix, a new potent and long acting LH-RH antagonist. International Journal of Peptide and Protein Research 43: 264–270
43. Teutsch G, Philbert D 1994 History and perspectives of antiprogestins from the chemists point of view. Human Reproduction 9(Suppl 1): 12–31
44. Kloosterboer HJ, Deckers GH, Schoonen WGEJ 1994 Pharmacology of two new very selective antiprogestogens: Org 31710 and Org 31806. Human Reproduction 9: 47–52
45. Kloosterboer HJ, Deckers GH, De-Gooyer ME, Dijkema R, Orlemans EOM, Schoonen WGEJ 1995 Pharmacological properties of a new selective antiprogestogen: Org 33628. Annals of the New York Academy of Science 761: 192–201

6. Chemical synthesis

John A. Edwards M. R. Henzl

Introduction

Since their discovery, steroid hormones used in therapy have affected more facets of human life than most other endocrine or therapeutic agents. These compounds have revolutionized the practice of medicine and have made an important inroad in an array of medical disciplines, such as dermatology, immunology, oncology and others. Synthetic estrogens and progestogens were the first pharmacological agents to be used by healthy individuals in a social context, namely for family planning. Estrogens, either synthetic or natural, given in sophisticated delivery systems to domestic animals, have played an important role in humankind's never ending quest for securing an adequate supply of food.

The possibilities of application of steroids, and specifically estrogens and progestogens, in so many and diversified areas of medicine provided the first major challenge to the synthetic chemist: to produce safe and effective compounds in quantities sufficient to meet the clinical needs. This challenge was augmented by the need to make steroids economically affordable.[1] The second major challenge for the chemist was to produce compounds with highly specific biological actions that would exceed those of the natural steroids.

The steroid molecule is one of nature's marvels of economy: by attaching relatively simple chemical groups to the skeleton of a tetracyclic molecule (cyclopentanophenanthrene) and by switching the double bonds within and between the individual rings, the steroid-producing organs create hormones affecting diverse biological activities ranging from mineral, glucose and protein metabolism to reproduction. In addition, each hormonal entity is multifaceted in nature: besides its primary function, it displays one or more secondary activities, e.g. the same estrogen molecule affects female reproduction and bone mineral metabolism. Sometimes it is difficult to declare one function as primary and another as secondary. Continuing with the example of estrogens, sexual maturation is their most explicit function during adolescence, however, during the menopausal years the clinician is interested more in the bone sparing effects.[2]

The extreme flexibility of the steroid molecule confronted modern chemists with a formidable task to produce compounds with substantially enhanced biological potency and to dissociate the multiple activities of a steroid molecule in order to obtain agents with a specifically targeted activity. In the domain of reproductive medicine, this goal was achieved with only a few compounds. Molecules of synthetic progestogens are grossly similar to other steroids and their functions can cross over or, under certain circumstances, one of their functions can be exaggerated. However, increasing the primary function of a hormone is not unlimited since it may be accompanied by the rise of another, undesired activity. Norgestrel, differing from norethindrone only by a methyl group on C-18, is a more potent progestogen, but displays more androgenicity and HDL-decreasing effects.[3]

Desogestrel and gestodene are derivatives of norgestrel. Modifications of the parent molecule are minor; nevertheless, they enhance progestational activity and enable reduction of both progestogen and estrogen content in combination oral contraceptives. These third generation progestogens may be associated with a small increase in risk of thromboembolism[4] and if so, what is the decisive molecular change that triggers the processes leading to this serious complication? Is it merely that they are slightly less anti-estrogenic than the second generation progestogens? On the other hand, the small increase in demonstrated thromboembolic risk could be explained just by the fact that 'higher-risk' women are using these third generation pills.

These and similar questions have reopened the enquiry into the relationship between the structure of the molecule and its biological function. Admittedly, over the years we have gained a considerable insight into the structure-function relationship; however our knowledge about the structure-adverse events relationship has been limited. To elucidate the molecular basis of steroid adverse events is perhaps the ultimate challenge facing modern biochemists which they can meet successfully only with close involvement of biologists and clinicians. The modern tools of molecular biology will hopefully make this task attainable.

Where does the clinician stand *vis-à-vis* these problems and what can he/she do? At the introduction of any new steroid, and indeed any new drug, clinicians should demand full disclosure of the biological profile of the compound with stress on indicators of adverse events. The pharmaceutical industry has the duty to follow up by basic and clinical investigations any hint of prospective adverse events, particularly with compounds such as oral contraceptives that are given for other than purely therapeutic purposes, sometimes for prolonged periods.

The foundations of the modern steroid industry were laid in the 1930s with the discovery and structure elucidation of the sex hormones and the corticosteroids. The availability of these unique agents in pure form for research purposes was extremely limited, the early sources being mammalian glandular tissues and urinary extracts.[5]

Early chemical investigations aimed at the identification of suitable raw materials for the production of these hormones centered on the abundant cholesterol (Fig. 6.1). Various laboratories in the United States and Europe demonstrated that the oxidation of a suitably protected cholesterol derivative followed by deprotection produced a complex mixture from which androstenolone was isolated as the principal product. Although androstenolone was obtained in low yield (*c* 7 g from

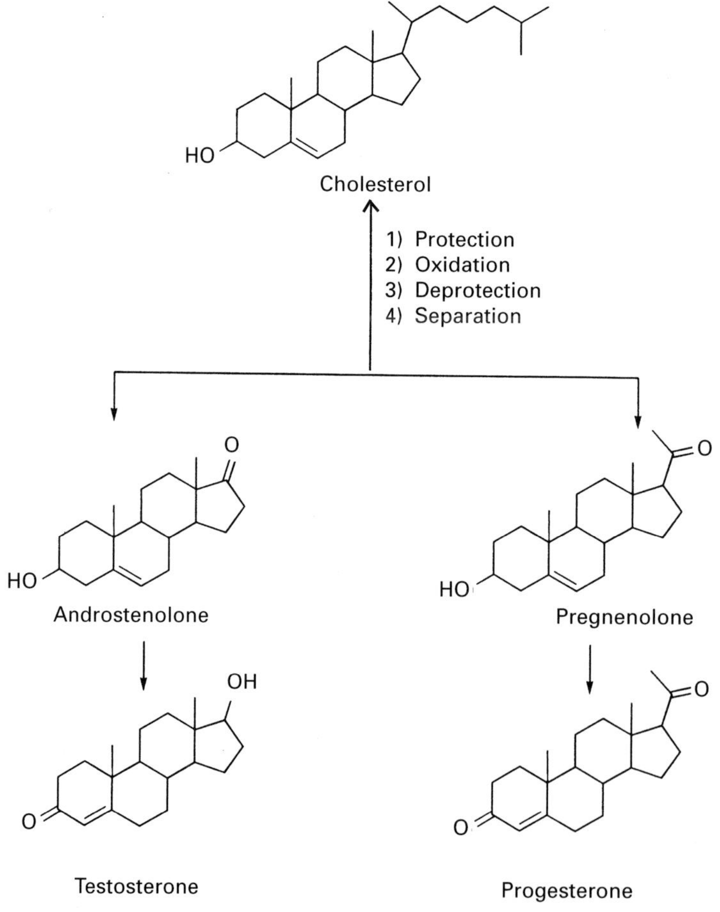

Fig. 6.1 Derivation of steroid hormones from cholesterol.

1 kg of cholesterol) this process was commercialized by several companies in Europe. Chemical methods were also devised from converting androstenolone to testosterone.[6] Progesterone was prepared in one step from pregnenolone, obtained as a minor product from the oxidation of cholesterol or by a lengthy degradation sequence from bovine bile acids or plant sterols.[7]

Despite these modest advances, costs remained excessive, the price of progesterone being of the order of US$180 per gram, and supplies were insufficient for broad therapeutic usage.[8] Clearly, new synthetic methodologies were required to solve the supply program in order to promote the growth and development of this important field of hormone research. In this chapter, aspects of the work which led to the solution of this critical problem will be described. In addition, representative examples of the technology, which was developed over nearly five decades for the industrial scale synthesis of estrogens and progestogens, will be provided. Brief mention will also be made of the chemistry employed for the synthesis of various stilbenes, triphenylethylenes and raloxifene. Because of the enormity of the field, reference will be made to only a few of the most important technical achievements.

STEROID HORMONE DEVELOPMENT

Structure and Nomenclature

The steroid molecule numbering system is illustrated in Fig. 6.2 with the structure of progesterone. It should be noted that this system is consistent throughout the estrane, androstane, pregnane and cholestane series of steroid derivatives in the examples in Fig. 6.2.

Compounds which are racemic or d,l- mixtures will be indicated throughout the text by the expression (±). Totally synthetic intermediates which have been resolved and possess the same absolute configuration as the natural steroids will be identified as (+) or (–), depending upon the sign of the optical rotation. The fact that the naturally occurring steroids and products derived therefrom are optically active will not be indicated in the discussion.

Production of steroid hormones from plant sources

The diosgenin breakthrough

The technological breakthrough which revolutionized the young steroid industry was made by the American chemist Russell Marker during the course of an investigation on the naturally occurring steroid sapogenins conducted at Pennsylvania State University. In an elegant series of studies carried out in the late 1930s, Marker succeeded in elucidating the structure of diosgenin and a host of related compounds (Fig. 6.3)[9]. In addition, he succeeded in effecting the three-step conversion of diosgenin to the C21 pregnane derivative neosterol acetate[9] which he then

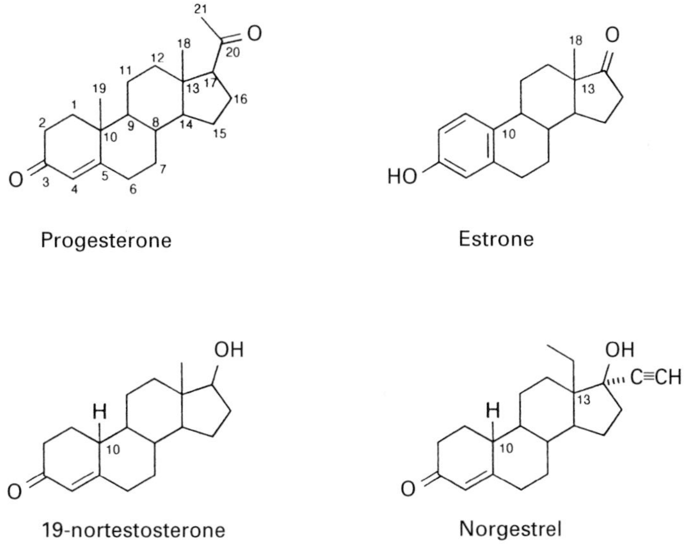

Progesterone

Estrone

19-nortestosterone

Norgestrel

Fig. 6.2 Steroid molecule numbering convention, using progesterone as an example.

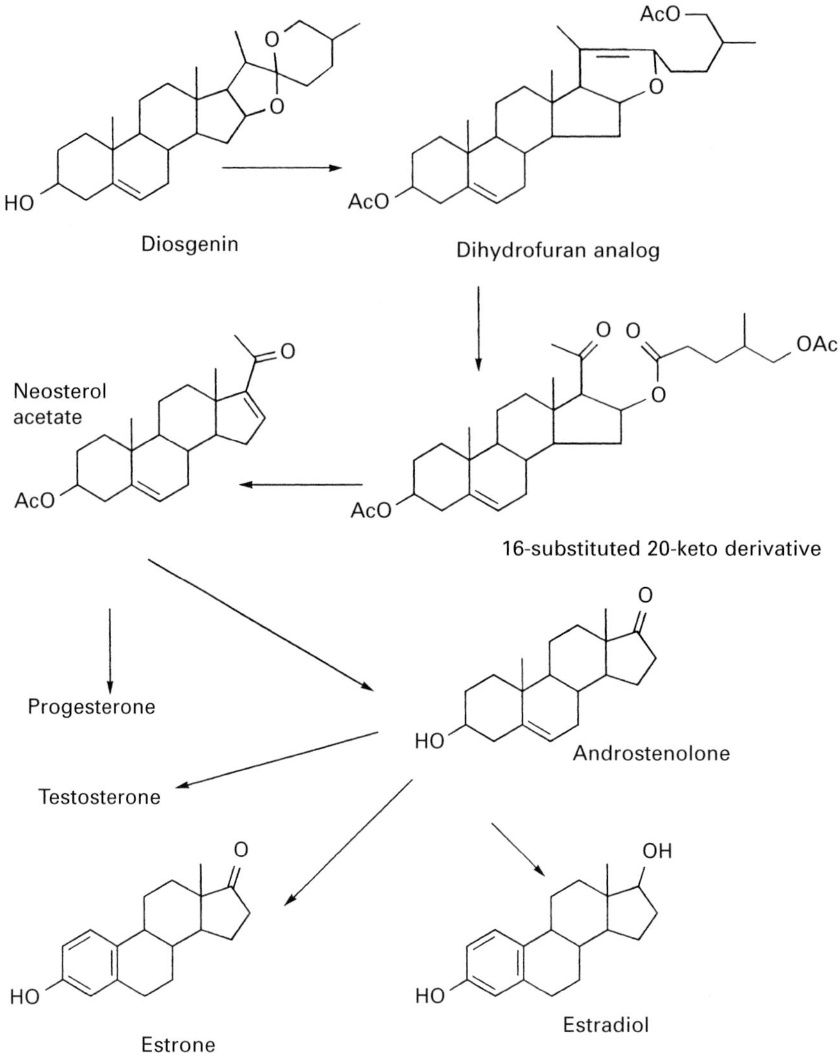

Fig. 6.3 Diosgenin and related compounds.

transformed into progesterone in three additional steps.[10]

Marker immediately recognized the industrial potential of this discovery and since he lacked a practical source of diosgenin he undertook a series of botanical expeditions to the southern United States and Mexico in search of plants bearing commercially useful concentrations of this sapogenin. He achieved success during a visit to the state of Vera Cruz in Mexico, with the discovery of a plant of the genus *Dioscorea* which yielded up to 5% by weight of diosgenin. The stage was set for the industrial development of this technology and the company Syntex was established for this purpose in Mexico City in 1944. The key reaction of the Marker process, shown in Fig. 6.3, is the first step, whereby diosgenin is heated with acetic anhydride at 180–200°C. This results in cleavage of the spiroketal unit to give a dihydrofuran analog which upon oxidation is severed to produce a 16-substituted 20-keto derivative. Base treatment then removes the six carbon fragment at C16 to furnish the key intermediate neosterol acetate.[10]

During the first year of operation at Syntex several kilograms of progesterone were produced at a cost of US$80 per gram. Under the leadership of George Rosenkranz, who succeeded Marker as technical director in 1945, a novel process was developed for transforming neosterol acetate into androstenolone. Improved methods were also discovered for the synthesis of testosterone, estrone and estradiol from androstenolone. Thus by the late 1940s all of the major sex hormones became available from an abundant plant source.[8]

Two significant events then occurred which made a major impact on the Mexican steroid industry. The first was the discovery of the remarkable antiinflammatory properties of cortisone by Hensch and Kendell in 1949.[11] Progesterone became an important starting material for the manufacture of cortisone and hydrocortisone and industrial requirements for progesterone shifted from kilogram to ton quantities. By 1951 the price of progesterone had fallen to US$0.48 per gram, prompted by the increased industrial demand for this hormone and increased efficiency in process technology.[8]

The second event which accelerated the growth of the steroid industry in Mexico was the discovery of the oral progestational agent norethindrone in 1951 and the subsequent development of this substance and the related norethynodrel for oral contraceptive purposes.[12,13] The process for the industrial production of these compounds commenced with estrone, which was obtained from diosgenin in a multistep sequence. Aspects of the technology employed for the synthesis of the 19-norsteroids will be disussed in the next section.

The successful implementation of the diosgenin technology at the industrial level shifted the locus of steroid production from Europe to Mexico. Indeed, by the early 1960s over 50% of all steroids produced throughout the world originated from Mexican diosgenin. By 1973 the annual production of diosgenin employed for the synthesis of corticosteroids, sex hormones and oral contraceptives totaled 1175 metric tons.[14] The period 1960–75 marked the golden age of steroids in Mexico. Thereafter a gradual and ultimately precipitous decline occurred in this industry, prompted by economic, political and technological developments.

Stigmasterol Route

In the search for a source of progesterone other than diosgenin, chemists from the Upjohn Company focused their attention on the phytosterol stigmasterol. This substance is a constituent of soybean oil and was recognized by many investigators as an attractive starting material for the following reasons: (a) stigmasterol is abundantly available from a reproducible plant source; (b) it contains a double bond between C22 and C23 which provides a point of attack for the oxidative removal of the side chain.[9] The Upjohn researchers developed novel methodology for the isolation of stigmasterol, which constitutes 20% of soybean oil.[15] The residue from this process contains the side chain saturated sterol sitosterol as a principal constituent and this substance was stockpiled over the years at the Upjohn plant despite its apparent lack of immediate utility. An efficient industrial scale process was developed by the Upjohn chemists which afforded progesterone in five chemical steps from stigmasterol.[16] This technology made a major impact on the world price of progesterone which fell from US$0.29 to US$0.19 per gram by the late 1950s.[17]

First generation progestogens: a fundamental innovation in the chemical synthesis of steroids

19-norsteroids

The technology that made possible the synthesis of the 19-norprogestational agents was discovered in 1948 by Arthur J. Birch, an Australian chemist working at Oxford University. Birch's initial studies, published in 1944, confirmed an earlier literature report that monobenzenoid systems (e.g. toluene, methoxybenzene) were reduced by sodium and ethanol in liquid ammonia to dihydro products of unassigned structure. Birch identified the products of these reductions as the 2,5-dihydro derivatives and he then undertook a series of investigations to explore the scope of this reduction process in synthesis.[18] A target of interest was the unknown 19-norsteroid system, which he reasoned should be obtainable from estradiol by the metal/ammonia reduction. Indeed the potential of this chemistry for the preparation of 19-norsteroids was demonstrated by Birch with a practical synthesis of 19-nortestosterone starting with estradiol 3-glyceryl ether (Fig. 6.4). Thus reduction of estradiol 3-glyceryl ether with potassium metal and ethanol in liquid ammonia furnished an acid sensitive dihydro derivative which was cleaved with very mild acid to the unconjugated ketone. Treatment of either dihydro derivative or unconjugated ketone with stronger acid provided the desired 19-nortestosterone.[18] Birch did not pursue his studies on the synthesis of other 19-norsteroids because of limited resources. Since 19-nortestosterone exhibited *c.* 20% of the androgenic potency of the parent hormone the National Research and Development Corporation in Britain expressed no interest in patenting either 19-nortestosterone or the metal/ammonia reduction process on Birch's behalf. However, the latter process proved to be of immense utility in synthetic organic chemistry and has been

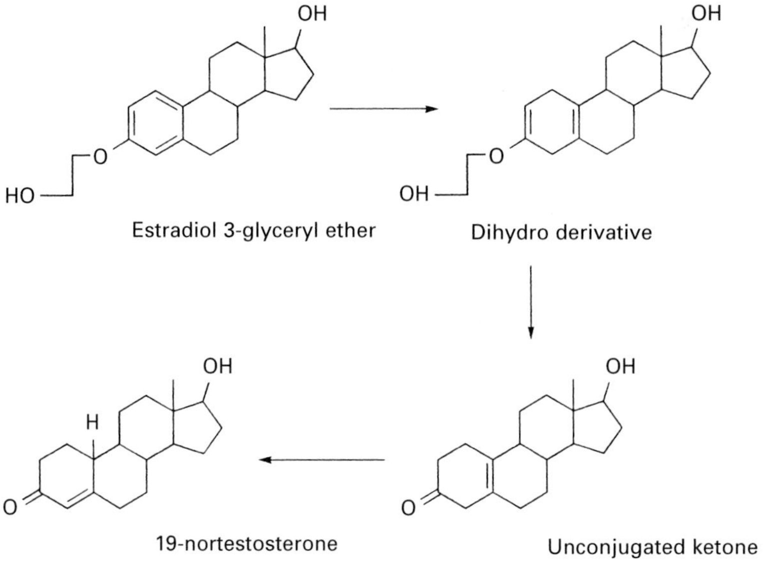

Estradiol 3-glyceryl ether → Dihydro derivative → Unconjugated ketone → 19-nortestosterone

Fig. 6.4 Synthesis of 19-nortestosterone.

appropriately named the Birch reduction in honor of its discoverer.

The technology was now in hand for the synthesis of norethindrone, the first potent progestational agent active by the oral route (Fig. 6.5). This was accomplished by Djerassi, Rosenkranz and Miramontes at Syntex in late 1951.[13] The closely related norethynodrel was prepared by F.B. Colton at G.D. Searle and Co. in 1953.[13] Both of these agents were approved by the United States Food and Drug Administration in 1957 for the treatment of menstrual disorders.[13] Norethynodrel was the agent selected by Pincus, Rock and Garcia for their classical studies carried out in Puerto Rico which demonstrated the clinical effectiveness of a 17α-ethynyl-19-norsteroid for controlling human fertility.[19] The first industrial processes employed for the preparation of norethindrone and norethynodrel are outlined in Fig. 6.5. Both processes commenced with estrone methyl ether, which was subjected to a modified Birch reduction to produce the dihydro derivative. The Syntex route proceeded from the dihydroderivative to 19-norandrostenedione in two steps and thence to norethindrone via a three step protection (at C3), ethynylation (at C17) deprotection sequence.[12] The Searle route proceeded from the dihydro derivative via oxidation to the 17-ketone followed by ethynylation at C17 and mild hydrolysis.[20]

Several 19-norsteroids related to norethindrone have been developed over the years for contraceptive purposes. These included norethindrone acetate (Syntex/Schering AG), the 3-desoxy analog lynestrenol (Organon) and the A-ring reduced 3β-acetoxy analog ethynodiol diacetate (Searle).[21] Compounds of the norgestrel series constitute another important family of 19-norsteroids which exhibit high progestational activity by the oral route. It is of interest to note that norgestrel was the first 19-norsteroid to be produced by total synthesis and marketed as a racemic mixture.

17α-acetoxyprogesterone analogs

The finding that 17α-acetoxyprogesterone (Fig. 6.6) exhibited oral progestational activity prompted a number of laboratories to explore this lead.[22] Three of the most important compounds developed in this series include 6α-methyl-17α-acetoxyprogesterone [medroxyprogesterone acetate (MPA)], its 6-dehydro analog (megestrol acetate) and 6-chloro-6-dehydro-17α-acetoxyprogesterone (chlormadinone acetate). The first synthesis of MPA, reported by an Upjohn group, started with 17α-hydroxyprogesterone which was readily available from neosterol acetate or pregnenolone.[23] 17α-Hydroxyprogesterone was first converted to the 3,20-bisketal epoxide which furnished the 6β-methyl homolog upon treatment with methyl Grignard. This compound was then transformed into MPA in four conventional steps. Megestrol acetate was first described by Ringold et al from Syntex and was prepared in one step from MPA by chloranil

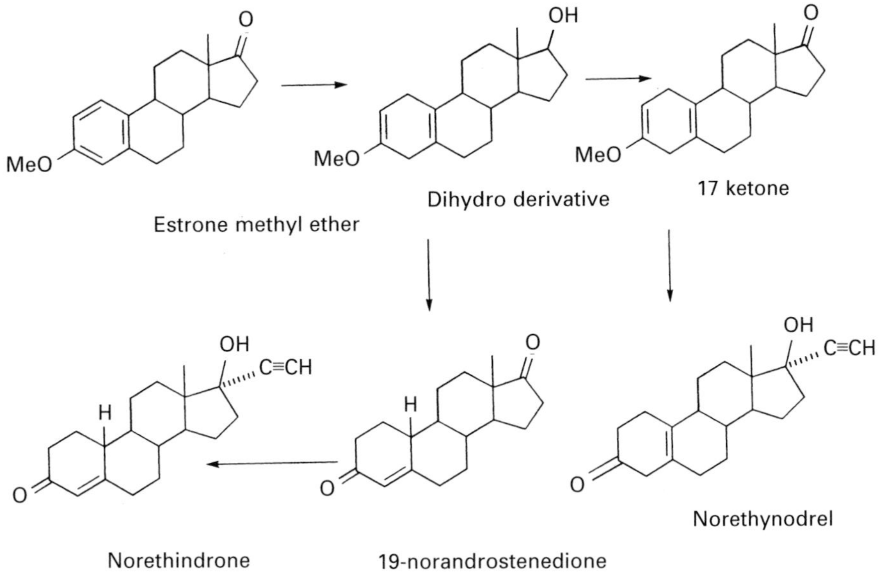

Estrone methyl ether

Dihydro derivative

17 ketone

Norethindrone

19-norandrostenedione

Norethynodrel

Fig. 6.5 Synthesis of norethindrone.

oxidation.[24] Chlormadinone acetate, another Syntex discovery, was one of the most potent progestational agents prepared in the acetoxyprogesterone series. Its synthesis was accomplished in four steps starting with 17α-acetoxyprogesterone.[25]

A new breakthrough: total synthesis of 19-norsteroids

The processes that have been described thus far fall into the category of partial syntheses. The advantages of this approach are due to the fact that plant-sourced starting materials such as diosgenin and stigmasterol possess the same tetracyclic ring system and absolute configuration as the mammalian steroid hormones. More specifically, the stereochemistry at carbons 8, 9, 10, 13 and 14 are the same in diosgenin, stigmasterol, testosterone and progesterone. Thus intermediates such as neosterol acetate and pregnenolone became cost effective relays for the transformation of diosgenin and stigmasterol into biologically active progestogens and estrogens.[14]

An important event took place in the 1970s which had a significant impact on the steroid industry. This was the decision by the Government of Mexico to nationalize the collection of *Dioscorea* root and to impose controls on the production of diosgenin. This decision, coupled with increased production costs and a dwindling supply of the root, resulted in a five-fold increase in the price of diosgenin to over US$120 per kg by 1976.[14] Because of these developments and the political uncertainties existing in Mexico at the time, the major steroid manufacturers gradually abandoned Mexico as a preferred source for steroid intermediates. Much of the industry shifted from a diosgenin to a soy sterol-based technology, and as a consequence of rising costs, total synthesis became a viable alternative for the production of steroids.

There are many problems associated with the development of a cost effective total synthesis of steroids on the industrial scale. Thus efficient methods must be devised for constructing the tetracyclic ring system and for controlling the stereochemistry at the ring junctions. Since the product of a total synthesis is a racemic or d,l-mixture, a resolution is required to separate the inactive enantiomer from its biologically active counterpart. It is essential that the resolution be conducted at an early stage of the synthesis so that the unwanted stereoisomer is not carried through the entire process, thereby adding substantially to the cost of the final product.

The challenge of developing a novel total synthesis of steroids has attracted the attention of organic chemists in academic and industrial laboratories for over half a century. Because of this effort, significant advances have been made in the development of new synthetic methods and many unique total syntheses of steroids have been developed over the years. One

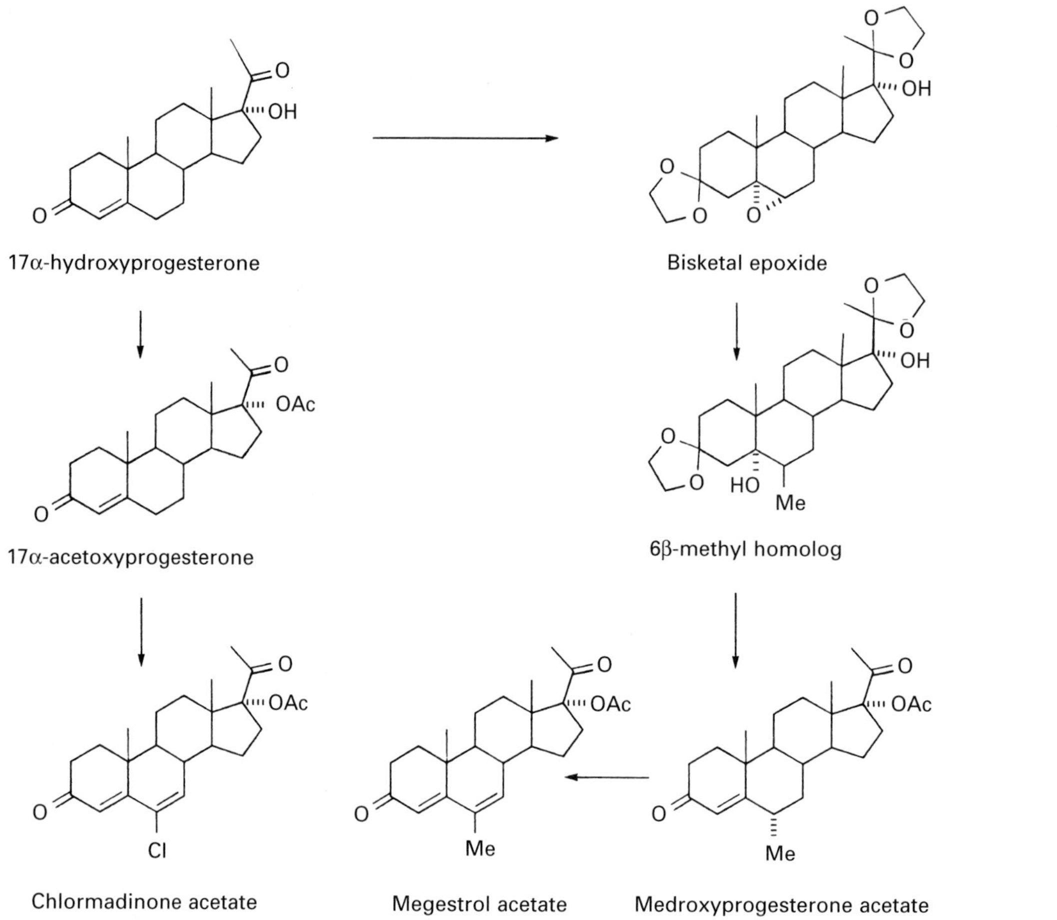

Fig. 6.6 Synthesis of medroxyprogesterone acetate.

of the first successful industrial total syntheses of a 19-norsteroid was due to the pioneering work of Leon Velluz and coworkers at Roussel UCLAF in France.[26] The Roussel process started with the readily available 2-methylclopentane-1,3-dione which was transformed in two steps into a bicyclic diketopropionic acid derivative. This substance was resolved with (−)-ephedrine to produce the (+)-enantiomer, which has the same absolute stereochemistry as the natural steroids. After two additional steps, the B and A rings were constructed in sequential fashion to yield 19-nortestosterone. Transformation of the latter into norethindrone followed established methodology. The Roussel process provided an alternative source of norethindrone and related products and convincingly demonstrated the value of total synthesis for the manufacture of these complex molecules. However, this process has the disadvantage of being linear in nature with each ring being added in sequential fashion. Indeed, starting with 2-methylcyclopentane-1, 3-dione, 11 chemical steps are required to make 19-nortestosterone.

An important advance in the development of a shorter convergent total synthesis of steroids was due to H. Smith and colleagues at Manchester University.[27,28] This process started with two monocyclic intermediates, which represent the A and D rings of the steroid tetracycle and furnished racemic estradiol methyl ether in four chemical steps. A second, more efficient synthesis of estradiol methyl ether and 19-nortestosterone as racemic mixtures, was developed independently by the Russian chemists Torgov and Ananchenkov[29] and H. Smith and collaborators[28] (Fig. 6.7). The starting vinyl carbinol, obtained in four steps from petroleum-based β-naphthol, is the precursor for the A and B rings of the steroid nucleus. Alkylation of 2-methylcyclopentane-1,3-dione (R=Me) with the vinyl carbinol in the presence of a trace of base furnished the intermediate

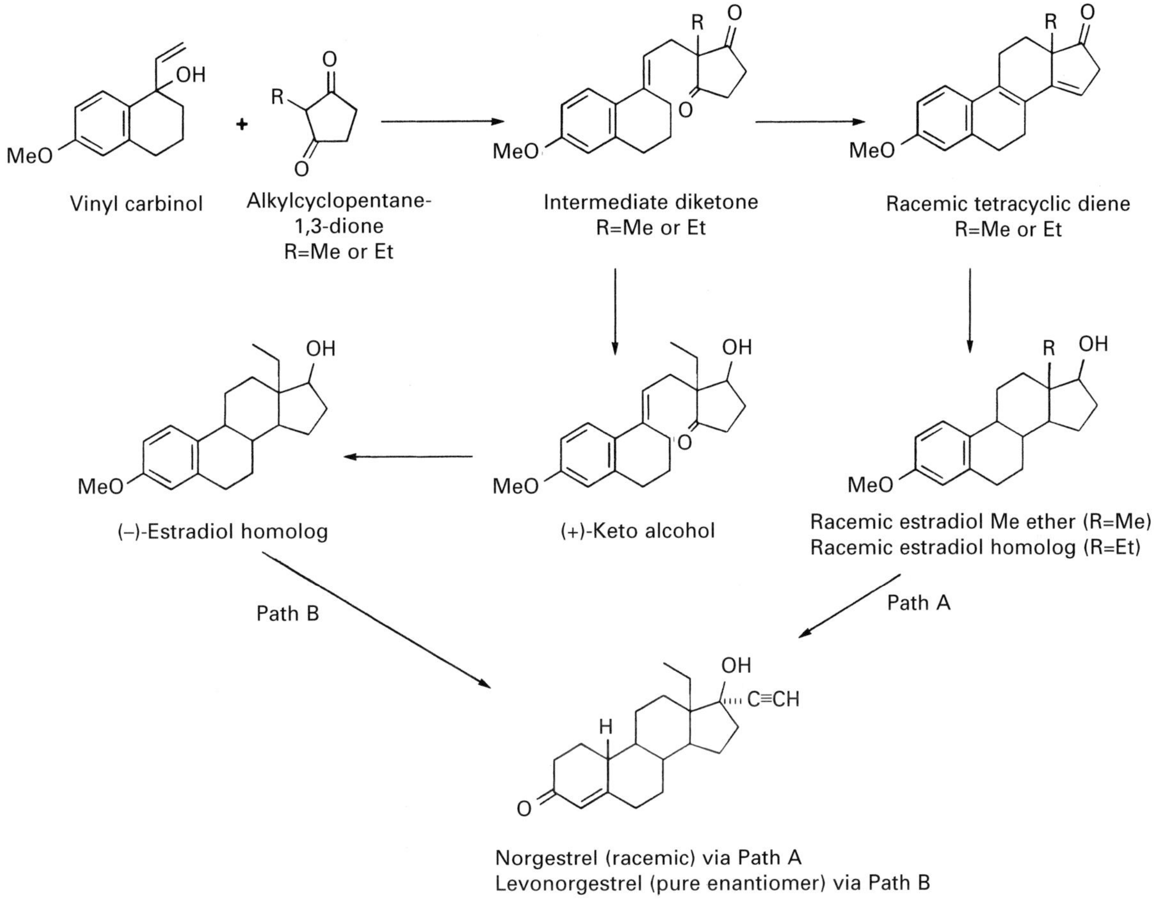

Fig. 6.7 Synthesis of norgestrel and levonorgestrel.

diketone (R=Me) in good yield. Exposure of the latter compound to acid gave the racemic tetracyclic diene (R=Me), identical to the diene made by the first Smith synthesis. Catalytic hydrogenation followed by metal-ammonia reduction afforded racemic estradiol methyl ether (R=ME) which was transformed into racemic 19-nortestosterone in two additional chemical steps.

The Torgov-Smith process is an exceptional contribution to the field of steroid synthesis. Its distinguishing features include:

(a) readily available starting materials
(b) shortness — six chemical steps to (±)-19-nortestosterone starting with vinyl carbinol and cyclopentanedione intermediates
(c) high efficiency
(d) adaptability to large scale operations

The Roussel process requires 11 steps to make (±)-19-nortestosterone starting from the same cyclopentanedione intermediate.

Second generation progestogens: norgestrel and levonorgestrel

The steroid chemist has also employed total synthesis to prepare novel compounds which are inaccessible from intermediates derived by partial synthesis. A striking illustration of this approach is H. Smith's discovery of norgestrel.[27,28] This substance, which is a racemic mixture and bears an ethyl group at C-13, was prepared by the Smith and Torgov-Smith routes starting with 2-ethylcyclopentane-1,3-dione. The latter route is highlighted in Fig. 6.7 and proceeds via intermediate diketone, racemic tetracyclic diene, racemic estradiol homolog, wherein R=Et, and path A to norgestrel. This agent was superseded in the marketplace by the optically pure levonorgestrel. Entry to the latter enantiomer was gained by classical resolution of racemic estradiol homolog (R=Et) followed by established chemistry. Alternatively, microbial reduction of intermediate diketone (R=Et) with

Saccharomyces uvarum[30] furnished the (+)-keto alcohol which could be elaborated to levonorgestrel via (–)-estradiol homolog and path B. The success of levonorgestrel underscores the contribution that total synthesis has made in the discovery and chemical production of steroids. Indeed, pharmaceutical compositions containing levonorgestrel presently make up the largest selling oral contraceptive product lines in the world.[18]

Third generation progestogens: norgestimate, gestodene and desogestrel

Compounds which comprise the third generation progestogens are related to levonorgestrel and include norgestimate, gestodene and desogestrel (Figs 6.8, 6.9). Norgestimate is the oxime of levonorgestrel acetate.[31] Studies in women indicate that the metabolite 17-deacetylated norgestimate participates in the pharmacological response to norgestimate. Levonorgestrel, another metabolite, binds to serum SHBG and albumin; its contribution to the pharmacological activity of norgestimate is probably limited.[32a,b,c]

From a chemical perspective, gestodene and desogestrel differ from levonorgestrel because of the increased complexity of their syntheses. In contrast to levonorgestrel, gestodene possesses a carbon-carbon double bond between positions 15 and 16. This unsaturated linkage is introduced by base-promoted

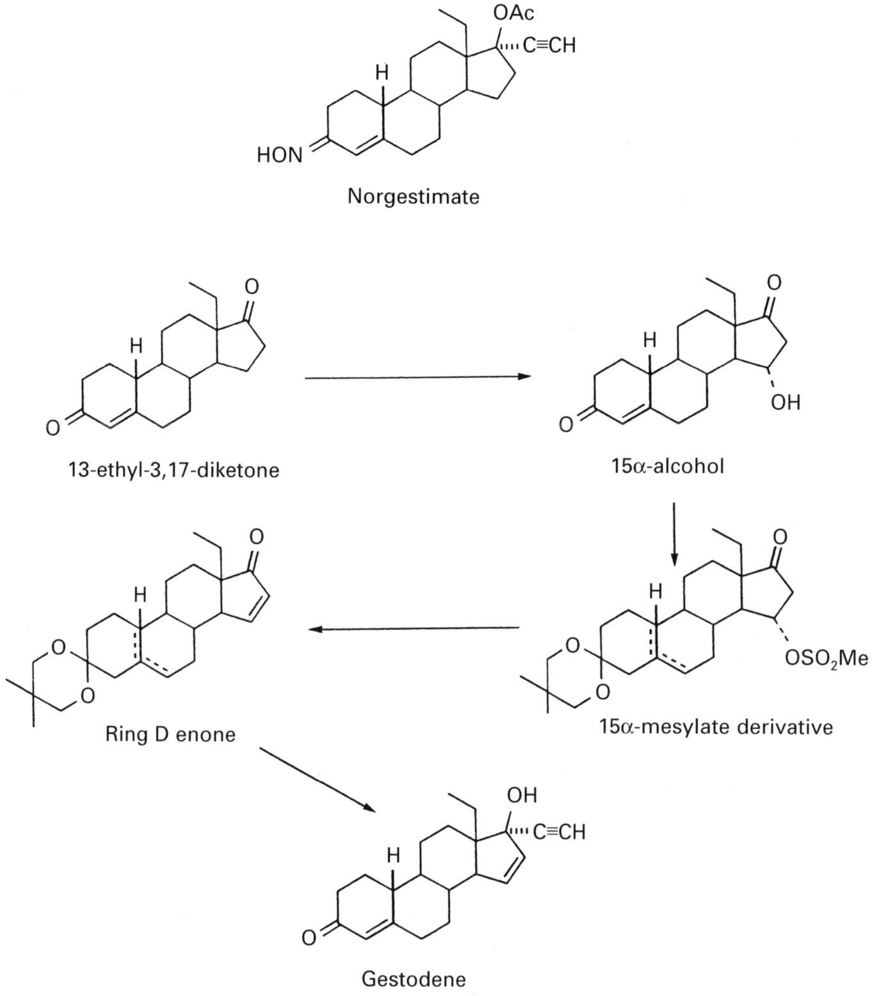

Fig. 6.8 Synthesis of gestodene.

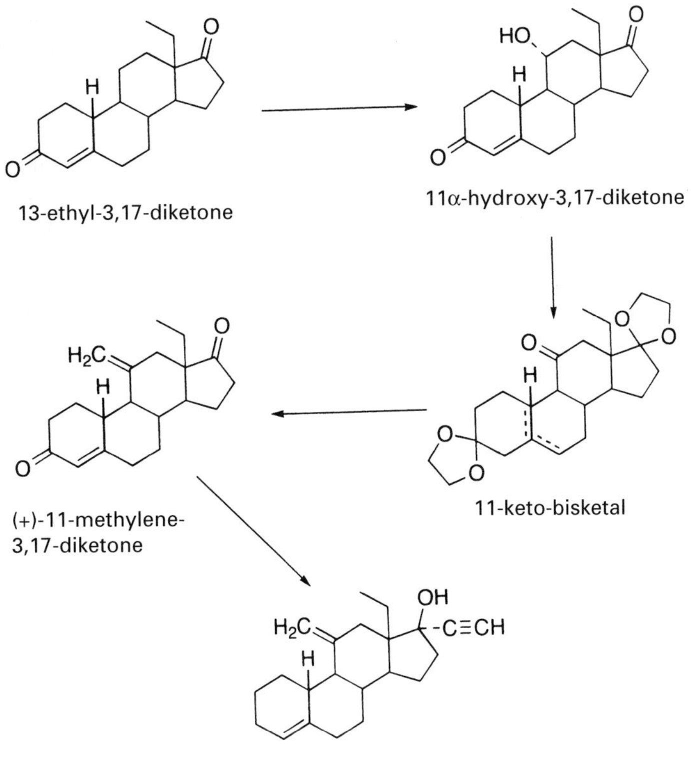

13-ethyl-3,17-diketone

11α-hydroxy-3,17-diketone

11-keto-bisketal

(+)-11-methylene-3,17-diketone

Desogestrel

Fig. 6.9 Synthesis of desogestrel.

elimination of a 15α-mesylate derivative with the precursor 15α-alcohol being prepared by microbiological hydroxylation of the 13-ethyl-3,17-diketone with cultures of *Penicillium raistrickii* (Fig. 6.8). The resulting ring D unsaturated ketone was transformed into gestodene in two steps. The process is described in a US Patent issued to Schering AG.[33] Although the starting 13-ethyl-3, 17-diketone was prepared by total synthesis, no optical rotations were reported for the compounds described in the Schering patent.

Desogestrel was discovered by chemists at Organon and, like lynestrenol, it lacks a carbonyl group at C-3. It also has the unique feature of bearing an exomethylene group at position 11. The process for the preparation of desogestrel also required a microbiological hydroxylation step in order to introduce the oxygen functionality at C-11 required for the methylenation step (Fig. 6.9).[34] Thus microbial fermentation of the 13-ethyl-3,17-diketone with *Rhizopus nigricans* furnished the 11α-hydroxy-3,17-diketone which was converted to the suitably protected 11-keto-bisketal in two steps. Application of standard methylenation chemistry followed by removal of the ketal protecting groups provided the (+)-11-methylene-3,17-diketone, from which desogestrel was obtained in three steps employing conventional methodology. The processes employed for the preparation of gestodene and desogestrel are several steps longer than the levonorgestrel process and consequently these third generation progestogens are more costly to produce than levonorgestrel.

Microbial Application to Partial Synthesis

Despite their abundance in nature, cholesterol and sitosterol were viewed as unsuitable starting materials for the production of steroid intermediates because of the difficulty associated with removing their respective saturated C-8 and C-10 side chains by chemical methods. In the 1960s several laboratories showed that a variety of microorganisms could be employed for effecting the latter transformation. Indeed, two microbiological processes were developed and commercialized by companies in Japan and the United

States for the production of androst-4-ene-3,17-dione and its 1,2-dehydro analog from cholesterol and sitosterol using mutants derived from *Mycobacterium* species.[35,36] The Upjohn Company has also employed microbiological methods for the production of a host of steroid intermediates from sitosterol, the sterol accumulated as a byproduct of stigmasterol production.[37] In addition, Upjohn microbiologists discovered mutants of *Mycobacterium fortuitum* which degraded sitosterol to the diketopropionic acid in good yield (Fig. 6.10).[38] By employing Upjohn sourced diketopropionic acid and by streamlining the latter stages of the Roussel process, a Syntex group developed a very efficient synthesis of norethindrone.[39] A key feature of the Syntex route was the use of the mixed anhydride intermediate for coupling with the C-5 Grignard reagent to produce the tricyclic diketone after treatment with base. 19-Norandrostenedione (NAD) was obtained from the latter diketone in two steps. Direct ethynylation of NAD then furnished norethindrone. This process has the advantage of commencing with an optically active starting material derived from an abundant natural source and it is several steps shorter than the Roussel synthesis. In recent years it has become the preferred method for the large scale production of norethindrone.

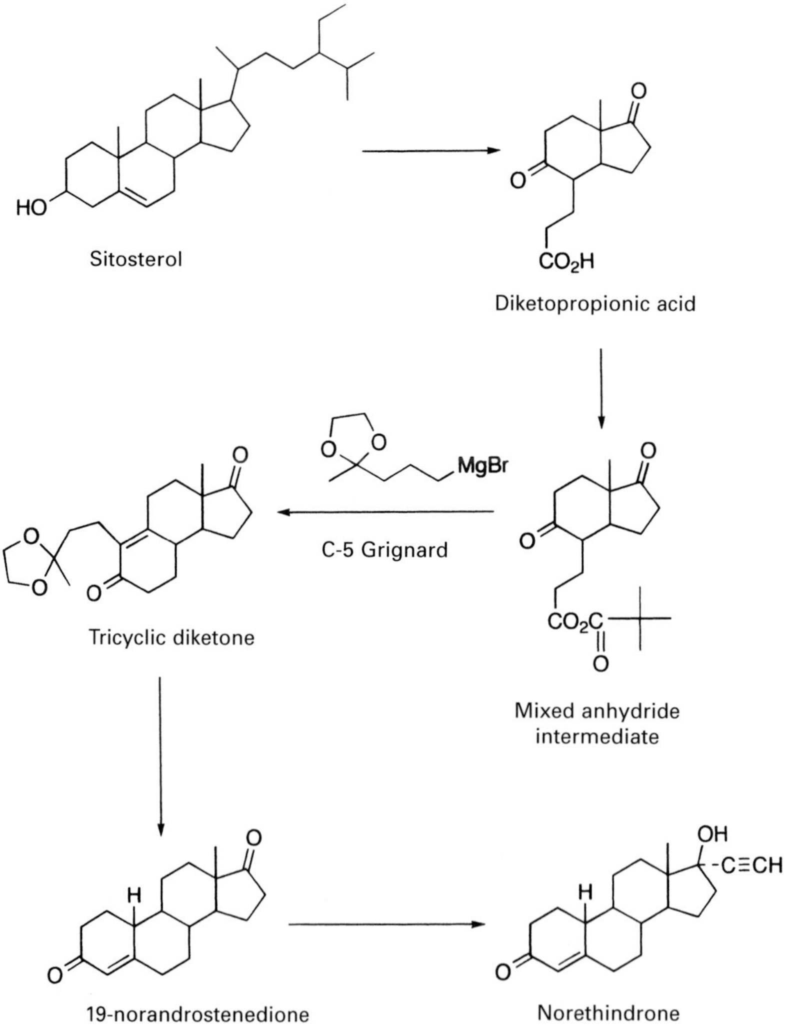

Sitosterol

Diketopropionic acid

MgBr

C-5 Grignard

Tricyclic diketone

Mixed anhydride intermediate

19-norandrostenedione

Norethindrone

Fig. 6.10 Partial synthesis of norethindrone starting with sitosterol.

Estrogens and antiestrogenic compounds

Estrogenic steroids

The discovery of 17α-ethynyl estradiol (Fig. 6.11) was the most significant advance to occur in the field of estrogenic steroids following the early work which led to the establishment of the structures of these hormones.[40] The 17α-ethynyl group was shown to impart high oral activity to the estradiol molecule and 17α-ethynyl estradiol and its methyl ether (mestranol) have been employed for many years as the estrogenic components of the combined estrogen-progestogen oral contraceptives. The first successful processes for the production of estrone and estradiol were partial syntheses and involved pyrolytic elimination of the C-19 methyl group from ring A doubly or triply unsaturated 3, 17-diketoandostrane derivatives.[41,42] These processes suffered from low throughput and modest yields. In a later innovation, the C-19-methyl elimination/aromatization process was achieved by treatment of 1,4-dien-3-one with lithium metal and biphenyl followed by acid workup to produce estrone in approximately 75% yield.[43] Ethynyl estradiol and mestranol were prepared by ethynylation of their 17-ketone precursors with potassium acetylide.[40] In the area of total synthesis, the Torgov-Smith process has provided one of the most efficient routes to the estrogenic steroids. This technology has been discussed previously (Fig. 6.7).[28,29]

The stilbene system and its manipulation: from highly potent estrogens to antiestrogens

The history of the synthetic estrogens had its beginning in the late 1930s with the discovery of diethylstilbestrol (DES) by Robinson and Dodds (Fig. 6.12).[44] Although DES and several of its congeners enjoyed widespread clinical usage at one time, these agents are of little interest today. The triphenylethylenes, which evolved from the DES system, form another unique family of synthetic estrogens and antiestrogens. Chlortrianisine was an early example of an estrogenic triphenylethylene in which the ethyl groups of DES have been replaced by phenyl and chloro groups.[45] Addition of a substituent bearing a basic nitrogen to one of the phenyl groups in the triphenylethylene system produced a significant effect on biological activity. Thus, clomiphene proved to be an impeded estrogen in the rat and it also inhibited the effects of concurrently administered estrone in this animal. Clomiphene has been marketed as a mixture of *cis* and *trans* geometrical isomers.

In 1965 chemists at ICI in England prepared the *cis* and *trans* isomers of 1-(p-dimethylamino-

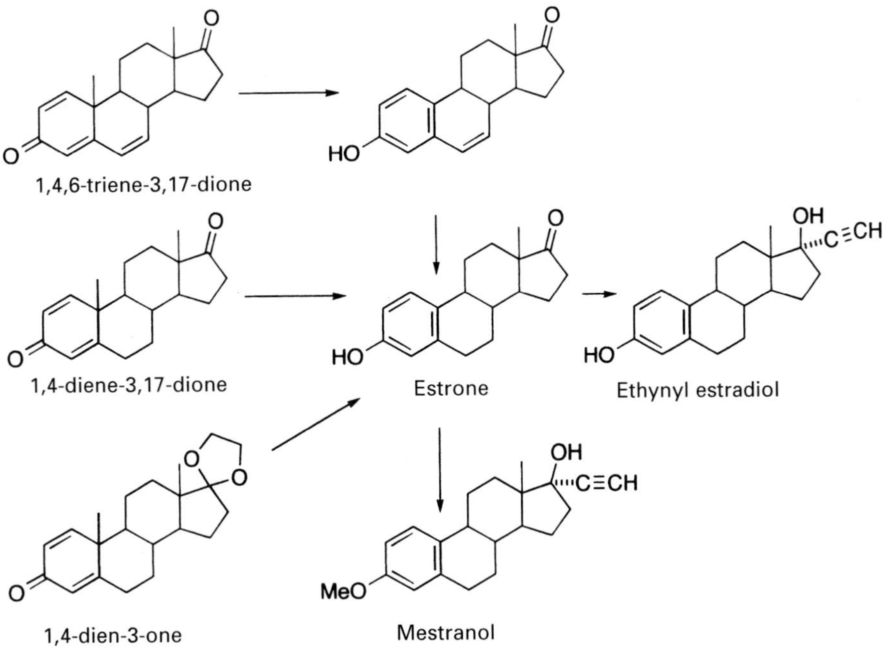

Fig. 6.11 Synthesis of ethynyl estradiol and its methyl ether, mestranol.

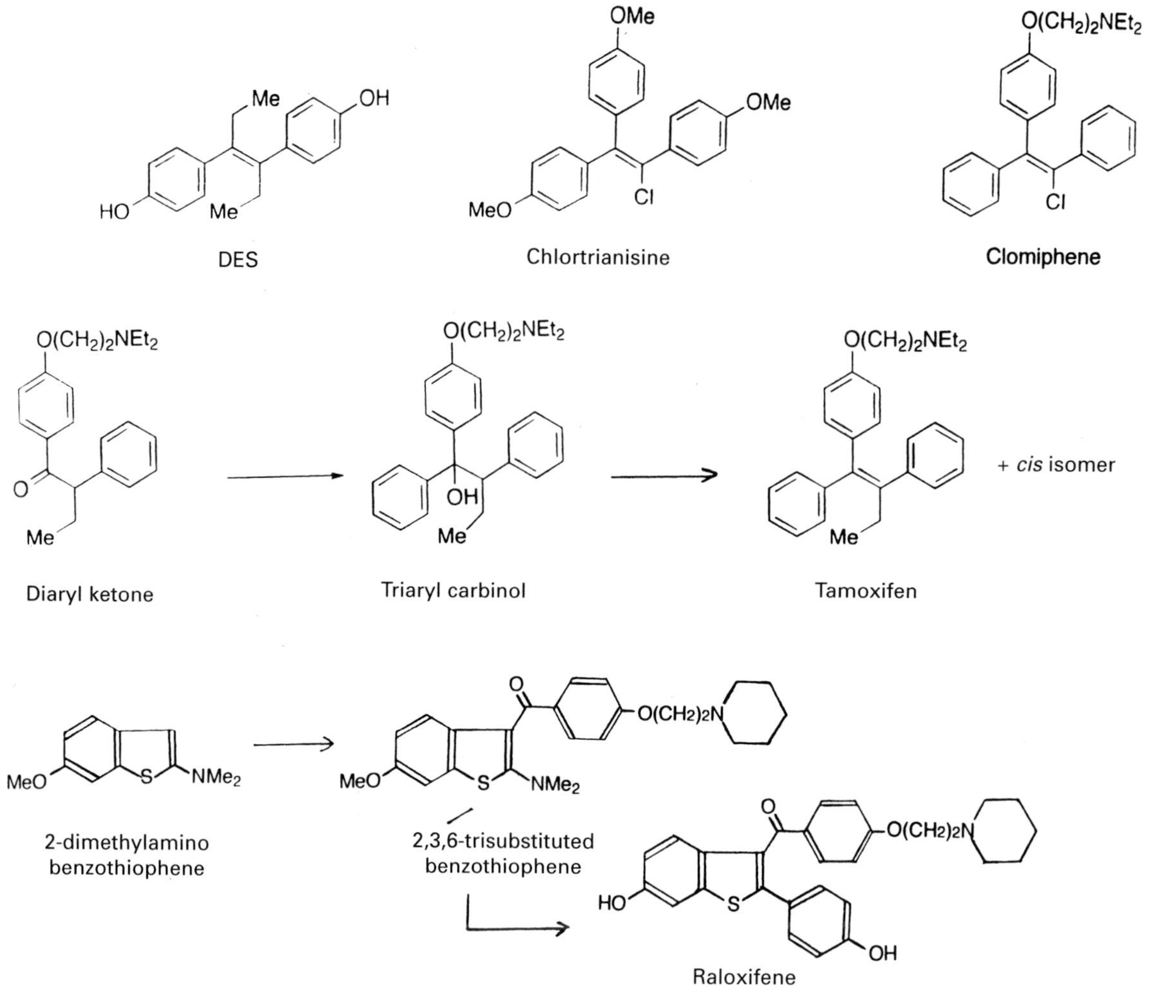

Fig. 6.12 Synthesis of tamoxifen and raloxifene.

ethoxyphenyl)-2-ethyl-1,2-diphenylethylene. It was reported that the *cis* isomer exhibited classical estrogenic activity whereas the *trans* isomer (tamoxifen) manifested antiestrogen effects in the rat (see Fig. 6.12). Tamoxifen has been employed in the treatment of breast cancer for many years. The discovery of raloxifene has added a new and exciting chapter to the story of the synthetic estrogens. With raloxifene, the diphenylethylene unit has been incorporated into a benzothiophene ring system and the third phenyl ring has been appended to the heterocycle by means of a carbonyl group. Raloxifene exhibits antiestrogen effects in breast and uterine tissues and it stimulates bone growth.[47] The compound was recently approved for the treatment of osteoporosis by the US Food and Drug Administration.

Unlike the steroids, compounds of the triphenylethylene series are relatively simple molecules and their syntheses were achieved by standard chemical methods. This is illustrated with the synthesis of tamoxifen and its *cis* isomer, which was achieved by treatment of the diaryl ketone with phenyl Grignard to produce the triaryl carbinol, followed by dehydration. The individual isomers were isolated from the resulting mixture by fractional crystallization.[48]

The synthesis of raloxifene commenced with the 2-dimethylaminobenzothiophene which was converted to the 2,3,6-trisubstituted benzothiophene by acylation with the appropriately 4-substituted benzoyl chloride. Treatment of the latter substance with 4-anisyl Grignard followed by cleavage of the methyl ether groups furnished raloxifene.[47]

Conclusion

After many years of clinical experience, levonorgestrel and norethindrone remain the most widely employed progestogens in oral contraceptive preparations. Total synthesis and partial synthesis in combination with microbiology have proved to be the most efficient and cost effective modern technologies for the production of levonorgestrel and norethindrone respectively. The estrogens are produced by total synthesis.

In the 17α-acetoxyprogesterone series, MPA and megestrol acetate continue as important therapeutic modalities, the former as an injectable contraceptive and the latter as a palliative for ovarian and breast cancer. These important progestogens will continue to be prepared by partial synthesis for some time to come since cost effective total synthesis processes have not yet been developed for this class of compounds.

Finally, it is of interest to note that the current price of bulk progesterone in the United States is in the US$0.50 per gram range which, after 35 years, is only about 2.6 times the price charged for this substance in the late 1950s.[49] This modest increase in the cost of progesterone over a span of nearly four decades provides striking testimony to the remarkable effectiveness of the technology which has been developed over the years for the production of steroids on the industrial scale.

REFERENCES

1. Henzl MR 1995 Synthetic sex steroids. In: Adashi EY, Rock J, Rozenwaks Z (eds) Reproductive endocrinology, surgery and technology. Lippincott-Raven, Philadelphia & New York; pp 585–604
2. Henzl MR 1996 Safety of modern contraceptives. Lancet 347: 257–258
3. Kraus RM, Tribble DL 1993 Oral contraceptives and plasma lipoprotein metabolism. In: Shoupe D, Haseltine P (eds) Contraception. Springer Verlag, New York pp 34–41
4. Weiss N 1995 Third-generation oral contraceptives: How risky? Lancet 346: 1570
5. Fieser LF, Fieser M 1975 Steroids. Reinhold Publishing Corp., New York, Chs 15, 16, 17, 19 (excellent account of early developments in steroid field)
6. Fieser LF, Fieser M 1975 Steroids. Reinhold Publishing Corp., New York, pp 504–515
7. Fieser LF, Fieser M 1975 Steroids. Reinhold Publishing Corp., New York, pp 542–546
8. Rosenkranz G 1992 From Ruzicka's terpenes in Zurich to Mexican steroids via Cuba. Steroids 57: 409–418
9. Marker RE, Rohrmann E 1939 The structure of the side chain of sarsasapogenin. Journal of the American Chemical Society 61: 846–851
10. Marker RE, TsukamotoT, Turner DL 1940. Diosgenin. Journal of the American Chemical Society 62: 2525–2532
11. Hench PS, Kendall EC, Slocumb CH, Polley HF 1949 Proceedings of Staff Meetings at the Mayo Clinic 24:18
12. Djerassi C, Miramontes L, Rosenkranz G, Sondheimer F 1954 Synthesis of 19-nor-17α-ethynyltestosterone and 19-nor-17α-methyltestosterone. Journal of the American Chemical Society 76: 4092–4094
13. Djerassi C 1981 The politics of contraception. WH Freeman, San Francisco, pp 247–252
14. Lenz GR 1983 Encyclopedia of chemical technology, J. Wiley, New York, ch 21, pp 645–729
15. Poulos A, Greiner JW, Fevig GA 1969 Ind Eng Chem 53: 949–962
16. Herr ME, Heyl FW 1952 Enamine derivatives of steroidal carbonyl compounds. Journal of the American Chemical Society 74: 3627–3630
17. Fieser LF, Fieser M 1975 Steroids. Reinhold Publishing Corp., New York, p 556
18. Birch AJ 1995 To see the obvious. American Chemical Society, Washington, pp 96–105
19. Rock J, Pincus G, Garcia CR 1956 Effects of certain 19-norsteroids on the normal human menstrual cycle. Science 124: 891–893
20. Colton FB 1955 US Patent 2,725,389 (Nov 29)
21. Djerassi C 1966 Steroid oral contraceptives. Science 151: 1055–1061
22. Goldzieher JW, Peterson WF, Gilbert RA 1958 Comparison of endometrial activities in man of anhydrohydroxyprogesterone and 17α-acetoxyprogesterone, a new oral progestational compound. Annals of the New York Academy of Sciences 713: 722–726
23. Babcock JC, Gutsell ES, Herr ME et al 1958 6α-Methyl-17α-hydroxyprogesterone 17-acylates; a new class of potent progestins. Journal of the American Chemical Society 80: 2904–2905
24. Ringold HJ, Ruelas JP, Batres E, Djerassi C 1959 6-Methyl derivatives of 17α-hydroxyprogesterone and of Reichstein's substance 'S'. Journal of the American Chemical Society 81: 3712–3716
25. Ringold HJ, Batres E, Bowers A, Edwards J, Zderic J 1959 6-halo progestational agents. Journal of the American Chemical Society 81: 3485–3486
26. Velluz L, Mathieu J, Nominé G 1966 Contraceptive compounds and total synthesis of steroids. Tetrahedron Supplement 8, Part III: 495–505
27. Smith H, Hughes GA, Douglas GT et al 1963 Totally synthetic (±)-13-alkyl-3-hydroxy and methoxygona-1,3, 5(10)-trien-17-ones and related compounds. Experientia XIX: 394
28. Smith H, Hughes GA, Douglas GA et al 1964 Totally synthetic hormones, Part II, 13β-alkylgona-1,3, 5(10)-triene, 13β-alkylgon-4-en-3-ones and related compounds. Journal of the American Chemical Society 4472–4492
29. Ananchenko SN, Torgov IV 1963 New synthesis of estrone, d,l,8-isoestrone and d,l-19-nortestosterone. Tetrahedron Lett 1553–1558

30. Rufer C, Kosmol H, Schroder E et al 1967 Total synthesis of optically active steroids III; total synthesis of optically active 13-ethylgonane derivatives. Annals of Chemistry 702: 141–148
31. Schroff AP 1977 US Patent 4,027,019 (May 13)
Hahn DW, Allen GO, McGuire JL 1976 Norgestimate: the progestational component of a new combination oral contraceptive. Pharmacologist 18: 250
32a. McGuire JL, Philips A, Hahn DW et al 1990 Pharmacologic and pharmacokinetic characteristics of norgestimate and its metabolites. Am J Obstet Gynecol 163: 2127–2131
32b. Philips A, Hahn DW, McGuire JL 1990 Relative binding affinity of norgestimate and other progestins for human sex hormone-binding globulin. Steroids 55: 373–375
32c. Fotherby K 1995 Levonorgestrel: clinical pharmacokinetics. Clin Pharmacokinet 28: 203–215
33. Hofmeister H, Wiechert R, Annen K et al 1978 US Patent 4,081,537 (May 28)
34. Van den Breck JJ 1975 US Patent 3,927,046 (Dec 16)
Van den Breck JJ, van Bokhoven C, Hobbelen PMJ et al 11-alkylidene steroids in the 19-nor series. Rec Trav Chem 95: 35–39
35. Arima K, Nagsawa N, Bae M et al 1969 Agricultural Biology Bulletin 33: 1636
36. Marsheck WJ, Kraychy S, Muir RD 1972 Applied Microbiology 23: 72
37. Wovcha MG, Antosz JF, Knight JC et al 1978 Biochem Biophys Acta 531: 308–321
38. Biggs CB, Pyke TR, Wovcha MG 1977 US Patent 4,062,729 (Dec 13)
39. Cooper GF, Van Horn AR 1981 A short efficient synthesis of 19-norandrost-4-ene-3,17-dione. Tet Letters 22: 1479–1482
40. Inhoffen HH, Logemann W, Hohlweg W, Serini A 1938 Structure–activity relationships of selective estrogen receptor modulators: modifications to the 2-arylbenzothiophene core of raloxifene. Chem Ber 71: 1024
41. Hershberg EB, Rubin M, Schwenk E 1950 Synthesis of estrone from androstadienone. Journal of Organic Chemistry 15: 292–300
42. Kaufman S, Pataki J, Rosenkranz G et al 1950 Contribution to the bromination of Δ^4-3-ketosteroids and a new partial synthesis of the natural estrogens. Journal of the American Chemical Society 72: 4531–4544
43. Dryden HL, Webber GM, Wieczorek JJ 1964 The reductive aromatization of steroidal dienones. A new method for the production of estrone. Journal of the American Chemical Society 86: 742–743
44. Dodds EC, Goldberg L, Lawson W, Robinson R 1938 Estrogenic activity of alkylated stilbestrols. Nature 142: 34
45. Lednicer D, Mitscher LA 1977 Organic chemistry of drug synthesis. Wiley Interscience, New York, pp 100–107
46. Harper MJK, Walpole AL 1966 Contrasting endocrine activities of *cis* and *trans* isomers in a series of substituted triphenylethylenes. Nature 212: 87
47. Grese TA, Cho S, Finley DR, Alexander GG, Jones CD et al 1997 Investigations in the sexual hormone series. Journal of Medicinal Chemistry 40: 146–167
48. Bedford GR, Richardson DN 1966 Preparation and identification of *cis* and *trans* isomers of a substituted triphenylethylene. Nature 212: 733–734
49. Yates D 1996 Personal communication, The Upjohn Company

SECTION 3

Physiology

CONTENTS

7. Biosynthesis and secretion of ovarian and adrenal steroids

Stephen G. Hillier

Introduction

The principal steroid secretory glands in nonpregnant women are the ovaries and adrenals. The ovaries mainly produce sex steroids — estrogens (C_{18}), androgens (C_{19}) and progestogens (C_{21}) — that govern reproduction through their actions in the reproductive tract and on the secondary sexual tissues. The adrenals undertake high rates of synthesis and secretion of C_{21} glucocorticoids and mineralocorticoids upon which the entire physiology of the organism depends. This chapter surveys current understanding of the regulation of steroid hormone formation by the ovaries and adrenals, highlighting cellular mechanisms that give rise to the distinctive endocrine functions of these glands.

STEROIDOGENIC PATHWAYS

Cholesterol synthesis

All steroidogenic cells use cholesterol as a precursor for steroid hormone synthesis. Cholesterol is obtained both by *de novo* synthesis from acetate and uptake of lipopoteins from the extracellular milieu.[1] The rate-limiting enzyme in cholesterol synthesis is 3-hydroxy-3-methylglutaryl coenzyme A reductase (HMG-CoA reductase). HMG-CoA exists in phosphorylated (inactive) and nonphosphorylated (active) forms, and its net activity increases in response to tropic stimulation of steroid synthesis.[2]

Cholesterol uptake

Tissues that undertake sustained high rates of steroid synthesis require exogenous precursor cholesterol taken up from circulating lipoproteins by receptor mediated and non-receptor mediated means, as well as from the plasma membrane itself.

Steroidogenic cells express LDL receptors responsible for taking up most of the cholesterol used for steroidogenesis. LDL receptors located on microvilli bind circulating LDL, to form LDL–receptor complexes that are internalized in clathrin coated vesicles. LDL is separated from its receptor, which is recycled back to the plasma membrane in receptorsomes.[2,3] Within the cell, LDL is degraded by lysozomal activity into cholesteryl esters, which are stored in lipid droplets until they are hydrolyzed by acid lipase to release free cholesterol. Cholesteryl ester hydrolysis is activated by protein kinase A and catalyzed by cholesteryl esterase. The esterase is similar, if not identical, to hormone-sensitive lipase in adipocytes, where an analogous lipolytic mechanism occurs.[4]

HDL also provides cholesterol to steroidogenic cells through several mechanisms including binding of HDL to HDL receptors on the cell membrane, where sterol esters are liberated by lipases and transferred directly into the cell. HDL-bearing apolipoprotein E (apo E) can also be metabolized by endocytosis via the LDL pathway through association with the LDL (B/E) receptor.[2]

C_{21} steroid synthesis

The steroidogenic machinery of all steroid secretory tissues is similar, differing only with respect to the level of expression of the particular steroidogenic enzymes that underpin the characteristic endocrine function of each gland (Fig. 7.1). Common to all is the conversion of C_{27} cholesterol to C_{21} pregnenolone, which is the immediate precursor for ovarian (progesterone) and adrenal (cortisol and aldosterone) hormone synthesis. The enzyme responsible for this step is cholesterol sidechain cleavage, a steroidogenic cytochrome P450 (P450scc) located in the inner mitochondrial membrane.[5–6]

Although P450scc catalyzes the critical metabolic step in steroid hormone synthesis, acute steroidogenic responses to tropic hormone stimulation are rate-

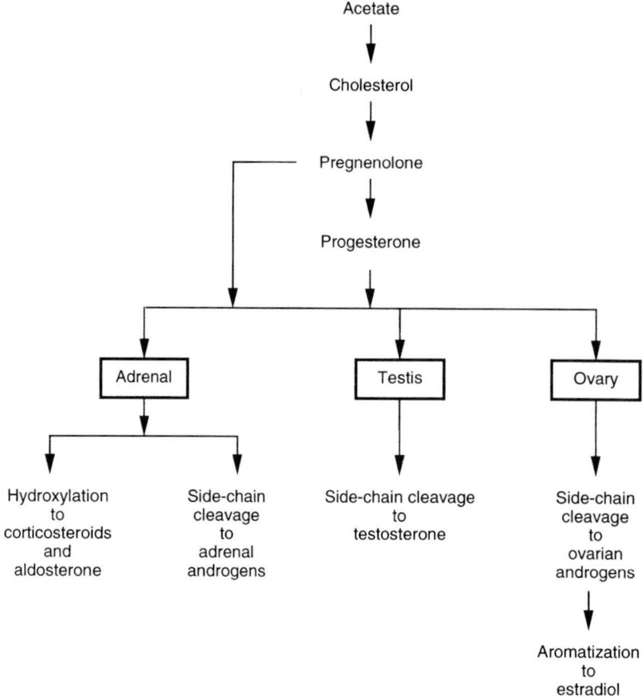

Fig. 7.1 The unified concept of steroid hormone synthesis. Characteristic steroid secretory functions of the ovary, testis and adrenal gland are shown: the pathway from acetate to progesterone is common to all.[1]

limited by cholesterol delivery to the inner mitochondrial membrane.[2,3] The intracellular movement of cholesterol is influenced by the cytoskeleton[7] and carrier proteins such as sterol carrier protein 2 (SCP2), which is a basic 13 kDa protein that facilitates the movement of cholesterol from lipid droplets to mitochondria. Within mitochondria, other factors govern the availability of cholesterol as a P450scc substrate. A 30 kDa phosphorylated protein termed steroidogenic acute regulatory protein (StAR),[8] which has been located to the inner mitochondrial membrane, appears to be indispensable to steroidogenesis in the adrenals and gonads. The StAR gene has been shown to be mutated and nonfunctional in individuals with congenital lipoid adrenal hyperplasia — an autosomal recessive disorder characterized by impaired synthesis of all adrenal and gonadal steroid hormones.[9,10] The mitochondrial benzodiazepine receptor also appears to be a key factor in the flow of cholesterol into mitochondria to permit the initiation of steroid hormone synthesis.[11]

The cholesterol sidechain cleavage reaction occurs in association with an electron transport system located in the inner mitochondrial membrane, consisting of ferroprotein reductase (adrenodoxin reductase or ferrodoxin reductase) and an iron sulfur protein shuttle (adrenodoxin or ferrodoxin), which carries electrons to P450scc. The reaction sequence entails three catalytic cycles, each of which consumes one molecule of NADPH and one molecule of oxygen.[2,5]

The subsequent metabolic fate of pregnenolone is tissue-dependent. Both ovary and adrenal cortex express microsomal 3β-hydroxysteroid dehydrogenase/Δ^{5-4} isomerase (3βHSD) activity, which converts pregnenolone to progesterone. In the ovary, progesterone is a major secreted hormone as well as an essential substrate for the synthesis of androgen and estrogen (see below). In the adrenal cortex, progesterone is the substrate for cortisol and aldosterone synthesis, as we shall now consider.

Adrenal

The major glucocorticoid produced by the adult adrenal cortex is cortisol, synthesized in zona fasiculata and zona reticularis cells via metabolism of C_{21}

pregenolone along the metabolic route illustrated in Fig. 7.2. The mineralocorticoid aldosterone is produced in the zona glomerulosa mainly through alternative metabolism of the cortisol precursor, corticosterone. Cholesterol stores in zona glomerulosa cells are significantly less than in zona fasciculata/reticularis cells, reflecting a reliance of glomerulosa cells on underlying fasciculata cells for the provision of aldosterone precursors (Fig. 7.3B).[12]

The steroidogenic enzymes important for corticosteroid synthesis are cytochrome P450s that hydroxylate precursor molecules at C21 (P450C21) and C11 (P45011β), to produce cortisol. Final hydroxylation at the C18 position (P450 aldo), gives rise to aldosterone. Each of these P450 enzymes is expressed in a cell-specific manner, consistent with the intraglandular site(s) of hormone synthesis (Table 7.1).[6] Both P45011β and P450aldo are located at the inner mitochondrial membrane, whereas P450C21 is microsomal. Steroidogenic intermediates presumably therefore shuttle back and forth across the inner mitochondrial membrane as steroid hormone synthesis occurs.

Hydroxylation at C17 can occur at any stage along the pathway from pregnenolone to cortisol, catalyzed by mitochondrial P450C17. This enzyme, common to ovary and adrenal, also cleaves the bond between C17 and C21 of C_{21} steroids to produce C_{19} steroids, explaining how both glands are able to produce androgens (see below).[13]

Ovary

The major C_{21} steroid hormone produced by the ovaries is progesterone, since ovarian cells minimally express P450C21, P45011β or P450aldo (Table 7.1).[6] Rates of ovarian pregnenolone synthesis and metabolism to progesterone are intrinsically linked to the follicular lifecycle (see below),[14] being maximal during the luteal phase of the menstrual cycle when progesterone secretion is the major endocrine function of the ovaries.

C_{19} steroid synthesis

Both adrenals and ovaries synthesize and secrete C_{19} steroids through the metabolism of C_{21} substrates by P450C17 (see above). In the ovaries, since P450C11β is absent, progesterone and pregnenolone are the main C_{21} substrates available for the C17–C20 lyase reaction catalyzed by P450C17. Consequently, the major ovarian C_{19} steroids produced by the ovary are androstenedione and dehydroepiandrosterone (DHA). Since DHA is also a substrate for ovarian 3βHSD activity, androstenedione can be produced by both the Δ^4 (progesterone → androstenedione) and Δ^5 (pregnenolone → DHA → androstenedione) routes of synthesis.[5]

In the adrenal cortex, large amounts of 11-oxy-C_{21} steroids, such as deoxycorticosterone (DOC) and corticosterone, as well as pregnenolone and progesterone, are available as P450C17 substrates.

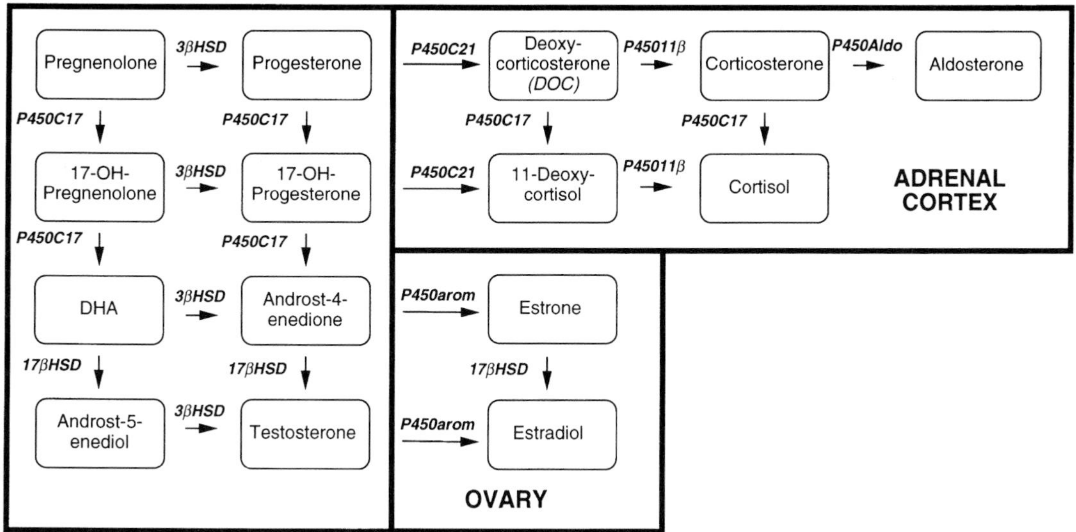

Fig. 7.2 Metabolic steps in steroid hormone synthesis, highlighting the roles of steroidogenic cytochrome P450 enzymes and steroid dehydrogenases mentioned in the text.[6]

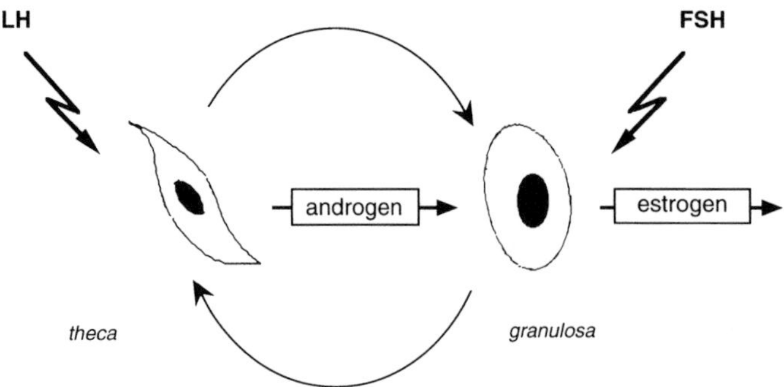

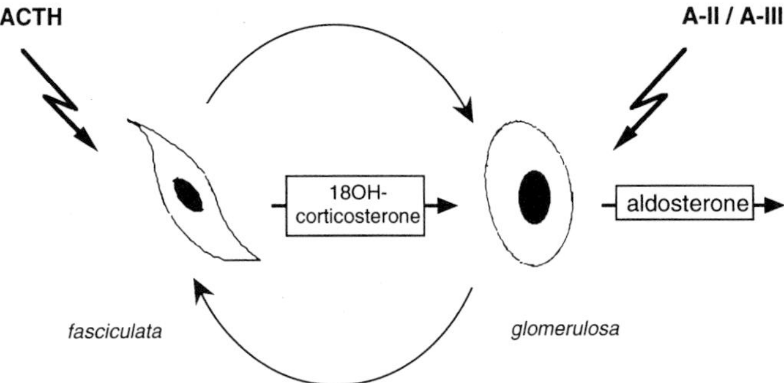

Fig. 7.3 Cell–cell interactions in steroid hormone synthesis. In the ovarian follicle (A) androgens produced by LH-stimulated thecal cells (sites of P450C17 expression) are substrates for estrogen formation in FSH-stimulated granulosa cells (sites of P450arom expression).[48, 49] In the analogous adrenal model (B), it is proposed that 18-hydroxycorticosterone (18OH-corticosterone) produced by ACTH-stimulated adrenal fasciculata cells (sites of P45011β expression) is available for metabolism to aldosterone in glomerulosa cells (sites of P450aldo expression), regulated by AG-II and AG-III.[68] Paracrine feedback loops (curved arrows), involving steroidal and nonsteroidal factors, coordinate the tropic regulation of steroidogenesis in both glands.

Table 7.1 Cell specific localization of steroidogenic cytochrome P450 enzymes in the adrenal gland and ovary, showing the major steroid hormone produced by each cell type.[6]

Cell type	P450scc	P45011β	P450aldo	P450C21	P450C17	P450arom	Hormone
Adrenal cortex							
Z. glomerulosa	+	–	+	+	–	–	aldosterone
Z. fasciculata	+	+	–	+	+	–	cortisol + 'adrenal' androgens
Z. reticularis	+	+	–	+	+	–	cortisol + 'adrenal' androgens
Ovary							
Follicle:							
Theca	+	–	–	–	+	–	'ovarian' androgens
Granulosa	+	–	–	–	–	+	estradiol > progesterone
Corpus luteum:							
Theca-lutein	+	–	–	–	+	–	androstenedione
Granulosa-lutein	+	–	–	–	–	+	progesterone > estradiol

Thus the adrenal gland produces 11-oxy-C_{19} steroids, such as 11-hydroxyandrostenedione.[15] Further modification of the C_{19} molecule occurs through reversible reduction of the oxy residue at C17, catalyzed by microsomal 17β-hydroxysteroid dehydrogenase (17βHSD),[16] yielding testosterone (ovary and adrenal) or 11-hydroxytestosterone (adrenal), depending on substrate availability.

C_{18} steroid synthesis

Estrogen synthesis depends crucially on the expression of the microsomal cytochrome P450 aromatase enzyme (P450arom) that aromatizes the A-ring of 4-ene-C_{19} substrates to yield C_{18} products: estrone (from androstendione) and estradiol (from testosterone).[17] The reaction consumes three molecules of molecular oxygen and six reducing equivalents from NADPH. The first two oxidations occur at the C19 carbon yielding 19-hydroxy and 19-oxo androgen intermediates. However, the mechanism of the third oxidation, which results in cleavage of the C10–C19 bond to yield the C_{18} estrogen molecule has yet to be determined.[18]

Increased expression of P450arom by granulosa cells is a hallmark of preovulatory follicular development (see below).[18] P450arom is minimally expressed in adrenal cells, explaining why estrogen is not a major adrenal hormone.[6] DHA sulfate, DHA and androstenedione secreted by the adrenal gland are however precursors for the formation of active androgens and estrogens in peripheral tissues, as discussed below.

OVARIAN STEROID SYNTHESIS

Cellular sites

The type and amount of steroid secreted by the ovaries are intrinsically related to follicular development. The major ovarian steroidogenic cell types are follicular granulosa and thecal cells and their luteinized derivatives, granulosa-lutein and theca-lutein cells (Table 7.1).[14,19,20] Thecal cells express P450scc and P450C17. Being vascularized, they are constantly exposed to blood-borne LDL cholesterol and can therefore undertake androgen (androstenedione>DHA synthesis) at all stages of antral follicular development and in the corpus luteum, regulated by luteinizing hormone (LH). Granulosa cells remain steroidogenically inert until activated by FSH during antrum formation, when they increasingly express P450arom and P450scc, but not P450C17 (see below). The granulosa cell layer of the preovulatory follicle remains avascular until ovulation and corpus luteum formation, when neovascularization occurs. Luteinized granulosa cells then become exposed to blood-borne LDL cholesterol, such that high rates of progesterone synthesis commence in the corpus luteum.

Before ovulation, the preovulatory follicle synthesizes mainly estrogen, rate-limited by the availability of theca-derived androgen for use as a P450arom substrate (see below). Follicles that become nonovulatory due to inadequate stimulation by FSH (see below) undergo atresia[21] and involute to leave pockets of theca-derived secondary interstitial cells in the stroma. Stromal interstitial cells continue to express P450C17 and synthesize androgens after the menopause, when folliculogenesis ceases. This has implications for ovarian steroid secretion in older women, as discussed below.

Tropic regulation

Ovarian steroid synthesis is subject to primary tropic regulation by the gonadotropins, follicle stimulating hormone (FSH) and LH, which are secreted by the anterior pituitary gland in response to stimulation by luteinizing hormone releasing hormone (LHRH).

FSH and LH regulate the expression of the P450 steroidogenic enzymes necessary for ovarian steroidogenesis. Gonadotropin receptors are members of the seven-transmembrane domain G-protein coupled superfamily of signaling molecules that activate cAMP-mediated postreceptor signaling. Hormone binding to the extracellular receptor domain stimulates adenylyl cyclase and activation of cAMP-dependent protein kinase, which relays the extracellular stimulus to the cell nucleus where the transcription of cAMP-responsive genes is enhanced.[14,20]

FSH receptors are expressed by granulosa cells and LH receptors by thecal cells at all stages of preantral and antral follicular development. Activation of the FSH receptor by FSH is essential for follicular growth to proceed beyond the stage of antrum formation, at which stage FSH becomes a granulosa cell 'survival' factor. FSH-responsive genes also govern the onset of steroidogenesis (e.g. P450scc and P450arom), responsiveness to LH (e.g. LH receptor) and paracrine/autocrine signaling (e.g. inhibin/activin subunits) (see below).[14,20]

Granulosa cell P450arom and P450scc respond differentially to FSH during preovulatory follicular development. In dose–response studies using isolated granulosa cells, relatively low concentrations of FSH or extracellular cAMP maximally stimulate P450arom activity, whereas P450scc requires exposure to high concentrations of cAMP for full activation.[14,22,23] P450arom and P450scc are thus regarded as 'low-tone' and 'high-tone' cAMP-response genes, respectively. The key to their differential response to FSH (cAMP) presumably resides in the upstream promoter regions that regulate their transcription in granulosa cells.[24,25]

Granulosa cell LH receptors induced by FSH are functionally coupled to P450scc and P450arom via cAMP-mediated postreceptor signaling. Other postreceptor mechanisms activated by LH include Ca^{++}/inositol lipid hydrolysis and tyrosine kinase signaling but the primary intracellular drive for steroidogenesis comes from intracellular cAMP.[14]

During late preovulatory development when granulosa cells become fully mature, LH is a more effective stimulus to granulosa cell cAMP formation than FSH.[14,22,23] This may be due to an increased density of LH receptors per cell and/or more efficient coupling of LH receptor molecules to cAMP formation. Either way, the ovulation-inducing LH surge triggers the increased expression of a panel of high-tone cAMP response genes, that lead to terminal granulosa cell differentiation and ovulation.[26] This gene panel includes prostaglandin endoperoxide synthase-2 (necessary for prostaglandin formation),[27] interleukins and interleukin receptors,[28] neurotropin receptors,[29] proteases involved in tissue remodeling[30,31] and factors necessary for both the production of progesterone (P450scc, StAR)[10] and intrafollicular progesterone action (progesterone receptor).[32,33]

Paradoxically, at the time of follicular rupture, when progesterone secretion by the newly forming corpus luteum is only starting to increase, granulosa-lutein cells in the human corpus luteum are already capable of undertaking maximal rates of progesterone synthesis *in vitro*.[34] As the corpus luteum develops and progesterone secretion increases, granulosa-lutein cell steroidogenic potential declines. A similar decline in steroidogenic enzyme (P450scc, 3βHSD) mRNA levels occurs in the corpus luteum of macaque monkeys.[35,36] Thus the degree of vascularization of the corpus luteum, which is most extensive in the midluteal phase, seems to be of overriding importance to the rise in progesterone secretion that occurs during the early luteal phase in the face of declining steroidogenic potential at a cellular level. This would serve to supply luteal cells of diminishing steroidogenic capacity with the increased amounts of blood-borne LDL-cholesterol necessary to sustain high rates of progesterone synthesis.[34] The recent discovery of the StAR protein that regulates cholesterol utilization in highly steroidogenic cells, such as luteal cells,[10] raises the question if this factor might play a major role in the control of progesterone secretion by the human corpus luteum.

Paracrine regulation

Locally produced steroidal and nonsteroidal factors modify FSH action and thereby bring about increased sensitivity of the maturing follicle to gonadotropins.[20] Autocrine factors thought most likely to affect FSH action *in vivo* include insulin-like growth factors (IGFs)[35–39] and members of the TGF-β family of growth/differentiation factors,[40,41] including inhibin, activin[42,43] and a newly discovered germ cell derived factor (GDF-9).[44] Paracrine factors that operate reciprocally to influence FSH action on granulosa cells include theca-derived growth factors[20] and androgens.[45,46] The granulosa cell androgen receptor (AR) that mediates paracrine androgen action is developmentally regulated by FSH. Immunocytochemical studies of the AR content of nonhuman primate and rat ovaries reveals AR to be present mainly in the granulosa cells of preantral and early-intermediate antral follicles, disappearing in the preovulatory follicle. *In vivo* experiments on immature female rats confirm that granulosa cell AR mRNA levels are *negatively* regulated by FSH.[47] A current working hypothesis is that negative regulation of the granulosa cell AR by FSH is part of the intraovarian mechanism that determines which follicle(s) becomes dominant and hence secretes estrogen in the normal menstrual cycle.

Once granulosa cells in the preovulatory follicle begin to express P450arom in response to stimulation by FSH, they utilize androgen produced by LH-stimulated thecal cells as an estrogen precursor — hence, the so-called 'two cell, two gonadotropin' mechanism of estrogen synthesis (Fig. 7.3A).[48,49] *In vitro* studies on isolated granulosa and thecal cells (human, nonhuman primate and rat) and whole follicles (rat) reveal that FSH stimulates granulosa cells to produce a factor(s) that upregulates LH-stimulated thecal P450C17 mRNA expression and androgen synthesis during preovulatory follicular maturation.[50] Growth/differentiation factors implicated in this positive feedback loop are inhibin and insulin-like growth factors (IGF-I and IGF-II).[20] Although physiological (intrafollicular) concentrations of IGF-I and IGF-II augment LH-stimulated human thecal androgen production *in vitro*, their effects are greatly enhanced by the additional presence of inhibin.[51] Thus paracrine inhibin may be of particular importance to the maintenance of follicular dominance in the human menstrual cycle.

Dynamics

Ovarian steroid secretion is entrained to a woman's reproductive status through its intrinsic link to folliculogenesis. During the reproductive years, circulating sex steroid levels undergo regular cyclic changes that correspond to stage of follicular and luteal development during menstrual cycles.

Menstrual cycle

In normal ovulatory cycles, ovarian estradiol secretion begins to rise during the midfollicular phase, reaching a maximum of 300–400 µg per day during the late follicular phase when the preovulatory follicle is fully mature, at which time it is the source of >90% of circulating estradiol. Around the time of ovulation, estradiol secretion briefly declines as luteinization commences, rising to a second peak during the midluteal phase.

Progesterone secretion begins to rise at around the beginning of the midcycle LH surge, reaching a peak of ~25 mg per day at the midluteal phase. In the absence of pregnancy, the secretion progressively declines thereafter as functional luteolysis sets in, heralding the next cycle.[52] The rising concentration of 17-hydroxyprogesterone in plasma during the follicular phase reflects the development of the Graafian follicle and, in the luteal phase, the corpus luteum. The corpus luteum is also the major source of 20α-dihydroprogesterone in blood.[53]

Androstenedione is the major androgen secreted by the adult ovary. Androstenedione and, to a much lesser extent, testosterone are synthesized by ovarian follicles throughout their most active phase of antral growth. During the follicular phase of the human menstrual cycle, the ovary contributes about 30% of the total blood androstenedione. The adrenal accounts for the rest, as revealed by the decline in circulating androstenedione levels that occurs in response to adrenal suppression with dexamethasone.[53] At midcycle the ovarian contribution rises to about 60% due to the increased synthesis and secretion of the steroid in the preovulatory follicle (see above).[52] The ovary also secretes small amounts of testosterone, but most of the testosterone in blood is derived by peripheral metabolism of androstenedione.[53]

Age

With age, the number of follicles in the ovaries gradually declines until the menopause is reached, when ovulation ceases. Once devoid of preovulatory follicles or corpora lutea, the ovaries cease to synthesize estrogen, and blood levels of estrogen decline. However, the postmenopausal ovary continues to secrete androstenedione and small amounts of testosterone, which are synthesized in secondary interstitial tissue. Occasionally, there is evidence of stromal hyperplasia and ovarian androgen secretion associated with circulating testosterone levels in the male range, which results in hirsutism and virilization. It is assumed that the low blood estrogen levels present in postmenopausal women are mainly derived from the extraglandular conversion of adrenal androstenedione, since castration of postmenopausal women does not reduce estrogen levels whereas adrenalectomy following castration does.[53] However, long-term suppression of pituitary gonadotropin secretion in postmenopausal women by treatment with a LHRH agonist causes a significant reduction in circulating testosterone and estradiol levels, indicating a continued dependence of ovarian androgen secretion on gonadotropic stimulation after the menopause.[54]

ADRENAL STEROID SYNTHESIS

The adult adrenal cortex possesses three morphologically distinct regions in which steroid hormone biosynthesis occurs.[55] The outer zona glomerulosa is the exclusive site of P450aldo expression, which catalyzes all of the steps between DOC and aldosterone (the 'late' aldosterone pathway). The inner fasciculata and reticularis zones do not measurably express P450aldo and are therefore unable to synthesize aldosterone. However, they do express P45011β, which catalyzes 11β- and 18-hydroxylation with the formation of cortisol and 18-hydroxycorticosterone, the immediate precursor of aldosterone (Fig. 7.3B).[6] 18-hydroxycorticosterone is a weak mineralocorticoid produced mainly in the zona glomerulosa, secretion of which parallels aldosterone.[55]

Tropic regulation

The principal tropic regulators of adrenal steroid synthesis are adrenocorticotropin (ACTH) and angiotensin-II (A-II). ACTH regulates both glucocorticoid and mineralocorticoid secretion while under normal physiological conditions AII mainly stimulates aldosterone production.[55–57]

ACTH

Pituitary ACTH secretion is under neuroendocrine regulation, mediated by corticotropin-releasing hormone (CRH) and other hypothalamic releasing factors such as vasopressin (AVP). Neural stimuli, e.g. due to stress, evoke hypothalamic CRH and AVP synthesis and release, which in turn stimulate the synthesis and secretion of ACTH. Glucocorticoids produced in response to ACTH exert negative feedback regulation of CRH, AVP and ACTH production, completing the adrenal-hyothalamo-pituitary feedback loop.[58,59]

Consistent with the ability of ACTH to stimulate both cortisol and aldosterone formation, ACTH receptors are expressed by all three steroidogenic cell types of the adrenal cortex, being most abundant on fasciculata cells.[60] The ACTH receptor gene is a member of the melanocortin gene subfamily, which also encode seven-transmembrane domain G-protein coupled receptors that activate cAMP-mediated postreceptor signalling. PKA activity is essential for acute ACTH stimulation of steroidogenesis, which depends on enhanced availability of cholesterol for the side chain cleavage reaction catalyzed by P450scc, similar to LH stimulation of thecal androgen synthesis and luteal progesterone synthesis. Longer term stimulation is mainly due to increased transcription of the genes encoding steroidogenic P450 enzymes.[5,6]

Angiotensin

Aldosterone secretion is mainly regulated by the actions of A-II and A-III on the zona glomerulosa. These vasopressive peptides are products of a proteolytic cascade in which angiotensinogen is hydrolyzed by renal renin to A-I, which is then converted, mainly in the lung, to A-II by angiotensin converting enzyme (ACE). Angiotensin-II is then further hydrolyzed to A-III. The rate-limiting factor in this process is the circulating renin level, which is mainly regulated by blood pressure. Reduced blood pressure (e.g. due to hemorrhage, increase in potassium intake, decrease in sodium intake, dehydration, upright posture, etc.) increases the circulating renin level, leading in turn to increased A-II, which acts directly via specific angiotensin receptors on glomerulosa cells to increase P450aldo mRNA levels and synthesis of aldosterone. Conversely, the raising of blood pressure (e.g. due to peripheral vasoconstriction, high salt intake, etc.) reduces the circulating renin level and thereby suppresses aldosterone production. Aldosterone feeds back to increase sodium resorption and plasma volume, thereby reducing renal arteriolar blood pressure and negatively regulating renin production.[55]

Binding of A-II and A-III to angiotensin receptors on glomerulosa cells activates calcium-dependent protein kinase signaling through increased inositol lipid metabolism.[56] A primary mode of angiotensin action is to stimulate intramitochondrial cholesterol transport, mediated by intracellular Ca^{++}. Potassium ions can also modulate the expression of key steroidogenic enzymes in adrenal cells through the Ca^{++} signaling pathway without involvement of the protein kinase A or protein kinase C pathways, highlighting the complexity of the postreceptor mechanisms that regulate adrenal steroidogenesis.[61]

Adrenal fascicular and reticular cells also express angiotensin receptors and A-II up-regulates ACTH receptor mRNA expression in these cells. A-II enhances basal and ACTH responsive steroid hormone synthesis in human adrenal fasciculata-reticularis cells *in vitro*, but under normal physiological conditions ACTH is the major tropic regulator of steroidogenesis in these cells *in vivo*.[62]

Paracrine regulation

Adrenal steroid production is subject to local modulation, similar to ovarian steroidogenesis (Fig. 7.3B).[5] The adrenal medulla influences steroid secretion by the cortex through the release of catecholamines[55,63] and regulatory peptides such as pituitary adenylate cyclase activating peptide (PACAP).[64] The action of epinephrine is mediated via G-protein coupled β-adrenergic receptors located on steroidogenic cells throughout the adrenal cortex, leading to cAMP mediated increases in the formation of P450scc, P450C17, P450C21 and P45011β mRNAs.[6,65] PACAP appears selectively to stimulate aldosterone rather than cortisol production through the PACAP stimulated production of catecholamines by medullary chromaffin cells that are scattered in cortical tissue, especially in the zona glomerulosa. Reciprocal cortical control of medullary catecholamine production is also thought to occur, mediated by nervous transmission and/or glucocorticoids secreted by the cortex.[63]

Adrenal sympathetic innervation profoundly influences steroidogenesis.[65] The zona glomerulosa and subcapsular regions are innervated by axons containing neuropeptides (e.g. neuropeptide-Y and AVP) and catecholamines that acutely influence steroid synthesis. Cortical and medullary cells are also closely interwoven with chromaffin cells containing catecholamines and diverse regulatory peptides capable of modulating steroidogenesis.[66]

AVP receptors are present on human fasciculata and glomerulosa cells, and AVP containing cells are present in both cortex and medulla. Direct stimulation of cortisol secretion by AVP in normal human adrenocortical tissue occurs through activation of V1 receptors. AVP has been shown to be equipotent with AG-II in stimulating aldosterone secretion, phosphoinositide turnover and Ca^{++} mobilization in glomerulosa cell-enriched cultures. AVP and AG-II also stimulate cortisol secretion and inositol phosphate formation in fasciculata cells. Thus AVP is likely to be a potent paracrine modulator of adrenal steroid secretion in man.[67]

A two cell mechanism of aldosterone synthesis has been suggested to operate in the adrenal, analogous to the cellular control of estrogen synthesis in the ovary (Fig. 7.3B).[68] Since 11β-OHase activity is confined to the inner cortical zones, whereas aldosterone synthase is expressed exclusively in glomerulosa cells, 18-hydroxycorticosterone synthesized in the inner zonal cells is presumed to serve as the substrate for aldosterone synthesis in the glomerulosa.[68]

AG-II is also a potential paracrine modulator of steroidogenesis, since adrenal tissue contains a complete renin-angiotensin system and locally produced AG-II has been demonstrated.[69] An intra-adrenal kallikrein-kinin system has been documented, with evidence for the role of bradykinin in the acute regulation of adrenal steroid secretion.[70] These and many other substances implicated in the paracrine regulation of adrenal steroidogenesis — including IGFs,[5,71] heparin-binding growth factors,[72] interleukins,[73] endothelins,[74] TGF-βs,[75] TNF-α,[76] etc. — also serve analogous functions in the ovarian paracrine system.

Dynamics

Adrenal steroids are secreted in episodic bursts reflecting the pattern of ACTH secretion by the pituitary gland, which is in turn influenced by diurnal rhythm, stress and glucocorticoid feedback through the hypothalamo-adrenal-pituitary axis.[55]

Diurnal rhythm

Episodic ACTH pulses increase in amplitude during sleep to a maximum around the time of waking and then decline throughout the day to minimum during the evening, giving rise to the characteristic diurnal rhythm in plasma cortisol concentrations. Androgen production by ACTH-responsive adrenal cells follows a similar pattern, with peak concentrations in blood at around 08.00 h.[77]

Stress

Stress activates the adrenal-pituitary axis through central pathways that stimulate hypothalamic secretion of CRH, AVP and other neuropeptides that stimulate pulsatile ACTH secretion.[78] Hypophyseal factors come more into play in acute stress. The extent to which CRH and/or AVP initiate ACTH release appears to depend on the type of stress inflicted. AVP is implicated as the main mediator of the stress response to strenuous exercise, electroconvulsive therapy, alcohol and infection, whereas both AVP and CRH are implicated in other situations (e.g. myocardial infarction). Because of the many stress situations in which ACTH pulses in peripheral blood coincide with AVP but not CRH, it has been suggested that AVP provides the signal for ACTH release to the pituitary, while CRH sets the gain.

Feedback regulation

Glucocorticoids act on the hypothalamus to inhibit CRH secretion and on the pituitary to inhibit CRH stimulated ACTH release. Thus, patients with adrenal insufficiency (e.g. Addison's disease) have chronically elevated plasma ACTH levels, whereas in those with adrenal excess (e.g. Cushing's syndrome) or in receipt of glucocorticoid therapy, ACTH is suppressed. Acute falls in cortisol elicit increases in ACTH release without corresponding changes in peripheral blood CRH or AVP levels, indicating that cortisol feedback operates acutely at the pituitary level.[55,78]

STEROID ACTION AND METABOLISM

Steroid hormones circulate in plasma bound to proteins (sex hormone binding globulin, corticosteroid binding globulin, albumin, etc.) that regulate the proportion of total hormone available for action and/or metabolism at target sites in the periphery. The classic model of steroid action entails delivery to cells containing specific receptors that influence transcriptional events in the nucleus, as discussed in chapters 11 and 12. Action via this mode depends both on the amount of hormone secreted and the extent to which a particular steroid is metabolized to more or less active forms within target cells and elsewhere in the periphery. This chapter concludes with a brief survey of the contribution of peripheral metabolism to ovarian and adrenal steroid endocrinology.

Progesterone

Progesterone secreted by the corpus luteum acts classically via nuclear progesterone receptors in endometrial cells to promote the morphological and secretory changes necessary for pregnancy. Most progesterone in extrahepatic sites is degraded to 5α-reduced progesterone metabolites that bind only weakly to the progesterone receptor.[79] The endometrium contains steroid metabolizing enzymes capable of inactivating progesterone, including 20-hydroxylase, 5α-reductase and 5β-reductase. Progesterone itself stimulates 17βHSD activity in the uterus, and may thereby influence estrogen action on the uterus (see below).[80] About one tenth of secreted progesterone occurs in urine as pregnanediol glucuronide, formed by glucoronidation in the liver. Assay of urinary pregnanediol provides a simple and effective means of detecting ovulation.[81]

Pregnenolone, progesterone and their reduced or sulfated metabolites have also been termed 'neurosteroids' because they are synthesized by glial cells within the central nervous system where they may modulate neurotransmission.[82] Progesterone is also synthesized by Schwann cells in the peripheral nervous system, where it promotes myelin formation during nerve regeneration.[83]

Androgens

Androgens in women are essential intermediates in the synthesis of estrogen. The major circulating C_{19} steroids in women are DHA sulfate, DHA and androstenedione, of which >90%, ~50% and ~50%, respectively, are of adrenal origin. An additional 30% of DHA comes from peripheral metabolism of DHAS. DHA is not itself an androgen but it can be metabolized to androstenedione and testosterone and thence to estrogens in peripheral tissues expressing 3βHSD, 17βHSD and aromatase. During pregnancy DHA sulfate produced by the fetal adrenal is the principal precursor of placental estrogen production.[15,55] In the human liver and adrenal, there is a single hydroxysteroid sulfotransferase that catalyzes the transformation of DHA to DHAS, the most abundant circulating steroid in humans. This enzyme also catalyzes the sulfation of a series of other 3β-hydroxysteroids, as well as cholesterol.[84]

3βHSD catalyzes the transformation of Δ^5-3β-hydroxysteroids into corresponding Δ^4-3-oxo-steroids, which is an obligate step in the biosynthesis of ovarian and adrenal steroids (see above). The dehydrogenization and isomerization reactions are catalyzed by a single polypeptide chain. Two human 3β-HSD genes have been characterized to date. The type I 3βHSD gene is predominantly expressed in placenta and peripheral tissues, while type II is the form that is mainly expressed in the adrenals and ovaries.[85]

During the follicular phase of the menstrual cycle, about two thirds of testosterone comes from peripheral metabolism of androstenedione by 17βHSD. 17βHSD is an enzyme family that catalyzes the interconversion of 17β-hydroxy and ketone groups of C_{18} and C_{19} steroids and thus plays a role in the activation/inactivation of androgens as well as estrogens (see below) in the periphery.[16] To date, five types of 17βHSD have been identified that catalyze the same reaction with variable substrate specificity. In intact cells, types II, IV and V preferentially catalyze the oxidative reaction, whereas types I and III preferentially catalyze the reductive reactions.[86]

Testosterone and androstenedione are further subject to 5α-reduction at peripheral sites, notably in skin where locally produced 5α-DHT mediates the stimulatory action of testosterone on hair growth via interaction with AR in the pilosebaceous units.[87] Hypersecretion of androgens by the adrenals and ovaries and increased peripheral 5α-reduction of testosterone — individually or collectively — are causes of hirsutism in women, frequently in association with PCOS.[88,89]

Δ^4-3-oxo steroids other than androgens are also substrates for 5α-reductases, including progesterone (see above) and corticosteroids. However, whereas androgenic potency is enhanced by 5α-reduction, in these cases hormonal potency is generally diminished.[90]

Testosterone and androstendione of adrenal and ovarian origin are also substrates for estrogen formation in peripheral tissues expressing P450arom. In premenopausal women, the highest levels of aromatase activity are normally found in the preovulatory follicle and, during pregnancy, the placenta. However, aromatase is also expressed at low levels in peripheral adipose tissues, muscle, bone, brain and skin.[15,17,53] Low circulating levels of estrogen persist after the menopause through the peripheral aromatization of adrenal androstenedione.

Formation of androgenic conjugates, glucuronides and sulfates, occurs mainly in the liver, with the exception of DHAS which arises largely from adrenal steroidogenesis (see above). Androstanediol glucuronide, androsterone glucuronide and androsterone sulfate circulate in concentrations several orders of magnitude higher than the active androgens testosterone and 5α-DHT. Thus measurement of urinary conjugated androgens can provide clinical marker of peripheral 5α-reductase activity in hyperandrogenic women.[91]

Estrogens

The major form of 17βHSD expressed in the ovary (also in placenta, brain and breast) is the type I, which has a preference for C_{18} substrates and preferentially catalyzes 17β-reduction. Thus estradiol is the major secreted ovarian estrogen even though androstenedione is the major ovarian androgen available for aromatization.[16]

Secreted estradiol has direct effects on target cells containing estrogen receptors in the reproductive tract, breast, skin, brain, bone and elsewhere. Formation and degradation of estrogens also occurs in target tissues through the concerted actions of aromatase (see above), sulfatase, sulfotransferase and 17βHSD.

Levels of estrone, estradiol and their sulfates in breast cancer tissues are many times higher than those found in blood. Sulfatase and 17βHSD activities in such tumors may generate locally active estrogen levels through the hydrolysis and reduction of circulating estrone sulfate, possibly contributing to the development of certain types of estrogen responsive cancer in postmenopausal women.[92,93]

Catecholestrogen formation also occurs to a limited extent within the ovaries[94] and estrogen target tissues such as breast and brain.[95] Catecholestrogens can inhibit the inactivation of catecholamines by catechol-*O*-methyl-transferase, and 2-hydroxylation is thought to provide a direct link between estrogens and catecholaminergic function in the central nervous system. However, the extent to which catecholestrogens are involved in estrogen action at other sites is controversial.

Estradiol is reversibly oxidized to estrone (17βHSD) followed by hydroxylation at C2, to produce 2-hydroxyestrogens (catecholestrogens), or at C16α, to produce 16α-hydroxyestrone. 16α-hydroxyestrone is reduced to estriol by 17βHSD.[96] Glucuronidation and sulfation of estrogen metabolites occurs mainly in liver, and estrone sulfate is quantitatively the major circulating estrogen in both pre- and postmenopausal women.[97] Measurements of urinary estrone-3-sulfate levels in conjunction with urinary pregnanediol-3-glucuronide (see above) afford a simple and convenient method for tracking follicular development and luteal function during the menstrual cycle.[83]

Corticosteroids

Peripheral oxidation/reduction of the oxygen function at C11 profoundly affects adrenal steroid physiology. Although mineralocorticoid and glucocorticoid receptors bind cortisol with similar affinities, the approximately 100-fold higher level of cortisol relative to aldosterone that circulates in blood does not cause aldosterone-like effects (i.e. hypertension). This is mainly due to the action of 11βHSD in aldosterone-selective tissues such as the kidney, which protects the mineralocorticoid receptor from 'seeing' cortisol by converting it to inactive cortisone.[98] Congenital absence of 11βHSD or its inhibition by liquorice permits cortisol access to the receptor and acts as a corticosteroid, causing hypertension.[99] The presence of 11βHSD in the same cells that express the mineralocorticoid receptor may constitute an autocrine mechanism for protecting aldosterone-responsive cells against hyperstimulation by cortisol.[100]

The type 2 11βHSD isoform that is expressed in kidney and other mineralocorticoid target tissues such as salivary gland and rectal colon is also expressed in placenta, where it may protect the developing fetus against cortisol excess or may play a role in the ontogeny of fetal adrenal steroidogenesis. A second (type 1) 11βHSD is expressed predominantly in adult glucocorticoid target tissues, including brain, pituitary, gonads, liver and lung. *In vitro*, type 1 11βHSD has a higher affinity for cortisone than cortisol, suggesting that its role *in vivo* is reductive, generating cortisol from cortisone. The two 11βHSD isoforms are encoded by separate genes and are members of the short chain alcohol deydrogenase superfamily, although they share little (<15%) homology with each other.[101] Ovarian 11βHSDs may serve physiological functions through locally modulating the effects of glucocorticoids[102,103] or alternative steroidal substrates[104] on steroidogenesis and gametogenesis.

Hepatic inactivation of corticosteroids mainly involves reduction of the Δ^4 double bond and the 3-ketone group, followed by conjugation (mainly glucuronidation) primarily at the 3α position. Tetrahydrocortisol, tetrahydrocortisone and their corresponding C20-reduced metabolites (cortols and cortolones) account for approximately 80% of the cortisol metabolites found in urine. Tetrahydroaldosterone glucuronidated at the 3-oxo position is the major urinary metabolite of aldosterone.[55]

Conclusion

This chapter has only surveyed the bare essentials of steroid hormone synthesis and secretion by the ovaries and adrenals. It has necessarily ignored testicular steroid synthesis. Steroids also have wide ranging roles beyond their classic reproductive functions. They influence the cardiovascular, nervous, skeletal and immune systems and also have roles in cancer and the cell cycle. A challenge to scientists and clinicians is to further unravel the molecular basis of steroid synthesis and action, in order to develop improved therapeutic strategies based on these ubiquitous bioregulatory substances.

REFERENCES

1. Ryan KJ 1972 Steroid hormones and prostaglandins. In: Ryan KJ, Benirschke K (eds) Principles and management of human reproduction. WB Saunders, Philadelphia, pp 4–27
2. Strauss JF III, Miller WL 1991 Molecular basis of ovarian steroid synthesis. In: Hillier SG (ed) Ovarian endocrinology. Blackwell Scientific Publications, Oxford, pp 25–72
3. Strauss JF III, Ohba T, Holt JA, Sugawara T 1995 Metabolic diseases reveal important loci for control of intracellular cholesterol movement in steroidogenesis. In: Fujimoto S, Hsueh AJW, Strauss JF III, Tanaka T (eds) New achievements in ovarian research. Frontiers in Endocrinology 13: 261–266
4. Servetnick DA, Brasaemle DL, Gruia Gray J, Kimmel AR, Wolff J, Londos C 1995 Perilipins are associated with cholesteryl ester droplets in steroidogenic adrenal cortical and Leydig cells. Journal of Biological Chemistry 270: 16970–16973
5. Miller WL 1988 Molecular biology of steroid hormone synthesis. Endocrinology Reviews 9: 295–318
6. Omura T, Morohashi K 1995 Gene regulation of steroidogenesis. Journal of Steroid Biochemistry and Molecular Biology 53: 19–25
7. Hall PF 1995 The roles of microfilaments and intermediate filaments in the regulation of steroid synthesis. Journal of Steroid Biochemistry and Molecular Biology 55: 601–605
8. King SR, Ronen-Fuhrmann T, Timberg R, Clark BJ, Orly J, Stocco DM 1995 Steroid production after in vitro transcription, translation, and mitochondrial processing of protein products of complementary deoxyribonucleic acid for steroidogenic acute regulatory protein. Endocrinology 136: 5165–5176
9. Sugawara T, Lin D, Holt JA, Martin KO, Javitt NB, Miller WL, Strauss JF III 1995 Structure of the human steroidogenic acute regulatory protein (StAR) gene: StAR stimulates mitochondrial cholesterol 27-hydroxylase activity. Biochemistry 34: 12506–12512
10. Lin D, Sugawara T, Strauss JF III, Clark BJ, Stocco DM, Saenger P, Rogol A, Miller WL 1995 Role of steroidogenic acute regulatory protein in adrenal and gonadal steroidogenesis. Science 267: 1828–1831
11. Thomson I, Fraser R, Kenyon CJ 1995 Regulation of adrenocortical steroidogenesis by benzodiazepines. Journal of Steroid Biochemistry and Molecular Biology 53: 75–80
12. Ogishima T, Suzuki H, Hata J-I, Mitani F, Ishimura Y 1992 Zone-specific expression of aldosterone synthase cytochrome P-450 and cytochrome P-45011β in rat adrenal cortex: histochemical basis for functional zonation. Endocrinology 130: 2971–2977
13. Yanase T 1995 17α-hydroxylase/17,20-lyase defects. Journal of Steroid Biochemistry and Molecular Biology 53: 153–157
14. Richards JS 1994 Hormonal control of gene expression in the ovary. Endocrinology Reviews 15: 725–751
15. Parker CR Jr 1993 Control of adrenal androgen production in normal development and aging. Seminars in Reproductive Endocrinology 11: 313–317
16. Andersson S, Geissler WM, Parel S, Wu L 1995 The molecular biology of androgenic 17β-hydroxysteroid dehydrogenases. Journal of Steroid Biochemistry and Molecular Biology 53: 37–40
17. Simpson ER, Mahendroo MS, Means GD, Kilgore MW, Hinshelwood MM, Graham-Lorence S, Amarneh B, Ito Y, Fisher CR, Michael MD, Mendelson CR, Bulun SE 1994 Aromatase cytochrome P450, the enzyme responsible for estrogen biosynthesis. Endocrinology Reviews 15: 342–355
18. Korzekawa KR, Trager WF, Mancewicz J, Osawa Y 1993 Studies on the mechanism of aromatase and other cytochrome P450 mediated deformylation reactions. Journal of Steroid Biochemistry and Molecular Biology 44: 375–387
19. Magoffin DA, Erickson GF 1994 Control systems of theca-interstitial cells. In: Findlay J (ed) Molecular biology of the female reproductive system. Academic Press, London, pp 39–65
20. Hillier SG 1994 Hormonal control of folliculogenesis and luteinization. In: Findlay J (ed) Molecular biology of the female reproductive system. Academic Press, London, pp 1–37
21. Hsueh AJW, Billig H, Tsafriri A 1994 Ovarian follicular atresia: a hormonally controlled apoptotic process. Endocrinology Reviews 15: 707–724
22. Yong E, Baird DT, Hillier SG 1992 Mediation of gonadotrophin-stimulated growth and differentiation of human granulosa cells by adenosine 3′,5′-monophosphate: one molecule, two messages. Clinical Endocrinology 37: 51–58
23. Yong EL, Hillier SG, Turner M, Baird DT, Ng SC, Bongso A, Ratnam SS 1994 Differential regulation of cholesterol side-chain cleavage (P450scc) and aromatase (P450arom) enzyme mRNA expression by gonadotrophins and cyclic AMP in human granulosa cells. Journal of Molecular Endocrinology 12: 239–249
24. Clemens JW, Lala DS, Parker KL, Richards JS 1994 Steroidogenic factor-1 binding and transcriptional activity of the cholesterol side-chain cleavage promoter in rat granulosa cells. Endocrinology 134: 1499–1508

25. Morohashi K, Hatano O, Nomura M et al 1995 Function and distribution of a steroidogenic cell-specific transcription factor, Ad4BP. Journal of Steroid Biochemistry and Molecular Biology 53: 81–88
26. Tsafriri A, Dekel N 1994 Molecular mechanisms in ovulation. In: Findlay JK (ed) Molecular biology of the female reproductive system. Academic Press, London, pp 207–258
27. Morris JK, Richards JS 1995 Luteinizing hormone induces prostaglandin endoperoxide synthase-2 and luteinization in vitro by A-kinase and C-kinase pathways. Endocrinology 136: 1549–1558
28. Adashi EY, Kokia E, Hurwitz A 1994 Potential relevance of cytokines to ovarian physiology. In: Findlay JK (ed) Molecular biology of the female reproductive system. Academic Press, London, pp 83–99
29. Dissen GA, Hirschfield AN, Malamed S, Ojeda SR 1995 Expression of neurotrophins and their receptors in the mammalian ovary is developmentally regulated: changes at the time of folliculogenesis. Endocrinology 136: 4681–4692
30. Carmeliet P, Schoonjans L, Kieckens L, Ream B, Degen J, Bronson R, De Vos R, van den Oord JJ, Collen D, Mulligan RC 1994 Physiological consequence of loss of plasminogen activator gene function in mice. Nature 368: 419–425
31. Smith GW, McGrone S, Petersen SL, Smith MF 1995 Expression of messenger ribonucleic acid encoding tissue inhibitor of metalloproteinase-2 within ovine follicles and corpora lutea. Endocrinology 136: 570–576
32. Park-Sarge O-K, Mayo KE 1994 Molecular biology of endocrine receptors in the ovary. In: Findlay JK (ed) Molecular biology of the female reproductive system. Academic Press, London, pp 153–205
33. Natraj U, Richards JS 1993 Hormonal regulation, localization and functional activity of the progesterone receptor in granulosa cells of rat preovulatory follicles. Endocrinology 133: 761–769
34. Fisch B, Margara RA, Wintston RM, Hillier SG 1989 Cellular basis of luteal steroidogenesis in the human ovary. Journal of Endocrinology 122: 303–311
35. Bassett SG, Little-Ihrig LL, Mason JI, Zeleznik AJ 1991 Expression of messenger ribonucleic acids that encode for 3β-hydroxysteroid dehydrogenase and cholesterol side-chain cleavage enzymes throughout the luteal phase of the macaque menstrual cycle. Journal of Clinical Endocrinology and Metabolism 72: 362–366
36. Ravindranath N, Little-Ihrig L, Benyo DF, Zeleznik AJ 1992 Role of luteinizing hormone in the expression of cholesterol side-chain cleavage cytochrome P450 and 3β-hydroxysteroid dehydrogenase, Δ^{5-4} isomerase messenger ribonucleic acids in the primate corpus luteum. Endocrinology 131: 2065–2070
37. Adashi E, Resnick CE, Hurwitz A, Ricciarelli E, Hernandez ER, Roberts CT, Leroith D, Rosenfeld R 1991 Insulin-like growth factors: the ovarian connection. Human Reproduction 6: 1213–1219
38. Hernandez ER, Hurwitz A, Vera A, Pellicer A, Adashi E, LeRoith D, Roberts CTJr 1992 Expression of the genes encoding the insulin-like growth factors and their receptors in the human ovary. Journal of Clinical Endocrinology and Metabolism 74: 419–425
39. Erickson GF, Nakatani A, Liu XJ, Shimasaki S, Ling N 1994 Role of insulin-like growth factors (IGF) and IGF binding proteins in folliculogenesis. In: Findlay JK (ed) Molecular biology of the female reproductive system. Academic Press, London, pp 101–151
40. Dorrington J, Chuma AV and Bendell JJ 1988 Transforming growth factor-β and follicle stimulating hormone promote rat granulosa cell proliferation. Endocrinology 123: 353–359
41. Matzuk MM 1995 Functional analysis of mammalian members of the transforming growth factor-β superfamily. Trends in Endocrinology and Metabolism 6: 120–127
42. Li Ronghao, Phillips DM, Mather JP 1995 Activin promotes ovarian follicle development in vitro. Endocrinology 136: 849–856
43. Miró F, Hillier SG 1996 Modulation of granulosa cell deoxyribonucleic acid synthesis and differentiation by activin. Endocrinology 137: 464–468
44. Incerti B, Dong J, Borsani G, Matzuk MM 1994 Structure of the mouse growth/differentiation factor-9 gene. Biochemical Biophysics Acta [Molecular Cell Research] 1222: 125–128
45. Hillier SG 1987 Intrafollicular paracrine function of ovarian androgen. Journal of Steroid Biochemistry 27: 351–357
46. Fitzpatrick SL, Richards JS 1991 Regulation of cytochrome P450 aromatase messenger ribonucleic acid and activity by steroids and gonadotropins in rat granulosa cells. Endocrinology 129: 1452–1462
47. Tetsuka M, Whitelaw PF, Bremner WJ, Millar MR, Smyth CD, Hillier SG 1955 Developmental regulation of androgen receptor in rat ovary. Journal of Endocrinology 145: 535–543
48. Armstrong DT, Goff AK, Dorrington JH 1979 In: Midgley AR, Sadler WA (eds) Ovarian follicular development and function. Raven Press, New York, pp 169–182
49. Hillier SG, Whitelaw PF, Smyth CD 1994 Follicular oestrogen synthesis: the 'two-cell, two-gonadotrophin' model revisited. Molecular and Cellular Endocrinology 100: 51–54
50. Smyth CD, Miró F, Whitelaw PF, Howles CM, Hillier SG 1993 Ovarian thecal/interstitial androgen synthesis is enhanced by a follicle stimulating hormone-stimulated mechanism. Endocrinology 133: 1532–1538
51. Nahum R, Thong KJ, Hillier SG 1995 Metabolic regulation of androgen production by human thecal cells. Human Reproduction 10: 75–81
52. Baird DT 1977 Synthesis and secretion of steroid hormones by the ovary *in vivo*. In: Zuckerman S, Weir BJ (eds) The ovary, vol III, 2nd edn. Academic Press, London, pp 305–307
53. Ross GT 1985 Disorders of the ovary and female reproductive tract. In: Wilson JD, Foster DW (eds) Williams textbook of endocrinology, 7th edn. WB Saunders, London, pp 206–257
54. Dowsett M, Cantwell B, Anshumala L, Jeffcoate SL, Harris A 1988 Suppression of postmenopausal ovarian steroidogenesis with the luteinizing hormone-releasing hormone agonist Gosrelin. Journal of Clinical Endocrinology and Metabolism 66: 672–677

55. Orth DN, Kovacs WJ, DeBold CR 1990 In: Wilson JD, Foster DW (eds) Williams textbook of endocrinology, 8th edn. WB Saunders, London, pp 489–619
56. Hartigan JA, Green EG, Mortensen RM, Menachery A, Williams GH, Orme-Johnson NR 1995 Comparison of protein phosphorylation patterns produced in adrenal cells by activation of cAMP-dependent protein kinase and Ca-dependent protein kinase. Journal of Steroid Biochemistry and Molecular Biology 53: 95–101
57. Rainey WE, Bird IM, Mason JI 1994 The NCI-H295 cell line: a pluripotent model for human adrenocortical studies. Molecular and Cellular Endocrinology 100: 45–50
58. Orth DN 1992 Corticotropin-releasing hormone in humans. Endocrinology Reviews 13: 164–191
59. Vamvakopoulos NC, Chrousos GP 1994 Hormonal regulation of human corticotropin-releasing hormone gene expression: implications for the stress response and immune inflammatory reaction. Endocrinology Reviews 15: 409–420
60. Mountjoy KG, Robbins LS, Mortrud MT, Cone RD 1992 The cloning of a family of genes that encode the melanocortin receptors. Science 257: 1248–1251
61. Bird IM, Mathis JM, Mason JI, Rainey WE 1995 Ca^{2+} regulated expression of steroid hydroxylases in H295R human adrenocortical cells. Endocrinology 136: 5677–5684
62. Lebrethon MC, Jaillard C, Defayes G, Begeot M, Saez JM 1994 Human cultured adrenal fasciculata-reticularis cells are targets for angiotensin II: effects on cytochrome P450 cholesterol side-chain cleavage, cytochrome P450 17α-hydroxylase, and 3β-hydroxysteroid dehydrogenase messenger ribonucleic acid and proteins and on steroidogenic responsiveness to corticotropin and angiotensin II. Journal of Clinical Endocrinology and Metabolism 78: 1212–1219
63. Einer-Jensen N, Carter AM 1994 Local transfer of hormones between blood vessels within the adrenal gland may explain the functional interaction between the adrenal cortex and medulla. Medical Hypotheses 44: 471–474
64. Neri G, Andreis PG, Prayer-Galetti T, Rossi GP, Malendowicz LK, Nussdorfer GG 1996 Pituitary adenylate cyclase activating peptide enhances aldosterone secretion of human adrenal gland: evidence for an indirect mechanism, probably involving the local release of catecholamines. Journal of Clinical Endocrinology and Metabolism 81: 169–173
65. Ehrhart-Bornstein M, Bornstein SR, Gonzalez-Hernandez J, Holst JJ, Waterman MR, Scherbaum WA 1995 Sympathoadrenal regulation of adrenocortical steroidogenesis. Endocrinological Research 21: 13–24
66. Wolfensberger M, Forssmann WG, Reinecke M 1995 Localization and coexistence of atrial natriuretic peptide (ANP) and neuropeptide Y (NPY) in vertebrate adrenal chromaffin cells immunoreactive to TH, DBH and PNMT. Cell and Tissue Research 280: 267–276
67. Guillon G, Trueba M, Joubert D, Grazzini E, Chouinard L, Cote M, Payet MD, Manzoni O, Barberis C, Robert M, Gallo-Payet N 1995 Vasopressin stimulates steroid secretion in human adrenal glands: comparison with angiotensin II effect. Endocrinology 136: 1285–1295
68. Vinson GP, Teja R, Ho MM, Puddefoot JR 1995 A two cell type theory for aldosterone biosynthesis: the roles of 11β-hydroxylase and aldosterone synthase, and a high capacity tightly binding steroid carrier for 18-hydroxydeoxycorticosterone in rat adrenals. Journal of Endocrinology 144: 359–368
69. Ganong WF 1994 Origin of the angiotensin II secreted by cells. Proceedings of the Society of Experimental Biology and Medicine 205: 213–219
70. Malendowicz LK, Macchi C, Nussdorfer GG, Markowska A 1995 Investigations on the possible involvement of bradykinin in the acute regulation of the secretion from rat adrenal cortex. Biomedical Research 16: 433–437
71. Han VKM 1996 The ontogeny of growth hormone, insulin-like growth factors and sex steroids: molecular aspects. Hormone Research 45: 61–66
72. Ho MM, Vinson GP 1995 Endocrine control of the distribution of basic fibroblast growth factor, insulin-like growth factor I and transforming growth factor β1 mRNAs in adult rat adrenals using nonradioactive in situ hybridization. Journal of Endocrinology 144: 379–387
73. Gonzalez-Hernandez JA, Bornstein SR, Ehrhart-Bornstein M et al 1995 IL-1 is expressed in human adrenal gland in vivo. Possible role in a local immune-adrenal axis. Clinical and Experimental Immunology 99: 137–141
74. Rossi G, Belloni AS, Albertin G et al 1995 Endothelin-1 and its receptors A and B in human aldosterone-producing adenomas. Hypertension 25: 842–847
75. Naaman-Reperant E, Hales DB, Durand P 1996 Effect of transforming growth factor β-1 on the cholesterol sidechain cleavage system in the adrenal gland of sheep fetuses and newborns. Endocrinology 137: 886–892
76. Gonzalez-Hernandez JA, Ehrhart-Bornstein M, SpathSchwalbe E, Scherbaum WA, Bornstein SR 1996 Human adrenal cells express tumor necrosis factor-α messenger ribonucleic acid: evidence for paracrine control of adrenal function. Journal of Clinical Endocrinology and Metabolism 81: 807–813
77. Lachelin GCL, Barnett M, Hooper BR et al 1979 Adrenal function in normal women and women with the polycystic ovarian syndrome. Journal of Clinical Endocrinology and Metabolism 49: 892–898
78. Donald RA 1996 Regulation of ACTH secretion in man and other domestic animals. Journal of Endocrinology 148 (Suppl): S3
79. MacDonald PC, Dombroski RA, Casey ML 1991 Recurrent secretion of progesterone in large amounts: an endocrine/metabolic disorder unique to young women. Endocrinology Reviews 12: 372–401
80. Gurpide E 1991 Local metabolic regulation of endometrial responses to hormones and drugs. In: Hochberg RB, Naftolin F (eds) The new biology of steroid hormones. Raven Press, New York, pp 89–100
81. Robel P, Young J, Corpéchot C et al 1995 Biosynthesis and assay of neurosteroids in rats and mice: functional correlates. Journal of Steroid Biochemistry and Molecular Biology 53: 355–360
82. Koenig HL, Schumacher M, Ferzaz B et al 1995 Progesterone synthesis and myelin formation by Schwann cells. Science 268: 1500–1503

83. Collins WP 1983 Biochemical approaches to ovulation prediction and detection and the location of the fertile period in women. In: Jeffcoate SL (ed) Ovulation: methods for its prediction and detection. John Wiley, Chichester, pp 49–66
84. Durocher F, Morissette J, Dufort I, Simard J, Luu-The V 1995 Genetic linkage mapping of the dehydroepiandrosterone sulfotransferase (STD) gene on the chromosome 19q13.3 region. Genomics 29: 781–783
85. Mason JI 1993 3β-hydroxysteroid dehydrogenase and its regulation. In: Mornex R, Jaffiol C, Leclere J (eds) Progress in endocrinology (Proceedings of the Ninth International Congress of Endocrinology). Parthenon, Carnforth, Lancs, pp 509–513
86. Zhang Y, Dufort I, Soucy P, Labrie F, Luu-The V 1995 Cloning and expression of human type V 17β-hydroxysteroid dehydrogenase. Program and abstracts, 77th Annual Meeting of the Endocrine Society. Endocrine Society Press, Bethesda, Md, Abstract P3–614
87. Wilson JD, Russell DW 1994 Steroid 5α-reductase: two genes/two enzymes. Annual Reviews of Biochemistry 36: 25–61
88. Steingold K, De Ziegler D, Cedars M et al 1987 Clinical and hormonal effects of chronic gonadotropin-releasing hormone agonist treatment in polycystic ovarian disease. Journal of Clinical Endocrinology and Metabolism 65: 773–778
89. Azziz R 1993 Adrenocortical dysfunction in androgen excess. Seminars in Reproductive Endocrinology 11: 353–358
90. Milewich L, Mendonca BB, Arnhold I et al 1995 Women with steroid 5α-reductase 2 deficiency have normal concentrations of plasma 5α-dihydroprogesterone during the luteal phase. Journal of Clinical Endocrinology and Metabolism 80: 3136–3139
91. Rittmaster RS 1994 Androgen conjugates as a measure of hyperandrogenism. Seminars in Reproductive Endocrinology 12: 45–50
92. Pasqualini JR, Chetrite G, Nguyen B-L et al 1995 Estrone-sulfate sulfatase and 17β-hydroxysteroid dehydrogenase activities: a hypothesis for their role in the evolution of human breast cancer from hormone dependence to hormone independence. Journal of Steroid Biochemistry and Molecular Biology 53: 407–412
93. Reed MJ, Purohit A, Duncan LJ et al 1995 The role of cytokines and sulphatase inhibitors in regulating oestrogen synthesis in breast tumours. Journal of Steroid Biochemistry and Molecular Biology 53: 413–420
94. Dehennin L, Blacker C, Reifsteck A, Scholler R 1984 Estrogen 2-,4-,6- or 16 hydroxylation by human follicles shown by gas chromatography-mass spectrometry associated with stable isotope dilution. Journal of Steroid Biochemistry 20: 465–471
95. Weisz J 1991 Metabolism of estrogens by target cells: diversification and amplification of hormone action and the catecholestrogen hypothesis. In: Hochberg RB, Naftolin F (eds) The new biology of steroid hormones. Raven Press, New York, pp 101–112
96. Lipsett MB 1986 Steroid hormones. In: Yen SCC, Jaffe RB (eds) Reproductive endocrinology, 2nd edn. WB Saunders, Philadelphia, pp 140–153
97. Loriaux DL, Ruder HJ, Lipsett MB 1971 The measurement of estrone sulfate in plasma. Steroids 18: 463–472
98. Funder JW 1995 Mineralocorticoid receptors and hypertension. Journal of Steroid Biochemistry and Molecular Biology 53: 53–56
99. White PC, Curnow KM, Pascoe L 1994 Disorders of steroid 11β-hydroxylase isozymes. Endocrinology Reviews 15: 421–438
100. Edwards CRW, Walker BR, Benediktsson R, Seckl JR 1993 Apparent mineralocorticoid excess syndromes. In: Mornex R, Jaffiol C, Leclere J (eds) Progress in endocrinology (Proceedings of the Ninth International Congress of Endocrinology). Parthenon, Carnforth, Lancs, pp 487–490
101. Stewart PM 1995 11β-hydroxysteroid dehydrogenase isoforms. Program and abstracts, 77th Annual Meeting of the Endocrine Society. Endocrine Society Press, Bethesda, Md, Abstract S23–3
102. Michael AE, Cooke BA 1994 A working hypothesis for the regulation of steroidogenesis and germ cell development in the gonads by glucocorticoids and 11β-hydroxysteroid dehydrogenase. Molecular and Cellular Endocrinology 100: 55–63
103. Tetsuka M, Thomas FJ, Thomas MJ, Anderson RA, Mason JI, Hillier SG 1997 Differential expression of messenger ribonucleic acids encoding 11β-hydroxysteroid dehydrogenase types 1 and 2 in human granulosa cells. Journal of Clinical Endocrinology and Metabolism 82: 2006–2009
104. Hillier SG 1994 Cortisol and oocyte quality. Clinical Endocrinology 40: 19–20

8. Metabolism of estrogens and progestogens

C. Longcope

Introduction

In this chapter I will address the transport and metabolism of natural and synthetic estrogens and progestogens. The estrogens include the natural estrogens estradiol, estrone, estrone sulfate, estriol, catechol estrogens and the synthetic ethinyl estradiol. The progestogens include the natural progesterone and the synthetics medroxyprogesterone acetate, norethindrone and norgestrel.

TRANSPORT OF ESTROGENS (Tables 8.1 & 8.2)

Natural estrogens

Estradiol, similar to many other 17-hydroxy steroids, circulates in the blood bound to sex hormone-binding globulin (SHBG), to albumin and unbound or free.[1] As shown in Table 8.1, there is more estradiol bound to albumin than to SHBG and only a small amount circulates as unbound.[1] Estrone and estriol are mainly bound to albumin or unbound. The catechol estrogen, 2-hydroxy estrone, is present in the blood in such small amounts[2] that its protein-binding would be unimportant. However, 2-methoxy-estradiol binds strongly to SHBG; whether this strong binding is of physiological importance is uncertain.[3] Estrone sulfate circulates bound only to albumin or unbound,[4] but its binding to albumin is an order of magnitude stronger than that of the other estrogens, and this stronger binding appears to have a major effect on its metabolism, as noted below.

Synthetic estrogens

While both ethinyl estradiol and its 3-methoxy derivative, mestranol, are 17β-hydroxy estrogens, they do not bind to SHBG but circulate unbound or bound to albumin.[5] Thus the addition of the 17α-ethinyl group appears to interfere with the binding of estradiol to SHBG. It is interesting that the addition of a 17α-ethinyl group to dihydrotestosterone does not interfere with its binding to SHBG.[6]

Table 8.1 Estrogen transport in the circulation: percentage of estrogen bound to sex hormone-binding globulin (SHBG), albumin or unbound.[1]

Estrogen	SHBG	Albumin	Free
Estradiol	37.3	60.8	1.8
Estrone	16.3	80.1	3.6
Estriol	1.1	90.7	8.1

Table 8.2 Relative binding affinities (RBA)[5] of estrogens to sex hormone-binding globulin.[1]

	RBA*
Estradiol	49
Ethinyl estradiol	8
Mestranol	<0.1
2-methoxyestradiol	200

*RBA relative to testosterone = 100

METABOLISM OF ESTROGENS

Natural estrogens

Metabolic clearance rates (MCR) (Table 8.2)

The metabolic clearance rate is defined as the volume of blood, or plasma, cleared of a substance in unit time.[7] It is a function of the extraction of the substance and the blood flow through tissues[7] and is, therefore, dependent in part on the protein-binding of the substance. In general, binding to SHBG appears to influence the MCR of a steroid more than the binding to albumin, with estrone sulfate as a major exception.

The MCR for estradiol is in the range of 1300 L/day for women, and is slightly greater than the estimated splanchnic plasma flow and reflects a degree of extrahepatic metabolism.[8,9] The splanchnic extraction, however, is only 64%[10] so that the binding of estradiol to SHBG does effect its metabolism. Although the liver is the organ responsible for most of the metabolism, adipose tissue and muscle[11] as well as other tissues contribute to the MCR.[7] Thus obese subjects, having a marked increase in the amount of adipose tissue, will have a much greater MCR for estradiol than normal weight subjects.[12,13] There appears to be little change in the MCR of estradiol through the menstrual cycle,[8] although there may be an increase in the periovulatory period.[14] There does appear to be a slight decline in the MCR with age, but not associated with the menopause.[15]

The MCRs of estrone and estriol are in the range of 2100–2200 L/day[8,16] and these MCRs are greater than that of estradiol and greater than estimated splanchnic plasma flow, reflecting their lack of binding to SHBG and also their extrahepatic metabolism. The MCRs of these estrogens are similar when measured in the follicular and luteal phases of the cycle, but the MCR of estrone may increase in the periovulatory phase.[14] The MCR for estrone is positively correlated with weight,[12,13] but the effect of obesity on the MCR of estriol has not been reported.

The MCR for 2-hydroxy estrone in women, 39 125 L/day[2,17,18] is greater than for any steroid studied and is far greater than splanchnic flow and cardiac output. This mean value is derived from data obtained by infusions of 2-hydroxy estrone and of ^{3}H-2-hydroxy estrone.[2,17] This indicates that there is extensive metabolism within the circulation and reflects the very active metabolism by red blood cells.[19] These cells contain the enzyme O-methyl catechol transferase that catalyzes the conversion of 2-hydroxy estrone to 2-methoxy estrone. It is because of the rapid metabolism of 2-hydroxy estrone to 2-methoxy estrone by this enzyme that the MCR for 2-hydroxy estrone is so great. Because of this high MCR it is doubtful whether circulating concentrations of 2-hydroxy estrone concentrations are measurable.[2] The MCR of 2-hydroxyestradiol is also high, 12 000–29 000 L/day[18] but the MCRs of 2-methoxy estrone and 2-methoxy estradiol are considerably less at 2 470 L/day[20] and 1 670 L/day[18] respectively.

The MCR of estrone sulfate is lower than that of other estrogens and is in the range of 150 L/day.[21,22] This low MCR is due in large part to the relatively strong binding and high capacity of albumin for estrone sulfate. It is also possible that the renal tubular reabsorption of steroid sulfates, in contradistinction to glucuronide conjugates, is great enough to influence the MCR of the sulfates.[23]

In hyperthyroidism the MCR of estradiol is decreased,[24,25] but that of estrone is unaltered.[26] In hypothyroidism, the MCR of estrone is decreased, but data for estradiol are not available.[27] When estradiol is given by mouth the MCR is increased to a mean value of 12 800 L/day.[28] This increase is due to the rapid splanchnic metabolism of the estradiol.

Conversion rates (Table 8.3)

As originally defined by Gurpide[29] the rho value $[\rho]^{prec,prod}_{BB}$ is the percent of a precursor entering the blood which re-enters the blood as product. The $[\rho]^{estradiol,estrone}_{BB}$ is 17% whereas the reverse $[\rho]^{estrone,estradiol}_{BB}$ is 4%.[7] Thus, the 17β-hydroxy steroid dehydrogenase activity favors the oxidative reaction. The conversion of both estrone and estradiol to estriol is very low, both $< 0.4\%$, as measured in blood.[16] The conversion of estrone to 2-hydroxy estrone is difficult to measure because of the very rapid metabolism of the product, leading to concentrations below the baseline of the method.[17]

Conjugation

Estrone and estradiol are rapidly converted to estrone sulfate and the concentration of the latter reflects this rapid and extensive conversion. The $[\rho]^{estrone,estrone\ sulfate}_{BB}$ is 40% and the $[\rho]^{estradiol,estrone\ sulfate}_{BB}$ is 42%. The back conversions or hydrolysis of estrone sulfate to estrone and estradiol are relatively small, 15% and 3% respectively.[21,22]

The conversions to the circulating glucuronides are not well studied and few data are available. However, glucuronidation of estrogens does occur but the

Table 8.3 Metabolic clearance rates (MCR) of estrogens.

Estrogen	MCR (L/day)	Reference
Estradiol	1350	55
Estrone	2210	55
Estriol	2100	16
2-hydroxy estrone	39 125	2,17,18
2-hydroxy estradiol	12 200	18
2-methoxy estrone	2470	20
Estrone sulfate	146	21, 22
Ethinyl estradiol	1070	30
Mestranol	1120	30

circulating levels of glucuronide conjugates appear to be low in comparison to the sulfates.

Synthetic estrogens

Metabolic clearance rates

The MCR of ethinyl estradiol is 1080 L/day and that of mestranol, 3-methoxy ethinyl estradiol is 1100 L/day.[30] Although neither of these estrogens is bound to SHBG, and their binding to albumin is weak, their MCRs are lower than other estrogens with similar binding properties. It should be noted that these studies were done administering the compounds intravenously. The MCRs would probably be considerably greater if measured after *per os* administration. The presence of the 17α-ethinyl group may interfere with the oxidation of the 17β-hydroxy to the 17-ketone.

Conversion rates

There is conversion of mestranol to ethinyl estradiol and the values for this conversion range from 23% as measured in plasma.[30,31] However, the conversion is close to 100% when measured using urinary metabolites of mestranol and ethinyl estradiol after the administration of [^{3}H]-mestranol *per os*.[31] Thus much of the conversion occurs in pools not in equilibrium with the blood pool. There does not appear to be any back conversion of ethinyl estradiol to mestranol.

Conjugation

Ethinyl estradiol can be sulfated and appear in the blood as ethinyl estradiol sulfate.[32] Thus, after the administration of ethinyl estradiol there is a rapid appearance of ethinyl estradiol sulfate in the circulation, and its concentration will eventually exceed that of ethinyl estradiol. Mestranol already is conjugated at the 3 position so must be hydrolyzed to ethinyl estradiol before any further conjugation can occur at the 3 position.

URINARY EXCRETION

Natural estrogens

Estradiol, estrone, estriol and the catechol estrogens all appear in the urine as a glucuronide or sulfate conjugate. The major conjugate in the urine is the glucuronide and much less will be as the sulfate,[28] the reverse of the pattern in the circulation. After the administration of either estradiol or estrone, 3-methoxy 2-hydroxy estrone glucuronide is the major urinary estrogen conjugate with lesser amounts of 2-hydroxy estrone glucuronide.[28] The 16α-hydroxy compounds are present, but in smaller amounts than the catecholamines and, again, primarily as the glucuronide conjugate. Estriol, estradiol and estrone glucuronide and sulfates are present, but at lower concentrations. There is little if any 17α-estradiol excreted by men or women.

Synthetic estrogens

After the administration of ethinyl estradiol there is slow excretion in the urine and only about 40% will appear in five days, mostly conjugated as a glucuronide, but there is some excretion as a sulfate while <2–6% appeared as unconjugated ethinyl estradiol.[33,34] There is metabolism to 2-hydroxy and 2-methoxy-17α-ethinyl estradiol and 2-hydroxy-17α-ethinyl estradiol-3-methyl ether.[33] There would appear to be little de-ethinylation to estradiol or estrone.[31] Up to 20% of administered ethinyl estradiol may be excreted in the feces.[34]

Mestranol is also excreted slowly, primarily as ethinyl estradiol glucuronide.[35] Since there is conversion of mestranol to ethinyl estradiol in the body, the same metabolites will be found in the urine after mestranol administration as after ethinyl estradiol.

TRANSPORT OF PROGESTOGENS

Progesterone

In the circulation progesterone is bound to cortisol binding globulin (CBG), to albumin and is also unbound or free.[1] Progesterone also binds to α1-acid glycoprotein (orosomucoid), but this binding does not appear to be of major import,[36] except possibly in pregnancy.[37] Because cortisol binds to CBG and is present at far higher concentrations than is progesterone, the binding of progesterone to CBG is also not of major import. Another protein, progesterone binding protein (PBP), is found in certain rodents, but does not occur in humans.[38]

Synthetic progestogens

The synthetic progestogens, derivatives of 19-nortestosterone, norgestrel and 17-acetoxy medroxyprogesterone, all circulate unbound or bound to albumin.[5] In addition there is a variable amount of binding to SHBG, but this binding is generally not of major import for any of the synthetic progestogens, except for levonorgestrel.[39]

METABOLISM OF PROGESTOGENS

Progesterone

Metabolic clearance rates (Table 8.4)

The MCR for progesterone ranges from 2100–2500 L/day depending, to some extent, on methodology[40,41] and indicates that the binding of progesterone to CBG does not influence its metabolism to any extent. As for other steroids, most of the clearance occurs in the liver[42] but other tissues, including the uterus, metabolize progesterone.[43,44] The MCR of progesterone does not vary through the menstrual cycle, and the mean value was reported as 2510 L/day.[41] This value was higher than that found in pregnancy (2020 L/day[45]) and in ovariectomized women (2170 L/day[40]). The decrease in pregnancy was attributed, in part, to decreased splanchnic clearance secondary to an increase in the CBG binding of progesterone.[45]

A metabolite of progesterone, 20α-hydroxy pregn-4-en-3-one was noted to have a MCR of 2260 L/day.[41]

Synthetic progestogens

Metabolic clearance rates

The MCR for norethynodrel was reported as 30 L/day after intravenous administration.[46] The MCR for norethindrone is in the range of 500 l/day in nonusers.[47] In women who take norethindrone in an oral contraceptive, the MCR has been reported to be increased to 700 L/day.[47] The MCR for medroxyprogesterone acetate has been reported as 21 L/day/kg, which would extrapolate to about 1200 L/day in a 60 kg woman.[48] It should be noted that all the MCRs for synthetic progestogens were measured after intravenous injection and not after oral administration.

Most synthetic progestogens, except levonorgestrel, are not bound strongly to a serum globulin and their MCRs are less than one half that of progesterone.

Table 8.4 Metabolic clearance rates (MCR) of progesterone and synthetic progestogens.

Progestogen	MCR (L/day)	Reference
Progesterone	2510	41
Norethynodrel	30	46
Norethindrone	500	47
Medroxyprogesterone acetate	1200	48

Thus, the difference in the structures between the synthetic and the natural progestogens affect the metabolism to a major degree. The MCR of levonorgestrel appears to increase slightly in the first few months after the insertion of levonorgestrel rods:[49] whether this is due to an effect on SHBG is uncertain.[39,49]

Pathways of metabolism

Progesterone

Progesterone is converted primarily via the 5α-reductase pathway but there is also conversion to the 5β-reduced compounds and to 20α-hydroxy pregn-4-en-z-one. As detailed by MacDonald et al,[50] 50% of the metabolism of progesterone occurs in the liver and there are equal amounts of 5α- and 5β-reduced compounds formed. However, 50% of the metabolism of progesterone occurs in extrahepatic tissues and, of this, 80% is via 5α-reduction; thus, 40% of progesterone metabolism occurs in extrahepatic tissues via 5α-reduction. Of the total metabolism, 10% occurs via 20α-reduction, primarily in extrahepatic tissues.[41]

There is conversion of a small amount of progesterone to desoxycorticosterone (DOC) by peripheral tissues. The conversion of progesterone to DOC is highly variable between women and can result in physiologically relevant levels of DOC, especially in the luteal phase of the cycle and in pregnancy.[50]

Synthetic progestogens

The 19-nortestosterone compound, norethynodrel, is reduced at the 3 position to 3α- and 3β-hydroxy compounds with the $\Delta^{5(10)}$ double bond retained. There is also some conversion to the 3α- and 3β-hydroxy compounds with reduction of the double bond.[51,52] Norethindrone is also reduced to the 3α- and 3β-hydroxy compounds with reduction of the Δ^4 double bond.[52] For neither of these compounds is there extensive de-ethynylation. The major circulating form of both after oral administration appears to be the sulfate, and there is little aromatization of either compound.[52]

There is extensive, but slow, conversion of levonorgestrel to the 3α, 5β-reduced compounds but some 3α, 5α-tetrahydrolevonorgestrel is also formed[52] as well as 16β-hydroxynorgestrel.[53] D-norgestrel-3-oxime-17 acetate (Norgestimate) is extensively converted to norgestrel and then further metabolized.[54] There are little data on the pathway of metabolism of medroxyprogesterone acetate in the circulation.

URINARY EXCRETION

Progesterone

Although percentage conversions of plasma progesterone to its circulating metabolites have been carried out, the extent of urinary excretion of these metabolites remains uncertain.[50] There is some fecal excretion but this will explain the apparent failure to account for the excretion of all the metabolites. Most of the urinary excretion is in the form of glucuronide conjugates with much less in the sulfated form.

Synthetic progestogens

The synthetic progestogens are metabolized as described previously. The metabolites are then excreted in the urine, primarily conjugated in the glucuronide form but also as the sulfate. De-ethinylation is not a major pathway, and while some progestogens and their metabolites are excreted in the feces, this also is not a major pathway.

REFERENCES

1. Dunn JF, Nisula BC, Rodbard D 1981 Transport of steroid hormones: binding of 21 endogenous steroids to both testosterone-binding globulin and corticosteroid-binding globulin in human plasma. Journal of Clinical Endocrinology and Metabolism 53: 58–68
2. Kono S, Brandon DD, Merriam GR, Loriaux DL, Lipsett MB 1980 Low plasma levels of 2-hydroxyestrone are consistent with its rapid metabolic clearance. Steroids 36: 463–472
3. Dunn JF, Merriam GR, Eil C, Kono S, Loriaux DL, Nisula BC 1980 Testosterone-estradiol binding globulin binds to 2-methoxyestradiol with greater affinity than to testosterone. Journal of Clinical Endocrinology and Metabolism 51: 404–406
4. Rosenthal HE, Pietrzak E, Slaunwhite WR Jr, Sandberg AA 1972 Binding of estrone sulfate in human plasma. Journal of Clinical Endocrinology and Metabolism 34: 805–813
5. Pugeat MM, Dunn JF, Nisula BC 1981 Transport of steroid hormones: interaction of 70 drugs with testosterone-binding globulin and corticosteroid-binding globulin in human plasma. Journal of Clinical Endocrinology and Metabolism 53: 69–75
6. Cunningham R, Tindall DJ, Lobl TJ, Campbell JA, Means AR 1981 Steroid structural requirements for high affinity binding to human sex steroid binding protein (SBP). Steroids 38(3): 243–262
7. Baird DT, Horton R, Longcope C, Tait JF 1969 Steroid dynamics under steady-state conditions. Recent Progress in Hormone Research 25: 611–664
8. Longcope C, Layne DS, Tait JF 1968 Metabolic clearance rates and interconversions of estrone and 17β-estradiol in normal males and females. Journal of Clinical Investigation 47: 93–106
9. Hembree WC, Bardin CW, Lipsett MB 1969 A study of estrogen metabolic clearance rates and transfer factors. Journal of Clinical Investigation 48: 1809–1819
10. Longcope C, Sato K, McKay C, Horton R 1984 Aromatization by splanchnic tissue in men. Journal of Clinical Endocrinology and Metabolism 58: 1089–1093
11. Longcope C, Pratt JH, Schneider SH, Fineberg SE 1976 In vivo studies on the metabolism of estrogens by muscle and adipose tissue of normal males. Journal of Clinical Endocrinology and Metabolism 43: 1134–1145
12. Kirschner MA, Ertel N, Schneider G 1981 Obesity, hormones and cancer. Cancer Research 31: 3711–3717
13. Longcope C, Baker S 1993 Androgen and estrogen dynamics: relationships with age, weight and menopausal status. Journal of Clinical Endocrinology and Metabolism 76: 601–604
14. Longcope C, Bourget C, Meciak PA, Okulicz WC, McCracken JA, Hoberg LM, Padykula HA 1988 Estrogen dynamics in the female rhesus monkey. Biology and Reproduction 39: 561–565
15. Longcope C 1990 Hormone dynamics at the menopause. Annals of the New York Academy of Science 592: 21–30
16. Flood C, Pratt JH, Longcope C 1976 The metabolic clearance and blood production rates of estriol in normal, non-pregnant women. Journal of Clinical Endocrinology and Metabolism 42: 1–8
17. Longcope C, Femino A, Flood C, Williams KIH 1982 Metabolic clearance rate and conversion ratios of 3H-2-hydroxyestrone in normal men. Journal of Clinical Endocrinology and Metabolism 54: 347–380
18. Kono S, Merriam GR, Brandon D, Loriaux DL, Lipsett MB, Fujino T 1983 Radioimmunoassay and metabolic clearance rate of catecholestrogens, 2-hydroxyestrone and 2-hydroxyestradiol in man. Journal of Steroid Biochemistry 19: 627–633
19. Bates GW, Edman CD, Porter JC, MacDonald PC 1977 Metabolism of catechol estrogen by human erythrocytes. Journal of Clinical Endocrinology and Metabolism 45: 1120–1123
20. Longcope C, Flood C, Femino A, Williams KIH 1983 Metabolism of 2-methoxyestrone in normal men. Journal of Clinical Endocrinology and Metabolism 57(2): 277–282
21. Longcope C 1972 The metabolism of estrone sulfate in normal males. Journal of Clinical Endocrinology and Metabolism 34: 113–122
22. Ruder HJ, Loriaux L, Lipsett MB 1972 Estrone sulfate: production rate and metabolism in man. Journal of Clinical Investigation 51: 1020–1033
23. Kellie AE, Smith ER 1957 Renal clearance of 17-oxo steroid conjugates found in human peripheral plasma. Biochemistry Journal 66: 490–495
24. Southren AL, Olivo J, Gordon GG, Vittek J, Brener J, Rafii F 1974 The conversion of androgens to estrogens in hyperthyroidism. Journal of Clinical Endocrinology and Metabolism 38: 207–214

25. Ridgway EC, Longcope C, Maloof F 1975 Metabolic clearance and blood production rates of estradiol in hyperthyroidism. Journal of Clinical Endocrinology and Metabolism 41: 491–497
26. Ridgway EC, Maloof F, Longcope C 1982 Androgen and oestrogen dynamics in hyperthyroidism. Journal of Endocrinology 95: 105–115
27. Longcope C, Abend S, Braverman LE, Emerson CH 1990 Androstenedione and estrone dynamics in hypothyroid women. Journal of Clinical Endocrinology and Metabolism 70: 903–907
28. Longcope C, Gorbach S, Goldin BM, Woods M, Dwyers J, Warman J 1985 The metabolism of estradiol: oral compared to intravenous administration. Journal of Steroid Biochemistry 23: 1065–1070
29. Gurpide E, Mann J, Lieberman S 1963 Analysis of open systems of multiple pools by administration of tracers at a constant rate or as a single dose as illustrated by problems involving steroid hormones. Journal of Clinical Endocrinology and Metabolism 23: 1155–1176
30. Longcope C, Williams KIH 1975 The metabolism of synthetic estrogens in non-users and users of oral contraceptives. Steroids 25: 121–133
31. Longcope C, Williams KIH 1977 Ethynylestradiol and mestranol: their pharmacodynamics and effects on natural estrogens. In: Garattini S, Berendes HW (eds) Pharmacology of steroid contraceptive drugs. Raven Press, New York, p 89
32. Bird CE, Clark AF 1973 Metabolic clearance rates and metabolism of mestranol and ethinylestradiol in normal young women. Journal of Clinical Endocrinology and Metabolism 36: 296–302
33. Abdel-Aziz MT, Williams KIH 1970 Metabolism of radioactive 17α-ethinylestradiol by women. Steroids 15: 695–710
34. Reed MJ, Fotherby K, Steele SJ 1972 Metabolism of ethynyloestradiol in man. Journal of Endocrinology 55: 351–361
35. Williams KIH 1970 The metabolism of radioactive 17α-ethynylestradiol 3-methyl ether (Mestranol) by women. Steroids 13(4): 539–544
36. Westphal U 1986 Steroid-protein interactions III. α1-Acid Glycoprotein (AAG, orosomucoid). Springer-Verlag, Berlin, pp 26–44
37. Steingold KA, Matt DW, Dua L, Anderson TL, Hodgen GD 1990 Orosomucoid in human pregnancy serum diminishes bioavailability of the progesterone antagonist RU 486 in rats. American Journal of Obstetrics and Gynecology 162(2): 523–524
38. Westphal U 1986 Steroid-protein interactions II. Progesterone-binding globulin (PBG). Springer-Verlag, Berlin, pp 138–198
39. Fotherby K 1995 Levonorgestrel: clinical pharmacokinetics. Clinical Pharmacokinetics 28: 203–215
40. Little B, Tait JF, Tait SAS, Erlenmeyer F 1966 The metabolic clearance rate of progesterone in males and ovariectomized females. Journal of Clinical Investigation 45(6): 901–912
41. Lin TJ, Billiar RB, Little B 1972 Metabolic clearance rate of progesterone in the menstrual cycle. Journal of Clinical Endocrinology and Metabolism 35: 879–886
42. Little B, Billiar RB, Bougas J, Tait JF 1973 The splanchnic clearance rate of progesterone in patients with cardiac disease. Journal of Clinical Endocrinology and Metabolism 36: 1222–1229
43. Little B, Billiar RB, Longcope C, Jassani M 1979 Uterine metabolism of gonadal steroids during the menstrual cycle. American Journal of Obstetrics and Gynecology 135: 957–964
44. Billiar RB, Takaoka Y, Reddy SP, Hess D, Longcope C, Little B 1981 Specific tissue metabolism of progesterone in vivo in the anesthetized female rhesus monkey during the follicular and luteal phase of the menstrual cycle. Endocrinology 108: 1643–1648
45. Lin TJ, Lin SC, Erlenmeyer F, Kline IT, Underwood R, Billiar RB, Little B 1972 Progesterone production rates during the third trimester of pregnancy in normal women, diabetic women, and women with abnormal glucose tolerance. Journal of Clinical Endocrinology and Metabolism 34: 287–297
46. Laumas KR, Murugesan K, Hingorani V 1971 Disappearance in plasma and tissue uptake of radioactivity after an intravenous injection of [6,7-3H] norethyndorel in women. Acta Endocrinologica 66(3): 385–400
47. Mahesh VB, Mills TM, Lin TJ et al 1977 Metabolism, metabolic clearance rate, blood metabolites, and blood half-life of norethindrone and mestranol. In: Garattini S, Berendes HW (eds) Pharmacology of steroid contraceptive drugs. Raven Press, New York, pp 117–130
48. Gupta C, Musto NA, Bullock LP et al 1977 In vivo metabolism of progestins II. Metabolic clearance rate of medroxyprogesterone acetate in four species. In: Garattini S, Berendes HW (eds) Pharmacology of steroid contraceptive drugs. Raven Press, New York, pp 131–136
49. Croxatto HB, Diaz S, Miranda P, Elamsson K, Johansson EDB 1981 Plasma levels of levonorgestrel in women during longterm use of Norplant. Contraception 23: 197–209
50. MacDonald PC, Dombroski RA, Casey ML 1991 Recurrent secretion of progesterone in large amounts: an endocrine/metabolic disorder unique to young women? Endocrine Reviews 12(4): 372–401
51. Cook CE, Twine ME, Tallent CR, Wall ME, Bressler RC 1972 Norethyndorel metabolites in human plasma and urine. Journal of Pharmacology and Experimental Therapeutics 183(1): 197–205
52. Breur H 1977 Metabolic pathways of steroid contraceptive drugs. In: Garattini S, Berendes HW (eds) Pharmacology of steroid contraceptive drugs. Raven Press, New York, pp 73–88
53. Sisenwine SF, Kimmel HB, Liu AL, Ruelius HW 1973 Urinary metabolites of dl-norgestrel in women. Acta Endocrinologica 73: 91–104
54. Alton KB, Hetyei NS, Shaw C, Patrick JE 1984 Biotransformation of norgestimate in women. Contraception 29: 21–29
55. Baird D, Horton R, Longcope C, Tait JF 1968 Steroid prehormones. Perspectives in Biology and Medicine 11: 384–421

9. Feedback mechanisms

David T. Baird

Introduction

During reproductive life, cyclic ovarian function depends on a tightly controlled feedback system involving the ovary, hypothalamus and anterior pituitary. Two steroids which are secreted by the ovary (estradiol and progesterone) have a major role in regulating the secretion of gonadotropins by the anterior pituitary gland. Loss of ovarian function, for example, at the menopause or by surgical castration results in a large increase in the release of follicle stimulating hormone (FSH) and luteinizing hormone (LH) due to an absence of the inhibitory effects of ovarian hormones. In the last decade basic research has improved our understanding of the mechanisms of this feedback system. The identification in 1985 of inhibin confirmed that the ovary secreted a protein hormone which was not a steroid which selectively suppressed the secretion of FSH.

In this chapter I shall discuss the physiology of the control of normal ovarian function and the way in which estrogens and progestogens which are used for therapeutic purposes influence the secretion of gonadotropins.

SOURCE AND SYNTHESIS OF OVARIAN STEROIDS

Both progesterone and estradiol were originally isolated and their structures determined from extracts of ovarian tissue and/or follicular fluid.[1] The theca cells of the Graafian follicle synthesize progesterone from cholesterol which is delivered from the blood bound to low density lipoprotein (LDL).[2] Under the influence of the enzymes P_{450}, 17,20 lyase and 17-hydroxylase, progesterone is converted to androstenedione and testosterone which are then subsequently converted to estrone and estradiol by the enzyme P_{450} aromatase.[3] We now know that aromatase is exclusively located in the granulosa cells of the Graafian follicle which are dependent on a supply of androgen precursor synthesized by the theca cells. Aromatase activity is stimulated by FSH, receptors for which are located exclusively in the granulosa cells of the follicle. In contrast, LH receptors are present on theca cells of all antral follicles but are only found on the granulosa cells of mature preovulatory follicles when they reach about 10 mm diameter. Thus, both gonadotropins stimulate the synthesis of estradiol: FSH by ensuring an adequate aromatase activity and LH by stimulating the theca cells to produce abundant amounts of androgen precursor. In the follicular phase of the cycle the dominant follicle is the major source of estradiol and accounts for about 90% of the estradiol in blood.[4]

Following ovulation, the corpus luteum becomes vascularized and secretes increasing amounts of progesterone. In contrast to the situation in most mammals, the corpus luteum of primates secretes, in addition, large amounts of estradiol (and inhibin).[5,6] Immunostaining for aromatase is confined to granulosa lutein cells while 17α-hydroxylase is found in the theca lutein cells.[7] It is likely, therefore, that the synthesis of estradiol by the corpus luteum in women involves an interaction between the two cell types similar to that which occurs in the follicle.

Inhibin is a dimeric glycoprotein which was originally isolated from follicular fluid and has the property of selectively suppressing FSH.[8,9] The two subunits (α and β) are joined noncovalently by disulfide bonds. Two different β subunits termed β_A and β_B have been identified and, hence, two different inhibin molecules, i.e. $inhibin_A$ and $inhibin_B$. Inhibin is synthesized by the granulosa cells of the follicle and the granulosa lutein cells of the corpus luteum. The relative amounts of $inhibin_A$ and $_B$ in serum varies depending on the stage of the cycle.[10] (Fig. 9.1). $Inhibin_B$ levels rise in early and midfollicular phase of the cycle and fall by midcycle, with a short-lived peak occurring at the time of ovulation. In contrast, the concentration of $inhibin_A$ rises in the late follicular

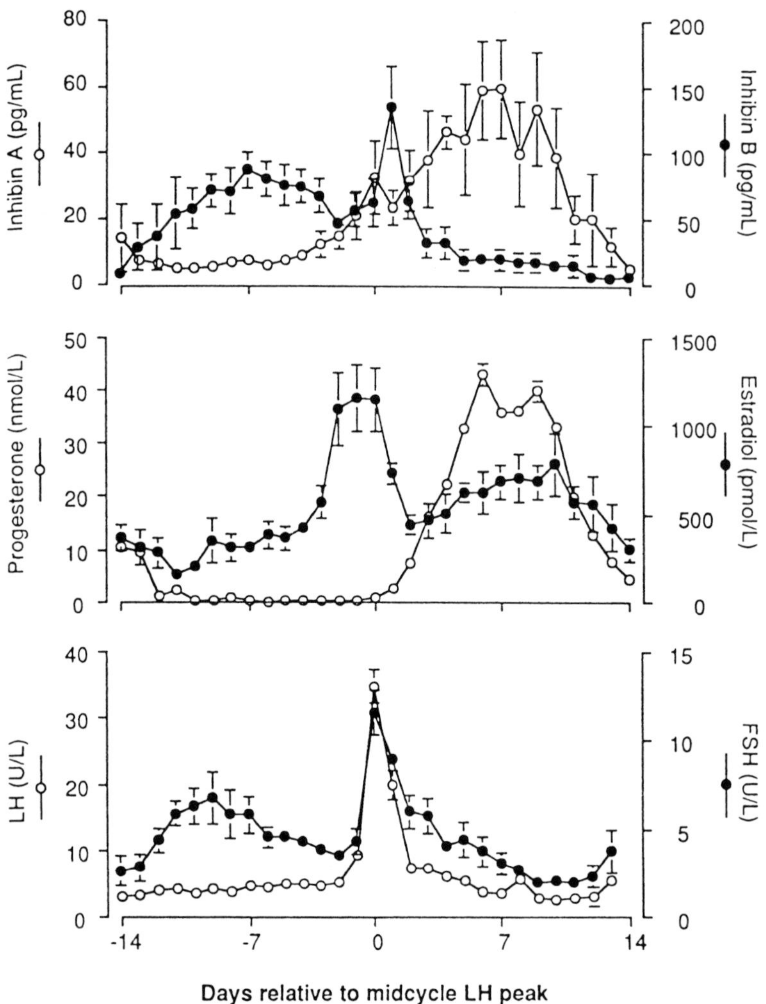

Fig. 9.1 Concentration of inhibin A and B and pituitary and ovarian hormones throughout the menstrual cycle. (Reproduced with permission[10])

phase of the cycle with a peak synchronous with the midcycle LH peak. Following ovulation, the concentration rises in parallel with the increased secretion of estradiol and progesterone by the corpus luteum. The levels of inhibin$_B$ remain low throughout the luteal phase.

In summary, the ovary is the source of three hormones which are involved in the control of secretion of gonadotropins, i.e. estradiol, progesterone and inhibin. Over 90% of these hormones arise either from the follicle which will ovulate or the corpus luteum, so that at all stages of the cycle the dominant structure has unique control of the signals which regulate the secretion of gonadotropins.

GONADOTROPINS

FSH and LH are both dimeric glycoproteins synthesized by specialized cells (gonadotrops) in the anterior pituitary gland. They share a common α subunit which is joined to the hormone specific β subunit by noncovalent bonds. Both gonadotropins are heavily glycosylated, with oligosaccharide side chains making up to 30% of FSH. Under physiological conditions there are over 30 different isoforms of FSH and LH which contain variable amounts and type of oligosaccharides. The heavily glycosylated acidic forms are cleared from the circulation more slowly than the more basic forms, which are favored by an estrogenic environment such as occurs at midcycle.[11]

The synthesis of FSH and LH is dependent on gonadotropin releasing hormone (GnRH) secreted by the hypothalamus.[12] This decapeptide is released from a network of GnRH neurones in the basal hypothalamus directly into the capillaries of the hypothalamic hypophyseal portal system. The secretion occurs in response to a synchronized burst of neuronal activity which occurs approximately every 60 minutes. GnRH interacts with receptors on the cell membrane of the gonadotrops and transduces the signal to the nucleus by a second messenger system that involves the phosphoinositol pathway.[12] The mechanism by which transcription and translation of the message to synthesize FSH or LH occurs is not entirely understood. It is necessary that GnRH is delivered to the anterior pituitary in a pulsatile fashion because continuous exposure to GnRH leads to down regulation of the receptor and decline in the secretion of gonadotropins.

The synchronous discharge of GnRH neurones occurs approximately every hour in the castrate animal. Hence, in the absence of feedback effects of ovarian hormones, LH and FSH are secreted in a series of hourly pulses which are reflected as a rise in the concentration in peripheral venous blood.[13,14] The pulses of FSH are more difficult to identify than those of LH because of its longer half-life (about 12 hours). Moreover, the relative amounts of FSH and LH secreted by the pituitary gonadotroph vary depending on the frequency of GnRH secretion. When GnRH pulses are infrequent, as in puberty, relatively more FSH than LH is released. In contrast, in the late follicular phase of the cycle, pulses of LH predominate as the GnRH pulses approach one per hour.

In summary, the hypothalamus seems to have the ability to generate a synchronized burst of neuronal activity about once per hour, in the absence of negative feedback. The activity of this so called 'pulse generator' is modulated by ovarian hormones which result in changes in both the frequency and amplitude of the signal.

FEEDBACK EFFECTS OF OVARIAN HORMONES

Receptors for both estradiol and progesterone are present in both the anterior pituitary and the hypothalamus and, hence, both are potential sites for the feedback effects of ovarian steroids,[15] which can be either negative or positive. *Negative* feedback involves suppression of FSH or LH or both. *Positive* feedback describes the ability of estradiol to stimulate the release of LH and FSH. Whether estradiol exerts negative or positive feedback depends on timing, dose and duration as well as interaction with progesterone. Although receptors for inhibin have not yet been isolated, the bulk of evidence suggests that inhibin acts virtually exclusively at the level of the anterior pituitary to inhibit the synthesis of FSH.

In a series of classic experiments in the rhesus monkey, Knobil and colleagues established that estradiol, when given in doses which reproduced the concentration observed during the follicular phase of the cycle, initially caused suppression of the concentration of FSH and, to a lesser extent, LH.[16] After a period of at least 36 hours, the concentration of LH rose above the initial value and eventually a discharge of LH similar to that seen during the preovulatory surge was observed (positive feedback). Subsequently detailed experiments in women have confirmed this dual feedback action of estradiol.[17] During the negative feedback phase, there is a decrease in the amplitude of LH pulses without any change in frequency, suggesting that either estradiol decreases the amount of GnRH discharged per pulse or that sensitivity of the anterior pituitary to GnRH is diminished.

The changes in secretion of GnRH in response to estradiol have been studied directly in experimental animals in which hypothalamic hypophyseal portal blood can be sampled. In the rat and the sheep, no reduction in secretion of GnRH into the hypothalamic hypophyseal portal blood occurs immediately following the injection of estradiol[18,19] (Fig. 9.2). These findings suggest that at least in these species the acute negative feedback effect of estradiol is due to diminished response of the anterior pituitary to GnRH. How far these experimental findings can be extrapolated to the follicular phase of the ovarian cycle of the intact animal is uncertain. The follicular phase of the sheep is characterized by the occurrence of frequent pulses of LH of low amplitude although there is no corresponding reduction in the amplitude of GnRH pulses. These findings suggest that during the follicular phase estradiol exerts an inhibitory effect by decreasing the sensitivity of the anterior pituitary to GnRH.

The positive feedback response to estrogen is essential to maintain ovarian cyclicity. *Positive* feedback can only be provoked by estradiol if the anterior pituitary has been primed with GnRH pulses of high frequency, such as are found during the follicular phase of the cycle. In the rhesus monkey, once the pituitary has been so primed, exposure to an adequate dose of estrogen for an appropriate time will provoke an LH surge even in the absence of continued

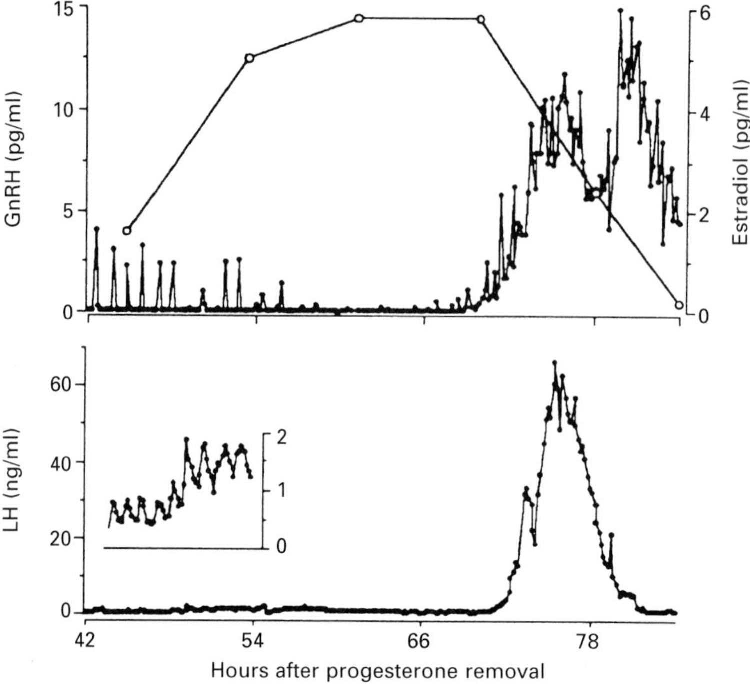

Fig. 9.2 Concentration of GnRH and LH in hypophyseal portal blood during the follicular phase of the sheep oestrous cycle. Note the increased secretion of GnRH during the LH surge. (Reproduced with permission[19])

exposure to pulsatile GnRH.[20] These findings, together with the observation that there is virtual cessation of electrical activity in the basal hypothalamus at midcycle,[21] have led Knobil to hypothesize that in the rhesus monkey the principal site of action of the positive feedback effect of estradiol is the anterior pituitary. Support for this hypothesis has come from experiments using potent antagonists of GnRH injected at different stages of the follicular phase.[22] Secretion of estradiol and cessation of follicular development occurs promptly after injection of GnRH antagonist in the early or midfollicular phase of the cycle. However, when the antagonist is injected in the late follicular phase within two days of expected ovulation, an LH surge and ovulation still occur in approximately half the animals. These findings are compatible with the suggestion that in this species once the anterior pituitary has been adequately primed by GnRH, estradiol alone is sufficient to provoke a discharge of LH. An alternative explanation is that the antagonist is no longer capable of blocking the action of endogenous GnRH, increased amounts of which are released at this time.

How do these findings in experimental animals apply to women? When women with hypogonadotrophic hypogonadism are treated with exogenous pulsatile GnRH, a spontaneous LH surge and ovulation occurs without any change in the frequency of GnRH pulses.[23] Indeed, a recent study reported in abstract demonstrated that the dose of GnRH per pulse (but not the frequency) could be dropped by a factor of three during the late follicular phase without compromising the incidence of ovulation.[24] However, the frequency of GnRH pulses required to ensure that an LH surge occurs (one pulse every 60–90 minutes) is similar to that which occurs normally in the late follicular phase of the cycle. If the frequency drops below that then an LH surge does not occur even although follicular development is stimulated.[25,26]

In summary, these findings suggest that in women, estradiol can provoke an LH surge without any change in the frequency or amount of GnRH secreted by the hypothalamus if the pituitary is primed with GnRH. However, it is still possible that under physiological circumstances, increased amounts of GnRH are secreted during the LH surge. Recent publications have demonstrated that the LH surge can always be prevented or aborted by the injection of potent antagonists of GnRH in the late follicular phase of the cycle.[22] In an elegant study, Dubourdieu et al demonstrated that following injection of GnRH antagonist (Nal-Glu) in the periovulatory period, there was an immediate fall in the concentration of LH and estradiol and ovulation was inhibited.[27] Injection of exogenous estradiol in amounts which were similar to the maximum secreted by the preovulatory follicle failed to elicit an LH surge. Taken together, these results strongly suggest that in women (in contrast to monkeys) continued secretion of GnRH is required during the estradiol induced preovulatory LH surge. It is not possible at the moment to determine whether there is an increase in GnRH secretion into hypothalamic hypophyseal portal blood during the LH surge in women, as has been found in other species, although there are three publications reporting an increase in immunoactive GnRH in peripheral venous blood at midcycle.[28,29,30]

Progesterone also acts at both hypothalamus and pituitary. In the absence of estrogen, progesterone has very little effect on the concentration of FSH or LH, presumably because of a relative lack of progesterone receptors, the synthesis of which are stimulated by estrogen. Following estrogen priming, progesterone reinforces the negative feedback effect of estrogen.[20] During the luteal phase of the cycle there is a marked slowing of the frequency of LH pulses due to the effect of progesterone at the hypothalamus.[31] Due to the negative feedback effect of both estradiol and progesterone secreted by the corpus luteum, the levels of FSH and LH reach their lowest values of the cycle in the luteal phase.[14]

Although progesterone predominantly has a suppressive effect on LH secretion, paradoxically small amounts can enhance the positive feedback effect of estradiol. Thus, administration of progesterone to menopausal women treated with estrogen provokes an immediate discharge of LH.[32] This action of progesterone in facilitating the positive feedback effect of estradiol probably has physiological relevance during the menstrual cycle. The small amounts of progesterone which are secreted by the preovulatory follicle 2–3 days prior to ovulation are sufficient to sensitize the anterior pituitary to estrogen and help amplify the positive feedback signal.[33,34] Administration of the progesterone antagonist, mifepristone, in the immediate preovulatory period, prevents or delays the LH surge, an effect which can be overcome by progesterone.[35] The fact that mifepristone exerts this inhibitory effect on positive feedback, even in women with hypogonadotrophic hypogonadism in whom follicular development is induced with exogenous

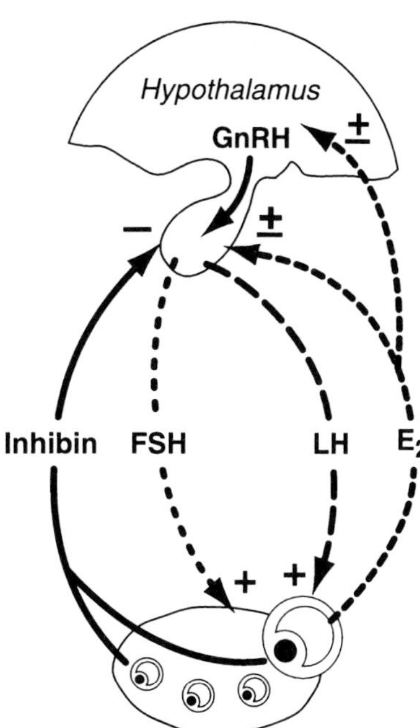

Fig. 9.3 Diagramatic representation of the hypothalamic-pituitary-ovarian axis in women during the follicular phase. Estradiol feeds back at both the hypothalamus and anterior pituitary to inhibit the secretion of FSH and LH (negative feedback). Under certain conditions it can provoke the discharge of LH (positive feedback). Inhibin arising from both dominant and small antral follicles suppresses the synthesis and release of FSH by the anterior pituitary.

pulsatile GnRH, strongly suggests an action at the anterior pituitary, as in the rhesus monkey.[36,37]

In summary, both estradiol and progesterone exert positive and negative feedback effects on the hypothalamic-pituitary unit (Fig. 9.3). Estradiol is the principal hormone responsible for regulating the important fluctuations in the concentrations of FSH which occur throughout the ovarian cycle. In the follicular phase of the cycle, the rising levels of estradiol secreted by the dominant follicle suppress the secretion of FSH, probably acting mainly at the level of the anterior pituitary. In the luteal phase the secretion of estradiol (and inhibin) by the corpus luteum suppresses the secretion of FSH to levels below which initiation of growth of small antral follicles (< 5 mm) into the active growth phase ceases.

DEVELOPMENT OF OVARIAN FUNCTION AT PUBERTY

The ovary is formed during early fetal life (7–10 weeks gestation) by migration of the primitive germ cells from the dorsal endoderm of the yolk sac to the genital ridge of the coloemic cavity.[38] Primordial oocytes divide by mitosis and then the chromosomes are reduced to the haploid number by meiosis and become arrested during the diplotene phase of the first meiotic division. By seven months of fetal life, oogenesis ceases and no further germ cells are formed.

The fetal pituitary secretes FSH by 12–14 weeks gestation, coincidental to the onset of folliculogenesis, and by birth the fetal ovary already contains several small antral follicles. In early infancy the concentration of FSH, LH and estradiol rises slowly indicating some stimulation of follicular development. After two years of age the concentration of gonadotrophins and estradiol decline and remain low until the onset of puberty at about 10–12 years.[39,40]

The mechanisms involved in the suppression of ovarian activity during infancy have been the subject of much experimental research.[41] Cyclical ovarian activity can be induced in prepubertal monkeys by the administration of pulses of GnRH every hour.[42] Ovarian cyclicity ceases when the treatment with GnRH is stopped. Similar results can be obtained by the pulsatile administration of N-methyl D-aspartic acid (NMDA), which activates the discharge of GnRH neurones.[43] Together, these results demonstrate all the components of the hypothalamic-pituitary ovarian axis, necessary to maintain cyclical ovarian activity, are present in the prepubertal animal but that the activity of the hypothalamic neurones is suppressed. In agonadal girls, e.g. Turner's syndrome, the concentrations of FSH and LH, which are raised for the first 2–3 years after birth, fall to low levels during childhood and only rise to castrate levels at the time of expected puberty (10–14 years).[44] These observations demonstrate that the hypothalamic-pituitary system has the potential to operate at a level similar to that found in adult women, even in early infancy, but that during childhood its activity is suppressed.

The mechanism by which this suppression of the activity of the hypothalamic GnRH neurones is achieved in childhood is not fully understood. Studies in the rhesus monkey have demonstrated that the full complement of GnRH neurones which have migrated from the olfactory plaque are already present in the hypothalamus at birth. Recent data in prepubertal girls demonstrate that small frequent pulses of LH of very low amplitude occur throughout childhood. These findings suggest that during childhood the GnRH pulse generator discharges at a rate similar to that seen in the adult (every 60–120 minutes) but that the amount of GnRH secreted is so low that it has very little effect on the secretion of FSH and LH. With the onset of puberty the amplitude of LH pulses increase initially at night and, hence, follicular development and a rise in the secretion of estradiol occurs. Ovulation does not occur until hourly pulses of LH occur throughout the 24 hours such that the secretion of estradiol by the preovulatory follicle is sufficient to provoke a discharge of LH (positive feedback).

The mechanism by which the activity of the hypothalamus is activated has been the subject of much speculation. The most plausible explanation at present is that it is due to removal of some inhibitory influence. Neurones from many other parts of the brain, e.g. hippocampus, anamygdala and locus ceruleus, project to the medial-basal hypothalamus and could be the source of inhibitory signals.[45] Support for this view comes from the finding that electrolytic lesions in the anterior hypothalamus can provoke precocious puberty in the rat and some children with brain lesions or hydrocephalus enter puberty at an early age.[46] Although neuroactive substances such as natural opioids, γ-aminobutyric acid (GABA) and serotonin have all been suggested as potential mediators of these inhibitions, there is no direct experimental proof that the onset of puberty *in vivo* is due to their removal.

In many animals, reproductive function is suppressed during seasonal anestrus by a mechanism involving recognition of a change in photoperiod and transduced through the secretion of melatonin by the pineal.[47,48] Precocious puberty has been described in some girls with pineal tumors, suggesting an involvement of this system. Puberty is delayed in girls who are significantly underweight due to malnutrition or excessive exercise.[49] It is difficult to accommodate all these observations with a single all-encompassing explanation for the control of reproductive function. Rather they may suggest that a number of factors (metabolic, hormonal and neuronal) can influence the activity of the GnRH neurones which results in a change in the frequency and amplitude secretion of GnRH and, hence, LH and FSH from the anterior pituitary.

SYNTHETIC STEROIDS

Estrogens and progestogens are used widely for a variety of indications in reproductive medicine, e.g. contraception, hormone replacement and treatment of hormone dependent conditions such as endometriosis, fibroids, etc.[50] Synthetic steroids exert their action by binding to the same receptors as endogenous steroids. However, many synthetic progestogens are derivatives of C-19 androgens and, hence, bind to the androgen receptor with varying degrees of affinity. For this reason, and because there is a degree of homology between the androgen, progestogen and glucocorticoid receptors, synthetic progestogens often have biological effects which are not found in native progesterone.[51]

Stilbestrol was the first synthetic steroid to be synthesized but has now been largely superseded by other preparations. Ethinyl estradiol, which is the principal estrogen used in combination with a progestogen in the combined oral contraceptive pill, is a very potent estrogen which is active orally. The presence of the methyl group at C-17 impairs metabolism so that its half-life after oral or systemic administration is about 12 hours. In common with all estrogens in large doses, it suppresses the secretion of both FSH and LH.[52] FSH appears to be particularly sensitive to the negative feedback effects of ethinyl estradiol and doses as low as 10 μg per day will cause a significant suppression of FSH concentration in menopausal women. The minimum dose of ethinyl estradiol combined with a progestogen which will suppress FSH and, hence, follicular development in women with intact ovaries is between 20–30 μg per day. Although the progestogen enhances the negative feedback effect of ethinyl estradiol, the degree of suppression of FSH appears to depend more on the amount of estrogen than progestogen.[53]

In contrast to its effect when combined with a progestogen, small doses of ethinyl estradiol alone have little if any effect on the concentration of LH. In one study a dose of 80 μg per day was given to women for a period of 15 days.[54] The concentration of FSH was depressed significantly while the mean concentration of LH remained unchanged, although there was considerable fluctuation from day to day. This effect of unopposed estrogen is similar to that observed during the follicular phase of the menstrual cycle when the concentration of LH rises slightly while that of FSH is significantly suppressed. Although inhibin probably contributes to this, secretion of estradiol by the dominant follicle exerts a selective suppression of FSH and, hence, ensures the demise of other secondary antral follicles which could be potential candidates for ovulation.

A range of other synthetic and natural estrogens which are used in hormone replacement therapy are less potent than ethinyl estradiol. There is no evidence that their mode of action is any different from estradiol or ethinyl estradiol, i.e. they bind with high affinity to the estrogen receptor. The degree of estrogenicity and the biological effect does vary depending on dose and route of administration. Estradiol is inactive if given by mouth, except if it is micronized and given in large amounts, because it is metabolized in the gut and liver. Routes which avoid first pass through the liver, e.g. vaginal, subcutaneous implantation or cutaneous patches, have less effect on the synthesis of proteins by the liver, e.g. sex hormone-binding globulin. Moreover, the hepatic metabolism of the steroid is reduced and, hence, more is available at peripheral target organs. With all these variables, it is difficult to make a valid comparison of the relative potencies of the different preparations with respect to their different biological effects.

While synthetic estrogens have biological effects which are very similar to that of estradiol, the effect of synthetic progestogens are more complicated. Synthetic progestogens are either derivatives of natural progesterone, e.g. medroxyprogesterone acetate, or C-19 androgens, e.g. norethisterone, the structures of which have been modified to impair metabolic degradation. Natural progesterone inhibits the secretion of LH by slowing the frequency of LH pulses but has very little effect on the secretion of FSH. In contrast, most synthetic progestogens alone, if given in large enough doses, suppress the secretion of both gonadotropins as well as enhancing the negative feedback effects of estrogen.[55] For example, norethisterone in doses of 10 mg per day inhibits ovulation by suppressing LH and FSH. In contrast, at 1 mg per day, the dose used in one current progestogen only minipill, cyclical ovarian activity with normal fluctuations in the concentration of gonadotropins occurs. Even larger doses of 10–20 mg per day completely inhibit ovarian activity by suppressing FSH and LH to a level below which the development of antral follicles ceases.

The reason why synthetic progestogens have a feedback effect on gonadotropins different from that of natural progesterone is not entirely clear. It has been suggested that some synthetic 19-nor steroids are metabolized to compounds which are estrogenic.[56] A more plausible explanation is that synthetic progestogens bind to a greater or lesser degree to the androgen as well as the progesterone receptor. Administration of testosterone to women suppresses FSH and LH, although how much of this effect is due to aromatization to estradiol is not known. It seems likely that the effect on secretion of gonadotropins of a particular compound will be determined by dose, route of administration and its metabolism and whether it is combined with estrogen, as well as the relative binding affinity to the steroid receptors.

Conclusion

Cyclical ovarian activity is dependent on the interplay between the secretion of pituitary gonadotropins and ovarian steroids. Estradiol and progesterone can both inhibit or stimulate the secretion of FSH and LH, depending on dose and duration; inhibin suppresses the secretion of FSH and is probably responsible for maintaining the overall level of FSH within physiological limits. In contrast, the fluctuations in FSH throughout the cycle are more likely to be due to variation in the secretion of estradiol by the dominant follicle or corpus luteum. Synthetic estrogens and progestogens have profound effects on the secretion of gonadotropins, which can be used for pharmacological manipulation of reproductive function, e.g. inhibition of ovulation. Current evidence suggests that synthetic steroids exert their action by interacting with the same receptors as those used by the natural ligands, estradiol and progesterone.

REFERENCES

1. Corner GW 1951 Our knowledge of the menstrual cycle, 1910–1950. Lancet i: 919–923
2. Hillier SG 1991 Cellular basis of follicular endocrine function. In: Hillier SG (ed) Ovarian endocrinology. Blackwell Scientific Publications, Oxford, pp 73–106
3. Strauss JF, Miller WL 1991 Molecular basis of ovarian steroid synthesis. In: Hillier SG (ed) Ovarian endocrinology. Blackwell Scientific Publications, Oxford, pp 25–72
4. Baird DT, Fraser IS 1975 Concentration of oestrone and oestradiol 17β in follicular fluid and ovarian venous blood of women. Clinical Endocrinology 4: 259–266
5. McLachlan RL, Robertson DM, Healy DL, Burger HG, De Kretser DM 1987 Circulating immunoactive inhibin during the human menstrual cycle. Journal of Clinical Endocrinology and Metabolism 65: 954–961
6. Reddi K, Wickings EJ, McNeilly AS, Baird DT, Hillier SG 1990 Circulating bioactive follicle stimulating hormone and immunoactive inhibin levels during the normal human menstrual cycle. Clinical Endocrinology 33: 547–557
7. Sasano H, Okamota M, Mason JI, Simpson ER, Mendelson CR, Sasano N, Silverberg SG 1989 Immunolocalization of aromatase, 17α-hydroxylase and side chain cleavage cytochromes P_{450} in the human ovary. Journal of Reproduction and Fertility 85: 163–169
8. Burger HG, Igarashi M 1988 Inhibin: definition and nomenclature, including related substances. Journal of Clinical Endocrinology and Metabolism 66: 885–886
9. Baird DT, Smith KB 1993 Inhibin and related peptides in the regulation of reproduction. Oxford Reviews of Reproductive Biology 15: 191–232
10. Groome NP, Illingworth PJ, O'Brien M, Roger PAI, Rodger FE, Mather JP, McNeilly AS 1996 Measurement of dimeric inhibin B throughout the human menstrual cycle. Journal of Clinical Endocrinology and Metabolism 81: 1401–1405
11. Padmanabhan V, Lang LL, Sonstein J, Kelch RP, Beitins IZ 1988 Modulation of serum follicle-stimulating hormone bioactivity and isoform distribution by estrogenic steroids in normal women and in gonadal dysgenesis. Journal of Clinical Endocrinology and Metabolism 67: 465–473
12. Hotchkiss J, Knobil E 1995 The hypothalamic pulse generator: the reproductive core. In: Adashi EY, Rock JA, Rosennacks Z (eds) Reproductive endocrinology, surgery and technology. Lippincott-Raven Press, Philadelphia, pp 123–162
13. Conn PM 1995 Gonadotropin-releasing hormone action. In: Adashi EY, Rock JA, Rosennacks Z (eds) Reproductive endocrinology, surgery and technology. Lippincott-Raven Press, Philadelphia, pp 163–179
14. Yen SSC, Tsai CC, Naftolin F, Vandenberg G, Ajobar L 1972 Pulsatile patterns of gonadotropin release in subjects with and without ovarian function. Journal of Clinical Endocrinology and Metabolism 34: 671–675
15. Sprangers SA, West NB, Brenner RM, Bethea CL 1989 Regulation and location of estrogen and progestin receptors in the pituitary of steroid-treated monkeys. Endocrinology 124: 1462–1470
16. Knobil E 1974 On the control of gonadotropin secretion in the rhesus monkey. Recent Progress in Hormone Research 30: 1–36
17. Liu JH, Yen SSC 1983 Induction of midcycle gonadotropin surge by ovarian steroids in women: a critical evaluation. Journal of Clinical Endocrinology and Metabolism 57: 797–802
18. Clarke IJ 1987 GnRH and ovarian hormone feedback. Oxford Reviews of Reproductive Biology 9: 54–95
19. Moenter SM, Caraty A, Locatelli A, Karsch FJ 1991 Pattern of gonadotropin-releasing hormone (GnRH) secretion leading up to ovulation in the ewe: existence of a preovulatory GnRH surge. Endocrinology 129: 1175–1182
20. Knobil E, Plant TM, Wildt L, Belchetz, PE, Marshall G 1980 Control of the rhesus monkey menstrual cycle: permissive role of hypothalamic gonadotropin-releasing hormone. Science 207: 1371
21. O'Byrne KT, Thalabard J-C, Grosser PM, Wilson RC, Williams CL, Chen M-D, Ladendorf D, Hotchkiss J, Knobil E 1991 Radiotelemetric monitoring of hypothalamic gonadotropin-releasing hormone pulse generator activity throughout the menstrual cycle of the rhesus monkey. Endocrinology 129: 1207–1214
22. Fraser HM, Bouchard P 1994 Control of preovulatory luteinizing hormone surge by gonadotropin-releasing hormone antagonists: prospects for clinical application. Trends in Endocrinology and Metabolism 5: 87–93
23. Leyendecker G, Wildt L, Hansmann M 1980 Pregnancies following chronic intermittent (pulsatile) administration of Gn-RH by means of a portable pump ('Zyklomat') — a new approach to the treatment of infertility in hypothalamic amenorrhea. Journal of Clinical Endocrinology and Metabolism 51: 1214–1216
24. Martin KA, Smith JA, Taylor AE, Crowley WF, Hall JE 1996 Reduced GnRH at the midcycle surge in the human: evidence from a GnRH deficient model. Program of Abstracts: International Congress of Endocrinology, San Francisco, June 12–13, No. OR 13-5
25. Belchetz PE, Plant TM, Nakai Y, Keogh EJ, Knobil E 1978 Hypophyseal responses to continuous and intermittent delivery of hypothalamic gonadotropin releasing hormone (GnRH). Science 202: 631–633

26. Filicori M 1994 Use of GnRH and its analogs in the treatment of ovulatory disorders: an overview. In: Filicori M, Flamigni C (eds) Ovulation induction. Excerpta Medica, Amsterdam, pp 239–243
27. Dubourdieu S, Charbonnel B, d'Acremont MF, Carreau S, Spitz IM, Bouchard P 1994 Effect of administration of a GnRH antagonist (Nal-Glu) during the preovulatory period: the luteinizing hormone surge requires the secretion of GnRH. Journal of Clinical Endocrinology and Metabolism 78: 343–347
28. Macacara J, Seyler LE Jr, Reichlin S 1972 Luteinizing hormone releasing factor activity in peripheral blood from women during the mid cycle luteinizing hormone ovulatory surge. Journal of Clinical Endocrinology and Metabolism 34: 271–278
29. Arimura A, Kastin AJ, Schally AV 1974 Immunoreactive LH releasing hormone in plasma: mid cycle elevation in women. Journal of Clinical Endocrinology and Metabolism 38: 510–513
30. Elkind-Hirsch K, Ravnikar V, Schiff I, Tulchinsky D, Ryan KJ 1982 Determinations of endogenous immunoreactive luteinizing hormone-releasing hormone in human plasma. Journal of Clinical Endocrinology and Metabolism 54: 602–607
31. Bäckström CT, McNeilly AS, Leask R, Baird DT 1982 Pulsatile secretion of LH, FSH, prolactin, oestradiol and progesterone during the human menstrual cycle. Clinical Endocrinology 17: 29–42
32. O'Dell WD, Swerdloff RS 1968 Progestogen-induced luteinizing and follicle stimulating hormone surge in post-menopausal women: a simulated ovulatory peak. Proceedings of the National Academy of Science, USA 61: 529–536
33. Hoff JD, Quigley ME, Yen SSC 1983 Hormonal dynamics at mid cycle: a re-evaluation. Journal of Clinical Endocrinology and Metabolism 57: 792–796
34. Djahanbakhch O, McNeilly AS, Warner PM, Swanston IA, Baird DT 1984 Changes in plasma levels of prolactin, FSH, oestradiol, androstenedione and progesterone around the pre-ovulatory surge of LH in women. Clinical Endocrinology 20: 463–472
35. Batista MC, Cartledge TP, Zellmer W, Nieman LK, Merriam GR, Loriaux DL 1992 Evidence for a critical role of progesterone in the regulation of the mid cycle gonadotropin surge and ovulation. Journal of Clinical Endocrinology and Metabolism 74: 565–570
36. Wildt L, Hutchison JS, Marshall G, Pohl CR, Knobil E 1981 On the site of action of progesterone in the blockade of the estradiol-induced gonadotropin discharge in the rhesus monkey. Endocrinology 109: 1293–1294
37. Batista MC, Cartledge TP, Zellmer AW, Nieman LK, Loriaux DL, Merriam GR 1994 The antiprogestin RU 486 delays the mid cycle gonadotropin surge and ovulation in gonadotropin-releasing hormone cycles. Fertility and Sterility 62: 28–34
38. Peters H, McNatty KP (eds) 1980 The development of the ovary in the embryo. In: The ovary: a correlation of structure and function in mammals. Granada, London & New York, pp 1–11
39. Kaplan SL, Grumbach MM, Aubert ML 1976 The ontogenesis of pituitary hormones and hypothalamic factors in the human fetus: maturation of central nervous system regulation of anterior pituitary function. Recent Progress in Hormone Research 32: 161–243
40. Faiman C, Winter JSD, Reyes FI 1976 Patterns of gonadotropins and gonadal steroids throughout life. Clinical Obstetrics and Gynecology 3: 467–483
41. Grumbach MM, Roth JC, Kaplan SL, Kelch RP 1974 Hypothalamic regulation of puberty: evidence and concepts derived from clinical research. In: Grumbach MM, Grave GD, Mayer FE (eds) The control of the onset of puberty. Wiley, New York, pp 115–116
42. Wildt L, Marshall G, Knobil E 1980 Experimental induction of puberty in the infantile female rhesus monkey. Science 207: 1373–1374
43. Plant TM, Gay VL, Marshall GR, Arslan M 1989 Puberty in monkeys is triggered by chemical stimulation of the hypothalamus. Proceedings of National Academy of Science in USA 86: 2506–2510
44. Conte FA, Grumbach MM, Kaplan SL 1988 A diphasic pattern of gonadotropin secretion in patients with the syndrome of gonadal dysgenesis. Journal of Clinical Endocrinology and Metabolism 40: 670–674
45. Barraclough CA, Wide PM 1982 The role of catecholamines in the regulation of pituitary luteinizing hormone and follicle stimulating hormone secretion. Endocrinology Reviews 3: 91–119
46. Weinberger LM, Grant FC 1941 Precocious puberty and tumours of the hypothalamus. Archives of Internal Medicine 67: 762–792
47. Lincoln GW, Short RV 1980 Season breeding: nature's contraceptive. Recent Progress in Hormone Research 36: 1–52
48. Arendt J 1986 Role of the pineal gland and melatonin in seasonal reproductive function in mammals. Oxford Review of Reproductive Biology 8: 266–320
49. Frisch RE, Gutz-Welbergen AN, McArthur JW 1981 Delayed menarche and amenorrhoea of college athletes in relation to onset of training. Journal of the American Medical Association 246: 1559–1564
50. Speroff L, Glass RH, Kase NG (eds) 1989 Steroid contraception. In: Clinical gynecologic endocrinology and infertility. Williams & Wilkins, Baltimore, pp 409–449
51. Klopper A 1971 Endocrinological effects of oral contraceptives. Clinics in Endocrinology and Metabolism 2: 489–502
52. Nillius SJ, Wide L 1970 Effects of oestrogen on serum levels of LH and FSH. Acta Endocrinologica 65: 583–594
53. Smith SK, Kirkham RJE, Arce BB, McNeilly AS, Loudon NB, Baird DT 1986 The effect of deliberate omission of Trinordial® or Microgynon® on the hypothalamic-pituitary-ovarian axis. Contraception 34: 513–522
54. Swerdloff RS, O'Dell WD 1969 Serum luteinizing and follicle stimulating hormone levels during sequential and non-sequential contraceptive treatment of eugonadal women. Journal of Clinical Endocrinology and Metabolism 29: 157–163
55. Diczfalusy E, Goebelsmann U, Johannisson E, Tillinger K-G, Wide L 1969 Pituitary and ovarian function in women on continuous low dose progestogens; effect of chlorminone acetate and norethisterone. Acta Endocrinologica 62: 679–693
56. Brown JB, Blair HA 1960 Urinary oestrogen metabolites of 19-norethisterone and its esters. Proceedings of the Royal Society of Medicine 53: 431–432

10. The normal menstrual cycle; changes throughout life

Robert Norman Greg Phillipson

Introduction

The menstrual cycle involves the coordination of many events by the hypothalamic-pituitary-ovarian axis (see ch. 9) and is readily influenced by physiological and pathological changes that occur during the lifetime of the woman. Absolute concentrations and relative patterns of release of gonadotropin releasing hormone (GnRH) from preoptic neurons are under the influence of a variety of neurotransmitters in the hypothalamus which ultimately alter the response of pituitary gonadotropes via its pulsatile secretory pattern. The resulting gonadotropins, follicle stimulating hormone (FSH) and luteinizing hormone (LH), are also influenced by the existing steroid milieu and provide the communication with the ovaries by well characterized intra-ovarian events to synchronize elements of the menstrual cycle (see ch. 9). Estradiol and progesterone feedback loops can be either stimulatory or inhibitory to gonadotropin release.

The menstrual cycle can be divided into three stages, although there is obviously a continuum between the various phases. The follicular phase, in which recruitment, growth and maturation of the Graafian follicle occurs in concert with paracrine and autocrine regulators, is variable in length (see below). Ovulation is the period during which the final maturation and release of the mature oocyte occurs, while the luteal phase is that time during which progesterone secretion initially predominates to promote optimal endometrial development for implantation, and in the later stages that in which the tissue fails to produce sufficient steroid to maintain endometrial integrity. The histological changes in the endometrium have been well investigated and together with the physiological changes are graphically shown in Fig. 10.1. Important intracellular mediators in menstruation are reviewed in chapter 14.

The purpose of this chapter is to review the highlights of the menstrual cycle from a clinical perspective and show the variations that occur across the reproductive lifespan. Many of the detailed processes are covered in other sections of the volume and will only be described in outline in this chapter.

ASPECTS OF THE MATURE MENSTRUAL CYCLE FROM A PRACTICAL PERSPECTIVE

Clinical

Cycle patterns and length

The first day of menstrual cycle is defined as the commencement of menstrual bleeding and the last as that on the day prior to the subsequent menstrual bleeding. Therefore cycle length is the time period between the first and the last day. Duration of the menstrual period is the length of time over which bleeding occurs. The amount of flow is the volume and intensity of menstrual blood loss.

Harlow and Ephross[1] have reviewed the literature on cycle length, duration of bleeding and amount of flow and their data are summarized in Tables 10.1 and 10.2. It is clear that the classical model of a 28 day cycle with 14 days of follicular and luteal phases is an approximation of the real pattern. While most cycles tend to fall in the range of 26–34 days, postmenarchal and premenopausal cycles tend to deviate from this pattern. Münster et al[2] have suggested that the usual cycle length decreases from a range of 23–35 days in the 15–19 year age group to 23–30 days in the 40–44 year age group (5th–95th centiles), as shown in Fig. 10.2. According to their data, only 0.5% of regular menstruating women have a cycle length less than 21 days and 0.9% a length greater than 35 days. However, nearly one third of all women reported a variation in their menstrual cycle of more than 14 days, with at least one cycle less than 21 days in 18% and at least one cycle greater than 35 days in 29%. Variation in blood loss is difficult to quantitate in population studies. Matsumoto et al[3] reported that duration of

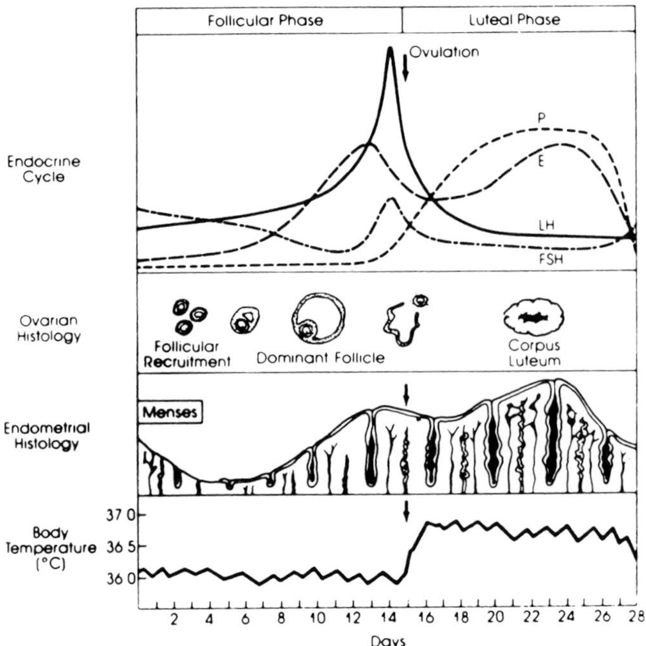

Fig. 10.1 The hormonal, ovarian, endometrial and basal body temperature changes and relationship throughout the normal menstrual cycle. (From Carr BR, Wilson JD 1987 Disorders of the ovary and female reproductive tract. In: Braunwald E, Isselbacher KJ, Petersdorf RG, Wilson JD, Martin JB, Anthony SF (eds) Harrison's principles of internal medicine, 11th ed. New York McGraw-Hill.)

Table 10.1 Menstrual cycle length (days) by age: results of four studies.[1]

	Treloar et al 1967		Vollman 1977		Chiazze et al 1968	Matsumoto et al 1962	
	Person-year mean	Range (5–95%)	Mean	Range (5–95%)	Mean (15–45 day cycles)	Mean	Range (10–90%)
Postmenarche							
Year 1	36.9	18.3–83.1	35.0	17.8–76.5			
Year 2	34.1	18.4–63.5	31.2	19.9–57.5			
Year 5	31.2	21.7–40.4	30.1	19.9–48.5			
Age (year)							
20	30.1	22.1–38.4	29.0	19.7–39.2			
20–24					29.1	31.0	26–38
25	29.8	22.7–37.1	30.7	23.6–43.5			
25–29					28.5	31.3	26–37
30	29.3	22.5–35.4	29.6	23.1–39.4			
30–34					28.0	30.1	25–36
35	28.2	22.3–33.4	29.1	22.8–36.4			
35–39					27.3	29.4	25–35
40	27.3	21.8–32.0	27.3	22.0–33.6			
40–44					26.9		
45			28.3	20.1–39.8			
Premenopause							
5 years	28.4	17.8–38.8					
2 years	43.5	15.4–80.0					
1 year	57.1	14.9–∞					

(From Harlow SD, Ephross SA 1995 Epidemiology of menstruation and its relevance to women's health. Epidemiologic Reviews 17(2): 265–286.)

Table 10.2 By-women probabilities of transition in cycle length from cycle t to cycle $t+1$ (144 women contributed, 1082 cycle pairs).

Length of cycle t (days)	Total number of transitions	Length of cycle $t+1$ (days)					
		<17	17–25	26–34	35–43	44–59	>59
<17	14	0.09	0.41	0.25	0.19	0.06	0.00
17–25	207	0.02	0.18	0.65	0.09	0.06	0.00
26–34	708	0.01	0.18	0.65	0.10	0.03	0.03
35–43	103	0.03	0.10	0.65	0.16	0.03	0.03
44–59	33	0.04	0.07	0.66	0.10	0.06	0.07
>59	17	0.04	0.25	0.40	0.07	0.21	0.04

(From Harlow SD, Ephross SA 1995 Epidemiology of menstruation and its relevance to women's health. Epidemiologic Reviews 17(2): 265–286).

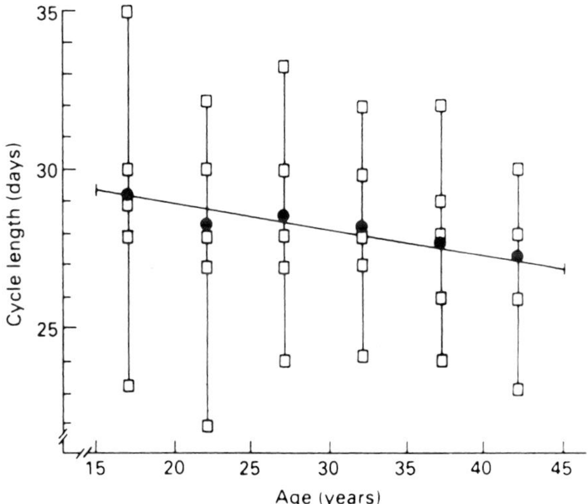

Fig. 10.2 Usual menstrual cycle length in 1988 by age. The mean (●) and the 5th, 25th, 50th, 75th and 95th centile values are shown (□). Regression line ($r = 0.23$, $P = 0.0001$).[2]

bleeding in ovulatory cycles was between 2–12 days (mean 4.6±1.3 days) with the heaviest flow on day 2. Women over 35 years bleed 0.5 days less than younger women and appear to have lighter flow. After menarche and before menopause, menstrual periods are more frequently disturbed with perimenopausal women experiencing heavier periods. Cycles following a recent pregnancy are also considerably different compared to the standard population-based models.

The luteal phase is more consistent than the follicular phase. Lenton et al[4] indicated that follicular phase length was significantly decreased from a mean of 14 days to less than 11 days in women of age 40–44 years compared with those of 18–24 years. When the luteal phase was defined as the days following but not including the LH peak up to the day before the onset of menstruation, approximately 5% of cycles revealed an abnormally short luteal phase of less than 9 days with a normal luteal phase duration of 14 days (95% CI 11–17 days). In all cycles where the follicular phase was less than 9 days the endocrinology of the luteal phase was assessed as abnormal, whereas only 22% of those luteal phases of 11 days and 2% of those of 12 days were assessed as abnormal.[5] Sherman and Korenman[6] have shown that a shorter follicular phase occurs in perimenopausal women associated with a shorter average menstrual cycle. These observations are not universally accepted: others have demonstrated that there was no difference in the mean cycle length in different age groups although older women displayed a prolonged follicular phase attributable to a reduced growth rate of the dominant follicle and an increased time taken from the onset of menses until the selection of the dominant follicle.[7]

While age is clearly a major determinant of menstrual variability, geographical and ethnic differences may play an important role in the length of the cycle. The biological variability may relate to weight, diet and physical exercise. There is a suggestion of an increased cycle length variation in lower socio-economic groups with a correlation between lower educational status and longer cycle lengths[8] although this could be influenced by nutrition and stress in disadvantaged groups. Weight, diet, physical activity, stress and environmental chemicals are also known to have a significant influence on the endocrine control of the menstrual cycle. Women who are well below their ideal body weight tend to become amenorrheic but resume menstruation when the body mass is restored to normal. Obesity is associated with loss of periods, with weight loss and change in body fat leading to menstruation. Other alleged influences on cycle length include photoperiod, noise and pheromones.

Cervical mucus

Following menstruation the mucus is thick, opaque and of minimal quantity. Secretion increases in the follicular phase and a peak is obtained shortly before ovulation. The quality of the mucus also changes, becoming thin and watery with spinnbarkeit demonstrable. When dried and examined under the light microscope, preovular mucus also exhibits arborization (ferning). The nature of mucus quickly changes and again becomes thick with lack of ferning during the secretory phase of the cycle. The thinning and alteration of mucus quality near ovulation permits spermatozoa to pass through the cervix in the most fertile time of the menstrual cycle. The increased sodium chloride content contributes to the ferning effect while increased secretion of estrogen in the follicular phase alters cervical vascularity and edema. The increase in cervical mucus may be as much as 10–20 times that of the early follicular phase. At the time of ovulation the external cervical os is seen to be patulous with a diameter often in excess of 3 mm. Cervical mucus assessment and cervical dilatation are useful clinical indicators of estrogen status and the stage of the menstrual cycle. There is little or no data on age or weight-related changes in cervical mucus.

Vaginal changes

The histological changes of the vaginal epithelium are like those of the cervix, also useful as indicators of the estrogen status. Infection of the vagina may however alter the reliability of both these factors and should be excluded. Exfoliative cytology of the vaginal epithelium along with simple observation demonstrates the changes of the menstrual cycle. Early in the follicular phase the epithelium of the vagina is thin and pale when low circulating estrogen levels are present. The epithelium thickens in direct response to the rising estrogen levels and there is an increase in the mature cornified epithelial cells. The early pallor changes to a more dusky appearance. With maximum estrogen levels, large numbers of superficial cells exfoliate and a vaginal smear stains pink with Papanicolaou at this time. In the luteal phase the number of superficial cells decreases and progesterone induces an increase in the intermediate epithelial cells and polymorphonuclear cells. A vaginal smear at this time may stain either pink or blue with Papanicolaou stain.

Temperature changes

A thermal shift from the basal temperature by at least 0.3°C is established on day +2 following the LH peak in almost all ovular women and is sustained for at least 11 days. Although basal body temperature is useful to indicate the approximate time of ovulation and permits assessment of the follicular and luteal phase length, the relationship between temperature, the LH peak and ovulation varies.[9] Alterations in temperature were previously attributed to alterations in progesterone concentration but more recent theories have suggested that the changes in luteal phase interleukin 1β and tumor necrosis factor are more important. Pregnancy, visualization of the ovarian stigma at laparoscopy or collapse of the follicle on ultrasound provide reliable evidence of ovulation.

Mittelschmerz

Women may report midcycle pain. Ultrasound studies have indicated that this pain is best described as preovulation pain and is reported several hours prior to the anticipated ovulation. Ultrasound and laparoscopic studies confirm the presence of the dominant follicle on the side of the pain. Local peritonism due to the loss of blood, ovulation or leakage from the early corpus luteum may also produce subsequent abdominal discomfort.[5,10,11]

Fecundity ranges and ovulation

One method of assessing changes in reproductive physiology across the lifetime of a woman is the study of fecundity (the biological capacity for reproduction) or fertility (the actual production of offspring). Several publications have described age-related changes in fertility in populations not using birth control methods, showing marked decreases in fertility as women get older.[12] Fecundity is more useful to examine the true reproductive potential and reflects a woman's ability to conceive as well as her ability to sustain the pregnancy to viability. Apparent fecundability decreases from 22 years of age, but much of this change may be due to decreased coital frequency. Figure 10.3 shows the variation in pregnancy rates where 2193 donor sperm cycles were used in which insemination was similar between different ages. Cumulative pregnancy rates were consistently lower in women aged 31–35 years than in women aged 30 or less, and sharply lower in women over 35. These differences indicate age-related changes in the reproductive physiology of the women involved. Figure 10.4 reflects the true effects of age on fecundability. Evidence from *in vitro* fertilization cycles where similar numbers of oocytes and embryos can be replaced in women of differing ages suggests an oocyte

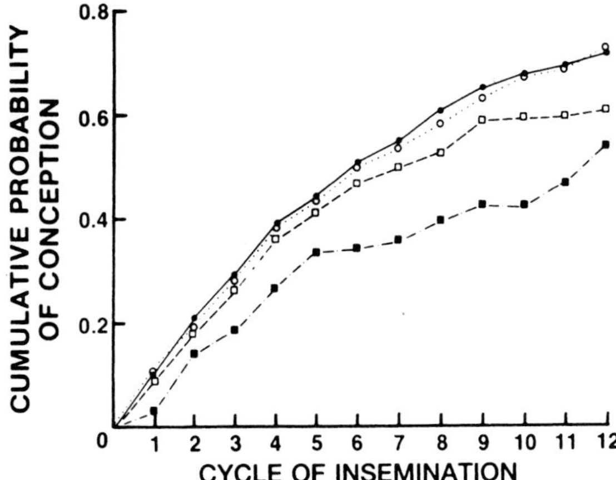

Fig. 10.3 Cumulative pregnancy rates following artificial insemination with donor sperm in four age groups of French women: ≤25 years (●), 26–30 years (○), 31–35 years (□), and ≥36 years (■).[12]

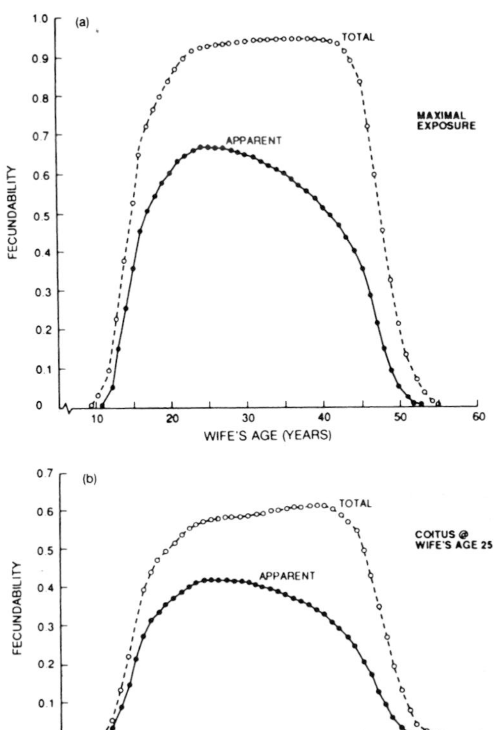

Fig. 10.4 Model predictions of age-specific total and apparent fecundability when coital frequency is held constant and parameters of female reproductive physiology are allowed to vary. (a) Maximal exposure or daily intercourse. (b) Coital frequency held constant at the level observed in married US women age 25.[12]

aging factor as the predominant mechanism of this loss of fecundability. The use of donor oocytes from young women implanted into women who are over 40 years confirms this suggestion, although there is some evidence of a partial endometrial factor contributing to age-related infertility.

Anatomical

Ovary

The primordial germ cells arise in the endoderm of the embryo and migrate to the genital ridge. At the 5th week of gestation mitotic activity is evident in the oogonia although the gonads remain undifferentiated until the 7th week of fetal life, following which time the primitive ovary can be differentiated from the testis. During this period intense mitotic activity increases the number of oogonia to over several million cells and meiotic division and concurrent apoptosis begins. Steroidogenesis in the ovary commences with oogonia evident in the developing ovarian cortex by week 8 of fetal development. There is development of primary oocytes with the maximal number of germ cells peaking at approximately 7 million at the 5th—6th month of gestation. From midgestation a rapid and massive loss of germ cells leaves fewer than 1–2 million cells at birth. Atresia continues throughout childhood and approximately 400 000 oocytes are present at the time of menarche. Only a few remain at menopause. The physiological causes are unknown although the processes of apoptosis are likely to be the underlying final event. The rate of atresia is increased in individuals when they are 45X karyotype so that often only a streak ovary remains at birth.

Meiosis commences following the completion of oogonia formation, halts at the first reduction division of the diplotene stage and does not resume until the time of onset of ovulation. The arrested primordial follicles comprise of a single layer of granulosa cells, a basement membrane separating the follicle from the interstitial tissue and the primary oocyte arrested at the pachytene step of the diplotene stage.

Uterus

The endometrium undergoes histological changes in the follicular, ovulation and luteal phases of the menstrual cycle. As the corpus luteum regresses and progesterone secretion decreases, menstrual bleeding occurs. Only the basal layer remains after menstruation and the endometrium is thin. The superficial layer of compact epithelial cells and spongiosa intermediate layer respond to the increased estrogen secretion during the follicular phase. In this proliferative phase the endometrial glands develop from the straight and narrow glands within the compact stroma. All elements of endometrium respond to estrogen; however the glands remain straight but become longer and the epithelial cells become tall and columnar. Basal nuclei appear and there is an increase in the total number of stromal cells. Infiltration of blood vessels occurs as stromal cells become loosely packed and with rising progesterone secretion the follicular endometrium becomes a secretory luteal phase pattern. The glands become tortuous and convoluted and the epithelial cell lining changes, with the basal nuclei moving towards the centre and the formation of subnuclear vacuoles. The lumina of the glands secrete a glycogen rich fluid with dilatation evident at day 24 of a 28 day cycle. The further increase in stromal gland size completes the edematous histological appearance. The spiral endometrial arterioles become more coiled with each day of the luteal phase. With regression of the corpus luteum the endometrium is no longer maintained and constriction of the spiral arteries occurs. Necrosis, bleeding and shedding of the endometrium ensues. The deeper basal layer remains and the cycle begins again.

Breasts

In utero transplacental estrogens interact with the rudimentary epithelial-stromal unit to induce duct penetration into the fat pad of the breast. Ductal elongation and branching occurs during puberty under the influence of estrogen, growth hormone, oxytocin and paracrine factors. Estrogen-dependent stem cells give rise to both epithelial and myoepithelial cells. During pregnancy lobuloalveolar differentiation is the final stage of breast development necessary for lactation. Several placental and maternal hormones and regulating factors are involved.

Menstrual cycle changes reflect these physiological responses to a much lesser degree. During the luteal phase proliferation of the mammary epithelial cells occurs in response to the increase in progesterone in the presence of estrogen. Secretion onto the alveoli and ductal lumen also occurs. Apoptosis follows during the follicular phase.[13] The above changes along with vascular and lymphatic congestion may result in a 20% increase in breast volume during the luteal phase. This volume increase combined with increased skin sensitivity prior to menstruation is responsible for luteal phase breast discomfort. Premenstrual breast engorgement decreases with the fall in progesterone levels.[14]

Endocrine and immune system

Blood

Hormonal events alter on a daily basis throughout the menstrual cycle as measured by the principal hormones detected in the peripheral circulation: LH and FSH from within the gonadotrope in the anterior pituitary gland, the two principal ovarian steroids 17β estradiol (E_2) and progesterone (P) and the circulating ovarian protein inhibin (INH) from the granulosa cells. Although they are not usually measured clinically, other hormones show menstrual cyclicity, including ovarian androgens, estrone and 17 hydroxy progesterone. The rise in FSH occurs in the late luteal phase and the early follicular phase and leads to the recruitment of gonadotropin dependent follicles. The midfollicular decrease in FSH coincides with the process of single follicle selection whereby only the largest follicle has developed sufficient FSH receptors to survive the decrease in circulating bioactive gonadotropin. The neuroendocrine events of the menstrual cycle are difficult to assess by simple methods. Rises in estradiol and inhibin concentrations reflect the increasing size and function of the dominant follicle and are useful clinical markers for monitoring spontaneous or induced ovulation. A protein known as gonadotropin surge attenuating factor (GnSAF) also changes to allow alterations in hypothalmic pituitary function. At a size of 18 mm or more, the leading follicle is able to produce E_2 at a level and rate of change that triggers a massive and immediate release of LH known as the ovulatory gonadotropin surge. The endocrine events that occur in the follicle and corpus luteum are described in chapter 7.

E_2 arises in the granulosa layer from the aromatization of androgenic precursors derived from the thecal cells from developing follicles in the follicular phase and luteinized granulosa cells in the corpus luteum. Small amounts of progesterone are also secreted by the developing follicle and administration of antiprogesterone agents such as mefipristone prevents ovulation. Progesterone is produced maximally when the corpus luteum is well developed in the midluteal phase. The pattern of progesterone and estradiol secretion in the luteal phase reflects the lifespan of the corpus luteum. The major endocrine events of the menstrual cycle are reflected in the circulating hormone concentrations as shown in Fig. 10.1.

Urine

The important changes in blood hormones can also be detected in the urine using either 24 hour urine collections or early morning specimens. Total urinary estrogen measurements reflect estrogen conjugates such as glucuronides and sulphates while progesterone activity is best reflected by pregnanediol concentrations.

Metcalf et al[15] used urinary hormones to study the effects of age distinct from approaching menopause. Luteal phase lengths were equal in young and older women although absolute levels tended to be lower in women 40–55 years. They also demonstrated that anovulation was common in young women (12–17 years, 43–60% and over the age of 40 years, 12–15%). Urinary FSH and LH can also be detected readily although two site immunoassays are preferred to eliminate the detection of biologically inactive subunits and fragments. These urinary assays are relatively simple, available as kits and are valuable for daily sampling which cannot be obtained easily from clinical populations. Urine hormones reflect those in the blood and hence will show prolonged cycles at the extremes of reproductive life, such as at puberty and perimenopause.

Saliva

The above benefits for urine samples also apply to saliva, although specimen collection may not always be as easy as implied. The detection of LH and FSH in saliva is much more questionable. This method of assessing the cycle has not achieved widespread acceptance but is particularly useful for long-term or population studies of sex steroid levels. For example, Vuorento and Huhtaniemi[16] have studied the effects of adolescence on the luteal phase characteristics in a population of Finnish girls by measuring daily salivary progesterone. Compared to a mature fertile control population, they showed that between a third and a quarter of all cycles were anovulatory in young teenagers while luteal phase length tended to be shorter and the percentage of girls not achieving the range of peak progesterone values were greater in the younger women. This type of data emphasize the time required for reproductive maturity to be achieved following menarche. There have been similar studies comparing reproductive maturity in adolescents of different ethnic and cultural background, investigating whether early or late onset of menarche is involved in the prevalence of various endocrine-related disorders such as breast cancer.

Immune function

Immune responsiveness differs considerably between females and males in many species, including humans. Women have higher plasma IgM levels than men and this becomes significant at puberty when estrogen concentrations increase. Autoimmune disease is more common in women and these diseases are modulated by gonadal steroids. Estrogen and progestogens have marked effects on immune cell function *in vitro* and immune cells play an important role in the cyclical changes on the female genital tract. For instance, there are dramatic influxes of leucocytes into the ovary at the time of ovulation and into the uterus at menstruation. While many studies do not show differences in circulating immune cells throughout the menstrual cycle, larger investigations have suggested that certain T-lymphocyte subsets are inversely correlated with estrogen levels with the lowest counts just prior to ovulation. Secreted adhesion molecules such as intercellular adhesion molecules fluctuate throughout the cycle and there are documented variations in cytokines such as interleukin 1, tumor necrosis factor and granulocyte macrophage colony stimulating factor.

Ultrasound

Ultrasonography of the reproductive organs has been studied for more than two decades initially with transabdominal transducers and more recently with transvaginal assessment. Detail of the normal cyclic changes of the uterus, the endometrium and ovaries are all well documented. The uterus can be examined in the longitudinal plane to demonstrate the depth of the uterus and the endometrial thickness defined as the interface from the anterior junction between the endometrium and myometrium to the posterior junction (this represents both layers of the endometrium). The volume of the ovaries, follicles and the uterus may also be calculated. Such measurements can be made serially throughout the menstrual cycle and correlated to the hormonal events.

Uterine

The correlation between endometrial thickness on ultrasound and serum estradiol concentration is variable due to a wide variation in the serum E_2 concentrations in the late follicular phase. Although the total uterine volume increases during a menstrual cycle there is little clinical utility in this measurement and as it correlates well with endometrial thickness, the latter is the easier and more clinically useful parameter. The appearances of the endometrial ultrasound begin as a thin linear echo in the central position of the uterus from day one until seven days prior to the LH surge of the menstrual cycle. The growth of endometrial thickness is regular from seven days prior to ovulation (Fig. 10.5). From six days prior to the LH surge the linear echogenic pattern changes with the appearance of three hyperechogenic lines separated by two hypoechogenic layers. It is at this stage that the endometrial thickness is usually 7 mm. From five days prior to LH surge through to two days prior to the LH surge the hypoechogenic layers gradually increase in thickness and coincide with the increase in serum estradiol concentration. The mean thickness of the endometrium increases from 7–11 mm and the leading follicle increases from the mean of 11–18 mm diameter. At the time of ovulation, three lines of reflectivity are distinct in the endometrium with a mean thickness of 12 mm. Following ovulation there is further increase in the echogenicity of two endometrial layers but without further increase in the endometrial thickness. By seven days following the LH surge peak the two central endometrial layers have increased in hypoechogenicity to a degree that the three hypoechogenic lines are barely visible and the endometrial thickness remains constant. The endometrial thickness is greater both on the day of ovulation and in the midluteal phase in older aged women with regular menstrual cycles (2–3 mm greater in women aged 37–45 compared to those 21–25 years (Fig. 10.6)).

The above descriptions correspond to the development of estrogen-induced proliferation of the endometrium. The hypoechogenic layers correspond to the proliferation of endometrial stroma with loose connective tissue glands and vessels. The three echogenic lines are thought to represent the

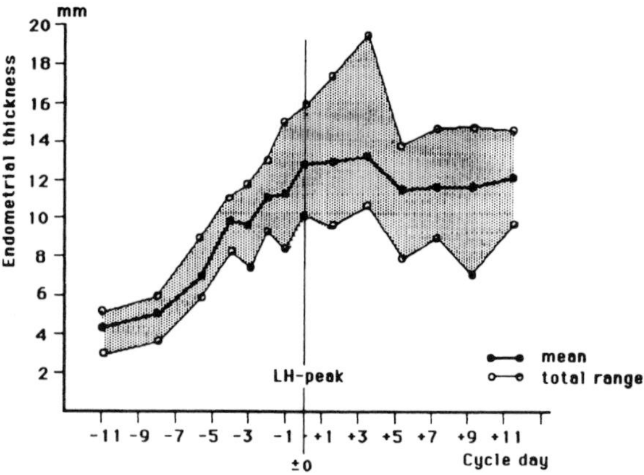

Fig. 10.5 The endometrial thickness (mm) measured by transvaginal ultrasound, presented as the mean and the total range, in 16 women during an ovulatory cycle. Each point on the curve represents a minimum of six observations.[17]

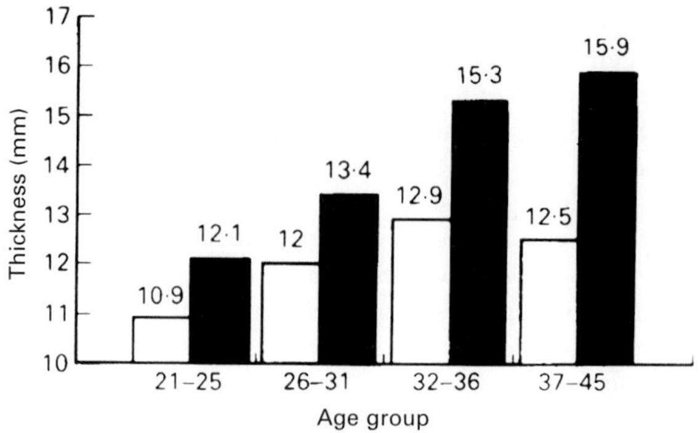

Fig. 10.6 Maximum luteal phase endometrial thickness and the endometrial thickness on the day of ovulation in women of different ages.[7]

myoendometrial borders in the luminal surfaces of the two opposing endometrial surfaces with a narrow uterine cavity intervening. In the postovulatory phase progesterone induced changes of the endometrium are characterized ultrasonographically by the increased echogenicity associated with the increased density of the endometrial layers and increased secretory activity in the glands along with increased vascularity of the stroma. There has been some disagreement amongst investigators as to whether the maximum endometrial thickness is reached at ovulation with subsequent thickness maintained or whether further growth occurs until the midluteal phase. Histologically the endometrial height is roughly that of the preovulatory phase of the cycle.

It has been suggested that the texture and thickness of the endometrium is of prognostic value in fertility treatment. Features most predictive are thought to be the thickened endometrium of more than 10 mm with the presence of the three described echogenic lines in the mid part of the menstrual cycle. These are in fact the findings seen in natural menstrual cycles and they support the hypothesis that this finding is more conducive for embryo implantation. A negative prognostic value has been suggested for endometrial hypoechogenicity prior to ovulation. This has not been observed consistently in normal menstrual cycles.[17]

Ovarian

The follicular growth pattern was described early in the 1980s and remains one of the reliable indicators of a normal menstrual cycle.[17,18] The dominant follicle at the time of ovulation may range from 14–29 mm in diameter, but on the day of the LH peak is usually over 17 mm in diameter. There is a significant correlation between the diameter of the follicle and the serum estradiol concentration so that either measure can be used in monitoring of a cycle for purposes of infertility investigation, timing of intercourse or planning events during ovarian stimulation for ovulation induction or *in vitro* fertilization.

Ovulation occurs equally between the right and the left ovary and although up to three or four smaller follicles may be evident in the ovary containing the dominant follicle or in the contralateral ovary, the changes in these follicle sizes are less than that observed in the dominant follicle. Once ovulation occurs the loss of the dominant follicles can be demonstrated ultrasonographically within 48 hours, as well as later development of the corpus luteum with its irregular internal echoes.[18] Following ovulation most women have a measurable increase in Pouch of Douglas fluid for up to five days. Fitzgerald[7] confirmed that even in prolonged follicular phase cycles in older women there was no difference in the mean follicular growth rate assessed on ultrasound during the three days prior to ovulation, although there was a significant reduction in the mean follicular diameter recorded prior to ovulation in women in the 37–45 year age group. This was in spite of equivalent estradiol levels compared to those with younger women.

Doppler blood flow

Pulsed-color Doppler ultrasonography has increased the capabilities of transvaginal ultrasonography to assess the hormonal effects on the endometrium and correlate these with vascular flow of the uterine arteries. Pulsatility and resistance indices can be calculated using Doppler flow studies and these parameters fluctuate across the menstrual cycle reflecting the expected increases in flow and reduced resistance to blood flow to the developing follicle and the newly derived corpus luteum. The pulsatility index is much lower on the side of the ovary bearing the developing corpus luteum, suggesting reduced downstream impedance or increased blood flow. In the uterus, the suggestion has been made that Doppler predicts the chances of successful implantation during assisted reproduction. While this technology holds much promise for the assessment of blood flow patterns, there does not appear to be a good correlation with peripheral hormone measurements.

Guanes et al[19] have studied the effect of age on color Doppler ultrasound and did not find any alteration in older compared to younger women.

Psychological and neurological

Libido

There is unresolved controversy regarding the possibility of changes in libido, frequency of intercourse and sexual arousal across the menstrual cycle. Increased activity and libido have been described in the preovulatory period but have not been confirmed in all studies. The relationship of sexual interest and activity to the secretion of androgens also remains unresolved. Testosterone tends to be higher in the late follicular phase but does not show marked variations throughout the cycle. More convincing evidence is emerging of a 'testosterone deficiency syndrome' in the peri- and postmenopausal stages of life. Various publications[20,21] have proposed the view that response to androgens indicates that androgens are important in sexuality and general health of women before and after the menopause. Emotional and environmental situations are also extremely important in determining the intensity and enthusiasm for erotic involvement.

Weight, stress and exercise

Many anovulatory patients provide a history of emotional or work related stress and the physiological response may be a result of altered hypothalamic endorphins or other neurotransmitters. Exercise can also induce hypothalamic amenorrhea, especially in those women who participate in athletics, gymnastics or ballet. In some cases the onset of menarche can be delayed by as much as 2–3 years. However the return of the menstrual cycle and progression of pubertal stages coincides with periods of rest or reduction of activities. The higher the levels of activities that are combined with a lower body weight (less than 20% body fat or 10% below ideal body weight) the more the likelihood of menstrual cycle irregularity. Swimmers and cyclists have lower rates of irregularity despite similar training intensities. The additional stress of competition may also contribute as the incidence of amenorrhea is significantly higher in competitive athletes compared to the other participants with similar activity levels in noncompetitive sports. Endocrine abnormalities occurring include prolonged menstrual cycles, loss of the LH surge, luteal phase dysfunction or amenorrhea. A significant risk of osteopenia or reduction in bone density may result in stress fractures. Gonadotropin secretion in patients with bulimia and anorexia nervosa is similar to that in other forms of hypothalamic amenorrhea. However with recovery to a normal body weight as many as 30% of previously anorexic patients remain anovulatory.[22]

A study of 166 women aged 17–19 years showed active dieting to lose weight reduced the total duration of menstrual bleeding by approximately half a day compared to those already at a low weight adjusted for height. Those who did little or no exercise had a slightly longer duration of menstrual bleeding by about half a day.[1] Measurements of body dimensions and relationships with subcutaneous fat tissue showed a mild influence of body type on the length and regularity of the menstrual cycle.[23]

Physiological alterations through life

Neonatal

Some vaginal discharge or frank bleeding may occur within days of birth as high estrogen concentrations in the neonate are cleared and the hyperplastic endometrium is shed. Any further bleeding in the neonate or young child is pathological and needs investigation. LH, FSH and E_2 levels tend to be very low in children until rising concentrations of the gonadotropins herald the start of puberty.

Puberty

Final maturation of ovarian follicles only commences during puberty under the influence of FSH and LH which regulate follicular development. When puberty nears, the GnRH pulse generator activity increases, initially at night in association with sleep. The first sign of this increase is seen in the LH immunoactivity in urine voided in the morning (Fig. 10.7). The resulting increase in estrogen secretion around the age of nine years promotes further increase of the pulsatile release of LH with eventual ovulation and subsequent menarche. Following this initial ovulation the gonadotropin concentrations are similar during both day and night time with adult values. Ovarian function is also controlled by several peptide and protein hormones and growth factors produced within the

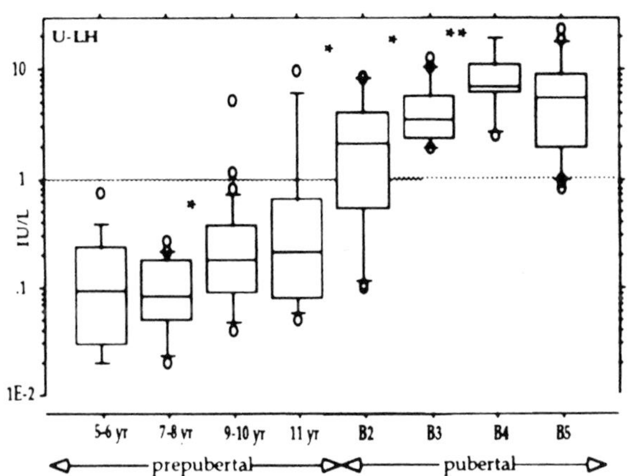

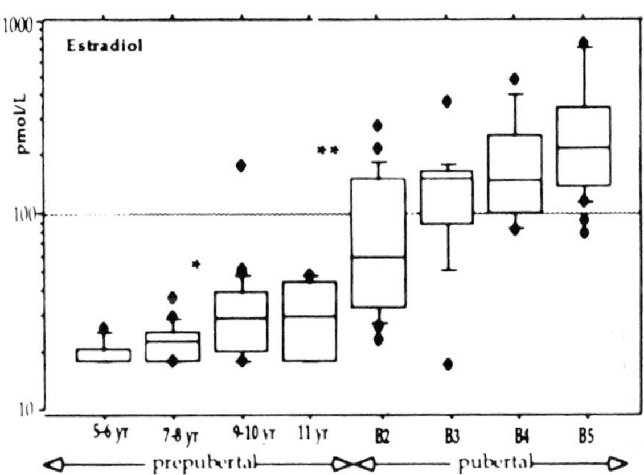

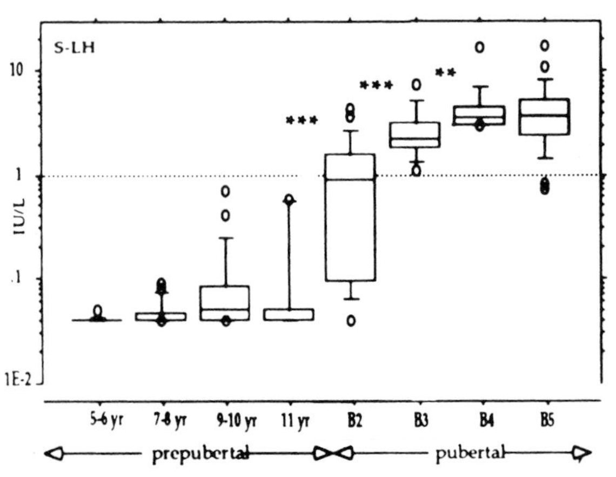

Fig. 10.7 Distribution pattern of urinary and serum LH and estradiol levels in female children from all pubertal stages; subjects (prepubertal) were divided into five age groups. The lines within the boxes show the median values (the 50th percentiles). The lower and upper limits of the boxes correspond to the 25th and 75th percentiles, whereas the notches represent the 10th and 90th percentiles. Outliers are separately plotted. Asterisks denote statistically significant differences between hormone levels in consecutive age groups or pubertal stages. *, $P<0.05$; **, $P<0.01$; ***, $P<0.001$; blank, not significant. (From Demir A, Voutilainen R, Juul A et al 1996 Increase in first morning voided urinary luteinizing hormone levels precedes the physical onset of puberty. Journal of Clinical Endocrinology and Metabolism 81(8): 2963–2967.)

ovary: the effect of changing age and sex steroids on these introvarian regulators is not known. Well described physical and anatomic changes of puberty occur, usually classified as described by the Tanner scale. The first changes are evident in young girls aged 10–11 years and follow the increase in adrenal androgens from approximately 6–8 years of age and the appearance of pubic and axillary hair (Fig. 10.8).

The age of menarche is determined by general health, genetic, socio-economic and nutritional factors. There has been a decrease in the mean age of menarche at a rate of four months per decade over the last 100 years in the United States, generally attributable to alteration in nutritional status. There appears to be a critical combination of weight, body water and body fat required for the hypothalamic response that leads to gonadotropin increased secretion. The critical weight is thought to be around 48 kg and this is supported by the earlier menarche observed in obese girls. Chronic disease, malnutrition and high levels of activity observed in athletes and dancers have been noted to delay menarche. For the first few years after menarche menstrual cycles are often irregular due to anovulation.

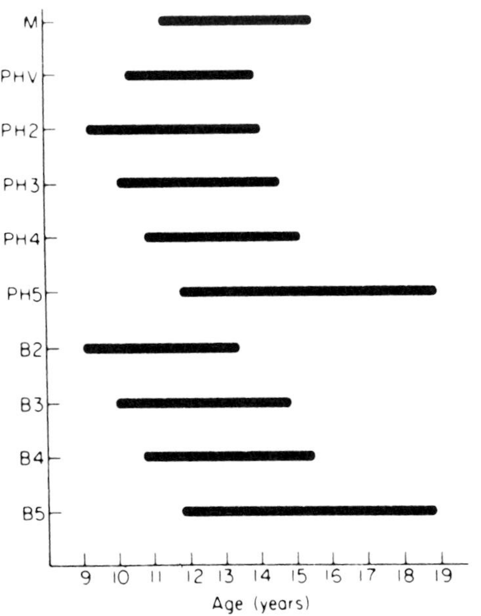

Fig. 10.8 Range of ages within which Western European girls reach various stages of puberty. M = menarche; PHV = peak height velocity; PH2, PH3, etc. = pubic hair stages; B2, B3, etc. = breast stages. (From Dewhurst J, de Swiet M, Chamberlain GVP (eds) 1986 Basic science in obstetrics and gynaecology: a textbook for MRCOG Part 1. Churchill Livingstone, Edinburgh, p 179).

The course of puberty can be disturbed in true precocious puberty, where the normal sequence of pubertal development occurs, but at an early age with an increased secretion of gonadotropins and ovulatory menstrual cycles. In precocious pseudopuberty there is increased estrogen formation with subsequent feminization without ovulation, although there may be intermittent menstrual bleeding. Estrogen secreting tumors or androgen secreting tumors (with subsequent conversion of estrogens at extra glandular sites) occur. Breast budding prior to the age of eight without accompanying estrogen secretion or premature bone maturation is likely to be due to temporary increase in the sensitivity to circulating estrogens or temporary increase in estrogen secretion. Premature adrenarche or pubarche in isolation without any other pubertal secondary sexual development with normal adrenal androgen levels may also occur, and like premature thelarche is self limiting. The assessment of sexual precociousness involves a careful history and physical examination and may include the determination of bone age and assessment of long bone epiphyses, and a thorough work-up to exclude serious or treatable causes.

Pregnancy

The onset of pregnancy results in sustained high concentrations of progesterone initially and later very high levels of estradiol. This suppresses ovulation and amenorrhea is the norm for pregnancy. FSH and LH secretion is suppressed to low levels from the time of implantation (see ch. 22).

Postpartum

Initially the hypothalmic-pituitary-ovarian axis remains suppressed as a result of the changes in pregnancy. In the absence of prolonged lactation, the first menstrual cycle returns within a few weeks and ovulation occurs within months (Fig. 10.9). Breast feeding allows for high prolactin values to be sustained as a result of suckling and nipple stimulation and this delays the recovery of the pulsatile secretion of GnRH and consequentially FSH and LH. The degree of breast feeding and avoidance of supplementary feeding of the baby determines the return of cyclical ovarian activity and hence, fertility.[24] Interpregnancy birth intervals in populations not using modern birth control methods are largely determined by lactation habits and breast feeding remains the single most important regulator of fertility today. These issues are fully addressed in chapter 23.

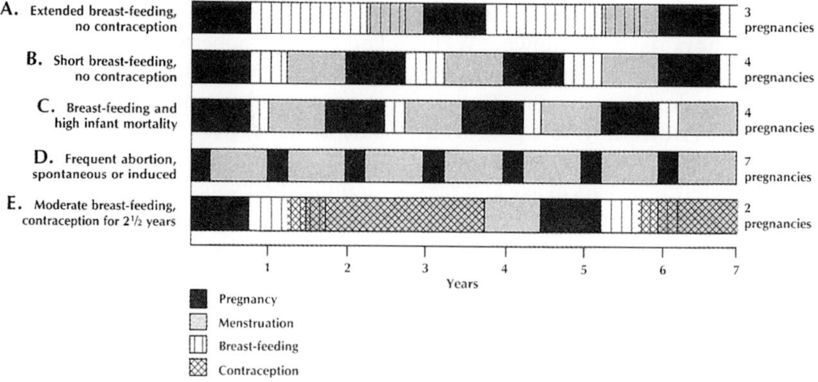

Fig. 10.9 The bars illustrate different patterns of breast feeding and contraception and their impact on fertility. Model A depicts a traditional society without contraception, where breast feeding lasts for two years and postpartum amenorrhea for 18 months; as a result about three pregnancies occur in seven years. In model B, with much shorter breast feeding, and model C, with high infant mortality, the interval between pregnancies is shorter and about four pregnancies occur in seven years. Frequent abortion, whether spontaneous or induced, means as many as seven pregnancies in seven years (model D). In model E, where breast feeding lasts 18 months and contraception begins at six months and lasts for 30 months, about two pregnancies would occur in seven years, with an interval of three and a half years between them. Too many pregnancies, closely spaced, can be harmful to maternal and child health. (From Breast feeding, fertility and family planning. Population Reports 1981; 1(24): J-541.)

Perimenopausal

Menopause is defined as the final episode of menstrual bleeding and has often been used synonymously with the climacteric, which more properly describes the transition from ovulatory menstrual cycles to beyond the last episode of menstrual bleeding. The climacteric represents a progressive loss of ovarian function, endocrine somatic and psychological changes. The median age of menopause is 50–51 years; preceding the menopause the path of menstrual cycles is variable but the interval between menses becomes longer. The postmenopausal ovaries reduce in size with only interstitial (stromal cells) evident histologically. As the ovaries become fibrous the uterus and tubes shrink and the body of the uterus reduces to a greater extent than the cervix. The ratio of the body to cervix may reduce to 1:1 or even smaller. As the vaginal epithelium contains glycogen and lactic acid is no longer produced, the vaginal pH becomes alkaline. Most of these changes can be reversed by therapeutic estrogen administration.

The striking endocrine changes associated with the perimenopause and menopause have been described in detail in chapter 48, Reame et al[25] and Klein et al[26] have all studied groups of women through the menopausal transition and have demonstrated great variability in endocrine patterns with early perimenopausal changes in perimenstrual FSH secretion and LH pulsatility throughout the cycle while estradiol secretion is initially maintained (Figs 10.10, 10.11). The endocrine changes became more pronounced when menstrual cycles became irregular.

Serum levels of testosterone are marginally less in the postmenopausal woman, with production rates decreasing from 200 μg to 150 μg per day. Serum androstenedione also falls following the menopause; extraglandular (mainly adipose tissue) estrogen formation is the major pathway of estrogen synthesis as estradiol synthesis reduces to very low levels and estrone becomes the principal estrogen. The climacteric symptoms of vasomotor instability (hot flashes), atrophy of urogenital epithelium and dermis may ensue as a consequence of estradiol withdrawal. Reduction in breast tissue and osteoporosis are common as a later effect.

Endometrial urogenital epithelial and vaginal mucosal histological changes are observed predominantly as a thinning and atrophy. Reduced circulating estrogen significantly reduces bone mineralization and absorption. At this time there is an increase in the urinary calcium:creatinine ratio and phosphate:creatinine ratio. With the subsequent cardiovascular changes, all lipid levels rise, with only a minimal increase in the protective HDL cholesterol. The development of osteoporosis is multifactorial with

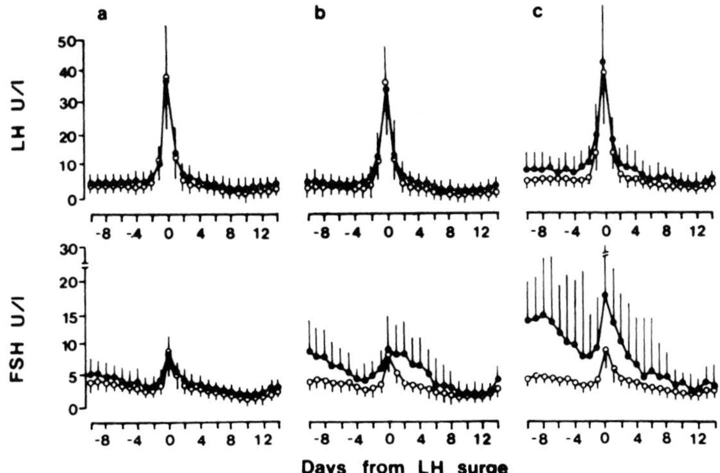

Fig. 10.10 Comparison of the daily geometric mean concentrations of LH and FSH (with 68% confidence intervals) in 41 women aged 24–35 years (○—○, the control group, profiles repeated in each section) with (a) 19 women aged 36–40 years; (b) 18 women aged 41–45 years, and (c) 16 women aged 46–50 years (all shown as ●-●). (From Lee SJ, Lenton EA, Sexton L, Cooke ID 1988. The effect of age on the cyclical patterns of plasma LH, FSH, oestradiol and progesterone in women with regular menstrual cycles. Human Reproduction 3(7): 851–855.)

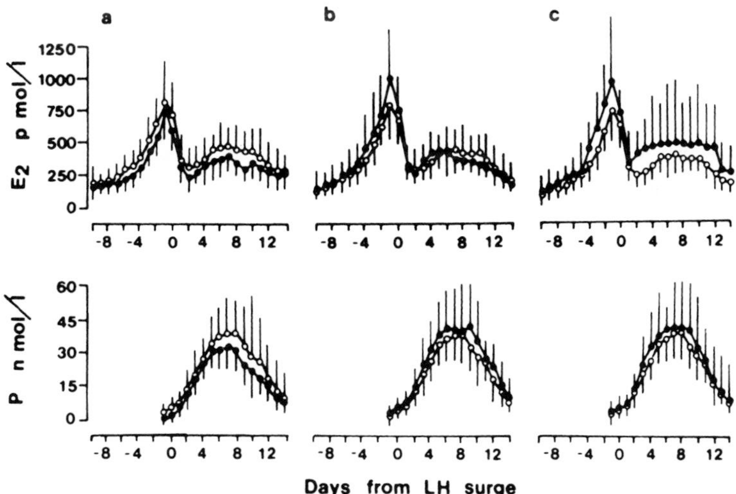

Fig. 10.11 Comparison of the daily geometric mean concentrations of estradiol (E_2) and progesterone (P) (with 69% confidence intervals) in 41 women aged 24–35 years (○—○, the control group, profiles repeated in each section) with (a) 19 women aged 36–40 years; (b) 18 women aged 41–45 years and (c) 16 women aged 46–50 years (all shown as ●—●). (From Lee SJ, Lenton EA, Sexton L, Cooke ID 1988. The effect of age on the cyclical patterns of plasma LH, FSH, oestradiol and progesterone in women with regular menstrual cycles. Human Reproduction 3(7): 851–855.)

calcium intake, smoking and general activity all contributing. However, the estrogen deprivation resulting from premature ovarian failure or bilateral oophorectomy also leads to the early onset of osteoporosis. Hence there is a close relationship between lower estrogen, circulating estrone levels and a later development of osteoporotic symptoms and signs. Nervousness, irritability, anxiety, sleep disorders and depression or other climacteric symptoms have an indirect relationship to estrogen deprivation.

Conclusion

Anatomical, clinical, biochemical and emotional relationships are heavily dependent not only on the stage of the menstrual cycle at which they are studied, but fluctuate significantly across the lifespan. Apart from several years of childhood and the years that follow cessation of periods at the menopause, the female reproductive system as reflected in the menstrual cycle is always in a stage of change. Clinical and laboratory observations need to reflect this in all interactions and measurements that are carried out.

REFERENCES

1. Harlow SD, Ephross SA 1995 Epidemiology of menstruation and its relevance to women's health. Epidemiologic Reviews 17(2): 265–286
2. Münster K, Schmidt L, Helm P 1992 Length and variation in the menstrual cycle — a cross-sectional study from a Danish county. British Journal of Obstetrics and Gynaecology 99(5): 422–429
3. Matsumoto S, Nogami Y, Ohkuri S 1962 Statistical studies on menstruation: a criticism on the definition of normal menstruation. Gunma Journal of Medical Science 11: 294–318
4. Lenton EA, Landgren BM, Sexton L, Harper R 1984 Normal variation in the length of the follicular phase of the menstrual cycle: effect of chronological age. British Journal of Obstetrics and Gynaecology 91(7): 681–684
5. Lenton EA, Landgren BM, Sexton L 1984 Normal variation in the length of the luteal phase of the menstrual cycle: identification of the short luteal phase. British Journal of Obstetrics and Gynaecology 91(7): 685–689
6. Sherman BM, Korenman SG 1975 Hormonal characteristics of the human menstrual cycle throughout reproductive life. Journal of Clinical Investigation 55: 699–706
7. Fitzgerald CT, Seif MW, Killick SR, Elstein M 1994 Age related changes in the female reproductive cycle. British Journal of Obstetrics and Gynaecology 101(3): 229–233
8. Jeyaseelan L 1993 Correlates of menstrual cycle length in south Indian women: a prospective study. Human Biology 65(4): 627–634
9. Baumann JE 1981 Basal body temperature: unreliable method of ovulation detection. Fertility and Sterility 36(6): 729–733
10. Hann LE, Hall DA, Black EB 1979 Mittelschmerz. Sonograph demonstration. JAMA 241: 2731–2732
11. Marinho AO, Sallam HN, Goessens L, Collins WP, Campbell S 1982 Ovulation side and occurrence of Mittelschmerz in spontaneous and induced ovarian cycles. British Medical Journal 284: 632
12. Wood JW 1989 Fecundity and natural fertility in humans. In: Milligan SR (ed) Oxford review of reproductive biology. Oxford University Press, Oxford; pp 61–109
13. Dickson RB 1996 Biochemical control of breast development. In: Harris JR, Morrow M, Lippman ME, Hellman S (eds) Diseases of the breast. Lippincott Raven, Philadelphia, pp 15–25
14. Brumsted JR, Riddick DH 1990 The endocrinology of the mammary gland. In: Hindle WH (ed) Breast disease for gynecologists. Connecticut, Appleton & Lange, pp 21–28
15. Metcalf M, Skidmore D, Lowry G, Mackenzie J 1983 Incidence of ovulation in the years after the menarche. Journal of Endocrinology 97: 213–219
16. Vuorento T, Huhtaniemi I 1992 Daily levels of salivary progesterone during menstrual cycle in adolescent girls. Fertility and Sterility 58(4): 685–690
17. Bakos O, Lundkvist Ö, Bergh T 1993 Transvaginal sonographic evaluation of endometrial growth and texture in spontaneous ovulatory cycles — a descriptive study. Human Reproduction 8(6): 799–806
18. Kerin JF, Edmonds DK, Warnes GM et al 1981 Morphological and functional relations of Graafian follicle growth to ovulation in women using ultrasonic, laparoscopic and biochemical measurements. British Journal of Obstetrics and Gynaecology 88(2): 81–90
19. Guanes PP, Remohi J, Gallardo E, Valbuena D, Simon C, Pellicer A 1996 Age does not affect uterine resistance to vascular flow in patients undergoing oocyte donation. Fertility and Sterility 66(2): 265–270
20. Davis SR, Burger HG 1996 Androgens and the postmenopausal woman. Journal of Clinical Endocrinology and Metabolism 81: 2759–2763
21. Sands S, Studd J 1995 Exogenous androgens in postmenopausal women. American Journal of Medicine 98: 576–579
22. Liu JH 1995 Hypothalamic-pituitary disorders. In: Keye WR, Chang RJ, Rebar RW, Soules MR (eds) Infertility: evaluation and treatment. Philadelphia, WB Saunders, pp 154–167
23. Kirchengast S 1994 Intercorrelations between menstrual cycle patterns and body dimensions in Austrian women. Journal of Biosocial Science 26(2): 207–216
24. Kennedy KI, Visness CM 1992 Contraceptive efficacy of lactational amenorrhoea. Lancet 339: 227–230
25. Reame NE, Kelche RP, Beitins IZ, Yu MY, Zawacki CM, Padmanabhan V 1996 Age effects of follicle stimulating hormone and pulsatile luteinizing hormone secretion across the menstrual cycle of premenopausal women. Journal of Clinical Endocrinology and Metabolism 81(4): 1512–1518
26. Klein NC, Battaglia DE, Fujimoto VY, Davis GS, Bremner WJ, Soules MR 1996 Reproductive aging: accelerated ovarian follicular development associated with a monotropic follicle stimulating hormone rise in normal older women. Journal of Clinical Endocrinology and Metabolism 81(3): 1038–1045

11. Action of estrogen and progesterone at the cellular level

Sophie Christin-Maitre Nathalie Chabbert-Buffet
Philippe Bouchard

Introduction

The female sex steroid 17β estradiol plays a crucial role in the development of feminine secondary sexual characteristics as well as in the female reproductive cycle, fertility and maintenance of pregnancy. Progesterone is the main luteal hormone. Although the existence of estrogen (ER) and progesterone (PR) receptors has been suggested for more than 30 years, ER and PR were only identified in the 1970s. Since the cloning of the human estrogen receptor cDNA in 1985 and the cloning of the human progesterone receptor cDNA in 1987, a lot has been learned about the molecular details of steroid hormone action. However, many additional steps remain to be elucidated, for instance the activation of the native receptor, the transcriptional activity of the hormone-receptor complex and the role of phosphorylation in these events. A recent striking finding is the existence of ligand-independent steroid effects, the presence of cross-talk and interactions between peptides and steroid receptors, as well as the discovery of a new class of ER (ERβ) which increases the scope of action of estrogens. In this chapter we shall:

1. Describe the structural characteristics of ER and PR
2. Review the cascade of events following hormone binding to its receptor and the transcription of target genes
3. Discuss the different ways by which estradiol and progesterone action can be regulated at a cellular level
4. Describe some of the 'nonclassical pathways of hormone action'
5. Describe the ER and PR mutations reported thus far in mice and men
6. Describe the action of estrogen and progesterone antagonists in the cell which illustrate the role of estradiol and progesterone
7. Report some of the nongenomic steroid effects on the cell membrane and the effect of estradiol on the cell cycle.

ESTROGEN AND PROGESTERONE RECEPTORS

Estrogen and progesterone receptors (ER, PR) are members of a superfamily of related proteins (intracellular receptors) that mediate the nuclear effects of steroid hormones, thyroid hormone and vitamin D.[1] Retinoic acid receptors α, β and γ, retinoid X receptors (RXR), as well as peroxisome proliferator activated receptors (PPARS), have also joined this family. The cloning of such receptors has led to the discovery of many related molecules. However, some members are still 'orphans' in that their ligands are unknown at present.

ER and PR were first identified in the 1970s, despite their existence having been suggested for some time before this.[2] The cloning of the human estrogen receptor (hER) cDNA was reported in 1985,[3] and the cloning of the human progesterone receptor (hPR) cDNA in 1987.[4] The human ER and the chicken PR gene have been characterized: they are both composed of eight exons. As shown in Figure 11.1, the hER molecule is composed of 595 amino acids and the hPR of 769 amino acids for isoform A and 933 for isoform B. Several mRNAs have been described for ER. Six to eight mature cytoplasmic messenger mRNAs have been described for the hPR in breast cancer cell lines. PR and ER both have the specific capability of hormone binding, DNA binding and gene activation. As with many other members of this superfamily, ER and PR are ligand-inducible transcription factors.[5,6]

Functional domains of the receptors

The receptor sequence can be divided into functional domains. As shown in Figure 11.1, these domains have

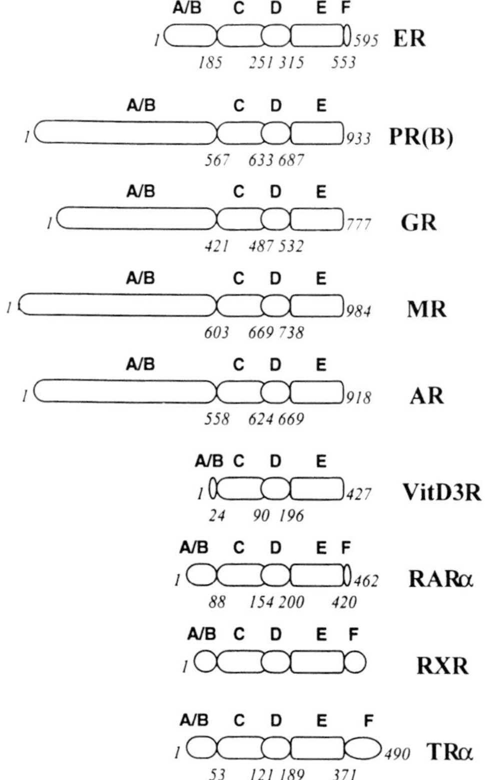

Fig. 11.1 The superfamily of nuclear receptors and the nuclear receptor functional domains A/B (NH2 region), C (DNA binding domain or DBD), D (hinge region), E (ligand binding domain or LBD), F (C terminal region).[9]

been schematically divided into an N terminal region ('A/B region'), a DNA binding domain ('C region'), a hinge region ('D region') and a ligand binding domain ('E region'). Furthermore, ER contains a C terminal region ('F region'). The DNA binding domain and the ligand binding domain exhibit the highest degree of evolutionary conservation.

The ligand binding domain (LBD) is located within the carboxyl terminus of the receptor. In PR, ER, glucocorticoid (GR) and vitamin D receptors, deletion of amino acids from the C terminus, insertional mutations or point mutations result in the loss of hormone binding activity. The LBD is very sensitive to single amino acid mutations anywhere in the region. Therefore, it has not been possible to more closely define the ligand binding domain by site directed mutagenesis. However, deletion of the C terminal portion of PR results in constitutive gene activation *in vivo*. The hypothesis is therefore that the ligand binding domain functions as a repressor of receptor function *in vivo*; hormone binding would reverse this transrepression. To define the role of the hormone binding domain, chimeric proteins were created in which hormone and DNA binding domains from different receptors were exchanged. A hybrid molecule composed of the hGR (glucocorticoid receptor) DNA binding domain and ER LBD behaves in an estrogen-responsive manner. Furthermore, when GR hormone binding domain is attached to the N terminal portion of the same receptor, transcriptional activation remains dependent on dexamethasone. The function of the hormone binding domain is then relatively independent of its position in the protein.

The LBD tridimensional structure of the human nuclear receptor RXR-γ has recently been reported.[7] RARs and RXRs also belong to the nuclear receptor superfamily. RARs are activated by both isomers of retinoic acid, all *trans* (t-RA) and 9 *cis* retinoic acid (9c-RA), whereas only 9c-RA binds to and activates RXRs. A ligand binding pocket has been identified. This would allow 9c-RA to interact with different functional modules. The folding of RXR-αLBD can be described as an antiparallel α-helical sandwich. A search for potential binding pockets for 9c-RA revealed two large hydrophobic cavities. The authors suggest that the three dimensional structure of the RXR LBD could correspond to a prototypic fold with structural modules that appear to be conserved within the nuclear receptor superfamily. The ligand seems to be located deeply inside the LBD folding. More detailed information on the tridimensional structure of ER and PR should be available in the near future.

The DNA binding domain (DBD) is highly conserved among the steroid receptor family.[8] Using PR as a standard for steroid receptors, the degree of identity in this region is 91, 91, 82 and 56% for the glucocorticoid receptor (GR), mineralocorticoid (MR), androgen (AR) and ER, respectively. This domain consists of 66–68 amino acids and includes nine perfectly conserved cysteines. As shown in Figure 11.2, it forms two zinc fingers. Positive identification of zinc in the finger structures was reported for GR using extended x-ray absorption fine structure and visible light spectroscopies. Each finger is composed of four cysteines which coordinate one zinc molecule. Zinc is required for DNA binding *in vitro*. Each of the zinc fingers is encoded by a separate exon of the receptor gene. The loop of the finger consists of 12–13 amino acids, and there is a link region of 15–17 amino acids between the two fingers. Using site-directed mutagenesis, specific amino acids required for DNA binding were identified. Mutants of the chicken progesterone receptor missing either of the two fingers do not bind to DNA *in vitro*. Finger swapping experiments have demonstrated that the amino-

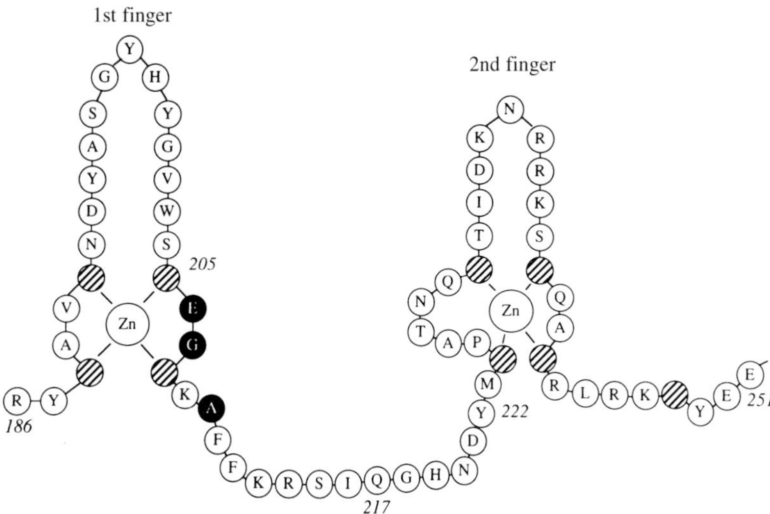

Fig. 11.2 The two human estrogen receptor zinc fingers.[9]

terminal zinc finger determines target gene specificity. Selective mutation of individual amino acids identified the response residues not within the zinc finger, but in the root of the finger. This region has been called P box. In ER, three residues have been identified to be necessary for specific binding of the receptor to DNA. As shown in Figure 11.2, these residues are Glu, Gly and Ala.[9] Furthermore, mutation of a single lysine in this region blocks transcription although it does not interfere with binding. Binding of the receptor to DNA is then a prerequisite of hormone action but is not sufficient for transactivation. The three dimensional structures of the DBD of ER have been determined by nuclear magnetic resonance (NMR), and the structures of the DNA complexes of ER DBD have been determined by x-ray crystallography.[10] The DBD is made of two subdomains, each composed of the motif: zinc domain–helix–extended region. The zinc domain contains the zinc ion, which is coordinated by four cysteine residues. The α-helices start between the third and fourth cysteines in the zinc region and are followed by extended regions.

The amino-terminal region of the receptor is a hypervariable region with low homology between receptors. The epitopes of most antibodies that have been raised against steroid receptors are located in this hypervariable region.

Transactivation sequences

Different regions of steroid receptors have been fused to a reporter gene. After measuring the transcription induced by these constructions, the receptor regions have been called 'Transcription Activating Function' (TAF or AF). As shown in Figure 11.3, three *transactivation sequences* (AF-1, AF-2 and AF-3) have been identified so far. AF-1 has been localized to a 91 amino acid region within the NH2 terminus of PR. AF-2 is contained within the C terminal ligand binding domain. AF-1 and AF-2 surround the DNA binding domain. A third activation domain (AF-3) has been recently identified[11] and is located in the hPR, in the unique N terminal segment of the B isoform. Sartorius et al have constructed a series of hPR expression vectors encoding the B upstream segment (BUS) fused to isolated downstream functional domains of the receptors AF-1 and AF-2.[11] Depending on the promoter of the cell tested, AF-3 can activate transcription autonomously or it can functionally synergize with AF-1 or AF-2. Autonomous AF-3 function can be suspected in hormone-resistant breast cancers and in tissue-specific agonist-like effects of hormone antagonists.

For hER, a mutant deprived of the N terminal region is able to initiate transcription in Hela cells nearly as well as the wild type receptor. On the contrary, a hER mutant lacking a C terminal region has a very low transcriptional activity. Therefore, ER AF-2 is more active than ER AF-1. The N terminal region of ER is less important than the C terminal region to induce transcription, at least in Hela cells. On the contrary, for chicken PR (cPR), the A/B region in the N terminal region is the most important transactivator and acts in synergism with the E region.

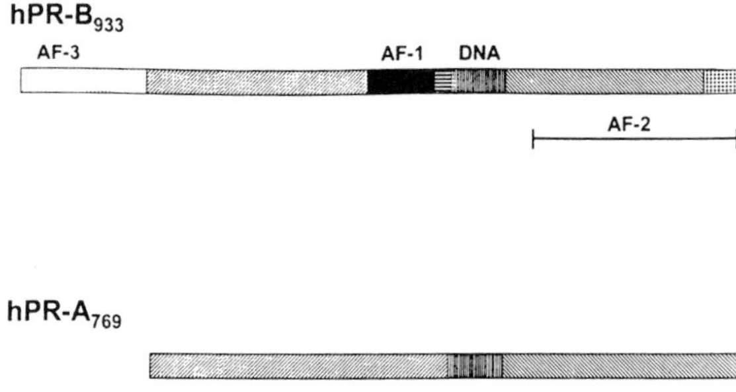

Fig. 11.3 The transactivation domains of the progesterone receptors AF-1, AF-2 and AF-3 which exist in progesterone receptor isoform B.

AF-1 and AF-2 activities vary according to the cell type and the promoter tested.

The F domain of the estrogen receptor

The F domain of the hER is a sizable 42 amino acid C terminal region. Montano et al have described a role for the F domain of the ER in modulating the magnitude of gene transcription by estrogen and antiestrogen, such as trans-hydroxytamoxifen and ICI 164,384.[12] The transcriptional activity of the full-length wild type human ER and ER lacking the F domain (δ F ER) was studied by transient transfection in different cell types. In Chinese hamster ovary (CHO) cells, the antiestrogens were more effective antagonists of E2-stimulated transcription by δ F ER than by wild type ER. By contrast, in Hela cervical cancer cells and 3T3 fibroblasts cells, δ F ER exposed to E2 is much less effective in stimulating transcription than wild type ER. In these cells, antiestrogens are less potent in suppressing E2-stimulated transcription by ER lacking the F domain.

Isoforms of PR

The human progesterone receptor (hPR) occurs as two distinct forms within target cells, hPR-A and hPR-B, of 94 and 114 kD respectively. As shown in Figure 11.3, hPR-B contains a 164 amino acid extension of the N terminal region.[13] hPR-B is 933 amino acids in length. Both forms of PR are derived from a single gene as a consequence of alternate initiation of transcription from distinct promoters. These variants exist in many species except in the rabbit. *In vitro*, hPR-A and hPR-B binding affinities for the hormone or for DNA are identical; however, the biological activity of hPR-A and hPR-B receptors are not. In most cells, hPR-B behaves as a transcriptional activator of progesterone-responsive genes, whereas hPR-A functions as a transcriptional inhibitor of all steroid hormone receptors. McDonnell et al have suggested that transcriptional activation and repression by PR are mediated by two separate pathways within the cell.[14] It thus appears that hPR-A inhibits hER transcriptional activity.[15] In many tissues, the two isoforms of hPR are often found in equimolar amounts. However, primary breast tumor contained a range of PR isoform, in which PRA exceeded hPR-B in 76% of cases. New data suggest that hPR-A to hPR-B ratios are developmentally or hormonally regulated.

Isoforms of ER

ERβ: a novel estrogen receptor

Recently, several groups have reported the identification of a cDNA encoding a separate subtype of ER named ERβ (ERα being the classical ER).[16,17] Rat and human clones were identified from rat prostate and human testis.[18] ERβ has a similar affinity for estradiol as ERα. Most ligands tested have a rather similar relative affinity to both subtypes. Interestingly, plant derived estrogens bind preferentially to ERβ.

Both ERα and ERβ show high conservation of the amino acid sequence in the ligand binding domain. DNA binding domains are identical (they differ by only one amino acid). However, the A/B domains are very different, suggesting different transcriptional activation: ERβ seems to be a weak transactivator. It is present in significant quantity in the ovary, testis and prostate. It is also present in the brain, bone and blood vessels. ERα remains the predominant subtype in the uterus and pituitary. The different ER subtypes remain to be studied. It is also possible that part of the estrogenic effect is mediated through heterodimerization of ERα and ERβ.

Novel isoforms of estrogen receptors have also been identified in vascular smooth muscle cells (VSMC). Reverse transcriptase-polymerase chain reaction using specific primers for rat ER cDNA was performed from RNA of rat VSMC.[19] Three isoforms of ER as well as the wild-type were identified. These ER mRNA isoforms lacked the region corresponding to exon 4, exon 4 and 5, and exon 3 and 4. ER isoform lacking exon 4 and 5 has an inhibitory effect on normal estrogen action when it is cotransfected with the wild-type ER. This isoform could be a potential inhibitor of estrogen action in vascular smooth muscle cells.

CLASSICAL HORMONE-RECEPTOR INTERACTIONS

Nuclear localization

In the absence of hormone, PR and ER are located in the nucleus of target cells. Enucleation experiments and immunohistochemical studies with monoclonal antibodies (mAbs) against ER and PR have revealed that receptor molecules are exclusively located in the nucleus.[20,21,22] On the contrary, the GR and MR seem to be either cytoplasmic or both cytoplasmic and nuclear in the absence of hormone and migrate to the nucleus in the presence of hormone.

ER and PR are synthesized in the cytoplasm and have been shown to shuttle continuously between the nucleus and the cytoplasm. Both nuclear import and export occur through the nuclear pore.

Import of the receptor into the nucleus

Active transport into the nucleus requires nuclear localization signals (NLSs) among the protein. NLSs are short basic sequence motifs, rich in arginines and lysines. The first to be described is the SV40 (Simian Virus) large T-antigen signal. These NLSs are recognized by NLS binding proteins (NBPs) which are intermediates between the protein going into the nucleus and the nuclear pore. NLSs have been identified in the sequence of PR[23,24] and ER.[25] Using subcellular localization of different mutants of rabbit PR (rPR), Guiochon-Mantel et al[24] demonstrated that the main NLS is a stretch of amino acids located in the hinge region around position 638–642. This PR-NLS has some similarities to the NLS present in SV40 large T antigen. This putative signal is called NLS1. It acts in the absence of hormone, therefore it is constitutive.

Using *in vitro* mutagenesis, a second NLS (NLS2) has been identified in the second zinc finger. This second NLS is hormone-dependent. The first NLS or NLS1 in the hinge region is more potent than NLS2. The integrity of both signals is necessary for the entry in the nucleus of a cytoplasmic protein such as β galactosidase.

The translocation of PR in the nucleus is not dependent on the integrity of the cytoskeleton. Different treatments were used to destroy the three cytoskeletal networks: nocodazole to disrupt the microtubules, demecolcine to induce the disappearance of the microtubules and the collapse of the intermediate filaments and cytochalasin B to disrupt the actin-containing microfilaments.[26] None of these compounds prevented the hormone dependent transfer of a wild type PR or of a mutant deleted with the nuclear localization signal, into the nucleus. In addition, they did not slow down or delay the transfer. Therefore, the cytoskeletal network does not seem to be important for the transfer. The NLSs and their interaction with the elements of the nuclear pore seem to be the major determinants of receptor traffic in the cells.

For hER, a 48 amino acid fragment located in the hinge region between the DNA and hormone binding regions mediates efficient nuclear localization of a β galactosidase fusion protein. This fragment contains three basic stretches. None of these stretches is by itself an NLS.

Export of the receptor from the nucleus

Studies using transient heterokaryons have also shown that ER[27] and PR are not confined to the nucleus. PRs are capable of bidirectional transfer through the nuclear envelope. A mouse L-cell line permanently expressing PR was fused with human 293 cells devoid of PR receptors. PR was present in human 293 cell nuclei 12 hours after the fusion.[28] Another group used PR-expressing Cos-1 cells and PR negative NIH3T3 cells to generate the heterokaryons.[29] In the presence or absence of hormone, cPRs migrate to NIH3T3 nuclei. Studies of different PR mutants have shown that PR NLS mediates both inward and outward movements of PR from the nucleus. Furthermore, Guiochon-Mantel et al[30] have grafted the nuclear localization signals of the progesterone receptor or the SV 40 large tumor antigen onto a cytoplasmic protein such as β galactosidase. These additions were shown to impart to the protein the ability to shuttle between the nucleus and the cytoplasm. Furthermore, when the NLS is grafted onto β galactosidase, this nuclear fusion protein is able to exit from the nucleus in the absence of ATP synthesis. On the contrary, microinjected proteins devoid of a nuclear localization signal are unable to exit from the nucleus.

The same nuclear localization signals are thus involved in both the inward and the outward movement of proteins through the nuclear membrane. However, the receptor constantly diffuses out of the nucleus and is being actively reimported into the nucleus, as shown by studies using transfection in energy depleted cells.[30] In other words, the nuclear import of the receptor requires energy while the nuclear export does not.

Hormone binding

The mode of hormone penetration in the cell is still controversial. Diffusion through the cell membrane was an accepted paradigm until recently. In fact, hormone penetration probably involves membrane transporters. Hormone binding to its receptor induces a conformational change in the receptor. This modification then initiates the cascade of events leading to 'activation' and transcription.

Activation of the receptors

In the absence of specific ligands, steroid receptors are inactive *in vivo*. The addition of hormone to cells or to hormone-deficient animals results in the rapid transformation of the inactive receptor to an active state. Unactivated steroid receptors associate a variety of proteins, either directly or indirectly. Hsp90 or heat shock protein 90 is the most widely recognized receptor-associated protein. Seven other proteins have been reported so far in purified progesterone receptor complexes. They include hsp70, p60, p23 and three large immunophilins: the FK506-binding proteins FKBP52 (also called p59 or hsp56) and FKBP54, and the cyclosporin A-binding protein CyP40.[31] Finally a 48 kDa protein (also called p48) has been found to be a transient component of progesterone receptor complexes. Smith et al have proposed a pathway for PR assembly:[32] Hsp 70 binds to free PR, followed rapidly by an intermediate PR complex containing hsp90, p60 and hsp70. The protein p48 was identified as an additional player in the early stages of PR activation. The complex lacks hsp70, p60 and p48 but contains hsp90, any one of the large immunophilins, and p23. This mature form is very stable. In the absence of progesterone, PR from dissociated mature complexes cycles back through the assembly pathway.

ER also associates with hsp90 via sequences of its ligand binding domain, although the interaction is rather weak.

Dimerization of the receptor

Interaction of progesterone with PR induces a receptor dimerization. Tsai et al first demonstrated *in vitro* that the DNA-bound PR dimerized.[33] Further studies proved that dimerization also occurred *in vivo*.[23] Three forms of dimers can be produced (A:A, A:B, B:B). The activated dimers can bind to DNA by the DNA binding region. They bind DNA with high affinity and are in a conformation which can direct gene transcription. The hER hormone binding domain dimerizes *in vitro* independently of ligand activation.[34] Furthermore, recent studies have demonstrated that ER mutants unable to bind 17β estradiol can form heterodimers *in vivo* and bind DNA as effectively as wild type ER.[35] These ER mutants are not functionally inactive as they are able to suppress the activity of wild type ER when they are coexpressed. X-ray crystallographic studies have demonstated more recently that the ER DNA-binding domain binds to DNA as a homodimer.[10] Interestingly the discovery of ERβ allows us to speculate that ERβ and ERα may form heterodimers. ERβ in addition to its specific effects may therefore regulate ERα action.

DNA binding

Dimers interact with specific DNA regulatory regions of target genes. Those regions are enhancer-like elements involved in the regulation of gene transcription. These *cis* elements are called hormone responsive or regulatory elements (HRE). They are often located in the 5′ flanking region, upstream of the transcription start site. HRE are sequences of 15 base pairs. Their structure is palindromic.[36] One receptor binds per half site. Three classes of HREs have been identified: the progesterone/glucocorticoid response element (PRE), the estrogen response element (ERE) and thyroid hormone response element (TRE) sequence. The sequence of the progesterone responsive element is also identical to the androgen receptor (ARE) and the mineralocorticoid receptor responsive (MRE) element. Although the sequence is identical for different ligands, different conditions are necessary according to each receptor to optimalize the receptor binding to its responsive element. As shown in Figure 11.4, ERE has a two base pair difference from PRE. HREs often exist as multiple copies. The region is then called hormone responsive units (HRU). Dimers enhance each other's activities: the binding of one dimer facilitates the binding of the second dimer.

Estrogen-responsive genes typically contain one or more copies of the consensus ERE or an imperfect ERE which deviates from the consensus sequence by one or more nucleotides. Although these imperfect EREs confer estrogen responsiveness to target genes, they are typically less potent activators of transcription than the consensus ERE.[37]

Transcription

Transcription studies are presently a major goal in this field of research. The mechanism by which receptor-DNA interaction promotes changes in gene transcription is not well understood. The ligand-induced receptor conformation is capable of recruiting general transcription factors. Protein-protein interactions with basal transcription factors or with

GRE/PRE/ARE/MRE	5'	**A G A A C A** N N N **T G T A C C**	3'
ERE	5'	N **G G T C A** N N N **T G A C C** N	3'
TRE	5'	**G G G T C A T G A C A G**	3'
RARE	5'	**A G G T C A T G A C C T**	3'

Fig. 11.4 HER (hormone estrogen responsive) element compared to the other HREs (hormone responsive element).

intermediary coactivators are involved. They form a complex and this initiates transcription by RNA polymerase II.[38]

Steroid receptors directly alter the rate of transcription by affecting the stability of the preinitiation complex. As shown in Figure 11.5, transcriptional activation of the gene involves RNA polymerase II and its associated general transcription factors (TF). At least eight cofactors have been identified (TFIIA, B, C, D, E, F, G, H and J). TFIID containing the TATA binding function associates with the TATA box of the gene promoter, just upstream of the transcription start site. This complex is stabilized by the binding of TFIIB, which is followed by the association of RNA polymerase II and general factors TFIIE and TFIIF with the promoter complex. These protein-protein interactions between the receptor and TFIIB are at least partially responsible for the induction of transcription. The initial transcript is processed and exported to the cytoplasm as messenger RNA with a polyadenylated tail. The messenger RNA is translated into protein by ribosomes. In some cases, a negative gene regulation may occur as progesterone and estrogen can decrease the transcription of specific genes.

Moreover, different interactions with coactivators or corepressors occur to enhance inductive or repressive functions of receptors. Some of those factors are reviewed below.

DNA bending

Studies have been performed to study the ER-induced bending of its target DNA or the PR-induced bending of its target DNA because DNA bending may be coupled to transcription as a mechanism with which to facilitate contact of upstream activators with other factors in the transcriptional apparatus. Steroid receptor-mediated bending of DNA has been demonstrated for thyroid hormone receptor, RXR, ER[39,40,41] and PR.[42] ER and PR cause a directional bend toward the major groove of the DNA helix. Interestingly, PR-B, which is a generally stronger transcriptional activator, induces a larger distortion of

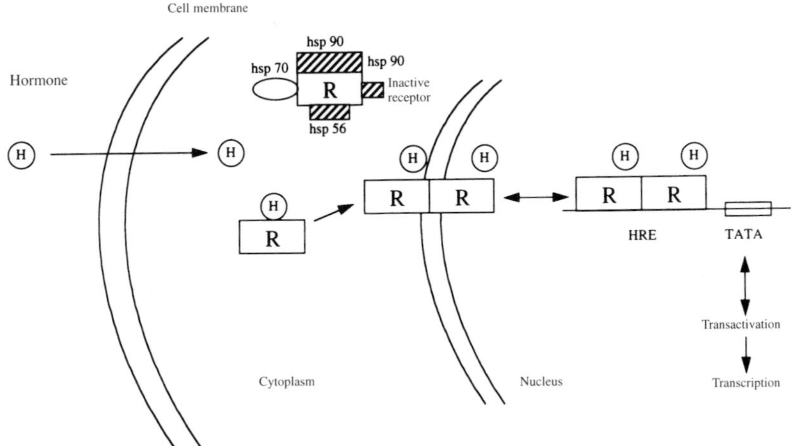

Fig. 11.5 Cellular mode of progesterone action showing the different steps: hormone binding, receptor dimerization, binding to HRE (hormone responsive element).

target DNA than PR-A. Although DNA bending may be a general property of the steroid receptor family, there is no direct functional evidence for DNA bending and transcriptional activation. Studies by Nardulli et al[39,40] have shown that three factors are important in transcription activation of estrogen-responsive genes: the affinity of ER for the ERE, the location of an ERE within the promoter and the magnitude and orientation of DNA bends induced by binding of ER or other proteins.

In summary, as shown in Figure 11.5, estradiol and progesterone act mainly through their respective receptors. The hormone penetrates into the cell, induces hsps dissociation from the receptor and a conformational change of the hormone-receptor complex, called 'activation'. Receptors dimerize and bind to hormone responsive elements on the promoter of the targeted genes. By this process, proteins are inhibited or synthesized under the control of the steroid receptors. However, this cascade of events is more complex as it involves different potential steps of regulation.

REGULATION OF ESTRADIOL AND PROGESTERONE ACTION

Synergism

Synergism can occur in a target gene to enhance transcription. The first type of synergism is *homologous*. For instance, a very strong synergism occurs when two PREs exist in the promoter of the activated gene. If only one PRE exists, progesterone enhances a reporter gene activity by 60 fold. If two PREs exist and are close to each other, the reporter gene activity is enhanced by 6000 fold. In such a case, the affinity of the progesterone receptor is 100 times higher for two PREs in tandem than for a single PRE.

The second type of synergism is *heterologous*. Some cases of synergism have been described with two different types of HREs, for instance ERE and PRE. This type of synergism acts probably by an interaction with a protein implied in the initiation of transcription.

Cofactors

The nuclear receptor-activated gene transcription is mediated by different cofactors which are coactivating or silencing mediators. Multiple factors have been shown to interact with steroid receptors in a ligand-dependent manner. The existence of such proteins has been suggested by the fact that the overexpression of a receptor can inhibit the signal induced by another receptor linked to its appropriate HRE. This phenomenon is called the 'squelching effect'. For instance ER overexpression inhibits progesterone stimulation of a progesterone target gene.

Different factors modulating ER and PR transcription have been identified such as Estrogen Receptor-Associated Protein 160 (ERAP-160), Steroid Receptor Coactivator-1 (SRC-1), a 140 kDa Receptor Interacting Protein (RIP140). ERAP-160 has been shown to form a complex with ER.[43,44,45] It correlates with the ability of ER to activate transcription *in vivo*. It may be a mediator of the estrogen-dependent AF-2 transactivation by ER. SRC-1 is another coactivator identified recently.[46] SRC-1 enhancement of hPR transactivation occurs through a ligand-bound receptor. SRC-1 also enhances estrogen ER, GR and TR. It is not a general coactivator for all classes of transactivators as it does not enhance the transcriptional activity of CREB (Cyclic Responsive Element Binding Protein). Coexpression of SRC-1 reversed the ability of ER to squelch activation by hPR. SRC-1 encodes a coactivator that is required for full transcriptional activity of the steroid receptor superfamily. Different transcriptional mediators/intermediary factors (TIFs), TIF1 and TIF2, have been recently isolated and cloned.[47,48] TIF2 could be a mediator of AF-2. It exhibits partial sequence homology with SRC-1. RIP140 interacts *in vitro* with the wild type receptor. It modulates transcriptional activation by ER.[44] CREB-binding protein (CBP) or the related P300 protein has been shown to trigger RNA polymerase II and thus transcription.[49] The nuclear receptors interact directly through their ligand-binding domains and hormone binding greatly stimulates this interaction.

Phosphorylation of the receptor

Post-translational modification of receptors is a possible mechanism by which receptor function can be regulated. The phosphorylation-dephosphorylation process has been proposed to be a control mechanism for the regulation of hormone binding, DNA binding and transactivation. Phosphorylation is enhanced during ligand-dependent activation in cells. The level of phosphorylation seems to contribute to the transactivation potential of the receptor.[50]

For cPR, three phosphorylation sites have been identified: serine 211, serine 260 and serine 530. Ser 211 and 260 belong to the A/B region, Ser 530 belongs to region D. In a basal state the phosphorylation levels are 20%, 20% and 2% for Ser 211, 260 and 530 respectively. When progesterone is added, the level of phosphorylation is increased to 35%, 35% and 35% respectively. Hyperphosphorylation is however not necessary for the binding, activation or down-regulation of PR. Phosphorylation could rather be involved in modulating the activity of the receptor. A nuclear kinase could be involved in the phosphorylation of the receptor in the nucleus.

For ER, data are more conflicting according to the species or the cellular type studied. ER could be phosphorylated on Tyr residues. A nuclear phosphatase would dephosphorylate ER. On the other hand, a cytosolic kinase could phosphorylate Tyr residues and would enhance binding of estrogen to ER. Other studies have suggested that mice uterine ER are phosphorylated on Ser residues. The phosphorylation of hER serine residue at position 118 is required for full activity of the ER activation function 1. Studies by Kato et al have shown that this phosphorylation occurs through the Ras-MAPK cascade of the growth signalling pathways.[51] This phosphorylation modulates the activity of AF-1.

Chromatin structure

Gene activation causes changes in chromatin structure. Proteins from the chromatin open or close regions of DNA and chromatin shifts from a condensed state to a less dense structure. ER can induce DNAse I hypersensitive sites around its response elements.[52] Emerging data suggest that additional nuclear/chromatin factors also confer specificity to steroid receptor-DNA interactions (SR-DNA). These proteins have been termed 'acceptor proteins'. When they are bound to DNA, they generate 'chromatin acceptor sites'. However, direct SR-DNA interactions could also occur on these sites. Landers and Spelsberg have proposed a model for the terminal part of the cascade of events following the hormone-receptor complex binding.[53] In summary, the hormone-receptor complex binds to the nuclear acceptor sites located on primary steroid regulatory elements in the 5′ flanking region of regulatory genes. Within a given target cell, many regulatory genes would be divided into several classes. The protein product of these genes would participate in many events in the cell. The protein product could regulate:

1. Membrane and cytoplasmic activities
2. Post-transcriptional regulation, such as changes in chromatin structure and RNA processing
3. Nuclear events involving the transcription of structural genes.

Tissue-specific regulation

Studies by Shupnik et al have found different tissue-specific forms of ER mRNA in the rat.[54] Furthermore, there is a tissue-specific regulation of these forms in normal rat tissues. For instance, pituitary and liver ER mRNAs are regulated positively with E_2. In contrast, ER mRNA is regulated negatively by E_2 in the uterus.

NONCLASSICAL PATHWAYS OF ESTRADIOL AND PROGESTERONE ACTION

Ligand-independent pathway for activation of steroid receptors

In the apparent absence of added hormone to cells in culture, transactivation by receptor occurs if stimulators of kinase activity or inhibitors of phosphatase activity are added.[50] Furthermore, dopamine or growth factors can enhance transcription of cPRA, cPRB and hER target genes in the absence of their respective ligand. Single amino acid mutations of the cPR and hER were performed in the C terminal regions of the receptor. A normal response to steroids occurred but the ligand-independent activation by dopamine was abolished. The author's hypothesis to explain such an inhibition is a structural change of the receptor. EGF and TGF-α are also capable of activating or transactivating ER in the absence of estrogen. It seems that the steroid receptor can be activated via a chemical signal originating from the plasma membrane. The hypothesis given by O'Malley et al[50] is that dopamine or growth factors bind to their membrane receptors. Protein kinases are then stimulated and enhance receptor phosphorylation. The degree of phosphorylation then induces the receptor transactivation.

Alternative pathway of ER action

An alternative to the classical pathway of ER action, and which involves the binding of ER to EREs, has been recently described.[55,56,57] ER appears to be able to stimulate transcription from a transfected promoter that contains an AP-1 site, the cognate binding site for the transcription factors Jun and Fos. This enhancement of transcription is believed to involve protein-protein interactions and not protein-DNA interactions because it is partly independent of the ER DNA binding domain. However, the exact mechanism by which transcription is enhanced is still unknown.

ER AND PR MUTATIONS

To elucidate the mechanisms of steroid action, at least two different approaches can be used: the identification of receptor mutations in animal models or in patients, or the use of an agonist or antagonist of the steroid studied. For androgens, studies have been facilitated by the occurrence of mutations in the androgen receptor described both in rodents as well as in humans (in the form of the clinical syndrome of androgen insensitivity (AIS)).[58,59] ER and PR mutations have been recently designed in mice. A single case of ER gene mutation has been described in a man.

Estrogen receptor gene mutation

The lack of known mutations in the ER gene suggested that such mutations would be lethal. However, homologous recombination has been used to disrupt expression of the mouse ER gene.[60] Furthermore, a case of a mutation of the ER gene has been recently reported in a young male.[61] The phenotype was confirmed in a man with a mutation on the aromatase gene.[62]

ER knock-out mouse

The mouse ER gene was disrupted[63] by inserting a 1.8 kb neomycin sequence in exon 2. Heterozygote mice had half the level of ER protein compared to wild-type animals. Both male and female animals survived to adulthood with normal external phenotypes. As expected, females are infertile and demonstrate hypoplastic uteri and hyperemic ovaries with no apparent corpora lutea. Males are also infertile with atrophy of the testes and seminiferous tubule dysmorphogenesis. However, prenatal development of the reproductive tracts of both sexes appear to be independent of an ER-mediated response. Both sexes show a decrease in skeletal bone density.

ER mutation in the human

The only reported case so far of a mutation in the ER gene, has been described in a 28-year-old male (Fig. 11.6).[61] This patient was 204 cm high. He was fully masculinized and presented to the clinic with severe genu valgum. He had a decrease in bone age and low bone density. His sperm count was 25 million but it had low viability of 16%. DNA analysis using single-strand conformation analysis (SSCA) detected a mutation in both copies of the ER gene in exon 2 at codon 157 (C→T). This nucleotide change introduces a premature stop codon. Therefore, the ER protein is truncated. Interestingly, the human mutation occurs in a similar region of the protein as the experimental disruption created in the mice. The patient's parents, who are heterozygous for the mutation, show no clinical abnormalities. This case report is very important as it demonstrates that a mutation in the ER gene is not lethal in the human species. Furthermore, it illustrates that estrogen plays a very important role in epiphyseal closure and bone density even in the male.

Mutation of ER in tumors

A mutant ER was identified that contains a point mutation in the N terminal region.[64] This B-variant estrogen receptor occurs naturally in women and has been linked to decreased estrogen binding and spontaneous abortion. In breast tumors, variant ER messenger RNAs have been identified.[65] Furthermore, an ER variant, missing part of the hormone binding domain, was identified in human breast tumors.[66] It

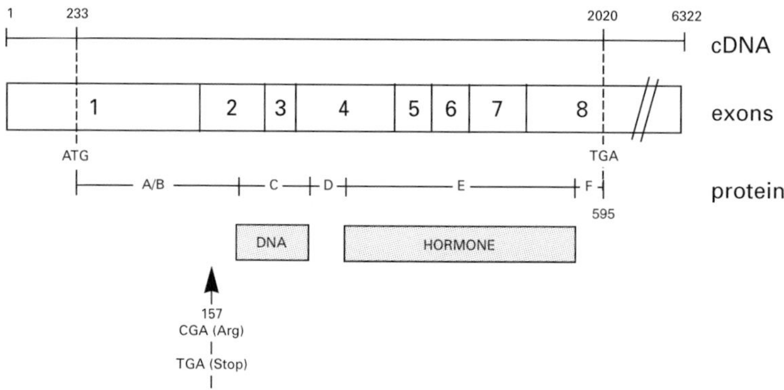

Fig. 11.6 The human estradiol receptor cDNA with the only mutation described in the human (CGA→TGA in exon 2).[61]

inhibited wild-type estrogen receptor function and could be involved in the development of hormone-resistant breast cancer.

Progesterone receptor gene mutation

A mouse model carrying a null mutation of the PR gene has been designed by Lydon et al, using embryonic stem cell/gene targeting techniques.[67] Male and female embryos homozygous for the PR mutation developed normally to adulthood. However, the adult female PR mutant displayed significant defects in all reproductive tissues. The mice were unable to ovulate; they presented uterine hyperplasia and inflammation and their mammary glands were small. Furthermore, the mice were unable to exhibit sexual behavior.

This mouse model illustrates a very important role of progesterone not only in maintaining pregnancy, but in achieving diverse reproductive events.

No clinical case has been reported so far of a mutation in PR in the human species.

PROGESTERONE AND ESTRADIOL ANTAGONISTS

A different way to further elucidate the mode of action of estradiol and progesterone is to study estradiol and progesterone antagonists.

Progesterone antagonists

RU486 (mifepristone) and ZK98299 (onapristone) are progesterone antagonists derived from 19-nortestosterone. Both interact with the PR ligand binding domain. Mifepristone has a high affinity for PR and yet forms an abortive complex. The antagonists competively inhibit progesterone binding but allow receptor dimerization. Their modes of action are still controversial. The main hypothesis is that they probably act by blocking PR-mediated signal transduction downstream of DNA binding.[68,69] Studies by Allan et al demonstrated that progesterone and mifepristone induce distinct conformational changes within the receptor protein at the carboxyl terminus of the receptor.[70] Vegeto et al studied hPR mutants in yeast, recognizing agonists or antagonists.[71] One of the mutants contained a carboxyl terminus truncation of 54 amino acids. This truncation converted all the known antiprogestogens into progestogens. From those studies it can be concluded that the C terminal region of PR contains a transcriptional inhibitory function that prevents transcriptional activity in the absence of hormone. Secondly, studies by Onate et al suggest that the inability of the antagonist-bound receptor to interact efficiently with SRC-1 leads to the *in vivo* biological consequence of hormonal antagonism.[46]

Estradiol antagonists (selective estrogen receptor modulators or SERM)

Tamoxifen, raloxifene (nonsteroidal) and ICI 164,384 (steroidal) represent the main antiestrogens. They inhibit E_2 induced activation of ERE-containing genes to various extents. However, some of these molecules have a tissue-selective activity and agonistic effects. This explains why the term SERM has been used instead of antiestrogen. For instance, tamoxifen acts as an agonist of ER in some tissues, such as uterus, liver and bone, and as an antagonist in other tissues, notably breast. The agonist activity is attributed to its ability to stabilize DNA binding and to activate AF-1. Its antagonist activity is due to competitive inhibition of the estradiol-dependent activation of AF-2. Estradiol and tamoxifen induce different conformations of the hormone binding domain region of ER and AF2. Furthermore, inhibition of receptor dimerization or interaction with cofactors could be involved in the antagonist activity. For instance, ICI 164,384 and ICI 182,780 are unable to promote ER-ERAP 160 complex formation. This interaction could explain the inhibition of transcription.[43]

Furthermore, tamoxifen is a potent activator of promoters regulated by AP-1 sites.[72] AP-1 sites are binding sites for jun and fos. Tamoxifen is an agonist of AP-1 dependent transcription. This agonism for AP-1 sites is cell specific: it occurs in uterine but not in breast cell lines. Therefore, it parallels tamoxifen agonism *in vivo*.

A recent study has identified an estrogen response element activated by metabolites of 17 β estradiol and raloxifene.[73] This could explain why certain key estrogen regulatory events in bone appear to be mediated through pathways independent of EREs.

New types of antagonists

A new type of antagonists are oligonucleotides. Single-stranded oligonucleotides bind specific nucleotide sequences with high affinity. 'Antisense' oligonucleotides hybridize to specific messenger RNA sequences and therefore inhibit translation. Antisense oligonucleotides to the progesterone receptor are currently being studied in the female rat.

A second type of oligonucleotides are triplex-forming oligonucleotides. These single-stranded DNA molecules bind to DNA and form triple-helix structures. A triplex-forming oligonucleotide directed to two PREs has been recently studied by Ing et al.[74] *In vivo* it inhibits progesterone receptor binding and transactivation.

NONGENOMIC EFFECTS OF STEROID ON THE CELL

Steroid hormones have been demonstrated to have nongenomic effects. These rapid membrane effects are opening of ionic channels, membrane receptor aggregation or changes in protein phosphorylation status. They have been first described for progesterone on frog oocytes and then in spermatozoa and neurons. *Xenopus laevis* oocytes constitute a well-documented case of steroid action at the level of the membrane.[75] Progesterone effect is related to an increase in intracellular calcium concentration. The calcium increase can be generated from a rapid release of Ca^{2+} from intracellular stores or from an influx of extracellular Ca^{2+}.[76] The vasomotor effects of estrogen may be related to blockade of the cell membrane voltage-dependent calcium channels, resulting in inhibition of extracellular Ca^{2+} mobilization and flux. The putative mediators of this nongenomic action could be membrane ER. For instance, in cultured rat osteoblasts, a cell surface receptor for estrogens, possibly coupled to phospholipase C via G protein, has been described.[77] Progesterone was identified as a major component of the follicular fluid for inducing the acrosome reaction. These rapid biological effects have been attributed to a sperm cell-surface receptor.[78] The existence of 'cross-talk' between membrane and genomic effect remains an open question.

Steroids can be modulators of neurotransmitter receptors such as $GABA_A$ receptor isoforms, glutamate, glycine, acetylcholine and opioid receptors. The physiological significance of these modulations is uncertain.

ESTRADIOL EFFECTS ON THE CELL CYCLE

It is well known that estradiol exerts growth-promoting effects on some breast cancers *in vivo*, as well as on breast cancer cell lines *in vitro*.

Estradiol action on the cell cycle

Cyclins and cyclin-dependent kinases

Estrogens are known to regulate cell cycle progression and cyclin expression in receptor-bearing breast cancer cell lines. Foster investigated the role of estrogen on the activity of cyclin-dependent kinases in breast cancer cells.[79] Cyclin-dependent kinases (Cdk) act to regulate the transition between G1 and S-phase in mammalian cells. Cdk activation depends upon binding with cyclins and site-specific phosphorylation by Cdk-activating kinases. Estradiol at physiological concentrations elicited Cdk2 and Cdk4-associated kinase activities. Estradiol effects were inhibited by the antiestrogen ICI 182,780. Therefore, estradiol regulates G1 progression in MCF-7 cells through direct effects upon Cdk activation, Rb phosphorylation and by inducing elimination of Cdk inhibitors.

Proto-oncogenes

Estrogens regulate expression of nuclear proto-oncogenes including c-fos, c-jun and c-myc.[80] 17β estradiol mimics ligand activity of the c-erbB2 proto-oncogene product.[81] The c-erbB2 proto-oncogene, also called neu, encodes a transmembrane glycoprotein. This protein product is overexpressed in many adenocarcinomas, including mammary carcinomas. Ligand-dependent activation of the kinase activity is thought to contribute to tumor progression. Estrogen can activate the kinase activity of ErbB2.

Conclusion

Steroids act through a cascade of events implying the ligand binding to its own receptor. However, new pathways of activation have been recently unraveled. They imply growth factors, steroid-DNA interactions and nongenomic mechanisms of action, possibly mediated through membrane receptors. Major progress is needed in understanding the 'cross-talk' between ligand-dependent and ligand-independent transactivation. Furthermore, greater understanding of the tissue specificity of estrogen and progesterone action would provide new tools to design hormonal treatment. Puzzling questions remain concerning the cell specificity of estradiol and progesterone action. For instance, estrogen elicits actions specific to various cells and target tissues, although the estrogen receptor protein present in all tissues appears identical. A better understanding of the molecular details of steroid hormone agonist and antagonist activities should provide, in the near future, new contraceptive pills, new hormonal replacement therapy, new pills for medical pregnancy termination and new treatments for breast cancer.

REFERENCES

1. Evans RM 1988 The steroid and thyroid hormone receptor superfamily. Science 240: 889–895
2. Jensen EV, Jacobsen HI 1962 Basic guides to the mechanism of estrogen action. Recent Progress in Hormone Research 18: 387–414
3. Walter P, Green S, Greene G, Krust A, Bornert JM, Jeltsch JM et al 1985 Cloning of the human estrogen receptor cDNA. Proceedings of the National Academy of Science, USA 82: 7889–7893
4. Misrahi M, Atger M, d'Auriol L, Loosfelt H, Meriel C, Fridlansky F et al 1987 Complete amino acid sequence of the human progesterone receptor deduced from cloned cDNA. Biochemical and Biophysical Research Communications 143: 740–748
5. Carson-Jurica MA, Schrader WT, O'Malley BW 1990 Steroid receptor family: structure and functions. Endocrine Reviews 11: 201–220
6. Ing NH, O'Malley BW 1995 The steroid hormone receptor superfamily: molecular mechanisms of action. In: Weintraub BD (ed) Molecular endocrinology: basic concepts and clinical correlations. Raven Press, New York, pp 195–215
7. Bourguet W, Ruff M, Chambon P, Gronemeyer H, Moras D 1996 Crystal structure of the ligand-binding domain of the human nuclear receptor RXR-γ. Nature 375: 377–382
8. Zilliacus J, Wright APH, Carlstedt-Duke J, Gustafsson JA 1995 Structural determinants of DNA-binding specificity by steroid receptors. Molecular Endocrinology 9: 389–400
9. Combarnous Y 1996 Mécanismes d'action des médiateurs à récepteurs nucléaires. In: Biochimie des communications cellulaires, 2nd edn. Editions Lavoisier Technique & Documentation. Paris, France pp 167–219
10. Schwabe JWR, Chapman L, Finch JT, Rhodes D 1993 The crystal structure of the estrogen receptor DNA-binding domain bound to DNA: how receptors discriminate between their response element. Cell 75: 567–578
11. Sartorius CA, Melville MY, Hovland AR 1994 A third transactivation function (AF3) of human progesterone receptors located in the unique N-terminal segment of the B-isoform. Molecular Endocrinology 8: 1347–1360
12. Montano MM, Muller V, Trobaugh A, Katzenellenbogen BS 1995 The carboxy-terminal F domain of the human estrogen receptor: role in the transcriptional activity of the receptor and the effectiveness of antiestrogens as estrogen antagonists. Molecular Endocrinology 9: 814–825
13. Kastner P, Turcotte B, Stropp U, Tora L, Gronemeyer H, Chambon P 1990 Two distinct estrogen-related promoters generate transcripts encoding the two functionally different human progesterone receptor forms A and B. EMBO J 9: 1603–1614
14. McDonnell DP 1995 Unraveling the human progesterone receptor signal transduction pathway. Insights into antiprogestin action. TEM 6: 133–138
15. Wen DX, Xu YF, Mais DE, Goldman ME, McDonnell DP 1994 The A and B isoforms of the human progesterone receptor operate trough distinct signaling pathways within target cells. Molecular and Cell Biology 14: 8356–8364
16. Mosselman S, Polman J, Dijkema R 1996 ERβ: identification and characterization of a novel human estrogen receptor. FEBS 392: 49–53
17. Kuiper GGJM, Enmark E, Pelto-Huikko M, Nilsson S, Gustafsson JA 1996 Cloning of a novel estrogen receptor expressed in rat prostate and ovary. Proceedings of the National Academy of Science, USA 93: 5925–5930
18. Kuiper GGJM, Carlsson B, Grandien K, Enmark E, Häggblad J, Nilsson S, Gustafsson JA 1997 Comparison of the ligand binding specificity and transcript tissue distribution of estrogen receptors α and β. Endocrinology. 138: 863–870
19. Inoue S, Hoshino S, Miyoshi H, Akishita M, Hosoi T, Orimo H, Ouchi Y 1996 Identification of a novel isoform of estrogen receptor, a potential inhibitor of estrogen action in vascular smooth muscle cells. Biochemical and Biophysical Research Communications (United States) 219: 766–772
20. King WJ, Greene GL 1984 Monoclonal antibodies localize estrogen receptor in the nuclei of target cells. Nature 307: 745–749
21. Perrot-Applanat M, Logeat F, Groyer-Picard MT, Milgrom E 1985 Immunocytochemical study of mammalian progesterone receptor using monoclonal antibodies. Endocrinology 116: 1473–1484
22. Welshons WV, Lieberman ME, Gorski J 1984 Nuclear localization of unoccupied oestrogen receptors. Nature 307: 747–749
23. Guiochon-Mantel A, Loosfelt H, Lescop P, Sar S, Atger M, Perrot-Applanat M, Milgrom E 1989 Mechanisms of nuclear localization of the progesterone receptor: evidence for interaction between monomers. Cell 57: 1147–1154
24. Guiochon-Mantel A, Lescop P, Christin-Maitre S, Loosfelt H, Perrot-Applanat M, Milgrom E 1991 Nucleo-cytoplasmic shuttle of the progesterone receptor. EMBO J 10: 3851–3859
25. Ylikomi T, Bocquel MT, Berry M, Gronemeyer H, Chambon P 1992 EMBO J 11: 3681–3694
26. Picard D, Kumar V, Chambon P, Yamamoto KR 1990 Signal transduction by steroid hormones: nuclear localization is differentially regulated in estrogen and glucocorticoid receptors. Cell Regulation 1: 291–299
27. Perrot-Applanat M, Lescop P, Milgrom E 1992 The cytoskeleton and the cellular traffic of the progesterone receptor. Journal of Cell Biology 119: 337–348
28. Dauvois S, Danielan PS, White R, Parker MG 1992 Antiestrogen ICI 164,384 reduces cellular estrogen receptor content by increasing its turnover. Proceedings of the National Academy of Science, USA 89: 4037–4041
29. Chandran UR, DeFranco DB 1992 Internuclear migration of chicken progesterone receptor, but not Simian virus-40 large tumor antigen, in transient heterokaryons. Molecular Endocrinology 6: 837–844
30. Guiochon-Mantel A, Delabre K, Lescop P, Milgrom E 1994 Nuclear localization signals also mediate the outward movement of proteins from the nucleus. Proceedings of the National Academy of Science, USA 91: 7179–7183
31. Smith DF, Toft DO 1993 Steroid receptors and their associated proteins. Molecular Endocrinology 7: 4–11

32. Prapapanich V, Chen S, Nair SC, Rimerman RA, Smith DF 1996 Molecular cloning of human p48 – a transient component of progesterone receptor complexes and an Hsp70-binding protein. Molecular Endocrinology, 10: 420–431
33. Tsai SY, Carlstedt-Duke J, Weigel NL, Dahlman K, Gustafsson A, Tsai MJ, O'Malley BW 1988 Molecular interactions of steroid hormone receptor with enhancer element: evidence for receptor dimer formation. Cell 55: 361–369
34. Salomonsson M, Häggblad J, O'Malley BW, Sitbon GM 1994 The human estrogen receptor hormone binding domain dimerizes independently of ligand activation. Journal of Steroid Biochemistry and Molecular Biology 48: 447–452
35. Zhuang Y, Katzenellenbogen BS, Shapiro DJ 1995 Estrogen receptor mutants which do not bind 17β-estradiol dimerize and bind to the estrogen response element *in vivo*. Molecular Endocrinology 9: 457–466
36. Beato M 1989 Gene regulation by steroid hormones. Cell 324: 335–344
37. Nardulli AM, Romine LE, Carpo C, Greene GL, Rainish B 1996 Estrogen receptor affinity and location of consensus and imperfect estrogen response elements influence transcription activation of simplified promoters. Molecular Endocrinology 10: 694–704
38. Zawel L, Reinberg D 1993 Initiation of transcription by RNA polymerase II: a multistep process. Progress in Nuclear Acids Research and Molecular Biology 44: 69–108
39. Nardulli AM, Greene GL, Shapiro DJ 1993 Human estrogen receptor bound to an estrogen response element bends DNA. Molecular Endocrinology 7: 331–340
40. Nardulli AM, Shapiro DJ 1992 Binding of the estrogen receptor DNA-binding domain to the estrogen response element induces DNA bending. Molecular and Cell Biology 12: 2037–2042
41. Sabbah M, Le Ricousse S, Redeuilh G, Beaulieu EE 1992 Estrogen receptor-induced bending of the Xenopus vitellogenin A2 gene hormone response element. Biochemical and Biophysical Research Communications 185: 944–952
42. Prendergast P, Pan Z, Edwards DP 1996 Progesterone receptor-induced bending of its target DNA: distinct effects of the A and B receptor forms. Molecular Endocrinology 10: 393–407
43. Halachmi S, Marden E, Martin G, MacKay H, Abbondanza C, Brown M 1994 Estrogen receptor-associated proteins: possible mediators of hormone-induced transcription. Science 264: 1455–1458
44. Cavaillès V, Dauvois S, Danielian PS, Parker MG 1994 Interaction of proteins with transcriptionally active estrogen receptors. Proceedings of the National Academy of Science, USA 91: 10009–10013
45. Cavaillès V, Dauvois S, L'Horset F, Lopez G, Hoare S, Kushner PJ, Parker MG 1995 Nuclear factor RIP140 modulates transcriptional activation by the estrogen receptor. EMBO J 14: 3741–3751
46. Onate SA, Tsai SY, Tsai M-J, O'Malley BW 1995 Sequence and characterization of a coactivator for the steroid hormone receptor superfamily. Science 270: 1354–1357
47. Le Douarin B, Zechel C, Garnier JM, Lutz Y, Tora L, Pierrat B et al 1995 The N-terminal part of the ligand-dependent activation function (AF-2) of nuclear receptors is fused to B-raf in the oncogenic protein T18. EMBO J 9: 2020–2033
48. Voegel JJ, Heine MJS, Zechel C, Chambon P, Gronemeyer H 1996 TIF2, a 160 kDa transcriptional mediator for the ligand-dependent activation function AF-2 of nuclear receptors. EMBO J 15: 3667–3675
49. Chakravarti D, La Morte VJ, Nelson MC, Nakajima T, Schulman IG, Juguilon H, Montminy M, Evans RM 1996 Role of CBP/P300 in nuclear receptor signalling. Nature 383: 99–102
50. O'Malley, Schrader WT, Mani S, Smith C, Weigel NL, Conneely OM, Clark JH 1995 An alternative ligand-dependent pathway for activation of steroid receptors. Recent Progress in Hormone Research 50: 333–347
51. Kato S, Endoh H, Masuhiro, Kitamoto T, Uchiyama S, Sasaki H et al 1995 Activation of the estrogen receptor through phosphorylation by mitogen-activated protein kinase. Science 270: 1491–1494
52. Pham TA, Elliston JF, Nawaz Z, McDonnell DP, Tsai MJ, O'Malley BW 1991 Antiestrogen can establish nonproductive receptor complexes and alter chromatin structure at target enhancers. Proceedings of the National Academy of Science USA 88: 3125–3129
53. Spelsberg TS, Lauber AH, Sandhu NP, Subramaniam M 1996 A nuclear matrix site of progesterone receptor in the avian c-myc gene promoter. Recent Progress in Hormone Research 51: 63–96
54. Shupnik MA, Gordon MS, Chin WW 1989 Tissue-specific regulation of rat estrogen receptor mRNAs. Molecular Endocrinology 3: 660–665
55. Umayahara Y, Kawamori R, Watada H, Imano E, Iwana N, Morishima T et al 1994 Estrogen regulation of the insulin-like growth factor I gene transcription involves an AP-1 enhancer. Journal of Biological Chemistry 269: 16433–16442
56. Philips A, Chalbos D, Rochefort H 1993 Estradiol increases and anti-estrogens antagonize the growth factor-induced activator protein-1 activity in MCF7 breast cancer cells without affecting c-fos and c-jun synthesis. Journal of Biological Chemistry 268: 14103–14108
57. Gaub MP, Bellard M, Scheuer I, Chambon P, Sassone CP 1990 Activation of the ovalbumin gene by the estrogen receptor involves the fos-jun complex. Cell 63: 1267–1276
58. Wilson JD, Griffin JE, Leshin M, MacDonald PC 1900 In: Stanbury JB (ed) The metabolic basis of inherited diseases. McGraw-Hill, New York, pp 1001–1026
59. Patterson MN, McPhaul MJ, Hughes IA 1994 Clinical endocrinology and metabolism: hormones, enzymes and receptors Baillière Tindall, London, 8(2): 379
60. Korach KS, Couse JF, Curtis SW, Washburn TF, Lindzey J, Sean Kimbro KS 1996 Estrogen receptor gene disruption: molecular characterization and experimental and clinical phenotypes. Recent Progress in Hormone Research 51: 159–188
61. Smith EP, Boyd J, Frank GR, Takahashi H, Cohen RM, Specker B et al 1994 New England Journal of Medicine 331: 1056–1061
62. Morishima A, Grumbach MM, Sipson ER et al 1995 Aromatase deficiency in male and female siblings caused by a novel mutation and the physiological role of estrogens. Journal of Clinical Endocrinology and Metabolism 80: 3689–3698

63. Lubahn DB, Moyer JS, Golding TS, Couse JF, Korach KS, Smithies O 1993 Alteration of reproductive function but not prenatal sexual development after insertional disruption of the mouse estrogen receptor gene. Proceedings of the National Academy of Science, USA 90: 11162–11166
64. Lehrer S, Sanchez M, Song HK et al 1990 Oestrogen receptor B-polymorphism and spontaneous abortion in women with breast cancer. Lancet 335: 622–624
65. Dotzlaw H, Alkhalaf M, Murphy LC 1992 Characterization of estrogen receptor variant mRNAs from human breast cancers. Molecular Endocrinology 6: 773–784
66. Fuqua SAW, Fitgerald SD, Allred DC 1992 Inhibition of estrogen receptor action by a naturally occurring variant in human breast tumors. Cancer Research 52: 483–486
67. Lydon JP, De Mayo FJ, Funk CR, Mani SK, Hughes AR, Montgomery CA Jr et al 1995 Mice lacking progesterone receptor exhibit pleiotropic reproductive abnormalities. Genes and Development 9: 2266–2278
68. Guiochon-Mantel A, Loosfelt H, Ragot T, Bailly A, Atger M, Misrahi M, Perricaudet M, Milgrom E 1988 Receptors bound to antiprogestin form abortive complexes with hormone responsive elements. Nature 336: 695–698
69. Horwitz K 1992 The molecular biology of RU486: is there a role for antiprogestins in the treatment of breast cancer? Endocrine Reviews 13: 146–163
70. Allan GF, Leng X, Tsai ST et al 1992 Hormone and antihormone induce distinct conformational changes which are central to steroid receptor activation. Journal of Biology Chemistry 267: 513–519
71. Vegeto E, Allan GF, Schrader WT, Tsai MJ, McDonnell DP, O'Malley BW 1992 The mechanism of RU 486 antagonism is dependent on the conformation of the carboxy-terminal tail of the human progesterone receptor. Cell 69: 703–713
72. Webb P, Lopez GN, Uht RM, Kushner PJ 1995 Tamoxifen activation of the estrogen receptor/AP-1 pathway: potential origin for the cell-specific estrogen-like effects of antiestrogens. Molecular Endocrinology 9: 443–456
73. Yang NN, Venugopalan M, Hardikar S, Glasebrook A 1996 Identification of an estrogen response element activated by metabolites of 17β estradiol and raloxifene. Science 273: 1222–1224
74. Ing NH, Kessler DJ, Murphy D, Jayaraman K, Zendegui JG, Hogan ME, O'Malley BW, Tsai MJ 1993 In vivo transcription of a progesterone-responsive gene is specifically inhibited by a triplex-forming oligonucleotide. Nucleic Acids Research 21: 2789–2796
75. Baulieu EE, Robel P 1995 Non-genomic mechanisms of action of steroid hormones. Ciba Foundation Symposium 24–42
76. Tesarik J, Mendoza C 1995 Nongenomic effects of 17β-estradiol on maturing human oocytes: relationship to oocyte development potential. Journal of Clinical Endocrinology and Metabolism 80: 1438–1443
77. Lieberherr M, Grosse B, Kachkache M, Balsan S 1993 Cell signaling and estrogens in female rat osteoblasts: a possible involvement of unconventional nonnuclear receptors. Journal of Bone Mineral Research 8: 1365–1376
78. Blackmore PF, Neulen J, Lattenzio F, Beebe SJ 1991 Cell-surface binding sites for progesterone mediate calcium uptake in human sperm. Journal of Biological Chemistry 266: 18655–18659
79. Foster JS, Wimalasena J 1996 Estrogen regulates activity of cyclin-dependent kinases and retinoblastoma protein phosphorylation in breast cancer cells. Molecular Endocrinology 10: 488–498
80. Schuchard M, Lander JP, Sanohu NP, Spelsberg TC 1993 Steroid hormone regulation of nuclear proto-oncogenes. Endocrine Reviews 14: 659–669
81. Matsuda S, Kadowaki Y, Ichino M, Akiyama T, Toyoshima K, Yamamoto T 1993 17β-estradiol mimics ligand activity of the c-erb B2 protooncogene product. Proceedings of the National Academy of Science, USA 90: 10803–10807

12. The molecular basis for the development of estrogen, and progesterone agonists and antagonists

Donald P. McDonnell   Brandee L. Wagner

Introduction

The biological activity of estrogen and progesterone within endocrine tissues, such as the uterus, mammary gland and the central nervous system, has been well documented.[1] However, the identification of estrogen (hER) and progesterone receptors (hPR) in 'nonclassical' target tissues indicated that estrogen and progesterone have activities other than those directly related to reproduction. This is particularly evident for estrogen where epidemiological and clinical evidence supports a role for this hormone as an osteoprotective agent in postmenopausal women.[2] In addition to preservation of bone, estrogen replacement therapy has also been shown to be associated with a sharp reduction in the risk of cardiovascular disease (CVD) associated with menopause.[3] It is not known how estrogen (or progesterone) manifest their biological activity in these specific systems. However, the application of molecular and genetic approaches to study hPR and hER action has generally assisted in the development of novel steroid receptor modulators which will likely be used in the management of CVD and osteoporosis as well as reproductive disorders and hormone dependent cancers.

THE ESTROGEN AND PROGESTERONE RECEPTORS AND THEIR GENETIC CONTROL

The biological activity of estrogen and progesterone are manifest through high affinity receptors located within the nuclei of target cells. The human α-estrogen receptor (hER) exists as a single 65 kDa protein within target cells.[4] Recently, a β-form of the estrogen receptor has been cloned, and this has variable expression in different tissues. It is briefly discussed in Chapter 11. The described differences between the ER subtypes in relative ligand binding affinity and tissue distribution could contribute to the selective action of ER agonists and antagonists in different tissues. Although other variant mRNAs which could potentially encode hER variants have been identified, their biological significance has not yet been determined.[5] The human progesterone receptor (hPR) also occurs as two distinct forms within target cells, hPR-A and hPR-B, of 94 and 114 kDa, respectively.[6] Both the A and B forms of hPR are derived from a single gene as a consequence of alternate initiation of transcription from distinct promoters.[7]

These receptors are members of a large superfamily of nuclear proteins which mediate the biological actions of steroids, thyroid hormone and the vitamins D and A.[8] In addition, this family also includes a large number of 'orphan' receptors for which ligands have not yet been identified.[9] Analysis of the sequence of these receptor cDNAs, coupled with extensive studies of the biological activities of a great number of receptor mutations, have indicated that these proteins share the same overall structural organization (for review see references 8, 10). They contain a 300 amino acid ligand binding domain at the carboxyl terminus, and a centrally located DNA binding domain of 66–68 amino acids. The amino terminus is the most divergent domain and appears mainly to be involved in making contact with the general transcription machinery.[7,11–15] Although the precise location of the sequences required for transactivation within this domain have not yet been identified it has been proposed that in hER a single transactivation function (TAF) is located within this region,[11,15,16] as is the case for the A-isoform of hPR.[15] Within hPR-B, an additional sequence, B-upstream sequence (BUS), seems to be required for maximal transcriptional activity.[17,18]

Transcriptional regulation by estrogen and progesterone receptors

The overall mechanism of action of steroid hormone receptors is similar.[19,20] This general mechanism is discussed below, followed by a consideration of the specific aspects of hER and hPR action which may be different. In the absence of hormone, the steroid hormone receptors reside in the nucleus of target cells in a latent form associated with a high molecular weight complex comprising heat shock protein 90 (hsp90), hsp72, hsp59 and possibly other proteins[21–23] (Fig. 12.1). The precise stoichiometry of the individual components within the receptor/heat shock complex is difficult to determine, however it is generally considered that only a single receptor molecule exists in each oligomeric complex.[24] The role of heat shock proteins in steroid receptor action is unknown, however they may be involved in assisting the folding of the nascent receptor peptide or in maintaining the receptor in a transcriptionally inactive state in the absence of hormone.[25–27] It is currently thought that the reversible binding of the steroid ligand defines a conformational modification of receptor structure which releases the receptor from the hsp complex.[23] Although all the steroid hormone receptors have been shown to be associated with hsp90, it is likely that its role in the biology of each receptor is different. For instance, it has been shown that hsp90 is required for the formation of a hormone binding competent form of glucocorticosteroid receptor[28] but does not appear to be required for correct folding of the hER binding domain.[29] Very little is known of the role of the other heat shock proteins which are associated with the untransformed receptor.[21,30]

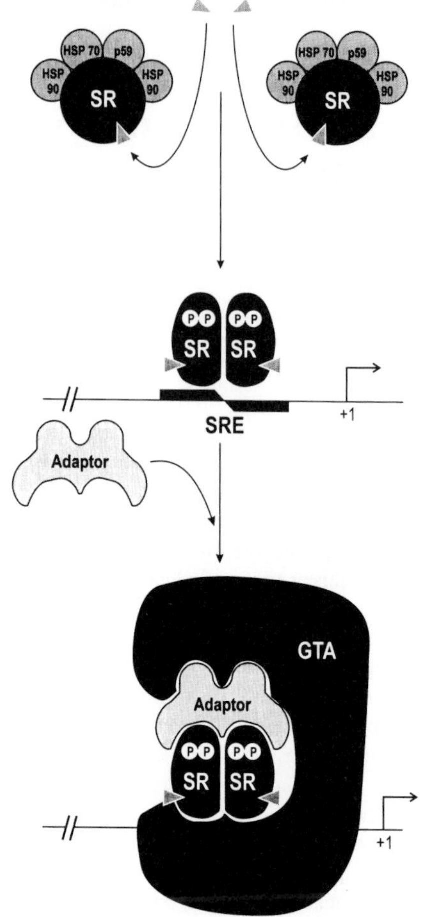

Fig. 12.1 The mechanism of action of steroid hormones. Steroid hormones exert their effects on gene transcription via specific intracellular receptor proteins. Genetic and biochemical evidence suggests that signal transduction to the nucleus occurs in a series of distinct steps. The details of the model are discussed in the text. In brief, hormone enters the cell passively where it encounters its cognate receptor (SR) in a complex with heat shock proteins. The binding of ligand initiates a cascade of molecular events, including phosphorylation, dimerization, nuclear translocation, interaction with specific DNA response elements (SREs) and recruitment of adaptor proteins which allow the steroid receptor to productively interact with the general transcription apparatus (GTA). The transcriptional effects of the hormone on RNA polymerase activity are determined ultimately by the cellular and promoter contexts of the receptor bound to DNA.

Initiation of the progesterone receptor mediated signal transduction pathway

Interaction of progesterone with hPR initiates the signal transduction cascade by promoting displacement of heat shock proteins[31] and facilitating the formation of stable receptor dimers. In cells where hPR-B and hPR-A are coexpressed, three distinct types of dimer (A:A, A:B, B:B) can form. The relative concentration of each dimer pair formed is directly proportional to the expression level of hPR-A and hPR-B.[31,32] The activated receptor dimers are then capable of interacting with high affinity with specific progesterone response elements (PREs) located within target gene promoters.[33] In addition to promoting the formation of receptor dimers, the interaction of receptor with hormone facilitates an increase in the overall phosphorylation state of hPR.[34–36] This appears to occur in two discrete steps: one phosphorylation event occurring upon displacement of heat shock proteins and the second occurring following the association of the receptor with DNA.[35,36] As yet, a specific role for phosphorylation is unknown.

Initiation of the estrogen receptor mediated signal transduction pathway

The association of ER with specific DNA sequences in the regulatory regions of target genes is a prerequisite step in its signal transduction pathway. However, the role of hormone in promoting these receptor-DNA interactions is controversial.[37] Whereas it is generally accepted that hormone is required under most circumstances to promote a high affinity association of ER with DNA in intact cells,[37–40] analysis of ER-DNA interactions *in vitro*, as accessed by electromobility shift assay, indicates that hormone is not required for specific DNA binding.[41] This issue has been complicated further by studies which showed that transfection of an ER-expression vector into mammalian Hela cells, in the absence of ligand, was sufficient to activate target gene transcription.[42] It is possible that this type of ligand independent activation occurs as a consequence of receptor overexpression, however it does suggest that in some cell and promoter contexts ER may interact with DNA and regulate gene transcription in a ligand independent manner.

ER and hPR as transcription factors

In the last few years significant advances in defining the mechanism of transcriptional regulation by RNA polymerase II has been achieved[43] providing insights which are likely to enhance our understanding of steroid hormone action. Briefly, eukaryotic transcription relies on a complex network of protein-protein interactions which occur between proteins bound at specific DNA sites within a particular promoter. These regulatory sequences are located near the start site of transcription (core promoter) and at remote positions upstream or downstream thereof (enhancer). The core promoter, which is required for basal transcription, consists of the initiation site at +1 and the TATA box around −25.[44] This promoter element anchors the general transcription machinery and, under appropriate stimulation, recruits RNA polymerase to the promoter. Hormone activated ER and hPR assist in the assembly of the general transcription apparatus at target gene promoters by binding at DNA sequences at positions in the proximal promoter, or at the remote enhancers,[45] permitting their interaction with the general transcription machinery. The precise mechanism by which ER and hPR alter transcription by RNA polymerase II is unknown. However, it has been shown that transcriptionally active hPR potentiates target gene transcription, in a reconstituted system *in vitro*, by stabilizing the preinitiation complex.[46] Additionally, the demonstration that hER and hPR contact the general transcription factor TFIIB[47] indicates that at least part of the receptors ability to regulate target gene transcription is as a result of a direct interaction with the general transcription apparatus. In addition to these direct interactions, the hormone activated receptor can contact the general transcription machinery through intermediary adaptor proteins. Since it is likely that these adaptors are differentially expressed in target cells it is possible that their level of expression could influence the cellular sensitivity to hormones or impart upon the transcription machinery the ability to distinguish between agonist and antagonist activated receptor.[16,48] Recently, candidate adaptor proteins which interact specifically with agonist but not antagonist activated hER and hPR have been identified and cloned.[49–52] The precise role of these proteins in steroid hormone action and their effect on receptor pharmacology is currently under investigation.

Steroid hormone receptor antagonists

The preceding discussion has outlined the recent advances which have been made in understanding the molecular mechanism of action of progesterone and estrogen. In addition, however, this work has assisted in the definition of the molecular mechanism of action of antiestrogens and antiprogestogens. From this work two models for receptor antagonism have evolved. Specifically, antihormones could function in a competitive manner to block the access of the endogenous ligands to their receptor. Consequently, the steroid receptor (SR) would remain in an unactivated, latent state within the cell (Fig. 12.2A).[1] Alternatively, antihormones could function as 'pseudoagonists' by mimicking some of the actions of agonists, but ultimately pushing the SR down a transcriptionally nonproductive pathway. As a result of this interaction, the 'inactive' receptor (Fig. 12.2B) may have additional activities, such as competing with the agonist activated SR for DNA binding sites and/or for components of the transcriptional machinery. The pharmacological implications of these two types of antagonists are likely to be different.[53] Given our current understanding of antihormone action, the second model more likely explains the mechanism of action for most known steroid receptor antagonists.

Antagonism of progesterone receptor function

All the currently available antiprogestogens interact directly with the hormone binding domain of hPR, competitively inhibiting progesterone binding. With one exception (ZK98299; Onapristone), interaction of the receptor with these antihormones is sufficient to promote high affinity interactions of the receptor with

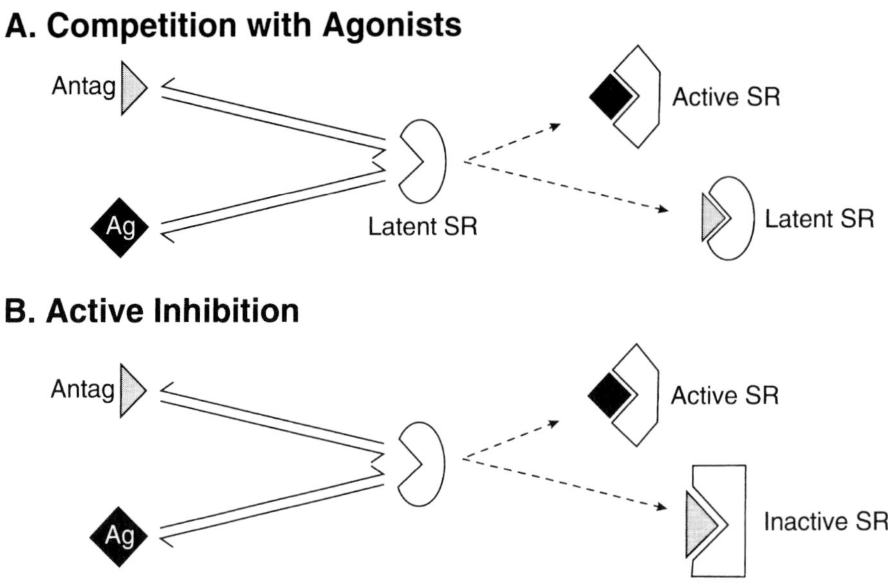

Fig. 12.2 Potential mechanisms of action of steroid hormone receptor antagonists. In the absence of hormone, the steroid receptor resides in an inactive complex in the nuclei of target cells. Hormone binding to the receptor initiates a cascade of events which result ultimately in the alteration of the rate of transcription of a target gene. Given what we know of the signal transduction pathway of sex steroids, it is likely that at least two types of antagonist can be developed. One class of antagonist could competitively interact with the receptor and block access to agonists. This passive type of inhibition would maintain the receptor in a 'latent state', while the antagonist is physically bound to the receptor. Alternatively, inhibition could be more 'active'. In this mode antagonists would behave as pseudoagonists, mimicking some of the effects of agonists. Thus, the antagonist would convert the receptor (SR) from a latent form to one which is 'inactive'. This form of the receptor is likely to have additional inhibitory activities by competing with hormone activated SR for DNA binding sites and ultimately by associating nonproductively with the general transcription apparatus. All but one of the currently available antihormones appear to function as 'active inhibitors' or 'pseudoagonists'.

target DNA sequences.[54,55] The mechanism of action of ZK98299 is distinct in that it binds to receptor but does not promote the formation of a high affinity hPR-DNA complex when assayed *in vitro*. One possible interpretation of this result is that ZK98299 prevents receptor dimerization, a requisite step for DNA binding. Based on these observations it has been concluded that processes which operate downstream of DNA binding are primarily responsible for distinguishing agonist from antagonist activated PR.[16,48,56,57] Consequently, the antiprogestogens have been classified as type I, which prevent DNA binding, and type II, which appear to deliver the receptor to DNA (Fig. 12.3). In addition, unlike Onapristone (type I), the type II antiprogestogens appear to exhibit partial agonist activities under some experimental conditions. Recently, however, the type I antiprogestogen ZK98299 has been found to have a lower ED_{50} than most of the other type II antiprogestogens, suggesting that the distinction between type I and type II antiprogestogens is not a mechanistic distinction but reflects a difference in affinity. This possibility is in agreement with data from Milgrom's laboratory which demonstrate that *in vivo*, at concentrations of ligand which saturate the receptor, ZK98299 is functionally identical to other antiprogestogens.[58] Irrespective of these results, however, the current basis for classifying hPR antagonists is whether they prevent (type I) or promote (type II) the association of receptor with DNA *in vitro* (using the nomenclature of Klein-Hitpass).[54]

Although both agonists and antagonists interact with the ligand binding domain of hPR, it has been determined by receptor mutagenesis that the sequences within this domain, required for agonist and antagonist binding, are overlapping but distinct.[59,60] In support of this hypothesis, a mutant hPR (hPR-UP-1) in which the carboxyl 54 amino acids were deleted, was

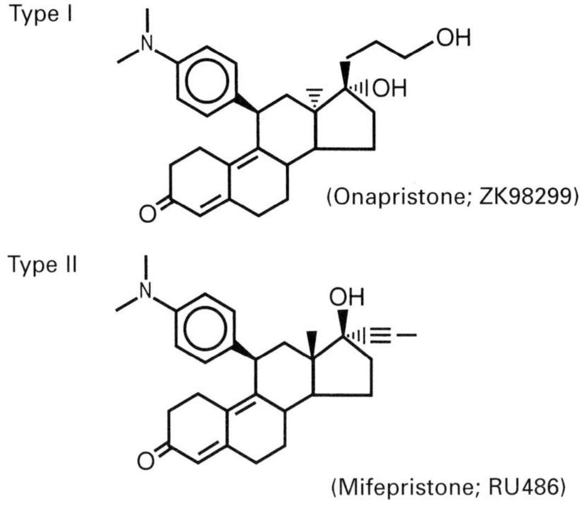

Type I

(Onapristone; ZK98299)

Type II

(Mifepristone; RU486)

Fig. 12.3 Classification of antiprogestogens. *In vitro* analysis reveals two distinct types: type I prevent or impair receptor/DNA interactions; type II interfere with a required process following DNA binding.

identified. Interestingly, antagonists, but not agonists, can bind this mutant receptor. In addition, it was observed that on this mutant the antiprogestogen RU486 could function as a potent agonist. In a separate series of studies, Benhamou et al identified amino acids within the PR-ligand binding domain which when mutated disrupted antagonist but not agonist binding.[59] Together this information indicated that the sequences required for progesterone and RU486 binding were distinct. In addition, it indicates that the carboxyl tail of hPR may be part of a functional unit which, in the absence of hormone, maintains the receptor in a transcriptionally inactive form. We have recently extended these studies and have demonstrated that a third class of ligands, mixed agonists, interact with the ligand binding domain in a manner distinct from agonist and antagonists.[61] Thus, we have concluded that the biology of a given hPR-ligand can be predicted based upon how it interacts with the receptor.[48,60,62]

An important clue to understanding how the cellular transcriptional machinery distinguishes between hPR ligands was provided by the elegant studies of Allan et al.[62] By performing limited protease digestion of *in vitro* synthesized hPR in the absence or presence of ligands, it was demonstrated that progesterone and the antagonist RU486 induce distinct conformational changes within the receptor protein. Using specific monoclonal antibodies, this conformational change was shown to occur at the extreme carboxyl terminus of the receptor.[60,62] In keeping with this theme, Wagner et al were able to show that the hPR mixed agonists, which interact in a unique manner with the receptor, induce an alteration within receptor structure distinct from that induced by agonists or antagonists.[61] Consequently, a link has been established between the structure of the ligand-receptor complex and resulting biology. This is an extremely important observation as it suggests that it may be possible to develop tissue (or process) specific hPR-modulators by selecting for compounds which induce or promote the formation of different receptor conformations which interface differently with cell and promoter specific factors.

Using the information gained from the biochemical and genetic experiments detailed above, we have developed a working model to explain the mechanism by which hPR distinguishes between different ligands (Fig. 12.4). In this model we propose that the C terminal region of hPR acts as a transcriptional repressor. This event results from either inter- or intramolecular interactions. We propose that interaction of hPR with either an agonist, an antagonist or a mixed agonist results in unique conformational changes within the receptor, all of which permit displacement of heat shock proteins. However, only the agonist, and to a lesser extent the partial agonist induced conformations, can overcome the effect of the inhibitory tail domain and effect a productive association of the receptor with the transcription apparatus. Although confirmation of this hypothesis will likely require crystallographic information, the observations we have made indicate that *different* ligands interacting with hPR in *different* ways can yield *different* biologies.

Antagonism of estrogen receptor function

Some of the most commonly used antiestrogens, both in therapy and experimental endocrinology, are shown in Figure 12.5. Using a combination of *in vitro* and *in vivo* methodologies these compounds have been classified into different mechanistic categories. Among these compounds are found both steroidal (ICI164,384) and nonsteroidal antiestrogens (tamoxifen).[16,48,63,64] The antiestrogen ICI164,384 is steroidal in nature and was originally developed as an affinity ligand for hER. It was subsequently determined that the addition of the large 7α-alkyl sidechain to the steroid nucleus permitted its interaction with the receptor and its subsequent activity as an antiestrogen. The biology of this class of antiestrogens has been studied extensively as they represent the first compounds developed which are

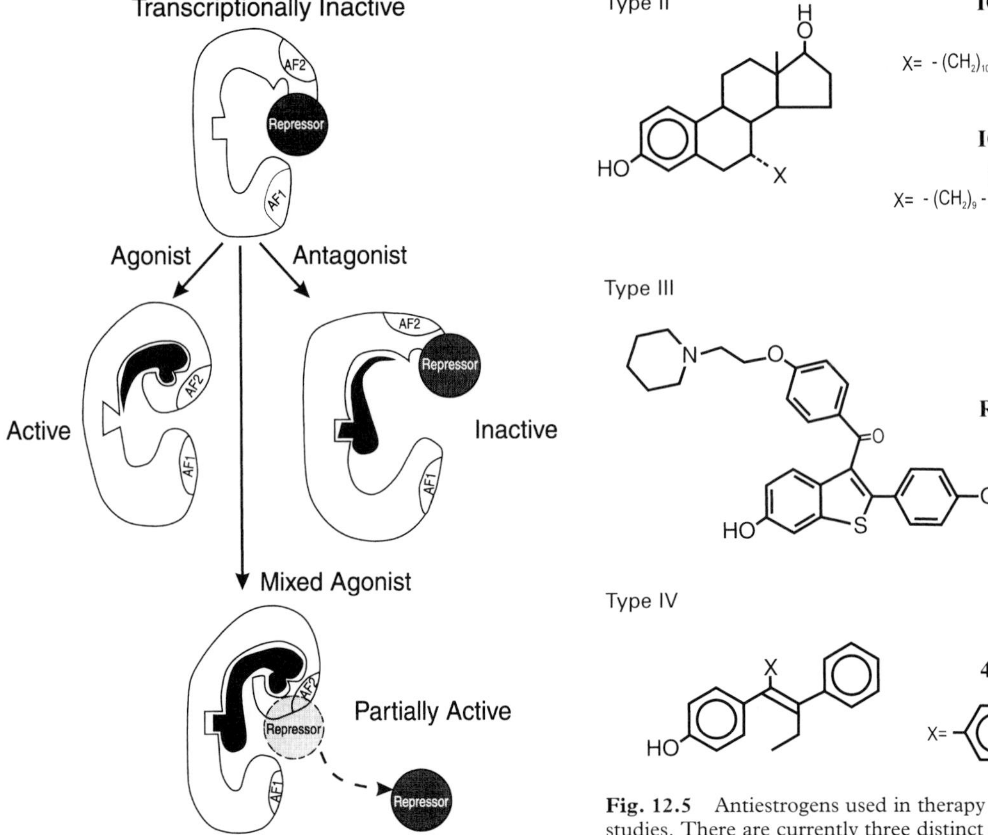

Fig. 12.4 The mechanism of action of hPR agonists and antagonists. Based on information which has been published (and referenced in the text) and additional data presented in this review, we propose the following model to explain how the cell distinguishes between PR agonists and antagonists. In the unliganded state PR is in a transcriptionally inactive conformation and consequently is associated with a putative repressor protein. Agonists bind to the more C terminal portion of the receptor and thereby induce a structural change in the receptor which results in a transcriptionally active receptor, possibly due to the removal of the repressor protein and/or by inducing a structural change in the activation domains producing a more productive conformation for transactivation. Antagonists, which bind to the more N terminal part of the HBD induce a different conformation in the receptor, in which the C terminus is not pulled in towards the receptor. The conformational change induced by antagonists may be insufficient to cause the removal of the repressor or allow activation by either AF1 or AF2. Mixed agonists can bind to both the C terminal and N terminal regions of the HBD inducing a new conformation that is different from those induced by either agonists or antagonists. The mixed agonist conformation allows some partial activity, but does not allow full agonistic activity. This may be the result of continued but less stable association with the repressor.

Fig. 12.5 Antiestrogens used in therapy and experimental studies. There are currently three distinct classes recognized: type II, where no partial agonist activity is observed; type III, which are antagonist in most tissues but agonist in bone; type IV, which are agonist in uterus and bone.

devoid of hER partial agonist activity. The other widely used antiestrogens are the triphenylethylenes, such as tamoxifen or droloxifene, and the benzothiophene derived compound, raloxifene. These compounds are unusual in that they function as hER antagonists in most tissues whereas in some cell and promoter contexts they manifest partial agonist activity. In particular, these compounds exhibit antiestrogenic activities in the breast whereas they manifest estrogenic actions in bone and in the cardiovascular system. The molecular basis for this action has been studied in extensive detail and will not be reviewed further here.[16,41,47,48,56,65]

The mechanism of action of the different antiestrogens is slowly being unraveled. The steroidal antiestrogen ICI164,384 is a pure antiestrogen both *in vivo* and *in vitro*. It has been postulated that ICI164,384 blocks hER function by impairing receptor dimerization.[41,63,66] However, whether or not effective binding of hER to DNA can occur following exposure to ICI164,384 remains controversial. It has been shown that the stability of hER dimers may vary depending on the cellular source of hER[67] and the experimental conditions used to test receptor dimers-DNA interaction. These differences may explain why some investigators have been unable to show any effects of ICI164,384 on hER-DNA interactions[68] but do not explain why in several *in vivo* systems DNA binding is accomplished by these compounds. Unlike ICI164,384, the benzothiophene (raloxifene) and triphenylethylene (tamoxifen)-derived antiestrogens clearly deliver hER to DNA. In most circumstances this activity can lead to antagonism of hER activity.[16,48,65] However, the agonist/antagonist activity of these latter compounds is influenced by cell and promoter context. Using a series of novel *in vitro* models, molecular criteria which clearly distinguish hER agonists from partial agonists and additionally classify the known hER antagonists into three functionally distinct categories have been derived. The behavior of known agonists and antagonists suggests that these classifications are related to distinct ligand induced structural alterations within hER. A model outlining these classifications is shown in Figure 12.6. It is proposed that hER exists in an equilibrium between an inactive and an active state, such that in the absence of ligand the inactive conformation is preferred. Interaction of hER with 17β-estradiol stabilizes the complex in a conformation which facilitates transactivation. The relative agonist/antagonist balance of other hER modulators is determined by the intermediate conformation promoted by the particular compound. Adopting the convention established by Klein-Hitpass et al, which was originally used to classify antiprogestogens, it is now proposed that compounds which prevent hER/DNA interactions are called type I antiestrogens.[54] Unlike the case of hPR, a type I antiestrogen has not yet been defined.

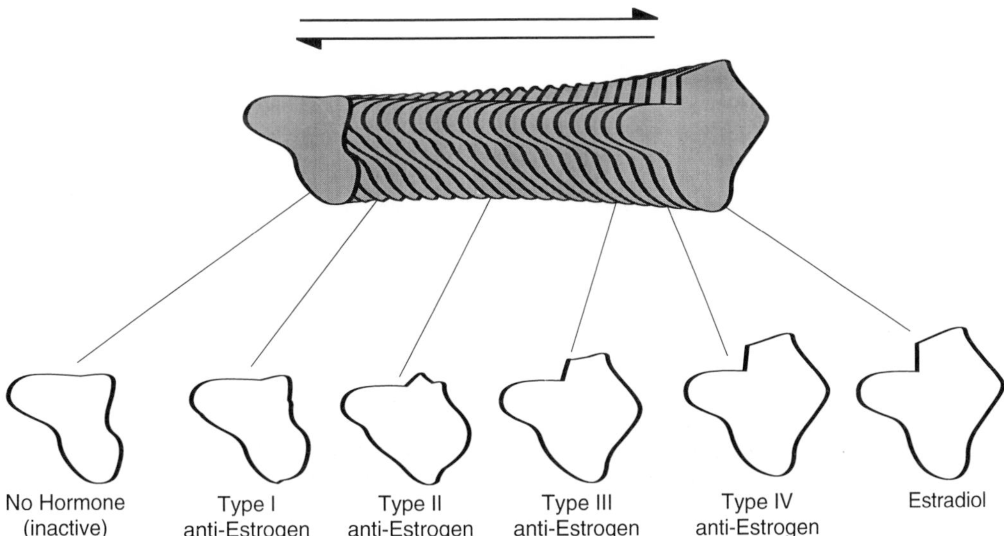

Fig. 12.6 Hormones and antihormones stabilize distinct conformational states within hER. It is likely that hER can exist in the cell in multiple conformations which represent the inactive state, the active state and several intermediate states, and that ligands exert their biological activities by stabilizing specific ER structures. These distinct conformations could result as a consequence of the ability of compounds to freeze the receptor in a specific conformation by blocking a processive interchange from inactive to active (as shown). Alternatively, the compounds can promote the establishment of unique receptor conformations which result as a consequence of specific ligand-receptor interactions. Based on the nomenclature established by Klein-Hitpass[54] and the findings of our study, we have divided the known antiestrogens into distinct classes represented by ICI164,384 (type II), raloxifene (type III) and 4-hydroxytamoxifen (type IV) respectively. Although we have been unable to demonstrate the existence of a type I antiestrogen (a compound which prevents receptor/DNA association), conceptually it is likely that such a compound will be discovered. The intense efforts to identify novel ER modulators make it likely that additional types of antiestrogen may emerge in the future.

Based on this nomenclature it is proposed that ICI164,384 is a type II antiestrogen that induces a conformation which is closest to that of the inactive receptor. The hER antagonist raloxifene, which can function as a partial agonist under restricted conditions, is a representative member of type III antiestrogens. Finally, 4OH-T (and other triphenylethylene derived antiestrogens) represent type IV antiestrogens which stabilize hER in a conformation which allows it to exhibit transcriptional activity on a limited subset of hER responsive genes.[16,48] Currently, this model demonstrates that the known antiestrogens can be divided into three distinct classes. As new chemicals are identified, it is possible that additional classes of antagonist may be discovered.

Conclusion

The information obtained from these and related studies will impact our understanding of the cellular mechanisms which distinguish between hormone agonists and antagonists. In addition, it provides a series of molecular tools with which to predict the *in vivo* biological activity of novel hER and hPR modulators. The remaining frontiers are to define the mechanism(s) by which the cellular transcription machinery distinguishes agonist from antagonist activated steroid receptors. The genetic tools currently available and the ability to reconstitute hER/hPR activity *in vitro* will assist greatly in the resolution of this issue.

REFERENCES

1. Clark JH, Peck EJ 1979 Female sex steroids: receptors and function, 1st edn. Monographs on Endocrinology, vol. 14. Springer-Verlag, New York
2. Barzel US 1988 Estrogens in the prevention and treatment of postmenopausal osteoporosis. American Journal of Medicine 85: 847–850
3. Eaker ED, Chesebro JH, Sacks FM, Wenger NK, Whisnant JP, Winston M 1993 Cardiovascular disease in women. Circulation 88: 1999–2009
4. Greene GL, Gilna P, Waterfield M, Baker A, Hort Y, Shine J 1986 Sequence and expression of human estrogen receptor complementary DNA. Science 231: 1150–1154
5. Fuqua SAW, Chamness GC, McGuire WL 1993 Estrogen receptor mutations in breast cancer. Journal of Cellular Biochemistry 51: 135–139
6. Horwitz KB, Alexander PS 1983 In situ photolinked nuclear progesterone receptors of human breast cancer cells: subunit molecular weights after transformation and translocation. Endocrinology 113: 2195–2201
7. Kastner P, Krust A, Turcotte B et al 1990 Two distinct estrogen-regulated promoters generate transcripts encoding the two functional different human progesterone receptor forms A and B. EMBO J 9: 1603–1614
8. Mangelsdorf DJ, Thummel C, Beato M et al 1995 The nuclear receptor superfamily: the second decade. Cell 83: 835–839
9. Laudet V, Hänni C, Coll J, Catzeflis F, Stéhelin D 1992 Evolution of the nuclear receptor gene superfamily. EMBO J 11(3): 1003–1013
10. Mangelsdorf DJ, Evans RM 1995 The RXR heterodimers and orphan receptors. Cell 83: 841–850
11. Danielian PS, White T, Hoare SA, Fawell SE, Parker MG 1993 Identification of residues in the estrogen receptor that confer differential sensitivity to estrogen and hydroxytamoxifen. Molecular Endocrinology 7: 232–240
12. Danielsen M, Northrop JP, Jonklaas J, Ringold GM 1987 Domains of the glucocorticoid receptor involved in specific and nonspecific deoxyribonucleic acid binding, hormone activation and transcriptional enhancement. Molecular Endocrinology 1: 816–822
13. Dobson ADW, Conneely OM, Beattie W et al 1989 Mutational analysis of the chicken progesterone receptor. Journal of Biological Chemistry 264(7): 4207–4211
14. Hollenberg S, Evans R 1988 Multiple and cooperative trans-activation domains of the human glucocorticoid receptor. Cell 55: 899–906
15. Tasset D, Tora L, Fromental C, Scheer E, Chambon P 1990 Distinct classes of transcriptional activating domains function by different mechanisms. Cell 62: 1177–1187
16. Tzukerman MT, Esty A, Santiso-Mere D et al 1994 Human estrogen receptor transcriptional capacity is determined by both cellular and promoter context and mediated by two functionally distinct intramolecular regions. Molecular Endocrinology 8: 21–30
17. Sartorius CA, Melville MY, Hovland AR, Tung L, Takimoto GS, Horwitz KB 1994 A third transactivation function (AF3) of human progesterone receptors located in the unique N-terminal segment of the B-isoform. Molecular Endocrinology 8: 1347–1360
18. Meyer M-E, Quirin-Stricker C, Lerouge T, Bocquel M-T, Gronemeyer H 1992 A limiting factor mediates the differential activation of promoters by the human progesterone receptor isoforms. Journal of Biological Chemistry 267: 10882–10887
19. Beato M, Herrlich P, Schutz G 1995 Steroid hormone receptors: many actors in search of a plot. Cell 83: 851–857
20. O'Malley BW, Schrader WT, Mani S et al 1995 An alternative ligand-independent pathway for activation of steroid receptors. Recent Progress in Hormone Research 50: 333–347
21. Pratt WB 1990 Interaction of hsp90 with steroid receptors — organizing some diverse observations and presenting the newest concepts. Molecular and Cellular Endocrinology 74(1): C69–C76
22. Smith DF, Faber LE, Toft DO 1990 Purification of unactivated progesterone receptor and identification of novel receptor-associated proteins. Journal of Biological Chemistry 265(7): 3996–4003
23. Bagchi MK, Tsai S-Y, Tsai M-J, O'Malley BW 1991 Progesterone enhances target gene transcription by receptor free of heat shock protein hsp90, hsp56, and hsp70. Molecular and Cell Biology 11: 4998–5004

24. Renoir JP, Radanyi C, Jung-Testas I, Faber LE, Baulieu EE 1990 The nonactivated progesterone receptor is a nuclear heteroligomer. Journal of Biological Chemistry 265: 14402–14406
25. Cadepond F, Schweizergroyer G, Segardmaurel I et al 1991 Heat shock protein-90 as a critical factor in maintaining glucocorticosteroid receptor in a nonfunctional state. Journal of Biological Chemistry 266(9): 5834–5841
26. Pratt W, Scherrer L, Hutchison K, Dalman F 1992 A model of glucocorticoid receptor unfolding and stabilization by a heat shock protein complex. Journal of Steroid Biochemistry 41(3–8): 223–229
27. Kost SL, Smith DF, Sullivan WP, Welch WJ, Toft DO 1989 Binding of heat shock proteins to the avian progesterone receptor. Molecular and Cell Biology 9(9): 3829–3838
28. Picard D, Khursheed B, Garabedian MJ, Fortin MG, Lindquist S, Yamamoto KR 1990 Reduced levels of hsp90 compromise steroid receptor action in vivo. Nature 348: 166–168
29. Bohen SP 1995 Hsp90 mutants disrupt glucocorticoid receptor ligand binding and destabilize aporeceptor complexes. Journal of Biological Chemistry 270: 29433–29438
30. Smith DF, Toft DO 1993 Steroid receptors and their associated proteins. Molecular Endocrinology 7(1): 4–11
31. DeMarzo AM, Beck CA, Onate SA, Edwards DP 1991 Dimerization of mammalian progesterone receptors occurs in the absence of DNA and is related to the release of the 90-kDa heat shock protein. Proceedings of the National Academy of Science, USA 88: 72–76
32. Edwards D, Kühnel B, Estes P, Nordeen S 1989 Human progesterone receptor binding to mouse mammary tumor virus deoxyribonucleic acid: dependence on hormone and nonreceptor nuclear factor(s). Molecular Endocrinology 3: 381–391
33. Bagchi MK, Elliston JF, Tsai SY, Edwards DP, Tsai M-J, O'Malley BW 1988 Steroid hormone-dependent interaction of human progesterone receptor with its target enhancer element. Molecular Endocrinology 2: 1221–1229
34. Bagchi M, Tsai M-J, O'Malley B, Tsai S 1992 Analysis of the mechanism of steroid hormone receptor-dependent gene activation in cell-free systems. Endocrine Reviews 13(3): 525–535
35. Takimoto G, Tasset D, Eppert A, Horwitz K 1992 Hormone-induced progesterone receptor phosphorylation consists of sequential DNA-independent and DNA-dependent stages: analysis with zinc finger mutants and the progesterone antagonist ZK98299. Proceedings of the National Academy of Science, USA 89: 3050–3054
36. Takimoto GS, Horwitz KB 1993 Progesterone receptor phosphorylation: complexities in defining a functional role. Trends in Endocrinology and Metabolism 4: 1–7
37. McDonnell DP, Nawaz Z, O'Malley BW 1991 In situ distinction between steroid receptor binding and transactivation at a target gene. Molecular and Cell Biology 11: 4350–4355
38. Pham TA, Elliston JF, Nawaz Z, McDonnell DP, Tsai M-J, O'Malley BW 1991 Antiestrogen can establish non-productive complexes and alter chromatin structure at target enhancers. Proceedings of the National Academy of Science, USA 88: 3125–3129
39. Pham TA, Hwung Y-P, McDonnell DP, O'Malley BW 1991 Transactivation functions facilitate the disruption of chromatin structure by estrogen receptor derivatives in vivo. Journal of Biological Chemistry 266: 18179–18187
40. Pham TA, Hwung Y-P, Santiso-Mere D, McDonnell DP, O'Malley BW 1992 Ligand-dependent and independent functions of the transactivation regions of the human estrogen receptor in yeast. Molecular Endocrinology 6: 1043–1050
41. Dana SL, Hoener PA, Wheeler DL, Lawrence CL, McDonnell DP 1994 Novel estrogen response elements identified by genetic selection in yeast are differentially responsive to estrogens and antiestrogens in mammalin cells. Molecular Endocrinology 8: 1193–1207
42. Tzukerman M, Zhang HK, Hermann T, Wills KN, Graupner G, Pfahl M 1990 The human estrogen receptor has transcriptional activator and repressor functions in the absence of ligand. New Biology 2: 613–620
43. Tjian R, Maniatis T 1994 Transcriptional activation: a complex puzzle with a few easy pieces. Cell 77: 5–8
44. Smale ST 1994 Core promoter architecture for eukaryotic protein-coding genes. In: Conaway RC, Conaway JW (eds) Transcription: mechanisms and regulation, vol. 3. Raven Press, New York, pp 63–81
45. Mitchell PJ, Tjian R 1989 Transcriptional regulation in mammalian cells by sequence-specific DNA binding proteins. Science 245: 371–378
46. Klein-Hitpass L, Tsai SY, Weigel NL et al 1990 The progesterone receptor stimulates cell-free transcription by enhancing the formation of a stable preinitiation complex. Cell 60: 247–257
47. Ing N, Beekman J, Tsai S, Tsai M-J, O'Malley B 1992 Members of the steroid hormone receptor superfamily interact with TFIIB (S300-II). Journal of Biological Chemistry 267: 17617–17623
48. McDonnell DP, Clemm DL, Herman T, Goldman ME, Pike JW 1995 Analysis of estrogen receptor function in vitro reveals three distinct classes of antiestrogens. Molecular Endocrinology 9: 659–669
49. Onate SA, Tsai S, Tsai M-J, O'Malley BW 1995 Sequence and characterization of a coactivator for the steroid hormone receptor superfamily. Science 270: 1354–1357
50. Cavaillès V, Dauvois S, L'Horset F et al 1995 Nuclear factor RIP140 modulates transcriptional activation by the estrogen receptor. EMBO J 14(15): 3741–3751
51. Le Douarin B, Zechel C, Garnier J-M et al 1995 The N-terminal part of TIF1, a putative mediator of the ligand-dependent activation function (AF-2) of nuclear receptors, is fused to B-raf in the oncogenic protein T18. EMBO J 14(9): 2020–2033
52. Kamei Y, Xu L, Heinzel T et al 1996 A CBP integrator complex mediates transcriptional activation and AP-1 inhibition by nuclear receptors. Cell 85: 403–414
53. McDonnell DP 1995 Unraveling the human progesterone receptor signal transduction pathway: insights into antiprogestin action. Trends in Endocrinology and Metabolism 6: 133–138
54. Klein-Hitpass L, Cato ACB, Henderson D, Ryffel GU 1991 Two types of antiprogestins identified by their differential activation in transcriptionally active extracts from T47D cells. Nucleic Acids Research 19: 1227–1234

55. Bocquel M-T, Ji J, Ylikomi T et al 1993 Type II antagonists impair the DNA binding of steroid hormone receptors without affecting dimerization. Journal of Steroid Biochemistry and Molecular Biology 45: 205–215
56. McDonnell DP, Clemm DL, Imhof MO 1994 Definition of the cellular mechanisms which distinguish between hormone and antihormone activated steroid receptors. Seminars in Cancer Biology 5: 503–513
57. McDonnell DP, Vegeto E, O'Malley BW 1992 Identification of a negative regulatory function for steroid receptors. Proceedings of the National Academy of Science, USA 89: 10563–10567
58. Delabre K, Guiochon-Mantel A, Milgrom E 1993 In vivo evidence against the existence of antiprogestins disrupting receptor binding to DNA. Proceedings of the National Academy of Science, USA 90: 4421–4425
59. Benhamou B, Garcia T, Lerouge T et al 1992 A single amino acid that determines the sensitivity of progesterone receptors to RU486. Science 255: 206–209
60. Vegeto E, Allan GF, Schrader WT, Tsai M-J, McDonnell DP, O'Malley BW 1992 The mechanism of RU486 antagonism is dependent on the conformation of the carboxy-terminal tail of the human progesterone receptor. Cell 69: 703–713
61. Wagner BL, Pollio G, Leonhardt S et al 1996 16a-substituted analogs of the antiprogestin RU486 induce a unique conformation in the human progesterone receptor resulting in mixed agonist activity. Proceedings of the National Academy of Science, USA in press.
62. Allan GF, Leng X, Tsai S-T et al 1992 Hormone and antihormone induce distinct conformational changes which are central to steroid receptor activation. Journal of Biological and Chemistry 267: 19513–19520
63. Fawell SE, White R, Hoare S, Sydenham M, Page M, Parker MG 1990 Inhibition of estrogen receptor-DNA binding by the 'pure' antiestrogen ICI164,384 appears to be mediated by impaired receptor dimerization. Proceedings of the National Academy of Science, USA 87: 6883–6887
64. Wakeling AE, Dukes M, Bowler J 1991 A potent specific pure antiestrogen with clinical potential. Cancer Research 51: 3867–3873
65. Berry M, Metzgar D, Chambon P 1990 Role of the two activating domains of the oestrogen receptor in the cell-type and promoter-context dependent agonistic activity of the anti-oestrogen 4-hydroxytamoxifen. EMBO J 9: 2811–2818
66. Dauvois S, Danielian PS, White R, Parker MG 1992 Antiestrogen ICI164,384 reduces cellular estrogen receptor content by increasing its turnover. Proceedings of the National Academy of Science, USA 89: 4037–4041
67. Arbuckle N, Dauvois S, Parker M 1992 Effects of antioestrogens on the DNA binding activity of oestrogen receptors in vitro. Nucleic Acids Research 20: 3839–3844
68. Martinez E, Wahli W 1989 Cooperative binding of estrogen receptor to imperfect estrogen-responsive DNA elements correlates with their synergistic hormone-dependent enhancer activity. EMBO J 8(12): 3781–3791

13. Effects of estrogen and progesterone on the endometrium

Hilary O.D. Critchley David L. Healy

Introduction

The endometrium is distinctive in both form and function. The important roles of the endometrium are implantation and, in the absence of pregnancy, a rapid ability to regenerate and repair.[1] There are morphological characteristics of the endometrium specific to the prevailing endocrine environment. In the absence of sex steroid exposure (e.g. after menopause) endometrium is inactive. Estrogen and progesterone act upon the endometrium via their respective receptors to initiate either directly or indirectly appropriate changes in structure responsible for the required functional end-points, implantation, regeneration and repair.

ENDOCRINE SEX STEROID CHANGES DURING NORMAL MENSTRUAL CYCLE

Throughout reproductive life the endometrium responds in a cyclical manner to endocrine stimuli. In women, estradiol and progesterone, mainly of ovarian origin, are secreted in a sequence of events which commences with folliculogenesis and proceeds to extrusion of a mature ovum and transformation of the follicle into a corpus luteum. During menses, levels of both estradiol and progesterone are low. Thereafter, the first half of the menstrual cycle (proliferative phase) is estrogen dominated and characterized by a progressive increase in circulating estradiol from the developing Graafian follicle.

The latter half of the cycle (secretory phase) is progesterone dominated. Progesterone is essential for the establishment and maintenance of pregnancy in all mammalian species. Luteal cells display an increasing ability to synthesize progesterone in large quantities, and to a lesser extent they also synthesize estradiol.

During the first three days after ovulation, circulating estradiol and progesterone levels are low, but reach a peak by day 8 or 9 postovulation. If conception fails to occur, they first gradually and then precipitously decline 10–12 days after ovulation. The corpus luteum lifespan is about 14 days in women. Its regression begins a few days earlier and is heralded by a progressive or precipitous decline in progesterone secretion.[2] The functional lifespan of the corpus luteum is dependent on luteinizing hormone (LH) support.[3] Regression of the corpus luteum is pivotal in regulating the menstrual cycle as it permits follicular development and the ovulatory surge of pituitary gonadotrophins in the subsequent cycle. With the decline in function of the corpus luteum, ovarian steroid secretion falls and menstrual bleeding follows. The fall in estradiol and inhibin production from the corpus luteum results in a rise in gonadotrophin release and a new cycle is initiated. Hence, 'the menstrual cycle is a repetitive expression of the operation of the hypothalamo-pituitary-ovarian system with associated structural and functional changes in the target tissues of the reproductive tract'.[3]

Morphological changes over the menstrual cycle

Accurate dating of the endometrium is essential in order to interpret the response of the endometrium to its steroid environment.[4,5] Ideally, the endometrial appearances should be related to the date of ovulation. Previously it was only possible to make reference to the date of the last menstrual period. However, since the availability of immunoassay, more precise dating with reference to timing of ovulation has been possible.[5] It is widely accepted that if histological dating is more than two days ahead of histological appearances, then the endometrium is advanced: if more than two days behind, it is retarded (i.e. out of phase). As a consequence of such descriptions much controversy over endometrial dating has arisen, which may well be the result of imprecise methodology.[5]

Maximum precision will be achieved if chronological dating is based on determination of the LH surge[6] or time of ovulation defined ultrasonically.

A yet superior method is morphometric analysis, which provides a quantitative description of endometrial structure.[7,8,9] Li et al[8] assessed endometrial biopsies from normal fertile women which were precisely dated by the LH surge (chronological dating). All biopsies were exposed to a total of 17 morphometric measurements which were analysed to show that of these, only five measurements are necessary to achieve a reliable correlation. These features are the volume fraction of the gland occupied by gland cells, predecidual reaction, luminal secretion, pseudostratification and glandular mitoses.[5] The detailed study by Johannisson et al[10] documented statistically that the endometrium was a good marker for luteal phase estradiol and progesterone function.

The normal endometrium

The endometrium is composed of two layers: a basal layer, from which the endometrium regenerates after menstrual shedding, and an overlying functional layer. The depth of the latter varies during the menstrual cycle. It is maximal in the late proliferative or midsecretory phase and shallowest immediately postmenstruation. It is absent in the postmenopausal years.[1] The functional layer has a classic response to ovarian sex steroid stimulation. Cyclic changes are demonstrated in all components: glandular, vascular and stromal, in anticipation of implantation of a blastocyst. In the absence of conception, menstruation ensues. The basal layer constitutes the reserve cell layer of the endometrium and provides the source for cyclic regeneration of the functional layer.

The endometrial stroma is composed of mesenchymal cells, collagen and a delicate network of reticulin fibers, embedded in a ground substance. The stroma provides support for the endometrial glands and has a rich blood supply. There are two types of blood vessel within the endometrium. The spiral arteries, which are steroid responsive, are coiled and extend throughout the full thickness of the endometrium. The straight arteries supply the basal layer and are involved in the process of menstruation. Blood vessels in this basal layer are not influenced by hormonal changes.

Histological changes in the normal endometrium during the menstrual cycle

The classic description of the sequence of cyclic endometrial changes was published in 1950 by Noyes and colleagues.[4] Three phases of the endometrial development are recognized: a preovulatory or proliferative phase, a postovulatory or secretory phase and a menstrual phase.

Menstrual phase

The menstrual cycle commences with the first day of blood flow. The upper two thirds of the endometrium are shed. Early menstrual endometrium exhibits focal areas of subepithelial necrosis with subsequent glandular collapse and necrosis. As menses cease a typical shallow dense endometrium remains that is composed of the basal layer and residual deeper functional layer. From the third day of the cycle regeneration commences in glands and stromal elements.[1]

Proliferative phase

This commences from the fourth day of the cycle until ovulation. The changes evident in the endometrium are a consequence of rising estradiol levels. Initially the regenerating glands are tall and tubular, the stroma is compact and the gland to stroma ratio is low.[1] The epithelium lining the glands is composed of low columnar cells with a basally situated nucleus. The stromal cells have large nuclei surrounded by indistinct cytoplasm.[4] The characteristic features of the proliferative phase are mitoses, evident in glands and stroma (Fig. 13.1). As ovulation approaches, the epithelial cells become tall, columnar and pseudostratified. Thus the surface epithelium, previously thin and cuboidal, assumes a columnar appearance.[1] Scanning electron microscopy of the surface epithelium 4–8 days postmenstrually reveals closely placed dome-shaped cells mixed with ciliated cells in an approximate 30:1 ratio (Fig. 13.2). The number of ciliated cells increase in number as ovulation approaches.[11]

Secretory phase

Endometrial changes from ovulation until the onset of menses reflect the response to estradiol and progesterone exposure. Total endometrial thickness is limited to its preovulatory extent and consequently there is progressive tortuosity of glands and enhanced coiling of the spiral arteries. Three subsidiary phases are described: early, mid and late secretory. The early secretory phase (days 1–4 postovulation) is distinguished by the appearance of clear subnuclear vacuoles in all of the cells of at least 50% of the glands. This feature is pathognomonic for ovulation,[1] appearing 24–36 hours after the event (Fig. 13.3). Mitoses cease to be seen in the glandular epithelium after the fourth postovulatory day. Subnuclear vacuoles may persist up to the sixth postovulatory day. The midsecretory phase is from 5–9 days after

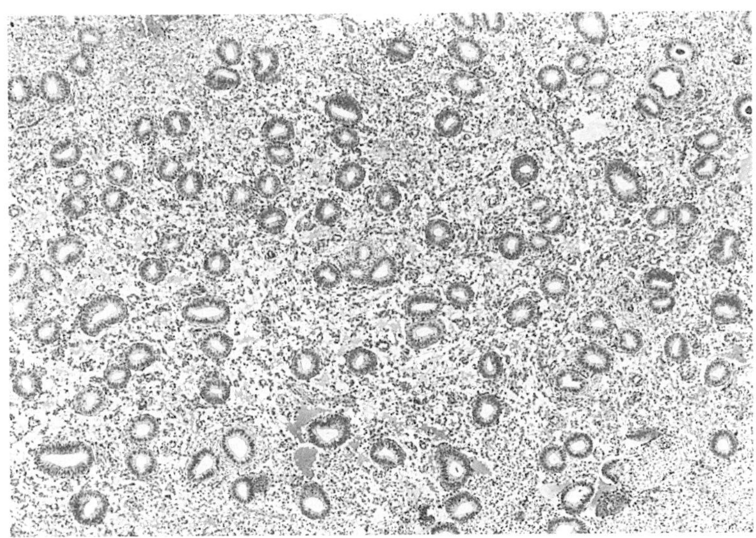

Fig. 13.1 Proliferative phase endometrium.[1]

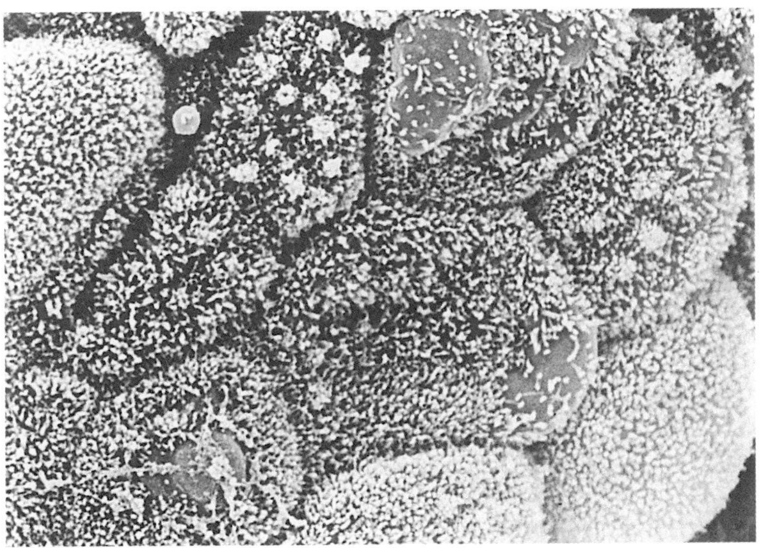

Fig. 13.2 Scanning electron micrograph of proliferative phase endometrium (day 8 of cycle). Dome shaped cells with a profuse array of short, occasionally branching, hair-like projections.

ovulation. Glandular secretions are copious and stromal edema is evident. Supranuclear vacuoles are no longer visible and the nuclei resume a basal position.[4] Stromal edema peaks on days 8–9 postovulation and spiral artery differentiation becomes apparent between the ninth and tenth postovulatory days.[1] Scrutiny with scanning electron microscopy (SEM) has revealed widening of gland orifices in the midsecretory phase.[15] Abundant ciliated cells occur close to the gland openings.

From midsecretory phase onwards ciliated cells then decrease in number and the cilia become shorter (Fig. 13.4). The period from day 10 postovulation until menses is described as the late secretory phase. It

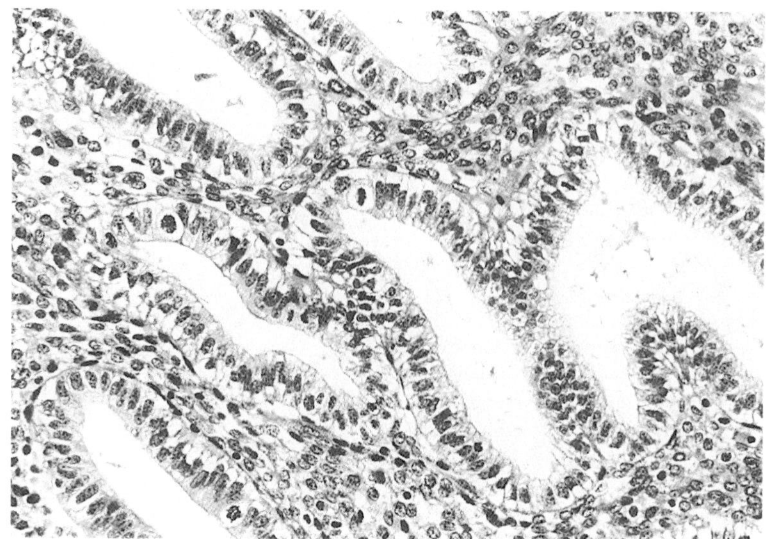

Fig. 13.3 Early secretory endometrium, 3rd postovulatory day. Subnuclear vacuoles are uniformly distributed.[1]

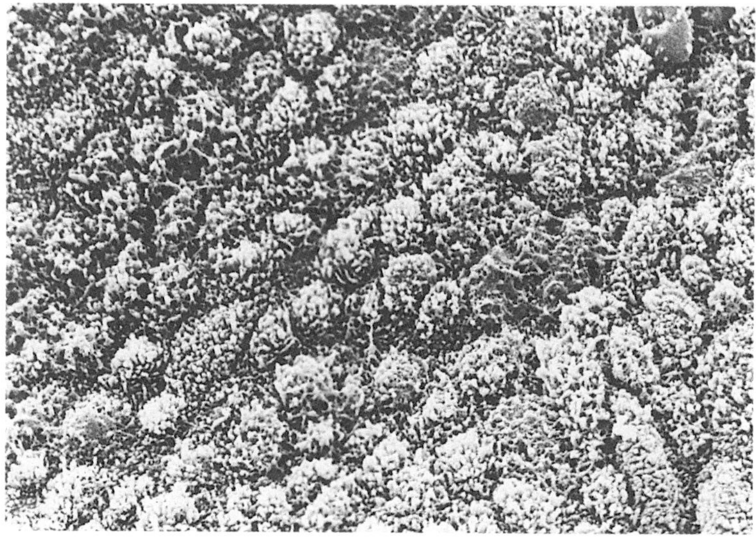

Fig. 13.4 Scanning electron micrograph of midsecretory phase endometrium (day 19 of cycle). Abundant hair-like microvilli cover the secretory cells.

is characterized by the progressive spread of predecidual change in the stroma, accompanied by regression of stromal edema and loss of endometrial height.[1] Initially, the predecidual change is evident around the spiral arteries but later is obvious around glands beneath the surface epithelium. Spiral arteries are particularly conspicuous (Fig. 13.5 & 13.6A,B). The glands have exhausted their secretions in the midsecretory phase and become tortuous, displaying a 'saw toothed' appearance.[1]

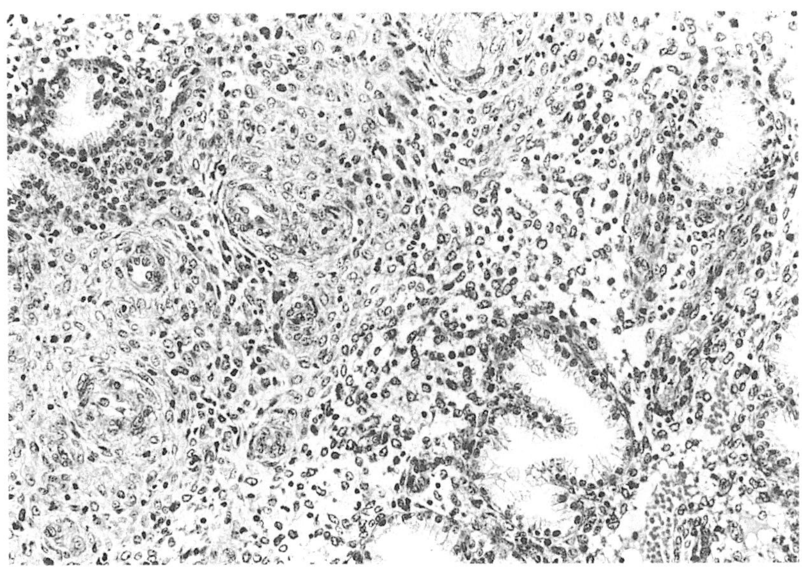

Fig. 13.5 Late secretory endometrium, 13th postovulatory day. Note the spiral arteriole is well muscularized and surrounded by a cuff of predecidualized stromal cells.[1]

Early decidual appearances

Successful implantation results in continued secretory activity and, indeed a hypersecretory appearance emerges.[1] Towards the end of the first trimester the glands become less active. Predecidual cells increase in size to become true decidual cells with pale nuclei, abundant cytoplasm and well defined borders (Fig. 13.7). Furthermore, SEM has demonstrated that ciliated cells disappear (Fig. 13.8). This is contrary to pseudodecidual tissue (Fig. 13.6A,B).[12]

Peri-implantation morphology

An ultrastructural marker of endometrial development, considered to signal the peri-implantation period in normal cycles, is the appearance on the apical surface of the luminal uterine epithelium of pinopodes.[13] Their precise function is unknown. In animal studies the formation of uterine pinopodes is dependent upon progesterone, and estrogen induces their regression.[14] In the human uterus the presence of epithelial pinopodes does not persist beyond 48 hours.[12,13] Pinopodes appear on day 19 of the cycle, are fully developed by day 20 and by day 21 most are regressing.[12,15]

Other features at the ultrastructural level, characteristic of the period when implantation may occur, include nuclear channel systems and giant mitochondria.[16] Nuclear channels are visualized in gland nuclei at day LH+4 and decrease in number from day LH+7. They are complex tubular systems with a lumen continuous with the perinuclear space (Fig. 13.9). Progesterone has been reported essential for nuclear channel formation, and *in vivo* and *in vitro*, exogenous estrogen has been observed to cause nuclear channels to disappear from gland cell nuclei.[16] Giant mitochondria have an unknown function (Fig. 13.10). They are thought to develop as a result of progesterone action on mitochondrial DNA.[16,17]

Leucocyte subpopulations in endometrium

The number and type of leucocytes in human endometrium and decidua varies during the menstrual cycle, with implantation and throughout pregnancy. It is thus likely that there is both an endocrine and paracrine control of leucocyte migration to and replication in this tissue.[18] Macrophages and lymphocytes form the major leucocyte subpopulations in the nonpregnant endometrial stroma. In the sheep,

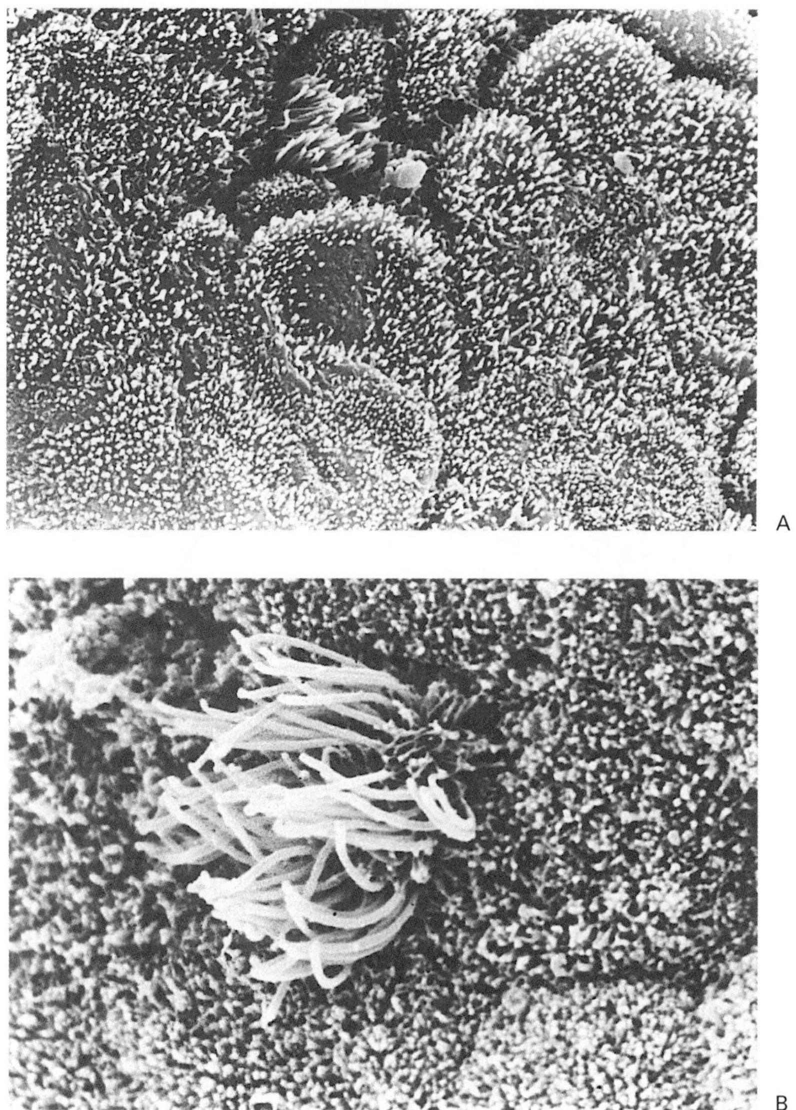

Fig. 13.6A Scanning electron micrograph of premenstrual phase endometrium. Ciliated cells remain evident. Nonciliated cells display a dome-shaped appearance. **B** Scanning electron micrographs of premenstrual endometrium (detailed view). Nonciliated cells with a microvillous cell surface. Detailed view of ciliated cell.

withdrawal of progesterone results in an influx of polymorphonuclear leucocytes.[19] Data pertaining to neutrophil subpopulations in human endometrium is scarce and there are no data on the mechanisms of recruitment. In 1987, Poropatich and colleagues,[20] reported the pattern of polymorphonuclear leucocytes during the normal menstrual cycle. Only small numbers were present throughout the cycle except immediately premenstrually and during menstruation. Neutrophils can synthesize and release a wide range of immunoregulatory cytokines and hence initiate and augment cellular and humoral immune responses.

Macrophages are an important component of endometrial tissue. About 20% of leucocytes in endometrium and decidua are macrophages[21] (Table 13.1). There is however some inconsistency in the

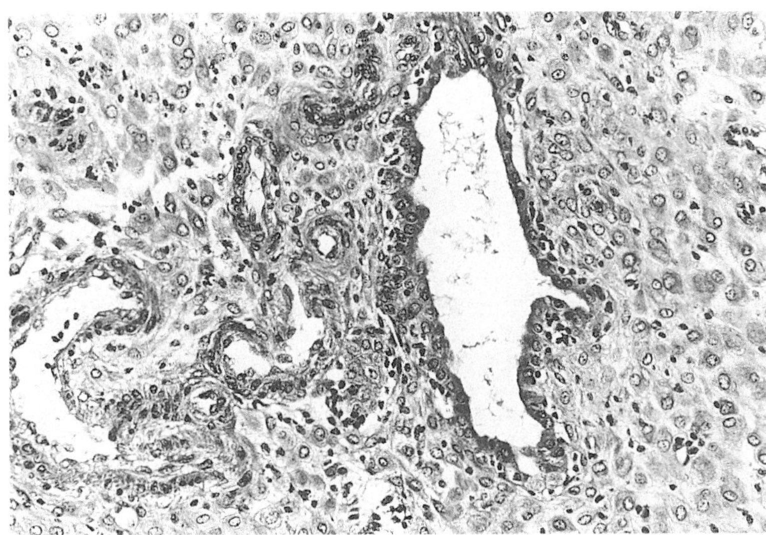

Fig. 13.7 Pregnancy endometrium. The stroma is decidualized and is infiltrated by a large number of darkly staining granulated lymphocytes. There is an exhausted secretory gland in the centre of the field and a cluster of thick-walled blood vessels lies to its left.

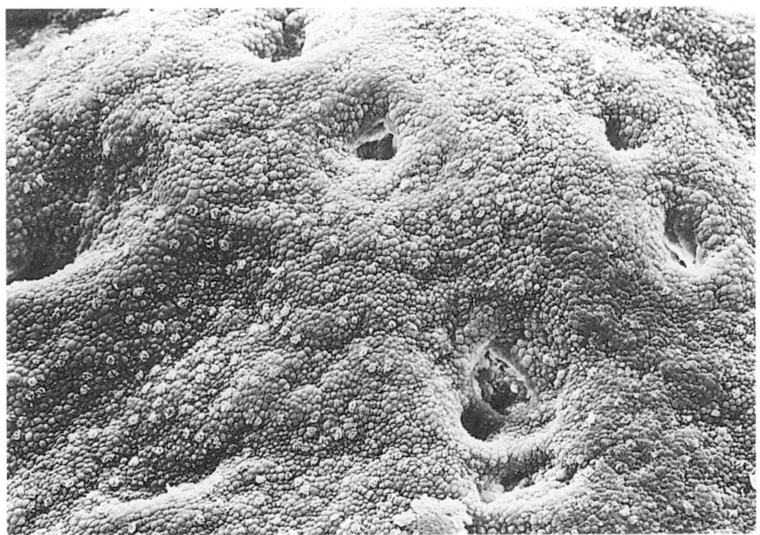

Fig. 13.8 Scanning electron micrograph of first trimester decidua (6 weeks gestation). Gland openings are clearly visible. Ciliated cells decrease in number.

literature concerning numbers and distribution of macrophages. This may reflect the surface markers utilized to identify macrophage populations and also whether or not the macrophages are activated. Bulmer and co-authors[22] described the presence of macrophages in the basal and functional layers throughout the cycle, failing to observe any fluctuation over the cycle and concluded that macrophage recruitment was not under hormonal control. In contrast, Kamat and Isaacson[23] have reported a premenstrual increase in endometrial macrophage populations. Klentzeris and colleagues[24] also reported

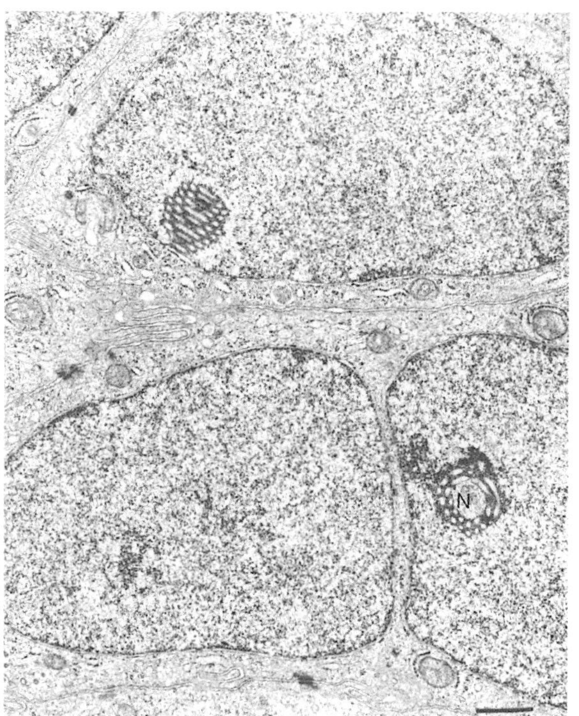

Fig. 13.9 Electron micrograph of human endometrium from day LH+6. Glandular epithelial cell nuclei are largely euchromatic and two nuclear channel systems (N) can be seen within the nuclei. Bar = 1 µm.

Fig. 13.10 Gland cells of human endometrium at about day LH+6 showing 'giant' mitochondria (M). Bar = 1 µm.

Table 13.1 Localization of leucocytes in uterine mucosa.[21]

	Nonpregnancy endometrium		Early decidua	
	Proliferative	Secretory	Basalis (trophoblast +)	Parietalis (trophoblast–)
Granulocytes				
Neutrophils	–	–/+	–/+	–
Eosinophils	–	–	–	–
Basophils	–	–	–	–
Lymphocytes				
B cells	–(+)	–(+)	–(+)	–(+)
T cells	+	+	+	+
NK cells (LGL)	+	+++	+++++	+++
Macrophages	+	+	+++	+

NK = natural killer; LGL = large granular lymphocyte

an increase in macrophage numbers in the late secretory phase (LH+10 to LH+13).

A population of phenotypically unusual lymphocytes (CD56+, CD16–, CD3–) have been reported to increase in the late luteal phase and cluster near glands and spiral arteries.[25] This cell population increases further in the first trimester of pregnancy, and numbers decline in the third trimester. These uterine leucocytes are granulated CD56+ NK (natural killer) like cells with a characteristic large granular lymphocyte morphology.[21] Their role is unknown, but a role in the implantation process has been postulated.

It also remains to be established whether the increases in this unique subpopulation of lymphocyte is a result of *in situ* proliferation or whether there is *de novo* peripheral migration from the circulation.[24,26] It would appear however that progesterone is essential for the appearance of CD56+ cells as their presence is only noted in ovariectomized women after treatment with both estrogen and progesterone. Estrogen replacement alone was insufficient.[21] In the absence of pregnancy, these unique cells undergo apoptosis prior to the influx of neutrophils characteristic of menstruation.[21] Loke and King[21] have suggested that uterine CD56+ cell survival may be progesterone dependent. These cells undergo apoptosis on day 26–27 of the menstrual cycle and in decidua of failing pregnancies, i.e. at a time of decreasing progesterone levels. Progesterone does not however induce proliferation of decidual CD56+ cells and these authors[21] state that the progesterone receptor has not as yet been colocalized on CD56+ cells.

Mast cells have been localized in human endometrium across all stages of the menstrual cycle. A recently published quantitative analysis of mast cell numbers has provided no evidence for major changes in number during the cycle, although changes in morphology, granule content and activation/degranulation was recognized premenstrually, during menses and in midsecretory endometrium. Eosinophils were demonstrated to accumulate just prior to and during menses. The authors[27] propose a functional role for these cell types in the context of endometrial remodeling since both contain potent local mediators (tryptase, chymase, histamine) and chemoattractants for eosinophils.

The major leucocyte components in the endometrium (nonpregnant and pregnant) are summarized in Table 13.1. These authors draw attention to the absence of data comparing leucocyte populations in the decidua basalis (trophoblast present) and decidua parietalis (trophoblast absent).

Estrogen and progesterone receptor localization over the normal menstrual cycle

There are two natural forms of the human progesterone receptor (PR). B-receptors (PR_B) are 933 amino acids in length and A receptors (PR_A) lack 164 amino acids from the N-terminus.[28] Recent data have indicated that PR isoforms change during the menstrual cycle. The PR_A:PR_B ratio appears to be greater premenstrually and immediately after menstruation.[29] Furthermore, the PR_B subtype appears to be differentially regulated in endometrial stroma.[30]

The PR is under dual control of estrogen and progesterone, which act sequentially to regulate cellular concentrations of progesterone receptor. The endometrial PR is increased by estrogen via an estrogen-mediated increase in PR mRNA levels and increased PR protein synthesis.[31] It is down regulated by its own ligand, progestogen, at the transcriptional and posttranscriptional levels.[32] In the human uterus high concentrations of progesterone result in an inhibition of estrogen actions. The reduction in estrogen receptor (ER) synthesis is due to progestogen mediated decrease in levels of ER mRNA.[31] Steroid hormones bind to specific upstream sequences (hormone response elements) in order to regulate transcription of hormone sensitive genes.[31] ER activation requires binding of a specific ligand and ligand binding is associated with dissociation of the heat-shock protein 90 (HSP90) and dimerization of the receptor.[33]

Lessey and colleagues in 1988[34] déscribed the estrogen and progesterone receptor distributions across the menstrual cycle from data based on ligand binding assays. These data revealed an increase in ER concentrations throughout the proliferative phase, peaking in the early secretory phase of the cycle; thereafter ER concentrations decline. A parallel but delayed rise in PR was also described with a decline in the secretory phase of the cycle. Ligand binding studies, however, give no indication of the tissue localization of sex steroid receptors.

The availability of monoclonal antibodies in recent years has made it possible to visualize the distribution of ER and PR across the normal menstrual cycle. Immunohistochemical studies have demonstrated the nuclear location of both the estrogen and progesterone receptors in the glands and stromal compartments of the endometrium (Fig. 13.11). In the secretory phase immunostaining for ER declines in both glands and stroma, although the glandular decline is slightly delayed compared to that in the stroma. The PR immunoreactivity is also marked in the nuclei of glands and stroma during the proliferative phase, but in the secretory phase this declines in the glandular component. A modest persistence of stromal staining remains, however, during the secretory phase.[34,35,36] It is interesting that the progesterone receptors have a specific localization in the perivascular regions of the stromal compartment (Fig. 13.12).

The immunohistochemical patterns of sex steroid receptor immunostaining in the normal endometrial cycle have been well described by Snijders and colleagues (Fig. 13.13).[35] A significant decline in estrogen and progesterone receptors was recorded in the glands with the transition from proliferative to

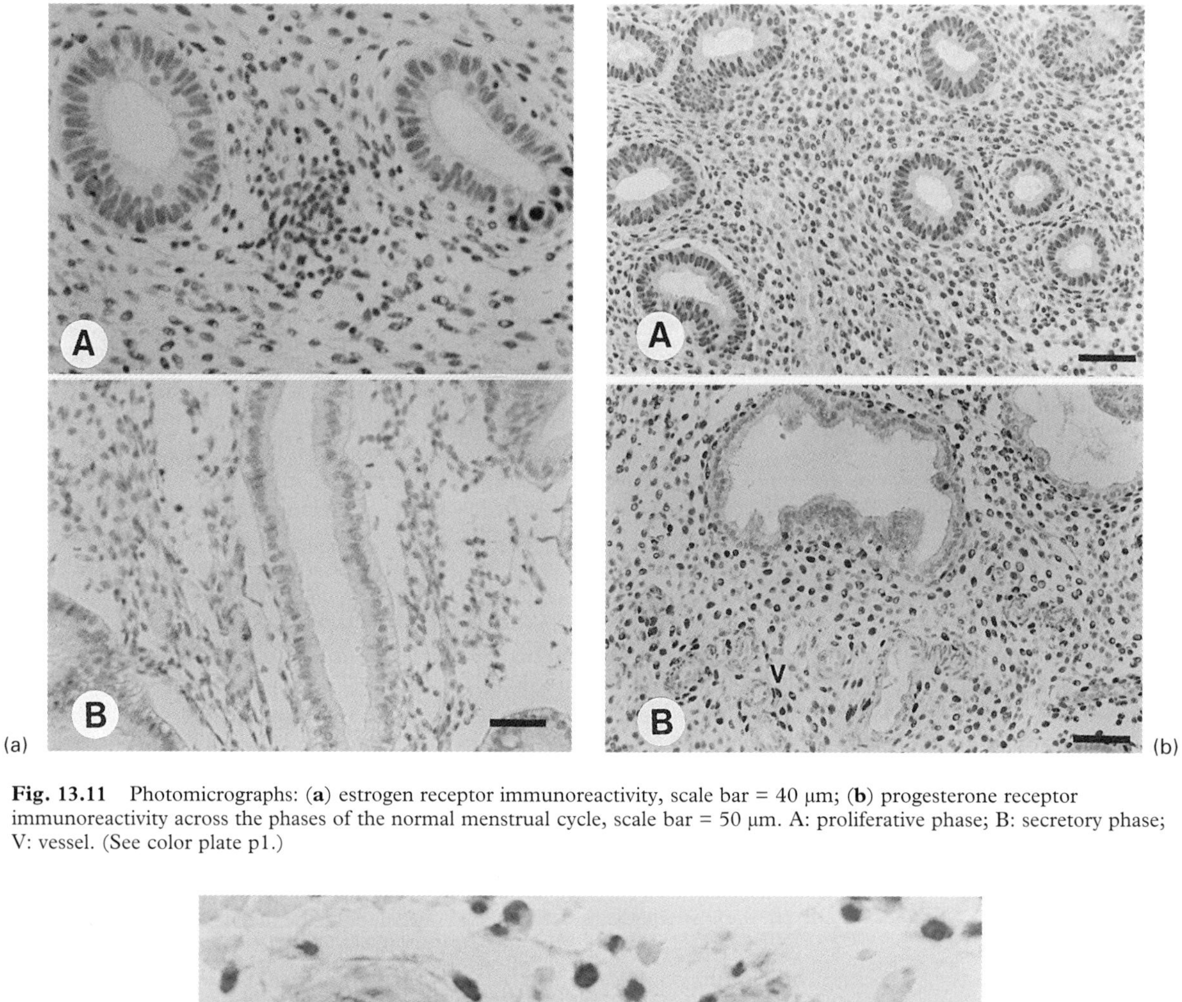

Fig. 13.11 Photomicrographs: (**a**) estrogen receptor immunoreactivity, scale bar = 40 μm; (**b**) progesterone receptor immunoreactivity across the phases of the normal menstrual cycle, scale bar = 50 μm. A: proliferative phase; B: secretory phase; V: vessel. (See color plate p1.)

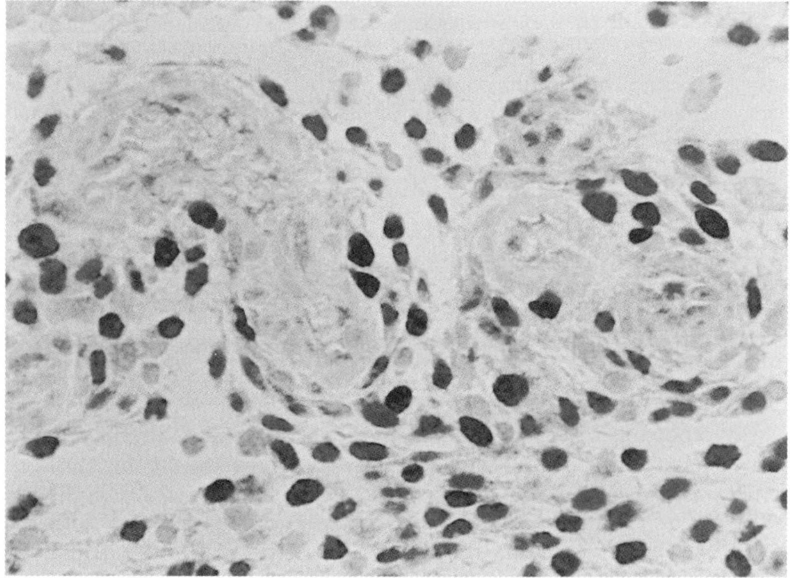

Fig. 13.12 Photomicrograph of late secretory phase endometrium demonstrating perivascular localization of progesterone receptor immunoreactivity. (See color plate p1.)

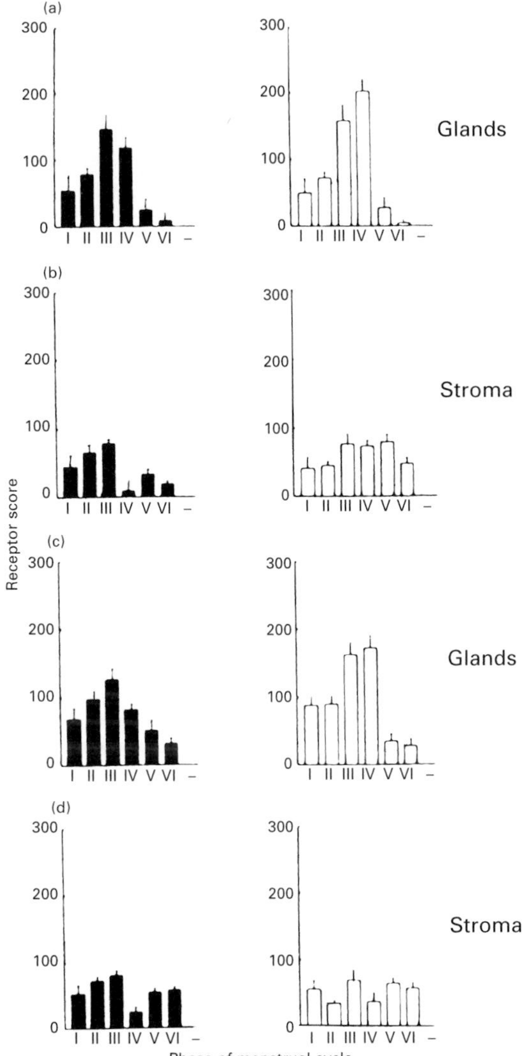

Fig. 13.13 Immunocytochemical estrogen (closed bars) and progesterone receptor (open bars) scores (mean +/– SEM) in (a) glandular epithelium functionalis; (b) stroma functionalis; (c) glandular epithelium basalis; (d) stroma basalis during the menstrual cycle phase I–VI (I–III = menstruation, early, late proliferative; IV–VI = early, mid, late secretory).[35]

secretory phase of the cycle. In the stromal compartment there was a similar decline in immunostaining in ER immunoreactivity but a persistence of PR immunostaining in the stroma. This particular publication differentiated between the functional and basal layers of the endometrium and it should be noted that in the glandular component both sex steroid receptors decline in the secretory phase of the cycle. There was no significant fall in ER or PR in the stromal compartment of the basal endometrium.

Following menopause, PR expression in the human uterus is characterized by moderate immunoreactivity of the glandular epithelium and only weak staining of the stromal compartment. ER expression is observed in both glandular epithelial and stromal cells of atrophic endometrium.[35]

ER and PR have been observed in the nonpregnant uterine vascular smooth muscle, but not in endothelium.[37] PR have however been reported in the endothelium in decidual tissue.[38] During pregnancy (4–38 weeks) PR are expressed in stromal cells and in the media of blood vessels. ER expression is negligible in the stromal compartment.

Relationships of sex steroid receptor patterns to endometrial function

Endometrial regeneration

New blood vessel formation (angiogenesis) is rare in adult tissues. The female reproductive tract is an exception, with blood vessel formation taking place during regeneration, development of spiral arterioles in the late secretory phase and at the time of placentation. Three peaks of regeneration have been described in endometrial tissue.[39,40] There is a period of endometrial regeneration immediately postmenstrually and also during the midproliferative phase of the cycle. These two peaks are considered to be estrogen related.[40,41] The third peak occurs during the secretory phase of the cycle and is progesterone related and involves the growth of spiral arterioles.[41] The presence of abundant estrogen receptor during the proliferative phase is consistent with the regenerative role of its ligand, estrogen. The persistence of stromal progestérone receptor provides support for a role for progestogen action in the stroma, i.e. directly or indirectly influencing development of the spiral arterioles.

Implantation

It has been considered that patterns of estrogen and progesterone receptor distribution may reflect endometrial maturation. The increase in both estrogen and progesterone steroid receptors do reflect estradiol action and the decline in both steroid receptors in the glandular compartment of endometrial tissue provides an index of progesterone activity. With successful implantation, there are features of steroid receptor localization particular to decidualized endometrium. Progesterone receptor expression remains constant in the stroma and perivascularly from 4–38 weeks gestation, and thus supports a role for progesterone in stromal decidualization. There is notable absence of both estrogen and progesterone receptors from the epithelial compartment of the decidua and estrogen receptor expression in the stroma is virtually undetectable (see earlier).

Effects of estrogen and progesterone upon local mediators within the endometrium

Since changes in sex steroid environment may directly or indirectly affect local mediators within the endometrium, a brief overview of what is known to date of steroid control of locally produced cytokines and growth factors intimately involved in proliferation and differentiation of various compartments of the endometrium (gland and stroma) now follows. The local actions of sex steroid and other hormones are critical to successful reproduction. However, some of the hormonal effects may result from the action of local mediators. The complex interactions of the network of uterine cells, i.e. epithelial, stromal, endothelial and cells of hemopoietic origin (lymphoid, macrophage, neutrophil) which are responsible for endometrial proliferation and differentiation, and menstrual shedding, require a well developed assembly of intercellular communication signals.[42,43] Many of the events in the human endometrium, such as menstrual shedding and abortion in early pregnancy, resemble inflammatory and regenerative processes. There is increasing evidence for the involvement of proinflammatory cytokines in normal uterine function.[42,43] Table 13.2 summarizes the putative roles of some local mediators (cytokines and growth factors) within the endometrium.

The insulin-like growth factors (IGFs) are considered to play an important role in both mitotic and differentiation events in the endometrium during the menstrual cycle and in early pregnancy.[42] The interleukins modulate cellular proliferation, induce the secretion of other cytokines and activate T-cells.[42] The IL-1 system (IL-1α, IL-1β, IL-1 receptor antagonist [an inhibitor] and IL-1 receptors) may be implicated in implantation.[46] IL-6 is present throughout the menstrual cycle but a definitive role in human endometrium has yet to be defined. The perivascular immunolocalization of IL-8 in endometrium[47] is consistent with its proposed biological role as a modulator of leucocyte vascular interactions. Interestingly, IL-1 (which facilitates IL-8 production) has been detected in endothelial cells of spiral vessels in endometrium.[45] TNF-α receptors are present in uterine cells and TNF-α has been implicated in angiogenesis, cell cytotoxicity and infection-induced preterm labour.[42] Epidermal growth factor (EGF) has been proposed as a mediator of estrogen actions in the uterus.[42]

Another important group of modulators of uterine function are the prostaglandins (PGs). There is good evidence that progesterone modulates PG activity in endometrium and decidua.[55,56] PGs are involved with the modulation of blood vessel tone and the transmigration of leucocytes. Furthermore, progesterone suppresses PG production in secretory endometrium.[57] It is likely that many of the local mediators (cytokines, growth factors and prostaglandins) referred to above may interact in some way with the leucocyte populations present within the uterus. These leucocyte populations may be stimulated or inhibited by local mediators as well as being the source of their production.

A growth factor in the maternal environment considered to play a critical role in regulating the development of the preimplantation embryo, is leukemia inhibitory factor (LIF).[58] Implantation failure in mice is associated with a null mutation in the LIF gene.[59] Preliminary evidence indicates that LIF synthesis is required by the uterus to undergo decidualization and by the blastocyst for implantation.[58]

Effects of estrogen and progesterone on endometrial prolactin production

Extrapituitary prolactin is synthesized and released from endometrial decidua. Identification of prolactin mRNA in decidua provides evidence for decidual prolactin being a functional molecule of endometrial origin.[60,61] The stimulation of prolactin secretion from endometrial cells by progesterone is dose-dependent and decidual production of prolactin in early pregnancy is the result of progesterone induced decidualization of stromal cells.[62] Recent literature has drawn attention to a possible angiomodulatory role for prolactin. Prolactin receptors have been identified in cells of the capillary endothelium and the immune system.[63,64] In human endometrium prolactin receptors are expressed in the glandular epithelium and decidualized stromal cells with a similar temporal expression to prolactin.[65]

Effects of estrogen and progesterone on endometrial cell adhesion molecules

Adhesion molecules expressed on endothelial cells have been shown to facilitate movement of leucocytes from

Table 13.2 Putative roles of local mediators within human endometrium.

Mediator	Mitogenic	Leucovascular epithelial interaction	Differentiation	Angiogenic	Chemotactic	Menstruation	Implantation
Growth Factors							
IGFs[42,44]	+		+				
EGF[42,51]	+						
TGFβ[52]	±			+			
bFGF[42,53]	+			+			
VEGF[54]				+			
LIF[58,59]							+
Cytokines							
IL-1 system[45,46]						+	+
IL-6[42,43]						+	+
IL-8[47,48,49]		+		+	+		
IFNγ[42]		+					
TNFα[42,50]				+			
Other mediators							
PGS[55,56]		+			+		

IGF = insulin-like growth factor; EGF = epidermal growth factor; TGFβ = transforming growth factor β; bFGF = basic fibroblast growth factor; VEGF = vascular endothelial growth factor; LIF = leukaemia inhibitory factor; IL = interleukin; IFNγ = interferonγ; TNFα = tumour necrosis factor α; PG = prostaglandin

peripheral blood into tissues. Intercellular adhesion molecule-1 (ICAM-1, CD54) and platelet endothelial cell adhesion molecule (PECAM, CD31) have both been implicated in the binding of leucocytes to endothelial cells. Tawia et al[66] have demonstrated low ICAM-1 expression in endothelial cells during the proliferative and secretory phases of the menstrual cycle (possible constitutive expression) and an increased expression menstrually, coinciding with an influx of leucocytes (possible expression after stimulation).

All cells express integrins on their surface. The integrins are members of a larger family of cell adhesion proteins, important for cellular differentiation, motility or attachment.[67] Integrins undergo changes in their expression in endometrial cells during the menstrual cycle and early pregnancy.[67] Integrin expression is regulated by growth factors and cytokines and expression in the endometrium is likely to be steroid hormone regulated. In certain infertility states, abnormal integrin expression has been reported.[68] Abnormal integrin expression may influence endometrial receptivity. Lessey and Castelbaum[67] have recently described the correlation between integrin expression, progesterone and progesterone receptor changes during the cycle. The co-expression of integrin subunits α4 and β3 coincides with 'putative maximal endometrial receptivity' when implantation may occur. With increasing levels of progesterone and loss of epithelial progesterone receptor there is a correlation with the appearance of β3 and loss of α4 subunits. These authors suggest that the loss of either component might result in receptivity defects.

Effects of pharmacological modulation of the steroid environment of the endometrium

Steroid withdrawal

Withdrawal of steroids from the endometrium has been shown to have fascinating effects on endometrial function and has thus shed light on mechanisms maintaining control of normal endometrial function.

Antiprogestogens are progesterone receptor antagonists that block the action of progesterone at its receptor and thus have provided the opportunity to explore new methods of contraception.[69] Effects of the antiprogestogen mifepristone (RU486) administered in the luteal phase depend upon dose and stage of the cycle. In the early luteal phase, secretory development of the endometrium is retarded without affecting the function of the corpus luteum and cycle length.[70] In contrast, administration in the mid and late luteal phases results in bleeding with or without luteolysis and hence normal menstruation is disrupted.[8,71]

Evidence of progesterone antagonism in the endometrium after antiprogestogen administration is the increase in cell proliferation (as identified by the cell proliferation marker Ki 67), particularly within the glands.[72] Progesterone normally inhibits proliferative activity within the endometrium. An important progesterone regulated enzyme in human endometrium is 17β hydroxy steroid dehydrogenase (17βHSD). In endometrium, progesterone and synthetic progestogens (*in vivo* and *in vitro*) increase the oxidation of 17β estradiol to estrone. The enzyme 17βHSD is localized in the glandular epithelium and demonstrates an antiestrogen action of progesterone (conversion of 17β estradiol to biologically weak/inactive estrone).[73] 17βHSD is shown to be antagonized by antiprogestogen administration.[74] The progesterone dependent enzyme, 15-hydroxy prostaglandin dehydrogenase is also inhibited by administration of antiprogestin in the early luteal phase.[72]

The local tissue response to withdrawal of progesterone, for example as might occur at menstruation, shows many features characteristic of an inflammatory response[48] (release of prostaglandins, increased permeability of blood vessels and an abundance of leucocytes in the endometrium). A significant increase in macrophages is observed in decidua following antiestrogen (RU486) administration *in vivo*.[75]

Estrogenic effects on the endometrium may be antagonized by pure antiestrogens. Dowsett and colleagues[76] have described the effects of a pure antiestrogen compound (ICI 182780) upon parameters of endometrial function. They have demonstrated significant antiproliferative effects on glandular epithelium with this compound.

Continuous steroid exposure

It has been reported[77] that short term administration of synthetic progestogens decrease the progesterone receptor content of both epithelium and stroma in pre- and postmenopausal women. By contrast, endometrium exposed to long term subdermal levonorgestrel (Norplant) exhibits a significant increase in stromal progesterone receptor immunoreactivity compared with control endometrium at all stages across the menstrual cycle.[36] The mechanism by which this observation may be explained, and whether the observed increase in stromal progesterone receptor immunoreactivity is associated with an increased number or concentration of functional progesterone receptors, is as yet unknown.

A contrasting situation is observed in endometrium exposed to intra-uterine delivery of levonorgestrel (levonorgestrel-releasing intra-uterine system, LNG-IUS). A reduced estrogen and progesterone receptor immunoreactivity has been observed after continuous local intra-uterine levonorgestrel exposure.[78]

Pekonen and colleagues[79] have also reported differences in endometrial response to local uterine and subdermal continuous delivery of levonorgestrel. This group observed that intra-uterine levonorgestrel was a potent stimulator of stromal cell IGFBP-I production, whereas subdermal delivery of levonorgestrel did not produce such an effect. Herewith, therefore, are cited two independent observations on endometrium function where continuous exposure to a progestogen is influenced by the delivery route. This is most likely to reflect the dose-dependency of the effects of levonorgestrel. The levonorgestrel intra-uterine system produces endometrial levonorgestrel levels 1000 times higher than serum levels, which are of the same order of magnitude with subdermal implants.[79] Data such as these are providing a unique opportunity to understand mechanisms controlling endometrial function.

Conclusion

The endometrium is unique in form and function in order to ensure an appropriate response to endocrine stimuli, these being estrogen and progesterone. We are still some way, however, from fully understanding the mechanisms which are responsible for the control of normal endometrial function. There are lines of evidence to indicate that there is a complex interplay between the component parts of the endometrium, these being the glands, stroma, vasculature and the immune cell population. It is likely that this interplay is orchestrated by numerous cytokines and growth factors acting at either a paracrine or autocrine level. The initial elements in the system, however, from which a cascade of local events is initiated, are most likely estrogen and progesterone. Only when the mechanisms regulating normal endometrium are understood will light be shed on the requirements for orderly menstruation, appropriate regeneration and successful implantation. Future research endeavors will no doubt focus upon a better understanding of the complex interaction between the endocrine system and local mechanisms within this fascinating target tissue.

Acknowledgments We are grateful to Mr C Gilpin (Biological Sciences Electron Microscope Unit,

University of Manchester, UK) for providing the scanning electron micrographs of human endometrium and decidua. We also wish to acknowledge Dr M A Warren (Dept of Biomedical Sciences, University of Sheffield, UK) and Dr T-C Li (Jessop Hospital for Women, Sheffield, UK) for the ultrastructural photographs of endometrium. Thanks are due to Dr C H Buckley (Dept of Gynaecological Pathology, University of Manchester, UK) for providing the histological photographs of endometrium and decidua. We acknowledge Mr Tom McFetters for assistance with the illustrations and Mrs Vicky Watters for secretarial support.

REFERENCES

1. Buckley CH, Fox H 1989 Biopsy pathology of the endometrium. In: Gottlieb L, Neville AM, Walker F, (eds) Biopsy pathology series. Chapman and Hall Medical, London
2. Gautray JP 1981 Menstrual cycle: some uncertain aspects. In: de Brux J, Mortel RB, Gautray JP (eds) The endometrium: hormonal impacts. Plenum Press, New York, pp 1–13
3. Yen SSC 1991 The human menstrual cycle: neuroendocrine regulation. In: Yen SSC, Jaffe RB (eds) Reproductive endocrinology, pathophysiology and clinical management. WB Saunders Co., Harcourt Brace Jovanovich Inc. Philadelphia, London, 273–308
4. Noyes RW, Hertig AT, Rock J 1950 Dating the endometrial biopsy. Fertility and Sterility 1: 3–25
5. Li T-C, Cooke ID 1989 Chronological and histological dating of the endometrial biopsy. Contemporary Reviews in Obstetrics and Gynaecology 1: 266–272
6. Li T-C, Rogers AW, Lenton EA, Dockery P, Cooke ID 1987 A comparison between two methods of chronological dating of human endometrial biopsies during the luteal phase and their correlation with histologic dating. Fertility and Sterility 48: 928–932
7. Johannisson E, Parker RA, Landgren BM, Diczfalusy E 1982 Morphometric analysis of the human endometrium in relation to peripheral hormone levels. Fertility and Sterility 38: 564–571
8. Li T-C, Rogers AW, Dockery P, Lenton EA, Thomas E, Cooke ID 1988 The effects of progesterone receptor blockade in the luteal phase of normal fertile women. Fertility and Sterility 50: 732–742
9. Dockery P, Li T-C, Rogers AW, Cooke ID, Lenton EA, Warren MA 1988 An examination of the variation in timed endometrial biopsies. Human Reproduction 3: 715–720
10. Johannisson E, Landgren BM, Rohr HP, Diczfalusy E 1987 Endometrial morphology and peripheral hormone levels in women with regular menstrual cycles. Fertility and Sterility 48: 401–408
11. Ferenczy A, Richart RM, Agate FJ, Purkerson ML, Dempsey EW 1972 Scanning electron microscopy of the human endometrial surface epithelium. Fertility and Sterility 23: 515–521
12. Martel D, Malet C, Gautray JP, Psychoyos A 1981 Surface changes of the luminal uterine epithelium during the human menstrual cycle: a scanning electron miscroscope study. In: de Brux J, Mortel R, Guatray JP (eds) The endometrium: hormonal impacts. Plenum Press, New York, pp 15–29
13. Nikas G, Drakakis P, Loutradis D et al 1995 Uterine pinopodes as markers of the 'nidation window' in cycling women receiving exogenous oestradiol and progesterone. Human Reproduction 10: 1208–1213
14. Martel D, Monier MN, Roche D, Psychoyos A 1991 Hormonal dependence of pinopode formation at the uterine luminal surface. Human Reproduction 6: 597–603
15. Psychoyos A, Nikas G 1994 Uterine pinopodes as markers of uterine receptivity. Assisted Reproduction Review 4: 26–32
16. Li T, Warren MA, Hill CJ, Saravelos H 1994 Morphology of the human endometrium in the peri-implantation period. Annals of the New York Academy of Sciences 734: 169–184
17. Dockery P, Li T, Rogers AW, Cooke ID, Lenton EA 1988 The ultrastructure of the glandular epithelium in the timed endometrial biopsy. Human Reproduction 3: 826–834
18. Lea R, Clark DA 1991 Macrophages and migratory cells in endometrium relevant to implantation. Baillières Clinical Obstetrics and Gynecology 5: 25–59
19. Staples L, Heap RB, Wooding FBP, King GJ 1983 Migration of leukocytes into the uterus after removal of ovarian progesterone during early pregnancy in the sheep. Placenta 4: 339–350
20. Poropatich C, Rojas M, Silverberg SG 1987 Polymorphonuclear leukocyes in the endometrium during the normal menstrual cycle. International Journal of Gynecological Pathology 6: 230–234
21. Loke YW, King A 1995 Uterine mucosal leucocytes. In: Loke Y, King, A (eds) Human implantation, cell biology and immunology. Cambridge University Press, Cambridge, p 103
22. Bulmer JN, Lunny DP, Hagin SV 1988 Immunohistochemical characterisation of stromal leucocytes in nonpregnant human endometrium. American Journal of Reproductive Immunology and Microbiology 17: 83–90
23. Kamat BR, Isaacson PG 1987 The immunocytochemical distribution of leukocytic subpopulations in human endometrium. American Journal of Pathology 127: 66–73
24. Klentzeris LD, Bulmer JN, Warren A, Morrison L, Li T-C, Cooker ID 1992 Endometrial lymphoid tissue in the timed endometrial biopsy. Morphometric and immunohistochemical aspects. American Journal of Obstetrics and Gynecology 167: 667–674
25. King A, Loke YW 1990 Uterine large granular lymphocytes: a possible role in embryonic implantation? American Journal of Obstetrics and Gynecology 162: 308–310

26. Marzusch K, Ruck P, Geiselhart A, et al 1993 Distribution of cell adhesion molecules on CD56++, CD3–, CD16– large granular lymphocytes and endothelial cells in first trimester human decidua. Human Reproduction 8: 1203–1208
27. Jeziorska M, Salamonsen LA, Woolley DE 1995 Mast cell and eosinophil distribution and activation in human endometrium throughout the menstrual cycle. Biology of Reproduction 53: 312–320
28. Tung L, Mohamed MK, Hoeffler JP, Takimoto GS, Horwitz KB 1993 Antagonist-occupied human progesterone B receptors activate transcription without binding to progesterone response elements and are dominantly inhibited by A receptors. Molecular Endocrinology 7: 1256–1265
29. Mangal R, Wiehle RD, Poindexter III AN, Hilsenrath RE, Weigel NL 1995 Uterine progesterone receptor A and B subunits change in the cycle. Journal of the Society for Gynecological Investigation 2 (Abstract 0104)
30. Wang H, Critchley HOD, Kelly RW, Shen D, Baird DT 1998 Progesterone receptor subtype B is differentially regulated in human endometrial stroma. Molecular Human Reproduction 4: 407–412
31. Clarke CL, Sutherland RL 1990 Progestin regulation of cellular proliferation. Endocrine Reviews 11: 266–301
32. Chauchereau A, Savouret JF, Milgrom E 1992 Control of biosynthesis and post-transcriptional modification of progesterone receptor. Biology of Reproduction 46: 174–177
33. Baulieu E 1994 Mechanisms of action of steroid hormones and antihormones; a mini-overview. In: Chwalisz K, Garfield, RE (eds) Basic mechanisms controlling term and preterm birth. Ernst Schering Research Foundation, Berlin, Heidelberg, New York, London, 89–95
34. Lessey BA, Killam AP, Metzger DA, Haney AF, Greene GL, McCarty KS 1988 Immunohistochemical analysis of human uterine estrogen and progesterone receptors throughout the menstrual cycle. Journal of Clinical Endocrinology and Metabolism 67: 334–340
35. Snijders MPML, de Goeij AFPM, Debets-Te Baerts MJC, Rousch MJM, Koudstaal J, Bosman FT 1992 Immunocytochemical analysis of oestrogen receptors and progesterone receptors in the human uterus throughout the menstrual cycle and after the menopause. Journal of Reproduction and Fertility 94: 363–371
36. Critchley HOD, Bailey DA, Au CL, Affandi B, Rogers PAW 1993 Immunohistochemical sex steroid receptor distribution in endometrium from long-term subdermal levonorgestrel users and during the normal menstrual cycle. Human Reproduction 8: 1632–1639
37. Perrot-Applanat M, Groyer-Picard MT, Garcia E, Lorenzo F, Milgron E 1988 Immunocytochemical demonstration of estrogen and progesterone receptors in muscle cells of uterine arteries in rabbits and humans. Endocrinology 123: 1511–1519
38. Wang JD, Fu Y, Shi WL 1992 Immunohistochemical localization of progesterone receptor in human decidua of early pregnancy. Human Reproduction 7: 123–127
39. Rogers P, Abberton K, Susil B 1992 Endothelial cell migratory signal produced by human endometrium during the menstrual cycle. Human Reproduction 7: 1061–1066
40. Goodger (Macpherson) A, Rogers P 1994 Endometrial endothelial cell proliferation during the menstrual cycle. Human Reproduction 9: 399–405
41. Ferenczy A, Bertrand G, Gelfand M 1979 Proliferation kinetics of human endometrium during the normal menstrual cycle. American Journal of Obstetrics and Gynecology 133: 859–867
42. Giudice L 1994 Growth factors and growth modulators in human uterine endometrium: their potential relevance to reproductive medicine. Fertility and Sterility 61: 1–17
43. Tabibzadeh S 1991 Human endometrium: an active site of cytokine production and action. Endocrine Reviews 12: 272–290
44. Murphy LJ, Murphy LC, Freisen HG 1987 Estrogen induces insulin-like growth factor I expression in the rat uterus. Molecular Endocrinology 1: 445–450
45. Simon C, Piquette GN, Frances A, Polan ML 1993 Localisation of interleukin-1 type receptor and interleukin-1B in human endometrium throughout the menstrual cycle. Journal of Clinical Endocrinology and Metabolism 77: 549–555
46. Simon C, Frances A, Lee BY, et al 1995 Immunohistochemical localization, identification and regulation of the interleukin-1 receptor antagonist in the human endometrium. Human Reproduction: Molecular Human Reproduction 10: 2472–2477
47. Critchley HOD, Kelly RW, Kooy J 1994 Perivascular expression of chemokine interleukin-8 in human endometrium: a preliminary report. Human Reproduction 9: 1406–1409
48. Kelly RW 1994 Pregnancy maintenance and parturition; the role of prostaglandin in manipulating the immune and inflammatory response. Endocrine Reviews 15: 684–706
49. Koch A, Polverini P, Kunkel S et al 1992 Interleukin-8 as a macrophage-derived mediator of angiogenesis. Science 258: 1798–1801
50. Hunt JS, Chien HL, Hu XL, Tabibzadeh SS 1992 Tumor necrosis factor-α messenger ribonucleic acid and protein in human endometrium. Biology of Reproduction 47: 141–147
51. Haining RE, Cameron IT, van Papendorf C et al 1991 Epidermal growth factor in human endometrium: proliferative effects in culture and immunocytochemical localization in normal and endometriotic tissues. Human Reproduction 6: 1200–1205
52. Clark DA 1992 Cytokines and uterine bleeding. In: Alexander NJ, d'Arcangues C (eds) Steroid hormones and uterine bleeding. AAAS Press, Washington, pp 263–275
53. Folkman J, Klagsbrun M 1987 Angiogenic factors. Science 235: 442–444
54. Charnock-Jones D, Sharkey A, Rajput-Williams J et al 1993 Identification and localization of alternately spliced mRNAs for vascular endothelial growth factor in human uterus and steroid regulation in endometrial carcinoma cell lines. Biology of Reproduction 48: 1120–1128
55. Cheng L, Kelly RW, Thong K, Hume R, Baird DT 1993 The effect of mifepristone (RU486) on prostaglandin dehydrogenase in decidual and chorionic tissue in early pregnancy. Human Reproduction 8: 705–709

56. Cheng L, Kelly R, Thong KJ, Hume R, Baird D 1993 The effect of mifepristone (RU486) on the immunohistochemical distribution of prostaglandin E and its metabolite in decidua and chorionic tissue in early pregnancy. Journal of Clinical Endocrinology and Metabolism 77: 873–877
57. Abel MH, Baird DT 1980 The effect of 17B estradiol and progesterone on prostaglandin production by human endometrium maintained in organ culture. Endocrinology 106: 1599–1606
58. Stewart C 1994 The role of leukaemia inhibitory factor (LIF) and other cytokines in regulating implantation in mammals. Annals of the New York Academy of Sciences 734: 157–165
59. Stewart C, Kaspar P, Brunet C et al 1992 Blastocyst implantation depends on maternal expression of leukaemia inhibitory factors. Nature 359: 76–79
60. Healy DL, Salamonsen L, Moon J, Cameron IT, Findlay JK 1990 Human endometrial prolactin. In: d'Arcangues C, Fraser IS, Newton JR, Odlind V (eds) Contraception and mechanisms of endometrial bleeding. Cambridge University Press, Cambridge, pp 213–221
61. Wu W-X, Brooks J, Millar MR, Ledger WL, Saunders PT, Glasier AF, McNeilly AS 1991 Localization of the site of synthesis and action of prolactin by immunocytochemistry and in situ hybridization within the human utero-placental unit. Journal of Molecular Endocrinology 7: 241–247
62. Wu W-X, Glasier A, Norman J, Kelly R, Baird D, McNeilly A 1990 The effects of the antiprogesterone mifepristone in vivo, and progesterone in vitro on prolactin production by the human decidua in early pregnancy. Human Reproduction 5: 627–631
63. Dardenne M, de Moraes M, Kelly P, Gagnerault M-C 1994 Prolactin receptor expression in human haematopoietic tissues analyzed by flow cytofluorometry. Endocrinology 134: 2108–2114
64. Clapp C, Weiner RI 1992 A specific high affinity saturable binding site for the 16 kilodalton fragment of prolactin on capillary endothelial cells. Endocrinology 130: 1380–1386
65. Jones RL, Critchley HOD, Brooks J, Jabbour HN, McNeilly AS 1998 Localization and temporal expression of prolactin receptor in human endometrium. Journal of Clinical Endocrinology and Metabolism 83: 258–262
66. Tawia SA, Beaton LA, Rogers PAW 1993 Immunolocalization of the cellular adhesion molecules, intercellular adhesion molecule-1 (ICAM-1) and platelet endothelial cell adhesion molecule (PECAM) in human endometrium throughout the menstrual cycle. Human Reproduction 8: 175–181
67. Lessey BA, Castelbaum AJ 1995 Integrins in the endometrium. Reproductive Medicine Review 4: 43–58
68. Lessey BA, Castelbaum AJ, Sawin SJ, Buck C, Schinnar R, Bilker W 1994 Aberrant integrin expression in the endometrium of women with endometriosis. Journal of Clinical Endocrinology and Metabolism 79: 643–649
69. Baird DT 1993 Potential contraceptive effects of antigestogens. In: Donaldson M, Dorflinger L, Brown SS, Benet LZ (eds). Clinical applications of mifepristone (RU486) and other antiprogestins. Proceedings of Institute of Medicine, National Academy of Sciences Committee on Antiprogestins: Assessing the Science. National Academy Press, Washington, pp 148–163
70. Swahn ML, Bygdeman M, Cekan S, Xing S, Masironi B, Johannisson E 1990 The effects of RU486 administered during the early luteal phase on bleeding pattern, hormonal parameters and endometrium. Human Reproduction 5: 402–408
71. Schaison G, George M, Lestrat N, Reinberg A, Baulieu EE 1985 Effects of the antiprogesterone steroid RU486 during midluteal phase in normal women. Journal of Clinical Endocrinology and Metabolism 61: 484–489
72. Cameron ST, Critchley HOD, Buckley CH, Kelly RW, Baird DT 1997 Effect of two antiprogestins (mifepristone and onapristone) on endometrial factors of potential importance for implantation. Fertility and Sterility 67: 1046–1053
73. Casey ML, MacDonald PC, Andersson S 1994 17β-hydroxysteroid dehyrogenase type 2: chromosomal assignment and progestin regulation of gene expression in human endometrium. Journal of Clinical Investigation 94: 2135–2141
74. Maentausta O, Svalander P, Gemzell-Danielsson K, Bygdeman M, Vihko R 1993 The effects of an antiprogestin, mifepristone, and an anti-estrogen, tamoxifen, on endometrial 17β hydroxysteroid dehydrogenase and progestin and estrogen receptors during the luteal phase of the menstrual cycle: an immunohistochemical study. Journal of Clinical Endocrinology and Metabolism 77: 913–918
75. Critchley HOD, Kelly RW, Lea RG, Drudy TA, Jones RL, Baird DT 1996 Sex steroid regulation of leucocyte traffic in human decidua. Human Reproduction 11: 2257–2262
76. Dowsett M, Howell R, Salter J, Thomas N, Thomas E 1995 Effects of the pure anti-estrogen ICI 182780 on estrogen receptors, progesterone receptors and K:67 antigen in human endometrium in vivo. Human Reproduction 10: 262–267
77. Lane G, King R, Whitehead M 1988 The effect of estrogens and progestogens on endometrial biochemistry. In: Studd J, Whitehead MJ (eds) The menopause. Blackwell, Oxford, pp 213–226
78. Critchley HOD, Wang H, Kelly RW, Gebbie AE, Glasier AF 1998 Progestin receptor isoforms and prostaglandin dehydrogenase in the endometrium of women using a levonorgestrel-releasing intra-uterine system. Human Reproduction (*in press*)
79. Pekonen F, Nyman R, Lahteenmaki P, Haukkamaa M, Rutanen EM 1992 Intrauterine progestin induces continuous insulin-like growth factor-binding protein-1 production in the human endometrium. Journal of Clinical Endocrinology and Metabolism 75: 660–664

14. Menstruation

P. A. Rogers

Introduction

Menstruation can be defined as the process whereby the superficial, or functionalis, layer of the endometrium is removed at the end of the luteal phase of a menstrual cycle in which a pregnancy has not been established. The evolutionary significance of menstruation remains a matter of some debate, although there is a reasonable amount of support for the concept that it is primarily a mechanism for removing the differentiated endometrial stromal cells from the uterus following a nonfertile cycle.[1] Regardless of the evolutionary reasons for menstruation, the spontaneous rupture of any vascular bed remains a highly unusual, and potentially lethal, event for an organism to undertake. For this reason alone, the mechanisms that control the onset, continuation and cessation of menstruation are of considerable interest. Clinically, a better understanding of the processes of normal menstruation is directly relevant to developing better treatments for disorders such as menorrhagia and a number of other menstrual problems. The aim of this chapter is to provide a brief overview of established knowledge of the mechanisms that control menstruation, and to outline a number of areas where current research shows promise of providing significant new information.

A SUMMARY OF TRADITIONAL AND CURRENT CONCEPTS ON THE EVENTS OF MENSTRUATION

Most of our current understanding of the vascular events during menstruation is still based on the remarkable series of observations using intraocular endometrial transplants in the rhesus monkey published by Markee over 50 years ago.[2] One to four days prior to the onset of bleeding, venous and arterial stasis occurs, sometimes accompanied by vasodilatation. Four to 24 hours prior to bleeding, vasoconstriction is also seen. About four days prior to menstruation leucocytic infiltration of the endometrium occurs. Menstrual bleeding usually commences from the wall of an arteriole or capillary once a previously constricted spiral arteriole relaxes and blood flow recommences. Approximately 70% of blood is lost in this way. Some blood cells also leave the capillary circulation by diapedesis (approximately 5% of blood loss), as well as by reflux from veins through previously formed breaks in the vasculature (approximately 25% of blood loss). Blood loss from a break in the endometrial vasculature during menstruation normally only lasts for 1–2 minutes before ceasing due to spiral arteriole vasoconstriction. Bleeding finally ceases with the growth of new capillaries and arterioles proximal to the occluded end of the existing spiral arteriole, allowing blood flow to recommence back into existing venules.

Routine histopathology provides the bulk of the most detailed information on the tissue and cellular events of menstruation in humans.[3] Premenstrually (postovulation days 11–13) the endometrial stroma is infiltrated by extravasated leucocytes. Normal menstruation lasts 4 ± 1 days, with 50% of the menstrual detritus being shed in the first 24 hours. Biopsies taken during the first two days of menstruation will usually contain relatively abundant amounts of shedding and degenerating functionalis. In contrast, the second half of the menstrual period is characterized by proliferation of the residual gland epithelium in the denuded basalis. Biopsies taken at this time usually provide scant material. Reepithelialization occurs by extension of the residual glandular epithelium over the denuded surface. Postmenstrual endometrial repair does not depend on oestrogen, since this process occurs regardless of circulating oestrogen levels. During the process of menstruation the endometrial blood vessels can range from a relatively normal appearance, through to a blocked lumen due to endothelial swelling and complete degeneration with ruptured walls and fibrinoid deposits. Menstrual bleeding is controlled primarily by vasoconstriction of the arterial segments in the basalis. The spiral arterioles of the functionalis lack elastin, and consequently it is thought they have limited ability to contract.

Hysteroscopy and microhysteroscopy are increasingly being used for diagnostic and operative procedures in gynecology, however there has been very little published on endometrial vascular changes during the normal menstrual cycle as visualized with these techniques. It has been reported that by the late secretory stage stromal oedema, the decidual response and glandular secretions combine to reduce or eliminate visualization of the spiral arterioles, leaving only the superficial capillary network visible.[4] During the premenstrual to menstrual phase small pools of blood collect near the endometrial surface prior to complete endometrial shedding.

There has been considerable interest in the process of hemostasis in menstrual endometrium, both because it has been recognized for some time that menstrual blood does not clot, and because a significant percentage of women with clotting disorders also suffer from excessive menstrual blood loss.[5] Hemostasis in menstrual endometrium differs from that in other parts of the body by the relative scarcity of hemostatic plugs and the complete intravascular localization of these plugs. Fibrin, a major component of hemostatic plugs, is broken down by fibrinolytic agents such as plasmin. Tissue plasminogen activator, which cleaves plasminogen to produce active plasmin, is elevated in late secretory and menstrual endometrium.[6] As a consequence, endometrial fibrinolytic activity is maximal on the first day of bleeding.[5] Thus it would seem that high levels of fibrinolytic activity are necessary for the tissue breakdown and emptying of the uterine cavity during menstruation. However, increased fibrinolytic activity can also threaten the normal equilibrium that exists between hemostatic plug formation and lysis, thus resulting in excessive menstrual blood loss.

Both prostaglandins E_2 and $F_{2\alpha}$ occur in human endometrium, with levels increasing through the secretory phase to a maximum at menstruation.[5] Large amounts of $PGF_{2\alpha}$, and smaller amounts of PGE_2, are found in menstrual fluid. Significantly higher levels of these prostaglandins are found in the endometrium of women with menorrhagia, and an inverse correlation has been demonstrated between the $PGF_{2\alpha}/PGE_2$ ratio in secretory endometrium and menstrual blood loss. Despite these and other observations that establish a strong connection between prostaglandins and specific mechanisms controlling menstruation, the precise relationship between prostaglandins and menstruation remains to be clarified.

It is well established in clinical practice that prostaglandin synthesis inhibitors, antifibrinolytic agents and progestogens can act to reduce menstrual blood loss in women suffering from menorrhagia.[7,8] This, and a range of other evidence, confirm the role of prostaglandins, fibrinolysis and progesterone (or its withdrawal) as mechanisms that play a central role in controlling menstruation. However, none of these treatments alone, or in combination, is capable of completely preventing menstruation, and it is not unusual for individual women to fail to respond at all to any one particular agent. Thus it would seem that the overall process of menstruation comprises a number of discrete steps, with no single mechanism within the endometrium being wholly responsible.

ROLE OF ESTROGEN AND PROGESTERONE IN THE CONTROL OF MENSTRUATION

In broad terms, it is well known that the sex steroids estrogen and progesterone control the menstrual process. In the nonfertile cycle, menstruation commences following a major fall in circulating levels of estrogen and progesterone during the latter part of the luteal phase. This process can be mimicked by withdrawal of exogenous hormones, or administration of progesterone antagonists such as RU486 at the appropriate time of the cycle. Local control of the menstrual process has been demonstrated by using crystalline estrone to produce continued growth of intraocular endometrial autotransplants in rhesus monkeys at the same time that menstruation was occurring in the uterus.[2] However, it can also be deduced that estrogen and progesterone withdrawal must act via secondary mechanisms to cause menstruation, since a number of other tissues with high levels of receptors for these two hormones, such as breast, oviduct and vagina, do not menstruate.

Estrogen has been shown to have numerous genomic and nongenomic affects on the vasculature in a wide range of studies.[9,10] To date over 20 genes with potential vascular actions have been identified which contain consensus repeats for the estrogen receptor, thus identifying them as targets for regulation by the estrogen–estrogen receptor bound complex. These studies have shown that estrogen, and to a lesser degree progesterone, can act on the vasculature both directly through nongenomic mechanisms, and also via receptors in smooth muscle cells, and possibly endothelial cells, to have a wide range of effects.

There is no evidence to date suggesting that absolute levels of circulating estrogen or progesterone correlate with either the duration of menstruation or the amount of blood lost. It has been hypothesized that one cause of excessive menstrual blood loss could be aberrations in the quantity or distribution of estrogen or progesterone receptors in the endometrium. This hypothesis is supported by the finding that solid phase immunoassay of endometrial nuclear and cytosolic extracts demonstrates significantly elevated estrogen and progesterone receptor levels in the late secretory phase in women with menorrhagia when compared to normal controls.[11] However, using immunohistochemical techniques to show endometrial stromal and glandular sex steroid receptor distribution, no differences were found between women with or without menorrhagia.[12]

While it seems likely that the actions of estrogen and progesterone on the endometrial glands and stroma play a role in orchestrating the local mechanisms that control menstruation, it is also important to consider the effects that these two hormones may exert directly on the endometrial vasculature. There has only been limited and somewhat contradictory mention of estrogen and progesterone receptor immunohistochemical staining in endometrial blood vessels. Some studies report that one or both receptor types cannot be demonstrated by immunohistochemistry in endometrial blood vessels at all.[13,14] However, whether this relates to just endothelial cells or includes other perivascular cells is not stated. Another study on progesterone receptors reported no expression in endometrial endothelial cells or vascular smooth muscle cells.[15] Others have reported absence of estrogen and progesterone receptors in endothelial cells but positive staining for some or all smooth muscle and predecidual cells around spiral arterioles.[16,17,18] In contrast to all the above reports, there has been one study showing that progesterone receptors are expressed in endothelial cells in decidual tissue taken from the 5th–9th weeks of pregnancy.[19]

In a recent study using double immunostaining protocols, a high degree of variability in the expression of estrogen and progesterone receptors in vascular smooth muscle in human endometrium was demonstrated, both from vessel to vessel within the same endometrium and between endometria from different women.[20] There was no statistically significant differences in expression of these two receptors at different stages of the menstrual cycle, or between women with or without menorrhagia. The lack of obvious variation in expression of either estrogen or progesterone receptors in vascular smooth muscle of the endometrium during the menstrual cycle raises an important issue as to the mechanisms which regulate their expression. Total endometrial estrogen and progesterone receptor content fluctuates during the menstrual cycle with peak levels at the periovulatory stage.[11,13] Using immunohistochemical methods, several workers have reported that glandular estrogen and progesterone receptors reach a peak around the late proliferative and early secretory stages of the cycle.[13,15,16,21,22] However, these same studies show a different pattern of expression for progesterone receptor (and to a lesser extent estrogen receptor) in the endometrial stroma, with relatively constant levels throughout the menstrual cycle and evidence for a reduction at the time of menstruation. In general terms, it is believed that estrogen will upregulate the expression of both estrogen and progesterone receptors, while progesterone acts to downregulate both of these receptors.[23,24] However, as stated above, this does not appear to be the case with estrogen or progesterone receptors in the endometrial stroma, and now also for these same receptors in vascular smooth muscle cells.

Vascular events during menstruation

Ultrastructural studies[25] have shown that in the late secretory phase of the nonpregnant cycle, the endometrial stroma and the vascular basal lamina show widespread degeneration prior to the onset of menstruation, with reduced cell-to-cell contacts. By contrast, endometrial endothelial cells appear to remain relatively intact, and in some instances show evidence of hypertrophy, at this time. These observations suggest that the cellular mechanisms initiating and controlling menstruation act differently on the endometrial stromal and/or epithelial cells compared with the blood vessels.

Throughout the normal menstrual process, the vascular bed shows constant signs of attempts to repair itself. High levels of endothelial cell proliferation have been demonstrated in menstrual endometrium,[26] correlating with the elevated levels of mRNA for vascular endothelial growth factor also found in menstrual endometrium.[27] However, there is also evidence to support the concept that endometrial blood vessels are specifically adapted for the menstrual process. For example, it has been shown that levels of the clotting factor, von Willebrand factor, are significantly reduced in endometrial endothelial cells at the time of menstruation.[28]

There is evidence that both the initiation, and regulation, of blood loss during menstruation is mediated primarily by the spiral arterioles.[2] Hence these specialized resistance arterioles, which develop over a relatively short time course during the secretory phase of the menstrual cycle, are an obvious focus for studies aimed at understanding menstrual disorders such as menorrhagia. Vascular smooth muscle cells provide the contractile force around arterioles that enables these vessels to regulate blood flow to the tissues. In a morphometric study using immunostaining of α-actin to identify vascular smooth muscle cells, it has been shown that total numbers of arterioles per unit volume of endometrium do not alter during the cycle.[29] In addition, once immunostaining was used to identify arterioles, it became apparent that a significant population of nonspiral, small arterioles were also present at all stages of the cycle in human endometrium. Another finding was that there were no differences in vascular smooth muscle cell α-actin immunostaining between women with and without menorrhagia.

Basement membranes play a major role in the structural and functional integrity of blood vessels. Just as endothelial cells can differ in structure, function and metabolic properties between and within different organs, so too can the composition of the underlying basement membrane alter. Studies of basement membrane composition in human endometrium reveal that the major components collagen IV, laminin and heparan sulphate proteoglycan are present throughout all stages of the menstrual cycle.[30] However, whereas the first two of these components appear to be in all vessels, and immunostain with equal intensity throughout the cycle, heparan sulphate proteoglycan is only apparent in approximately 55% of vessels, and its staining intensity is dramatically reduced in menstrual tissue. In addition, breaks and small gaps can be seen in both vascular and glandular basement membrane at the time of menstruation. Thus there is evidence in the endometrium for both vascular basement membrane heterogeneity and regulation during the menstrual cycle.

The female sex hormones have somewhat paradoxical vascular effects, being protective against cardiovascular disease, whilst increasing susceptibility to other vascular disorders such as migraine, Raynaud's phenomenom and primary pulmonary hypertension.[10] The cellular mechanisms behind these actions are incompletely understood, although there is evidence to support a number of different pathways. These include regulation of the endothelial derived vasodilator, nitric oxide, and the vasoconstrictor, endothelin. In addition, vascular eicosanoid metabolism, adrenergic responsiveness and calcium ion homeostasis can all be influenced by the sex steriods.[10] The relative roles of these different vascular mechanisms in the process of menstruation remain important issues for future investigation.

The potent vasoconstrictor endothelin is produced by endometrial endothelial and epithelial cells, with immunohistochemical studies showing peak levels in the mid–late secretory phase.[31] Endothelin is inactivated by neutral endopeptidase, which is predominantly located in the stromal cells and reaches maximal levels during the early to midsecretory phase. As of yet there is no direct evidence for a role for endothelin in the initiation or control of menstruation.

From observation of endometrial transplants in the anterior chamber of the eye in Rhesus monkeys, Markee reported[2] that venous and arterial stasis commenced 1–4 days prior to the onset of menstrual bleeding, and that vasoconstriction of the spiral arterioles occurred 4–24 hours before bleeding commenced. It was subsequently assumed that this lack of blood flow to the endometrium resulted in widespread tissue necrosis, thus explaining the vascular rupture and bleeding that occurred immediately after blood flow recommenced. It is unknown if similar vascular events occur prior to menstruation in humans, although limited evidence from blood flow analyses during the menstrual cycle have not shown any significant reduction in overall endometrial blood flow just prior to, or during, menstruation.[32] If localized short-term endometrial blood flow stoppages do occur prior to menstruation, then it is possible that ischemia reperfusion injury (IRI) could also contribute to tissue damage. Tissue damage during IRI results in part from the generation of reactive oxygen metabolites such as superoxide, hydrogen peroxide and hydroxyl radical, as oxygenated blood re-enters the tissue.[33] Reactive oxygen metabolites also serve to increase recruitment of neutrophils to postischemic tissues, and these cells in turn can mediate further tissue damage. Experiments using both free radical scavengers, such as superoxide dismutase, and antibodies to block neutrophil recruitment, have been successful in significantly reducing IRI.[33] Determining whether IRI plays a role in the process of menstruation, or in stimulating the endometrial neutrophil influx that occurs prior to menstruation, requires further investigation.

The hemoglobin content of menstrual discharge is greatly reduced compared to normal circulating blood. In a study of 28 women, the percentage contribution of blood to total fluid loss during menstruation was calculated as $36.1 \pm 3.6\%$.[34] It was suggested that the extra fluid content of menstrual discharge could be due to endometrial glandular secretions and tissue exudate during shedding. There are a number of mechanisms that could theoretically contribute to increased tissue exudate during menstruation. Increased microvascular permeability will result in increased tissue fluid, and can occur as a consequence of IRI,[33] or elevated vascular endothelial cell growth factor levels.[27] Blood leaving damaged vessels could have reduced hematocrit due to filtration effects either from partly formed fibrin clots, or partial blockage of capillaries due to endothelial cell hypertrophy or white blood cell accumulation and adhesion. The finding that menstrual hemoglobin levels are significantly lower in oral contraceptive users compared to intra-uterine contraceptive device users indicates that there are factors that can alter the fluid component of menstrual discharge independently of blood loss.[34]

NEW INSIGHTS INTO THE LOCAL CONTROL OF MENSTRUATION

Markee[2] reported that endometrial regression occurs 2–6 days prior to the commencement of bleeding, and that it was primarily due to fluid and tissue resorption. In addition, following manipulation of intraocular endometrial autotransplants in rhesus monkeys with exogenous estrone and progesterone, he concluded that, 'menstruation follows experimental procedures which induce rapid and extensive regression and that it is inhibited by those which cause growth or prevent the occurrence of rapid and extensive regression'. Recent advances in understanding of the mechanisms involved in tissue remodeling and programmed cell death, or apoptosis, have stimulated a new interest in the process of endometrial regression that precedes menstruation.

Apoptosis, or programmed cell death, plays a key role in the homeostatic maintenance of cell numbers.[36] Evidence for hormonally regulated mechanisms controlling endometrial apoptosis has recently been published,[37] using immunohistochemistry of the protein from proto-oncogene Bcl-2. Bcl-2, which prolongs cell survival by preventing apoptosis, is expressed primarily in gland cells during the proliferative stage, but disappears during the secretory phase. Endothelial cells were always Bcl-2 negative, although vascular smooth muscle cells from proliferative stage small arterioles and secretory stage spiral arterioles were positive. More recently, an immunohistochemical study of Bcl-2 distribution in human endometrium concluded that it was unlikely that Bcl-2 is important in prolonging endometrial cell survival when the luteal phase was prolonged by the use of exogenous human chorionic gonadotropin.[38] These authors made no comment about Bcl-2 distribution in relation to the endometrial vasculature.

Work in nonendometrial tissues and cells has shown that in addition to Bcl-2, which inhibits apoptosis, various homolog of Bcl-2 such as Bax and Bak can act to accelerate apoptosis under certain conditions. It has been suggested that the widespread tissue distribution of Bak mRNA supports the concept that apoptosis is controlled primarily by regulation of molecules such as Bcl-2 that inhibit apoptosis.[39] Investigation of these mechanisms in the endometrium and its vasculature is still in its infancy, despite the fact that a role in menstruation seems highly likely.

Matrix metalloproteinases (MMPs) are a family of neutral pH enzymes which degrade components of both interstitial and basement membrane extracellular matrix. Messenger RNA for proMMPs-1 and 3 is only detectable in normal endometrium perimenstrually and menstrually, although mRNA for its tissue inhibitors (TIMPs) -1 and 2 are present throughout the cycle.[35] Cultured endometrial stromal cells release MMPs -1, 2, 3 and 9, and progesterone withdrawal from cultures increases release of all four enzymes. *In vitro* release of MMPs -1, 3 and 9 is also stimulated by IL-9 and tumor necrosis factor α. Thus MMPs are strong candidates for a major role in the processes of endometrial regression and breakdown that are part of menstruation.

Cellular adhesion molecules play a crucial role in a range of biological processes, including maintenance of tissue integrity, cell–cell and cell substrate recognition, leucocyte recruitment and tissue remodeling.[40] As a dynamic tissue undergoing constant remodeling, the endometrium has received considerable recent attention as a model system for investigating adhesion molecules.[41,42,43] Intercellular adhesion molecule-1 (ICAM-1) is expressed primarily on endothelial cells throughout the menstrual cycle, with an increase in immunostaining at the time of menstruation.[41] ICAM-1 is not expressed by all vessels, although there is no apparent pattern in terms of veins, capillaries and arterioles as far as the staining is concerned. In contrast to ICAM, platelet endothelial cell adhesion molecule (PECAM) showed strong immunostaining on all blood vessels at all stages of the menstrual cycle. Based on these results, it appears that PECAM is expressed constitutively in the vasculature of human endometrium, and presumably plays some role in maintaining normal vessel integrity. Interestingly, it does not appear to change at the time of menstruation, when vessel breakdown occurs. In contrast, ICAM-1 expression appears to be increased at the time of menstruation, and presumably plays some role in that process.

Two ligands for ICAM-1 include lymphocyte function associated antigen-1 (LFA-1) and macrophage antigen-1 (Mac-1). Immunohistochemical studies of the distribution of these ligands in human endometrium (unpublished observations) demonstrated that LFA-1 occurred on cells dispersed throughout the endometrium, both within the stroma and the epithelium, as well as on clusters of cells also spread throughout the endometrium. In contrast Mac-1 only appeared on cells scattered throughout the stroma. It was not seen on cells within the epithelium, or on cells clumped together. Both LFA-1 and Mac-1 levels increased around the time of menstruation.

Other adhesion molecules that play a role in the trafficking of white blood cells from the vasculature into the endometrial tissues include vascular cell adhesion molecule-1 (VCAM-1), and E-selectin.[42] While it is clear that these, and other, vascular adhesion molecules play a central part in controlling the recruitment of different white blood cell populations to the endometrium, considerably more work is required before a full understanding of their role in the control of menstruation becomes clear.

Human endometrium contains a large population of leucocytes, which typically comprises about 70% endometrial granulated lymphocytes (eGLs), 20% macrophages and 10% lymphocytes. Some endometrial leucocytes that are positive for either leucocyte common antigen or CD3 have been reported as expressing estrogen receptors,[44] indicating that hormonal control may regulate their function. One to two days prior to the onset of menstruation the endometrium is infiltrated by increased numbers of polymorphonuclear leucocytes and granulocytes.[3] Prior to and during menstruation is also the only time that eosinophils are found in the endometrium.[45] The role of these cells in the menstrual process remains to be determined. Endometrial mast cells do not change in number during the menstrual cycle, however they do undergo extensive activation and/or degranulation just prior to and during menstruation,[45] suggestive of a role in tissue or vascular remodeling.

Integrins are a family of transmembrane glycoproteins that act as receptors for the extracellular matrix. They are heterodimeric complexes made up of α and β subunits, of which there are currently 19 known combinations.[43] To date there has been very little reported work on the role that integrins may play in controlling the endometrial vasculature during the menstrual cycle, despite the fact that they play a key role in controlling vascular integrity,[46] and more recent reports have identified a key role for $\alpha_v\beta_3$ in regulating angiogenesis.[47]

Growth factors can be defined as proteins that interact with specific cell membrane receptors to initiate intracellular signaling pathways that result in cell division. Many growth factors are pleiotrophic in action, and can promote cell differentiation as well as in some cases having inhibitory effects on mitogenesis. Cytokines include proteins that modulate a variety of cellular functions, including morphogenesis, chemotaxis, expression of epitopes, immunoregulatory function, etc. It is becoming increasingly clear that the endometrium expresses a large number of growth factors and cytokines, and that many of these are regulated during the menstrual cycle either directly or indirectly by estrogen and progesterone.[48,49] *In vitro* evidence indicates that many growth factors and cytokines can either be produced by, or have actions on, endothelial cells. However, the *in vivo* relevance of *in vitro* experiments should always be critically questioned, especially given the pleiotrophic nature of most of these proteins.

Predecidualization of the stromal cells surrounding the spiral arterioles commences approximately 8–9 days after ovulation. Decidual cells have metabolic functions related either to pregnancy, or if implantation does not occur, to menstrual breakdown of the endometrium.[3] The location of the metabolically active predecidual cells around the spiral arterioles suggests an intimate role for these cells in the menstrual process. A number of studies have demonstrated high levels of growth factor and cytokine expression around spiral arterioles in the secretory phase of the cycle.[50,51] Interleukin-1β has been demonstrated by immunohistochemical methods in endometrial endothelial cells throughout the menstrual cycle, and more strongly in spiral arterioles.[52] There is increased staining in the secretory phase compared to the proliferative phase. Interleukin-1 type 1 receptor is found only in glandular epithelial cells, providing evidence for a mechanism whereby the vasculature can directly modulate epithelial function. Other cytokines expressed by endometrial endothelial cells include interleukin-1α and interleukin-6.[49] Transforming growth factor α shows moderate to intense immunostaining round spiral arterioles during the secretory phase,[50] while tumor necrosis factor α mRNA is found in the vascular smooth muscle cells surrounding spiral arterioles and the protein in smooth muscle and endothelial cells.[53] One feature of many of these immunohistochemical and *in situ* hybridization studies is the variability in regional distribution of many proteins in the endometrium. This regional variability includes microvascular heterogeneity, and makes it critically important that the human endometrium is not considered as a homogeneous tissue when planning research studies or interpreting results.

Conclusion

Considerable research work remains to be done before the complex series of events that make up menstruation are fully understood. As a biological system for studying control of tissue regression and remodeling in the human, the process of menstruation provides unique opportunities. Many of the cellular mechanisms involved in menstruation occur in other individual tissues throughout the body, however in no other situation do these cellular systems activate spontaneously and with cyclical regularity. From a clinical viewpoint, disorders of menstruation remain a major challenge to modern gynecology. A better understanding of the physiology and pathology of the menstrual process is essential if new clinical treatments are to be devised for menstrual problems. Many current treatments are based on significant surgical procedures or systemic administration of hormones or drugs. With an improved understanding of local mechanisms controlling menstruation, one goal for the future will be to identify new agents that can be easily and conveniently administered through local delivery systems with minimal side effects and at a low cost.

REFERENCES

1. Finn CA 1994 The adaptive significance of menstruation: the meaning of menstruation. Human Reproduction 9: 1202–1207
2. Markee JE 1940 Menstruation in intraocular endometrial transplants in the rhesus monkey. Contributions to Embryology: Carnegie Institution 28: 223–308
3. Ferenczy A 1987 Anatomy and histology of the uterine corpus. In: Kurman RJ (ed) Blaustein's pathology of the female genital tract. Springer-Verlag, New York, pp 257–291
4. van Herendael BJ, Stevens MJ, Flakiewicz-Kula A, Hansch CH 1987 Dating of the endometrium by microhysteroscopy. Gynecological and Obstetrical Investigation 24: 114–118
5. Christiaens GCML, Sixma JJ, Haspels AA 1982 Hemostasis in menstrual endometrium: a review. Obstetrics and Gynecology Survey 37: 281–303
6. Koh SCL, Wong PC, Yuen R, Chua SE, Ng BL, Ratnam SS 1992 Concentration of plasminogen activators and inhibitor in the human endometrium at different phases of the menstrual cycle. Journal of Reproduction and Fertility 96: 407–413
7. van Eijkeren MA, Christiaens GCML, Scholten PC, Sixma JJ 1992 Menorrhagia. Current drug treatment concepts. Practical Therapeutics 43: 201–209
8. Fraser IS 1990 Treatment of ovulatory and anovulatory dysfunctional uterine bleeding with oral progestogens. Australian and New Zealand Journal of Obstetrics and Gynaecology 30: 353–356
9. Mendelsoln ME, Karas RH 1994 Estrogen and the blood vessel wall. Current Opinion in Cardiology 9: 619–626
10. White MM, Zamudio S, Stevens T et al 1995 Estrogen, progesterone and vascular reactivity: potential cellular mechanisms. Endocrine Reviews 16: 739–751
11. Gleeson N, Jordan M, Sheppard B, Bonnar J 1993 Cyclical variation in endometrial oestrogen and progesterone receptors in women with normal menstruation and dysfunctional uterine bleeding. European Journal of Obstetrics, Gynaecology and Reproductive Biology 48: 207–214
12. Critchley HOD, Abberton KM, Taylor NH, Healy DL, Rogers PAW 1994 Endometrial sex steroid receptor expression in women with menorrhagia. British Journal of Obstetrics and Gynecology 101: 428–434
13. Lessey BA, Killam AP, Metzger DA, Haney AF, Greene GL, McCarty KS 1988 Immunohistochemical analysis of human uterine estrogen and progesterone receptors throughout the menstrual cycle. Journal of Clinical Endocrinology and Metabolism 67: 334–340
14. Bergeron C, Ferenczy A, Toft DO, Schneider W, Shyamala G 1988 Immunocytochemical study of progesterone receptors in the human endometrium during the menstrual cycle. Laboratory Investigation 59: 862–869
15. Press MF, Udove JA, Greene GL 1988 Progesterone receptor distribution in the human endometrium. American Journal of Pathology 131: 112–124
16. Snijders MPML, de Goeij AFPM, Debets-Te Baerts MJC, Rousch JJM, Koudstaal J, Bosman FT 1992 Immunocytochemical analysis of estrogen receptors and progesterone receptors in the human uterus throughout the menstrual cycle and after the menopause. Journal of Reproduction and Fertility 94: 363–371
17. Perrot-Applanat M, Groyer-Picard MT, Garcia E, Lorenzo F, Milgrom E 1988 Immunocytochemical demonstration of estrogen and progesterone receptors in muscle cells of uterine arteries in rabbits and humans. Endocrinology 123: 1511–1519
18. Perrot-Applanat M, Deng M, Fernandez H, Lelaidier C, Meduri G, Bouchard P 1994 Immunohistochemical localization of estradiol and progesterone receptors in human uterus throughout pregnancy: expression in endometrial blood vessels. Journal of Clinical Endocrinology and Metabolism 78: 216–224
19. Wang J-D, Fu Y, Shi W-L, Zhu P-D, Cheng J, Qiao G-M, Wang Y-Q, Greene GL 1992 Immunohistochemical localization of progesterone receptor in human decidua of early pregnancy. Human Reproduction 7: 123–127
20. Rogers PAW, Lederman F, Kooy J, Taylor NH, Healy DL 1996 Endometrial vascular smooth muscle estrogen and progesterone receptor distribution in women with and without menorrhagia. Human Reproduction 11: 2003–2008

21. Critchley HOD, Bailey DA, Au LC, Affandi B, Rogers PAW 1993 Immunohistochemical sex steroid receptor distribution in endometrium from long-term subdermal levonorgestrel users and during the normal menstrual cycle. Human Reproduction 8: 1632–1639
22. Ben-Hur H, Mor G, Insler V, Blickstein I, Amir-Zaltsman Y, Kohen F 1995 Assessment of estrogen receptor distribution in human endometrium by direct immunofluorescence. Acta Obstetrica Gynecologica Scandinavica 74: 97–102
23. Nardulli AM, Katzenellenbogen BS 1988 Progesterone receptor regulation in T47D human breast cancer cells: analysis by density labeling of progesterone receptor synthesis and degradation and their modulation by progestin. Endocrinology 122: 1532–1540
24. Nardulli AM, Greene GL, O'Malley BW, Katzenellenbogen BS 1988 Regulation of progesterone receptor messenger ribonucleic acid and protein levels in MCF-7 cells by estradiol: analysis of estrogen's effect on progesterone receptor synthesis and degradation. Endocrinology 122: 935–944
25. Roberts DK, Parmley TH, Walker NJ, Horbelt DV 1992 Ultrastructure of the microvasculature in the human endometrium throughout the normal menstrual cycle. American Journal of Obstetrics and Gynecology 166: 1391–406
26. Goodger (Macpherson) AM, Rogers PAW 1994 Endometrial endothelial cell proliferation during the menstrual cycle. Human Reproduction 9: 399–405
27. Charnock-Jones DS, Sharkey AM, Rajput-Williams J et al 1993 Identification and localization of alternately spliced mRNAs for vascular endothelial growth factor in human uterus and estrogen regulation in endometrial carcinoma cell lines. Biology of Reproduction 48: 1120–1128
28. Au CL, Rogers PAW 1993 Immunohistochemical staining of von Willebrand factor in human endometrium during normal menstrual cycle. Human Reproduction 8: 17–23
29. Abberton KM, Taylor NH, Healy DL, Rogers PAW 1996 Vascular smooth muscle α-actin distribution around endometrial arterioles during the menstrual cycle: increased expression during the perimenopause and lack of correlation with menorrhagia. Human Reproduction 11: 201–207
30. Kelly FD, Tawia SA, Rogers PAW 1995 Immunohistochemical characterization of human endometrial microvascular basement membrane components during the normal menstrual cycle. Human Reproduction 10: 268–276
31. Marsh MM, Findlay JK, Salamonsen LA 1996 Endothelin and menstruation. Human Reproduction 11 Suppl 2: 83–89
32. Fraser IS, Peek MJ 1992 Effects of exogenous hormones on endometrial capillaries. In: Alexander NJ, d'Arcangues C (eds) Steroid hormones and uterine bleeding. AAAS Publications, Washington, pp 65–79
33. Zimmerman BJ, Granger DN 1994 Mechanisms of reperfusion injury. American Journal of Medical Science 307: 284–292
34. Fraser IS, McCarron G, Markham R, Resta T 1985 Blood and total fluid content of menstrual discharge. Obstetrics and Gynecology 65: 194–197
35. Salamonsen LA, Woolley DE 1996 Matrix metalloproteinases in normal menstruation. Human Reproduction 11 Suppl 2: 124–133
36. Schwartzman RA, Cidlowski JA 1993 Apoptosis: the biochemistry and molecular biology of programmed cell death. Endocrinology Review 14: 133–151
37. Gompel A, Sabourin JC, Martin A, Yaneva H, Audouin J, Decroix Y, Poitout P 1994 Bcl-2 expression in normal endometrium during the menstrual cycle. American Journal of Pathology 144: 1195–1202
38. Koh EAT, Illingworth PJ, Duncan WC, Critchely HOD 1995 Immunolocalization of bcl-2 protein in human endometrium in the menstrual cycle and simulated early pregnancy. Human Reproduction 10: 1557–1562
39. Kiefer MC, Brauer MJ, Powers VC, Wu JJ, Umansky SR, Tomei LD, Barr PJ 1995 Modulation of apoptosis by the widely distributed Bcl-2 homologue Bak. Nature 374: 736–739
40. Edelman GM, Crossin KL 1991 Cell adhesion molecules: implications for a molecular histology. Annual Review of Biochemistry 60: 155–190
41. Tawia SA, Beaton LA, Rogers PAW 1993 Immunolocalization of the cellular adhesion molecules, intercellular adhesion molecule-1 (ICAM-1) and platelet endothelial cell adhesion molecule (PECAM), in human endometrium throughout the menstrual cycle. Human Reproduction 8: 175–181
42. Tabibzadeh S, Kong QF, Babaknia A 1994 Expression of adhesion molecules in human endometrial vasculature throughout the menstrual cycle. Journal of Clinical Endocrinology and Metabolism 79: 1024–1032
43. Lessey BA, Castelbaum AJ 1995 Integrins in the endometrium. Reproductive Medicine Reviews 4: 43–58
44. Tabibzadeh SS, Satyaswaroop PG 1989 Sex steroid receptors in lymphoid cells of human endometrium. American Journal of Clinical Pathology 91: 656–663
45. Jeziorska M, Salamonsen LA, Woolley DE 1995 Mast cell and eosinophil distribution and activation in human endometrium throughout the menstrual cycle. Biology of Reproduction 53: 312–320
46. Dejana E, Raiteri M, Resnati M, Lampugnani MG 1993 Endothelial integrins and their role in maintaining the integrity of the vessel wall. Kidney International 43: 61–65
47. Brooks PC, Clark RAF, Cheresh DA 1994 Requirement of vascular integrin $\alpha_v\beta_3$ for angiogenesis. Science 264: 569–571
48. Giudice LC 1994 Growth factors and growth modulators in human uterine endometrium: their potential relevance to reproductive medicine. Fertility and Sterility 61: 1–17
49. Tabibzadeh S, Sun XZ 1992 Cytokine expression in human endometrium throughout the menstrual cycle. Human Reproduction 7: 1214–1221
50. Horowitz GM, Scott RT Jr, Drews MR, Navot D, Hofmann GE 1993 Immunohistochemical localization of transforming growth factor-α in human endometrium, decidua and trophoblast. Journal of Clinical Endocrinology and Metabolism 76: 786–792
51. Tabibzadeh S 1991 Ubiquitous expression of TNF-α cachectin immunoreactivity in human endometrium. American Journal of Reproductive Immunology 26: 1–4

52. Simon C, Piquette GN, Frances A, Polan ML 1993 Localization of interleukin-1 type I receptor and interleukin-1β in human endometrium throughout the menstrual cycle. Journal of Clinical Endocrinology and Metabolism 77: 549–555

53. Philippeaux M-M, Piquet PF 1993 Expression of tumor necrosis factor α and its mRNA in the endometrial mucosa during the menstrual cycle. American Journal of Pathology 143: 480–486

15. Effects of estrogen and progesterone on myometrium, cervix, fallopian tube, vagina and vulva

Robert P.S. Jansen

Introduction

The female reproductive tract — hollow and muscular in structure, 'oviductal' in purpose — connects the female celomic cavity to the exterior. In the human, the steroid-responsive female tract that develops from the paramesonephric, or Müllerian ducts is duplicated for the left and right fallopian tubes, but is generally fused and single for the uterus, cervix and upper vagina. The (always single) introitus and vulva are embryologically derived from androgen-dependent ectoderm and supporting mesoderm of the urogenital sinus, and will not be considered further here. Estrogen sensitivity has been claimed to be present in the Müllerian ducts during embryonic differentiation,[1] but an essential embryological role for estradiol is contradicted by indefatigable Müllerian development when fetal estrogen is absent, in congenital aromatase deficiency.[2] During pubertal maturation of the tract to adult dimensions, estradiol exerts a pronounced proliferative action on the immature fallopian tubes, uterus, cervix and vagina.

In the conducting of the reproductive process in adulthood, regional specialization of the tract allows ascent of sperm, provides the site for fertilization, and permits the interrupted transport of the gestated ovum to, ultimately, the exterior. The best-characterized estrogen and progestogen-responsive element in the mammalian tract is the epithelium of the primate endometrium[3] (see also Ch. 13). Endometrial epithelial responsiveness — estradiol-induced growth, progesterone-induced differentiation, periodic shedding — is, however, not typical of the tract's other tissues, where estradiol and progesterone act together more subtly. In particular, progesterone-induced destruction of progesterone responsiveness, dramatically evident in endometrial epithelium, is not seen elsewhere in the tract.

Endocrine events or processes are brought about when a hormone acts on a tissue that is sensitive to it through the display of hormone receptors. The process thus depends *quantitatively* on both the concentration of the hormone in the milieu and the concentration of specific receptor in the tissue; *qualitatively* on the differential display of receptors, receptor subtypes and varying intracellular responses to hormone receptor binding; and *temporally* to the sequential order and duration of the hormonal exposure, as well as to the interplay of nonsteroidal, water-soluble chemical signaling. Cyclical and pregnancy-related changes in estradiol and progesterone dominate the Müllerian tract, defining the endocrine base upon which reactions to peptide hormones as well as neurocrine, paracrine and autocrine influences can act. A short chapter can just give an overview of these processes and responses at an organ and tissue level. So far, too little research has been published on the isoforms of the estrogen receptor (ER) and progesterone receptor (PR) to make differential observations in non-endometrial reproductive tissues.

THE NATURE OF THE STEROID MILIEU

Estrogens, progestogens and other steroid hormones can reach the reproductive organs systemically or locally (respectively blood-borne or through diffusion across tissues). The only purely systemic route is exogenous, after oral, intramuscular or intravenous administration, when steroids must reach the tract just by way of its arterial blood supply.

Steroid production from the ovaries before and after ovulation results in quantitatively substantial and temporally characteristic circulating levels (see Ch. 10) but remember that local release of estradiol and progesterone into peritoneal fluid with ovulation causes concentrations bathing serosal surfaces to be orders of magnitude higher than those that reach these tissues arterially,[4] and they have a different time course, monomodal peaks occurring at midcycle for both estradiol and progesterone (see Fig. 15.1).

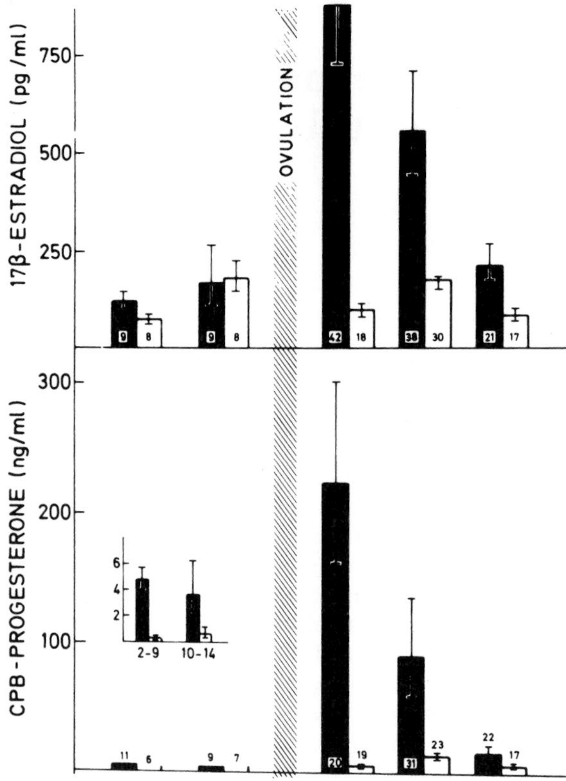

Fig. 15.1 Estradiol and progesterone concentrations in peritoneal fluid (solid bars) and plasma (open bars) through the ovarian cycle. Estradiol concentrations in peritoneal fluid increase dramatically with follicular rupture at ovulation; progesterone concentrations do too, but levels in peritoneal fluid are also higher than plasma levels in the follicular phase.[4]

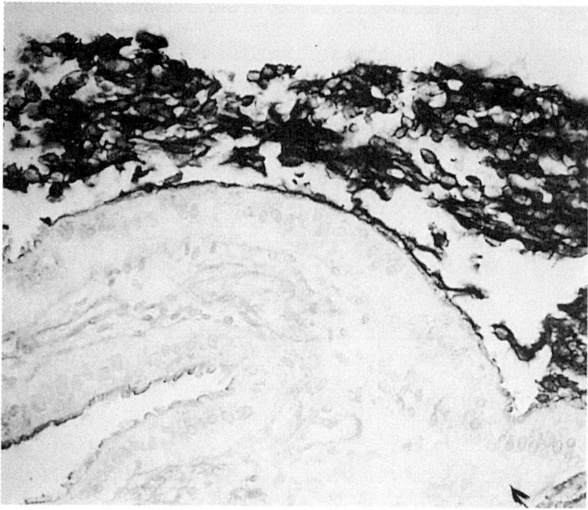

Fig. 15.2 Dark-staining cumulus tissue in the monkey fallopian tube lumen after ovulation. *In vitro* studies indicate that cumulus cells secrete estradoil and progesterone, which might thus have a direct effect on endosalpingeal function. High iron diamine reaction at pH 1.[3]

In the genital tract a disproportionately high concentration of steroid hormones is brought to paracrine action by diffusion into tissues immediately adjacent to the steroid source. This is seen during fetal development (when, for example, testosterone from the developing testis in male fetuses rescues the embryonic mesonephric duct ipsilaterally), during periods of cyclical ovarian activity (with intraperitoneal diffusion and with release from ovulated cumulus in the tubal lumen — see Fig. 15.2),[5] and during pregnancy (with diffusion from trophoblast implanted in the submucosa of the uterus).

Thus it can be seen that administration of steroids by vaginal application can have special advantages. The vaginal route is an increasingly utilized parenteral route of drug administration, partly because of good absorption characteristics and partly because a first-pass effect in the liver is avoided,[6] the venous absorption path being systemic, not portal. Vaginal absorption of exogenous sex steroids therefore usually produces very satisfactory circulating levels. But a local effect from direct diffusion through the tissues is now also recognized as important — and therapeutically exploitable — not just for topical action of sex steroids in the vaginal mucosa but for effects in the uterus too.[7]

FALLOPIAN TUBE

Structure and function

The fallopian tube's steroid-responsive tissues comprise the epithelial lining, or endosalpinx, and the muscular wall, or myosalpinx, both of which are in anatomical continuity with their uterine counterparts, the endometrium and myometrium.

Tubal ER and PR have immunological, sedimentation and binding characteristics similar to those of respective endometrial receptors.[8–10] In a nonhuman primate it has been shown that cytoplasmic ER is increased by estradiol and decreased by progesterone.[11] Also, as in the endometrium, progesterone enhances the oxidation and deactivation of estradiol to estrone through estradiol dehydrogenase.[12] Unlike among the endometrial glands, however, PR remains demonstrable in the endosalpinx and myosalpinx throughout the luteal phase.[8] Tubal epithelial steroid receptor concentrations increase down the tube, from low concentrations in the fimbrial ends to high estimated densities in the (relatively sparse) endosalpinx of the isthmus.[8,9,13–15]

The two main types of differentiated cell in the endosalpinx are the nonciliated *secretory cells* and *ciliated cells*.[14,15] Mature, differentiated cells are seen only under high estradiol conditions, namely at midcycle.[16] Mitosis is rare in the adult tube at any stage of the menstrual cycle, so there is little change in cell number. Under the prolonged influence of progesterone or progestogens, cells dedifferentiate, so that those that have lost their cilia are indistinguishable from those that have lost their secretory granules.

Under the influence of estrogen, ciliogenesis occurs in the endosalpinx if this phenomenon is not already maximal, and secretory cells mature. Secretion itself is estradiol-dependent, but in humans becomes maximal only with the particularly high levels of estradiol found in the tube at midcycle. The endosalpingeal ciliary beat, which qualitatively is directed to the uterus irrespective of hormonal milieu, may be maximal during a change from estradiol to progesterone dominance, as mitochondria then aggregate at cell apices adjacent to the ciliary bodies and impedance offered by estradiol-induced secretion disappears. Eventually, either continued exposure of ciliated cells to progesterone or prolonged deprivation of cells from estradiol causes atrophy of secretory cells and regression of ciliation.

The myosalpinx is arranged in sheets that tend to form, in the isthmus, an inner circular layer and an outer longitudinal layer; in the thin-walled ampulla the relatively sparse myosalpinx shows no layering.[17,18] Spontaneous muscle activity in the primate tube is estradiol-dependent.[19] Propagation is slow, because (unlike the myometrium, see below) only simple contacts and not gap junctions form between adjacent smooth muscle cells. Progesterone inhibits contractions. Under the influence of estradiol unopposed by progesterone, the adrenergically innervated isthmus constricts.[20]

Ovarian cycle

Studies on receptor turnover in the fallopian tube[9] indicate that there are slight but important differences between the fallopian tube and the endometrium, with receptor action and translation possibly occurring earlier in the tube.[15] During ovulation, which is generally a unilateral event, disproportionately ipsilateral steroid effects have been revealed in fallopian tube epithelial[13,15] and myosalpingeal[21] function (see Fig. 15.1). The active ovary thus creates around itself a steroid milieu different to the steroid environment provided by the adnexal arterial blood supply. With development of a Graffian follicle, peritoneal (and presumably tubal luminal) estradiol levels rise (see Fig. 15.3); with ovulation, an explosive increase in estradiol and progesterone takes place. Extruded cumulus and granulosa cells derived from the luteinized, steroid-producing follicular cells then enter the tube, where they continue to produce estradiol and progesterone.[5,22]

The thickness and general morphology of the human endosalpinx varies during the cycle, but the variations are less conspicuous than the changes the endometrium undergoes (see refs 14 & 15 for reviews). Secretory cells show the most conspicuous cyclical changes,[23] especially in the isthmus (Fig. 15.4). Early in the cycle, scanning electron microscopy (SEM) reveals that the apices of secretory cells have prominent microvilli and the cilia of ciliated cells appear discrete (Fig. 15.4A). With the high estrogen concentrations before, during and immediately after ovulation, apocrine secretion occurs and secreted

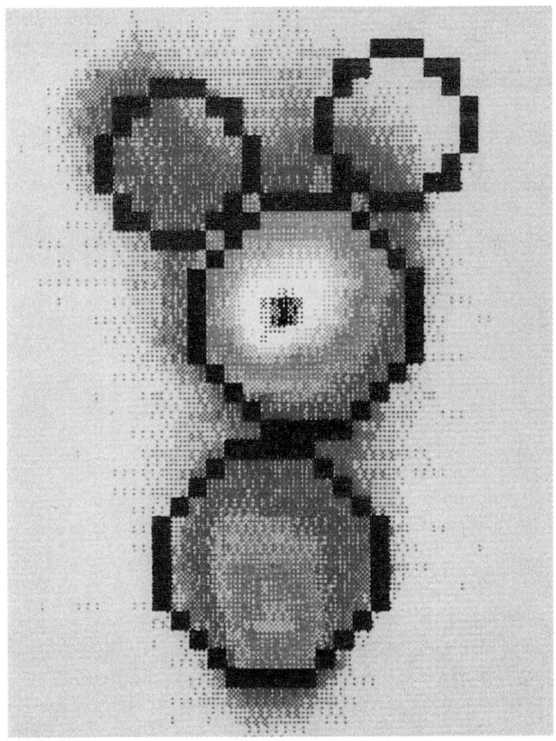

Fig. 15.3 Radioscintographic image of the distribution of technicium-labeled microspheres 16 minutes after placement in the cervix in the late follicular phase. Note that myosalpingeal contractions have resulted in preferential passage of spheres into the right fallopian tube (the left side of the figure), ipsilateral to the side of ovulation.[21] (See also color plate p2.)

material obscures the cilia (Fig. 15.4B). At this time, serous granules are evident in the apical cytoplasm of the secretory cells on transmission electron microscopy (TEM); in primates, however, endoplasmic reticulum vacuoles rather than serous granules seem to dominate the secretory process, apparently with direct release of glycogen and acid mucus glycoproteins.[24] Sperm ascent takes place during this time, with the secretion-laden isthmus functioning as a reservoir for sperm.[25]

The muscular isthmus under the influence of estradiol is in a state of contraction (Fig. 15.5A). Circular muscle tone is high;[20] cellular fluid content is high, causing high mural bulk and functional impedance;[26] and mucus glycoproteinaceous secretions occupy the lumen.[23,27,28] Any of these

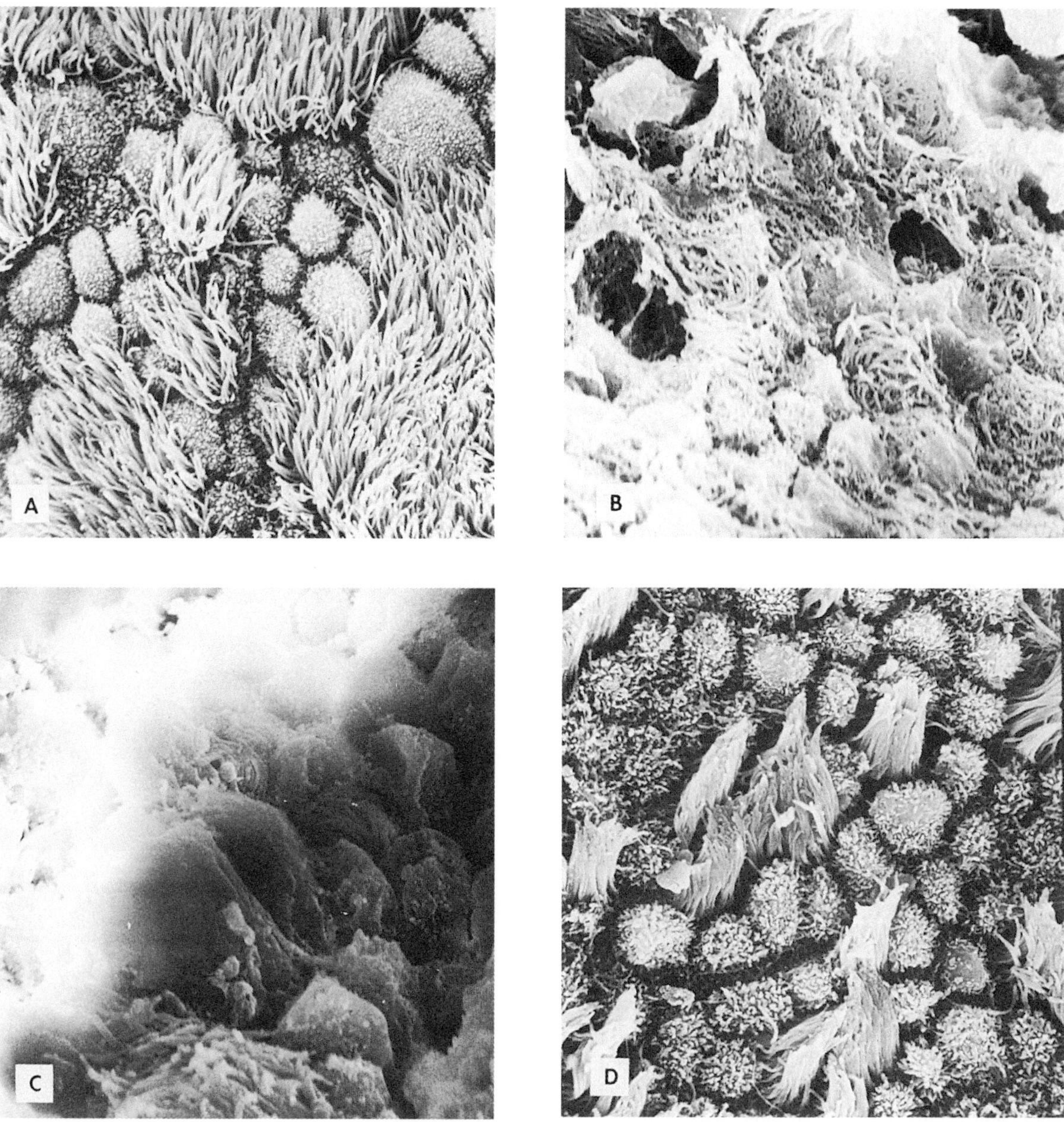

Fig. 15.4 (see overleaf)

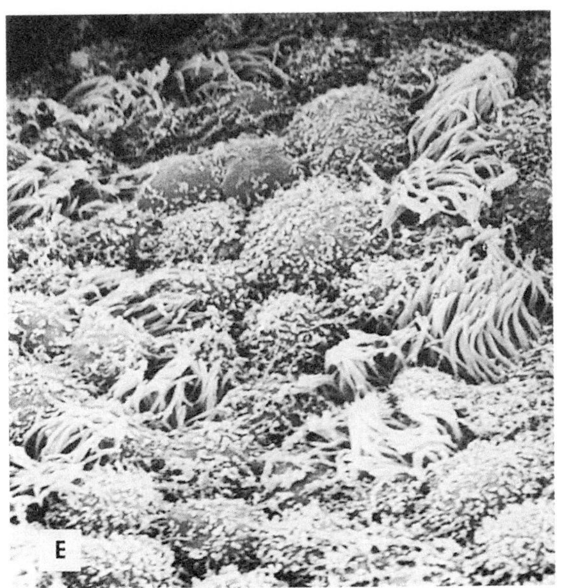

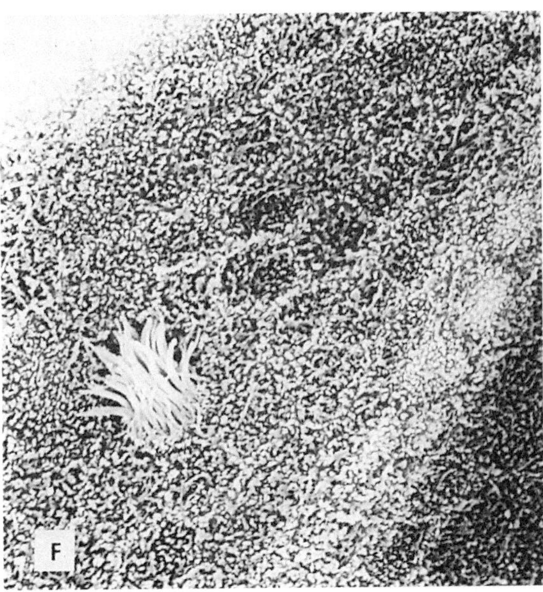

Fig. 15.4 Human fallopian tube isthmic mucosa and secretion visualized by scanning electron microscopy.[23] **A** Late menstrual phase. Early estrogen effect after recovery from progesterone effect. Secretory cells with surface microvilli lie among the ciliated cells. **B** Late follicular phase. Extracellular secretion produced under the influence of estradiol blankets the cell surfaces, so that cilia are indistinct. **C** Postovulation. Abundant extracellular secretion fills the isthmic lumen before progesterone action dominates. The ovum is confined to the ampullary isthmic junction at this time. **D** Four days after ovulation. Progesterone influence causes secretion to disappear and cilia to appear prominent at the time the fertilized ovum transits the isthmus. **E** Late luteal phase. Progesterone withdrawal causes a loss of hormonal support from the endosalpinx at the time menstruation starts in the uterus. **F** Prolonged progestrogen therapy (or pregnancy, or the postmenopause) leads to atrophy and deciliation.

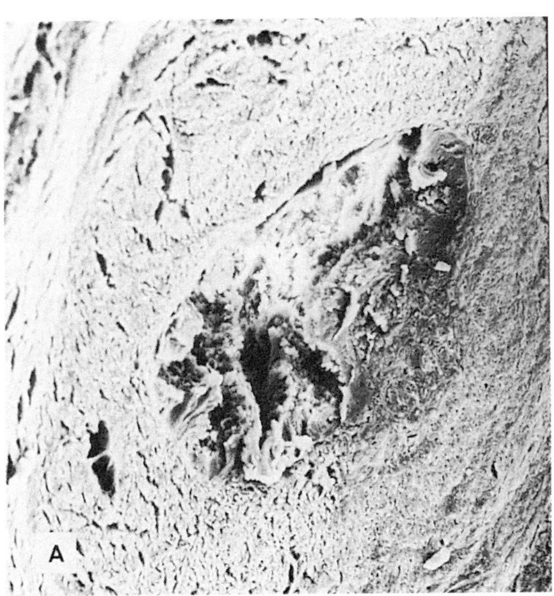

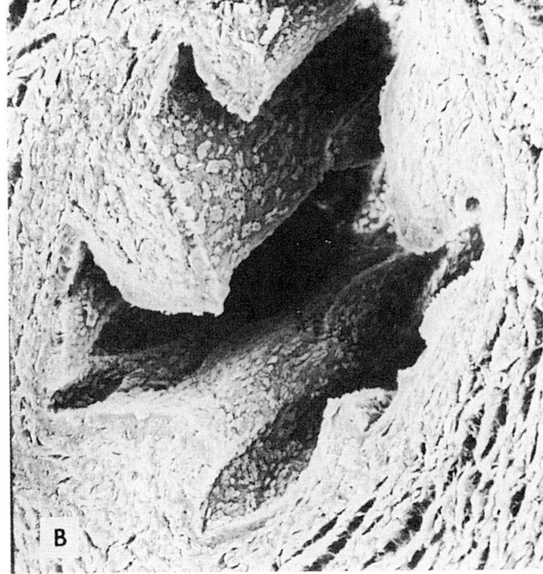

Fig. 15.5 Fallopian tube isthmic contraction (**A**) in the human under the unopposed action of estradiol, and relaxation (**B**) under the opposing influence of progesterone after ovulation. Low power scanning electron micrographs.[23]

estradiol-dependent phenomena could account for the transport delay the ovulated egg experiences when it reaches the ampullary-isthmic junction (AIJ), about 30 minutes after ovulation. Fixable luminal secretion persists through the time of ovulation (Fig. 15.4C) and for several days afterwards. Fertilization and the first cleavage divisions of the zygote take place at the AIJ.

As exposure to progesterone accumulates, secretion stops, granules are no longer seen on TEM; SEM shows cilia again to be conspicuous and unencumbered (Fig. 15.4D); the myosalpinx of the isthmus loses water-content and relaxes (Fig. 15.5B) and the fertilized egg transits the isthmus to reach the uterus.[14]

With the loss of hormonal support at the end of the luteal phase, numerous lysozomes are found in epithelial cell cytoplasm,[29,30] cilia give the SEM appearance of having lost vigour, and the nonciliated cells' microvilli are sparse (Fig. 15.4E).

Pregnancy

Deciliation of the endosalpinx occurs during pregnancy and, especially, in the pueperium[23,31] — as a result, presumably, of prolonged progesterone action and then estradiol and progesterone withdrawal.

Steroid contraception

Microdose levels of progestogen do not appreciably alter the numbers of ciliated and secretory cells in the human endosalpinx.[32] With prolonged higher doses of progestogen administration, atrophy and deciliation of the endosalpinx can be produced (Fig. 15.4F). Similar findings occur with estrogen and progesterone withdrawal after the menopause.

MYOMETRIUM

Structure and function

The myometrium is the most specialized region of the genital tract musculature. The bundles and sheets of smooth muscle cells constitute an interlacing network of substantial intricacy: attempts to distinguish layers of different orientation or composition have not produced a uniform view.[33] Ultrasound studies and MRI have delineated an anatomically and functionally distinct, coordinated layer immediately adjacent to the endometrial basalis, which shows substantial dependence on the steroidal environment.[34,35,36]

Molecular studies show that the myometrium's ER and PR are the same isoforms as those of the endometrium,[37,38] with generally similar steroidal control. Myometrial growth requires estradiol, as do the other tissues of the uterus, and myometrial ER is stimulated by estradiol and inhibited by progesterone. Unlike the case in endometrial glandular epithelium, however, PR expression is maintained in myometrial cells with prolonged exposure to progesterone, both in the ovarian cycle and in pregnancy.[39]

ER and PR levels in myomas are at least as high as those in normal myometrium[38,40] and there is evidence that both estrogen action[40] and progesterone action[41] are overexpressed. Estradiol and progesterone are both capable of promoting myoma growth.[42] The rate of smooth muscle cell mitosis in myomas peaks with the action of progesterone in the luteal phase.[43] Endocrine strategies designed to diminish myoma size must decrease the levels of both hormones (e.g. with GnRH-agonists)[44] or block PR as well as ER (e.g. with gestrinone or mifepristone).[45,46] Interestingly, the therapeutic use of the PR antagonist mifepristone to shrink myomas has been shown to *decrease* immunohistochemically identifiable PR receptor concentration in myomatous tissue,[46] consistent with the idea that progesterone maintains PR in myometrium and the opposite to what might be expected if, as in endometrial glands, progesterone caused destruction of PR.

The muscle layer of the genital tract is unique among smooth muscle tissues of the body in requiring estrogen for acquisition of spontaneous activity and rhythmicity. The action of progesterone on contractile activity of normal myometrium is determined by the extent to which the myometrium has been primed with estrogen. Progesterone's effect on estrogen-deprived myometrium is negligible, whereas the propagated electrical activity of stimulated strip of myometrium from an estrogen-treated rabbit can be changed, with progesterone treatment, to a pattern where only the immediate segment stimulated contracts.[47] Observations such as these in the 1970s led Csapo to propose that a 'progesterone block' occurs during pregnancy to enable uterine quiescence to last until the time of labor.[48,49] The extent to which smooth muscle cells of the myometrium act in concert to form a functional syncytium depends on the frequency with which gap junctions occur between the cells, a process favored by the withdrawal of progesterone (see below).

Estradiol and progesterone change the myometrium's response to the water soluble hormones and to drugs. In the myometrium, estrogen-dependent intracellular release of calcium ions, associated with calmodulin mediated stimulation of myosin ATPase, can be elicited by:

(a) Neurotransmitters and related drugs (e.g. noradrenalin or ergometrine acting on α-receptors, with inhibition by stimulation of adrenergic β-receptors)
(b) Water-soluble hormones (including prostaglandins and oxytocin; inhibition by relaxin)
(c) Spontaneously, especially in response to stretch. Unlike the case with endometrial glands, progesterone action can be maintained in the myosalpinx for weeks and months, as is seen in pregnancy.

Ovarian cycle

Myometrial expression of ER and PR, qualitatively and temporally, varies through the ovarian cycle with a comparable pattern to endometrial changes,[50] except that PR is maintained in the luteal phase despite exposure to progesterone;[39,51,52] ER densities fall during the luteal phase.

Transvaginal ultrasound scanning has led to characterization of a particularly steroid sensitive part of the nonpregnant uterus, the myometrium just deep to the endometrial basalis. Contractions of this slightly hypoechoic junctional zone of the myometrium[34,36] are thought to help propel sperm up to the fallopian tubes before ovulation and later perhaps to position the pre-embryo properly for implantation.[53] The waves require exposure to estrogen and probably correspond with contractions of the myometrium capable of rapidly transporting inert particles — and by implication sperm cells — from the cervix to the fallopian tubes. Radioscintigraphic studies using technetium-labelled albumin microspheres reveal an increasing frequency and intensity of such fundally directed waves as the follicular phase develops.[21] Ascent to the tubal isthmus of microspheres placed in the cervix at midcycle occurs within 60 seconds, with preferential direction to the tube ipsilateral to the dominant follicle (Fig. 15.1). The frequency and amplitude of myometrial contractions abates quickly as luteal levels of progesterone rise;[33] by the time of implantation, the uterus is quiescent, and especially resistant to the action of oxytocin, although oxytocin receptors in myometrium rise sharply during progesterone exposure.[54] Contraction frequency remains low until, with withdrawal of steroid support for the endometrium and the release there of $PGF_{2\alpha}$, the amplitude of contractions and their sensitivity to oxytocin rise considerably, as menstruation starts. Women with dysmenorrhea show an especially high prevalence of gap junctions between smooth muscle cells during this time.[55]

Cause and effect between the rise and fall of estradiol and progesterone exposure and these changes in myometrial activity are not in doubt in principle, but the pathways and intermediaries by which these steroids, especially progesterone, ultimately exert their actions are not entirely clear.

Pregnancy

The uterus enlarges in pregnancy from the transcriptional action of hormones and from the physical stimulus of the growing gestational sac, with an increase in uterine weight from 10–15 g to 800–1000 g brought about entirely by cellular hypertrophy (rather than by hyperplasia).[47] Estrogen is irrelevant to this growth, which is normal in pregnancy complicated by a lack of estrogen from aromatase deficiency.[2] It is thought that progesterone, even though produced by the submucosal trophoblast in substantial amounts, is insufficient alone to account for the hypertrophy,[47] and that other factors must operate; but it is not known to what extent the stimulus for hypertrophy is physical or to what extent trophoblastic somatotropic hormones might play a part.

As pregnancy progresses, the frequency of spontaneous uterine contractions is relatively high (~132/h) and the amplitude low (<10 mmHg).[33] After 14 weeks there is a gradual increase in amplitude — slow at first, and then, toward term, more quickly. Labor is characterized by regular, highly coördinated, high amplitude (50–100 mm) contractions with a frequency of 3–10 per 10 minutes.[56]

The mechanism by which myometrial activity is blocked prior to labor remains controversial in humans, although in species such as the rabbit progesterone has both the ability and the likely predominant role. In the rat, withdrawal of progesterone and the introduction of $PGF_{2\alpha}$ produces a precipitate and highly significant increase in the number, area and size of gap junctions, which by establishing direct cytoplasmic electrical contact between muscle cells transforms the myometrium into a functional syncytium, with contractions coordinated through most of the uterus. The situation in humans is complicated by the fact that, unlike the rabbit, (a) plasma progesterone concentrations do not fall in any indisputable manner prior to the onset of labor, and (b) even massive amounts of exogenous progesterone do not inhibit labor once it has begun. Human myometrium in labor, however, shows the same gap-junction-mediated generation of low-resistance pathways displayed by rodents and attributed there to withdrawal of progesterone.[49,57] Furthermore, myometrial PR densities detected immunocytochemically are lower at term than during preterm, and are lower in women in labor compared with those who are not, all of which is consistent with a progesterone-withdrawal role to the mechanism of onset of human labor; ER levels do not obviously change.[58]

Meanwhile, it is also true that there has been no exception to the rule that complete withdrawal of progesterone at any stage of human pregnancy — whether through luteectomy[48] or by PR blockade,[59,60,61] — promptly acts towards expelling the conceptus or fetus. So the etymological basis for the name 'progesterone' — the hormone that promotes pregnancy — remains firm for humans as well as for other mammals. These issues are discussed in more detail in Chapter 22.

CERVIX

There are three distinct steroid-sensitive tissues in the cervix: the *endocervix*, which shows characteristic changes through the ovarian cycle; the *cervical stroma*, which softens in pregnancy and especially in labor; and the *ectocervix*, with squamous epithelium comparable to that of the vagina (and discussed later).

Structure and function

The response of the endocervical mucosa to estrogen is among the more dramatic of endocrine reponses in the genital tract. The endocervix is lined by goblet-cell-like epithelium that secretes highly acidic mucus glycoproteins (acid MGPs) (Fig. 15.6). These cells show strong immunoreactivity for ER during all phases of the ovarian cycle.[52] Immunoreactive PR staining is strongest in the presence of unopposed estrogen, weaker with progesterone exposure and absent in atrophy.[62]

Under the unopposed influence of estrogen, the state of hydration of the 'bottle-brush'-like acid MGP molecules increases, converting the state of the endocervical secretions from a viscous gel to a more fluid sol, which in turn allows the mucus to be colonized and penetrated by spermatozoa (for review see reference 15). At other times, especially under the additional influence of progesterone in the luteal phase or during pregnancy, the mucus is viscous, and sperm are largely excluded from the higher parts of the genital tract.

The cervical stroma is also characterized by highly hydrated complex carbohydrates — the proteoglycans of the connective tissue ground substance. Although the stroma contains specific ER and PR, positive cells are sparse and comprise subepithelial cells and

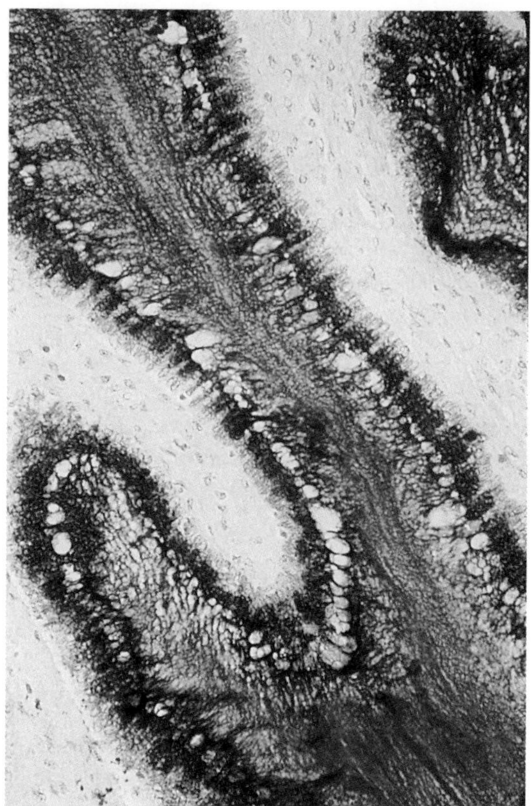

Fig. 15.6 Longitudinal section through the endocervical canal, showing the highly acidic mucus glycoproteins that result from the action of estradiol. Alcian blue. (See color plate P2.)

(sporadic) smooth muscle cells;[63] concentrations of stromal ER and PR both fall during pregnancy,[64] with a further fall during labor[65] (the PR levels, at least, thus mirroring changes seen in the myometrium, discussed earlier).

Ovarian cycle

Cyclical changes in cervical mucus are among the best known quantitative and qualitative alterations in genital tract steroid responsiveness that occur during the ovarian cycle. These changes consist of:

(a) An increase in volume
(b) A decrease in viscosity
(c) An increase in stretchiness (Spinnbarkheit)
(d) Acquisition of ferning (a crystallizing property exhibited when the mucus is allowed to dry on a microscope slide).

All of these changes take place with follicular development leading to ovulation and can be clinically

Table 15.1 Cervical score (after Insler et al[66]). Each parameter receives a score from 0–3; the maximum score under the unopposed influence of estradiol is 12.

Parameter	Score 0	1	2	3
Amount of mucus	None	Scant	Dribble	Cascade
Spinnbarkheit (stretchability)	None	Slight	Moderate	Pronounced
Ferning	Amorphous	Linear	Partial	Complete
Cervical os	Closed		Partly open	Gaping

quantifiable as a *cervical score*,[66] with points from 0–3 awarded for each of the four parameters (Table 15.1). With abundant estrogen exposure at midcycle or with exogenous estrogen administration, most women will have a score of at least 8,[67] ideally with full scores for stretchibility and ferning to correlate with good sperm penetrability. Modifications have been suggested to this method of cervical scoring to take into account mucus cellularity; the number of leukocytes is high in the early follicular and luteal phases, and low at midcycle.[68,69]

The biochemical basis for the cyclical changes in endocervical mucus — and hence the mechanism behind its rapid and substantial sensitivity to estrogen and progesterone action — is still not clear. There is no change in the general protein composition of mucus through the ovarian cycle. Basic considerations of mucus glycoprotein chemistry would predict increased sialic acid content and especially sulfation as a possible anionic explanation for the increased hydration seen at midcycle.[28,70] Histochemistry has not confirmed this prediction: although an increase in neutral and sialo-glycoproteins (stainable with cationic dyes at pH 2.5) has been demonstrated in the periovulatory phase, it is mucus in the secretory phase and mucus in immature and postmenopausal females that shows an apparent increase in sulfated glycoproteins (stainable with cationic dyes at pH 1.0).[71,72] This is the opposite to what might be expected, because the very low pK_a of sulfate groups ought to increase hydration at physiological pH, not decrease it. Definitive chemical analyses of carbohydrate moieties of the mucus glycoproteins in different estrogenic and progestogenic states have not been performed yet.

The cervical score has been used to predict the time of ovulation in the treatment of infertility, particularly with assisted insemination, when it serves as a bioassay of estrogen action unopposed by progesterone; however, although there is a direct and predictable relationship between circulating estradiol levels and cervical score for an individual, the correlation between the two is poor in a population.[67,73] A low cervical score can result from:

(a) A low amount of estrogen
(b) Antagonism of estrogen effect by progesterone, a progestogen or an anti-estrogen such as clomiphene
(c) Resistance of the cervix to the effects of estrogen due to temporary or permanent damage associated with either inflammation (associated with decreased concentrations of ER)[74] or destructive operations for cervical intraepithelial neoplasia.[15]

A reduced amount of responsive endocervical mucosa might in some cases still allow response to a pharmacological dose of estrogen, although the ovulation-inhibition action of such dosages of estrogen will necessitate concomitant gonadotropin therapy.[75]

Pregnancy

During the late luteal phase and especially during pregnancy, the cervix comes under the influence of the hormone relaxin as well as a prolonged and pronounced exposure to estradiol and progesterone. Relaxin is a polypeptide produced in large amounts by the (progesterone-dominated) decidua of the endometrium, especially in the third trimester of pregnancy, and is available for endocrine and paracrine action. Relaxin in pregnancy:

(a) Inhibits myometrial contractility, as described above
(b) Relaxes the pelvic ligaments in preparation for parturition
(c) Softens the fibromuscular tissue of the body of the cervix to permit dilatation during labor.[76]

Cervical softening seems to be accounted for by degradation and increased solubility of collagen and an alteration in the proteoglycan composition of the connective tissue ground substance, with a decline in concentration of small proteoglycans.[65]

Relatively high estrogen levels seem to be an absolute condition for the process of cervical softening, and the use of PR blocking drugs also induces this.[77] Whether these are direct effects or mediated by decidual or other proteins remains to be worked out. Whether the decrease in ER and PR concentrations seen in the cervical stroma in pregnancy[64,65] is a primary or a secondary event is also still to be determined.

Steroid contraception

Progestogen administration, with or without concomitant estrogen administration, causes mucus to become impenetrable to sperm within several hours — an important part of the contraceptive action of progestogen-only 'minipill' formulations as well as of the conventional combined estrogen-progestogen birth control pill.[78]

VAGINA

Structure and function

The vagina is unique in its displayed response to sex steroids, as it alone is lined by stratified squamous epithelium (Fig. 15.7). Estradiol is the active endogenous estrogen in the vagina, as elsewhere, and immunocytochemical studies on ER reveal staining of the basal and parabasal cells (see below), especially in the follicular phase.[79] Early binding studies for receptors could not demonstrate specific PR in human vaginal tissue.[80] Immunoreactive studies of the human ectocervix, the squamous epithelium of which is contiguous with that of the vagina, also reveal that ER is much more abundant than immunoreactive PR, which immunohistochemically is weak or absent throughout the ovarian cycle.[52,63] Konishi et al[81] could demonstrate PR in parabasal cells of the ectocervix in the luteal phase.

The transit time from basal and parabasal layers to the superficial layers of the epithelium is four days, irrespective of the steroidal milieu.[82] Estradiol then stimulates growth and maturation of the stratified epithelium to the point of 'cornification', with pyknosis

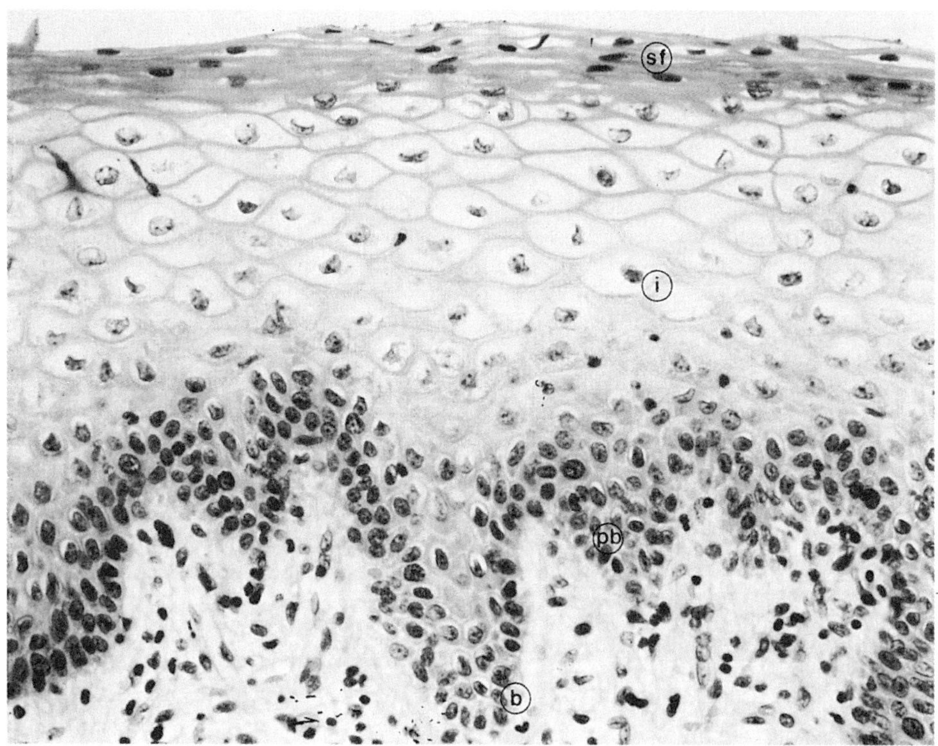

Fig. 15.7 Vaginal mucosa under the unopposed influence of estradiol, showing layers of squamous epithelium. Basal cells (**b**) line the basement membrane; adjacent cuboidal parabasal cells (**pb**) are desquamated under conditions of estrogen lack; flattened intermediate cells (**i**) with vacuolated nuclei are desquamated with moderate estrogen effect or under the influence of progesterone; superficial cells (**sf**) with pyknotic nuclei are desquamated under conditions of substantial and unopposed estrogen exposure.[3]

of nuclei, but normally falling short of the full keratinization that occurs in the dermis.[83,84] Estradiol-dependent mitosis takes place in the parabasal and basal cells, where ER is localized. Progesterone appears to inhibit maturation at the epithelium's midzone.

Ovarian cycle

The most superficial cells under an unopposed estrogen effect have pyknotic nuclei and contain keratin: they are cornified.[82,85] Historically it was this action in castrated female rats that defined the biological action of an estrogen in the Allen Doisy test, devised in the 1920s.[86] Progesterone prevents this final maturation and cornification. As the vaginal mucosa exfoliates its most superficial cells, staining for nuclear morphology and keratin content allows estimation of the relative numbers of pyknotic cells or the relative numbers of parabasal cells, intermediate cells and superficial cells to indicate the steroidal response status of the vagina (respectively called the *karyopyknotic index* and the *maturation index*) — except that a predominance of intermediate cells cannot enable a distinction to be made between moderate estrogen action and estrogen antagonized by progesterone or a progestogen. Parabasal cells dominate smears from prepubertal girls and estrogen-deficient postmenopausal women. Superficial cells dominate the smear only under the unopposed influence of estrogen; under prolonged and extreme estradiol influence, cells can become anuclear.

It is hard to imagine today just how important exfoliative cytology of the vagina was for estimating a woman's estrogen status a generation ago, before chemical estimations of estrogens in urine and then radioimmunoassays for estradiol in blood became available.

The vagina is kept moist during the reproductive years by secretions from the cervix and by transudation of fluid through the vaginal epithelium.[68] The cervical component of vaginal moisture is increased by estradiol, as mentioned above, but in women who have had a total hysterectomy it is clear that vaginal transudation is also increased by estrogens.[87] The mechanism of estrogen-induced vaginal transudation is thought to be an estrogen-dependent increase in vaginal mucosal bloodflow. Estrogen priming enables sexual arousal further to increase this bloodflow and transudation through neurocrine and paracrine mechanisms involving the release of vasoactive intestinal peptide and nitrous oxide.[88,89,90]

REFERENCES

1. Glatstein IZ, Yeh J 1995 Ontogeny of the estrogen receptor in the human fetal uterus. Journal of Clinical Endocrinology and Metabolism 80: 958–964
2. Morishim A A, Grumbach MM, Simpson ER, Fisher C, Qin K 1997 Aromatase deficiency in male and female siblings caused by a novel mutation and the physiological role of estrogens. Journal of Clinical Endocrinology and Metabolism 80: 3689–3698
3. Jansen RPS 1985 Endocrine consequences of female genital tract neoplasia. In: Shearman RP (ed) Clinical reproductive endocrinology. Churchill Livingstone, Edinburgh, pp 697–726
4. Koninckx PR, Heyns W, Verhoeven G, van Baelen H, Lissens WD, de Moor P, Brosens IA 1980 Biochemical characterization of peritoneal fluid in women during the menstrual cycle. Journal of Clinical Endocrinology and Metabolism 51: 1239–1244
5. Shutt DA, Lopata A 1981 The secretion of hormones during the culture of human preimplantation embryos with corona cells. Fertility and Sterility 35: 413–416
6. Katz E, Schran HF, Weiss BE, Adashi EY, Hassell A 1991 Increased circulating levels of bromocriptine after vaginal compared with oral administration. Fertility and Sterility 55: 882–884
7. Balasch J, Fabregues F, Ordi J, Creus M, Penarrubia J, Casamitjana R, Manau D, Vanrell JA 1996 Further data favoring the hypothesis of the uterine first-pass effect of vaginally administered micronized progesterone. Gynecological Endocrinology 10: 421–426
8. Amso NN, Crow J, Shaw RW 1994 Comparative immunohistochemical study of oestrogen and progesterone receptors in the Fallopian tube and uterus at different stages of the menstrual cycle and the menopause. Human Reproduction 9: 1027–1037
9. Pollow K, Inthraphuvasak J, Manz B, Grill H-J, Pollow B 1981 A comparison of cytoplasmic and nuclear estradiol and progesterone receptors in human fallopian tube and endometrial tissue. Fertility and Sterility 36: 615–622
10. Verhage HG, Akbar M, Jaffe RC 1980 Cyclic changes in cytosol progesterone receptor of human fallopian tube. Journal of Clinical Endocrinology and Metabolism 51: 776–780
11. Brenner RM, Resko JA, West NB 1974 Cyclic changes in oviductal morphology and residual cytoplasmic estradiol binding capacity induced by sequential estradiol-progesterone treatment of spayed rhesus monkeys. Endocrinology 95: 1094–1104
12. Wu CH, Mastroianni L, Mikhail G 1977 Steroid hormones in monkey oviductal fluid. Fertility and Sterility 28: 1250–1256
13. Flickinger GL, Elsner C, Illingworth DV, Muechler EK, Mikhail G 1977 Estrogen and progesterone receptors in the female genital tract of humans. Annals of the New York Academy of Science 286: 180–189
14. Jansen RPS 1984 Endocrine response in the fallopian tube. Endocrine Reviews 5: 525–551
15. Jansen RPS 1985 Endocrine response in the female genital tract. In: Shearman RP (ed) Clinical reproductive endocrinology. Churchill Livingstone, Edinburgh, pp 109–164

16. Verhage HG, Bareither ML, Jaffe RC, Akbar M 1979 Cyclic changes in ciliation, secretion and cell height of the oviductal epithelium in women. American Journal of Anatomy 156: 505–521
17. Daniel EE, Lucien P, Posey VA, Paton DM 1975 A functional analysis of the myogenic control systems of the human Fallopian tube. American Journal of Obstetrics and Gynecology 121: 1046–1053
18. Daniel EE, Posey VA, Paton DM 1975 A structural analysis of the myogenic control systems of the human Fallopian tube. American Journal of Obstetrics and Gynecology 121: 1054–1066
19. Fromm E 1985 Physiological assessment of oviductal motility — extraluminal telemetric subject evaluation. In: Harper MJK, Pauerstein CJ, Adams CE, Coutinho EM, Croxatto HB, Paton DM (eds) Ovum transportation and fertility regulation. Scriptor, Copenhagen, pp 107–125
20. Paton DM, Widdicombe JH, Rheaume DE, Johns A 1978 The role of the adrenergic innervation of the oviduct in the regulation of mammalian ovum transport. Pharmacology Reviews 29: 67–102
21. Kunz G, Beil D, Deininger H, Wildt L, Leyendecker G 1996 The dynamics of rapid sperm transport through the female genital tract: evidence from vaginal sonography of uterine peristalsis and hysterosalpingoscintigraphy. Human Reproduction 11: 627–632
22. McNatty KP, Smith DM, Makris A, Osathanondh R, Ryan KJ 1980 Steroidogenesis by the human oocyte-cumulus cell complex in vitro. Steroids 35: 643–651
23. Jansen RPS 1980 Cyclic changes in the human fallopian tube isthmus and their functional importance. American Journal of Obstetrics and Gynecology 136: 292–308
24. Jansen RPS, Bajpai VK 1983 Periovulatory glycoprotein secretion in the macaque fallopian tube. American Journal of Obstetrics and Gynecology 147: 598–608
25. Hunter RHF 1994 Modulation of gamete and embryonic microenvironments by oviduct glycoproteins. Molecular Reproduction and Development 39: 176–181
26. Hodgson BJ 1978 Post-ovulatory changes in the water content and inulin space of the rabbit oviduct. Journal of Reproduction and Fertility 53: 349–351
27. Jansen RPS 1978 Fallopian tube isthmic mucus and ovum transport. Science 201: 349–351
28. Jansen RPS 1995 Ultrastructure and histochemistry of estrogen-dependent acid mucus glycoproteins in the mammalian oviduct. Microscopy Research and Technique 32: 29–49
29. Hashimoto M, Shimoyama T, Kosaka M, Komori A, Hirasawa T, Yokoyama Y, Akashi K 1962 Electron microscopic studies on the epithelial cells of the human fallopian tube (Report I). Journal of the Japan Obstetrical Gynecologic Society 9: 200–209
30. Clyman MJ 1966 Electron microscopy of the human fallopian tube. Fertility and Sterility 17: 281–301
31. Andrews MC 1951 Epithelial changes in the puerperal fallopian tube. American Journal of Obstetrics and Gynecology 62: 28–37
32. Moghissi KS 1995 Endometrium and endosalpinx of women treated with microdose progestogens. Journal of Reproductive Medicine 14: 217–218
33. Finn CA, Porter DG 1975 The uterus. Elek Science, London, p 204
34. De Vries K, Lyons EA, Ballard G, Levi CS, Lindsay DJ 1990 Contractions of the inner third of the myometrium. American Journal of Obstetrics and Gynecology 162: 679–682
35. Turnbull LW, Rice CF, Horsman A, Robinson J, Killick SR 1994 Magnetic resonance imaging and transvaginal ultrasound of the uterus prior to embryo transfer. Human Reproduction 9: 2438–2443
36. Brosens JJ, de Souza NM, Braker FG 1995 Uterine junctional zone: function and disease. Lancet 346: 558–560
37. Parl FF, Schonbaum CP, Cox DL, Cavener DR 1987 Detection of estrogen receptor mRNA in human uterus. Molecular and Cellular Endocrinology 52: 235–242
38. Viville B, Charnock-Jones D, Sharkey A, Wetzka B, Smith SK 1997 Distribution of the A and B forms of the progesterone receptor messenger ribonucleic acid and protein in uterine leiomyomata and adjacent myometrium. Human Reproduction 12: 815–822
39. Lessey BA, Killam AP, Metzger DA, Haney AF, Greene GL, McCarty KS Jr 1988 Immunohistochemical analysis of human uterine estrogen and progesterone receptors throughout the menstrual cycle. Journal of Clinical Endocrinology and Metabolism 67: 334–340
40. Brandon DD, Erickson TE, Keenan EJ, Strawn EY, Novy MJ, Burry KA, Warner C, Clinton GM 1995 Estrogen receptor gene expression in human uterine leiomyomata. Journal of Clinical Endocrinology and Metabolism 80: 1876–1881
41. Brandon DD, Bethea CL, Strawn EY, Novy MJ, Burry KA, Harrington MS, Erickson TE, Warner C, Keenan EJ, Clinton GM 1993 Progesterone receptor messenger ribonucleic acid and protein are overexpressed in human uterine leiomyomas. American Journal of Obstetrics and Gynecology 169: 78–85
42. Rein MS, Barbieri RL, Friedman AJ 1995 Progesterone: a critical role in the pathogenesis of uterine myomas. American Journal of Obstetrics and Gynecology 172: 14–18
43. Kawaguchi K, Fujii S, Konishi I, Nanbu Y, Nonogaki H, Mori H 1989 Mitotic activity in uterine leiomyomas during the menstrual cycle. American Journal of Obstetrics and Gynecology 160: 637–641
44. Friedman AJ, Barbieri RL, Doubilet PM, Fine C, Schiff I 1988 A randomized, double-blind trial of a gonadotropin releasing-hormone agonist (leuprolide) with or without medroxyprogesterone acetate in the treatment of leiomyomata uteri. Fertility and Sterility 49: 404–409
45. Coutinho EM, Boulanger GA, Gonçalves MT 1986 Regression of uterine leiomyomas after treatment with gestrinone, an antiestrogen, antiprogesterone. American Journal of Obstetrics and Gynecology 155: 761–767
46. Murphy AA, Kettel LM, Morales AJ, Roberts VJ, Yen SCC 1993 Regression of uterine leiomyomata in response to the antiprogesterone RU 486. Journal of Clinical Endocrinology and Metabolism 76: 513–517
47. Heap RB, Perry J, Challis JRG 1975 Hormonal maintenance of pregnancy. In: Astwood E, Grey R (eds) Handbook of physiology, section 7, volume II, part 2. American Physiological Society, Baltimore, pp 217–260
48. Csapo AI, Pulkkinen M 1978 Indispensibility of the human corpus luteum in the maintenance of early pregnancy. Obstetric and Gynecologic Survey 33: 69–81

49. Garfield RE, Puri CP, Csapo AI 1982 Endocrine, structural, and functional changes in the uterus during premature labor. American Journal of Obstetrics and Gynecology 142: 21–27
50. Soules MR, McCarty KS Jr 1982 Leiomyomas: steroid receptor content. Variation within normal menstrual cycles. American Journal of Obstetrics and Gynecology 143: 6–11
51. Clarke CL, Sutherland RL 1990 Progestin regulation of cellular proliferation. Endocrine Reviews 11: 266–301
52. Snijders MPML, De Goeij AFPM, Debets-Te Baerts MJC, Rousch MJM, Koudstaal J, Bosman FT 1992 Immunocytochemical analysis of oestrogen receptors and progesterone receptors in the human uterus throughout the menstrual cycle and after the menopause. Journal of Reproduction and Fertility 94: 363–371
53. Ramsay P, Jansen RPS 1998 Ultrasonography of the normal pelvis. In: Anderson JC (ed) Gynecological imaging. Churchill Livingstone, London (in press)
54. Maggi M, Magini A, Fiscella A, Giannini S, Fantoni G, Toffoletti F, Massi G, Serio M 1992 Sex steroid modulation of neurohypophyseal hormone receptors in human nonpregnant myometrium. Journal of Clinical Endocrinology and Metabolism 74: 385–392
55. Garfield RE, Hayashi RH 1980 Presence of gap junctions in the myometrium of women during various stages of menstruation. American Journal of Obstetrics and Gynecology 138: 569–574
56. Caldeyro-Barcia R, Poseiro JJ 1965 The powers and the mechanism of labor. In: Greenhill JP (ed) Obstetrics. WB Saunders, Philadelphia, pp 278–304
57. Garfield RE, Hayashi RH 1981 Appearance of gap junctions in the myometrium of women in labor. American Journal of Obstetrics and Gynecology 140: 254–260
58. How H, Huang ZH, Zuo J, Lei ZM, Spinnato JA II, Rao CV 1995 Myometrial estradiol and progesterone receptor changes in preterm and term pregnancies. Obstetrics and Gynecology 86: 936–940
59. Couzinet B, Le Strat N, Ulmann A, Baulieu EE, Schaison G 1986 Termination of early pregnancy by the progesterone antagonist RU 486 (mifepristone). New England Journal of Medicine 315: 1565–1570
60. Frydman R, Baton C, Lelaidier C, Vial M, Bourget P, Fernandez H 1991 Mifepristone for induction of labour. Lancet 337: 488–489
61. Bygdeman M, Swahn M-L, Gemzell-Danielsson K, Gottlieb C 1994 The use of progesterone antagonists in combination with prostaglandin for termination of pregnancy. Human Reproduction 9 (suppl. 1): 121–125
62. Kupryjanczyk J 1991 Progesterone receptor expression in human cervix uteri. Zentralblatt für Pathologie 137: 346–348
63. Cano A, Monmeneu R, Serra V, Marzo C, Rivera J 1990 Expression of estrogen receptors, progesterone receptors, and an estrogen receptor-associated protein in the human cervix during the menstrual cycle and menopause. Fertility and Sterility 54: 1058–1064
64. Stjernholm Y, Sahlin L, Akerberg S, Elinder A, Eriksson HA, Malmström A, Ekman G 1996 Cervical ripening in humans: potential roles of estrogen, progesterone, and insulin-like growth factor-I. American Journal of Obstetrics and Gynecology 174: 1065–1071
65. Stjernholm Y, Sahlin L, Malmström A, Barchan K, Eriksson HA, Ekman G 1997 Potential roles for gonadal steroids and insulin-like growth factor I during final cervical ripening. Obstetrics and Gynecology 90: 375–380
66. Insler V, Melmed H, Eichenbrenner I, Serr DM, Lunenfeld B 1972 The cervical score. A simple semiquantitative method for monitoring of the menstrual cycle. International Journal of Gynaecology and Obstetrics 10: 223–228
67. McBain JC, Pepperell RJ 1980 Unexplained infertility. In: Peperrel RJ, Hudson B, Wood C (eds) The infertile couple. Churchill Livingstone, Edinburgh, pp 164–181
68. Moghissi KS 1979 The cervix in infertility. Clinics in Obstetrics and Gynecology 22: 27–42
69. Rezai P, Dmowski WP, Auletta F, Scommegna A 1979 Effect of oral estriol on cervical secretions and on ovulatory response. Fertility and Sterility 31: 627–633
70. Allen A 1978 Structure of gastrointestinal mucus glycoproteins and the viscous and gel-forming properties of mucus. British Medical Bulletin 34: 28–33
71. Wakefield EA, Wells M 1985 Histochemical study of endocervical glycoproteins throughout the normal menstrual cycle and adjacent to cervical intraepithelial neoplasia. International Journal of Gynecological Pathology 4: 230–239
72. Gilks CB, Reid PE, Clement PB, Owen DA 1989 Histochemical changes in cervical mucus-secreting epithelium during the normal menstrual cycle. Fertility and Sterility 51: 286–291
73. Zegers F, Lenton EA, Sulaiman R, Cooke ID 1981 The cervical factor in patients with ovulatory infertility. British Journal of Obstetrics and Gynaecology 88: 537–542
74. Kupryjanczyk J, Moller P 1988 Estrogen receptor distribution in the normal and pathologically changed human cervix uteri: an immunohistochemical study with use of monoclonal anti-ER antibody. International Journal of Gynecological Pathology 7: 75–85
75. Check JH 1980 Treatment of cervical factor with combined high-dose estrogen and human menopausal gonadotropins. Fertility and Sterility 33: 562–563
76. MacLennan AH, Grant P, Borthwick AC 1991 Relaxin and relaxin c-peptide levels in human reproductive tissues. Reproduction, Fertility and Development 3: 577–583
77. Uldbjerg N, Ulmsten U 1990 The physiology of cervical ripening and cervical dilatation and the effect of abortifacient drugs. Baillière's Clinical Obstetrics and Gynaecology 4: 263–282
78. Moghissi KS, Marks C 1971 Effects of microdose norgestrel on endogenous gonadotropin and steroid. Fertility and Sterility 22: 424–434
79. Sjoberg I, Rylander E, Von Schoultz B 1989 Menstrual variation of estrogen receptor content in vaginal tissue. Gynecologic and Obstetric Investigation 27: 48–51
80. van Haaften M, Wiegerinck MA, Poortman J, Haspels AA, Thijssen JH 1982 Progesterone receptors in human oestrogen target tissues. Maturitas 4: 57–66
81. Konishi I, Fujii S, Nonogaki H, Nanbu Y, Iwai T, Mori T 1991 Immunohistochemical analysis of estrogen receptors, progesterone receptors, Ki-67 antigen, and human papillomavirus DNA in normal and neoplastic epithelium of the uterine cervix. Cancer 68: 1340–1350

82. Averette HE, Weinstein GD, Frost P 1970 Autoradiographic analysis of cell proliferation kinetics in human genital tissues. American Journal of Obstetrics and Gynecology 108: 8–17
83. Ferenczy A, Guralnick MS 1979 Morphology of the human vagina. In: Beller FK, Schumacher GFB (eds) The biology of the fluids of the female genital tract. Elsevier/North Holland, New York, pp 3–12
84. Morse AR, Hutton JD, Jacobs HS, Murray MAF, James VHT 1979 Relation between the karyopyknotic index and plasma oestrogen concentrations after the menopause. British Journal of Obstetrics and Gynaecology 86: 981–983
85. Frost JK 1979 Gynecologic and obstetric clinical cytopathology. In: Novak ER, Woodruff J D (eds) Novak's gynecologic and obstetric pathology. WB Saunders, Philadelphia, pp 689–781
86. Terenius L 1971 The Allen-Doisy test for oestrogens reinvestigated. Steroids 17: 653–661
87. Perl JI, Milles G, Shimazato Y 1997 Vaginal fluid subsequent to panhysterectomy. American Journal of Obstetrics and Gynecology 78: 285–289
88. Helm G, Otteson B, Fahrenkrug J, Larsen J-J, Owman C, Sjöberg N-O, Stolberg B, Sundler F, Walles B 1981 Vasoactive intestinal polypeptide (VIP) in the human female reproductive. Biology of Reproduction 25: 227–234
89. Palle C, Bredkjaer HE, Fahrenkrug J, Otteson B 1991 Vasoactive intestinal polypeptide loses its ability to increase vaginal blood flow after menopause. American Journal of Obstetrics and Gynecology 164: 556–558
90. Hoyle CH, Stones RW, Robson T, Whitley K, Burnstock G 1996 Innervation of vasculature and microvasculature of the human vagina by NOS and neuropeptide-containing nerves. Journal of Anatomy 188: 633–644

16. Effects of estrogen and progesterone on the breast

William H. Hindle

Introduction

Researchers and health care providers for women are keenly interested in the effects of estrogen and progesterone on human female breast tissue. Current knowledge of these effects is limited due to the lack of an animal model with breasts that are anatomically and endocrinologically the same as in the human female. Direct observations have been limited to biopsy (aspiration and tissue), surgical specimens and autopsy material. Cancer and noncancer cell lines have been established but the cellular behavior and response *in vitro* may not reflect the actual *in vivo* activity. The frequency of incidence of breast cancer, with its predominate ratio of women to men, suggests a critical role of estrogen and progesterone in the carcinogenesis of breast cancer.

The effects of estrogen and progesterone upon the breast are species specific and site (end organ) specific. Thus, it cannot be assumed that our extensive knowledge of the effects of estrogen and progesterone on the endometrium can be empirically applied to the breast ductal epithelium. The process of development, function, epithelial proliferation and maturation of the human female breast is interminably multifactorial, and the physiologic and pathologic microbiology is infinitely complex. Hopefully, future research will be fundamentally revealing. Meanwhile, molecular biology data and evidence-based medicine focused on outcome, e.g. mortality and quality of life, give us the rational basis of clinical medical practice for the care of female breast disorders.

Embryology

During the fifth week of human fetal development, the symmetrical paired mammary ridges begin to form from ectodermal thickenings. The surface epithelium invaginates and coalesces to form the embryologic mammary buds during the seventh week. The buds canalize and penetrate the surrounding mesenchyme forming a complex branching ductal system (Fig. 16.1). At 20 weeks the surface areola forms. At birth, the female and male breasts are identical in development and function, to the extent that milky fluid is often secreted.

Anatomy

The branching ductal systems of the breast are configured in separate lobes, each of which has a single opening (galactophore) onto the nipple surface. Secretion of milk occurs in the terminal duct lobular units (TDLU), or acini, which are clustered into lobules connected to the galactophore by lactiferous ducts, with a dilated lactiferous sinus (ampula) emptying through a collecting duct into the nipple opening. The remainder of the breast is composed of adipose tissue, which constitutes the bulk of the volume of the breast, and connective tissue. With pregnancy, estrogen stimulates the increased size and pigmentation of the nipple and areola.

Physiology

The function of the breast is lactation. Technically, the breast tissue (particularly the TDLU) of nonlactating women of reproductive age is in a 'resting' state. However, there are cyclic (menstrual) physiologic changes which are not uniform throughout the breast. The essential hormonal and functional changes prior to lactation are illustrated in Figure 16.2. The rapid decrease in serum estrogen and progesterone immediately following delivery allows the elevation of serum prolactin and subsequent lactation. In addition, balanced levels of cortisol, growth hormone, insulin and thyroxine are essential for lactation.[1]

In animal studies, an intact functioning hypothalamic-pituitary-gonadal axis with balanced presence of estrogen, progesterone, prolactin, growth

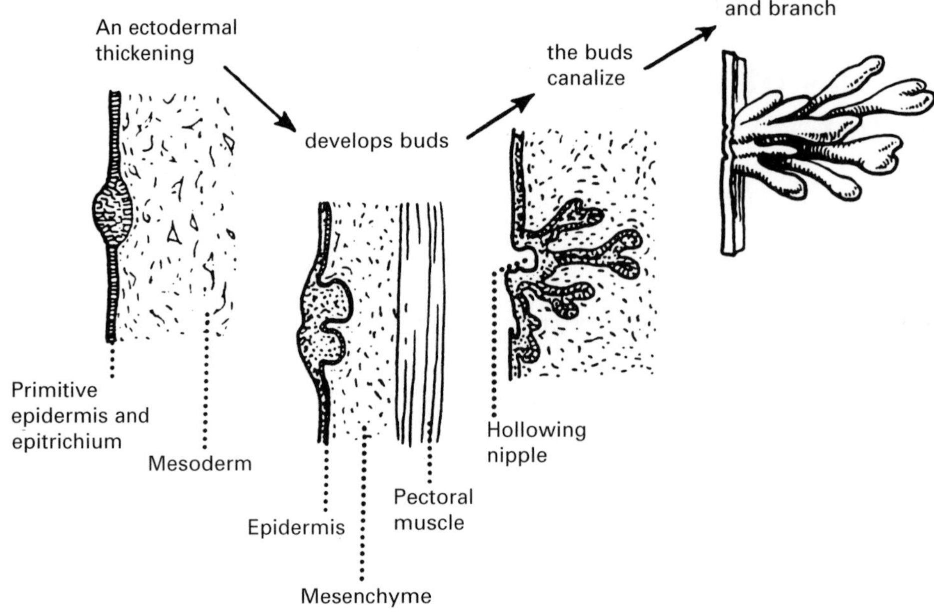

Fig. 16.1 Embryologic development of the female breast.[1]

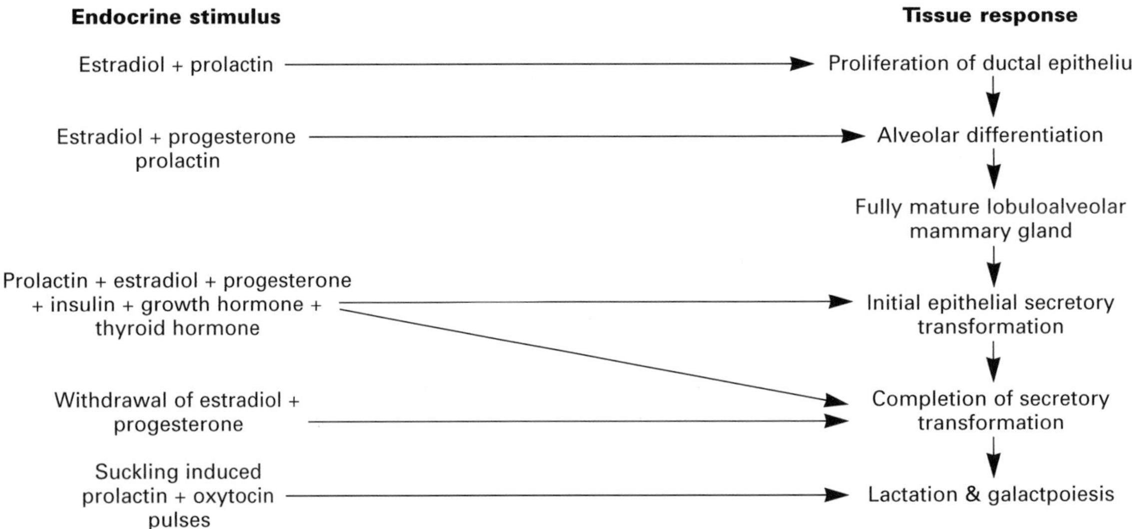

Fig. 16.2 Hormonal stimuli and the consequent anatomic and functional changes in the breast required for lactation.

hormone, insulin, cortisol and thyroxine have been shown to be essential for complete breast development.[2–5] In immature female monkeys, exogenous estradiol can induce complete breast development.[2]

Also in animal and tissue culture studies, estradiol has been shown to:

1. Have direct stimulating effect on the growth and differentiation of the ductal epithelium[6]
2. Initiate increasing mitotic activity in the ductal cylindrical cells
3. Stimulate ductal growth and breast connective tissue hyperplasia
4. Stimulate secretion of mucoid watery substance

and hyalinization of the periductal connective tissue
5. Increase the subcutaneous fat of the breast[6]
6. Increase the number of receptors for both estrogen and progesterone in the ductal epithelium.[7]

Estrogen can have a histamine-like effect on the microcirculation of the breast.[8] Enzymatic aromatase in the breast adipose tissue can convert circulating androgen precursors into estrogen (androstenedione to estrone).[9]

Progesterone has been shown in animal and tissue culture studies to:

1. Stimulate galactophore maturation
2. Stimulate acini development
3. Inhibit vasodilatation
4. Inhibit tissue edema
5. Inhibit ductal cellular differentiation
6. Inhibit estrogen induced ductal proliferation.

Although the results of *in vitro* human breast cancer cell line studies upon the proliferative effect of progesterone are conflicting,[10] Gomel found inhibition of proliferation of normal breast ductal cells by progestogens *in vitro*.[11]

Mauvais-Jarvis reviewed the published data on the antiproliferative effect of antiestrogen on normal human breast cells in culture and concluded with recommendations for clinical trials of progestogens and tamoxifen related compounds for the treatment of benign breast disorders and breast cancer prevention.[12]

The synergistic action of estrogen and progesterone stimulates distal ductal differentiation and acini development, and completes the differentiation of the TDLUs.[13] Estrogen and progesterone have antagonistic action (a) upon capillary permeability, and (b) in high concentrations, upon breast tissue cell division.

The influence of estrogen and progesterone on the protein expression of p53, ErbB-2 ($p185^{erbB-2}$), epidermal growth factor (EGF), and angiogenic factor platelet-derived endothelial cell growth factor/ thymidine phosphorylase is unresolved.[14]

Epithelial estrogen receptors (ER) and progesterone receptors (PR)

Khan reviewed the literature on ER and PR in benign breast epithelium and tabulated (a) the ER and PR positivity rates and ER labelling index (quantitative comparison of ER levels by percent positive nuclei) for normal breast tissue (Table 16.1), (b) positivity rates during natural menstrual cycles and on oral contraceptive therapy (Table 16.2), and (c) ER positivity in benign breast disease (Table 16.3).[15]

Schmitt reported high proliferation rates in ER positive ductal cells of hyperplastic breast epithelium (vs ER negative ductal cells) in contrast to higher rates in ER negative malignant ductal epithelial cells (vs ER positive malignant cells).[16]

Puberty

Pubertal growth of the female breast begins with the anatomical breast bud development which correlates with increasing plasma estradiol levels.[17] The proliferation of ductal, myoepithelial and stromal cells is stimulated by estrogen. Progesterone and estrogen stimulate the secretory TDLU and the distal ductules. Further ductal and lobular development occurs at

Table 16.1 Estrogen and progesterone receptor (ER, PR) positivity rates and mean labelling index (LI) for normal breasts.[15]

			ER		PR	
Author	No. of patients	Population	% pos*	Mean LI	% pos*	Mean LI
Ligand binding						
Feherty	41	Benign disease	0	0	–	–
Witliff	22	Normal/benign[a]	0	0.74[b]	–	–
Netto	104	Cancer	13.5%	<7.3 fm/mg[c]	15.4%	<5.4 fm/mg[c]
Silva	56	Normal	–			
Histochemical			16			
Petersen	18	Reduction		7%	–	–
Ricketts	143	Normal	43–56%[e]	–	81–84%[e]	–
Khan[d]	120	Case control	55%	15.6[c]	87%	24

*% pos: percent samples categorized as positive; [a]six samples from cancer containing breasts; [b]calculated by assuming all values <1 fm mg = 0; [c]mean LI of positive samples only; [d]data on controls; [e]positivity threshold altered to include all samples with any positive cells.

Table 16.2 Positivity rates for estrogen and progesterone receptor (ER and PR) with natural menstruation and oral contraceptive use.[15]

		Natural cycle				Oral contraceptives			
		Follicular		Luteal		Follicular		Luteal	
Author	No. of patients	ER	PR	ER	PR	ER	PR	ER	PR
Soderqvist	42	68%	80%	32%	80%				
Silva*	53	36%	28%	15%	10%				
Battersby	158	61%	76%	34%	71%	34%	59%	17%	81%
Williams†	216	3.9	12.1	†	†	†	†		
Markopulos	69	60%		0					

*Positivity defined as levels >3 fm/mg protein; †mean ER and PR labeling index is reported. Data are presented in four week categories, with significant differences in week 2.

Table 16.3 Benign breast disease and estrogen receptor (ER) positivity.[15]

Reference	No. of patients	Population	No proliferation, ER positive total	Hyperplasia
Girling	79	Benign disease	3/7	12/24
Fabris	150	Benign disease	Heterogeneous	Homogenous
Jacquemier[a]	27	High risk	0/14	11/13
			14.5 fm/mg	31.5 fm/mg
Jacquemier[b]	100	Benign disease		
premenopausal	68		6%[c]	12–24%[c,d]
postmenopausal	8		26%[c]	22%[c]
Gianni	97	Benign disease	No relationship of ER with proliferation	

[a]Data in fm/mg cytosol protein reflect mean ER levels in each category, measured by the DCC assay; [b]seven cases of carcinoma *in situ* included in the original paper are not shown here; [c]mean % ER positive cells in normal epitheium; [d]several categories of histologic lesion with varying degrees of proliferation. DCC = dextran coated charcoal.

menarche, influenced by increased cyclic estrogen and progesterone.[17]

Changes with the menstrual cycle

The histologic changes in breast tissue have been correlated with the menstrual cycle.[18–20] Under the influence of estrogen and progesterone, vascular and lymphatic congestion produce increased volume of the breast during the late luteal phase. There can be as much as a 40% increase in breast volume.[21] Increased mitotic activity of the nonglandular tissue accompanying the vascular congestion during this late luteal phase, when the progesterone effect is dominant, has also been described.[22]

Vogel has quantitated the changes in the breast histology correlated with the phase of the menstrual cycle (Table 16.4).[18] Similar descriptions of changes in the breast histology during the menstrual cycle have been reported.[19,20,23] Though both estrogen and progesterone are active throughout the menstrual cycle, it is presumed that the histologic changes in the follicular phase are related to estrogen dominance and the changes in the luteal phase to progesterone dominance. The importance of the precise estrogen/progesterone ratios has yet to be elucidated. The measured ER levels are highest during the follicular phase and drop considerably during the luteal phase, whereas the PR levels are relatively constant throughout the menstrual cycle.[24,25]

Menstrual/hormone effect on epithelial proliferation

In 1981, when reporting on the morphologic changes in the epithelial and stromal tissues of women (n=90) undergoing subcutaneous mastectomy or reduction mammoplasty, Vogel et al noted epithelial cell mitotic activity during day 3–7 of the menstrual cycle with minimal activity during day 8–14 and no detectable mitotic activity at other times.[18] These findings are in contrast to other *in vivo* studies of epithelial proliferation and mitotic activity.[19,20,23,26,27]

Table 16.4 Morphologic criteria for phase assignment.

Phase secretion	Days	Stroma	Lumen	Epithelium: Cell types	Epithelium: Orientation of epithelial cells	Epithelium: Mitoses	Epithelium: Active
I Proliferative	3–7	Dense, cellular	Tight	Single, predominant pale eosinophilic cell	No stratification apparent	Present: average 4/10 HPF	None
II Follicular	8–14	Dense, cellular, collagenous	Defined	1. Luminal columnar basophilic cell 2. Intermediate pale cell 3. Basal clear cell with hyperchromatic nucleus (myoepithelial)	Radial around lumen	Rare	None
III Luteal	15–20	Loose, broken	Open with some secretion	1. Luminal basophilic cell 2. Intermediate pale cell 3. Prominent vacuolization of basal clear cell (myoepithelial)	Radial around lumen	Absent	None
IV Secretory	21–27	Loose, edematous	Open with secretion	1. Luminal basophilic cell 2. Intermediate pale cell 3. Prominent vacuolization of basal clear cell (myoepithelium)	Radial around lumen	Absent	Active apocrine secretion from luminal cell
V Menstrual	28–2	Dense, cellular	Distended with secretion	1. Luminal basophilic cell with scant cytoplasm	Radial around lumen	Absent	Rare

Reproduced with permission from Harris JR (1991) Breast disease, 2nd edn. Lippincott, Philadelphia

In the same year (1981) Ferguson and Anderson evaluated the epithelial cell multiplication (mitosis and cellular deletion [apoptosis]) in 90 breast tissue samples without evidence of histologic pathology from 83 women undergoing reduction mammoplasty or biopsy of nonmalignant lesions.[26] All the women were having regular menstrual cycles (17 were on oral contraceptive therapy). The day of the menstrual cycle was calculated to a 28 day equivalent utilizing the date of the last menstrual period before, and the beginning of the menstruation following, the surgical procedure.

The observations were based on an average of 50 lobules. The results are depicted in Figures 16.3 and 16.4. The highest mitotic activity per lobule was at day

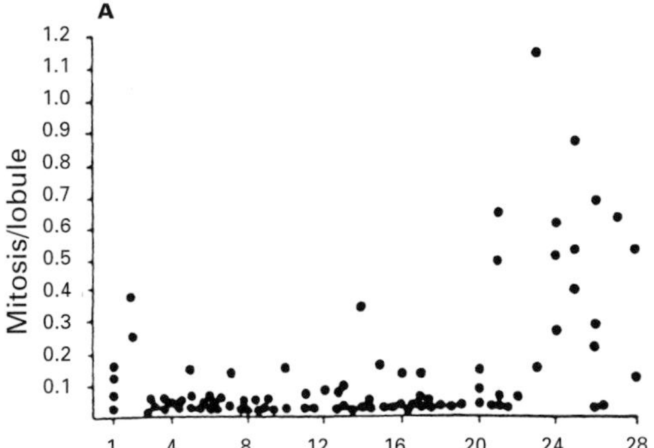

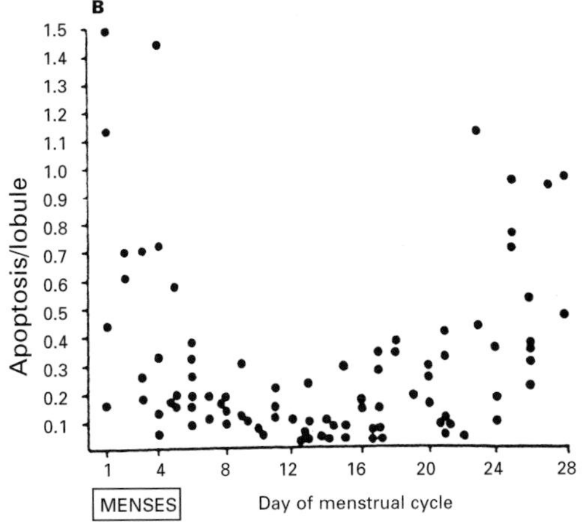

Fig. 16.3 The mitotic (A) and apoptotic (B) frequences for 90 breast samples plotted against day of the menstrual cycle.[26]

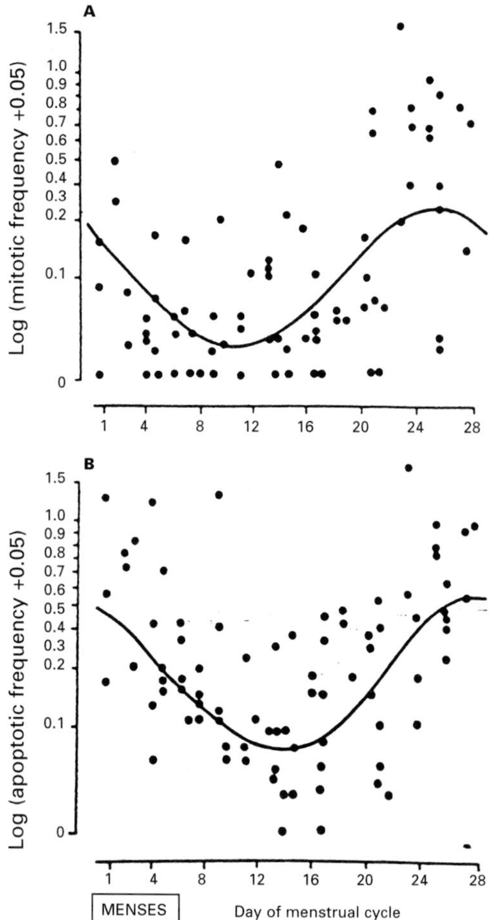

Fig. 16.4 The log of the transformed values for the mitotic (A) and apoptotic (B) frequencies plotted against day of the menstrual cycle, along with the fitted curves for the average sinusoidal variation.[21]

25 (95% confidence limits days 23–26). The highest frequency of apoptosis was at day 28 (95% confidence limits day 26–day 1). The difference between the two peaks was statistically significant at $P<0.01$. The lobular mitotic activity closely correlates with combined progesterone/estrogen peak (days 22–24). There was no change in mitotic activity detected at the estrogen ovulatory peak.

This investigation was extended by Anderson, Ferguson and Rabb in 1982 to include 125 samples from 116 women of whom 23 were on oral contraceptive therapy.[27] The material and methods were the same as previously described[26] as were the peaks of mitosis levels at day 25 and apoptosis levels at day 28 observed in the lobules. The peak levels in the ductules were day 24 for mitosis and day 27.5 for apoptosis. The log of the transformed values and curves for the average sinusoid variation are almost identical to Figure 16.5. The subset analysis for women aged <25, 25–34, and >34 years is presented in Figure 16.5. Flattening of the curve for apoptosis for women >34 years was noted. Otherwise, the age subset curves were not significantly statistically different. Evaluation for nulliparous women compared to parous women revealed no consistent differences. After adjustments for age, no difference was found in the subsets of women on combined oral contraceptive therapy (COC) compared to the women not on COC. The authors state: 'Yet a search for other [than estrogen/progesterone] stimulants is encouraged by our observed persistence of responses at a time of

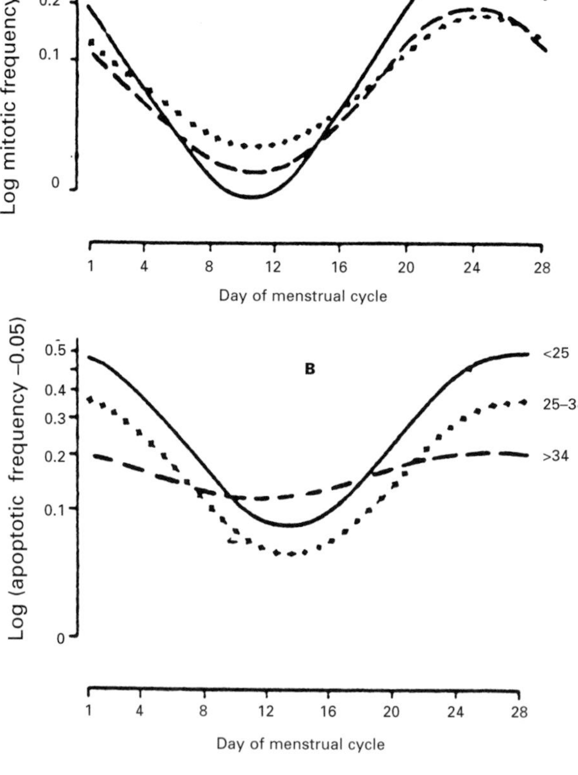

Fig. 16.5 The fitted curves for the average sinusoidal variation of the log of the transformed values in the different age groups for the mitotic (A) and apoptotic (B) frequencies, plotted against the day of menstrual cycle. Age groups: <25: —; 25–34: ++++ > 34: – – –.[26]

suppressed ovarian steroid-hormone levels with oral-contraceptive use ...'. When the mitosis and apoptosis levels for women with and without fibroadenomas present in the breast issue were compared, there was a trend to higher peak levels of apoptotis in the 'fibroadenoma present' groups in all age categories. Comparison of the levels from specimens from the right and left breast revealed higher apoptosis levels from the right breast when compared to the left. Further subset analyses of laterality by age groups was inconclusive.

Chang et al, in a double blind randomized study reported in 1995, applied estrogen, progesterone, combined estrogen and progesterone or a placebo to the breast of premenopausal women (n=40) daily for 10–13 days prior to breast surgery for benign disease.[28] Plasma and tissue estrogen and progesterone concentrations were obtained. The proliferative activity of the epithelial cells was assessed by counting mitoses (mitotic index, MI) and by proliferating cell nuclear antigen (PCNA) immunostaining quantitative analyses. The results are given in Tables 16.5 and 16.6. The plasma hormone concentrations were minimally affected by hormone therapy except for some increase in progesterone levels with that treatment. The intraglandular hormone concentrations increased for each type of treatment vs placebo, with a lessening of the estrogen increase when combined with progesterone therapy. Both the MI and PCNA labeling index were increased with estrogen therapy and decreased with progesterone alone therapy. The combined estrogen/progesterone therapy resulted in lower levels than estrogen alone treatment. The authors suggest that shorter therapy may have given paradoxical results which would be consistent with some other reports. However, the results of long term hormonal therapy and trials involving postmenopausal women would be of particularly keen interest to clinicians.

Menopause and thereafter

With decreasing estrogen and progesterone levels, there is progressive involution of both the glandular (acini) and ductal breast tissues. Over time (years), this degeneration proceeds through hypoplasia to complete atrophy. The relative proportion of adipose tissue and to some extent stromal tissue, increases. However, with continued aging, the total volume of the breast decreases.[17]

Jacquemier, in studies of benign breast tissue, demonstrated a marked shift from the premenopausal PR dominant pattern to a dominant ER pattern after the menopause.[29] However, the expression of the receptor pattern is heterogeneous throughout the breast glandular tissue.

Conclusion

Estrogen and progesterone are essential for the development, maturation and function of the human female breast. The breast tissue, particularly the glandular portion, changes with the menstrual cycle. After the menopause, with its accompanying estrogen (and progesterone) deficiency, the glandular and ductal tissues atrophy. Although most studies of

Table 16.5 Intraglandular steroid concentration.[a]

Treatment	Placebo (n = 8)	P (n = 7)	E_2 (n = 9)	E_2 + P (n = 9)
P (ng/g)[b]	0.6 ± 0.3	66 ± 120[c]	2.1 ± 3.8[d]	41.2 ± 75.2[c,e]
E_2 (ng/g)[f]	0.5 ± 0.4	0.5 ± 0.7	91.0 ± 232.7[c,d]	35.5 ± 69.6[c,d]

[a]Values are mean ± SD; [b]conversion factor to SI unit, 3.180; [c]P < 0.05 versus placebo; [d]P < 0.05 versus P group; [e]P < 0.05 versus E_2 group; [f]conversion factor to SI unit, 3.671. Data from reference 28.

Table 16.6 Proliferation markers in normal lobular epithelial cells.[a]

Treatment	Placebo	P	E_2	E_2 + P
Mitosis/1000 cells	0.51 ± 0.24	0.17 ± 0.19[a]	0.83 ± 0.42[a,b]	0.52 ± 0.42[d]
PCNA (LI %)	7.8 ± 4.8	1.9 ± 0.8[a]	17.4 ± 6.4[a,b]	6.5 ± 4.4[c]

[a]Values are means ± SD; [b]P < 0.05 versus placebo; [c]P < 0.05 versus P group; [d]P < 0.05 versus E_2 group. Data from reference 28.

cycling (menstrual) women show the highest epithelial mitotic activity in the late luteal phase, the association of the mitotic activity with estrogen and progesterone is unclear. The effects of long-term exposure have not been studied. A consistent predominate effect of estrogen and/or progesterone upon the origin and biologic behavior of neoplasms in the human female breast has not been identified.

REFERENCES

1. Mishell DR 1991 Jr Endocrinology of lactation and the puerperium. In: Mishell DR Jr, Davajan V, Lobo RA (eds) Infertility, contraception and reproductive endocrinology. Blackwell Scientific, Cambridge, MA, pp 180–203
2. Klineberg DL, Niemann W, Flamm E, Cooper P, Babitsky G, Valensi Q 1985 Primate mammary development. Journal of Clinical Investigation 75: 1943–1950
3. Apter D 1980 Serum steroids and pituitary hormones in female puberty: a partly longitudinal study. Clinical Endocrinology 12: 107–120
4. Lyons WR, Lee LH, Johnson RE 1958 The hormonal control of mammary growth and lactation. Recent Progress in Hormone Research 14: 219–254
5. Topper YJ, Freeman CS 1980 Multiple hormone interactions in the developmental biology of the mammary gland. Physiological Review 60: 1049–1060
6. Porter JC 1974 Hormonal regulation of breast development and activity. Journal of Investigative Dermatology 63: 85–92
7. Mauvais-Jarvis P, Kuttenn F, Gompel A 1986 Estradiol/progesterone interaction in normal and pathologic breast cells. Annals of the New York Academy of Science 464: 152–167
8. Zeppa R 1969 Vascular response of the breast to estrogen. Journal of Clinical Endocrinology and Metabolism 29: 695–700
9. Perel E, Davis S, Killinger DW 1981 Androgen metabolism in male and female breast tissue. Steroids 37: 345–352
10. Clarke CL, Sutherland RL 1990 Progestin regulation of cellular proliferation. Endocrine Reviews 11: 266–301
11. Gompel A, Malet C, Spritzer P, Lalardrie J-P, Kuttenn F, Mauvais-Jarvis P 1986 Progestin effect on cell proliferation and 17β-hydroxysteroid dehydrogenase activity in normal human breast cells in culture. Journal of Clinical Endocrinology and Metabolism 63: 1174–1180
12. Mauvais-Jarvis P, Kuttenn F, Malet C et al 1988 Antiproliferative effect of antiestrogens on normal human breast cells in culture. In: Genazzani AR, Petraglia F (ed) Advances in gynecological endocrinology, vol I. Parthenon Publishing Group, New Jersey, pp 385–392
13. Jacobsohn D 1961 In: Kon S, Cowie AT (eds) The mammary gland and its secretion. Academic Press, New York, p 127
14. Fox SB, Westwood M, Moghaddam A, Comley M, Turley H, Whitehouse RM, Bicknell R, Gatter KC and Harris AL 1996 The angiogenic factor platelet-derived endothelial cell growth factor/thymidine phosphorylase is up-regulated in breast cancer epithelium and endothelium. British Journal of Cancer 73: 275–280
15. Khan SA 1995 Estrogen and progesterone receptors in benign breast epithelium. The Breast Journal 1: 251–261
16. Schmitt FC 1995 Multistep progression from an estrogen-dependent growth towards an autonomous growth in breast carcinogenesis. European Journal of Cancer 31: 2049–2052
17. Haagensen CD 1986 The normal physiology of the breasts. In: Haagensen CD (ed) Diseases of the breast WB Saunders, Philadelphia, pp 47–55
18. Vogel PM, Georgiade NG, Fetter BF et al 1981 The correlation of histologic changes in the human breast with the menstrual cycle. American Journal of Pathology 104: 23–34
19. Longacre TA, Bartow SA 1986 A correlative morphologic study of human breast and endometrium in the menstrual cycle. American Journal of Surgical Pathology 10: 382–393
20. Going JJ, Anderson TJ, Battersby S et al 1988 Proliferative and secretory activity in human breast during natural and artificial menstrual cycles. American Journal of Pathology 130: 193–204
21. Hamilton T, Rankin ME 1975 Changes in volume of the breast during the menstrual cycle. British Journal of Surgery 62: 660 (abstract)
22. Milligan D, Drife JO, Short RV 1975 Changes in breast volume during normal menstrual cycle and after oral contraceptives. British Medical Journal 4: 494–496
23. Potten CS, Watson RJ, Williams GT et al 1988 The effect of age and menstrual cycle upon proliferative activity in the normal human breast. British Journal of Cancer 58: 163–170
24. Soderquist G, Von Schoultz B, Tani E et al 1993 Estrogen and progesterone receptor content in breast epithelial cells from healthy women during the menstrual cycle. American Journal of Obstetrics and Gynecology 168: 874–879
25. Battersby S, Robertson BJ, Anderson TJ et al 1992 Influence of menstrual cycle, parity and oral contraceptive use on steroid hormone receptors in normal breast. British Journal of Cancer 65: 601–607
26. Ferguson DJ, Anderson TJ 1981 Morphological evaluation of cell turnover in relation to menstrual cycle in the resting human breast. British Journal of Cancer 44: 177–181
27. Anderson TJ, Ferguson DJ, Rabb GM 1982 Cell turnover in the resting human breast: influence of parity, contraceptive pill, age and laterality. British Journal of Cancer 46: 376–382
28. Chang K-J, Lee TTY, Linares-Cruz G, Fournier S, de Lignieres B 1995 Influences of percutaneous administration of estradiol and progesterone on human breast epithelial cell cycle in vivo. Fertility and Sterility 63: 785–791
29. Jacquemier JD, Rolland PH, Vague D, Lieutaud R, Spitalier JM, Martin PM 1982 Relationships between steroid receptor and epithelial cell proliferation in benign fibrocystic disease of the breast. Cancer 49: 2534–2536

17. Effects of estrogen and progesterone on the central nervous system

Tibor Polcz Tamas Horvath Frederick Naftolin

Introduction

The brain is a loose confederation of neuron-rich areas that develop along the most cranial part of the neural tube. These anatomical outpouchings and thickenings reflect evolutionary adaptation of the central nervous system. In humans these include the relatively large cerebral cortex, temporal lobe/hippocampus and hypothalamus. The overall appearance of the brain is defined as these structures are folded together as the neural tube is bent during development to fit in the cranial vault. The neurones of most brain areas and their functions are sensitive to estrogen or other sex steroids. The effects may be direct or indirect by means of connections from other estrogen-sensitive neurons. This chapter reviews basic mechanisms of sex steroid action in the brain and explores the effects of these hormones during development and adult life.

MECHANISM OF ACTION

Sex hormones and their metabolites have various actions on the brain (Table 17.1). These include direct and indirect effects on neurons, glia and vessels. Many of these effects require steroid receptor-mediated gene expression, transcription and translation, which may take hours or days to result in physiologic changes. But, other effects take only a fraction of a second when hormones act directly on ion channels, or several seconds to minutes when actions are coupled to second messengers and to the so called early-intermediate genes, such as c-Fos and Jun.

Effects on the function and integrity of neuronal synapses can result from any of these mechanisms. Traditionally, it is known that estrogen affects the concentration of enzymes involved in synthesis and catabolism of neurotransmitters, thereby shifting stimulatory/inhibitory balances of established neural networks. Examples include increased choline acetyltransferase production leading to increased synthesis of acetylcholine,[1] stimulation of neuronal nitric oxide (NO) synthase which produces the neuromodulator/neurotransmitter NO[2] and changes in the catabolism of serotonin by increasing the degradation of monoamine oxidase.[3] Each of these examples are related to specific brain functions such as memory, learning and mood, respectively.

On the other hand, steroid hormones also have synaptic actions that are much more rapid. For example, progesterone stimulates the release of dopamine in striatal tissue and the release of GnRH from hypothalamic neurons after binding to specific sites on the cell membrane to affect movement and autonomic functions, respectively. Other examples of rapid action are the alteration of potassium permeability in the postsynaptic membrane of medial amygdala neurons and the postsynaptic potentiation of non N-methyl-D-aspartate (NMDA) receptors in the CA1 neurons of the hippocampus by estrogen.[4] Synaptic transmission can also be modulated by estrogen effects on the Ca^{2+} transport mechanisms in nerve endings.[5] The potentiation of kainate-induced current in CA1 neurons by estrogen action on the G-protein coupled cAMP dependent phosphorylation pathway[6] is an example of second messenger mediated response. Of course, not all rapid hormonal effects are on the synapses. Our group has shown changes in hypothalamic neural endocytosis that occur within seconds of estrogen administration.

Effects on synaptic receptors may be regulated by transcriptional means to increase or reduce the number of receptors or by modulating their rapid responses. Examples of the latter are the effects of progesterone on oxytocin binding in the hypothalamus, estrogen-induced change of the dopamine receptors in the striatum from a high affinity to a low affinity state, progesterone inhibition of opioid receptor binding and the potentiation of gamma amino butyric acid (GABA) action on its receptor by progesterone metabolites.

Table 17.1 Effects of sex steroids on neurons.

A. Delayed action: Estrogen/progesterone	Genomic response mediated by steroid receptor
	Nerve growth and differentiation
	Modulation of intramembranous protein particles
	Cytoarchitectural changes
	Synaptologic changes in hypothalamus
Estrogen	Increased choline acetyl transferase synthesis
	Stimulates neuronal NO synthase
	Increased degradation of monoamine oxidase
	Increased number of NMDA sensitive receptors in hippocampus
B. Intermediate action:	Involves second messenger systems or early intermediate genes (e.g. c-Fos, Jun)
Estrogen	Increased G-protein coupled cAMP dependent kainate-induced ion current in CA1 neurones
C. Rapid action:	Direct action on cell membrane (e.g. ion channel, synaptic transmitters)
Estrogen	Modulation of dopamine receptor binding in striatum
	Increased K^+ permeability of postsynaptic membrane in amigdala neurones
	Postsynaptic potentiation of non-MNDA receptors in CA1 neurones
	Ca^{2+} transport mechanism in nerve endings
Progesterone	Stimulates release of dopamine in striatal tissue
	Stimulates release of GnRH from hypothalamic neurones
	Modulation of oxytocin receptor binding in the hypothalamus
	Inhibition of opioid receptor binding
	Potentiation of GABA
	Direct incorporation of steroids into cell membrane?

Sex steroids also influence actual synaptic connectivity in various ways. In addition to the above described pre- and postsynaptic changes of synaptic function, these hormones regulate changes in cellular morphology of neurons and glia. These changes take place during development as well as in adulthood. For example, estrogen has been shown to cause changes in the number of synapses in the hypothalamic arcuate nucleus of rats[7] and monkeys.[8] Physiological cytoarchitectural changes include a denervation-renervation cycle which is believed to play a role in the control of gonadotropins.[9]

Long term potentiation (LTP) of hippocampal neurons is a form of neuronal activation that is important in learning and memory. LTP is dependent on the number and shape of neuronal dendritic spines and is a form of neuronal synaptic plasticity. The mechanism of LTP also involves N-methyl-D-aspartate (NMDA)-sensitive glutamate receptors. Estrogen has been shown to increase the number and length of dendritic spines and the density of NMDA receptors in the hippocampus.

The properties of the cell membrane can also be altered by direct incorporation of steroid hormones. However, this may only be important when circulating hormone levels are high.

Neurons account for only 10% of the brain's cells. The rest are glial cells that play pivotal roles in fostering neuronal action. Sex steroids influence glial cell functions such as proliferation and myelin production during development and in response to damage. Furthermore, during the ovarian cycle, in part by influencing glial cell function, the fluctuating estrogen levels drive synaptic remodeling in the arcuate nucleus of the hypothalamus. The glia responds to estrogen by increasing its processes and increasing neuronal ensheathment[7] to cover the area of neuronal surfaces denuded during synaptic retraction in the arcuate nucleus. In addition, glial cells appear to be an important site of steroid hormone formation and metabolism. Some of these steroids have profound effects on neuronal function.

Although the effects of estrogen on the smooth muscle and endothelium of the vascular system are described elsewhere in more detail, it is important to point out the implications of such effects for the CNS. For example, estrogen has been found to protect against atherosclerotic vascular disease and perhaps stroke. It increases cerebral blood flow, which improves CNS function. Conversely, hypoestrogenic states are frequently associated with vascular spasms which may cause headaches and may even contribute to ischemic attacks in the nervous system.

In the following sections we discuss individual brain functions that are affected by the cellular actions described above.

BRAIN DEVELOPMENT

The development of the brain occurs in stages: cell migration, cell proliferation, differentiation, programmed cell death and synapse formation. There is little known about the effects of gonadal steroids during neuronal migration, but in animal models during determination of cell survival and development of connections between neurons, sex steroids have been shown to have an important regulatory role. Estrogen appears to act as an inducer and cofactor of neurotropins, such as nerve growth factor and brain derived neurotrophic factor.[10]

In rodents, brain sexual differentiation occurs during late fetal development and the perinatal period, therefore it is accessible to experimental study. We have found that whether sensitive parts of the brain are organized into a male or female phenotype for neuronal number and gonadotropin control depends on the exposure of the hypothalamus to estrogen. In females the brain is exposed only to basal amounts of estrogen during early development while males secrete testosterone that readily enters the brain and is converted to estrogen, which will determine the final cell number and synaptic organization of the hypothalamus. One result of this estrogen effect on the developing brain is that the synaptology of the hypothalamus supports the biphasic gonadotropin feedback in females but not in males. It is now apparent that many of the effects of androgens on the development of hypothalamus are in fact mediated by locally produced estrogen.

Since GnRH-producing neurons do not bind estrogen, in order to further define its regulatory mechanism, one needs to look at the effects of estrogen in the supporting neuronal network. The arcuate nucleus of the hypothalamus, which has an important role in controlling the biphasic feedback,[11] is also known to form and bind estrogen.[12] The ultrastructure of this nucleus, during the perinatal period, is characterized by poorly developed dendrites and axons, fewer number of synapses and extensive intercellular space. As the arcuate nucleus matures the intercellular space fills with neuronal processes and the number of synapses increases. These developmental changes can be greatly facilitated by administration of estrogen.[13] In vitro studies have also confirmed these stimulatory effects of estrogen on neuronal growth. The sex differences in the axosomatic synapses of arcuate nucleus neurons is preceded by differentiation of the neuronal membranes. These membranes contain intramembraneous protein particles (IMP) within the lipid bilayer which can be observed by the freeze-fracture technique. IMPs are believed to represent receptors or cell surface recognition molecules that are important in neuronal interactions such as synapsis formation and encapsulation by glia. There are clear sex differences in the number of IMPs within the membranes of neurons in the arcuate nucleus.[14] During sexual maturation, the changes in the IMPs correlate with changes in the synaptology of the arcuate nucleus.[15] While the sexually mature male maintains the same IMP count, in the adult female these characteristics will fluctuate in synchrony with the ovarian cycle. There is now sufficient evidence to say that estrogen exerts these effects on the synaptology and membrane characteristics not only during hypothalamic development but also during the reproductive period.

Hypothalamus

Autonomic functions

Different nuclei of the hypothalamus are responsible for the central regulation of several autonomic functions, including appetite, thermoregulation, sleep-wake cycles, vasomotor functions and reproduction. While all of these mechanisms were shown to be influenced by circulating gonadal steroids, the role of estradiol and progesterone is most understood regarding gonadotropin secretion.

As previously discussed, estrogen modifies hypothalamic structure and function during the development of the central nervous system. In rats and perhaps in primates the result of this is a permanent gender-specific change in the way the hypothalamus responds to estrogen in adulthood, providing the basis for the different, tonic vs cyclic patterns of gonadotropin release. Estrogen produced by the ovarian follicles causes synaptic separation and reapplication in the arcuate nucleus. The preovulatory estrogen surge changes the composition of neural membranes, increases the length of astrocytic processes and enhances glial ensheathment of presynaptic boutons. The result is a decrease in the presynaptic input into arcuate nucleus neurons. The arcuate nucleus contains β-endorphin neurons which project to and inhibit the activity of GnRH neurons. Stimulation of these β-endorphin neurons results in inhibition of GnRH neurons. They are also known to contain estrogen receptors, thus may contribute to the negative feedback mechanism of GnRH secretion. On the other hand, the positive feedback mechanism requires decreased inhibition of the GnRH neurons, e.g. by the β-endorphin neurons. This can be achieved by either decreasing the stimulatory catecholaminergic input to the β-endorphin neurons or increasing its GABA-ergic inhibitory input. This estrogen effect on synaptic plasticity is blocked by progesterone and dihydrotestosterone,[16] both of which can block positive feedback (Fig. 17.1). In rats, this recurrent estrogen-induced synaptic plasticity apparently has an

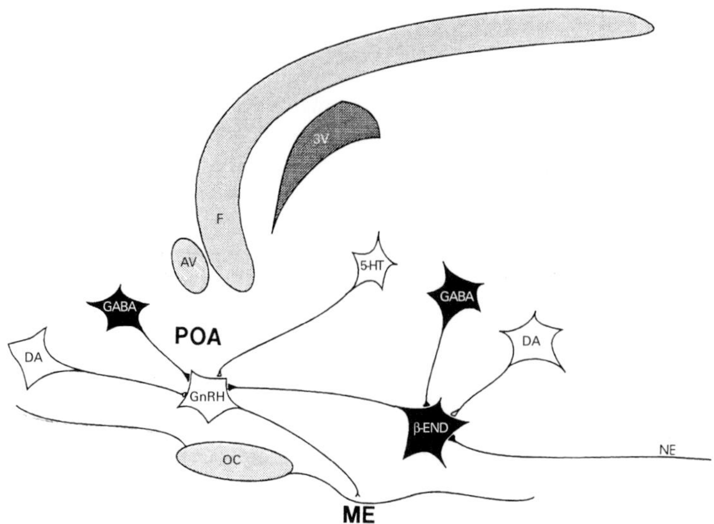

Fig. 17.1 Neurotransmitter systems involved in the regulation of GnRH secreting neurons. β-endorphin (β-END) and GABA-ergic cells have inhibitory actions. Other cells shown GnRH secreting (GnRH), serotoninergic (5-HT) and dopaminergic (DA) neurons. NE: norepinephrine innervation; f: fornix; 3V: third ventricle; OC: optic chiasm; AC: anterior commissure.

accumulating effect on the hypothalamus which ultimately results in permanent neural membrane composition and synaptologic changes leading to male-like, tonic gonadotrophin control. Exposure to high or repeated doses of estrogen has similar effects. This mechanism may play an important role in the aging of the reproductive CNS in primates (Fig, 17.2).

Hot flashes during menopause are also thought to be the result of altered peripheral vascular control, triggered in the CNS. Altered cyclic release of norepinephrine in the medial preoptic area of the hypothalamus may be the initial disturbance followed by inappropriate activation of other, e.g. heat regulation, centers. Hot flashes are the result of estrogen withdrawal. They do not develop if there was no prior estrogen exposure. For example, patients with gonadal dysgenesis do not get hot flashes if they never received estrogen replacement. Although we don't know the exact mechanism, this vasomotor regulatory problem has been effectively treated with estrogen replacement.

Sleep regulation

The effect of sex hormones on circadian rhythm was first observed in animals. A frequently observed phenomenon, the splitting of circadian rhythm into two independent components under constant light conditions, is inhibited by estrogen.[17] The organizing factor between the two separate oscillators in this case is probably the brain's central pacemaker, the suprachiasmatic nucleus (SCN) of the hypothalamus, which contains estrogen receptors. In ovariectomized rats the SCN shows different serotonin turnover during the light and dark phases of the day, however after estrogen treatment the opposite effect is observed.[18]

In humans the relationship between sleep and sex hormones can be observed in physiologic as well as in pathologic conditions. In temporal isolation experiments women show a sleep-wake cycle with a longer sleep component than that of men.[19] On the other hand menopause is associated with sleep disturbances including insomnia, frequent awakening and decreased sleep duration. Frequent awakening at night is associated with hot flashes, however awakening precedes the measurable changes in skin temperature and resistance suggesting that it is a result of direct central process, not the somatic symptoms. Studies of postmenopausal women found that women on estrogen had fewer awakenings, longer total REM sleep time and shorter sleep latency. Estrogen has been shown to reduce insomnia independent of hot flashes. Not surprisingly in estrogen deprived states such as after oophorectomy or during GnRH-analog treatment for premenopausal women, a frequently reported symptom is sleep disturbance. The association of sleep

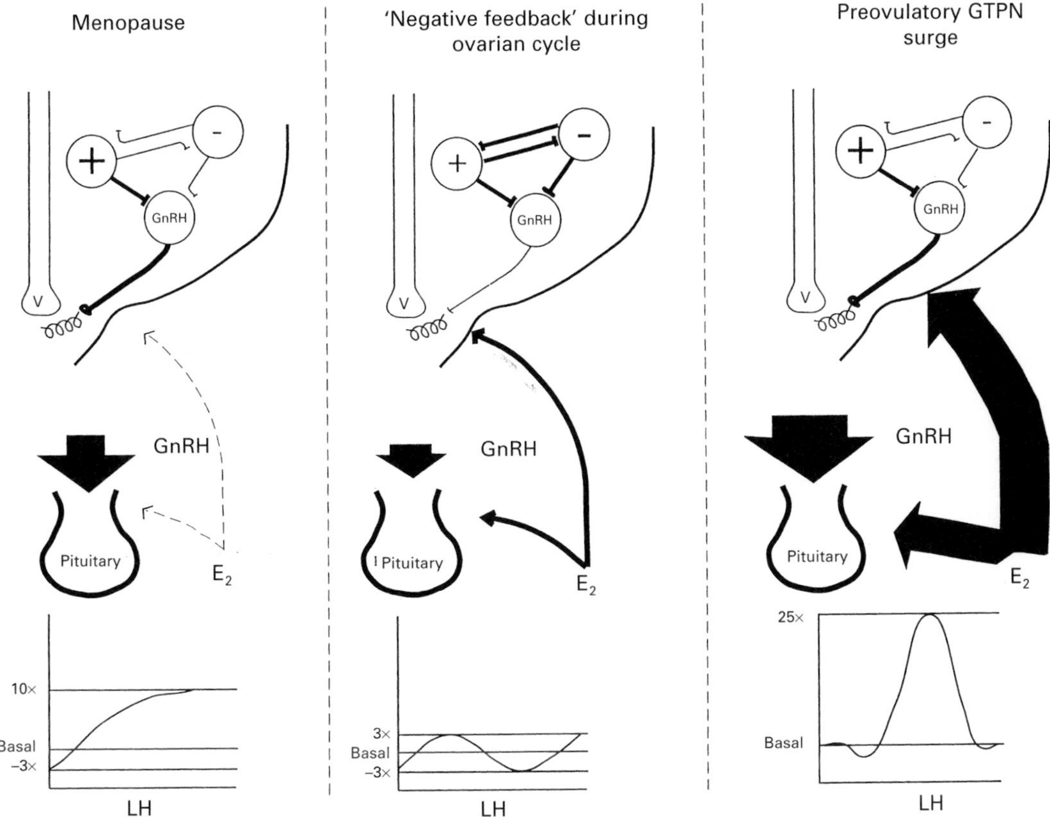

Fig. 17.2 A representation of the possible role of estrogen-induced synaptic plasticity in the control of gonadotrophins. The drawings compare menopause (open loop feedback), left frame, closed loop feedback during the follicular phase of the normal cycle, middle frame, with the preovulatory estrogen surge-induced changes in GnRH release which cause the pituitary gonadotrophins to rise, right frame. The low or modest levels of estrogen during the menopause and early follicular phase fail to sensitize the pituitary, but allow for neurotransmitter interactions at the hypothalamic level which maintain varying but basal levels of GnRH. As the follicular phase continues the estrogen levels rise, sensitizing the pituitary gland. This results in low GnRH and circulating gonatrophins and elevated estrogen (not pictured). After the period of inhibition of GnRH/gonatrophins the pituitary is massively sensitized but does not release gonatrophins because of the lowered GnRH due to increased inhibitory tone from i.e. endorphin neurons. On the preovulatory day, the estrogen rises in the blood asymptomically and this causes retraction of inhibitory synapses so that the GnRH levels return to baseline or slightly higher. The result is a massive release of gonatrophin (LH and FSH) from the sensitized pituitary gland gonatrophs. (See text for further detail.)

disorders with hot flashes indicate that the lack of estrogen during menopause may predominantly effect the hypothalamus where both the circadian rhythm and sleep-wake cycles are regulated. Gender differences in certain mental disorders point to the same direction. Seasonal affective disorder and rapid cycling bipolar disorder, both of which are associated with disturbances of the circadian rhythm, occur more frequently in women than in men. Women with bipolar disorders also show more episodes of depression and increased sleep than men who tend to have more manic episodes.

As early as in the 1950s exogenous progesterone was reported to have calming and even sleep inducing effects. This may be mediated by the more recently discovered modulatory action of progesterone on the inhibitory GABA receptor channel complex. Estrogen and progesterone may be protective against sleep-disordered breathing such as sleep apnea. Sleep apnea is a potentially serious disorder affecting not only mood, memory and higher mentation but also increasing the risk for myocardial infarction. It causes hypoxia and the subsequent acidosis may sensitize the cardiac muscle. At that point a sudden awakening associated with adrenalin surge may trigger acute coronary artery spasm and myocardial infarction. Premenopausal women have sleep-disordered breathing less commonly than men but this difference can not be seen after menopause. Women after oophorectomy also show fewer sleep-disordered breathing episodes when receiving hormone replacement therapy with progesterone or estrogen.[20] Progesterone has been observed to improve hypoxia associated with sleep apnea in some men. The mechanism of these actions is yet to be determined.

Sex steroids have direct and indirect effects on sleep. When studying these effects, it is important to recognize the other influences of these hormones, for example on anxiety, depression or vasomotor instability. Since they are related to sleep disturbances, any change in these conditions can effect sleep patterns. Conversely, disturbed sleep may contribute to the development or worsening of mood disorders.

Cortex

Temporal lobe

There are several mechanisms by which sex hormones can influence synaptic plasticity and long term potentiation of hippocampal neuronal functions, apparently the necessary physiologic changes of neurons involved in memory. The involved neurons are primarily located in the limbic system, with the hippocampus playing an essential role in this function. There have been an increasing number of studies reporting rapid, short term and long term effects of the sex steroids on these parts of the brain. The relationship between these hormones and memory can be observed on different levels and from different angles. On a cell neurophysiology level, experiments on acute brain slices involving the hippocampus have provided invaluable data, while on a clinical level, studies of hormone replacement therapy have been the major source of our information.

The stimulatory neurotransmitter glutamate and its NMDA sensitive receptor play a role in at least one form of long term potentiation of the neuron. In the hippocampus, estrogen was found to increase the density of NMDA agonist receptor/ion channel complex[21] and increase the density of dendritic spines specifically in CA1 neurones,[22] the area involved in memory. Some of the other mechanisms that influence neuronal functions and can effect memory are sex steroid hormone action on nerve growth as a cofactor of nerve growth factors,[23] modification of aging and stress related damage of neurons related to glucocorticoid induced disruption of glucose metabolism,[24] stimulation of cholinergic, monoaminergic and serotoninergic neurotransmitter systems, protection against free radicals[25] and vascular effects that improve blood flow. The latter action of estrogen may be particularly important in preventing the common infarctional dementia; however, more data are needed to prove this.

Alzheimer's disease is a noninfarctional form of dementia which might be influenced favorably by estrogen. In addition to the previously mentioned estrogen effects on the CNS, the proposed mechanisms include a decrease of the cerebral β-amyloid accumulation, an important pathologic abnormality in this disease. There is an increasing body of evidence from clinical trials and epidemiologic studies that estrogen has a role in preventing and/or delaying the onset of this disease.[26,27]

Estrogen has also been found to improve memory in postmenopausal women without dementia and in surgically menopausal women. It is important to recognize that memory is a complex function of the brain and the different forms of memory, e.g. short or long-term memory, are functions of separate systems. There are also differences based on the relation to the sensory systems, e.g. auditory, verbal, visual or spatial memory. There is overwhelming evidence that estrogen positively influences memory, however it is now becoming clear that this involves primarily verbal memory while visual or spatial memory, is unaffected. This effect is also more profound on short-term memory compared to long-term memory.

Cerebral cortex

In addition to memory, estrogen is known to affect other cognitive functions of the brain. Estrogen-responsive neurons are present in several areas of the brain that are known to play a role in higher mental functions, such as in the basal forebrain, hippocampus and amygdala. Sex hormone effects on cognitive functions in general share some of the basic underlying physiologic mechanisms that are involved in memory.

It appears that changes in cognition and higher mentation may be seen during the normal menstrual cycle, but these are generally subclinical and not of concern. In some cases there are extremes ranging from mood swings, mentation difficulties even to epilepsy. Estrogen, progesterone and androgen have all been implicated in several higher mental function disorders. These include phobias, sense of well being, libido and aggression.

Most of the clinical studies that found sex steroid effects on cognitive functions have been done on postmenopausal women. Reports of controlled studies were published as early as the beginning of the 1950s when, for example, estrogen was found to enhance certain cognitive functions measured by verbal IQ scores.[28] The number of publications has increased as hormone replacement therapy gained acceptance in clinical use during the next couple of decades. The overwhelming majority of studies report a positive effect of estrogen on some of the cognitive functions in postmenopausal women; nevertheless, a few reports found no relation or were inconclusive. The methodological concerns about these studies have been reviewed by others.[29,30] One of these factors that needs to be considered is the relation between sleep, mood disorders and cognitive functions. Estrogen effects anxiety and depression, both of which profoundly influence cognition. In more recent years Sherwin has published a series of elegant studies that considered many limitations of previous works on this subject. She has confirmed the observations of positive estrogen effect on cognition. It is again important to remember that the different components of cognition are not effected equally. Undoubtedly, studies will follow that address the effects of estrogen on other specific cognitive functions.

Mood

There is substantial evidence that sex steroids have a profound effect on mood and mood disorders. This relationship can be seen in physiologic states such as during the menstrual cycle or menopause and in patients with certain types of affective disorders. In the various clinical situations estrogen and progesterone were found to have different, frequently opposite effects on mood. To study the underlying mechanisms has been challenging, mainly because of the difficulty establishing a direct relationship between the effects of these hormones on a cellular level and the clinically observed changes in mood. The mechanisms that may be involved include the stimulatory effects of estrogen on nerve excitability and on the adrenergic system, stimulation of the serotoninergic system, which is believed to play a role in depression, and increased synthesis of NO that functions as a neuromodulator in the CNS. Progesterone and related neurosteroids are thought to exert their anxiolytic and hypnotic activities through enhancing GABA-mediated chloride currents which have inhibiting effect on nerve cells.

Several clinical studies reported a favorable response to estrogen replacement therapy for perimenopausal and postmenopausal women who were complaining of anxiety and depression while progesterone was found to have an opposite effect. It appears that estrogen has a dose related response in these cases. Severe depression has been treated successfully with large doses of estrogen,[31] however in most cases the usual doses of hormone replacement therapy will effectively alleviate depressive symptoms that are related to menopause.[32]

Another form of this disorder, thought to be related to falling sex hormone levels, can be observed sometimes in the postpartum period. In individuals suffering from postpartum depression there are no sex hormonal disturbances, but exogenous estrogen was found to significantly improve the course of the disease where other treatment modalities failed.[33] Possible involvement of NO is suggested on the basis of observations that NO is found in increased concentrations during estrogen replacement therapy[34] and during pregnancy.[35]

It is difficult to define the role of sex hormones in premenstrual syndrome (PMS) and in the depression associated with this disorder. Studies have failed to provide sufficient data to conclude which gonadal steroids are involved in PMS. For example, the previously suggested role of progesterone was questioned in a study of women with PMS who took the progesterone antagonist RU-486 with no apparent change in their symptoms.[36] It is important to remember, however, that progesterone and the other sex steroids also have nongenomic effects. It has been suggested that differences in the regulation of melatonin,[37] its precursor serotonin[38] and possibly the noradrenergic system may be responsible for the development of PMS in susceptible women. Some of the treatments suggested for PMS include suppression of endogenous gonadal steroid production by GnRH-agonist, giving exogenous progesterone and using drugs that increase serotonin levels in the CNS. Binding of the antidepressant imipramine to serotonin receptors was found to be enhanced by both estradiol and progesterone.[39]

The effects of gonadal steroids on sex drive can be observed in animal experiments and in clinical studies of hormone deprived individuals. Progesterone rapidly induces female mating behavior in previously estrogen treated rats, suggesting the involvement of a nongenomic action. In humans, it has long been known that some women after menopause or surgical removal of the ovaries have markedly reduced libido. The primary role of sex steroids, and androgens in particular, is apparent when women on hormone replacement therapy are compared to hormone-deprived controls. Treatment of these women with testosterone in addition to estrogen effectively restores libido and also contributes to the general feeling of well being. It is also known, however, that testosterone increases aggressive behavior. Suppression of testosterone levels may be used to treat aggressive criminal behaviors, e.g. in cases of criminal sex offenders. Loss of libido seems to be worse after oophorectomy than after menopause. This may be because the postmenopausal ovary continues to produce some androgens, although in a significantly reduced amount. The mechanisms by which testosterone increases sexual drive in women after ovariectomy and after menopause is still unclear.

Seizure disorder

Catamenial seizure is the most apparent clinical manifestation of the relationship between steroid hormones and seizure activity. These are seizures characteristically occurring during certain phases of the menstrual cycle, sometimes at midcycle (if the cycle is ovulatory) and frequently in the premenstrual period or during menstruation. The etiology of this disorder is believed to be related to the known effect of estrogen to increase nerve excitability and to lower seizure threshold. In contrast, progesterone has an inhibitory effect. As mentioned previously, estradiol increases the density of NMDA-sensitive glutamate receptor in the CA1 region of the hippocampus. This increase in the NMDA agonist receptor sites results in a higher sensitivity to the excitatory neurotransmitter glutamate. On the other hand, certain neurosteroid progesterone metabolites are known to act as potent allosteric modulators and direct activators of the inhibitory GABA-chloride channels, and accordingly they have a protective effect against seizures. Both progesterone and its metabolite 5 α-pregnan-3 alpha-ol-20-one have been shown to increase seizure threshold probably through both pre- and postsynaptic effects.

It is important to note that the sex steroids can have different effects on different parts of the nervous system, therefore seizure activities originating in these areas can respond to sex hormones differently. It has been observed in epilepsy-prone strains of mice that estradiol actually decreased the frequency of vestibular seizures which are associated with paroxysmal activity in temporal structures whereas oophorectomy produced a decrease in audiogenic seizure activity which is related to collicular and tegmental regions. Likewise the type of seizure, e.g. primary or secondary generalized and absence seizure may respond to sex hormones differently, as seen in the case of a patient with absence seizure which was exacerbated by progesterone.[40] Catamenial seizures, like other seizures, are treated with anticonvulsant drugs, however when they fail to control the disease progesterone may be used with success.[41] Addition of the antiestrogen clomiphene or the aromatase inhibitor testolactone may also result in improved control. Another therapeutic approach is to suppress the entire pituitary-gonadal axis by a GnRH analogue.[42]

Conclusion

Sex hormones directly and indirectly influence many brain functions such as sleep, mood, memory and other cognitive functions. Generally, the brain's responses to sex steroids depend on both the level of the sex steroid and presence of other regulatory substances, such as growth factors. Expression of the effects on brain functions can be characterized according to the reproductive status: development, puberty, reproductive life and the climacteric. Because the average woman lives about one third of her life after menopause, we have concentrated on this period to exemplify the sex steroid dependent functions of the brain.

Estrogen has been used widely for the prevention and treatment of disorders associated with menopause. Chief among these are vasomotor instability (hot flushes), sleep disorders and effects on cognitive function. There is considerable interest in possible effects of estrogen on mood, cognition and dystrophies such as Alzheimer's disease. Although the above entities may respond favorably to estrogen therapy, androgen replacement can also be beneficial, especially in the more profoundly androgen deficient surgical menopause. The beneficial effects of testosterone in conjunction with estrogen replacement are now being studied.

The topic covered by this chapter will probably be an area which undergoes significant changes in the next few years as we gain more insight in the different mechanisms by which sex hormones work in the CNS. A rapid evolution, if not revolution, is taking place in the way we look at the functions of individual neurons, glial cells and neuronal networks. This is, indeed the 'decade of the brain', and fundamental research into both sex steroids and brain function will contribute to better use of our therapeutic armamentarium and the development of new therapeutic strategies.

REFERENCES

1. Luine VN 1985 Estrogen increases choline acetyltransferase activity in specific basal forebrain nuclei and projection areas of female rats. Experimental Neurology 80: 484–490
2. Moncada S, Higgs EA 1993 The L-arginine nitric oxide pathway. New England Journal of Medicine 329: 2002–2012
3. Luine VN, McEwen BS 1977 Effect of estradiol on turnover of type A monoamine oxidase in brain. Journal of Neurochemistry 28: 1221–1227
4. Wong M, Moss RL 1992 Long-term and short-term electrophysiological effects of estrogen on the synaptic properties of hippocampal CAI neurons. Journal of Neuroscience 12(8): 321725
5. Nikezic G, Horvat A, Nedeljkovic N, Martinovic JV 1996 17 beta-estradiol in vitro affects Na-dependent and depolarization-induced Ca^{2+} transport in rat brain synaptosomes. Experimentia 52(3): 217–220
6. Gu Q, Moss RL 1996 17 beta-estradiol potentiates kainate-induced currents via activation of the cAMP cascade. Journal of Neuroscience 16(11): 3620–3629
7. Garcia-Segura LM, Baetens D, Naftolin F 1986 Synaptic remodeling in arcuate nucleus after injection of estradiol valerate in adult female rats. Brain Research 366: 131–135
8. Naftolin F, Leranth C, Perez J, Garcia-Segura LM 1993 Estrogen induces synaptic plasticity in adult primate neurons. Neuroendocrinology 57: 935–939
9. Horvath TL, Leedom L, Garcia-Segura LM, Naftolin F 1995 Estrogen-induced synaptic plasticity; implications for the regulation of gonadotrophins. In: Smith MS (ed) Current opinion in endocrinology and diabetes. Garcia-Segura, Naftolin 1986, pp 186–190
10. Miranda RC, Sohrabji F, Toran-Allerand D 1994 Interactions of estrogen with the neutrophins and their receptors during neural development. Hormones and Behavior 28(4): 367–375
11. Szenagothai J, Flerko B, Mess B, Halasz B 1962 Hypothalamic control of the anterior pituitary. Akademiai Kiado, Budapest, pp 40–58
12. Naftolin F, Ryan K, Davis I, Reddy V, Flores F, Petro Z, Kuhn M, White R, Takaoka Y, Wolin L 1975 The formation of estrogens by central neuroendocrine tissue. Recent Progress in Hormone Research 31: 295–319
13. Arai Y, Matsumoto A 1978 Synapse formation of the hypothalamic arcuate nucleus during postnatal development in the female rat and its modification by neonatal estrogen treatment. Psychoneuroendocrinology 3: 31–45
14. Garcia-Segura LM, Baetens D, Naftolin F 1985 Sex differences and maturational changes in arcuate nucleus neuronal plasma membrane organization. Developmental Brain Research 19: 146–149
15. Naftolin F, Maclusky NJ, Leranth C, Sakamoto HS, Garcia-Segura LM 1988 The cellular effects of estrogens on neuroendocrine tissue. Journal of Steroid Biochemistry 39: 195–207
16. Perez J, Luquin S, Naftolin F, Garcia-Segura LM 1993 The role of estradiol and progesterone in phased synaptic remodeling of the rat arcuate nucleus. Brain Research 608(1): 38–44
17. Thomas EMV, Armstrong SM 1989 Effect of ovariectomy and estradiol on unity of female rat circadian rhythms. American Journal of Physiology 257: R1241–R1250
18. Cohen IR, Wise PM 1988 Effects of estradiol on the diurnal rhythm of serotonin activity in microdissected areas of ovariectomized rats. Endocrinology 122: 2619–2625
19. Wever RA 1984 Sex differences in human circadian rhythms: intrinsic periods and sleep fractions. Experientia 40: 1226–1234
20. Pickett CK, Regensteiner JG, Woodard WD, Hagerman DD, Weil JV, Moore LG 1989 Progestin and estrogen reduce sleep-disordered breathing in postmenopausal women. Journal of Applied Physiology 66(4): 1656–1661
21. Weiland NG 1992 Estradiol selectively regulates agonist binding sites on the N-methyl-D-aspartate receptor complex in the CA1 region of the hippocampus. Endocrinology 131(2): 662–668
22. Gould E, Woolley C, Frankfurt M, McEwen B 1990 Gonadal steroids regulate dendritic spine density in hippocampal pyramidal cells in adulthood. Journal of Neuroscience 10: 1286–1291
23. Toran-Allerand CD, Miranda RC, Bentham WD, Sohrabji F, Brown EJ et al 1992 Estrogen receptors colocalize with low affinity nerve growth factor receptors in cholinergic neurons of the basal forebrain. Proceedings of the National Academy of Science 89: 4668–4672
24. Mizoguchi K, Tatshuhide T, De-Hua C, Tabira T 1992 Stress induces neuronal death in the hippocampus of castrated rats. Neuroscience Letters 138: 157–160
25. Subbiah MTR, Kessel B, Agrawal M, Rajan R, Abplanalp W, Rymaszewski A 1993 Antioxidant potential of specific estrogens on lipid peroxidation. Journal of Clinical Endocrinology and Metabolism 77: 1095–1097
26. Tang M-X, Jacobs D, Stern Y, Marder K, Schofield P, Gurland B, Andrews H, Mayeux R 1996 Effect of estrogen during menopause on risk and age at onset of Alzheimer's disease. Lancet 348: 429–432
27. Paganini-Hill A, Henderson VW 1994 Estrogen deficiency and risk of Alzheimer's disease in women. American Journal of Epidemiology 140: 256–261
28. Caldwell BM, Watson RI 1952 An evaluation of psychologic effects of sex hormone administration in aged women. Results of therapy after six months. Journal of Gerontology 7: 228–244
29. Sherwin BB 1996 Estrogen, the brain and memory. Menopause 3(2): 97–105
30. Tivis LJ 1996 Estrogen replacement therapy and cognitive functioning in postmenopausal women. Menopausal Medicine 4(2): 1–4
31. Klaiber EL, Broverman DM, Vogel W, Kobayashi Y 1979 Estrogen therapy for severe persistent depression in women. Archives of General Psychiatry 36: 550–554
32. Sherwin BB 1988 Affective changes with estrogen and androgen replacement therapy in surgically menopausal women. Journal of Affective Disorders 14: 177–187
33. Gregoire AJP, Kumar R, Everitt B, Henderson AF, Studd JWW 1996 Transdermal estrogen for treatment of severe postnatal depression. Lancet 347: 930–933
34. Roselli M, Imthurn B, Keller PJ et al 1995 Hypertension 25: 845–853

35. Lopez-Jaramillo P 1996 Estrogens and depression. Lancet 348: 135–136
36. Schmidt PJ, Nieman LK, Grover GN et al 1991 Lack of effect of induced menses on symptoms in women with premenstrual syndrome. New England Journal of Medicine 324: 1174–1179
37. Parry BL, Berga SL, Kripke DF et al 1990 Altered waveform of plasma nocturnal melatonin secretion in premenstrual depression. Archives of General Psychiatry 47: 1138–1146
38. Severino SK 1994 A focus on 5-hydroxytryptamine (serotonin) and psychopathology. In: Gold JH, Severino SK (eds) Premenstrual dysphorias: myths and realities. American Psychiatric Press, Washington, DC, pp
39. Kendall DA, Stancel GM, Enna SJ 1981 Imipramine: effect of ovarian steroids on modifications in serotonin receptor binding. Science 211: 1183
40. Grunewald RA, Aliberti V, Panayiotopoulos CP 1992 Exacerbation of typical absence seizures by progesterone. Seizure 1 (2): 137–138
41. Herzog AG 1995 Progesterone therapy in women with complex partial and secondary generalized seizures. Neurology 45(9): 1660–1662
42. Bauer J, Hocke A, Elger CE 1995 Catamenial seizures — an analysis. Nervenarzt 66(10): 760–769

18. Effects of estrogen and progesterone on bone

Bent Winding, Henrik L. Jørgensen, Claus Christiansen

Introduction

The effect of female sex hormones on the skeleton and calcium metabolism have been intensively investigated over the last 15–20 years. This interest has been stimulated by concern over the increasing incidence of osteoporosis and subsequent fragility fractures.[1] Osteoporosis occurs when the normally balanced processes of bone formation and bone resorption become unbalanced and resorption exceeds formation. These processes are complex and are influenced by a number of hormonal, metabolic and lifestyle factors. Although it has been clearly shown that hormone replacement therapy (HRT) prevents postmenopausal bone loss (Fig. 18.1)[2], the mechanisms by which estrogen influences bone metabolism are not, as yet,

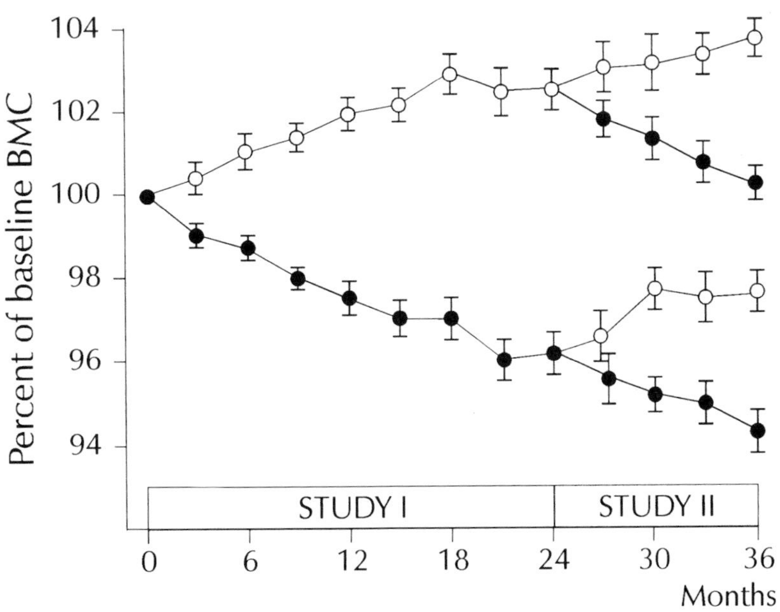

Fig. 18.1 Bone mineral content (BMC) at the lower forearm in early postmenopausal women (Study I), receiving either combined estrogen/progestogen treatment (●) or placebo (○). The women were rerandomized after two years (Study II): 50% of the HRT treated women were changed to placebo and 50% of the placebo treated women were changed to active treatment. Adapted with permission.[2]

completely understood. However, the identification of estrogen receptors in the bone resorbing cells, the osteoclasts,[3] as well as in the bone forming cells, the osteoblasts,[4,5] has now rendered molecular studies of the action of estrogens possible.

NORMAL SKELETAL HOMEOSTASIS

Bone morphology

The skeletal system, composed of bone and cartilage, is important for the protection of vital organs, e.g. heart, lungs, CNS and bone marrow. Further, the bones are important for the transduction of movements and as a reservoir of ions for the entire organism, especially calcium and phosphate. The basic constituents of bone, as in all connective tissue, are the cells and extracelluar matrix. The latter being composed of collagen type I fibers (90% of total proteins), noncollagenous proteins, crystals of hydroxyapatite ($Ca_{10}(PO_4)_6(OH)_2$) and glycoproteins and proteoglycans.

Bone cells

Osteoclast

Osteoclasts originate from the pluripotent hematopoietic stem cells. Mature osteoclasts, responsible for the active resorption of mineralized bone, are formed by fusion of mononuclear preosteoclasts and the total number of nuclei in the mature osteoclasts can be up to 100; normally there will be six to ten nuclei.

The shape and activity of osteoclasts are controlled by systemic hormones and locally released cytokines. Upon appropriate stimulatory impulse, the osteoclast will adhere to the bone surface by a cell-integrin-bone surface interaction, forming a tight seal between the cell and bone. The apical membrane adjacent to the bone surface will fold up creating the unique ruffled border, thereby greatly increasing the area of the apical membrane, allowing fast exchange of high amounts of materials between the cell and the extracelluar space.[6] The space between the cell and bone is called the resorption lacunae.

H^+ and bicarbonate are formed in the cytoplasm by hydration of CO_2, a process accelerated by carbonic anhydrase type II. Protons are actively pumped across the apical membrane into the resorption lacunae by H^+-ATPases and bicarbonate is exchanged for chloride ions across the basolateral membrane. The acidification of the resorption lacunae,[7] essential for the dissolution of hydroxyapatite crystal, is accompanied by the secretion of a range of proteinases concerting the degradation of demineralized matrix,[8] (Fig. 18.2, lower panel left).

Osteoblast

Osteoblasts originate from a mesenchymal stem cell and mature osteoblasts are responsible for the production of the bone matrix, composed of collagen, noncollagenous proteins and ground substance. The bone-forming osteoblasts, with one basal nucleus, have a cytoplasm rich in rough endoplasmic reticulum and Golgi complex, and a cellular membrane rich in alkaline phosphatases. Osteoblasts are always found in clusters of cuboidal cells lining a layer of unmineralized bone matrix (osteoid) that they have formed (Fig. 18.2, lower panel right).

Osteocytes originate from bone-forming osteoblasts that have been trapped into their own production of bone matrix, which later becomes calcified. They are connected to lining cells at the endosteal bone surfaces and to each other by small cellular extensions. Osteocytes have been hypothesized to serve as sensors to mechanical loading.

Bone remodeling

In the normal adult skeleton, bone is continuously renewed by osteoclastic resorption of old bone and osteoblastic formation of new bone.[9] The cells in the localized process of bone renewal constitute the bone remodeling units (BMU), where resorption always precedes bone formation (Fig. 18.2). The first event in bone remodeling involves recruitment of mature osteoclasts and generation of new osteoclasts from stem cells adjacent to the BMU. Osteoclasts will resorb a confined volume of old bone in the BMU. The resorption phase is terminated in an, as yet, undefined manner, with a cease in osteoclast activity followed by the reversal phase, where mononuclear macrophage-like cells might be involved in forming the 'cement line' on the cleaned bone surface. Bone-forming osteoblasts will follow the cement line with formation of demineralized matrix (osteoid). The BMU is completed by the mineralization of the osteoid, mainly by fixation of hydroxyapatite crystals to the collagen fibers. In the normal skeleton the volume of bone formed by osteoblasts equals the volume of bone resorbed by the osteoclasts (balanced remodeling).

EFFECT OF ESTROGEN ON BONE CELLS

During the past few years several *in vivo* and *in vitro* studies have been conducted in order to appreciate the

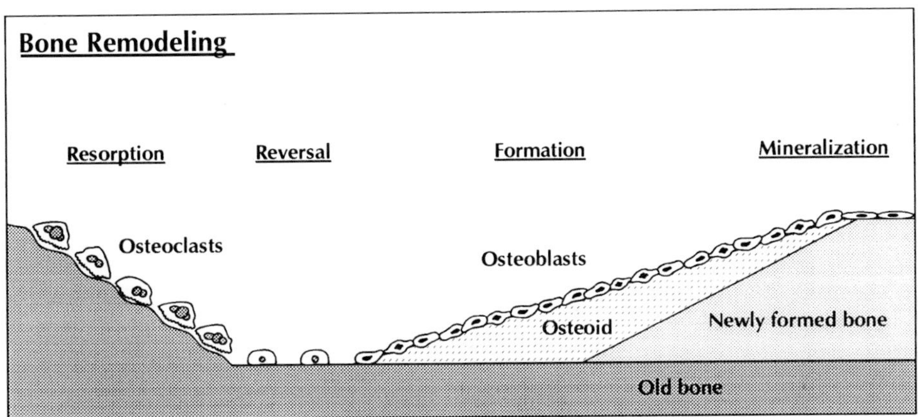

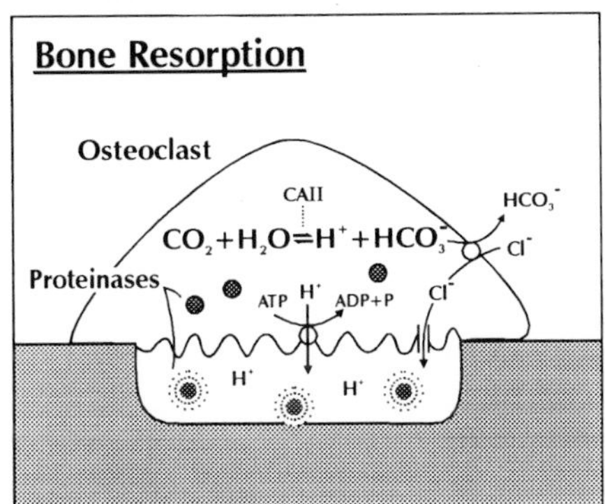

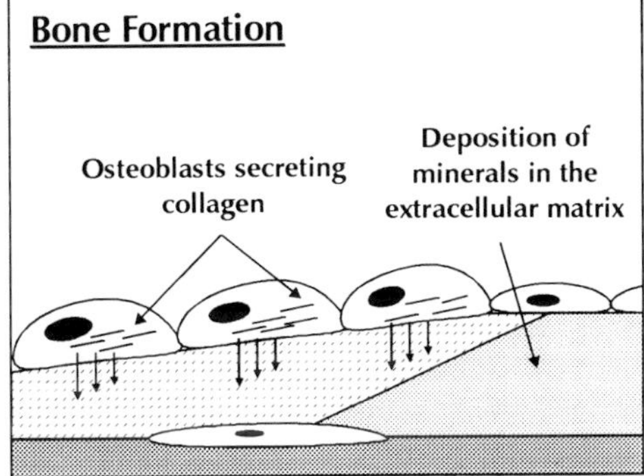

Fig. 18.2 Schematic drawing showing the steps in normal bone remodeling at bone surfaces. The resorption of bone is initiated by activation and formation of osteoclasts which adhere to the bone surfaces, forming erosion cavities. After resorption has been completed mononuclear macrophage-like cells clean the bone surface (reversal). Subsequently, osteoblasts will be activated forming a seam of collagen, noncollagenous proteins and ground substance (osteoid). The remodeling is completed by the mineralization of the osteoid, primarily by the deposition of hydroxyapatite crystals.

The lower panel shows two schematic drawings of osteoclastic bone resorption and osteoblastic bone formation. The degradation of old bone is accomplished by osteoclastic secretion of proteinases and protons into the resorption lacunae. New bone is produced by osteoblastic secretion of osteoid, which is subsequently mineralized.

mechanism involved in estrogen deficiency induced bone loss, associated with increased numbers of BMUs and resulting in imbalanced bone remodeling (Fig. 18.3)[10]. Using surgically induced (ovariectomy, OVX) estrogen deficiency in mice as an animal model for postmenopausal or surgically induced estrogen deficiency in the human, it has been possible to elucidate the role of different cytokines in imbalanced bone remodeling.[11,12,13]

In the OVX mice, a significant increase in the number of osteoclasts was found at the trabecular bone surfaces and bone resorption sites. The increase in osteoclast number and bone resorption could be prevented by treatment with estrogen and, perhaps more intriguingly, by treatment with inhibitors to interleukin-1 (IL-1) and tumor necrosis factor (TNF).[12,13] Furthermore, antibodies raised against interleukin-6 (IL-6) prevented an increase in the osteoclast number[11] but failed to affect bone loss.[13] IL-1, TNF and IL-6 are cytokines known as potent stimulators of osteoclastogenesis and bone resorption (IL-1 and TNF), but the studies using OVX mice provided us with the first line of evidence for the importance of cytokines in the accelerated osteoclastogenesis and bone loss after onset of estrogen deficiency *in vivo*.[11,12,13]

In humans, mRNA levels for IL-6 and IL-1 have been found to be increased in trabecular bone extracts

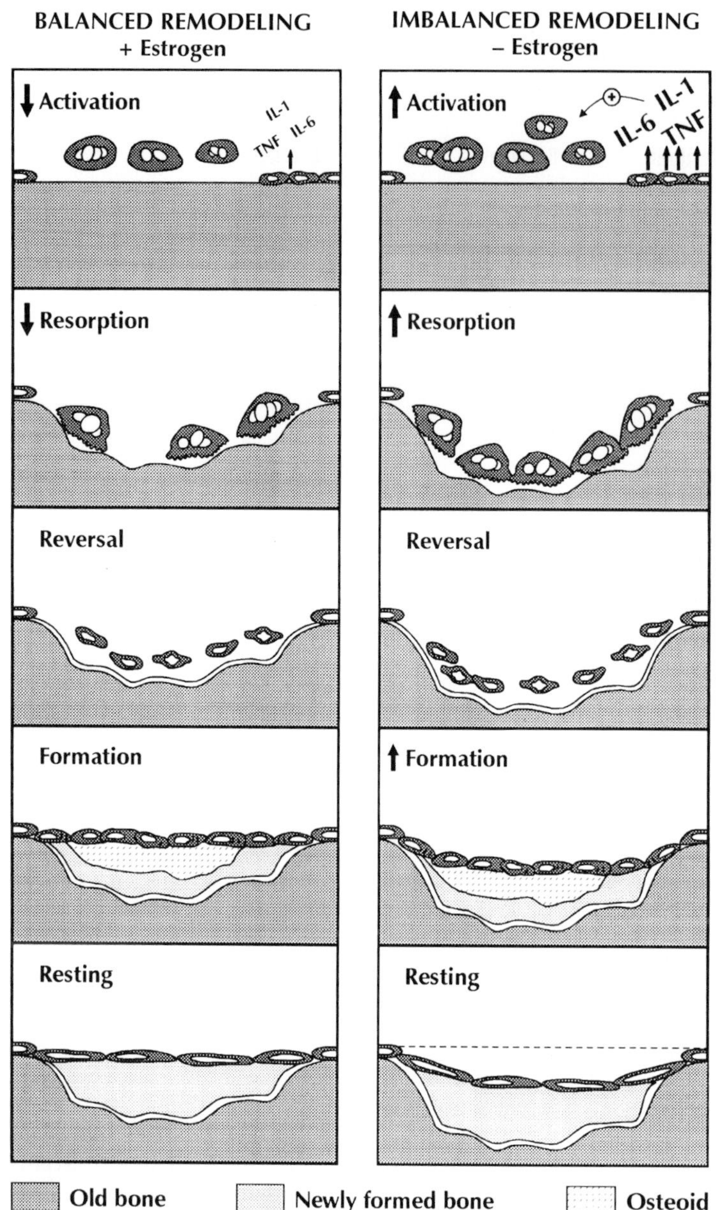

Fig. 18.3 Working model for balanced and imbalanced bone remodeling in premenopausal or estrogen-treated women and postmenopausal women, respectively. In balanced remodeling, the bone formation equals the bone resorption; in imbalanced remodeling, the accelerated bone resorption, induced at least partly by an increase in IL-1, TNF and IL-6 levels secreted by stromal cells, will be greater than bone formation. Adapted with permission.[10]

from postmenopausal women with osteoporotic fractures when compared with normal age-matched women without osteoporosis,[14] whereas the levels of IL-6 and IL-1 in serum have repeatedly been found to be unaffected by bone-status.[15,16] This further supports the view that estrogen acts directly on bone cells by an alteration of their synthesis and secretion of cytokines, which act as paracrine factors in the bone microenvironment and not as systemic 'hormones'.

Following the demonstration of estrogen receptors in both osteoblasts and osteoclasts,[3,4,5] numerous *in vitro* studies have been performed to reveal the biological and molecular role for estrogen in bone cell metabolism (Table 18.1). In purified avian and human-like osteoclast cultures, estrogen decreased bone resorption as well as lysosomal proteinase secretion when osteoclasts were cultured on thin slices of mineralized substrates;[17,18,19] osteoclast formation has also been found to be suppressed by estrogen treatment.[20,21] In both primary osteoblasts and cell lines with osteoblastic phenotype, estrogen has been found to increase the type I collagen synthesis and secretion[5,23] and the differentiation of cells, measured as cellular alkaline phosphatase activity.[24,25] The mitotic effect of estrogen is still controversial, as some studies demonstrate inhibition of cell proliferation while others find an increase or lack of effects on cell proliferation in response to estrogen treatment.[24,25,26] Both osteoblasts and bone-derived stromal cells are reproducibly found to decrease their level of IL-6 synthesis and secretion in response to estrogen,[27,28,29] whereas the production of transforming growth factor beta (TGF β) is increased.[5] The observed effects of estrogen, though, seem to be highly dependent on the cellular number of estrogen receptors and the experimental conditions used during the studies.[19]

Based on the *in vivo* and *in vitro* experiments conducted so far, estrogen may be considered as a bone-acting hormone with direct effects on both osteoclasts and osteoblasts. The antiresorptive effect of estrogen appears to be mediated through a direct inhibitory effect on osteoclasts[17,18,19] as well as an indirect effect mediated at least in part by the

Table 18.1 Effect of estrogen on bone cells *in vitro*.

Cell of origin	Cellular response	References
Avain osteoclasts	↓ resorption, ↓ lysosomal proteinases secretion	Oursler et al 1993[17], 1997[19]
Human osteoclastoma osteoclast-like cells	↓ resorption, ↓ lysosomal proteinases secretion	Oursler et al 1994[18]
Avain osteoclasts	↑ TGFβ secretion s.t ↓ TGFβ secretion 1.t.	Robinson et al 1996[22]
Murine calvaria	↓ osteoclast formation	Girasole et al 1992[27]
Mouse bone marrow cells	↓ PTH-stimulated osteoclast formation	Kaji et al 1996[21]
Rat Obl-like osteosarcoma cell line UMR-106	↓ proliferation ↑ differentiation	Gray et al 1987[24]
Rat and human Obl-like osteosarcoma cell lines ROS 17/2.8, HOS TE85	↑ type I procollagen mRNA ↑ TGFβ mRNA	Komm et al 1988[5]
Human Obl-like cell line BG688	↑ α,(I)-procollagen mRNA	Benz et al 1991[23]
Human, murine Obl-like cells	↓ IL-6 secretion ↓ IL-6 mRNA	Girasole et al 1992[27]
Human Obl-like cells	– proliferation – differentiation	Rickard et al 1993[26]
Mouse Obl-like cell line MC3T3-E1	↓ IL-6 production	Bellido et al 1993[28]
Human Obl-like cells	– proliferation ↑ differentiation	Verhaar et al 1994[25]
Human fetal Obl-like cell line hFOB	↓ IL-6 production	Kassem et al 1996[29]

↑ = increase; ↓ = decrease; – = no effect observed; s.t. = short term treatment; l.t. = long-term treatment; PTH = parathyroid hormone; TGFβ = transforming growth factor beta; Obl = osteoblast; IL-6 = interleukin-6.

suppression of IL-6, IL-1 and TNF release and the augmented TGF β release by osteoblast and other bone-derived stromal cells.[5,11,12,13,27,28,29,30]

Effect of estrogen on markers of bone remodeling

The rate of bone turnover can be indirectly assessed by the use of a number of biochemical markers. The major part of the organic bone matrix consists of type I collagen. When bone is resorbed, this collagen is degraded into smaller fragments and released into the extracellular fluid. These fragments are excreted into the urine and can be measured by a variety of assays as markers of bone resorption. However, specificity and clinical utility vary considerably between the different markers.

Osteoblasts produce small amounts of osteocalcin for incorporation into the bone matrix. A proportion of this escapes into the serum and can be measured as a marker of bone formation. Alkaline phosphatase, believed to reflect osteoblast differentiation, is less specific in itself, but newer bone specific assays have been developed.[31]

Figure 18.4 shows that the estrogen deficiency after menopause increases both bone formation and resorption, while HRT reverses this effect.[32] As can be seen from Figure 18.5, the level of bone remodeling (as measured by the markers) is reduced to postmenopausal levels after 12 months of HRT. Correspondingly, bone mass increased in the HRT group and decreased in the placebo treated group.[33]

It has been shown in a longitudinal study that biochemical markers of bone turnover can predict the rate of bone loss, making it possible to distinguish between 'fast bone losers' and 'slow bone losers'.[34]

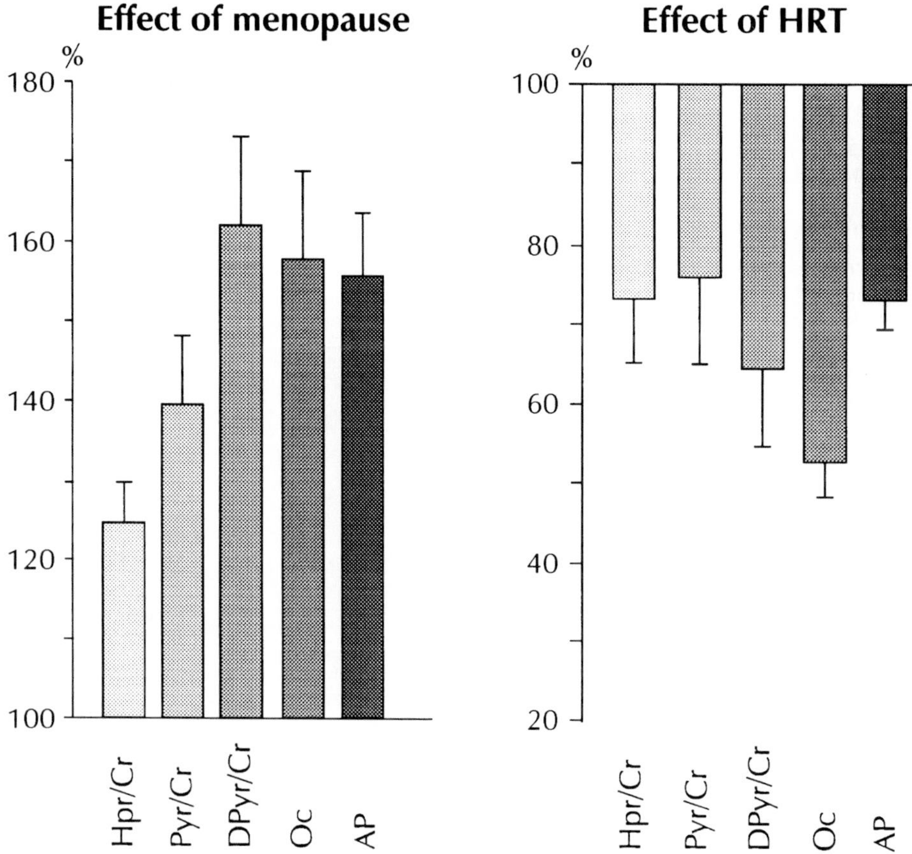

Fig. 18.4 This graph shows the effect of menopause and HRT, respectively, on three urinary markers of bone resorption (corrected for urinary creatinine excretion): hydroxyproline (Hpr/Cr), pyridinoline (Pyr/Cr), deoxypyridinoline (DPyr/Cr) and on two serum markers of bone formation: osteocalcin (Oc) and alkaline phosphatase (AP). Adapted with permission.[32]

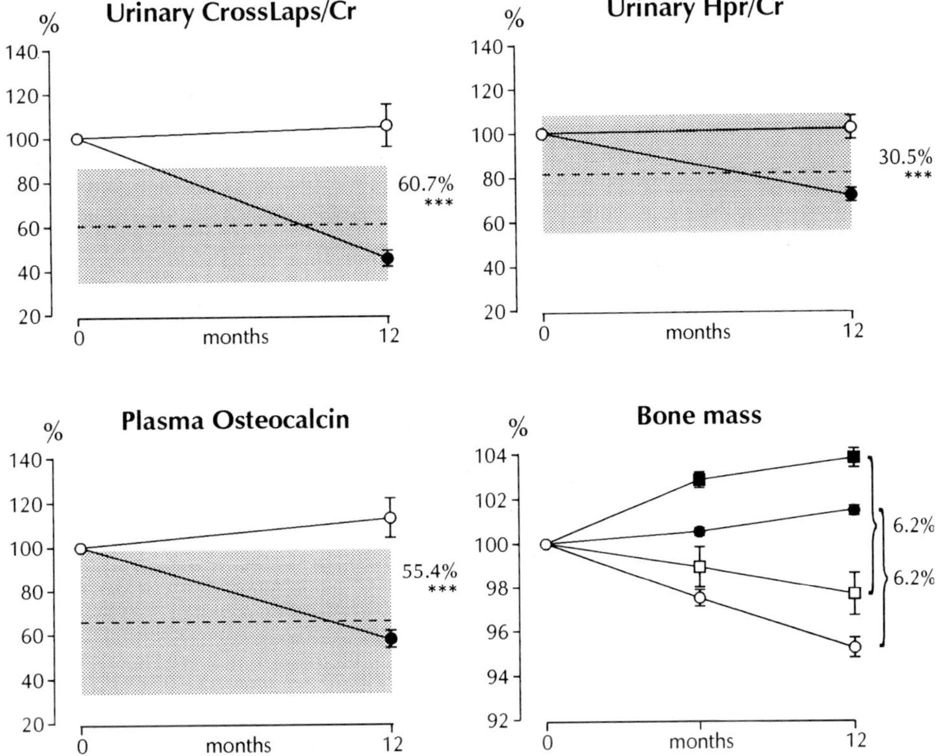

Fig. 18.5 Mean changes in the biochemical markers and forearm (●) and spinal (■) bone mass after 12 months of HRT (n=80, ●) or placebo (n=35, ○), expressed as a percentage of baseline values. The hatched areas represent the variation in premenopausal women. CrossLaps is a relatively new marker of bone resorption based on the measurement of degradation products of type I collagen crosslinks. Adapted with permission.[33]

Effect of estrogen on bone mass

Postmenopausal bone loss occurs in all parts of the skeleton, in areas with mainly trabecular bone as well as in areas with mainly cortical bone, and has been shown to be reversible through the use of HRT.[2,35,36]

The loss of bone mineral density seems to be most pronounced in the early postmenopausal years.[37] Thus, the greatest benefit from HRT is obtained if the treatment is instituted shortly after the menopause. HRT primarily decreases bone resorption and only secondarily decreases bone formation. Bone mineral density will therefore increase for some time after institution of HRT as the resorption lacunae are filled up, as can be seen in Figure 18.1. However, the rate of formation and resorption will eventually be balanced and the increase in bone mineral density will level off. Continuation of HRT after this point will result in a stabilization of the bone mineral density level. This effect persists for as long as therapy is provided and is lost when HRT is discontinued.

All estrogens appear capable of inhibiting bone loss, provided adequate doses are administered and adequate serum levels are obtained. The prevention of bone loss and, therefore, fractures will be dealt with in greater detail in chapter 54.

The effects of natural progesterone on bone

Although, there have not been many randomized clinical studies on the effect of progesterone on bone, there seems to be evidence for an important role of this hormone in human bone metabolism. Four clinical studies have found combined estrogen/progesterone therapy to be effective in preventing postmenopausal bone loss[38,39,40,41] and the combined therapy seems to be even more effective than when estrogen is administered alone.[40] This may best be explained by a remarkable uncoupling of formation and resorption is response to progesterone in favor of higher bone mass.[38]

The progesterone induced uncoupling have been confirmed in animals studies using the OVX/Sham operated rat and dog models.[42,43] Histomorphometry revealed that progesterone inhibited the increase in bone resorption parameters after OVX, whereas, the bone formation parameters remained elevated. At the moment several clinical trials are underway to further elucidate the role of progesterones in the human skeleton.

Conclusion

Several lines of evidence suggest that bone cell derived cytokines play a pivotal role in the imbalance in bone remodeling following postmenopausally or surgically induced estrogen deficiency (Fig. 18.3). In post-menopausal women, the observed increase in bone resorption, reflected in bone serum markers, is due to an increase in the number of BMU with an accelerated osteoclast activity within the single BMU. Although the bone formation will be partially increased, the volume of bone mass resorbed by osteoclasts will be greater than the bone mass formed by osteblasts. This results in an imbalanced bone remodeling with a net loss in bone mass every time a BMU has been completed. The process seems to be reversible as estrogen-therapy can reestablish balanced bone remodeling in estrogen-deficient women.

Acknowledgment The authors would like to thank Drs Bente J Riis and Jean-Marie Delais for valuable comments on the manuscript.

REFERENCES

1. Consensus Development Conference 1993 Diagnosis, prophylaxis and treatment of osteoporosis. Journal of the American Medical Association 94: 646–650
2. Christiansen C, Christensen MS, Transbol I 1981 Bone mass in postmenopausal women after withdrawal of oestrogen/gestagen replacement therapy. Lancet 1: 459–461
3. Oursler MJ, Osdoby P, Pyfferoen J, Riggs BL, Spelsberg TC 1991 Avian osteoclasts as estrogen target cells. Proceedings of the National Academy of Science, USA. 88: 6613–6617
4. Eriksen EF, Colvard DS, Berg NJ, Graham ML, Mann KG, Spelsberg TC, Riggs BL 1988 Evidence of estrogen receptors in normal human osteoblast-like cells. Science 241: 84–86
5. Komm BS, Terpening CM, Benz DJ, Graeme KA, Gallegos A, Korc M, Greene GL, O'Malley BW, Haussler MR 1988 Estrogen binding, receptor mRNA and biologic response in osteoblast-like osteosarcoma cells. Science 241: 81–84
6. Holtrop ME, Raisz LG 1979 Comparison of the effects of 1,25-dihyroxycholecalciferol, prostaglandin E_2 and osteoclast-activating factor with parathyroid hormone on the ultrastructure of osteoclasts in cultured long bones of fetal rats. Calcified Tissue International 29: 201
7. Baron R, Neff L, Louvard D, Courtoy PJ 1985 Cell-mediated extracellular acidification and bone resorption: evidence for a low pH in the resorbing lacunae and localization of a 100 kD lysosomal membrane protein at the osteoclast ruffled border. Journal of Cell Biology 101: 2210–2222
8. Delaissé JM, Boyde A, Maconnachie E, Ali NN, Sear CHJ, Eeckhout Y, Vaes G, Jones SJ 1987 The effects of inhibitors of cysteine-proteases and collagenase on the resorptive activity of isolated osteoclasts. Bone 8: 305–313
9. Parfitt AM 1979 Quantum concept of bone remodeling and turnover: implications for the pathogenesis of osteoporosis. Calcified Tissue International 28: 1–5
10. Christiansen C 1993 Can bone density be increased with estrogen therapy? In: Asch RH, Studd JWW (eds) Annual progress in reproductive medicine. Parthenon Publishing Group, USA, pp 283–290
11. Jilka RL, Hangoc G, Girasole G, Passeri G, Williams DC, Abrams JS, Boyce B, Broxmeyer H, Manolagas SC 1992 Increased osteoclast development after estrogen loss; mediation by interleukin-6. Science 257: 88–91
12. Kimble RB, Vannice JL, Bloedow DC, Thompson RC, Hopfer W, Kung VT, Brownfield C, Pacifici R 1994 Interleukin-1 receptor antagonist decreases bone loss and bone resorption in ovariectomized rats. Journal of Clinical Investigation 93: 1959–1967
13. Kitazawa R, Kimble RB, Vannice JL, Kung VT, Pacifici R 1994 Interleukin-1 receptor antagonist and tumor necrosis factor binding protein decrease osteoclast formation and bone resorption in ovariectomized mice. Journal of Clinical Investigation 94: 2397–2406
14. Ralston SH 1994 Analysis of gene expression in human bone biopsies by polymerase chain reaction: evidence for enhanced cytokine expression in postmenopausal osteoporosis. Journal of Bone and Mineral Research 9: 883–890
15. Khosla S, Peterson JM, Egan K, Jones JD, Riggs BL 1994 Circulating cytokine levels in osteoporotic and normal women. Journal of Clinical Endocrinology and Metabolism 79: 707–711
16. McKane WR, Khosla S, Peterson JM, Egan K, Riggs BL 1994 Circulating levels of cytokines that modulate bone resorption: effect of age and menopause in women Journal of Bone and Mineral Research 9: 1313–1318
17. Oursler MJ, Pederson L, Pyfferoen J, Osdoby P, Fitzpatrick LA, Spelsberg TC 1993 Estrogen modulation of avian osteoclast lysosomal gene expression. Endocrinology 132: 1373–1380
18. Oursler MJ, Pederson L, Fitzpatrick LA, Riggs BL, Spelsberg TC 1994 Human giant cell tumors of the bone (osteoclastomas) are estrogen target cells. Proceedings of the National Academy of Science, USA 88: 6613–6617
19. Pederson L, Kremer M, Foged NT, Winding B, Fitzpatrick LA, Oursler MJ 1997 Evidence of a correlation of estrogen receptor level and avian osteoclast estrogen responsiveness. Journal of Bone and Mineral Research 12: 742–752

20. Manolagas SC, Jilka RL, Girasole G, Passeri G, Bellido T 1993 Estrogen, cytokines and the control of osteoclast formation and bone resorption in vitro and in vivo. Osteoporosis International 3: 114–116
21. Kaji H, Sugimoto T, Kanatani M, Nasu M, Chihara K 1996 Estrogen blocks parathyroid hormone (PTH)-stimulated osteoclast-like cell formation by selectively affecting PTH-responsive cyclic adenosine monophosphate pathway. Endocrinology 137: 2217–2224
22. Robinson JA, Riggs BL, Spelsberg TC, Oursler MJ 1996 Osteoclasts and transforming growth factor-beta: estrogen-mediated isoform-specific regulation of production. Endocrinology 137: 615–621
23. Benz DJ, Haussler MR, Komm BS 1991 Estrogen binding and estrogenic responses in normal human osteoblast-like cells. Journal of Bone and Mineral Research 6: 531–541
24. Gray TK, Flynn TC, Gray KM, Nabell LM 1987 17β-estradiol acts directly on the clonal osteoblastic cell line UMR106. Proceedings of the National Academy of Science, USA 84: 6267–6271
25. Verhaar HJ, Damen CA, Duursma SA, Scheven BA 1994 A comparison of the action of progestins and estrogen on the growth and differentiation of normal adult human osteoblast-like cells in vitro. Bone 15: 307–311
26. Rickard DJ, Gowen M, MacDonald BR 1993 Proliferative responses to estradiol, IL-1α and TGFβ by cells expressing alkaline phosphatase in human osteoblast-like cell cultures. Calcified Tissue International 52: 227–233
27. Girasole G, Jilka RL, Passeri G, Boswell S, Boder G, Willians DC, Manolagas SC 1992 17β estradiol inhibits interleukin-6 production by bone marrow-derived stromal cells and osteoblasts in vitro: a potential mechanism for the antiresorptive effect of estrogens. Journal of Clinical Investigation 89: 883–891
28. Bellido T, Girasole G, Passeri G, Yu XP, Mocharla H, Jilka RL, Notides A, Manolagas SC 1993 Demonstration of estrogen and vitamin D receptors in bone marrow-derived stromal cells: up-regulation of the estrogen receptor by 1,25-dihydroxyvitamin-D3. Endocrinology 133: 553–562
29. Kassem M, Harris SA, Spelsberg TC, Riggs BL 1996 Estrogen inhibits interleukin-6 production and gene expression in a human osteoblastic cell line with high levels of estrogen receptors. Journal of Bone and Mineral Research 11: 193–199
30. Passeri G, Girasole G, Jilka RL, Manolagas SC 1993 Increased interleukin-6 production by murine bone marrow and bone cells after estrogen withdrawal. Endocrinology 133: 822–828
31. Rosalki SB, Foo AY 1984 Two new methods for separating and quantifying bone and liver alkaline phosphatase isoenzymes in plasme. Clinical Chemistry (July) 30(7): 1182–1186
32. Hassager C, Risteli J, Risteli L, Christiansen C 1994 Effect of the menopause and hormone replacement therapy on the carboxy-terminal pyridinoline cross-linked telopeptide of type I collagen. Osteoporosis International 4: 349–352
33. Bonde M, Qvist P, Fledelius C, Riis BJ, Christiansen C 1995 Applications of an enzyme immunoassay for a new marker of bone resorption (CrossLaps): follow-up on hormone replacement therapy and osteoporosis risk assessment. Journal of Clinical Endocrinology and Metabolism 80: 864–868
34. Christiansen C, Riis BJ, Rødbro P 1987 Prediction of rapid bone loss in postmenopausal women. Lancet 1: 1105–1108
35. Gotfredsen A, Nilas L, Riis BJ, Thomsen K, Christiansen C 1986 Bone changes occurring spontaneously and caused by oestrogen in early postmenopausal women: a local or generalized phenomenon? British Medical Journal 292: 1098–1100
36. Riis BJ, Christiansen C 1988 Measurement of spinal of peripheral bone mass to estimate early postmenopausal bone loss. American Journal of Medicine 84: 646–653
37. Nilas L, Christiansen C 1988 Rates of bone loss in normal women: evidence of accelerated trabecular bone loss after the menopause. European Journal of Clinical Investigation 18: 529–534
38. Christiansen C, Riss BJ, Nilas L, Rødbro P, Deftos L 1985 Uncoupling of bone formation and resorption by combined oestrogen and progestagen therapy in postmenopausal osteoporosis. Lancet 2: 800–801
39. Grey AB, Cundy TF, Reid IR 1994 Continuous combined oestrogen/prosgetin therapy is well tolerated and increases bone density at the hip and spine in post-menopausal osteoporosis. Clinical Endocrinology 40: 671–677
40. The Writing Group for the PEPI 1996 Effects of hormone therapy on bone mineral density: result from the postmenopausal estrogen/prosgetin interventions (PEPI) trial. JAMA 276: 1389–1396
41. Gallagher JC, Nordin EC 1975 Effects of oestrogen and progestogen therapy on calcium metabolism in post-menopausal women. Front Horm Res 3: 150–176
42. Barengolts EI, Gajardo HF, Rosol TJ, D'Anza JJ, Pena M, Botsis J, Kukreja SC 1990 Effects of progesterone on postovariectomy bone loss in aged rats. Journal of Bone and Mineral Research 5: 1143–1147
43. Karambolova KK, Snow GR, Anderson C 1986 Surface activity on the periosteal and corticoendosteal envelopes following continuous progestogen supplementation in spayed beagles. Calcified Tissue Internation 38: 239–243

19. Vascular effects of estrogen and progesterone

V.M. Miller G.C. Sieck
Y. Prakash L.A. Fitzpatrick

Introduction

Coronary artery disease is the most frequent cause of death among women in the United States. Epidemiological studies show that the incidence of coronary artery disease is lower in premenopausal women compared to age-matched men. However, the mortality from coronary artery disease is the same for postmenopausal women and age-matched men.[1,2] The reduced incidence of coronary artery disease in postmenopausal women who undergo estrogen replacement suggests that estrogen may provide protection against development of coronary artery disease.[3–6] Mechanisms by which estrogen exerts cardioprotection are beginning to be defined. Estrogen reduces serum low density lipoproteins and increases high density lipoproteins. However, these effects of estrogen on serum lipids may account for only 30% of the cardiovascular protection in women on estrogen replacement.[7] It is becoming clear that estrogen can alter all components of the vascular wall, including peripheral autonomic neurotransmission, through modulation of release, uptake and metabolism of norepinephrine at the nerve terminal.[8–10] This chapter will focus on how estrogen might affect vascular endothelium, smooth muscle and deposition of matrix proteins.

Distribution of estrogen receptors in the vascular wall

Receptors for sex steroids are present in endothelial and vascular smooth muscle cells.[11–14] The low density of estrogen receptors in atherosclerotic coronary arteries from premenopausal women compared to arteries free of disease[15] suggests that expression of estrogen receptors may be related to development of atherosclerosis. However, mechanisms affecting the nonhomogeneous distribution of these receptors are not clear.

Effects of estrogen on the endothelium

In response to blood-borne substances such as oxygen, cytokines and hormones, and mechanical forces such as pressure and shear stress, the vascular endothelium releases diffusible factors into the local environment which affect coagulation of blood, adhesion, and migration of leukocytes and the tone and proliferation of the underlying smooth muscle.[16] Estrogen increases adhesion, migration and proliferation of endothelial cells.[17] Rapid replacement of damaged endothelial cells with the subsequent release of anti-inflammatory and/or anti-proliferative cytokines from regenerated cells may limit direct effects of inflammatory processes on the smooth muscle in the vicinity of the injury.

Endothelium-derived factors can be classified as free radicals (nitric oxide and superoxide), metabolites of arachidonic acid (prostacyclin, thromboxane A_2, prostaglandins, hydroxyeicosatetraenoicacids (HETEs), epoxyeicosatrineonic acids (EETs)) or peptides (endothelins, angiotensins and natriuretic peptides like ANP and CNP, atrial and C-type natriuretic peptides, respectively).[18–24] Each factor may have multiple actions, and the actions of any given factor may antagonize those of other endothelium-derived factors. For example, nitric oxide inhibits contraction and proliferation of smooth muscle[20,25,26] while the endothelins promote contraction of smooth muscle and under some conditions, stimulate smooth muscle proliferation.[23,27] Therefore, modulation by sex steroid hormones of the ratio or balance between vasodilatory/antimitogenic and vasoconstrictor/promitogenic endothelium-derived factors may impact not only on vascular resistance but also on proliferative processes associated with coronary artery disease.

There is general agreement that estrogen replacement therapy to ovariectomized experimental animals or postmenopausal women increases release of endothelium-derived relaxing factor(s).[28–32] Estrogens may affect more than one endothelium-derived relaxing factor and the predominant factor affected by estrogen treatment may be specific for a particular vascular bed.

In support of estrogen affecting release of endothelium-derived nitric oxide are the observations that basal release of nitric oxide is greater in aorta of female rats and rabbits compared to male animals.[33] In addition, there is a positive and significant correlation among increases in estrogen and plasma concentrations of oxidized products of nitric oxide in women.[34,35] The mechanisms by which estrogens modulate production/release of nitric oxide from endothelial cells are unclear. Nitric oxide is produced enzymatically from L-arginine by the enzyme nitric oxide synthase.[36] There are three isoforms of the enzyme: Type I, neuronal; Type II, inducible; and Type III, endothelial.[37] The gene for Type III nitric oxide synthase does not contain the full palindrome for the estrogen receptor in the 5′ promoter region.[38] This does not preclude the possibility that half-palindrome regions could regulate the gene. Indeed, treatment of guinea pigs with estrogen increases mRNA for Type III enzyme in homogenates of brain and skeletal muscle.[38] Increases in mRNA for Type III enzyme are inhibited partially by the estrogen receptor antagonist tamoxifen, suggesting that there is estrogen receptor-mediated transcriptional regulation of the gene for this enzyme. These findings are consistent with increases in the amount of protein for endothelial nitric oxide synthase in cultured endothelial cells treated with estrogen.[39] However, these results are contrary to findings from experiments from our laboratory which indicate that mRNA for Type III enzyme is increased in ovariectomized compared to gonadally intact female pigs, and the amount of nitric oxide synthase measured by Western blot is the same in both groups.[40] Assessment of effects of exogenous estrogen compared to results obtained in animals with intact ovaries and the presence of other gonadal hormones may explain the differences in results.

Stimulation of muscarinic receptors on endothelial cells releases nitric oxide.[41] Endothelium-dependent relaxations to acetylcholine are increased within three minutes of acute infusion of estrogen into the coronary circulation of experimental animals and humans.[32,42] The time frame is not compatible with transcriptional activation of a gene and subsequent synthesis of enzyme. Therefore, estrogens may affect nitric oxide production/release by mechanisms other than synthesis of enzyme. For example, receptors for estrogen on the surface of endothelial cells may regulate intracellular calcium and other cofactors required for activity of endothelial nitric oxide synthase.[43,44] Alternatively, estrogens could increase the amount of nitric oxide by reducing lipid peroxidation and subsequent production of superoxide anion which could interact with nitric oxide to form peroxynitrite.[45]

In addition to direct increases in production of endothelium-derived relaxing factors, estrogen could increase endothelium-dependent relaxations indirectly through inhibition of production of endothelium-derived contractile factors. Support for this possibility is the observation that circulating concentrations of endothelin-1 decrease in male to female transsexuals.[46] Whether or not estrogens directly affect transcription of the gene for endothelin-1 is not known.

Messenger RNA for preproendothelin, the precursor for endothelin-1, is increased in aortic endothelial cells of ovariectomized female pigs compared to gonadally intact female and male pigs (Fig. 19.1). This could represent an indirect effect of decreased production of nitric oxide in the absence of estrogen, as nitric oxide decreases production of endothelin-1 in endothelial cells.[47,48]

Metabolism of arachidonic acid by cyclooxygenase results in multiple products which either stimulate (thromboxane, prostaglandin $F_{2\alpha}$) or inhibit (prostacyclin, prostaglandin $E_{1 \text{ or } 2}$) contractions of vascular smooth muscle.[19,49] Whether or not estrogen increases production of prostacyclin in endothelial cells depends upon the dose of estrogen, duration of treatment and anatomical origin of the tissue.[50]

Metabolism of arachidonic acid in endothelial cells can also occur through cytochrome P450, resulting in production of endothelium-derived hyperpolarizing factors.[21,51] Effects of estrogen on this enzyme have not been examined. Metabolism of arachidonic acid also occurs in smooth muscle cells. Therefore, actions of estrogen could affect responses to endothelium-derived factors indirectly through changes in the arachidonic acid pathway in the smooth muscle. For example, relaxations to adenosine diphosphate, a product released from aggregating platelets, are greater in femoral arteries of ovariectomized rabbits treated with estrogen when the endothelium is present. However in the presence of indomethacin, an inhibitor of cyclooxygenase, this potentiating effect to the endothelium is lost. This is probably due to inhibition of production of contractile prostanoids in the smooth muscle.[52]

It is unclear as to the extent to which progesterone antagonizes effects of estrogen on the endothelium. Endothelium-dependent relaxations to alpha$_2$-adrenergic stimulation are less in female dogs treated with estrogen and progesterone compared to

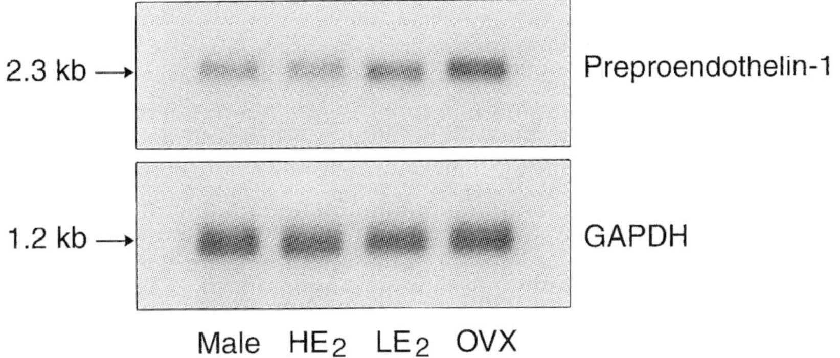

Fig. 19.1 Northern blot analysis of messenger RNA for preproendothelin in aortic endothelial cells from gonadally intact male, female (HE_2, serum estrogen >10 pg/ml; HE_2 serum estrogen <10 pg/ml) and ovariectomized (OVX) female pigs. Each lane contained the combined mRNA (1.5 μg/lane) from three separate animals. Intensity of bands for preproendothelin were compared to that for GAPDH to control for loading of mRNA onto the membrane. The intensity of band for preproendothelin was stronger in the ovariectomized female pigs compared to either gonadally intact male or female pigs.

relaxations from animals treated only with estrogen.[53] However, endothelium-dependent relaxations were not reduced in women receiving estrogen and progesterone compared to estrogen treatment alone.[54] Differences in concentrations of each replacement hormone may account for these disparate results. Alternately, if the presence of circulating hormones and mechanical stimulus of flow contributes to responses in the presence of estrogen and progesterone, *in vivo* responses would be lost when arteries are studied *in vitro*.

Effects of estrogen on vascular smooth muscle

Contraction

The final common pathway for activation of contraction in vascular smooth muscle is elevation of intracellular calcium. Intracellular calcium is elevated by influx of extracellular calcium through receptor-coupled or voltage-gated membrane channels and is decreased by efflux of intracellular calcium to the extracellular space by ion pumps. In addition, intracellular concentrations of calcium are regulated by release from and/or reuptake into the sarcoplasmic reticulum (Fig. 19.2). Estrogen may affect one or more of these mechanisms.

Regulation of receptor-coupled elevations in intracellular calcium may result from estrogen affecting protein synthesis and the number of membrane receptors.[55,56] Sex steroids also may affect receptor-coupled activation of calcium by regulating receptor affinity.[57] For example, affinity, but not the number, of

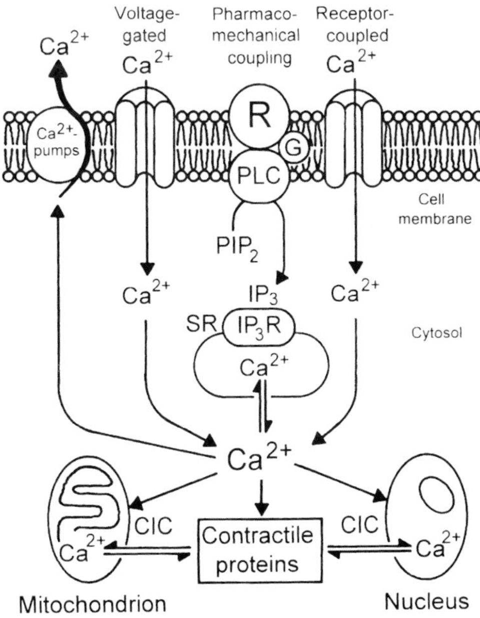

Fig. 19.2 Schematic of pathways by which intracellular calcium may be regulated in vascular smooth muscle cells. Sex steroid hormones may affect one or more of these intracellular mechanisms. Ca^{2+}, calcium; CIC, calcium stimulated calcium release; G, guanine nucleotide regulatory protein; IP_3, inosotol trisphosphate; IP_3R, inosotol receptor; PIP_2, phosphotidyl inositol biphosphate; PLC, phospholipase C; R, receptor; SR, sarcoplasmic reticulum.

receptors for the endothelium-derived contractile peptide endothelin-1 is increased in coronary arterial smooth muscle of female pigs when endogenous estrogen is high.[57] Since changes in the affinity of endothelin receptors cannot account for functional differences in contractions to endothelin-1 observed in coronary arteries of male and female pigs, other cellular mechanisms must be affected by the hormone. Estrogens may regulate intracellular calcium instead of altering the affinity of the contractile proteins to bind calcium.[58]

Several lines of evidence suggest that estrogens affect regulation of intracellular calcium through hyperpolarization of the smooth muscle cell membrane[59,60] and inhibition of voltage-gated calcium channels.[61] These latter effects require high concentrations of estrogen and are not associated with binding of estrogen to classical intracellular estrogen receptors.

Preliminary experiments from our laboratory suggest that estrogen also may regulate intracellular calcium through enhancement of calcium efflux. In freshly dissociated single coronary arterial smooth muscle cells contracted with endothelin-1 (0.1 μM), 17β-estradiol (10 nM) causes relaxation and rapid decrease in intracellular calcium in cells from sexually mature female but not ovariectomized animals (Fig. 19.3). The estrogen receptor antagonist ICI 182,780 blocks the reduction in intracellular calcium by estrogen in cells from gonadally intact females. Taken together, these data suggest that activation of an estrogen receptor reduces intracellular calcium. In cells contracted with endothelin-1, decreases in intracellular calcium by estrogen were observed even when voltage gated L-type calcium channels were blocked by nifedipine and calcium reuptake by the sarcoplasmic reticulum was blocked by thapsigargin. Under these conditions, estrogen-stimulated reductions in intracellular calcium were blocked by lanthanum, a nonspecific blocker of calcium influx and efflux. However, because inhibition of calcium influx alone with nifedipine did not alter the response to estrogen, antagonism of the response to estrogen by lanthanum may be due to inhibition of calcium efflux, either by

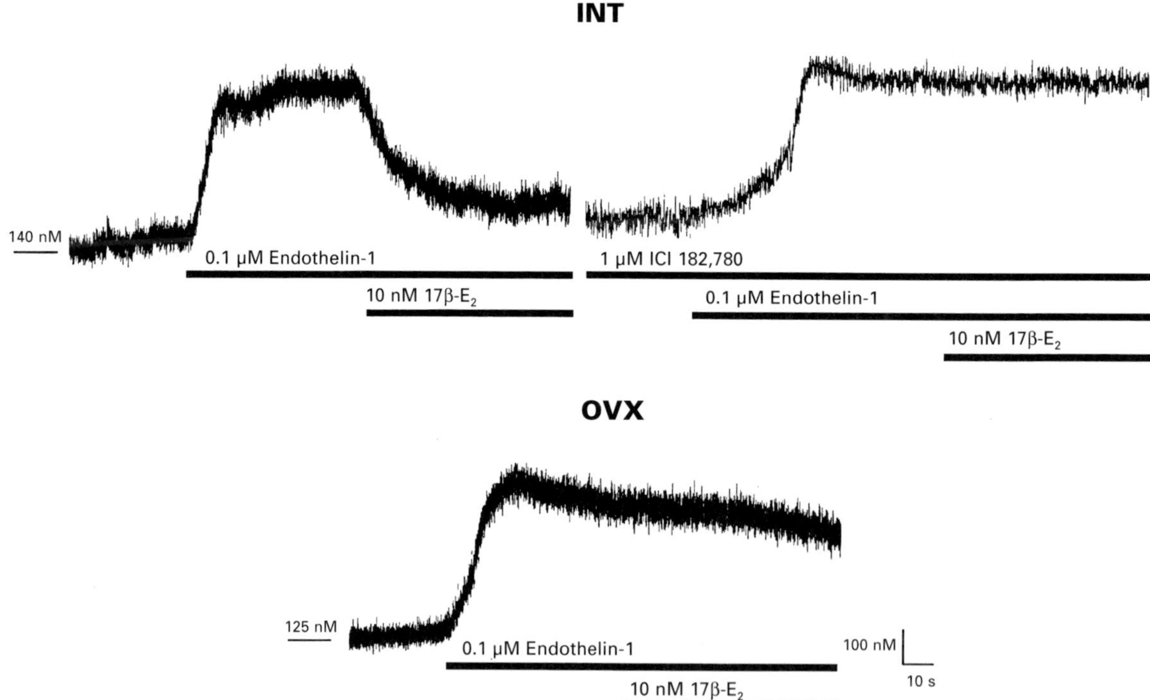

Fig. 19.3 Changes in intracellular calcium in fluo_3-loaded, freshly dispersed coronary arterial smooth muscle cells from sexually mature (INT, upper panel) and ovariectomized (OVX, lower panel) female pigs. Cells were exposed to endothelin-1 (0.1 nM) and the response allowed to stabilize. 17β-estradiol (10 nM 17β-E_2) was added acutely to the preparation. A rapid decrease in intracellular calcium was observed only in cells from sexually mature animals with intact ovaries. This decrease was blocked by the estrogen receptor antagonist ICI 182,780 (1 μM).

increasing activity of the plasma membrane calcium-activated ATPase pump or by enhancing sodium-calcium exchange.

Proliferation

In early atherosclerosis, smooth muscle cells are a dominant cell type as the tunica intima progresses to form a fibrofatty lesion.[62] Estrogen receptors are absent in regions of atherosclerotic plaque in women with coronary artery disease. Therefore, estrogen may limit progression of the fibrofatty lesion through inhibition of proliferation of smooth muscle by receptor-mediated processes.[15] Estrogen treatment also limits neointimal formation following arterial injury and transplant associated acceleration of atherosclerosis in humans and experimental animals.[63–66] These observations suggest that estrogen may inhibit in a general way proliferative processes associated with arterial injury.

Estrogen inhibits proliferation of smooth muscle cells cultured from sexually mature female but not gonadally intact male or ovariectomized female animals (Fig. 19.4).[67–69] The inactive form of estradiol, 17α-estradiol, does not inhibit proliferation of vascular smooth muscle cells from sexually mature female pigs, further pointing to the specificity of the effects of estrogen.[68] Autoradiographs of coronary arteries incubated with radiolabeled estradiol show silver grains both in the cytoplasm and over the nucleus, as would be predicted by the distribution of the hormone when binding to a receptor.[67] However, the variability with which the estrogen receptor antagonist tamoxifen blocks the antiproliferative effects of estrogen[67,69] may reflect that the drug acts as a partial estrogen receptor agonist.[70] Alternatively, vascular estrogen receptors may represent a different subclass of receptors than those found in uterine or breast tissue. The mechanism by which estrogen limits proliferation may involve regulation of immediate early response genes like C-myc.[71]

In mature female animals, another ovarian hormone, progesterone, also inhibited proliferation of cultured smooth muscle cells. However, effective concentrations required for inhibition by progesterone were greater (10^{-9} M) than those for estrogen (10^{-11} M).[68] These observations are inconsistent with studies in animals which suggest that progesterone may antagonize the antiproliferative effects of estrogen following arterial injury.[72] However, treatment with both progesterone and estrogen did not impact negatively on the regression of atherosclerotic plaque in cynomolgus monkeys[66] nor did simultaneous administration of estrogen and progestogen increase risk factors for heart disease in postmenopausal women.[73] These conflicting observations of progesterone added to estrogen treatment may point to differences in the sequence of events associated with intimal injury compared to atherosclerotic processes. Interactions among ovarian hormones may depend upon their relative concentrations, time of initiation of treatment relative to disease processes and duration of therapy.

Estrogen may also limit progression of atherosclerotic plaque formation through actions other than proliferation of smooth muscle including: cytokine-induced adhesion of leukocytes,[74] fibroblast migration,[75] and uptake/degradation of lipids.[76]

FEMALE

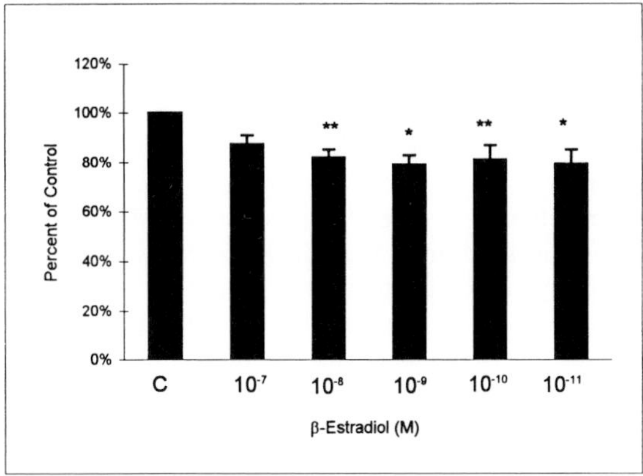

MALE

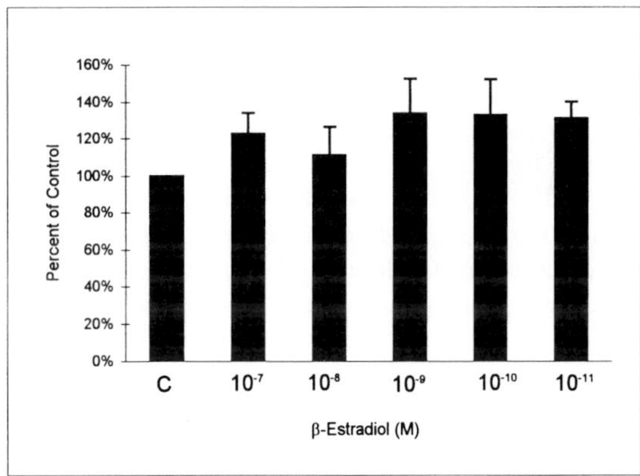

Fig. 19.4 Dose response of 17β-estradiol on thymidine incorporation in cultures of coronary arterial smooth muscle cells (VSMC) from sexually mature female (upper panel) and male (lower panel) pigs. VSMC were treated with 17β-estradiol at concentrations of 10^{-11}–10^{-7} M for 24 hours. *$P<0.005$ from control (C) by ANOVA. **=*P<..005*

Effects of estrogen on production of extracellular matrix

Coronary arterial calcification is common in patients with coronary artery disease and increases dramatically as a function of age. The onset and progression of calcification is poorly understood. However, new evidence suggests that pathologic calcification of atherosclerotic arteries shares features in common with normal bone, including expression of bone morphogenetic protein-2a,[77] Type I collagen,[78] phosphatases, calcium-binding phospholipids, matrix vesicles that serve as nucleators of crystal formation[79] and mineral deposits of crystal and hydroxyapatite.[77]

Human atherosclerotic coronary arteries were prepared undecalcified and mineralization was found within the plaque and adventitia suggesting that mineralization may play a major role in alterations in arterial compliance and elasticity (Fig. 19.5). Methyl methracylate-embedded sections of undecalcified atherosclerotic coronary arteries were stained for hydroxyapatite using Goldner's Masson-Trichome. Arteries without plaques showed no positive staining for hydroxyapatite. To determine the extent of calcification, undecalcified specimens were embedded in glycomethylacrylate and subjected to x-ray microradiographs. Calcified plaques contained a calcium to phosphate molar ratio of 1.55:1 to 1.70:1 which corresponds closely to the known ratio of 1.66:1 of hydroxyapatite in bone. In addition, the calcification was associated with osteopontin, a matrix protein involved in normal bone mineralization. Tissue surrounding osteopontin-positive plaque stained negative for osteopontin, as did arterial segments free of atheroma (Fig. 19.5).[80]

Noncollagenous proteins are synthesized and released in the extracellular space where they regulate the growth of hydroxyapatite crystals during the process of calcification in bone. Osteopontin is a complex protein associated with mineral binding and cell attachment.[81] It may regulate mineralization of the arterial wall because it has affinity for both calcium and hydroxyapatite. However, osteopontin may act as either a promoter or as an inhibitor of calcification in the atherosclerotic plaque.

Cell cultures of porcine coronary arterial smooth muscle express osteopontin as well as other non-collagenous matrix proteins such as osteocalcin, osteonectin, bone sialoprotein, decorin, biglycan and Type I collagen.[82] Dynamic changes in the matrix composition of atherosclerotic arteries may make the tissue more susceptible to calcification. The decrease in estrogens associated with menopause may represent one such condition which influences the extracellular matrix. Further studies are necessary to evaluate the influence of sex steroids on matrix production.

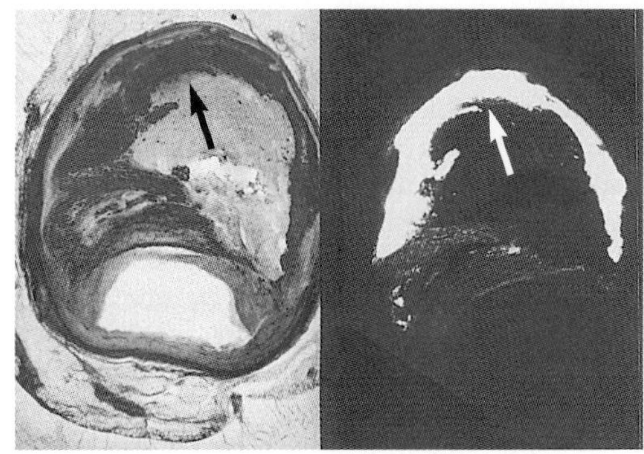

Fig. 19.5 Light microscopy cross section of an undecalcified human atherosclerotic coronary artery embedded in methylmethacrylate and stained with Goldner's Masson-Trichome (left panel) which is specific for hydroxyapatite (arrows). In areas of the artery not associated with atherosclerotic plaque, no hydroxyapatite was detected. Adjacent sections were not decalcified and examined for calcium deposits by x-ray microradiography (right panel). Deposits of mineral are apparent as radiodense images in the microradiograph (white area). The distribution of calcium was consistent with the distribution of hydroxyapatite.

REFERENCES

1. Furman RH 1968 Are gonadal hormones (estrogens and androgens) of significance in the development of ischemic heart disease? Annals of the New York Academy of Science 149: 822–833
2. Barrett-Connor E, Bush TL 1991 Estrogen and coronary heart disease in women. Journal of the American Medical Association 265(14): 1861–1867
3. Stampfer MJ, Colditz GA, Willett WC et al 1991 Postmenopausal estrogen therapy and cardiovascular disease: ten-year follow-up from the Nurses' Health Study. New England Journal of Medicine 325: 756–762
4. Stampfer MJ, Colditz GA 1991 Estrogen replacement therapy and coronary heart disease: a quantitative assessment of the epidemiologic evidence. Preventive Medicine 20: 47–63
5. Ettinger B, Friedman GD, Bush T, Quesenberry CP, Jr 1996 Reduced mortality associated with long-term postmenopausal estrogen therapy. Obstetrics and Gynecology 87(1): 6–12
6. Paganini-Hill A 1995 The risks and benefits of estrogen replacement therapy: leisure world. International Journal of Fertility and Menopause Studies 40(Suppl 1): 54–62

7. Samaan SA, Crawford MH 1995 Estrogen and cardiovascular function after menopause. Journal of the American College of Cardiology 26(6): 1403–1410
8. Hamlet MA, Rorie DK, Tyce GM 1980 Effects of estradiol on release and disposition of norepinephrine from nerve endings. American Journal of Physiology 239: H450–H456
9. Chan C-C, Kalsner S 1982 Termination of responses to sympathetic nerve stimulation and to noradrenaline in a perfused arterial preparation: the role of neuronal and extraneuronal uptake. Journal of Pharmacology and Experimental Therapeutics 222: 731–740
10. Du X-J, Dart AM, Riemersma RA, Oliver MF 1991 Sex difference in presynaptic adrenergic inhibition of norepinephrine release during normoxia and ischemia in the rat heart. Circulation Research 68: 827–835
11. Colburn P, Buonassisi V 1978 Estrogen-binding sites in endothelial cell cultures. Science 201: 817–819
12. Kim-Schulze S, McGowan KA, Hubchak SC, Cid MC, Martin MB, Kleinman HK, Greene GL, Schnaper HW 1996 Expression of an estrogen receptor by human coronary artery and umbilical vein endothelial cells. Circulation 94: 1402–1407
13. Bei M, Lavigne MC, Foegh ML, Ramwell PW, Clarke R. Specific binding of estradiol to rat coronary artery smooth muscle cells. Journal of Steroid Biochemistry and Molecular Biology 58(1): 83–88
14. Karas RH, Patterson BL, Mendelsohn ME 1994 Human vascular smooth muscle cells contain functional estrogen receptor. Circulation 89: 1943–1950
15. Losordo DW, Kearney M, Kim EA, Jekanowski J, Isner JM 1994 Variable expression of the estrogen receptor in normal and atherosclerotic coronary arteries of premenopausal women. Circulation 89: 1501–1510
16. Ralevic V, Lincoln J, Burnstock G, Ryan US, Rubanyi GM (eds) 1992 Endothelial regulation of vascular tone. Marcel Dekker, Inc, New York, ch 18, pp 297–328
17. Morales DE, McGowan KA, Grant DS, Maheshwari S, Bhartiya D, Cid MC, Kleinman HK, Schnaper HW 1995 Estrogen promotes angiogenic activity in human umbilical vein endothelial cells in vitro and in a murine model. Circulation 91: 755–763
18. Katusic ZS, Vanhoutte PM 1989 Superoxide anion is an endothelium-derived contracting factor. American Journal of Physiology 257: H33–H37
19. Miller VM, Vanhoutte PM 1985 Endothelium-dependent contractions to arachidonic acid are mediated by products of cyclo-oxygenase. American Journal of Physiology 248: H432–H437
20. Ignarro LJ 1989 Endothelium-derived nitric oxide: actions and properties. The FASEB Journal 3: 31–36
21. Campbell WB, Gebremedhin D, Pratt PF, Harder DR 1996 Identification of epoxyeicosatrienoic acids as endothelium-derived hyperpolarizing factors. Circulation Research 78: 415–423
22. Bunting S, Gryglewski R, Moncada S, Vane JR 1976 Arterial walls generate from prostaglandin endoperoxides a substance (prostaglandin X) which relaxes strips of mesenteric and coeliac arteries and inhibits platelet aggregation. Prostaglandins 12(6): 897–913
23. Yanagisawa M, Kurihara H, Kimura S, Tomobe Y, Kobayashi M, Mitsui Y, Yuzaki Y, Goto K, Masaki T 1988 A novel potent vasoconstrictor peptide produced by vascular endothelial cells. Nature 332: 411–415
24. Suga S, Itoh H, Komatsu Y, Ogawa Y, Hama N, Yoshimasa T, Nakao K 1993 Cytokine-induced C-type natriuretic peptide (CNP) secretion from vascular endothelial cells — evidence for CNP as a novel autocrine/paracrine regulator from endothelial cells. Endocrinology 133: 3038–4041
25. Garg UC, Hassid A 1989 Nitric oxide-generating vasodilators and 8-bromo-cyclic guanosine monophosphate inhibit mitogenesis and proliferation of cultured rat vascular smooth muscle cells. Journal of Clinical Investigation 83: 1774–1777
26. Assender JW, Southgate KM, Newby AC 1991 Does nitric oxide inhibit smooth muscle proliferation? Journal of Cardiovascular Pharmacology 17(Suppl 3): S104–S107
27. Dubin D, Pratt RE, Cooke JP, Dzau VJ 1989 Endothelin, a potent vasoconstrictor, is a vascular smooth muscle mitogen. Journal of Vascular Medicine and Biology 1: 150–154
28. Bell DR, Rensberger HJ, Koritnik DR, Koshy A 1995 Estrogen pretreatment directly potentiates endothelium-dependent vasorelaxation of porcine coronary arteries. American Journal of Physiology 268: H377–H383
29. Gisclard V, Miller VM, Vanhoutte PM 1988 Effect of 17β-estradiol on endothelium-dependent responses in the rabbit. Journal of Pharmacology and Experimental Therapy 244: 19–22
30. Williams JK, Shively CA, Clarkson TB 1994 Determinants of coronary artery reactivity in premenopausal female cynomolgus monkeys with diet-induced atherosclerosis. Circulation 90: 983–987
31. Lieberman EH, Gerhard MD, Uehata A, Walsh BW, Selwyn AP, Ganz P, Yeung AC, Creager MA 1994 Estrogen improves endothelium-dependent flow-mediated vasodilation in postmenopausal women. Annals of Internal Medicine 121: 936–941
32. Reis SE, Gloth ST, Blumenthal RS, Resar JR, Zacur Ha, Gerstenblith G, Brinker JA 1994 Ethinyl estradiol acutely attenuates abnormal coronary vasomotor responses to acetylcholine in postmenopausal women. Circulation 89: 52–60
33. Hayashi T, Fukuto JM, Ignarro LJ, Chaudhuri G 1992 Basal release of nitric oxide from aortic rings is greater in female rabbits than in male rabbits: implications for atherosclerosis. Proceedings of the National Academy of Science 89(23): 11259–11263
34. Hashimoto M, Akishita M, Eto M, Ishikawa M, Kozaki K, Toba K, Sagara Y, Taketani Y, Orimo H, Ouchi Y 1995 Modulation of endothelium-dependent flow-mediated dilatation of the brachial artery by sex and menstrual cycle. Circulation 92: 3431–3435
35. Kharitonov SA, Logan-Sinclair RB, Busselt CM, Shinebourne EA 1994 Peak expiratory nitric oxide differences in men and women: relation to the menstrual cycle. British Heart Journal 72: 243–245
36. Palmer RMJ, Rees DD, Ashton DS, Moncada S 1988 L-arginine is the physiological precursor for the formation of nitric oxide in endothelium-dependent relaxation. Biochemical and Biophysical Research Communications 153: 1251–1256
37. Marsden PA, Schappert KT, Chen HS, Flowers M, Sundell CL, Wilcox JN, Lamas S, Michel T 1992 Molecular cloning and characterization of human endothelial nitric oxide synthase. FEBS Letters 307: 287–293

38. Weiner CP, Lizasoain I, Baylis SA, Knowles RG, Charles IG, Moncada S 1994 Induction of calcium-dependent nitric oxide synthases by sex hormones. Proceedings of the National Academy of Science 91: 5212–5216
39. Hayashi T, Yamada K, Esaki T, Kuzuya M, Satake S, Ishikawa T, Hidaka H, Iguchi A 1995 Estrogen increases endothelial nitric oxide by a receptor-mediated system. Biochemical and Biophysical Research Communications 214(3): 847–855
40. Wang X, Barber DA, Lewis DA et al 1997 Gender and transcriptional regulation of NO synthase and ET-1 in porcine aortic endothelial cells. American Journal of Physiology 273(42): H1962–H1967
41. Palmer RMJ, Ferrige AG, Moncada S 1987 The release of nitric oxide by vascular endothelial cells accounts for the activity of EDRF. Nature 327: 524–526
42. Gilligan DM, Badar DM, Panza JA, Quyyumi AA, Cannon RO III 1994 Acute vascular effects of estrogen in postmenopausal women. Circulation 90: 786–791
43. Morley P, Whitfield JF, Vanderhyden BC, Tsang BK, Schwartz J 1992 A new, nongenomic estrogen action: the rapid release of intracellular calcium. Endocrinology 131: 1305–1312
44. Hayashi T, Ishikawa T, Yamada K, Kuzuya M, Naito M, Hidaka H, Iguchi A 1994 Biphasic effect of estrogen on neuronal constitutive nitric oxide synthase via Ca^{2+}-calmodulin dependent mechanism. Biochemical and Biophysical Research Communications 203: 1013–1019
45. Arnal JF, Clamens S, Pechet C, Negre-Salvayre A, Allera C, Girolami JP, Salvayre R, Bayard F 1996 Ethinylestradiol does not enhance the expression of nitric oxide synthase in bovine endothelial cells but increases the release of bioactive nitric oxide by inhibiting superoxide anion production. Proceedings of the National Academy of Science 93(9): 4108–4113
46. Polderman KH, Stehouwer CDA, van Kamp GJ, Dekker GA, Verheugt FWA, Gooren LJG 1993 Influence of sex hormones on plasma endothelin levels. Annals of Internal Medicine 118: 429–432
47. Boulanger C, Luscher TF 1990 Release of endothelin from the porcine aorta. Journal of Clinical Investigation 85: 587–590
48. Flowers MA, Wang Y, Stewart RJ, Patel B, Marsden PA 1995 Reciprocal regulation of endothelin-1 and endothelial constitutive NOS in proliferating endothelial cells. American Journal of Physiology 269(38): H1988–H1997
49. DeMey JG, Vanhoutte PM 1982 Heterogeneous behavior of the canine arterial and venous wall. Circulation Research 51: 439–447
50. Barber DA, Miller VM 1998 Endothelium-dependent vasoconstrictors. In: Estrogen and the Vessel Wall, edited by Rubanyi GM, Berkeley CA. Harwood Academic Publishers, pp 167–185
51. Harder DR, Campbell WB, Roman RJ 1995 Role of cytochrome P-450 enzymes and metabolites of arachidonic acid in the control of vascular tone. Journal of Vascular Research 32(2): 79–92
52. Miller VM, Gisclard V, Vanhoutte PM 1988 Modulation of endothelium-dependent and vascular smooth muscle responses by oestrogens. Phlebology 3: 63–69
53. Miller VM, Vanhoutte PM 1991 Progesterone and modulation of endothelium-dependent responses in canine coronary arteries. American Journal of Physiology 261: R1022–R1027
54. Gerhard MD, Tawakol A, Haley EA et al 1996 Long-term estradiol therapy with or without progesterone improves endothelium-dependent vasodilation in postmenopausal women. Circulation 94(8): I-279 (Abstract)
55. Freedman RR, Sabharwal SC, Desai N 1987 Sex differences in peripheral vascular adrenergic receptors. Circulation Research 61: 581–585
56. Gisclard V, Flavahan NA, Vanhoutte PM 1987 Alpha-adrenergic responses of blood vessels of rabbits after ovariectomy and administration of 17β-estradiol. Journal of Pharmacology and Experimental Therapeutics 240: 446–470
57. Barber DA, Sieck GC, Fitzpatrick LA, Miller VM 1996 Endothelin receptors are modulated in association with endogenous fluctuations in estrogen. American Journal of Physiology 271(40): H1999–H2006
58. Miller VM, Barber DA, Fenton AM, Wang X, Sieck GC 1996 Gender differences in response to endothelin-1 in coronary arteries: transcription, receptors and calcium regulation. Clinical and Experimental Pharmacology and Physiology 23: 256–259
59. Harder DR, Coulson PB 1979 Estrogen receptors and effects of estrogen on membrane electrical properties of coronary vascular smooth muscle. Journal of Cell Physiology 100: 375–382
60. White RE, Darkow DJ, Falvo Lang JL 1995 Estrogen relaxes coronary arteries by opening BK_{Ca} channels through a cGMP-dependent mechanism. Circulation Research 77: 936–942
61. Sudhir K, Chou TM, Mullen WL, Hausmann D, Collins P, Yock PG, Chatterjee K 1995 Mechanisms of estrogen-induced vasodilatation: in vivo studies in canine coronary conductance and resistance arteries. Journal of the American College of Cardiology 26: 807–814
62. Raines EW, Ross R 1993 Smooth muscle cells and the pathogenesis of the lesion of atherosclerosis. British Heart Journal 69(Suppl): S30–S37
63. Foegh ML, Asotra S, Howell MH, Ramwell PW 1994 Estradiol inhibition of arterial neointimal hyperplasia after balloon injury. Journal of Vascular Surgery 19(4): 722–726
64. O'Keefe JH, Kim SC, Hall RR, Cochran VC, Lawhorn SL, McCallister BD 1997 Estrogen replacement therapy after coronary angioplasty in women. Journal of the American College of Cardiology 29(1): 1–5
65. Foegh ML, Khirabadi BS, Nakanishi T, Vargas R, Ramwell PW 1987 Estradiol protects against experimental cardiac transplant atherosclerosis. Transplant Proceedings 19: 90–95
66. Adams MR, Kaplan JR, Manuck SB, Koritnik DR, Parks JS, Wolfe MS, Clarkson TB 1990 Inhibition of coronary artery atherosclerosis by 17-beta estradiol in ovariectomized monkeys. Lack of an effect of added progesterone. Arteriosclerosis 10(6): 1051–1057
67. Vargas R, Wroblewska B, Rego A, Hatch J, Ramwell PW 1993 Oestradiol inhibits smooth muscle cell proliferation of pig coronary artery. British Journal of Pharmacology 109: 612–617

68. Moraghan T, Antoniucci DM, Grenert JP, Sieck GC, Johnson C, Miller VM, Fitzpatrick LA 1996 Differential response in cell proliferation to beta estradiol in coronary artery vascular smooth muscle cells obtained from mature female versus male animals. Endocrinology 137: 5174–5177
69. Espinosa E, Oemar BS, Luscher TF 1996 17 beta-estradiol and smooth muscle cell proliferation in aortic cells of male and female rats. Biochemical and Biophysical Research Communications 221(1): 8–14
70. Jordan VC 1984 Biochemical pharmacology of antiestrogen action. Pharmacology Reviews 36: 245–257
71. Philips A, Chalbos D, Rochefort H 1993 Estradiol increases and anti-estrogens antagonize the growth factor-induced activator protein-1 activity in MCF7 breast cancer cells without affecting *c-fos* and *c-jun* synthesis. Journal of Biological Chemistry 268(19): 14103–14108
72. Levine RL, Chen S, Durand J, Chen Y, Oparil S 1994 Medroxyprogesterone attenuates estrogen-mediated inhibition of neointima formation after balloon injury of the rat carotid artery. Circulation 94: 2221–2227
73. The Writing Group for the PEPI Trial 1995 Effects of estrogen or estrogen/progestin regimens on heart disease risk factors in postmenopausal women. The postmenopausal estrogen/progestin interventions (PEPI) trial. Journal of the American Medical Association 273(3): 199–208
74. Caulin-Glaser T, Watson CA, Pardi R, Bender JR 1996 Effects of 17β-estradiol on cytokine-induced endothelial cell adhesion molecule expression. Journal of Clinical Investigation 98: 36–42
75. Shi Y, O'Brien JE, Fard A, Mannion JD, Wang D, Zalewski A 1996 Adventitial myofibroblasts contribute to neointimal formation in injured porcine coronary arteries. Circulation 94: 1655–1664
76. Wagner JD, Clarkson TB, St Clair RW, Schwenke DC, Shively CA, Adams MR 1991 Estrogen and progesterone replacement therapy reduces low density lipoprotein accumulation in the coronary arteries of surgically postmenopausal cynomolgus monkeys. Journal of Clinical Investigation 88(6): 1995–2002
77. Bostrom K, Watson KE, Horn S, Wortham C, Herman IM, Demer LL 1993 Bone morphogenetic protein expression in human atherosclerotic lesions. Journal of Clinical Investigation 91(4): 1800–1809
78. Murata K, Motoyama T 1990 Collagen species in various sized human arteries and their changes with intimal proliferation. Artery 17: 96–106
79. Tanimura A, McGregor D, Anderson H 1986 Calcification in atherosclerosis I. Human studies. Journal of Experimental Pathology 2: 261–273
80. Fitzpatrick LA, Severson A, Edwards WD, Ingram RT 1994 Diffuse calcification in human coronary arteries. Association of osteopontin with atherosclerosis. Journal of Clinical Investigation 94(4): 1597–1604
81. Butler W 1989 The nature and significance of osteopontin. Connective Tissue Research 23: 123–136
82. Severson A, Ingram R, Fitzpatrick LA 1995 Matrix proteins associated with bone calcification are present in human vascular smooth muscle cells grown *in vitro*. In Vitro Cellular Developmental Biology 31: 853–857

20. Estrogen and progesterone effects on nonreproductive tissues: urinary tract

S. Johnston   S. Stanton

Introduction

Our population is ageing, with ever increasing numbers of women entering the postmenopausal years. Furthermore, beyond menopause, women are living longer, with the average female life span now extending beyond 80 years. Since the menopause causes a hypoestrogenic state, those problems and diseases affected by estrogen deficiency must now receive increasing attention.

Urinary symptoms in the menopause include incontinence, urgency, frequency, nocturia, dysuria, and in some, recurrent urinary tract infections. These symptoms, while not life-threatening, can interfere significantly with quality of life. With varying success, exogenous estrogen replacement may improve these symptoms.

THE URINARY TRACT: BASIC CONSIDERATIONS

Embryology

Approximately two weeks after conception, the human embryo exists as a trilaminar disc, with mesoderm sandwiched between layers of ectoderm. Caudally, however, endoderm and ectoderm are tightly fused without intervening mesoderm to form the cloacal membrane (Fig. 20.1).

Concomitantly, the allantois is formed as an outpouching from the yolk sac. As the embryo grows and bends, the allantois is carried ventrally, along with the cloacal membrane. The hindgut of the embryo enlarges and receives the allantois, forming a terminal cavity, the cloaca. Mesoderm migrates around the cloaca, producing urethral folds laterally, and in the midline the genital tubercle from which the labia minora and clitoris derive.

In the fifth week of development, the cloaca becomes divided by the urorectal septum, a spur of mesoderm growing caudally between the hindgut and allantois. The primitive urogenital sinus and rectum are thus formed as compartments (Fig. 20.2). By this time, the mesonephric ducts have reached the urogenital sinus. Above these ducts, the primitive urogenital sinus differentiates to form the vesicourethral canal, from which the female bladder and proximal and midportions of the urethra later develop. Below the mesonephric ducts, the true urogenital sinus remains, from which the distal urethra, distal vagina and vestibule are derived. This common embryologic origin undoubtedly accounts for the similar hormonal responsiveness of these organs.

Functional anatomy

The urinary bladder is hollow muscular organ which functions as a reservoir for urine. It is lined by transitional epithelium, with detrusor smooth muscle beneath. Over most of the bladder, detrusor muscle fibers run in various directions, creating a web-like anatomy which permits uniform contraction upon emptying. In the base of the bladder is a triangular-shaped area, the trigone. It is here that both ureteric orifices and the internal urethral orifice are found. Distinct superficial and deep smooth muscle layers are present here, with the deep fibers fusing somewhat with detrusor fibers.

The urethra is a tubular structure 3–4 cm long, with a diameter of approximately 6 mm.[1] Distally, it is lined by a stratified squamous epithelium continuous with that of the vulva. Near the bladder neck, this epithelium becomes transitional, though it may undergo squamous metaplasia during the reproductive years.[2] Supporting the epithelium of the urethra is a submucosal layer containing abundant collagen and elastic fibers, as well as thin-walled veins and capillaries which are thought to be important in generating urethral resistance. The urethral smooth musculature lies beneath, comprised mainly of longitudinal fibers, with fewer circular fibers more

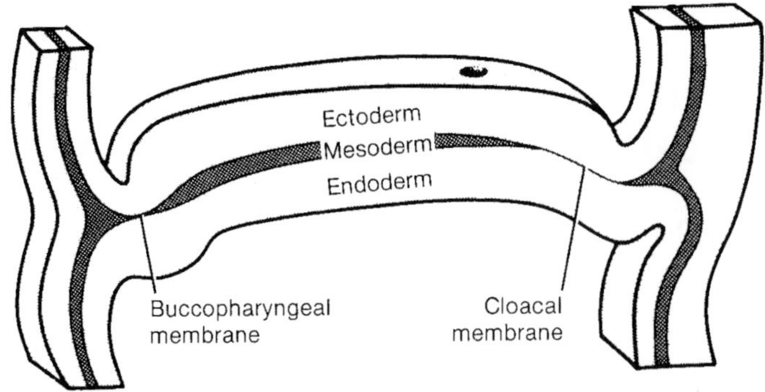

Fig. 20.1 Embryonic plate approximately one day after fertilization. Ectoderm and endoderm are separated from each other by mesoderm except in region of buccopharyngeal and cloacal membranes. (Courtesy of Gosling JA, Dixon J, Humpherson JR 1982 Functional anatomy of the urinary tract. Gower Medical Publishing Ltd, London)

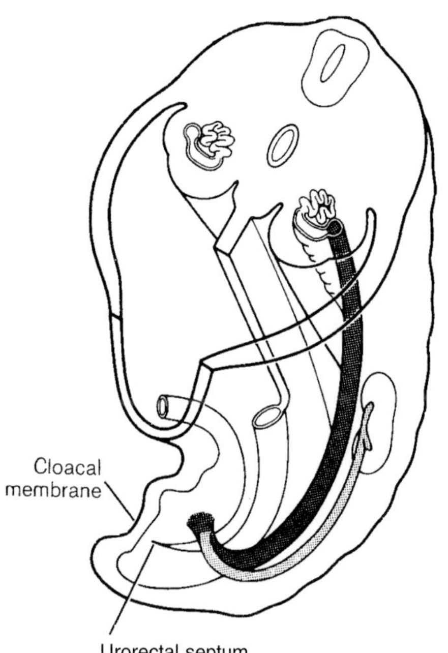

Fig. 20.2 Embryo approximately 32 days (8 mm crown–rump length) after fertilization. Definitive ureter and mesonephric duct share a common opening into partially divided cloaca. Cloacal membrane and urorectal septum are indicated. Note that ureter has induced formation of kidney from metanephrogenic blastema. (Courtesy of Gosling JA, Dixon J, Humpherson JR 1982 Functional anatomy of the urinary tract. Gower Medical Publishing Ltd, London)

peripherally. Together with the detrusor muscle of the trigone, this smooth muscle forms the internal urethral sphincter, at the bladder neck, though this sphincter is difficult to define well anatomically. Finally, striated muscle wraps around the urethra in band-like fashion (Fig. 20.3). Along with the skeletal muscle of the pelvic floor, this muscle forms the external (voluntary) urethral sphincter.

The pelvic floor, containing the levator ani muscles and fascia and the urogenital diaphragm, provides anatomic support for the bladder base and urethra, the uterus and vagina and the rectum, as well as the intra-abdominal contents above.

Estrogen and progesterone receptors

Animal work has demonstrated the presence of estrogen receptors in bladder and urethral tissues of the rabbit[3] and baboon,[4] but in the urethra only in dogs.[5]

In human studies, Iosif and colleagues have demonstrated the existence of high affinity estrogen receptors, similar to those in the vagina, in the female urethra and bladder,[6] though with concentrations considerably higher in the urethra than in the bladder.

Although progesterone receptors have been demonstrated in the urethra and bladder of estrogenized rabbits,[7,8] studies on human tissues, regardless of estrogen status, have not consistently documented their presence in either the bladder or the urethra.[6,9,10] If, indeed, progesterone receptors are present in the human urinary tract, their number is low. Although progesterone does reduce the number of estrogen receptors in endometrial tissue, it does not appear (at least in the rabbit) to decrease estrogen receptor numbers in the urethra.[11]

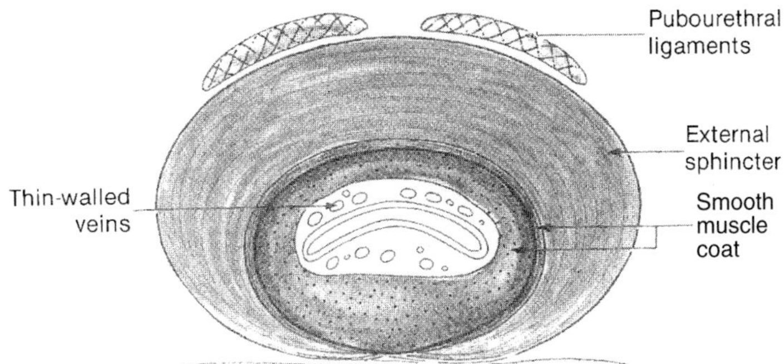

Fig. 20.3 Horizontal section of female urethra. Pubourethral ligaments lie anterior to striated urethral muscle, which forms external sphincter. Smooth muscle coat consists of relatively minor outer circular part and much thicker inner longitudinal component. Lamina propria contains numerous prominent thin-walled veins.

The continence mechanism

In order for continence to exist, intraurethral resistance must exceed the intravesical pressure at all times except during voiding. Both the internal and the external urethral sphincters contribute to this resistance, as do also mucosal and submucosal factors within the urethra itself.

Primary control over the bladder is exerted by the parasympathetic component of the autonomic nervous system, while at the bladder neck and urethra (i.e. the internal urethral sphincter), the sympathetic system predominates. α-adrenergic stimulation thus increases urethral resistance, and correspondingly, α blockade decreases it. Alone, however, the internal sphincter is weak, and unable itself to generate enough resistance to prevent urine loss. Thus, urethral resistance must be enhanced by other mechanisms.

The urethra and bladder neck, as proposed by Delancey,[12] are supported in sling like fashion by the anterior vaginal wall, which is itself supported by the pelvic floor musculature and endopelvic fascia. In the normal continent female, the internal urethral sphincter is supported as an intra-abdominal structure, and intra-abdominal pressure transmission to the bladder and proximal urethra is thus equal. Intraurethral resistance is in this way provided indirectly at the bladder neck. When the proximal urethra is not intra-abdominal, as in the situation of a cystourethrocele, pressure transmission is unequal, and stress incontinence may develop.

The external urethral sphincter maintains a resting tone and resistance at the level of the urethra, but either through voluntary or reflex control this can be enhanced when intra-abdominal pressure rises when urgency occurs to prevent incontinence. Fantl[13] has described this as a 'defence mechanism' to maintain continence when the internal sphincter fails.

Urethral resistance is additionally influenced by the 'mucosal seal mechanism,'[14] which incorporates the factors of urethral epithelial thickness, the degree of congestion of the submucosal vasculature, and the content of submucosal collagen and elastin.

Urethral resistance remains rather difficult to quantitate accurately. The urethral pressure profile has commonly been used, which generates clinical parameters including the maximal urethral closure pressure (MUCP), the functional urethral length, and the pressure transmission ratio (PTR). Of these, MUCP during stress is most important; it is this parameter that has been shown to change following successful surgery for genuine stress incontinence,[15,16,17] though even this has been questioned by some.[18]

Hormone action

Estrogen can act at several levels to promote urethral resistance and thus improve continence. In the rabbit urethra, estrogens have been shown to increase α-receptor sensitivity in the urethral smooth muscle.[19] Similarly, in humans, treatment for stress incontinence using estrogen and phenylpropanolamine in combination seems to have a synergistic result. Hilton and colleagues[20] in a double-blind, placebo controlled trial using estrogen with or without phenylpropanolamine in 60 postmenopausal women, found an objective improvement in stress incontinence in only those women who received combination therapy.

Estrogen administration has been shown to reduce descent of the bladder base observed using videocystourethrography,[21] and may thus play a role in maintaining musculofascial support to the urethra and pelvic floor. Rud and group[22] similarly hypothesized that the improvement in urethral pressure transmission they observed after estrogen treatment was due to improved function of the pelvic floor muscles and fascia. Bacho and Winandy[23] reported preliminary evidence showing improved pelvic floor tone and contractility in estrogen supplemented menopausal women as compared to menopausal women not receiving hormonal replacement, though their study numbers were small. Estrogen receptors have been demonstrated in high number in the vesicovaginal fascia.[24]

As noted previously, estrogen receptors are found in abundance in the epithelial and submucosal tissues of the urethra. In estrogen deficiency, there is thinning of both the vaginal and urinary tract epithelium.[6,10] Estrogen affects urethral cells by influencing the growth and maturation of squamous cells, a mechanism similar to that seen in the vagina. Administration of estrogens to postmenopausal women increases urethral pressure and mucosal thickness and blood vessel engorgement.[25] Furthermore, hypoestrogenism reduces the collagen content and impacts upon the mechanical properties of the skin.[26] Versi and coworkers showed that perineal skin collagen content was reflective of urethral collagen content.[27] At the level of the urethra, then, estrogen deficiency compromises the ability of the urethra to maintain an adequate mucosal seal and thus favors the development of urinary incontinence.

Fantyl and coworkers[28] have proposed that hypoestrogenism may reduce the sensory threshold of the lower urinary tract. They compared clinical and urodynamic variables in two groups of postmenopausal women, one group taking estrogen and one not. Women not supplemented experienced significantly more urge incontinence and nocturia. Interestingly, measures of urethral function (MUCP and functional length) were not different between groups.

Severe atrophy of the urethra can progress to urethral stricture formation,[29] with resultant voiding difficulty. It has thus been suggested that estrogen replacement therapy be used for both prevention and treatment of urethral stricture. Their rationale for estrogen use here is logical, though admittedly there are as yet no randomized, controlled data in the literature to support this use.

In the uterus, progesterone causes smooth muscle relaxation, so it can be expected that progesterone would have a similar relaxing effect on the bladder and urethra. There are, however, few (if any) progesterone receptors in the human bladder and urethra, so the influence of this steroid hormone on the urinary tract is not likely to be very important clinically. The effects on the urinary tract of progestogens have been most extensively studied during pregnancy, a high progesterone state. Investigation on pregnant animals has suggested that progesterone facilitates β-adrenergic activity in ureteral, and bladder tissues.[30,31] Such β-receptor mediated relaxation might also cause blunting of α-adrenergic activity,[32] with resultant urethral sphincter incompetence. However, these theoretical considerations have not been demonstrated clinically. No change in urethral closure pressure was seen by Van Geelen and associates[33] in their study of 43 pregnant women despite rising levels of 17-hydroxyprogesterone. The authors thus concluded that progesterone did not significantly alter urethral tone. Raz and colleagues[32] showed, in continent women, no change in the urethral pressure profile and no incontinence when a progestogen was added to postmenopausal hormone replacement therapy. Similar findings have been reported in both continent and stress incontinent women by Rud and group.[34] There is some contradictory evidence: Benness et al[35] did show an exacerbation of incontinence (by pad weight) during the progestogen phase of the cyclic hormone replacement in 10 of 14 menopausal patients. In total, however, the body of evidence to date does not support a significant role for progestogens in urinary tract function.

CLINICAL USES

Estrogens and genuine stress incontinence

For more than 50 years, estrogens have been used clinically in the management of genuine stress incontinence in females. Salmon and colleagues[36] in 1941 reported their results of intramuscular estradiol treatment in 10 postmenopausal women with stress incontinence and six patients with frequency, urgency and dysuria. In total, 12 patients experienced subjective improvement, with symptoms recurring in all following cessation of treatment. The subsequent development of urodynamics has provided an objective means of outcome assessment following estrogen administration, with increases in MUCP, functional urethral length and abdominal pressure transmission ratio occurring with estrogen, though these findings to date have been inconsistent.

Work in our own unit,[37] using 2 g daily of intravaginal conjugated estrogen for one month in postmenopausal women, demonstrated a significant improvement in symptoms of stress incontinence, urgency and frequency, with significantly improved pressure transmission to the urethra. Bergman et al[38] in a similar study showed a subjective improvement in urinary stress incontinence in estrogen supplemented women. Walter and coworkers[39] investigated 13 women with genuine stress incontinence by urodynamic assessment using estriol 4 mg/day or placebo for three months and showed an objective improvement in quantitative urine loss (via a one hour perineal pad test) in those receiving estrogen. Contradictory evidence however exists. In another study, Walter and colleagues[40] studied 29 postmenopausal women with urodynamically proven stress incontinence, randomizing them to either cyclic treatment with oral estradiol and estriol or placebo for four months. They noted improvement in urgency and urge incontinence with estrogen, but no improvement in stress incontinence, nor significant changes in MUCP nor functional urethral length between groups. Others have reported similar findings.

Problems with interpretation of the literature regarding estrogen on incontinence stem from the fact that only a handful of prospective double-blind, placebo-controlled studies exist, and even these have no standardization regarding diagnosis, treatment, nor outcome. Estrogens of different type have been administered in varying doses and routes among studies, to dissimilar patient groups. Several studies lack objective outcome measures, and are thus open to significant bias. In 1994, the Hormones and Urogenital Therapy Committee found in their review[41] only 23 trials appropriate for meta-analysis; they found an overall significant subjective improvement with estrogen therapy for the total group of *all* incontinent menopausal women, and for the subgroup comprising women with genuine stress incontinence alone. MUCP was significantly improved on meta-analysis by estrogen therapy, though no significant effect on quantitative urine loss was seen between groups. It may be the improvement in overall quality of life, rather than a direct improvement in urethral function, that accounts for effects seen with estrogens on urinary incontinence, as pointed out by the Committee.

Estrogens and urgency/urge incontinence

Little evidence exists in the literature with respect to the success of estrogen treatment of urgency or urge incontinence. Hilton and Stanton[37] have reported improvement in symptoms of urgency and frequency with intravaginal estrogen, and Walter[40] has similarly shown a subjective reduction in urgency and urge incontinence using oral estriol and estradiol. However, in a double-blind, placebo-controlled, multi-centre trial using oral estriol (3 mg/day) in the treatment of 64 postmenopausal women with either sensory urgency or detrusor instability,[42] Cardozo and colleagues were unable to demonstrate any significant benefit of estriol over placebo. Cardozo and Kelleher[43] later demonstrated that intravaginal 17β-estradiol was no better than placebo in treatment of urgency associated with either normal urodynamics or detrusor instability. While estrogen replacement may have some role in the treatment of stress incontinence, a definitive role for its use in urgency or urge incontinence has not yet been established.

Estrogens and urinary tract infection

After the menopause, lactobacilli growth in the vagina lessens, with a resultant rise in vaginal pH.[44] With the subsequent overgrowth in the vagina of enteric organisms, superficial vaginitis occurs, and urogenital epithelial thinning and lower urinary tract infections become more common. Earlier work suggested that estrogen replacement (oral estriol) could restore premenopausal vaginal flora in women with recurrent urinary tract infections, reducing the requirement for antibiotics by up to 16 times compared to those unsupplemented.[45] More recently, Raz and Stamm,[46] in a randomized, double-blind, placebo-controlled trial format, studied 93 postmenopausal women with a history of recurrent urinary tract infections. Participants received either intravaginal estriol 0.5 mg twice weekly or placebo, and were followed by serial urine culture. The incidence of urinary tract infection was significantly reduced in the estriol group, with lactobacilli re-appearing in the vaginal flora in 61% of the treated group. It thus seems that estrogen replacement therapy in postmenopausal women has an important prophylactic role for urinary tract infection.

Routes of administration

Estrogens can be administered orally, transdermally, subcutaneously or intravaginally. A variety of different forms are available, including conjugated estrogen, estradiol, estriol and estrone. To date, no clear benefit has been shown on urinary tract function from one route of administration over others. Tissue levels are higher in urinary tissues with vaginal application of estrogens, though the clinical significance of this has yet to be determined.

Conclusion

The female lower urinary and genital tracts have a common embryologic origin, and estrogen receptors have been found in the female urethra, and, in lesser number, in the bladder. While the effects of estrogen deprivation are seen in the urethra as well as in the vagina, the overall clinical benefit of estrogen replacement on urethral and bladder function is somewhat limited. Exogenous estrogen therapy enhances urethral resistance and possibly urethral support, and provides subjective improvement for incontinent menopausal women, especially those with genuine stress incontinence. True objective evidence of benefit on incontinence is still, however, lacking. Sensory urgency and bladder instability have not clearly been improved with estrogen replacement, leaving a small place for its use in the treatment of recurrent urinary tract infections in the menopause, where estrogen replacement significantly reduces the incidence of infection and allows recolonization of normal vaginal flora.

Progesterone receptors have not been reliably demonstrated in the lower urinary tract, nor has any clear clinical role for progestogens been established in the treatment of lower urinary tract dysfunction in the female.

REFERENCES

1. Gosling JA, Dixon JS 1991 Embryology and ultrastructure of the female lower urinary tract. In: Ostergard DR, Bent AE (eds) Urogynecology and urodynamics theory and practice, 3rd edn. Williams and Wilkins, Baltimore; pp 19–30
2. Carlile A, Davies J, Faragher E et al 1987 The epithelium in the female urethra: a quantitative study. Journal of Urology 138: 775
3. Urner F, Weil A, Herman WL 1983 Estradiol receptors in the urethra and bladder of the female rabbit. Gynecologic and Obstetric Investigation 16: 307
4. Weaker FJ, Heerbert DC, Sheridan PJ 1983 Autoradiographic demonstration of binding sites for oestradiol and dihydrotestosterone in the urinary tract of male and female baboons. Urological Research 11: 127
5. Schulze H, Barrack 1986 Immunocytochemical localization of estrogen receptors in the normal male and female canine urinary tract and prostate. Endocrinology 121: 1773
6. Iosif CS, Batra SC, Ek A, Astedt BI 1981 Estrogen receptors in the human female urinary tract. American Journal of Obstetrics and Gynecology 141: 817
7. Punnonen R, Lukola A, Puntala P 1983 Lack of estrogen and progestin receptors in the urinary bladder of women. Hormone and Metabolism Research 15: 464
8. Batra SC, Iosif CS 1985 Progesterone receptors in the female lower urinary tract. Journal of Urology 138: 1301
9. Wilson PD, Barker G, Barnard RJ, Siddle NC 1984 Steroid hormone receptors in the female lower urinary tract. Urology International 39: 5
10. Batra SC, Iosif CS 1983 Female urethra: a target organ for estrogen action. Journal of Urology 129: 418
11. Batra SC, Iosif CS 1989 Tissue specific effects of progesterone on progesterone and estrogen receptors in the female urogenital tract. Journal of Steroid Biochemistry 32: 35
12. DeLancey JOL 1992 Anatomy of the pelvis. In: Thompson JD, Rock JA (eds) TeLinde's operative gynecology, 7th edn. JB Lippincott, Philadelphia
13. Fantl A 1994 The lower urinary tract in women — effect of aging and menopause on incontinence. Experimentia Gerontologica 29 (3/4): 417
14. Wein AJ 1991 Practical uropharmacology. Urology Clinics of North America 18(2): 269–281
15. Kujansuu E, Kauppila A, Iahde S 1983 Correlation between urethrovesical anatomy and urethral closure function in female stress urinary incontinence before and after operation: urethrocystographic and urethrocystometric evaluation. Urology International 38: 19
16. Koonings PP, Bergman A, Ballard CA 1990 Low urethral pressure and stress incontinence in women: risk factor for failed retropubic surgical procedure. Urology 36: 245
17. Leach GE, Yip C, Donovan BJ 1987 Mechanism of continence after modified Pereyra bladder neck suspension. Urology 29: 328
18. Bergman A, Ballard CA, Koonings PP 1989 Comparison of three different surgical procedures for genuine stress incontinence: prospective randomized study. American Journal of Obstetrics and Gynecology 160: 1102
19. Levin RM, Shofer FS, Wein AJ 1980 Cholinergic, adrenergic and purinergic response of sequential strips of rabbit urinary bladder. Journal of Pharmacology and Experimental Therapeutics 212: 536
20. Hilton P, Tweddell AL, Mayne C 1990 Oral and vaginal estrogens alone and in combination with alpha adrenergic stimulation in genuine stress incontinence. International Urogynaecological Journal 12: 80
21. Cardozo LD 1990 Role of estrogens in the treatment of female urinary incontinence. Journal of the American Geriatric Society 38: 326
22. Rud T, Andersson KE, Asmussen M, Hunting A, Ulmsten U 1980 Factors maintaining the intraurethal pressure in females. Investigative Urology 17: 343
23. Bacho C, Winanady A 1992 Etude preliminaire de l'influence hormonale sur les differents parametres du plancher pelvien chez la femme en activite genitale sans hormonotherapie et chez la feme menopausee. Acta Urologica Belgica 60: 45–60
24. Rechberger T, Donica H, Baranowski W, Jakowicki J 1993 Female urinary stress incontinence in terms of connective tissue biochemistry. European Journal of Obstetrics, Gynecology and Reproductive Biology 49: 187–191
25. Miodrag A, Castleden CM, Vallance TR 1988 Sex hormones and the female urinary tract. Drugs 36: 491
26. Brincat M, Moniz CF, Kabalan S, Versi E, O'Dowd T, Magos AL, Montgomery J, Studd JW 1987 Decline in skin collagen content and metacarpal index after the menopause and its prevention with sex hormone replacement. British Journal of Obstetrics and Gynaecology 94: 126–129
27. Versi E, Cardozo L, Brincat M, Cooper D, Montgomery J, Studd JW 1988 Correlation of urethral physiology and skin collagen in postmenopausal women. British Journal of Obstetrics and Gynaecology 95: 147–152

28. Fantl JA, Wyman JF, Anderson RL, Matt DW, Bump RC 1988 Postmenopausal urinary incontinence: a comparison between non-estrogen-supplemented and estrogen-supplemented females. Obstetrics and Gynecology 71(6): 823–828
29. Smith PJB 1977 The menopause and the lower urinary tract – another case for hormone replacement therapy? The Practitioner 218: 1–4
30. Raz S, Zeigler M, Caine M 1972 Hormonal influences on the adrenergic receptors of the urethra. British Journal of Urology 44: 405
31. Zderic SA, Pizak JE, Duckett JW, Snyder HM, Wein AJ, Levin RM 1990 Effect of pregnancy on rabbit urinary bladder physiology: effect of extracellular calcium. Pharmacology 41: 124
32. Raz S, Zeigler M, Caine M 1973 The role of female hormones on stress incontinence. Presented at 26th Conference de la Societe International d'Urologie, Amsterdam, The Netherlands
33. van Geelen JM, Lemmens WAJG, Eskes TKAB, Martin LB 1982 The urethral pressure profile in pregnancy and delivery in healthy nulliparous women. American Journal of Obstetrics and Gynecology 144: 636
34. Rud T 1980 The effects of estrogens and progestogens on the urethral pressure profile in urinary continent and stress incontinent women. Acta Obstetrica Gynecologica Scandinavica 59: 265
35. Benness C, Gangar K, Cardozo L, Cuther A, Whitehead M 1991 Do progestogens exacerbate urinary incontinence in women on HRT? Neurology and Urodynamics 10(4): Abstract 25: 316
36. Salmon UJ, Walter RI, Geist SA 1941 The use of estrogens in the treatment of dysuria and incontinence in postmenopausal women. American Journal of Obstetrics and Gynecology 42: 845
37. Hilton P, Stanton SL 1983 The use of intravaginal oestrogen cream in genuine stress incontinence. British Journal of Obstetrics and Gynaecology 90: 940
38. Bergman A, Karram MM, Bhatia N 1990 Changes in urethral cystometry following estrogen administration. Gynecologic and Obstetric Investigation 29: 211
39. Walter S, Kjaergaard B, Lose G, Andersen JT, Heisterberg L, Jakobsen H, Klarskov P et al 1990 Stress urinary incontinence in postmenopausal women treated with oral estrogen (estriol) and alpha-adrenoreceptor stimulating agent: a randomized double-blind placebo controlled study. International Urogynaecological Journal 12: 74
40. Walter S, Wolf H, Barlebo H, Jansen H 1978 Urinary incontinence in postmenopausal women treated with oestrogens: a double-blind clinical trial. Urology International 33: 135
41. Fantl JA, Cardozo L, McClish DK 1994 Estrogen therapy in the management of urinary incontinence in postmenopausal women: a meta-analysis. First report of the Hormones and Urogenital Therapy Committee. Obstetrics and Gynecology 83(1): 12–18
42. Cardozo LD, Rekers H, Tapp A, Barnick C, Shepherd A, Schussler B et al 1993 Oestriol in the treatment of postmenopausal urgency — a multicentre study. Maturitas 18: 47
43. Cardozo LD, Kelleher CJ 1995 Sex hormones, the menopause and urinary problems. Gynecological Endocrinology 9: 75–84
44. Klutke JJ, Bergman A 1995 Hormonal influence on the urinary tract. Urology Clinics of North America 22(3): 629–639
45. Brandberg A, Mellstrom D, Samsioe G 1984 Low dose oral estriol treatment in elderly women with urogenital infections. Acta Obstetrica Gynecologica Scandinavica (140): 33
46. Raz R, Stamm W 1993 A controlled trial of intravaginal estriol in postmenopausal women with recurrent urinary tract infections. New England Journal of Medicine 329(11): 753–802

21. Effects of estrogen and progesterone on skin

M.P. Brincat M. Formosa

Introduction

In man, the skin forms a sheet-like single organ composed of a population of cells of diverse embryonic origins and potentialities. Under normal conditions these different cell types exist side by side in harmony as a complex mosaic.

A thin outer layer, the epidermis, is composed of keratin-producing cells (keratinocytes) of ectodermal origin intermingled with melanin-producing cells (melanocytes) which arise from a specialized embryonic ectodermal tissue, the neural crest. The dermis, is a stroma that forms the main bulk of the skin. It is intimately bound with the overlaying epidermis: finger-like processes, or dermal papillae, project upwards into corresponding recesses in the epidermis. In contrast with the epidermis, the dermis is relatively cellular and predominantly fibrous, containing blood vessels. Like all connective tissue (including bone) the dermis is of mesodermal origin. It also contains several structures derived from the embryonic ectoderm, e.g. sweat glands, hair follicles (Fig. 21.1).

Fibres of two main types are seen in the dermis; both are fibrous protein in nature. By far the largest amount by weight is collagen, with elastin fibres (2.5%) making up the remainder.[1] Collagen fibres are responsible for the main mass and resilience of the dermis. Collagen is disposed mainly parallel to the skin surface whereas elastin fibres form a subepidermal network and are only thinly distributed elsewhere in the dermis.

The dermis and the epidermis are nourished by blood vessels that derive from the subcutaneous layer. In the dermis they form relatively small channels (arterioles) which pass towards the under surface of

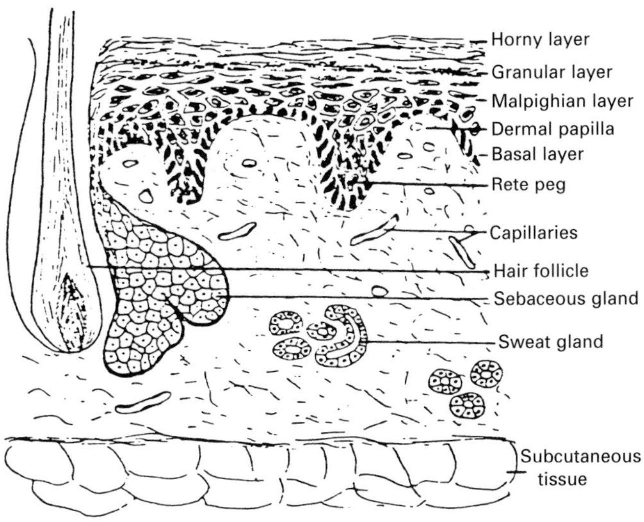

Fig. 21.1 Cross-section of the human skin demonstrating its normal structure.

the epidermis, forming a rich capillary network in the dermal papillae. It is these vessels that are involved in the menopausal flash, the most characteristic symptom of the menopause, affecting some 75% of all women in their first menopausal year[2] and still affecting 25% five years later.[3] Photoplethysmograph studies have shown that women suffering from postmenopausal flashes not only have abnormal peripheral (dermal) vascular behavior during a flash[4] but also always have abnormal peripheral (dermal) vascular control when not flashing.[5] This abnormal control response can be reversed with estrogen therapy.[5]

Other structures found in the dermis include veins, lymph vessels, sensory corpuscles and autonomic and sensory nerves. Hair follicles and their attendant muscles and cutaneous glands are also situated in this layer. Cells are scanty in the dermis although representatives of the reticuloendothelial system, including histocytes, fibrocytes and mast cells, are found.

With increasing postmenopausal age, the skin tends to become thinner. Albright[6] observed that the thin flaky skin of postmenopausal women reflected a generalized atrophy of connective tissues in the body (including bone, manifesting as osteoporosis). The deterioration in the condition of the skin after the menopause has been shown to be due to atrophy of the dermis. Women on hormone replacement therapy (HRT) have a higher dermal collagen content than women who receive no replacement therapy, indicating that it is a hormone-responsive decrease in the dermal collagen that is responsible for postmenopausal skin atrophy.

THE EFFECTS OF OVARIAN STEROIDS ON SKIN

Both estrogen and androgen receptors have been identified on dermal fibroblasts. Estrogens have been shown to enhance dermal water content, mucopolysaccharoid concentration and collagen content. All these factors together improve the quality and appearance of the skin of patients receiving HRT.

In animals, estrogens appear to alter the vascularization of the skin.[7] A change in the connective tissue of the dermis occurs and is reflected by increased mucopolysaccharide incorporation, hydroxyproline turnover and alterations in ground substance.[8] In addition to increased dermal turnover of hyaluronic acid, the dermal water content is enhanced with estradiol therapy.[9] Atrophy of the epidermis disappeared after treatment lasting six weeks, with the number of capillaries increasing and collagenous fibers appearing less fragmented. Both testosterone and estrogen ointments had similar effects on the skin of both sexes.[10] Rauramo[11] observed that oral estrogen therapy in castrated women caused thickening of the epidermis for three months and this persisted for six months.

Punnonen[12] used two different strengths of estrogen in castrated women, estriol succinate and the stronger estradiol valerate. Both caused statistically significant thickening of the epidermis after three months. While this thickness persisted with estradiol succinate, 34% of the patients on estradiol valerate subsequently acquired significant thinning of the epidermis. It was postulated that this was due to excessive dosage.

Mitotic activity in the epidermis

Studies into the effects of estrogens on mitotic activity in the epidermis provide conflicting results. Punnonen[12] claimed significantly higher mitotic activity in the epidermis in studies utilizing ^{3}H thymidine labeling *in vitro*, while Shahrad,[13] using the same labeling agent in his *in vitro* studies, claimed a depressor effect of estrogen on thymidine incorporation in the human epidermis. However Shahrad used pharmacologically high concentrations of estrone, raising the possibility that there may be an optimum dose of estrogen to yield the maximum beneficial results. Collagenous fibrils were less fragmented in the dermis of women treated with estrogens and Shahrad noted an increase in the number of capillaries in the dermis of these women.

Estrogens and skin dehydration

The production of mucopolysaccharides is a function of fibroblasts in the skin. Estrogens may increase the rate of collagen production by altering the polymerization of mucopolysaccharides.[14] Estrogens increase the hydroscopic qualities and reduce the adhesion of collagen fibers in connective tissues[15] and the dermis is one site in which estrogens work in this way. As noted above the dermal water content increases due to enhanced synthesis of dermal hyaluronic acid.[8]

In mice, hyaluronic acid content was shown to increase dramatically with administration of estrogens, with a close linear relationship existing between the increase in high molecular weight hyaluronic acid and the increase in tissue water.[8] Uzuka, also working with mice, reported similar findings to Grossman[8] and suggested that the stimulation of hyaluronic acid synthesis in mouse skin in response to estrogens is mediated through estrogen receptors and involves the induction of the enzyme hyaluronic acid synthetase.[16,17]

Collagen

Collagen constitutes approximately one third of the total mass of the body and 20% of its total protein. It is a major constituent of all connective tissues. Eighty-eight per cent of body collagen is found in the skin and in bones, the amount of collagen being almost equally shared between these two organ systems.

Connective tissue consists of an extracellular matrix and cellular elements. The extracellular matrix is composed of two classes of macromolecules, the collagens and the polysaccharide glycosaminoglycans (GAGs). GAG chains allow rapid diffusion of water molecules and are responsible for skin turgor. Collagen fibrils, on the other hand, resist tissue stretching. By weight, GAGs amount to less than 5% of the total fibrous protein, the rest is composed largely of collagen together with some elastin.[18] Although the bulk of the body collagen is remarkably stable, a fraction of the collagen in all tissues is continuously degraded and replaced, even in old age. Such change in overall collagen metabolism can be approximately followed by assaying the excretion of peptide-bound hyrdoxyproline in urine.[19,20] Changes in collagen metabolism can also be assayed by urinary assay of pyridinium cross-links. Two basic α chains have been identified in collagen (α 1 and α 2) each consisting of just over 100 amino acids in groups of three in the basic collagen triple-helix configuration. This very stable structure forms the basic building unit of collagenous structures. Proline and hydroxyproline constitute 20–25% of total amino acids in collagen.

Collagen changes, both in quality, type and amount, with age. For example, type III collagen is found in greater amounts in the skin of young animals. This indicates gene switching, comparable to the switch from fetal and embryonic hemoglobin to hemoglobin A. Growth of connective tissue involves an increased rate of collagen biosynthesis and this is reflected in an increased tissue level of intracellular posttranslational enzymes. Both the rates of translation and the levels of these enzymes decrease with age.[21]

Skin and bone share a common collagen: type I. Skin contains, in addition, the very similar type III collagen. Type I, which constitutes 90% of the total collagen in the body, is the most important.[18] It has been shown that skin collagen and skin thickness decrease with postmenopausal age and that this decrease is prevented by hormone replacement therapy. This finding suggests that the collagen decrease after the menopause is due to estrogen deficiency.[22] Evidence suggests that postmenopausal bone loss shares a common etiology: and that an overall decline in connective tissues affects most organs and occurs as a result of estrogen deficiency.

The epithelium of the vagina has the highest concentration of estrogen receptors in the body. After the menopause, the vagina sustains a decrease in vascularity and becomes thin, increasing its susceptibility to becoming inflamed and ulcerated. The cervix atrophies and retracts, while atrophy of the corpus results in a return to the 1:2 corpus/cervix ratio of childhood. Postmenopausal genital atrophy is associated with dyspareunia, apareunia and pruritus vulvae. All these symptoms improve with estrogen replacement therapy.

Skin thickness and collagen content

Studies have been carried out on the skin changes seen in various connective tissue and endocrine disorders. A brief review is presented below.

Black et al[23] and Shuster et al[24] looked at the relationship between skin thickness and skin collagen in systemic sclerosis, osteoporotics of mixed etiology and hirsute women and found a good correlation between the two. In a small study, Black et al[23] demonstrated changes in the collagen content and thickness of the skin in osteoporotics (mixed etiology) treated with androgens, when compared to osteoporotics who had not received this treatment. Shuster et al[22] found an increase in skin collagen in hirsute women, but the increase was not statistically significant. In scleroderma, Black et al[23] demonstrated a decrease in total collagen content and skin thickness in affected areas. In clinically normal areas, the skin thickness was decreased but the collagen content was not significantly altered. Arho[25] did not find any difference between skin thickness and collagen content in patients with scleroderma when compared to controls. He found a good correlation between skin thickness and collagen content in a number of patients with a variety of endocrine and collagen disorders. The conditions studied were acromegaly, rheumatoid arthritis, lupus erythematosus, scleroderma, prurigo Besnier, psoriasis and Cushing's syndrome. Patients with prurigo Besnier and scleroderma had normal skin collagen content. Acromegaly produced both thicker skin and a higher skin collagen content, whilst patients with Cushing's syndrome and those who had been treated with costicosteroids had thinner skin and a lower skin collagen content than normals.

Effects of age

Reports on skin collagen changes associated with age are conflicting. Shuster and Bottoms[26,27] showed that the best way of expressing skin collagen content was by measuring the collagen content of a skin biopsy per mm^2 of skin surface. This method takes into account the possibility of changes in the total mass of the dermis. They reported a reduction in total skin collagen with age, but this was not confirmed by Reed and Hall.[28] Shuster and Black[24] found that the amount of collagen present in skin was at all ages higher in males than in females. Hall[29] confirmed that skin collagen was higher in males than in females but once again could not significantly confirm the decline of skin collagen with age. The effects of the menopause and of hypo-estrogenism on skin collagen content has not received any attention to date.

Effects of corticosteroids

Several studies confirm that corticosteroid therapy or excess endogenous costicosteroids, as in Cushing's disease, reduces skin collagen content and skin thickness both in humans[25,29,30–32] and in animals (rats and mice).[31,33]

Effects of sex steroids

A study comparing patients treated with estradiol and testosterone implants (2–10 years duration of treatment) with untreated postmenopausal women found that the implant treated group had a significantly greater skin collagen content than the untreated group (Fig. 21.2). Optimum skin collagen was obtained after two years of an optimum estrogen regimen. Too high or too low estrogen levels give lower levels of collagen.[34] The same conclusions were reported in relation to the epidermis.[35]

The decline in skin collagen content after the menopause occurs at a much more rapid rate in the initial postmenopausal years. Some 30% of skin collagen is lost in the first five years following the menopause,[36] with an average decline of 21% per postmenopausal year over a period of 20 years. The increase in skin collagen content after six months of sex hormone therapy depends on the collagen content at the start of treatment.[36] In women with a low skin collagen content, estrogens are initially of therapeutic and later of prophylactic value; whereas in those with a mild loss of collagen in the early postmenopausal years estrogens are of prophylactic value only. Thus a deficiency in skin collagen can be corrected but not overcorrected.

Skin collagen content has been shown to have a strong correlation with skin dermal thickness measured radiologically.[36] Using 100 mg subcutaneous estradiol implants, significant increases in skin thickness and metacarpal index occurred over a one year period. Most of the increase occurred in the first six months.

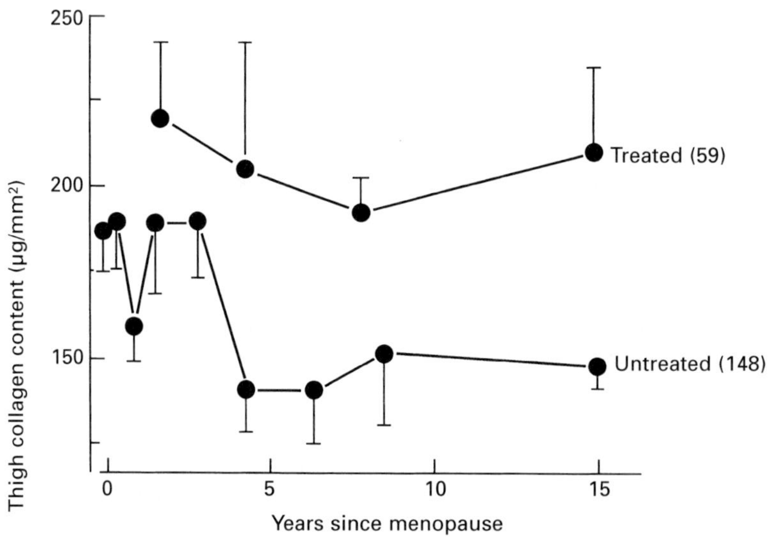

Fig. 21.2 Thigh skin collagen content (M±SE) with years since menopause in 148 untreated postmenopausal women and in 59 postmenopausal women who had been on sex hormone treatment for between 2–10 years.

These findings were irrespective of the woman's age, number of years since the menopause, original skin thickness or previous metacarpal index.

Collagen is therefore the key to changes in connective tissue after the menopause. Osteoporosis is being seen as a manifestation of an overall connective tissue disorder affecting various systems such as the skin, bone, the vascular system and the bladder. Several studies have shown skin thickness and skin collagen to be reduced after the menopause. Brincat and Castelo-Barcia[37,38,39] have shown that following the menopause skin collagen content and skin thickness are increased in women on HRT compared to age-matched women on no treatment. Prospective studies have also shown that skin thickness, skin collagen and bone mass increase in postmenopausal women who start estrogen replacement. The mechanical properties of postmenopausal skin have been shown to be improved with HRT and to reach premenopausal levels.[40] In this study, the mechanical properties of skin were defined by extensibility and elasticity measurements obtained using a computerized device. These parallel the skin collagen changes noted elsewhere. The mechanism by which increases in bone mass occur in women on estrogen replacement is still unclear. Likewise the relationship to the incidence of osteoporotic fractures needs further elucidation.

Our group carried out two studies which compliment each other.[40a] The first was a biophysical study which looked at differences in various bone density parameters and in skin thickness between a group of untreated postmenopausal women and a group of untreated postmenopausal women who had sustained an osteoporotic fracture. The second was a biophysical/biochemical study between a group of untreated postmenopausal women and a group of women who were receiving estrogen replacement therapy. Bone density and skin thickness measurements were obtained, and collagen marker studies were performed. The excretion of procollagen I C-end terminal peptides (PCICP) and pyridinium cross-links were also measured on random samples from within the study groups. Procollagen I C-end terminal peptide is produced as a result of enzymatic cleavage of procollagen. Bone collagen type I is therefore an index of osteoblastic activity, which in turn is an index of bone formation.

Pyridinium cross-links, pyridinoline and deoxypyridinoline are found mainly in type I bone collagen. After the collagen matrix is formed, the enzymatic action of lysyl oxidase causes the condensation of the amino acids lysine and hydroxylysine in adjacent collagen, resulting in the formation of the covalent crosslinks PYD and DPD. These crosslinks play an important part in the structure of collagen. In the process of bone resorption, collagen undergoes proteolytic degradation, releasing free forms of PYD and DPD into the circulation; these are cleared by the kidney and subsequently found in the urine. These crosslinks are therefore an index of osteoclastic activity, which in turn is an index of bone resportion.

Cross-links and procollagen peptide assays were not carried out in the osteoporotic group in this study since they had been so long postmenopausal that a steady state of excretion of markers would have been established for several years.

Skin thickness and bone density parameters were much lower in women who had sustained osteoporotic fractures compared to controls. Women with fractures had mean bone mass values that were some 20% below the mean values of controls (Fig. 21.3). Skin thickness varied within a narrower range (mean difference 4%) (Fig. 21.4) but significant differences between controls and women who had sustained an osteoporotic fracture were consistently noted.

When compared with women who had been on hormone replacement therapy (study B) the untreated postmenopausal controls had a decreased osteoclastic activity (pyridinium cross-links excretion) by a mean of 27.2%; osteoblastic activity (serum procollagen I C-end terminal peptide) was decreased by a mean of 11.3%. All these differences ($P<0.001$) indicated that bone remodeling had readjusted. The women on hormone replacement therapy had only been on therapy for a short time (mean six months) (Fig. 21.5), thereby implying that changes occurred rapidly. It is interesting to note that according to the above calculations, a mean positive change of 15.9% occurred in bone remodeling in women on HRT. This value is of the same order as the mean percentage change in bone mass that occurred when the same untreated group were compared to the treated group, particularly when L2–L4 measurements are compared. The treated group has a 16.1% higher mean L2–L4 bone density.

Topical estradiol gel has also been shown to increase skin collagen content as measured by skin hydroxyproline.[37] Skin blister fluids were assayed and an increase of both PICP and PMNP were found with the gel.

It has been postulated that HRT leads to an increase in bone mass by virtue of an increase in collagen levels. Indeed the observation that women on HRT had a higher dermal skin collagen content than those who were not on HRT[34] led to the idea that a similar increase in bone collagen was occurring in women on HRT. It was postulated that this increase in

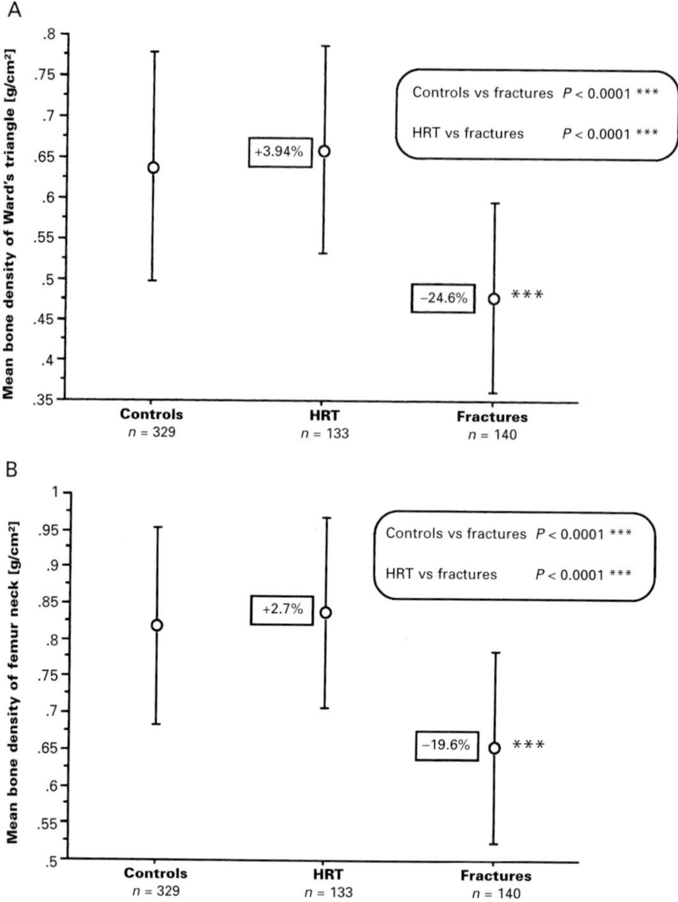

Fig. 21.3 Mean and standard deviations of **A** Ward's triangle and **B** femoral neck bone density in controls, hormone replacement therapy patients and fracture cases.

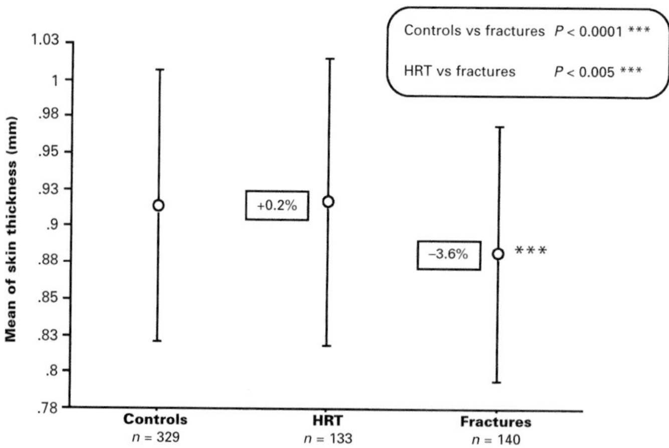

Fig. 21.4 Mean and standard deviations of skin thickness in controls, hormone replacement therapy patients and fracture cases.

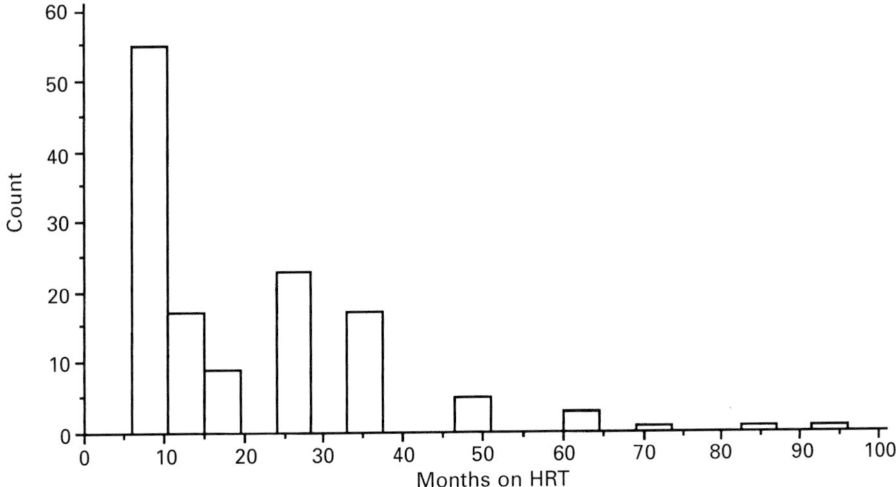

Fig. 21.5 Frequency distribution of months on hormone replacement therapy (HRT).

collagen and total collagen content was leading to an increase in bone strength and thus a diminution of osteoporotic fractures.[41]

The effect of the menopause and HRT on collagen markers (cross-links) has been studied.[42] The measurements of collagen markers in our study indicate that hormone replacement causes a readjustment of bone remodeling. As a consequence, a dramatic decrease in bone resorption (27.2%) occurs. There was a similar decrease in bone formation (11.3%). The overall mean change in bone markers was 15.9%, which was similar (16.1%) to the overall mean change in bone mass as measured using biophysical methods (L2–L4) in the same group of women (Fig. 21.6). This indicates that these markers are indeed sensitive and can be used in monitoring postmenopausal bone loss as well as in accurately titrating the response to treatment prophylactically when such treatment is used both prophylactically as well as when used therapeutically in the management of established osteoporosis (Fig. 21.7). It remains to be shown just how soon after treatment these collagen markers will change; cross-link excretion has been shown to characteristically decrease after six months of treatment.

Skin thickness

With increasing postmenopausal age, the skin tends to get thinner and this is reversed with adequate HRT. Albright[6] speculated that postmenopausal osteoporosis was part of a generalized connective tissue disorder, having observed that the skin of osteoporotic women was noticably thin, suggesting that the atrophy was more widespread than just in the bone matrix. McConkey et al[43] showed that the incidence of transparent skin on the dorsum of the hand was most common in women over 60 years of age and the prevalence of osteoporosis in women with transparent skin was 83%.

This implies that skin and bone changes associated with HRT after the menopause somehow mimic each other, as has been suggested in the more recent work outlined above. Some authors have failed to demonstrate short-term beneficial effects using topical or transdermal HRT but this is almost certainly a dose related problem since other authors were able to show beneficial skin changes using both topical (estradiol gel)[37] and estradiol implants.[36] Dermal thickness has been measured in most of these studies since this is the skin layer that contains most connective tissue. Subcutaneous tissue is an added variable and studies using Harpenden's callipers, for example, which include subcutaneous fat in the measurement have been conflicting.[42] The dermis itself, composed as it is of connective tissue and including the predominant protein collagen as well as elastin (small amounts) and glycosaminoglycans also has more than one variable that can be affected by HRT and the menopause. In rat work, for example,[14] castrated rats that were given estrogens had a 70% increase in their dermal content glycosaminoglycans after two weeks. Similar increases in women would lead to skin thickness increases that far outstrip that which would be expected from collagen content increases alone.

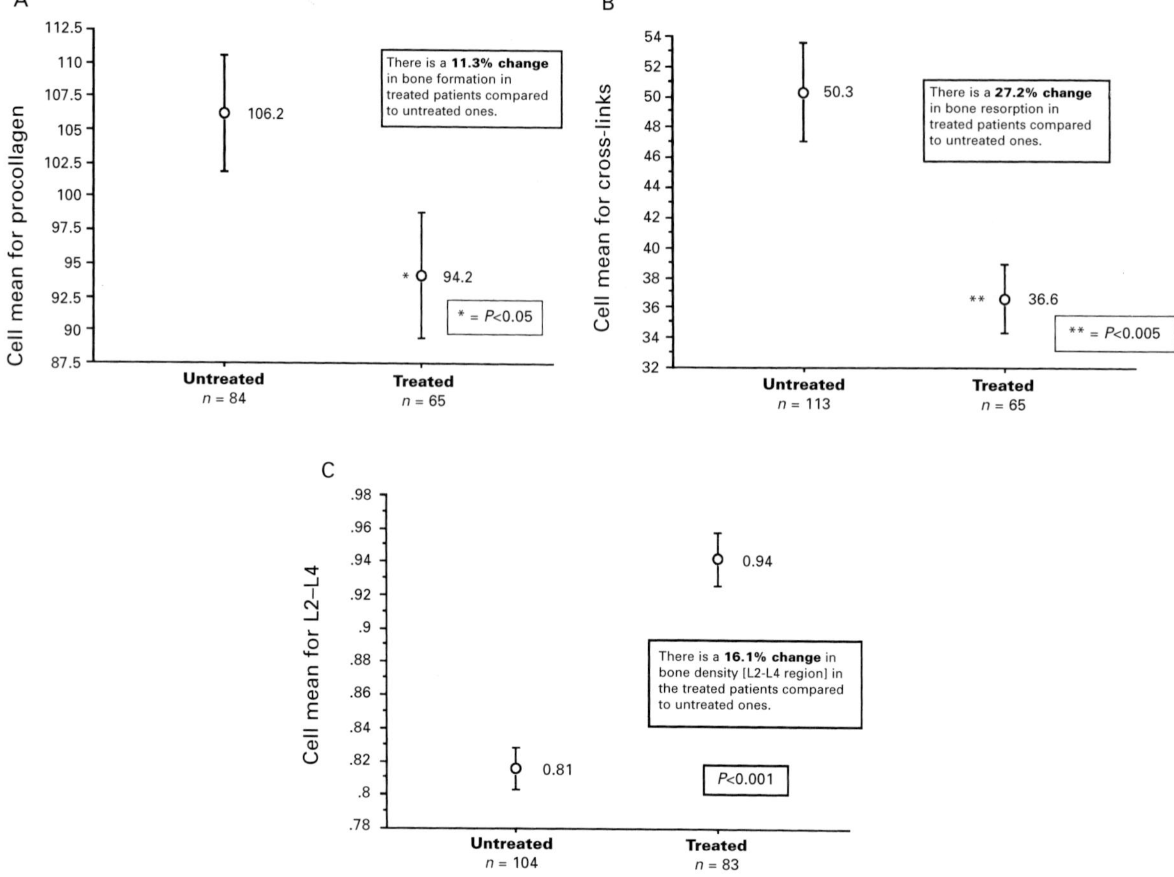

Fig. 21.6 Plot of mean **A** procollagen and **B** cross-links in untreated patients and in patients on hormone replacement therapy. **C** Plot of mean L2–L4 bone density in untreated patients and in patients on hormone replacement therapy.

PROGESTERONE AND PROGESTOGENS

In contrast to the relative wealth of information on the effects of estrogens on skin in postmenopausal women, there is very limited information on the effects of progesterone. There appears to be no information on the actual changes in skin thickness or composition with progesterone alone, or in combination with estrogens. On the other hand, synthetic progestogens may have effects on skin structures including sebaceous glands and hair, and this appears to depend on the degree of androgenicity of the individual progestogenic compound. For example, norethindrone (norethisterone) may sometimes increase sebum secretion, lead to acne formation and occasionally increase facial and body hair growth. Formal studies to look at the effects of different progestogens on skin composition and thickness, and function of specific skin structures such as hair and sebaceous glands after the menopause, are clearly needed.

Conclusion

The skin is one of the largest organs in the body. It is an old adage that skin is a manifestation of inner health. Its appearance, in terms of quality, elasticity, translucence and hydration, have important cosmetic implications, which affect the self-esteem of the individual.

The menopause has been shown to be a major event having profound effects on the skin and, similar to the effects on bone, causing rapid deterioration. This, can be prevented and even reversed with appropriate and adequate estrogen replacement. These effects have been demonstrated at all levels of the skin including the

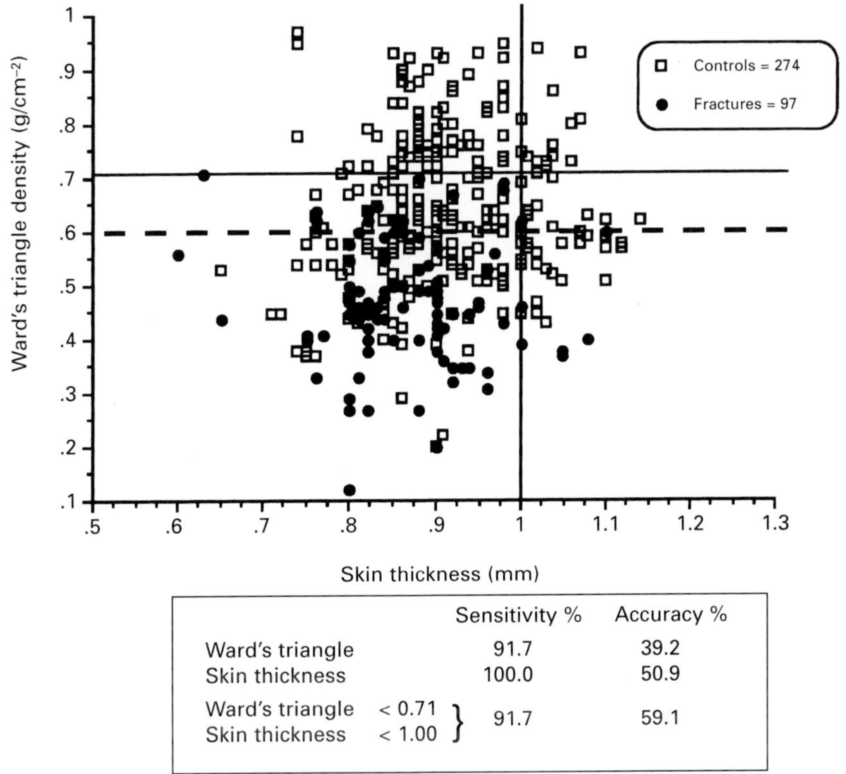

		Sensitivity %	Accuracy %
Ward's triangle		91.7	39.2
Skin thickness		100.0	50.9
Ward's triangle	< 0.71	91.7	59.1
Skin thickness	< 1.00		

Fig. 21.7 Scattergram of Ward's triangle bone density vs skin thickness.

epidermis, dermis (collagen and glycosaminoglycans content) and overall skin thickness. As a consequence, not surprisingly, the mechanical properties of the skin have been shown to derive beneficial effect with HRT after the degenerative effects which occur as a consequence of menopause. The skin contains some 40% of the total body collagen with a further 40% being present in bone. Bone changes after the menopause have been shown to parallel connective tissue changes and studies based on collagen marker studies have found that profound alterations in bone remodeling occur with HRT in postmenopausal women. This leads to a convincing argument that bone weakness leading to postmenopausal bone fractures is largely due to a connective tissue deficiency which may be mirrored by the individual's skin changes.

REFERENCES:

1. Bailey AJ, Etherington DJ 1980 Metabolism of collagen and elastin. In: Florkin M, Neuberger A, Van Dienen LLM (eds) Comprehensive biochemistry. Elsevier Scientific Publications, ch 5, pp 408–431
2. McKinlay SM, Jeffreys M 1974 The menopausal syndrome. British Journal of Preventive Medicine and Social Medicine 28: 108–115
3. Thompson B, Hart SA, Durno D 1973 Menopausal age and symptomatology in a general practice. Journal of Biosocial Science 5: 71–72
4. Sturdee DW, Wilson KA, Papili E, Croaker A 1978 Physiological aspects of the menopausal hot flush. British Medical Journal 2: 79–80
5. Brincat M, De Trafford JC, Lafferty K, Studd JWW 1984 Peripheral vasomotor control and menopausal flushing. A preliminary report. British Journal of Obstetrics and Gynaecology 91: 1107–1110
6. Albright F, Bloomberg E, Smith PH 1940 Postmenopausal osteoporosis. Transactions of the Association of American Physicians 55: 298–305
7. Goodrich SM, Wood JE 1966 The effect of oestradiol 17β on peripheral venous distensibility and velocity of venous blood flow. American Journal of Obstetrics and Gynecology 96: 407–412
8. Grosman M, Hindberg E, Schen J 1971 The effect of oestrogenic treatment on the acid mucopolysaccharide pattern in skin of mice. Acta Pharmacologica et Toxicologica 30: 458–464

9. Grossman N 1973 Studies on the hyaluronic acid protein complex, the molecular size of hyaluronic acid and the exchangeability of chloride in skin of mice before and after oestrogen treatment. Acta Pharmacologica et Toxicologica 33: 201–208
10. Goldzieher MA 1946 The effects of oestrogens on the senile skin. Journal of Gerontology 1: 196
11. Rauramo L, Punnonen R 1969 Wirking einer oralen estrogentherapie mit oestriolsuccinat auf die haut hastierter. Frauen Haut Gerchluts Kr 44(13): 463–470
12. Punnonen R 1973 Effect of castration and peroral therapy on skin. Acta Obstetrica Gynecologica Scandinavica 21(Suppl): 1–4
13. Shahrad P, Marks RA 1977 Pharmacological effect of oestrone on human epidermis. British Journal of Dermatology 97: 383–386
14. Boucek RS, Noble ML, Woessner JF Jnr 1959 Properties of fibroblasts. In: Page IM (ed) Connective tissue thrombosis and atherosclerosis. Academic Press, New York, pp 193–211
15. Danforth DM, Vers A, Breen M, Weinstein HC, Buckingham JC, Manalo P 1974 The effect of pregnancy and labour on the human cervix. Changes in collagen, glycoprotein and glycosaminoglycans. American Journal of Obstetrics and Gynecology 120: 641–651
16. Uzaka M, Makamiza K, Okta S, Mori Y 1980 The mechanism of oestrogen induced increase in hyaluronic acid biosynthesis with special reference to oestrogen receptors in the mouse skin. Biochemical Biophysics Acta 627: 199–206
17. Uzaka M, Makamiza K, Okta S, Mori Y 1980 Induction of hyaluronic acid synthetase by oestrogen in the mouse skin. Biochemical Biophysics Acta 627: 199–206
18. Alberts B, Bray D, Laws J, Raff M, Roberts M, Watson D 1983 Cell-cell adhesion and the extracellular matrix. In: Alberts B et al (eds) Molecular biology of the cell, vol 12. Garland Publishing, New York, pp 673–718
19. Kivirikko KI 1973 Urinary excretion of hydroxyproline in health and disease. International Review of Connective Tissue Research 5: 93–163
20. Krane SM, Kontrwitz FG, Byrne M et al 1977 Urinary excretion of hydroxylysine and its glycosides as an index of collagen degradation. Journal of Clinical Investigation 59: 819–827
21. Amen H, Crara J, Ryhanent et al 1973 Assay of protocollagen bysyl hydroxylase activity in the skin of human subjects and changes in the activities with age. Clinical Chim Acta 47: 289–294
22. Hall D 1981 Gerontology; collagen disease. Clinics in Endocrinology and Metabolism 2: 23
23. Black MM 1969 A modified radiographic method for measuring skin thickness. British Journal of Dermatology 1: 661
24. Shuster J, Black MM, McVitie E 1975 The influence of age and sex on skin thickness, skin collagen and density. British Journal of Dermatology 93: 639
25. Araho P 1972 Skin thickness and collagen content in some endocrine connective tissue and skin diseases. Acta Dermatologica Venerologica Stockholm 69(suppl): 1–48
26. Shuster S, Bottons E 1963 Senile degeneration of skin collagen. Clinical Science 25: 487–491
27. Shuster S, Bottons E 1963 Effect of ultraviolet light on skin collagen. Maturitas 199: 192–193
28. Reed VB and Hall DA 1974 In: Frische R, Hartmann F (eds) Connective tissues — biochemistry and pathophysiology. Spinger Verlag, Berlin, p 290
29. Hall DA, Reed FB, Noki G, Vince JD 1974 The relative effects of age and corticosteriod therapy on the collagen profiles of dermis from subjects with rheumatoid arthritis. Age and Ageing 3: 15–22
30. Castor CN, Baker BL 1950 The action of adrenocortical steroids on epidermis and connective tissue of the skin. Endocrinology 47: 234–241
31. Kirby JD, Munro DD 1976 Steroid induced atrophy in an animal and human model. British Journal of Dermatology 94: 111–119
32. Ferguson JK, Donald RA, Weston TS, Espina EA 1983 Skin thickness in patients with acromegaly and Cushing's syndrome and response to treatment. Clinical Endocrinology 18: 347–353
33. Smith QT 1962 Quantative studies on cutaneous collagen, procollagen and hexosamine in normal and cortisone treated rats. British Journal of Dermatology 38: 62–68
34. Brincat M, Moniz CF, Studd JWW et al 1983 Sex hormones and skin collagen content in postmenopausal women. British Medical Journal 287: 1337
35. Sharad P, Marks R 1977 A pharmacological effect of oestrone on human epidermis. British Journal of Dermatology 97: 383–386
36. Brincat M, Versi E, Moniz CF, Magos A, De Trafford J, Studd JWW 1987 Skin collagen changes in post-menopausal woman receiving different regimens of oestrogen therapy. Obstetrics and Gynecology 70(6): 840–845
37. Brincat M, Moniz CJ, Studd JWW, Darby A, Magos A, Emburey G, Versi E 1985 Long term effects of the menopause and sex hormones on skin thickness. British Journal of Obstetrics and Gynecology 92: 256–259
38. Brincat M, Moniz CF, Studd JWW, Darby AJ, Magos AL, Cooper D 1983 Sex hormones and skin collagen content in post-menopausal women. British Medical Journal 287: 1337–1338
39. Castelo-Barcia C, Pons F, Gratacos E, Fortuny A, Panrell JA, Gonzalez Merlo J 1994 Relationship between skin collagen and bone changes during ageing. Maturitas 18: 199–206
40. Pverard GE, Letawe L, Dowlati A, Pierard-Franchimant L 1995 Effect of hormone replacement therapy for menopause on the mechanical properties of skin. Journal of the American Society 43(6): 662–664

40a. Brincat M, Galea R, Muscat Baron Y, Xuerab A 1997 Changes in bone collagen markers and in bone density in oestrogen treated and untreated post-menopausal women. Maturitas 27: 171–177
41. Varila E, Rantala I, Ikarinem A, Risteli S, Rectala T, Okamen H, Punnonen R 1995 The effect of topical oestriol on skin collagen of postmenopausal women. British Journal of Obstetrics and Gynaecology 102: 985–989
42. Melton LJ, Wahner HW, Richelson LS, O'Fallon WM, Dunn WL, Riggs BC 1986 Osteoporosis and the risk of hip-fracture. American Journal of Epidemiology 124: 254–261
43. McConkey B, Fraser GR, Blight AJ, Whitely M 1963 Transparent skin and osteoporosis. Lancet 1: 693–695
44. Brincat M, Muscat Baron Y, Galea R 1995 Skin thickness, oestrogen use and bone mass in older women. Journal of the North American Menopause Society

22. Estrogen and progesterone during pregnancy and parturition

John R.G. Challis Steven J. Lye

Introduction

Many of the important metabolic and physiologic adjustments of pregnancy are dependent on the production and action of steroid hormones. In this chapter we consider changes that occur in two major groups of steroids, estrogen and progesterone, and their role in the regulation of myometria activity during pregnancy and at the time of birth.

Steroid hormones are derived from a common cholesterol precursor.[1] They are synthesized by dehydrogenases and cytochrome P450 enzymes which catalyze hydroxylation and oxidation-reduction reactions. The P450 enzymes are membrane bound, localized in either inner mitochondrial or endoplasmic reticulum membranes of cells in steroid synthesizing tissues. Commonly, the side chain cleavage of cholesterol (C-27) to form pregnenolone (C-21) is a major rate-limiting step in steroid synthesis. Conversion of pregnenolone to 17α hydroxy pregnenolone through the activity of the P450C17 (CYP17; 17α hydroxylase-17,20-lyase) enzyme is critical in the generation of 17α hydroxy corticosteroids such as cortisol, and in the production of androgens. We shall see that the lack of P450C17 in the human placenta allows conversion of pregnenolone to progesterone, through the activity of the 3β hydroxysteroid dehydrogenase (3β HSD) enzyme, but means that C-21 steroids cannot be converted to C-19 steroids *de novo*.

In the sheep, placental P450C17 expression is upregulated at term in response to prepartum activation of the fetal hypothalamic-pituitary-adrenal (HPA) axis, and increased cortisol secretion.[2] Thus, in term sheep placental tissue, the potential exists to convert cholesterol through to estrogen. In primates, however, P450C17 is not expressed in the placenta, even at term, and the biosynthesis of placental estrogen (C-18 steroid) is therefore dependent on the provision of C-19 steroid precursors from other sites, largely from the maternal and fetal adrenal gland.[3] Thus the fetus and placenta form a biochemically complementary unit in terms of steroid hormone synthesis, since the fetal adrenal cortex expresses abundant P450C17, but has little 3β HSD activity, whereas 3β HSD but not P450C17 is present in the placenta. This unit has been described as the 'fetoplacental unit' of steroid biosynthesis (Fig. 22.1).

PROGESTERONE

Progesterone has a major role during pregnancy in suppressing spontaneous myometrial contractility and in diminishing induced activity. Characteristically, myometrial excitability rises before parturition (see below), and this is associated with a decrease in the concentration of progesterone in the maternal peripheral circulation. In species where the ovary continues as the major source of progesterone throughout gestation, ovariectomy results in increased myometrial activity (so-called effect of 'withdrawal of the progesterone block' to the myometrium) that can be reversed by exogenous progesterone. In many species (e.g. sheep) where the placenta is the major source of progesterone during the second half of pregnancy, a decrease in placental progesterone output is reflected in a decrease in peripheral plasma progesterone concentrations. In primates, however, the position is somewhat different. Essentially, all studies have failed to demonstrate systemic progesterone withdrawal in late human pregnancy. In some subhuman primates, such as the rhesus monkey, maternal peripheral plasma progesterone concentrations clearly rise prepartum. The possibility that local (intra-uterine) changes in progesterone production or action occurs in these species has been raised as a possible explanation of this apparent discrepancy.[2,4]

Ovarian progesterone production predominates during the first 5–6 weeks of human pregnancy, and ovariectomy or administration of a progesterone

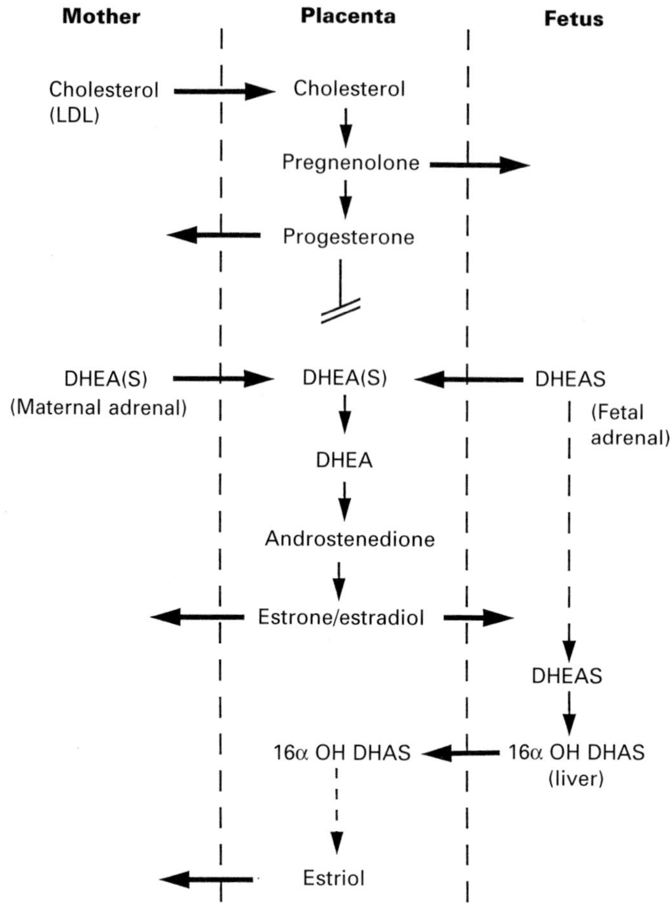

Fig. 22.1 Pathways of steroid production in mother, placenta and fetus during human pregnancy. LDL: low density lipoprotein; DHEA(S): dehydroepiandrosterone (sulphate).

receptor antagonist such as RU486 during this time leads to the evolution of myometrial contractility. After the sixth week of gestation, the placenta becomes the main site of progesterone synthesis, although ovarian progesterone production continues.[3] Maternal peripheral plasma progesterone concentrations rise progressively towards term. There is no significant change in the concentration of non-protein bound progesterone, nor in the ratio of total or free progesterone:estradiol in plasma. Concentrations of progesterone in amniotic fluid are lower than in maternal blood, and decline only gently during pregnancy. There is some evidence for a modest diurnal rhythm in maternal progesterone concentrations in women at 30–36 weeks of pregnancy.[5] Values were lower by 10–20% at the peaks of maternal cortisol concentrations. It is possible that this change reflects displacement from high affinity protein, such as transcortin (corticosteroid-binding globulin, CBG) by elevations in endogenous cortisol.

Alternatively, it has been proposed that this change in maternal progesterone reflects that component derived from placental utilization and conversion of pregnenolone sulphate of fetal adrenal origin. This explanation seems less likely, however, because progesterone levels are maintained in human pregnancy after fetal death, with anencephaly, or after administration to the mother of a synthetic corticosteroid, which does not bind to CBG.

It is generally considered that placental progesterone production depends on the availability of LDL-associated cholesterol, and adequate utero-placental blood flow.[3] Trophoblast tissue contains LDL receptors, and syncytiotrophoblast expresses 3β hydroxy steroid dehydrogenase Type II enzyme, as determined by immunohistochemistry and northern blotting. Uptake of LDL by trophoblast is enhanced by estrogen, an effect due to upregulation of LDL receptor expression.[6] In chorion, there was no formation of progesterone from LDL or free cholesterol, despite evidence for the presence of 3β HSD mRNA by northern blotting, and localization of immunoreactive 3β HSD Type II to trophoblasts by immunostaining. The paucity of estrogen receptor (ER) subtypes in this tissue may preclude any estrogenic effect.[7]

Alternatively, both chorion trophoblasts and syncytiotrophoblast could utilize pregnenolone or pregnenolone sulphate from plasma or amniotic fluid for progesterone synthesis. It has generally been considered that placental blood flow is the major regulator of placental progesterone output. However, maternal progesterone concentrations are lowered in patients with homozygous hypobetalipoproteinemia, showing the importance of substrate availability. Further, progesterone output in the placenta and/or membranes may be stimulated by analogs of cyclic AMP and activators of protein kinase A, including agonists.[2] These effects occur at the level of transcriptional control. Levels of mRNA encoding P450 SCC and adrenodoxin in cultured trophoblasts are augmented by addition of 8 bromo cyclic AMP to the cell.[8]

Catechol estrogens stimulate accumulation of progesterone by cultured trophoblasts; this effect was blocked by both phenoxybenzamine and propranolol, suggesting a nonspecific action through either α or β receptors. In the pregnant baboon, administration of the antiestrogen MER-25 leads to a fall in progesterone levels *in vivo*.[3] This drug resulted in a decrease in placental mitochondrial P450 SCC activity and LDL usage, supporting a stimulatory role for estrogen in placental progesterone biosynthesis. Presumably an effect of estrogen could also be mediated through an increase in uteroplacental blood flow. The failure to detect alterations in the circulating progesterone concentration in late pregnancy has led to the proposition that there might be local regulation of progesterone within the pregnant uterus, especially within the fetal membranes and decidua.[9] Term amnion and chorion exhibit 3β HSD activity with both dehydroepiandrosterone (DHEA) and pregnenolone as substrate.[9,10] Chorion was more active that amnion, although the cofactor requirements and substrate specificity for the enzyme were similar in both tissues. Activity of the enzyme was inhibited by several steroids, especially progesterone and 20α dihydroprogesterone (20α diHP). The abundance of 3βHSD mRNA in chorion/decidua was greater than in amnion but less than in the placenta. However, there was no difference in levels of 3βHSD mRNA in any one of amnion, chorion or placenta obtained from patients at term Cesarean section in the absence of labor, or after labor of spontaneous onset at term or preterm.[11,12] Thus, there is presently no evidence to support the possibility of changes in 3βHSD gene expression as a regulator of local or placental progesterone production at the time of labour.

There are also no changes in levels of the bioactive metabolite of progesterone, allopregnanolone (3α hydroxy-5α-pregnane-20-one) in maternal plasma at the time of labour.[12] This could provide an alternative to progesterone as the major progestational steroid. Western blotting has failed to reveal alterations in levels of progesterone receptor isoforms in myometrium at the time of parturition, although not all of the potentially interacting heat-shock proteins have been examined. In species such as the horse, progesterone can be metabolized to compounds which act as endogenous antagonists of progestational activity, but those pathways have not been fully explored in human tissues.

One interesting proposed mechanism for effective progesterone withdrawal is through the antagonism of progesterone action by a protein such as transforming growth factor β (TGFβ). Casey and MacDonald[13] reported that TGFβ antagonized the effect of progesterone on progestogen-responsive genes such as preproendothelin-1, connexin-43 and parathyroid hormone related peptide (PTHrP) in cultured endometrial stromal cells. Studies are required to determine levels and regulation of TGFβ expression, and of its receptor interaction in late pregnancy tissues.

Recent studies have clearly demonstrated a role for progesterone in inhibiting expression of contraction associated proteins (CAPs) in response to the stimulus of uterine stretch (see below).[14] Early *in vitro* experiments suggested that progesterone inhibited prostaglandin synthesis, through actions on the prostaglandin synthesizing enzymes. This does not appear to be a direct action, since nucleotide sequences that would serve as progesterone response elements have not been identified within the promotor regions of either the constitutively expressed prostaglandin synthase Type I (PGHS-I) or the inducible PGHS-II. Progesterone may, however, alter the rate of prostaglandin degradation through the enzyme 15-OH prostaglandin dehydrogenase (PGDH). PGDH activity in kidney and lung was increased by progesterone treatment. PGDH activity was decreased, and levels of PGE2 increased, in endometrium from women treated with RU486 in early pregnancy. Patel et al[15] were unable to demonstrate any effect of exogenous progesterone on PGDH activity or levels of PGDH mRNA in cultured chorion trophoblasts from term pregnancies. However, they reasoned that this result might be accounted for by high endogenous progesterone production, or by progesterone metabolism by the cells. In agreement with this, the synthetic progestogens R5020 and MPA did stimulate PGDH activity. Importantly, trilostane, an inhibitor of 3βHSD and of progesterone formation, reduced PGDH activity in chorion cells. This effect was overcome by addition of progesterone, suggesting clearly that one action of progesterone may be to regulate prostaglandin metabolism in the membranes, and that this effect could be due to steroid that is generated locally.

The evidence in support of changes in progesterone output by the ovary or placenta being critical in the control of parturition in subprimate species is substantial, and has been reviewed exhaustively. At the present time, however, it should be clear that equivalent information for primates remains unavailable.[2,3]

ESTROGENS

Estrogens have critical activities in the physiological changes that occur during pregnancy. It is clear that estrogens are involved in the stimulus to increased uterine blood flow during pregnancy, and in the accompanying maternal cardiovascular adaptations.[3] It is generally considered that estrogen stimulates growth and development of the pregnant uterus and production of contractile proteins. Clearly, estrogen is responsible, in large part, for the increased output of corticosteroid-binding globulin (CBG) from the maternal liver. This protein binds cortisol, providing an explanation for the apparent lack of Cushingoid characteristics in the mother, despite a relative maternal hypercortisolemia. In late pregnancy estrogens contribute to the environment that allows increased expression of a cassette of contraction-associated proteins, such as connexin-43, the oxytocin receptor, and choriodecidual oxytocin synthesis (see below).[16]

Maternal peripheral plasma concentrations of unconjugated estrone (E_1), estradiol 17β E_2) and estriol (E_3) rise progressively during gestation.[3,17] In plasma, E_2 predominates. In urine, E_3 is present in higher amounts, predominantly as glucuronide/sulphate conjugates. During the third trimester, maternal plasma estriol concentrations exhibit a diurnal pattern, with highest concentrations during the day and lowest concentrations at night. This rhythm is the opposite of that of maternal plasma cortisol. It is likely that the rhythm in maternal E_3 results from tonic rhythmic suppression of the fetal pituitary adrenal axis by maternally derived glucocorticoid, at least at this stage of gestation.[18]

Estrogen production in human pregnancy is dependent on the biochemical interdependence of anatomically distinct compartments: the fetus, the placenta and the maternal adrenal gland.[2,17] Specifically, the human placenta lacks P450C17 activity, and is therefore unable to convert C-21 steroids (such as progesterone) to C-19 steroids (androgens). However, the placenta expresses abundant aromatase activity and utilizes C-19 precursor steroids from other sources in the synthesis of estrogen (Fig. 22.1). The fetal zone of the fetal adrenal gland, which occupies 85% of the fetal adrenal cortex, has a relative deficiency of Type II 3βHSD. Therefore, the gland secretes predominantly Δ5- rather than Δ4- steroids. Because of the high sulphotransferase activity in the fetal adrenal, these compounds, predominantly dehydroepiandrosterone (DHA) are secreted as sulphoconjugates (DHAS). A high proportion of fetal DHAS moves directly to the placenta where it is ultimately converted to estrogen. Much of the fetal adrenal DHAS moves to the fetal liver where it is converted by a 16α hydroxylase enzyme to form 16α hydroxy DHAS. This compound then passes back to the placenta where it proceeds through hydrolysis, isomerase and aromatase steps to form a 16α hydroxy estrogen, estriol (E_3).

Approximately 50% of maternal plasma estrone (E_1) and estradiol (E_2) are derived from fetal adrenal precursors, with the remainder being derived from DHAS of maternal adrenal origin. However, approximately 90% of maternal estriol is derived from precursors formed in the fetus through 16α hydroxylation in the fetal liver. The maternal liver also metabolizes estrogen through the 16α hydroxylase pathway, and contributes to the remaining fraction.[17]

The human fetal adrenal is divided into medulla, an outer cortex and transitional zone that produces predominantly cortisol, and an inner fetal zone of the cortex that produces predominantly Δ5 steroids. In tissue culture these cells utilize LDL to derive cholesterol, and uptake of LDL by fetal adrenal cortical cells is promoted by treating them with ACTH. ACTH treatment of cultured cells also results in an increase in levels of ACTH receptor mRNA, as well as RNA transcripts encoding key steroidogenic enzymes. These observations are consistent with progressive maturation/activation of fetal hypothalamic-pituitary-adrenal (HPA) function, particularly during late gestation.

Measurements in the chronically catheterized fetal baboon and rhesus monkey have shown that the drive to fetal adrenal function likely comes from increasing concentrations of ACTH in the fetal circulation during the latter 20–30% of gestation. In turn, this drive is associated with increased levels of proopiomelanocortin (POMC) mRNA in the pars distalis of the fetal pituitary.[3] Similar observations have been made in domestic animal species, such as the sheep. Here, the fetus signals the onset of parturition through activation of the fetal HPA axis.[2,19] In fetal plasma there are increases in both ACTH and cortisol during the latter 15–20 days of pregnancy (term ~150 days). The rise in fetal plasma ACTH relates directly to an increase in levels of mRNA encoding POMC in the fetal pituitary pars distalis, and of CRH mRNA in the paraventricular nucleus of the fetal hypothalamus during late pregnancy. Mechanisms must be in place, *in vivo*, to assure that negative feedback by rising fetal cortisol does not shut off the drive from the fetal hypothalamus and the pituitary. These mechanisms include a reduction in glucocorticoid receptor number in the hypothalamus to diminish cortisol feedback on CRH expression and secretion; a concurrent increase in the high affinity corticosteroid-binding globulin (CBG) in the fetal circulation that maintains a relatively low free cortisol concentration until immediately before term; and isoforms of the enzyme 11β hydroxysteroid dehydrogenase in the placenta and fetal tissues, which determine the interconversion of cortisol to biologically inactive cortisone.

In the fetal rhesus monkey, plasma DHAS concentrations rise in late pregnancy with a time course that resembles closely that of cortisol in fetal sheep.[3] The increase in maternal estriol concentrations, which reflect fetal adrenal provision of C19 precursors for placental aromatization, shows a similar pattern in human gestation. Thus there appear to be fundamentally similar mechanisms between different species. In the monkey an additional, transitional zone of the fetal adrenal cortex, anatomically placed between the definitive and fetal zones, has been described. It is not clear yet whether a similar zone is present in the human fetal adrenal. This zone may give rise to the adult adrenal cortex. Its contribution of precursors for estrogen biosynthesis during pregnancy is unclear; and its major products are Δ4 steroids, especially cortisol.

The human fetal adrenal reaches its maximum size in the first trimester of pregnancy, and at about 10 weeks may be larger than the fetal kidney.[3,17] Eighty-five percent of the gland is occupied by the fetal zone of the cortex. This zone regresses postnatally. Eventually it disappears by about 12 months postpartum, as remodelling to form the zones of the mature adrenal occurs. The trophic factors responsible for these changes are unclear. Certainly, administration of synthetic glucocorticoids to pregnant monkeys and baboons results in reductions in fetal pituitary POMC mRNA levels, reduced plasma ACTH concentrations, and reductions in fetal adrenal cortical size, adrenal ACTH receptor mRNA levels and biological activity, and depletion of mRNA encoding steroidogenic enzymes. Maternal estrogen concentrations fall dramatically, an important point to note when betamethasone is being given to the patient at risk of preterm labor, and in whom serial urinary or salivary estriol measurements are components of clinical management.

In the human placenta, conversion of sulphoconjugated C-19 steroids to estrogen requires activities of sulphatase, 3βHSD, aromatase and 17βHSD enzymes.[17] Using immunohistochemistry these enzymes have been localized to the syncytiotrophoblast layer of the placental villi. Absence of sulphatase results in inability of the placenta to utilize sulphoconjugated precursors from the fetus, and leads to lowered estrogen concentrations in the mother. Although patients with placental sulphatase deficiency may progress to term, the development of uterine activity and cervical dilatation at labor is impaired. Placental sulphatase deficiency can be recognized clinically by very low maternal plasma or urinary estrogen concentrations, and failure of an exogenous oral dose of DHAS to be converted into estrogen (although free DHA is an adequate substrate for estrogen formation).

Placental type 1 3βHSD which catalyzes conversion of Δ5 to Δ4 steroids is associated with both mitochondrial and microsomal fractions of syncytiotrophoblast. Regulation of this enzyme by cyclic AMP (cAMP) and IGF was discussed above. Trophoblast cells express abundant IGF-1 and IGF-2. The actions of these growth factors on 3βHSD may be effected through similar mechanisms. Recent studies have characterized the P450arom, and shown that this belongs to a functionally related multigene family. P450arom is upregulated by cAMP and by activators of the protein kinase C pathway.

Thus output of estrogens by the placenta depends on the availability of precursors from both the mother and fetus, and from the activities of placental enzymes, including placental sulphatase. In conditions of anencephaly and fetal adrenal hypoplasia there are greatly reduced concentrations of estrogen in maternal plasma. Similarly, as discussed, administration of synthetic glucocorticoids into the maternal compartment results in transplacental transfer, and leads to suppression of fetal HPA function. Maternally-derived glucocorticoid suppresses fetal ACTH, reduces the supply of fetal adrenal precursors for placental aromatase, and maternal estrogens decrease. This effect is particularly marked for estriol synthesis, since E_3 is formed in the placenta from 90% fetal precursors. Endogenous glucocorticoids influence the fetal HPA in a similar manner. During the third trimester of pregnancy, maternal estriol concentrations are highest between 2200 and 0400 h, at the time when the endogenous rhythm of maternal cortisol concentration is at its nadir.[18] As maternal cortisol concentrations increase during the morning hours, so maternal estriol concentrations decrease. Interpretation of these results suggested that at physiologic concentrations maternal cortisol can cross the placenta and exert some level of negative feedback on the fetus.

In human pregnancy there is a substantial concentration gradient between cortisol concentrations in mother and fetus. The fetus is 'protected' from these high levels of maternal cortisol by the enzyme 11β HSD in the placenta.[20] In fact, there are two isoforms of 11β HSD: 11β HSD-1 and 11β HSD-2. These are separate gene products. 11β HSD-1 is more ubiquitous in distribution, and is present in chorion trophoblasts of the human fetal membranes, and in intermediate trophoblasts and endothelial cells of umbilical vessels in the floating villi. 11β HSD-1 operates at μM values of Km, and interconverts cortisol and cortisone in a bidirectional fashion. However it appears that 11β HSD-1 operates predominantly as a reductase, converting cortisone to cortisol. In the human fetal membranes, for example, cortisone affects expression of some genes such as 15-OH prostaglandin dehydrogenase, but only after conversion to cortisol through 11β HSD-1. 11β HSD-2 is localized to mineralocorticoid target tissues, where it operates as a unidirectional dehydrogenase at nM values of Km, converting cortisol to cortisone. Thus corticosteroid type-I (mineralocorticoid) receptors are protected from saturation by high levels of cortisol. 11β HSD-2 is expressed abundantly in human placenta and has been localized to syncytiotrophoblast.[21,22] Its expression and activity is stimulated by activation of cAMP, and decreased by progesterone and by nitric oxide. High levels of 11β HSD-2 in placental syncytiotrophoblast are believed to be important in metabolizing maternal cortisol to cortisone, and thereby diminishing excessive influences of maternally-derived corticosteroids on fetal growth and development.

Recent studies have shown an association between low levels of placental 11β HSD-2 and reductions in fetal birth weight. The level of 11β HSD may determine not only the extent to which maternal glucocorticoids affect HPA function in the fetus, but also be crucial in preventing long-term downregulation of fetal hippocampal corticosteroid (type II or type I) receptors (programming) in response to maternal corticoids. Synthetic glucocorticoids are generally less well metabolized by 11β HSD in the placenta, thus these compounds can be used to promote fetal development. However there is an increasing literature about their effects in decreasing fetal growth rates, and in producing permanent alterations of the set point for stress-induced HPA feedback and cortisol release in postnatal life.

Estrogens are also produced in the fetal membranes, although here aromatase activity is limited, and the major activity is estrogen sulphatase, utilizing estrone sulphate as precursor.[10] Estrone sulphatase activity is greatest in choriodecidual tissue, although it is present throughout the membranes. This activity is higher in tissues from patients at term spontaneous labour, compared to term elective Cesarean section. The V_{max} of the enzyme was also greater in tissue collected from patients in idiopathic preterm labour. There was no change in activity of the sulphatase converting DHAS to DHA in membranes, attesting to the specificity of the change in estrone sulphatase. Estrone sulphate was converted to estradiol in term human choriodecidua, indicating the presence of 17β HSD activity as well. These studies raise the possibility that local production of unconjugated estrogens may occur in the membranes from sulphoconjugated precursors at the time of labor. Estrone sulphatase has been localized by immunohistochemistry to chorionic trophoblasts. Further studies are clearly warranted on the regulation and expression of the potentially important enzyme at this site.

REGULATION OF MYOMETRIAL FUNCTION BY ESTROGEN AND PROGESTERONE

Pregnancy requires an extraordinary structural and functional remodeling of the myometrium. Not only must contractility be suppressed, only to be activated again at term, but a tremendous increase in uterine volume occurs to support the growth of the developing fetus. Estrogen and progesterone are the key hormones that orchestrate these changes, which allow the fetus to be maintained in the protective uterine environment until its physiologic organ systems have matured to an extent that it is capable of independent life. These steroids contribute both to the regulation of uterine growth and to the control of genes which directly or indirectly regulate contractility of this muscle.

Regulation of myometrial growth

Depending upon the species, the uterus can exhibit a 500–1000 fold increase in volume and >15 fold increase in weight — representing one of the most spectacular examples of organ growth in mammalian biology. Then, within days of birth, remodeling and regression occur as the nonpregnant form is re-established. Despite the fundamental nature of these alterations there is limited information as to the mechanisms that can produce such dramatic changes in uterine growth. The information that is available suggests that hormones and growth factors in combination with mechanical signals mediate these remarkable changes in uterine structure (Fig. 22.2).

The growth of the uterus represents a combination of hyperplasia and hypertrophy. There is some debate as to the contribution of each of these components as pregnancy progresses. However, our own preliminary data would support the view that early in pregnancy there is substantial hyperplasia, likely due to endocrine influence, whereas beyond the first third of pregnancy hypertrophy becomes a prominent factor due to fetal growth-induced stretch of the uterine wall. The mechanisms underlying this response, however, are not well understood. Growth factors and their receptors such as insulin-like growth factor (IGF-1), IGF-1 receptor, epidermal growth factor (EGF)/receptor, transforming growth factor (TGF), fibroblast growth factor (FGF), platelet-derived growth factor (PDGF) and vascular endothelial growth factor (VEGF) have been identified in uterine tissue, and expression of some of these is increased after estrogen treatment.[2]

Basic FGF increases DNA synthesis and cell proliferation in rat and human myometrial cells. Estrogen is generally considered to promote blood flow to the uterus, and studies in sheep support this proposition. However, uterine development and vascular adjustments do not appear to be rate-limiting

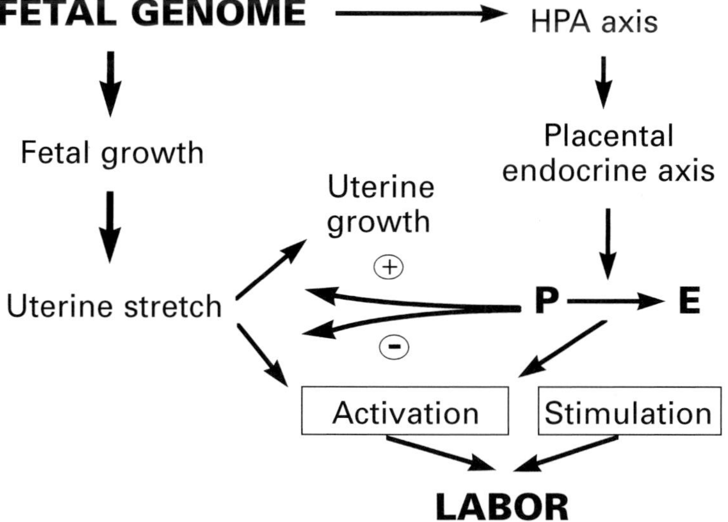

Fig. 22.2 A model for the fetal involvement in the onset of labor. The fetal genome regulates the onset of labour through two separate pathways: the classical endocrine pathway via activation of the HPA-placental axis and an increase in the E:P ratio, and a mechanical pathway mediated by stretch of the myometrium due to fetal growth. Both of these pathways act to increase the expression of genes that induce myometrial activation and stimulation. During pregnancy, the effect of stretch on myometrial expression of contraction-associated proteins is blocked by progesterone, thus supporting the maintenance of myometrial quiescence. We speculate that under the influence of progesterone, myometrial stretch promotes growth of the myometrium — an effect likely mediated by growth factors.

in pregnancies with sulphatase deficiency, or in anencephaly, so that it is difficult to suggest that high levels of estrogen are essential for these processes. Uterine activity is maintained in a relatively quiescent state during pregnancy despite the remarkable stimulus of uterine stretch. Studies in the rat suggest that this is attributable to interactions involving mechanical and endocrine inputs to the control of myometrial contractility.[14,23] When a small, 3 mm diameter vinyl tube was placed into the nonpregnant horn of unilaterally pregnant rats, it promoted an increase in the expression of contraction-associated proteins (CAPs). These include connexin-43, and the oxytocin receptor.[14,24] However, this response was seen only in animals at term (day 23) in which systemic withdrawal of progesterone had occurred. It was not present in animals at day 18 of gestation, in which there was no progesterone withdrawal. The vinyl tubes induced expression of mRNA encoding CAPs in nonpregnant ovariectomized animals, but this response was inhibited by concurrent administration of progesterone. Hence uterine stretch represents a potent stimulus to expression of those genes required for synchronous uterine activity at term, but this response can be blocked by progesterone, at least in experimental animals.

REGULATION OF MYOMETRIAL ACTIVITY BY STEROIDS

Throughout most of pregnancy the myometrium is unexcitable and relatively unresponsive to uterotonic agents such as oxytocin and prostaglandins (PGE, PGF). The myocytes are poorly coordinated. The muscle is not totally inactive, however, and low grade waves of contractile activity, lasting 5 to 8 minutes, associated with bursts of uterine electromyographic activity have been reported in several species.[25] These 'contractures' may be analogous to Braxton-Hicks contractions of the human uterus during gestation. They have little apparent effect on the cervix, and do not initiate labor. However, they may result in stimulus to the fetus (for example, as a result of transient utero-placental hypoperfusion and transient hypoxemia), and alter fetal behavioral state. In subhuman primates uterine contractile activity shows a marked diurnal rhythm, with increased activity during the hours of darkness. The magnitude of these activity excursions increases during the last 7–10 days of pregnancy in the rhesus monkey and correlates with rhythms in maternal oxytocin, before giving rise to labor.

We have considered it useful to regard uterine activity through late gestation as being divisible into at least four distinct phases.[2,4,16] These are phase 0 (quiescence), phase 1 (activation or preparedness), phase 2 (stimulation) and phase 3 (postpartum involution). There has been considerable discussion in the literature as to the nature of the agent(s) that initiate labor. Central to this discussion has been the definition of the initiation of labor itself. In our view, the transition from phase 0 to phase 1, quiescence to activation, is an appropriate time point for defining labor onset. However, we regard progression of labor as being divisible into two, time-dependent orderly steps, activation and stimulation. For optimal labor to occur, the uterus can only be stimulated after activation of myometrial function has taken place.

The relative quiescence of the uterus during pregnancy is likely maintained through the separate or combined activities of different inhibitors.[2,4] These include progesterone, relaxin, prostacyclin (PGI2), parathyroid hormone related peptide (PTHrP) and nitric oxide. Increased α-adrenergic tone and the potential to elevate intracellular cAMP characterize the vast majority of pregnancy. It is apparent that withdrawal of one or all of these influences could contribute to labor at term or preterm. The evidence, however, for 'withdrawal' in the sense of reduced synthesis, diminished circulating or local concentrations or antagonism of action remains circumspect for each of these agents.

The evolution of spontaneous contractile pattern with the initiation of labor is the manifestation of the transformation in phenotype of the myometrium. With the approach of labor, the muscle exhibits increased excitability, associated with a depolarization of the resting membrane potential. It also becomes highly responsive to uterotonic agents, and the smooth muscle cells increase markedly their electrical coupling. These changes collaborate to increase the effectiveness of uterotonic agents in generating high frequency contractions, and in ensuring that those contractions that are initiated rapidly spread to involve the entire uterus. We have called the increase in the capability of the myometrium to develop contractions 'myometrial activation'. Once the myometrium has undergone activation it can then undergo 'stimulation' in response to endocrine or paracrine uterotonins.[16] The combined effect of activation and stimulation is to enable the myometrium to generate the high frequency, high amplitude intense contractions required to assist dilation of the cervix and delivery of the fetus (Fig. 22.3).

As discussed earlier, the relative quiescence of the uterus during most of pregnancy has been attributed to a family of inhibitors, amongst which progesterone has

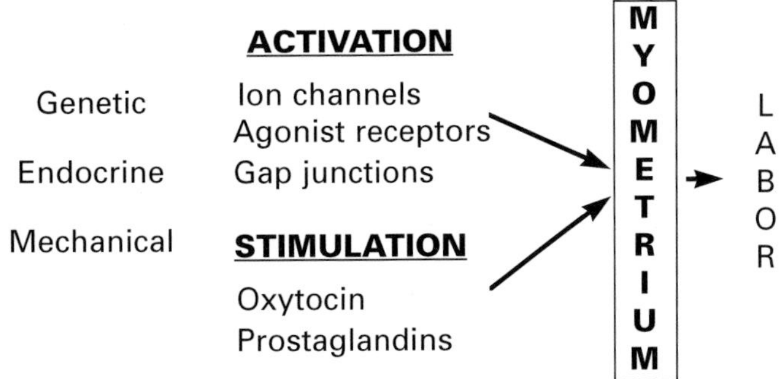

Fig. 22.3 Activation of the myometrium involves the increased expression of a cassette of genes encoding contraction-associated proteins (CAPs). These CAP genes include ion channels, receptors for uterotonic agonists and gap junctions. Together, these act to increase the excitability, responsiveness and coordination of myometrial contractility during labor. Once activated, the myometrium is able to respond effectively to the stimulation provided by the increased production of uterotonic agonists such as oxytocin and stimulatory prostaglandins. Activation and stimulation are controlled by the fetal genome through endocrine and mechanical pathways.

a preeminent position. In most species, administration of progesterone delays labor, reduces myometrial activity, attenuates coordination of contractions and reduces responsiveness to agonists. Progesterone achieves these effects on the myometrium through uncoupling of excitation-contraction and inhibition of the synthesis of agonist receptors, gap junctions or other contraction-associated proteins. In addition, progesterone suppresses production and formation of prostaglandins and blocks pituitary oxytocin release.[2] Progesterone also reduces the synthesis of CRH and lowers levels of CRH mRNA from intrauterine tissues including the placenta.[26]

Several recent studies have reported an association between increasing uterine activity and placental CRH expression. Maternal plasma CRH levels rise exponentially in normal pregnancies, are elevated in patients at risk of preterm labor and may be useful in discriminating between patients in true preterm labor from those who are not, but present in threatened preterm labor.[27] Regulation of CRH is clearly multifactorial, but appears to involve a balance between inhibition by NO and progesterone and stimulation by corticosteroids and cytokines.[28] Some workers have suggested that placental CRH output is essentially suppressed by progesterone, acting through glucocorticoid receptors. Elevations in cortisol at term displace progesterone thereby reducing its inhibitory effect — an outcome that appears as stimulation of CRH output by corticosteroids (exogenous or endogenous of fetal and/or maternal origin).

The vast majority of the physiologic actions of progesterone have been attributed to receptor-mediated regulation of genomic events.[2] In animals, maximal inhibitory effects of progesterone on the myometrium occur only after a delay of up to 48 hours. However, while the amplitude of contractions, cell-to-cell coupling and responsiveness to agonists is significantly reduced, low amplitude high frequency contractions remain, suggesting that myocyte excitability is not suppressed. By contrast, inhibitory uterotonins such as relaxin and PGI2 have an immediate effect on spontaneous uterine activity, but do not block responsiveness to stimulatory uterotonins. Nitric oxide would appear to function in a similar manner. These agents inhibit activity of myosin light chain kinase, either through mechanisms involving increasing cyclic nucleotides or through reductions in intracellular $[Ca^{2+}]$. Thus, progesterone acts in synergy with other agents to suppress spontaneous and stimulated uterine activity during pregnancy.

Estrogens act in many ways to antagonize the effects of progesterone. Exogenous estrogen increases responsiveness to oxytocin, upregulates choriodecidual oxytocin gene expression and enhances propagation of myometrial activity. The effects of estrogen on uterine activity are clearly illustrated in a recent series of experiments using the rhesus monkey.[29] In pregnant monkeys, maternal infusion of androstenedione (given as an estrogen precursor) accelerated the switch from contractures to contractions, and led to premature delivery. The effect of androstenedione was blocked by concurrent infusion of 4-OH androstenedione, an aromatase inhibitor. Thus the first result was not attributable to the administered androgen itself, but required conversion to estrogen. Infusion of estradiol itself, however, did not result in premature delivery. Several other groups had previously reported this result. The present authors ascribe the difference in effect between infused androstenedione and infused estradiol as being due to the necessity of generating estrogen locally in intrauterine tissues, presumably near to the myometrium. One anticipates that this interesting study will be extended to infusion of androgen into the fetus to mimic its physiologic site of production, as an obvious prerequisite to show that androgen of fetal origin, not just androgen infusion, results in premature delivery.

In species such as sheep, increased activity of the fetal HPA axis results in increased secretion of cortisol, rather than androgen, from the fetal adrenal gland.[19] Fetal cortisol acts on the placenta to increase expression and activity of placental P450C17. In turn, androgen can then be generated in the placenta through either the $\Delta 5$ pathway from pregnenolone or $\Delta 4$ pathway from progesterone.[2] The ovine placenta has abundant aromatase activity, and the androgen so formed is converted into estrogen. Thus this species has evolved a very nice mechanism by which the preparturient signal of fetal cortisol is utilized both for fetal organ maturation, and as initiator of parturition. Progesterone (P) output from the placenta falls as estrogen (E) increases, thereby effecting an increase in the E:P ratio. This, in turn, increases the state of activity of the myometrium during labor, but also contributes to the increased synthesis/release of stimulatory uterotonins such as prostaglandins and oxytocin. These agents act through receptor-mediated pathways to increase intracellular calcium, and hence activate the contractile elements.

Conclusion

Estrogen/progesterone: a molecular mechanism for labor

It is apparent that the myometrial phenotype switches from a state of relative quiescence, unresponsiveness and limited conductivity during pregnancy, to excitability, responsiveness and cell-to-cell coordination at term. It has been suggested that myometrial preparedness or 'activation' results from the orderly expression of genes encoding a cassette of contraction-associated proteins or CAPs (gap junctions, ion channels, uterotonin receptors).[14,16] Once activated, the myometrium can then respond to stimulation brought about by increased expression of endogenous uterotonins, such as oxytocin and prostaglandins (Fig. 22.3).

We suggest that this maintenance of myometrial quiescence during pregnancy and activation at labor requires both endocrine (provided by estrogen and progesterone) and mechanical inputs. As discussed above, increased tension within the myometrium due to stretch of the uterine wall from the growing fetus (or experimentally induced stretch) can increase the expression of myometrial CAPs. This stretch effect is modulated by the endocrine environment. During pregnancy stretch-induced expression of CAPs is blocked (probably due to the inhibitory action of progesterone). However, in the endocrine environment of labor (increased E:P ratio) the stretch-induced CAP expression is manifested.

The mechanisms by which this endocrine and mechanical regulation of myometrial CAP expression is achieved remain to be determined. However the synchronous expression of CAPs in association with the onset of labor suggests a role for a small number of transcription factors acting as master control genes. Sequence and functional analysis of the promoter region of the connexin-43 and oxytocin receptor genes reveal that while estrogen activates the promotor, there are no consensus palindromic estrogen response elements.[30] Further, the effect of estrogen on connexin-43 requires *de novo* protein synthesis.[31] The promotor regions of both of these genes contain AP-1 or fos/jun binding site sequences and these sequences appear to be highly conserved between species. Estrogen-induced upregulation of connexin-43 mRNA levels was associated in time with increases in c-fos and c-jun mRNA levels, in a fashion that would suggest a cause/effect relationship.[31] Fos mRNA is also increased in the rat myometrium during labor in association with increases in connexin-43 and the oxytocin receptor. Progesterone treatment of these rats blocked expression of each of these genes and blocked labor.[31] It is possible that CAP expression by stretch involves similar pathways. In nonpregnant rats stretch of one uterine horn induced an increase in c-fos mRNA; an effect that was blocked by progesterone (unpublished data). Moreover, *in vitro* stretch of myocytes has been reported to increase c-fos expression in several tissues. However, stretch can also activate multiple intracellular signaling pathways, leaving the mechanisms underlying this component of activation to be determined.

Thus these data suggest that in a uterine horn under tension an increase in the E:P ratio triggers a regulatory cascade in which one or more transcription factors, of which c-fos is a candidate member, orchestrate the expression of a cassette of CAPs in the myometrium. Activation is manifest as increased spontaneous activity, responsiveness and cell-to-cell coupling. The altered E:P ratio also contributes directly and indirectly to upregulation of stimulatory uterotonins. Activation and stimulation is therefore closely coordinated and eventuates in the generation of the high amplitude, high frequency contractions of labor.

REFERENCES

1. Lindzey J, Korach KS 1997 Steroid hormones. In: Conn PM, Melmed S (eds) Endocrinology: basic and clinical principles. Humana Press, Totowa, NJ, pp 47–62
2. Challis JRG, Lye SJ 1994 Parturition. In: Knobil E, Neill JD (eds) The physiology of reproduction, 2nd edn. Raven Press, New York, pp 985–1031
3. Pepe GJ, Albrecht ED 1995 Actions of placental and fetal adrenal steroid hormones in primate pregnancy. Endocrine Reviews 16: 608–648
4. Challis JRG, Gibb W 1996 Control of parturition. Prenatal and Neonatal Medicine 1: 283–291
5. Challis JRG, Sprague C, Patrick JE 1983 Relation between diurnal changes in peripheral plasma progesterone, cortisol and estriol in normal women at 30–31, 34–35, and 38–39 weeks of gestation. Gynecological and Obstetrical Investigation 16: 33–44
6. Simpson ER, Bilheimer DW, MacDonald PC, Porter JC 1979 Uptake and degradation of plasma lipoproteins by human choriocarcinoma cells in culture. Endocrinology 104: 8–16
7. Yeons MA, Besch NF, Besch PK 1981 Estradiol and progesterone binding in human term placental cytosol. American Journal of Obstetrics and Gynecology 141: 170–174
8. Pepe GJ, Waddell BJ, Albrecht ED 1989 Effect of estrogen on pituitary peptide-induced dehydroepiandrosterone secretion in the baboon fetus at midgestation. Endocrinology 125: 1519–1524
9. Gibb W, Riopel L, Lavoie JC 1988 Steroidogenesis and steroid-binding proteins in human fetal membranes. In: Mitchell BF (ed) Research in perinatal medicine (VI) — the physiology and biochemistry of human fetal membranes. Perinatology Press, Ithaca, NY, pp 29–47
10. Mitchell BF, Challis JRG 1988 Estrogen and progesterone metabolism in human fetal membranes. In: Mitchell BF (ed) Research in perinatal medicine (VI) — the physiology and biochemistry of human fetal membranes. Perinatology Press, Ithaca, NY, pp 5–28
11. Riley SC, Bassett NS, Berdusco ETM, Yang K, Leystra-Lantz C, Luu-The V, Labrie F, Challis JRG 1993 Changes in the abundance of mRNA for Type 1 3β-hydroxysteroid dehydrogenase/$\Delta^5 \rightarrow \Delta^4$ isomerase in the human placenta and fetal membranes during pregnancy and labor. Gynecological and Obstetrical Investigation 35: 199–203
12. Erb GE, Purdy RH, Lye SJ, Morrow RJ, MacLusky NJ 1997 Circulating and amniotic fluid sex steroid concentrations in human term pregnancy: does a change in steroid 5α-reduction signal the onset of labour? Steroids (in press).
13. MacDonald PC, Casey ML 1996 Preterm birth. Scientific American, Science and Medicine 3: 42–51
14. Ou Che-Wei, Orsino A, Lye SJ 1997 Expression of connexin-43 and connexin-26 in the rat myometrium during pregnancy and labor is differentially regulated by mechanical and hormonal signals. Endocrinology (in press)
15. Patel FA, Clifton VL, Challis JRG 1997 Regulation of prostaglandin dehydrogenase activity by cortisol in human term placenta and fetal membranes. 44th Annual Meeting of the Society for Gynecologic Investigation, San Diego, California, March 19–22, Abstr. 125
16. Lye SJ, Challis JRG 1989 Paracrine and endocrine control of myometrial activity. In: Gluckman PD, Johnston BM, Nathanielsz PW (eds) Advances in fetal physiology: reviews in honour of GC Liggins. Series title: Advances in perinatal medicine (VIII). Perinatology Press, Ithaca, NY, pp 361–375
17. Yen SSC 1994 Endocrinology of pregnancy. In: Creasy R, Resnik R(eds) Maternal fetal medicine — principles and practice, 3rd edn. WB Saunders, Philadelphia, pp 382–407
18. Patrick JE, Challis J, Campbell K, Carmichael L, Natale R, Richardson B 1980 Circadian rhythms in maternal plasma cortisol and estriol at 30–31, 34–35 and 38–39 weeks' gestational age. American Journal of Obstetrics and Gynecology 136: 325–334
19. Matthews SG, Challis JRG 1996 Regulation of the hypothalamo-pituitary-adrenocortical axis in fetal sheep. Trends in Endocrinology and Metabolism 7: 239–246
20. Brown RW, Chapman ICF, Edwards CRW, Seckl JR 1993 Human placental 11β-hydroxysteroid dehydrogenase: evidence for and partial purification of a distinct NAD-dependent isoform. Endocrinology 132: 2614–2621
21. Sun K, Yang K, Challis JRG 1997 Regulation of 11β-hydroxysteroid dehydrogenase type 2 by placental steroids and cyclic AMP pathway in cultured human placental trophoblasts. Biology of Reproduction (in press)
22. Sun K, Yang K, Challis JRG 1997 Glucocorticoid actions and metabolism in pregnancy: implications for placental function and fetal cardiovascular activity. Placenta (in press)
23. Lye SJ, Nicholson BJ, Mascarenhas M, MacKenzie L, Petrocelli T 1993 Increased expression of connexin-43 in the rat myometrium during labour is associated with an increase in the plasma estrogen:progesterone ratio. Endocrinology 132: 2380–2386
24. Ou C-W, Lye SJ 1997 Stretch is required to upregulate expression of the oxytocin receptor but not the prostaglandin F receptor in the rat myometrium during labour. Annual Meeting of the Society of Gynecologic Investigation, San Diego, California, March 19–22, Abstr. 029
25. Lye SJ 1997 Initiation of parturition. Animal Reproductive Science 42: 495–503
26. Challis JRG, Matthews SG, van Meir C, Ramirez MM 1995 The placental CRH-ACTH axis. Placenta 16: 481–502

27. Korebrits C, Ramirez MM, Watson L, Brinkman E, Bocking AD, Challis JRG 1998 Maternal corticotropin – releasing hormone is increased with impending preterm birth. Journal of Clinical Endocrinology and Metabolism 83: 1585–1591
28. Petraglia F, Florio P, Nappi C, Genazzani AR 1996 Peptide signaling in human placenta and membranes; autocrine, paracrine and endocrine mechanisms. Endocrine Reviews 17: 156–186
29. Mecenas CHA, Giussani DA, Owiny JR, Jenkins SL, Wu WX, Honnebier MBOM, Lockwood CJ, Kong L, Guller S, Nathanielsz PW 1996 Production of premature delivery in pregnant rhesus monkeys by androstenedione infusion. Nature, Medicne 2: 443–448
30. Lefebvre DL, Piersanti M, Bai X-H, Chen Z-Q, Lye SJ 1995 Myometrial transcriptional regulation of the gap junction gene, connexin-43. Reproduction and Fertility Developments 7: 603–611
31. Piersanti M, Lye SJ 1995 Increase in mRNA encoding the myometrial gap junction protein connexin-43 requires protein synthesis and is associated with increased expression of the AP-1 protein, C-FOS. Endocrinology 136: 3571–3578

23. Estrogens and progesterone in the post-partum period

P.J. Illingworth   A.S. McNeilly

Introduction

The interval after childbirth is an important time for women, when critical emotional and physiological changes are taking place. As well as recovery from the effects of pregnancy, there are also the profound endocrine and metabolic adaptations to breastfeeding. These effects are of vital importance, for as well as nourishment and prevention of infant infection, breastfeeding offers protection against further conception.[1] Indeed, it has been estimated that in many developing countries breastfeeding still prevents more pregnancies than all modern forms of contraception.[2] It is therefore imperative that artificial contraceptive strategies do not compromise this effect and indeed considerable attention has recently been given to identifying the conditions under which breastfeeding itself can be relied on as a method of contraception.[3–6] A detailed understanding of the mechanisms behind the endocrine changes of the postpartum period in general, and of lactational infertility in particular, is central to further developments in this area.

ACUTE CHANGES IN HORMONE CONCENTRATION FOLLOWING DELIVERY

In women, unlike many other species, the progesterone concentration remains elevated throughout pregnancy until separation of the placenta. However, following delivery, there is an abrupt decline in the concentration of placental hormones over the first two days (Fig. 23.1).[7,8,9] The fall in progesterone concentration leads directly to the initiation of lactogenesis.[10] The rapid decline in the concentrations of sex steroids and inhibin[7] suggest that during pregnancy the

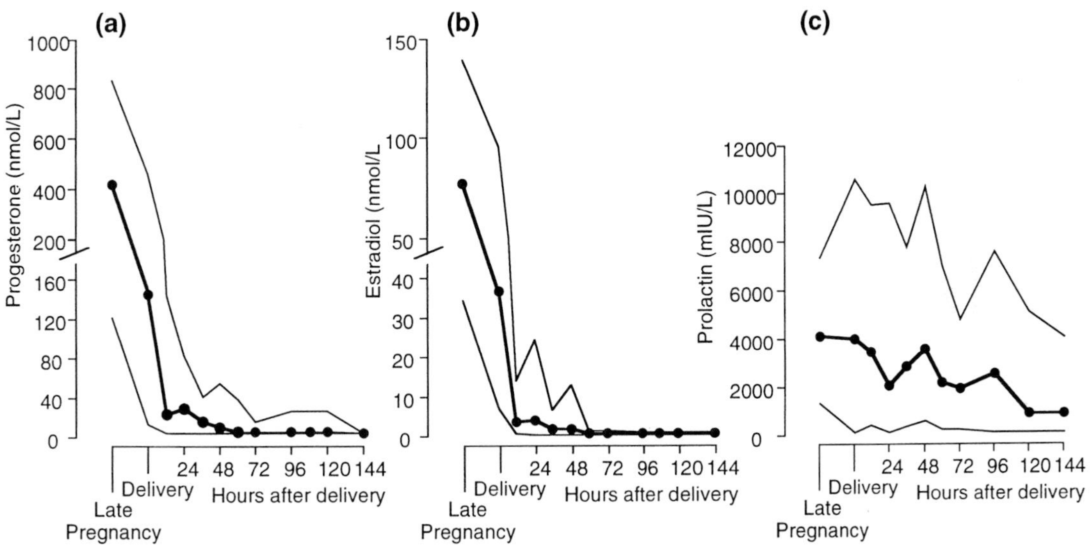

Fig. 23.1 Plasma concentrations of (**a**) progesterone (**b**) estradiol and (**c**) prolactin immediately before and for six hours after delivery in non-breastfeeding women (n=25).[8]

placenta is the principal source of these hormones. While the ovary has a luteinized appearance with multiple small follicles present,[11] it does not appear that these secrete significant amounts of hormone.

The circulating concentrations of pituitary gonadotropins are low throughout pregnancy. This is due to suppression at the pituitary level as the pituitary content of LH at term is less than 1% of normal.[12] The concentrations of both LH and FSH remain suppressed and unresponsive to GnRH for up to 10 days after delivery, even in bottle-feeding women. As the concentrations of placental steroids drop in bottle-feeding women, the FSH concentration starts to rise at approximately 15 days after delivery and reaches normal menstrual cycle concentrations by 28 days postpartum.[13,14] At the same time, LH pulses become re-established, but at random frequencies during the day.[15,16] However, for some time after delivery, the frequency and amplitude of these pulses remain less than that seen in the early follicular phase of the normal menstrual cycle.[16] Following delivery, the concentration of prolactin falls rapidly in nonlactating women, returning to normal values by 30 days postpartum.[16,17]

The gradual increase in gonadotropin secretion after delivery results in a resumption of ovarian activity and menses. However, in both breastfeeding and bottle-feeding women, the early menstrual cycles are often irregular and anovulatory (Fig. 23.2).[18] Indeed only two thirds of women ovulate during the first menstrual cycle[19] and in 80% of these women, the progesterone concentrations during the first luteal phase remain.[19,20] The mechanism for the inadequate corpus luteum in the early postpartum cycles remains unknown. In the absence of breastfeeding, the mean time to first ovulation is approximately 42 days[9,20,21] although ovulation has been noted as early as 27 days after delivery.[19]

EFFECTS OF LACTATION ON ESTROGEN AND PROGESTERONE SECRETION

Lactational amenorrhea

The suppression of fertility during breastfeeding is a physiological mechanism of fundamental importance. During breastfeeding, the suppression of ovarian activity and the consequent alterations in circulating concentrations of estradiol and progesterone are closely related to the feeding patterns used. Lactational amenorrhea is extended by prolonged breastfeeding[22] and is particularly related to an interaction between the frequency of suckling and the duration of individual feeds[18,23] although the relative contribution of these factors is not clear.[24] Conversely, disruption of the pattern of suckling by the early introduction of

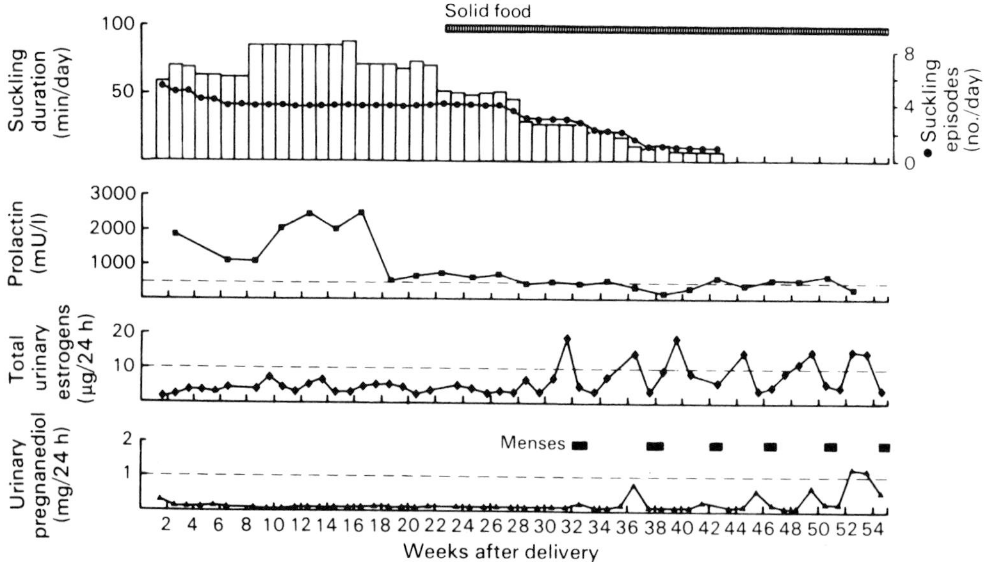

Fig. 23.2 Serial measurements of total suckling duration, plasma prolactin concentration, total urinary estrogens and urinary pregnanediol in a breastfeeding mother during lactation. As solid food is introduced, the suckling frequency diminishes and ovulation returns. It is notable that most of the early cycles are anovulatory.[18]

supplementary feeds, results in a shortening of the lactational amenorrhea.[23,24,25]

The feeding pattern does not, however, appear to be the only factor regulating the duration of lactational amenorrhea as large variations have been observed in the duration of lactational amenorrhea between different populations.[22] The explanation for the wide variations observed is not clear. One possibility which has been highlighted is the nutritional status of the mother.[26] However, while extremes of nutritional deprivation can undoubtedly affect the regulation of fertility, it does not appear that lesser degrees of nutritional variation exert a major effect on the duration of lactational amenorrhea.[26,27]

Changes in gonadotropin secretion

During breastfeeding, the alterations in gonadotropin concentration seen in the early postpartum period are continued. Despite suckling, the concentration of FSH in breast feeding women increases to within normal early follicular phase levels by 4–8 weeks gestation.[13,14,28,29] While the LH level rises after delivery, the mean concentration remains abnormally low for most of the lactational amenorrhea interval.[29,30] The response to GnRH is reduced in the very early post-partum period[31] but later in lactation high amplitude LH responses to GnRH have been reported.[32,33]

The abnormal gonadotropin secretion during lactational amenorrhea may be due to suppression of pulsatile GnRH release. The demonstration that administration of pulsatile GnRH to breastfeeding women results in both a return of ovarian activity[34] and subsequently full ovulation, if maintained for an adequate duration,[35] represents important evidence. The observation that both the pituitary and ovary are capable of responding to this treatment indicates that any direct effect of prolactin (or other lactation-induced factor) at these levels is likely to be of only limited importance.

Serial studies of 24 hour hormone secretion in breastfeeding women at different intervals after delivery, have provided detailed evidence of serial changes in the patterns of pulsatile LH release.[36] At four weeks after delivery, the majority of fully breastfeeding women studied had no detectable LH pulses and while LH pulses were detectable in most women by eight weeks post-partum, the pulse frequency remained grossly abnormal.[29] Low amplitude pulsatility has been detected in the plasma LH concentration soon after delivery[30] but the low amplitude of the pulses observed makes the physiologic significance of these pulses unclear. As lactation progresses, supplementary feeding is introduced and suckling declines, the frequency of LH pulses increases to near the frequency seen in the normal follicular phase (Fig. 23.2).[15] In contrast to these findings, recent studies in Chile[37] have reported apparently normal patterns of both frequency and amplitude of LH pulsatility, despite continuing anovulation. These women were, however, studied several months post-partum and it is possible that the different findings represent variations due to the differing breastfeeding patterns seen in extended lactation.

Neuroendocrine control

One critical question is the nature of the mechanism by which suckling behavior results in a suppression of GnRH pulsatility. In this respect, a number of possibilities have been proposed.

An enhancement of endogenous opioidergic tone in the hypothalamus is a strong candidate as detailed studies in other species, including rats and farm animals, have provided strong evidence for a role of enhanced opioidergic tone in post-partum anestrus in these species.[38] Four published studies have investigated this issue in women.[32,33,39,40] Tay[32] and Kremer[39] found no effects of naloxone on untreated women. Ishizuka[40] found no effects in the initial days post-partum but did demonstrate an increase in mean LH concentration when naloxone was administered after day 23. The administration of either the progestogen-only pill or exogenous estradiol, however, led to a marked responsiveness to naloxone.[32,33] Further support for a role of opioids has come from the demonstration of increased concentrations of the opioidergic agent β-casomorphin-8 in the cerebrospinal fluid of breastfeeding women.[41]

These findings can be interpreted in a number of ways. It is possible that as lactation becomes more advanced and the degree of opioid suppression less pronounced, the suppressant effects of endogenous opioids can now be overcome by an opioid antagonist such as naloxone. Alternatively, it may be that during the early stages of amenorrhea, opioids are not involved but during the later stages of lactation, a steroid-dependent opioid inhibition of GnRH pulsatility becomes an important component of lactational amenorrhea. In conclusion, while a role for opioids in lactational infertility appears likely, definitive evidence in support of this effect is still lacking.

The role of alterations in dopaminergic tone in lactational amenorrhea is even more complex. As prolactin is under predominantly inhibitory dopaminergic control, the high prolactin concentration during breastfeeding may reflect a reduced pituitary dopaminergic tone during breastfeeding. Indeed, the administration of dopamine antagonists to non-breastfeeding women results in an increase in prolactin concentration as well as an inhibition of ovulation, presumably through a central inhibition of GnRH pulsatility.[42] However, the further inhibition of dopaminergic action through the administration of dopamine antagonists to a group of breastfeeding women had no effect on either pulsatile or basal LH concentration.[32] Conversely, the administration of dopamine agonists is effective in the clinical treatment of pathologic hyperprolactinemia, resulting in a lowering of prolactin concentration as well as a return of fertility. However, as the administration of dopamine agonists to breastfeeding women is generally associated with a reduction or cessation of suckling, it is unclear whether the dopamine agonists themselves are responsible for the effects seen.

Prolactin

The concentration of prolactin increases progressively through pregnancy and remains high for up to three weeks post-partum even in the absence of suckling.[43] During breastfeeding, prolactin is released in response to the suckling stimulus of the baby with no evidence of release before the onset of nipple stimulation.[44] Prolactin is essential for milk production[43] but there is no close correlation between the plasma concentration of prolactin, either basal or following suckling, and the amount of milk produced.[45]

The role of prolactin in the mechanisms of lactational amenorrhea remains unclear. There is a clear association between a high plasma prolactin concentration and a prolonged duration of lactational infertility.[14,46,47] Conversely, a reduced prolactin concentration has been associated with an early return of fertility, and a negative correlation has been reported between the preovulatory estradiol rise and prolactin concentration. However the relationship between prolactin and fertility may be indirect. The prolactin concentration is closely related to the level of suckling activity,[26] which is likely to be the principal factor regulating normal LH secretion.

It is possible that prolactin exerts a direct negative effect on ovarian function.[48] The restoration of ovarian activity by pulsatile GnRH without a significant change in prolactin concentration makes a functionally important effect of prolactin on the ovary unlikely,[34,35] although a role in the etiology of the inadequate corpus luteum remains possible (see ch. 37). The administration of dopamine antagonists to induce hyperprolactinemia has the effect of suppressing fertility.[42] However, this may be due to a direct effect of the dopaminergic inhibition on LH secretion and thus coincidental to the changes in prolactin concentration.

Prolactin may act through a direct effect on the hypothalamus by an ultra short feedback loop. It has been shown that administration of prolactin to the third ventricle of rats and sheep[49] results in an increase in dopamine turnover and specific prolactin receptors have been demonstrated in the hypothalamus of the rat.

Prolactin exists in a number of different forms with varying bioactivities. No consistent changes have been observed in either the half-life[50] or the predominant molecular weight form (22 kDa) secreted during lactation.[51] Prolactin bioactivity (as measured by lymphocyte proliferation bioassay) has been found to be increased relative to immunoactivity in early lactation compared to late lactation[52] as well as in prolonged breast feeders. The physiological significance of this is however unclear.

Negative feedback effects of estradiol

A further possibility is that the pituitary and hypothalamus may exhibit enhanced sensitivity to the negative feedback effects of estradiol. This has previously been demonstrated using intramuscular estradiol benzoate.[53] More recently it has been shown that small increases in plasma estradiol concentration result in a significant change in the concentrations of both LH and FSH.[33] This was shown to be due to a direct effect on the hypothalamus, as the response of LH and FSH to a single bolus of GnRH was not suppressed. Other work has shown that the ability of higher dose estradiol to evoke an LH surge is also attenuated during breastfeeding.[53] Inhibins have been implicated in the control of FSH secretion but current data suggest that total inhibin immunoreactivity remains low during breastfeeding.[7] The effect of lactation on the concentrations of bioactive inhibin-A and inhibin-B remain unknown.

Ovarian function in the post-partum period

During lactational amenorrhea, ovulation is inhibited. Luteal structures are not seen and measurements of plasma progesterone as well as urinary pregnanediol excretion remain low. There is also a general suppression of ovarian activity.[34] Both the plasma estradiol concentration[14] and the urinary estrogen excretion[18,20,54] are generally reduced. However, ovarian scanning has revealed patterns of multifollicular development with large numbers of follicles evident at up to 8 mm in diameter, while in some women, larger follicles developed and produced estradiol but did not ovulate.[55] These follicles generally appeared to secrete little estradiol and while short-term elevations of estrogen secretion have been noted,[18,54] the concentration generally remains below that seen in association with a preovulatory follicle.

Taken together, these observations suggest that in women, as in some other species, follicle growth is reduced but not completely inhibited. It is possible that this arises as a result of the normal FSH concentration initiating follicular development while the abnormalities in LH pulsatility prevent further development and ultimately ovulation. Indeed, similar patterns of follicular development occur in hypogonadotropic women treated with pure FSH preparations lacking LH bioactivity. In any case, the result is that while ovulation is inhibited, the small prevulatory follicles may produce sufficient estradiol (and possibly inhibin-B)[56] to maintain inhibition of normal gonadotropin secretion through the enhanced sensitivity to estrogen feedback[33] of the hypothalamo-pituitary axis during lactation (Fig. 23.3).

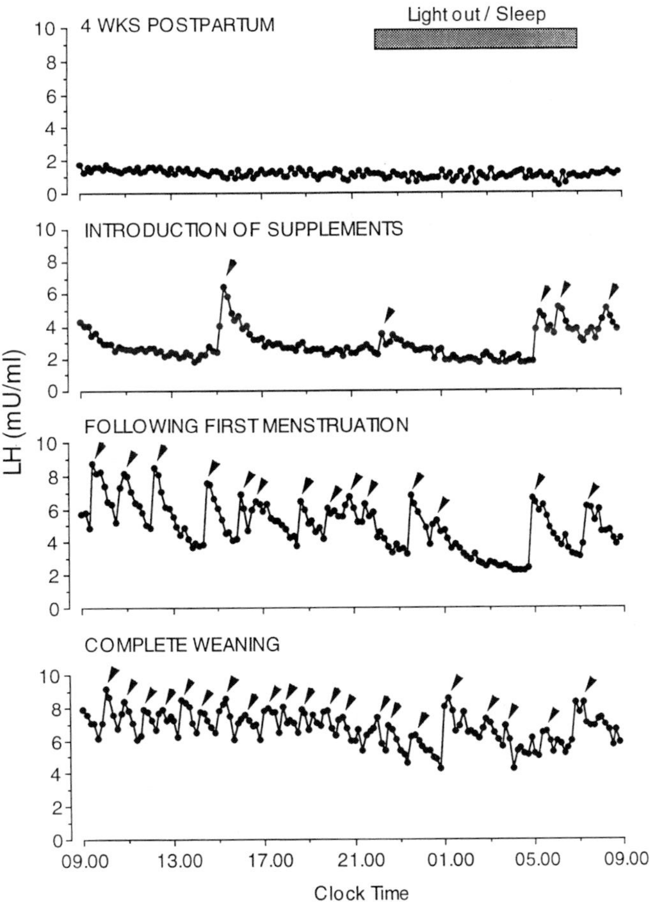

Fig. 23.3 Progressive return of the pulsatile pattern of LH secretion over 24 h periods at different stages in the return of normal ovarian activity in a breastfeeding woman. No follicles were present and at the introduction of supplements at 16 weeks only limited estradiol secretion was evident indicating the presence of a follicle. Follicle growth had resumed after first menses but was associated with an inadequate corpus luteum, while normal menstrual cycles resumed after weaning when the pulsatile pattern of LH release was normal.[36] ▼ indicates an LH pulse.

THE CONSEQUENCES OF HYPOESTROGENISM DURING LACTATION

The effects on maternal health of the altered concentrations of estrogens and progestogens during the post-partum period have not been clear. One critical issue is the possibility of osteoporosis due to the prolonged hypoestrogenic state. Several studies have demonstrated evidence of enhanced bone loss, particularly with prolonged feeding[57,58] which is not prevented by calcium ingestion[59] and there have been isolated case reports of osteopenic fractures during breastfeeding.[60] In addition, a further potential factor is the enhanced rate of bone resorption to provide calcium for breastmilk.[61] Changes in bone density seen during lactation appear to be more marked in the lumbar spine than in the radial spine.[57,62] However, these effects appear to be balanced by an increased rate of recovery of bone density following breastfeeding,[57,58] even if a subsequent pregnancy intervenes.[63] This effect may be due to an enhanced bone turnover during the recovery period. The enhanced bone turnover may be related to elevated concentrations of parathyroid hormone (PTH) seen in the weaning period,[58,59] possibly acting through an inhibition of renal calcium absorption. A complicating feature has been the demonstration of increased concentrations of PTH-related protein (PTH-rP) in both breastfeeding and pathologically hyperprolactinemic women. This protein originates from lactating mammary gland and pituitary adenomas. While it is thought to have effects on mammary gland blood flow and adverse effects on bone density, its physiological role in women is unclear.

The data on the cumulative effects of breastfeeding obtained from retrospective studies of postmenopausal women are generally reassuring. These data show either a weak effect,[64] no effect[62,65,66] or, indeed, a positive effect[62,67] on subsequent bone density or fracture risk. However, the multifactorial nature of these retrospective studies means that the power to detect the effect of an individual factor such as lactation is limited.

The extent of other effects of estradiol deficiency in the postpartum period are less clear. Despite one report of hot flushes in association with breastfeeding,[68] hypoestrogenic autonomic disturbances are uncommon at this time, probably due to central suppression of the hypothalamic processes involved. Mood swings are clearly a common and important feature of the immediate postpartum period, but their relationship to the steroid milieu is uncertain. While an association has been suggested between salivary hormone concentrations and postnatal mood changes,[69] no relationship has been established between plasma hormone concentrations and mood in lactating women.[70] Conversely, both estradiol and progesterone have been suggested as potential treatments for postnatal depression.[71,72] However the true value of such treatments has not been clearly established by adequate randomized trials and, in view of the potential side effects of estrogens and progestogens in the early post-partum days, they cannot be recommended on the presently available evidence.

CONTRACEPTION DURING THE POST-PARTUM PERIOD

Bottle-feeding women

In order to prevent early ovulation in bottle-feeding women, it has been recommended that contraception is used from 3–4 weeks after delivery, depending on risk factors for possible thromboembolism at this time. Apart from this consideration, bottle-feeding women's contraceptive needs are the same as those outside the post-partum period.

Breastfeeding women — the lactational amenorrhea method

While the overall effect of lactation on fecundity is beyond doubt, the extent to which a woman can rely on breastfeeding as her sole method of contraception has long been a source of controversy. A group of experts meeting at Bellagio calculated on the basis of the available data from 13 studies of ovulation rates and fecundity, carried out in eight countries, that if a woman is fully breastfeeding and amenorrheic, she ought to be able to expect 98% protection from pregnancy for up to six months.[3] These conclusions have been applied to the development of an algorithm for the Lactational Amenorrhea Method (LAM) of contraception.[73] Clinical trials have subsequently confirmed the contraceptive efficacy of this careful approach.[5,6]

Breastfeeding women — additional contraception

However, most women continue to opt for an additional method of contraception during breastfeeding. The principles of use of barrier methods or the intra-uterine contraceptive device are the same as in the nonlactating woman. Intra-uterine devices should be fitted at about six weeks post-partum.

Where a hormonal method of contraception is preferred, a progestogen-only method is generally advised as estrogen-containing contraceptives have the potential for an adverse effect on milk production. This effect appears to be dose-related for, while higher doses of estrogens clearly inhibit milk synthesis, the effect may be less-marked at lower doses.[74,75]

The use of any hormonal method is associated with concern about the potential for adverse effects of the hormone content of breastmilk at such a critical stage of infant development. The evidence relating to progestogen-only methods is however reassuring. Several detailed studies of infant development following the use of a progestogen-based method, including depot and orally active preparations, have no evidence of any adverse effect on breastmilk volume, infant growth or infant health.[76,77] Despite this, progestogen-based contraceptives should not generally be used in breastfeeding women before six weeks post-partum. As well as avoiding the possibility of harmful effects at the very early stages of infant life, such an approach also helps to reduce the likelihood of troublesome bleeding. In any case, a fully breastfeeding woman has no need for additional contraception before this time.

Similarly reassuring data are not available for estrogen-containing contraceptives. However, in the later months of breastfeeding, as the contraceptive protection decreases, many women may prefer to switch to an estrogen-containing preparation because of the greater contraceptive efficacy and the improved cycle control.

REFERENCES

1. Thapa S, Short RV, Potts M 1988 Breast feeding, birth spacing and their effects on child survival. Nature 335: 679–682
2. Short RV 1993 Lactational infertility in family planning. Annals of Medicine 25: 175–180
3. Kennedy KL, Rivero R, McNeilly AS 1989 Consensus statement on the use of breastfeeding as a family planning method. Contraception 39: 477–496
4. Kennedy KI, Parenteau-Carreau S, Flynn A, Gross B, Brown JB, Visness C. The natural family planning-lactational amenorrhea method interface: observations from a prospective study of breastfeeding users of natural family planning. American Journal of Obstetrics and Gynecology 165: 2020–2026
5. Kennedy KI, Visness CM 1992 Contraceptive efficacy of lactational amenorrhoea. Lancet 339: 227–230
6. Short R, Lewis PR, Renfree MB 1991 Contraceptive effects of extended lactation amenorrhoea: beyond the Bellagio consensus. Lancet 2: 715–717
7. Burger HG, Hee HPC, Mamers P, Bangah M, Zissimos M, McCloud PI 1994 Serum inhibin during lactation: relation to the gonadotrophins and gonadal steroids. Clinical Endocrinology 41: 771–777
8. West C, McNeilly AS 1979 Hormone profiles in lactating and nonlactating women immediately after delivery and their relationship to breast engorgement. British Journal of Obstetrics and Gynaecology 86: 501–506
9. Poindexter AN, Ritter MB, Besch PK 1983 The recovery of normal plasma progesterone levels in the postpartum female. Fertility and Sterility 39: 494–498
10. Cowie AT, Forsyth IA, Hart IC 1980 Hormonal control of lactation. Springer-Verlag, Berlin
11. Govan ADT 1970 Ovarian follicular activity in late pregnancy. Journal of Endocrinology 48: 235–241
12. dela Lastra M, Llados C 1977 Luteinizing hormone content of the pituitary gland in pregnant and nonpregnant women. Journal of Clinical Endocrinology and Metabolism 44: 921–923
13. Glasier A, McNeilly AS, Howie PW 1983 Fertility after childbirth: changes in serum gonadotrophin levels in bottle and breast feeding women. Clinical Endocrinology 19: 493–501
14. Delvoye P, Badawi M, Demaegd M, Robyn C 1978 Serum prolactin, gonadotrophins and estradiol in menstruating and amenorrhoeic women during two years of lactation. American Journal of Obstetrics and Gynecology 130: 635–640
15. Glasier A, McNeilly AS, Howie PW 1984 Pulsatile secretion of LH in relation to the resumption of ovarian activity post partum. Clinical Endocrinology 20: 415–426
16. Liu JH, Park KH 1988 Gonadotropin and prolactin secretion increases during sleep during the puerperium in nonlactating women. Journal of Clinical Endocrinology and Metabolism 66: 839–845
17. Glasier A, McNeilly AS, Howie PW 1984 The prolactin response to suckling. Clinical Endocrinology 21: 109–116
18. Howie PW, McNeilly AS 1982 Effect of breast feeding patterns on human birth intervals. Journal of Reproduction and Fertility 65: 545–557
19. Gray RH, Campbell OM, Zacur HA, Labbok MH, MacRae SL 1987 Postpartum return of ovarian activity in nonbreastfeeding women monitored by urinary assays. Journal of Clinical Endocrinology and Metabolism 64: 645–650
20. Howie PW, McNeilly AS, Houston MJ, Cook A, Boyle H 1982 Fertility after childbirth: postpartum ovulation and menstruation in bottle and breast feeding mothers. Clinical Endocrinology 17: 323–332
21. Gross BA, Eastman CJ 1985 Prolactin and the return of ovulation in breast feeding women. Journal of Biosocial Science (Suppl) 9: 25–42
22. Howie PW 1993 Natural regulation of fertility. British Medical Bulletin 49: 182–199
23. Gray RH, Campbell OM, Apelo R et al 1990 Risk of ovulation during lactation. Lancet 335: 25–29
24. Diaz S, Aravena R, Cardenas H et al 1991 Contraceptive efficacy of lactational amenorrhea in urban Chilean women. Contraception 43: 335–352

25. Howie PW, McNeilly AS, Houston MJ, Cook A, Boyle H 1981 Effect of supplementary food on suckling patterns and ovarian activity during lactation. British Medical Journal 283: 757–759
26. Lunn P 1985 Maternal nutrition and lactational infertility: the baby in the driving seat. In: Dobbing J (ed) Maternal nutrition and lactational infertility. Raven Press, New York, pp 41–64
27. Hennart P, Hofvander Y, Vis H, Robyn C 1985 Comparative study of nursing mothers in Africa (Zaire) and in Europe (Sweden): breast feeding behaviour, nutritional status, lactational hyperprolactinaemia and status of the menstrual cycle. Clinical Endocrinology 22: 179–187
28. Cholst IN, Wardlaw SL, Newman CB, Frantz AG 1984 Prolactin response to breast stimulation in lactating women is not mediated by endogenous opioids. American Journal of Obstetrics and Gynecology 150: 558–561
29. Tay CCK, Glasier A, McNeilly AS 1992 The 24 h pattern of pulsatile luteinizing hormone, follicle stimulating hormone and prolactin release during the first 8 weeks of lactational amenorrhoea in breastfeeding women. Human Reproduction 7: 951–958
30. Nunley WC, Urban RJ, Evans WS 1991 Preservation of pulsatile luteinizing hormone release during postpartum lactational amenorrhoea. Journal of Clinical Endocrinology and Metabolism 73: 629–636
31. Le Maire WJ, Shapiro AG, Riggall F, Yang NST 1974 Temporary pituitary insensitivity to stimulation by synthetic LRF during the postpartum period. Journal of Clinical Endocrinology and Metabolism 38: 916–918
32. Tay CCK, Glasier AF, McNeilly AS 1993 Effect of antagonists of dopamine and opiates on the basal and GnRH-induced secretion of luteinizing hormone, follicle stimulating hormone and prolactin during lactational amenorrhoea in breastfeeding women. Human Reproduction 8: 532–539
33. Illingworth PJ, Seaton J, McKinlay C, Reid-Thomas V, McNeilly AS 1995 Low dose transdermal oestradiol suppresses gonadotrophin secretion in breast-feeding women. Human Reproduction 10: 1671–1677
34. Glasier A, McNeilly AS, Baird DT 1986 Induction of ovarian activity by pulsatile infusion of LHRH in women with lactational amenorrhoea. Clinical Endocrinology 24: 243–252
35. Zinaman MJ, Cartledge T, Tomai T, Tippett P, Merriam GR 1995 Pulsatile GnRH stimulates normal cyclic ovarian function in amenorrheic lactating postpartum women. Journal of Clinical Endocrinology and Metabolism 80: 2088–2093
36. McNeilly AS, Tay CCK, Glasier A 1994 Physiological mechanisms underlying lactational amenorrhoea. In: Campbell KL, Wood JW (eds) Human reproductive ecology; interactions of environment, fertility and behaviour. New York Academy of Sciences, New York, pp 145–155
37. Diaz S, Cardenas H, Zepeda A et al 1995 Luteinizing hormone pulsatile release and the length of lactational amenorrhoea. Human Reproduction 10: 1957–1961
38. McNeilly AS 1994 Suckling and the control of gonadotropin secretion. In: Knobil E, Neill JD (eds) The physiology of reproduction, vol. 2, 2nd edn. Raven Press, New York, pp 1179–1212
39. Kremer JAM, Borm G, Schellekens LA, Thomas CMG, Rolland R 1991 Pulsatile secretion of luteinizing hormone and prolactin in lactating and nonlactating women and the response to naltrexone. Journal of Clinical Endocrinology and Metabolism 72: 294–300
40. Ishizuka B, Quigley MS, Yen S 1984 Postpartum hypogonadotrophinism: evidence for increased opioid inhibition. Clinical Endocrinology 20: 573–578
41. Nyberg F, Lieberman H, Lindstrom LH, Lyrenas S, Koch G, Terenius L 1989 Immunoreactive beta-casomorphin-8 in cerebrospinal fluid from pregnant and lactating women: correlation with plasma levels. Journal of Clinical Endocrinology and Metabolism 68: 283–289
42. Payne MR, Howie PW, Cooper W, Marnie M, Kidd L, McNeilly AS 1985 Sulpiride and the potentiation of progestogen only contraception. British Medical Journal 291: 559–561
43. Glasier A, McNeilly AS 1990 Physiology of lactation. Baillières Clinical Endocrinology and Metabolism 4: 379–395
44. McNeilly AS, Robinson ICAF, Houston MJ, Howie PW 1983 Release of oxytocin and prolactin in response to suckling. British Medical Journal 286: 257–259
45. Unvas-Moberg K, Widstrom AM, Werner S, Mattiesen AS, Winberg J 1990 Oxytocin and prolactin levels in breast-feeding women. Correlation with milk yield and duration of breast-feeding. Obstetrica Gynecologica Scandinavica 69: 301–306
46. Duchen MR, McNeilly AS 1980 Hyperprolactinaemia and long-term lactational amenorrhoea. Clinical Endocrinology 12: 521–527
47. Diaz S, Cardenas H, Brandeis A 1991 Early differences in the endocrine profile of long and short lactational amenorrhoea. Journal of Clinical Endocrinology and Metabolism 72: 196–201
48. McNeilly AS, Glasier A, Jonassen J, Howie PW 1982 Evidence for direct inhibition of ovarian function by prolactin. Journal of Reproduction and Fertility 65: 559–569
49. Curlewis JD, McNeilly AS 1991 Prolactin short-loop feedback and prolactin inhibition of luteinizing hormone secretion during the breeding season and seasonal anoestrus in the ewe. Neuroendocrinology 54: 279–285
50. Nunley WC, Urban RJ, Kitchin JD, Bateman BG, Evans WS, Veldhuis JD 1991 Dynamics of pulsatile prolactin release during the postpartum lactational period. Journal of Clinical Endocrinology and Metabolism 71: 287–293
51. Fonseca ME, Ochoa R, Moran C, Zarate A 1991 Variations in the molecular forms of prolactin during the menstrual cycle, pregnancy and lactation. Journal of Endocrinological Investigation 14: 907–912
52. Ellis LA, Picciano MF 1995 Bioactive and immunoreactive prolactin variants in human milk. Endocrinology 136: 2711–2720
53. Baird DT, McNeilly AS, Sawers RS, Sharpe RM 1979 Failure of estrogen-induced discharge of luteinizing hormone in lactating women. Journal of Clinical Endocrinology and Metabolism 49: 500–506
54. Fraser HM, Dewart PJ, Smith SK, Cowen GM, Sandow J, McNeilly AS 1989 Luteinizing hormone releasing hormone agonist for contraception in breast feeding women. Journal of Clinical Endocrinology and Metabolism 69: 996–1002

55. Flynn AM, Docker M, Brown JB, Kennedy KI 1991 Ultrasonographic patterns of ovarian activity during breastfeeding. American Journal of Obstetrics and Gynecology 165: 2027–2031
56. Groome NP, Illingworth PJ, O'Brien M et al 1996 Measurement of dimeric inhibin-B throughout the human menstrual cycle. Journal of Clinical Endocrinology and Metabolism 81: 1401–1405
57. Kalkwarf HJ, Specker BL 1995 Bone mineral loss during lactation and recovery after weaning. Obstetrics and Gynecology 86: 26–32
58. Kent GN, Price RI, Gutteridge DH et al 1990 Human lactation: forearm trabecular bone loss, increased bone turnover, and renal conservation of calcium and inorganic phosphate with recovery of bone mass following weaning. Journal of Bone and Mineral Research 5: 361–369
59. Cross NA, Hillman LS, Allen SH, Krause GF 1995 Changes in bone mineral density and markers of bone remodelling during lactation and postweaning in women consuming high amounts of calcium. Journal of Bone and Mineral Research 10: 1312–1320
60. Yamamoto N, Takahashi HE, Tanizawa T, Kawashima T, Endo N 1994 Bone mineral density and bone histomorphometric assessments of postpregnancy osteoporosis: a report of five patients. Calcified Tissue International 54: 20–25
61. Specker BL, Vieira NE, OBrien KO et al 1994 Calcium kinetics in lactating women with low and high calcium intakes. American Journal of Clinical Nutrition 59: 593–599
62. Feldblum PJ, Zhang J, Rich LE, Fortney JA, Talmage RV 1992 Lactation history and bone mineral density among perimenopausal women. Epidemiology 3: 527–531
63. Sowers M, Randolph J, Shapiro B, Jannausch M 1995 A prospective study of bone density and pregnancy after an extended period of lactation with bone loss. Obstetrics and Gynecology 85: 285–289
64. Berning B, Van Kuijk C, Schutte HE, Kuiper JW, Drogendijk AC, Fauser B 1993 Determinants of lumbar bone mineral density in normal weight, non-smoking women soon after menopause. A study using clinical data and quantitative computed tomography. Bone Minerals 21: 129–139
65. KritzSilverstein D, Barrett-Connor E, Hollenbach KA 1992 Pregnancy and lactation as determinants of bone mineral density in postmenopausal women. American Journal of Epidemiology 136: 1052–1059
66. Melton LJ, Bryant SC, Wahner HW et al 1993 Influence of breastfeeding and other reproductive factors on bone mass later in life. Osteoporosis International 3: 76–83
67. Hu JF, Zhao XH, Chen JS, Fitzpatrick J, Parpia B, Campbell TC 1994 Bone density and lifestyle characteristics in premenopausal and postmenopausal Chinese women. Osteoporosis International 4: 288–297
68. Marshall WM, Cumming DC, Fitzsimmons GW 1992 Hot flushes during breast feeding? Fertility and Sterility 57: 1349–1350
69. Harris B, Lovett L, Newcombe RG, Read GF, Walker R, RiadFahmy D 1994 Maternity blues and major endocrine changes: Cardiff puerperal mood and hormone study II. British Medical Journal 308: 949–953
70. Alder EM, Cook A, Davidson D, West C, Bancroft J 1986 Hormones, mood and sexuality in lactating women. British Journal of Psychiatry 148: 74–79
71. Dalton K 1994 Postnatal depression and prophylactic progesterone. British Journal of Family Planning 19: 10–12
72. Henderson A, Studd J 1995 Oestrogens and postnatal depression. Contemporary Reviews of Obstetrics and Gynaecology 7: 90–96
73. Labbok MH, Perez A, Valdes V et al 1994 The lactational amenorrhea method (LAM): a postpartum introductory family planning method with policy and program implications. Advances in Contraception 10: 93–109
74. Lonnerdal B, Forsum E, Hambraeus L 1980 Effect of oral contraceptives on composition and volume of breast milk. American Journal of Clinical Nutrition 33: 816–824
75. Nilsson S, Nygren K, Johansson EDB 1977 Megestrol acetate concentrations in plasma and milk during administration of an oral contraceptive containing 4 mg megestrol acetate to nursing mothers. Contraception 16: 615–623
76. Shaaban M, Abol-Oyoun M, Yousef AE et al 1994 Progestogen-only contraceptives during lactation: I. Infant growth. World Health Organization task force for epidemiological research on reproductive health; special programme of research, development and research training in human reproduction. Contraception 50: 35–53
77. Bathija H, Shaaban M, Abol-Oyoun M et al 1994 Progestogen-only contraceptives during lactation: II. Infant development. World Health Organization task force for epidemiological research on reproductive health; special programme of research, development and research training in human reproduction. Contraception 50: 55–68

24. Estrogen and progesterone in the fetus and neonate

Bruce R. Carr

Introduction

During human pregnancy, there are marked alterations in hormone secretion in the fetus as well as the mother. The formation of both estrogen and progesterone in the fetal-placental-maternal unit, as well as the transfer of steroid hormone between the mother and fetus, is complex. The purpose of this chapter is to discuss the source of estrogen and progesterone as well as provide hormone levels in plasma in the human fetus and neonate. Finally, the proposed physiologic role of estrogen and progesterone in the fetus will be discussed.

SOURCE OF ESTROGEN IN THE FETUS AND NEONATE

During human pregnancy, the rate of estrogen production and the levels of progesterone increase markedly.[1] The mechanism of the synthesis of estrogen in human pregnancy is unique (Fig. 24.1) The

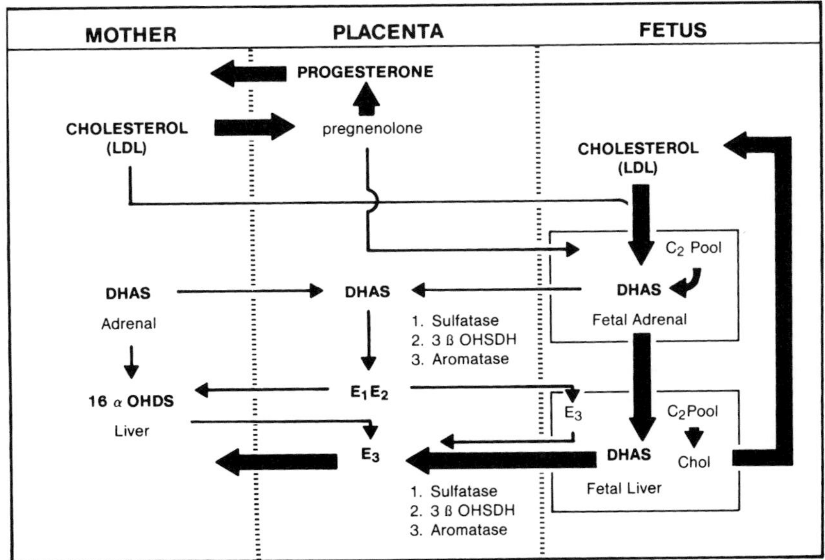

Fig. 24.1 Sources of estrogen biosynthesis in the maternal-fetal-placental unit. (LDL: low density lipoprotein; Chol: cholesterol; C_2 pool: carbon-carbon unit; DHEAS: dehydroepiandrosterone sulfate; E_1: estrone; E_2: estradiol-17β; E_3: estriol.) (From Carr BR, Gant NE 1983 The endocrinology of pregnancy-induced hypertension. Clinical Perinatology 10: 737. With permission of the WB Saunders Co.)

placenta cannot convert progesterone to estrogen directly due to a deficiency of 17-α hydroxylase (P450c17).[2] Thus, the placenta must rely on androgens (C-19 steroids) produced primarily by the fetal adrenal and to a lesser degree by the maternal adrenal. 17β-estradiol and estrone are synthesized by the conversion of dehydroepiandrosterone sulfate (DHEAS) from the adrenals of the fetus and mother. Near term, 40% of the 17β-estradiol and estrone is formed from maternal DHEAS and 60% from fetal DHEAS as precursor.[3] The placenta metabolized DHEAS to estrogens through placental sulfatase, Δ^5, 4 isomerase and 3β-hydroxysteroid dehydrogenase and aromatase enzymes. The principle source of DHEAS secreted by the fetal adrenal is derived from low density lipoprotein (LDL)-cholesterol which is synthesized by the fetal liver.[4] Since only 20% of fetal cholesterol is derived from the maternal compartment, and because fetal amniotic fluid cholesterol levels are negligible, the fetal liver has been proposed to provide adequate cholesterol as precursor for DHEAS secretion by the fetal adrenal.[5] Estriol is synthesized by the placenta from 16α-hydroxydehydroepiandrosterone sulfate (16α-OHDS) formed in the fetal liver from circulating DHEAS. At least 90% of urinary estriol in the maternal compartment is derived from the fetal adrenal gland.[3]

Near term the total production of estrogen by the placenta is about 100 mg per day and estriol represents about 60–70% of the total.[6] Of the estrogen produced, 75% is transferred to the maternal compartment and 25% to the fetus. The placenta contains high sulfatase activity, and thus placental content of estrogens consists of free or unconjugated estrogens.[7] After conversion of androgens to estrogens in the placenta occurs, the unconjugated estrogens are transferred to the fetus. The fetal tissues are high in sulfokinase activity and thus the majority of estrogen (60–80%) circulates in the form of sulfates.[8,9] In addition, estrogen transfer from the maternal to fetal compartment can occur but requires unconjugated estrogen. Furthermore, there appears to be a preferential selection of secretion of estradiol into the maternal circulation but estrone is secreted equally into both compartments. It has been proposed that the expression of placental 17β-hydroxysteroid dehydrogenase may play a role in the transfer of estradiol toward the maternal compartment.[10,11]

The fetal ovary is primarily involved in the formation of germ cells. Although the fetal ovary expresses aromatase activity, it is thought to contribute little if any to the estrogen pool of the fetus or mother.[12,13]

Plasma levels of estrogen in fetus and neonate

Estradiol and estrone levels (unconjugated form) are higher in the umbilical vein than in the umbilical artery and these values reflect the source of the estrogens (i.e. the placenta) entering the fetal compartment, as presented in Table 24.1.[14–18] However, the corresponding sulfated estrone and estradiol levels (conjugated form) are similar in both umbilical vein and artery. The levels of unconjugated estrone in fetal umbilical vein is 2–3 times higher than maternal plasma at term and 20 to 100 times higher than in nonpregnant women. However the levels of unconjugated estradiol are greater in maternal than fetal plasma, which reflects the preferential secretion of estradiol in the maternal compartment as discussed earlier. Estriol is the most abundant estrogen in fetal plasma. Of the unconjugated total estrogens in fetal plasma, 70–80% are in the form of estriol, and estriol sulfate comprises 90–95% of total estrogen sulfates.[17] The concentration of both unconjugated estriol and estriol sulfates are 4–8 times higher in fetal plasma than

Table 24.1 Estrogen levels in fetal and maternal plasma.[23]

Pregnancy in weeks		Unconjugated E_1 and E_2 nmol/L		Sulfated E_1 and E_2 nmol/L		Unconjugated and sulfated E_3 nmol/L	
		E_1	E_2	E_1S	E_2S	E_3unconjugated	E_3S
15–20	UA	0.5–1.1	0.2–0.4	5.5–7.3	1.3–2.5	2.8–3.7	32.8
	UV	1.6–4.9	1.1–1.2	2.8–9.6	1.4–1.8	10–26	42–110
	M	1.7	4.3	—	—	1.9	11.8
37–40	UA	1.5–7.6	1.1–4.9	1.5–6.1	1.1–2.6	119	260
	UV	8.3–13.3	4.3–8.5	2.0–8.1	1.6–3.4	121	417
	M	3.6–6.8	13.3–21.5	—	—	2	8

E_1: estrone; E_2: 17β estradiol; E_3: estriol; S: sulfate; UA: umbilical artery; UV: umbilical vein; M: maternal plasma. Results presented as range or mean values in nmol/L when available. See also refs 15–18.

Table 24.2 Plasma concentrations (nmol/L) of progestogens and estrogens (mean ± 1 SD) at birth and during infancy.[19]

		Progestogens		Estrogens	
		P_4	OHP	E_2	E_1
At birth: Mother		500–610	23.7 ± 6.9	64.5 ± 33.7	47.3 ± 21.9
Fetus: Cord vein[a]	M		56.4 ± 31[c]		
		1540 ± 985[b]		29.6 ± 14.7[b]	92.8 ± 24[b]
	F		70.8 ± 41		
Peripheral vein	M	12–32			
(0–2 hours)			12.7 ± 5.8[b]	1.4 ± 0.07[b]	4 ± 7.4[b]
	F	10–30			
Infancy					
4–8 days	M	0.75–3.5	3.2 ± 1.8	0.007–0.018	0.007–0.045
	F	0.2–6.5	2.9 ± 1.2	0.001–0.03	0.003–0.02
1–2 months	M	0.09–1.1	6.1 ± 2.4	0.001–0.041[c]	0.003–0.015
	F	0.05–0.9	3.2 ± 1.5	0.001–0.02	0.004–0.015
7–9 months	M	0.09–0.5	0.88 ± 0.63[c]	0.001–0.09	0.002–0.012
	F	0.12–0.8	1.82 ± 1.27	0.0015–0.01	0.0015–0.010
9–12 months	M	0.16–0.7	0.85 ± 0.66	0.001–0.009	ND–0.009
	F	0.11–0.8	1.30 ± 0.75	0.002–0.008	ND–0.01
Children: 1–2 years	M + F	0.1–0.5	0.77 ± 0.3	ND–0.03	ND–0.02
Adults: Male		0.3–0.6[c]	3.5–1.2[c]	0.09 ± 0.03[c]	0.15 ± 0.05
Female	FP	1.8 ± 0.34	1.3 ± 0.25	0.35 ± 0.18	0.16 ± 0.08
	LP	43 ± 13	7.4 ± 2	0.64 ± 0.38	0.33 ± 0.09[c]

[a]In most instances, mixed cord blood constituted mostly of venous blood; [b]Pooled M and Fl values, no sex difference; [c]Sex difference. P_4: progesterone; OHP: 17α-hydroxyprogesterone; E_2: estradiol-17β, E_3: estrone; M: males; F: females; ND: not detectable; FP: follicular phase; LP: luteal phase.

in the maternal plasma (Table 24.1), which reflects the greater sulfokinase activity in the fetus compared to the mother.

Immediately after birth, fetal plasma levels of estrogen fall rapidly (within two hours) and thereafter are essentially undetectable up to two years of life. This fall in estrogen levels is due to the withdrawal of the source of estrogen (the placenta) and lack of neonatal or childhood ovarian estrogen secretion (Table 24.2).[19]

SOURCE OF PROGESTERONE IN THE FETUS AND NEONATE

Progesterone levels also increase markedly during human pregnancy.[1] The principle source of progesterone secretion is from maternal LDL-cholesterol and the site of progesterone formation is the placenta.[2] In women with low or absent levels of LDL-cholesterol, plasma progesterone levels are significantly decreased.[20] There is minimal transfer of progesterone or precursor from the fetus to the maternal compartment. Progesterone formation by the placenta is independent of the fetus so that fetal distress or even death is not associated with a decline in progesterone levels in the maternal compartment.[2] Others have suggested that pregnenolone sulfate of fetal adrenal origin may provide a source of placental progesterone secretion.[21] However, since maternal progesterone levels do not decline with anencephaly (adrenal atrophy), fetal stress or even fetal death, as stated previously, there is little clinical importance for a fetal contribution to maternal progesterone. Of more importance to the theme of this chapter is the source of progesterone that circulates in the fetus and neonate. The principle source in the fetus is obviously placental secretion. Studies of infusion of radiolabelled progesterone in pregnant women revealed that only 4–10% of fetal progesterone is derived from the maternal compartment, thus 90–96% is from the placenta.[22] Once progesterone reaches the fetus it is metabolized by hydroxylations, reductions and conjugations, primarily in the fetal liver and adrenals. The progesterone concentrations and transfers between the maternal-placental-fetal unit are depicted in Figure 24.2. The concentration of progesterone is greatest in the placenta. Umbilical blood progesterone levels are 3–10 times that of maternal plasma and 2–10

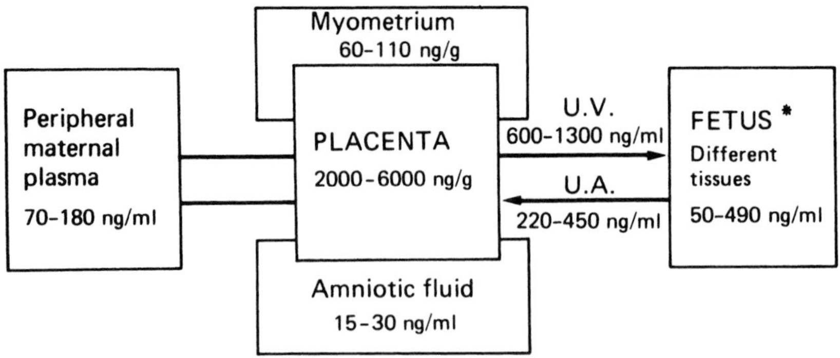

Fig. 24.2 Progesterone concentration in the maternal-placental-fetal compartments at term.[23] (UV: umbilical vein; UA: umbilical artery.)

times that of fetal tissues. Progesterone levels are lowest in the amniotic fluid.[23]

Plasma levels of progesterone in the fetus and neonate

Although the amount of progesterone delivered from the placenta to the mother is 8–10 times greater than to the fetus, because the volume of distribution is lower in the fetus, the concentration of progesterone in umbilical cord blood at term is greater than maternal blood (see Fig. 24.2, Tables 24.2 and 24.3).[19,23–25] Approximately 95% of progesterone in pregnant women and in cord blood of infants at term is bound to plasma proteins (mainly corticosteroid binding globulin). As seen in Table 24.3, the 20 dihydroxyprogesterone derivatives are the same in the fetal umbilical vein and artery, suggesting that these are derived from the placental compartment.[25] Hagemenas and Kittinger reported that the umbilical venous-arterial difference in progesterone levels was higher in the female fetus (828 ± 88 nmol/L) compared to male fetuses (570 ± 60 nmol/L).[26] However reasons for this difference are not readily explained.

Immediately following birth, and with separation of the placenta, progesterone levels in the blood of the newborn drop one hundred-fold within two hours. During the first few days of life the levels decrease another one hundred-fold and remain at the lower limits of detection throughout the remainder of infancy (Table 24.2).[19]

PROPOSED PHYSIOLOGIC ROLES OF ESTROGEN AND PROGESTERONE IN THE FETUS AND NEONATE

The physiologic roles of estrogen and progesterone during development of the human fetus has not been clearly delineated. Several hypotheses suggest that estrogen plays little if any role in female sexual development. However, estrogen receptors have been described in the fetal brain and aromatase activity has been reported, suggesting estrogen may play a role in brain gender development. However in spite of the extremely high levels of estrogen in fetal blood, the fetus remains relatively unresponsive, i.e. lacks breast budding, until late in gestation. This may be due to the fact that most of the estrogen is found in sulfated form

Table 24.3 Concentration of progesterone and 20-dihydro derivatives (20α- and 20β-dihydroprogesterone) in the maternal, placental and fetal compartments at term.[23]

	Maternal blood nmol/L	Placental tissue nmol/g	Placental blood nmol/L	UV nmol/L	UA nmol/L
Progesterone	129 ± 49	5060 ± 1435	723 ± 245	704 ± 227	324 ± 94
20α-dihydroprogesterone	15 ± 15	230 ± 158	24 ± 13	17 ± 3	17 ± 5
20β-dihydroprogesterone	1.7 ± 0.9	38 ± 30	1.0 ± 0.1	1.2 ± 0.3	2.6 ± 2.1

Mean values ± SD; UV: umbilical vein; UA: umbilical artery. See also ref. 25.

or other conjugates. Others have proposed a role of estrogen in stimulating prostaglandin release, leading to parturition.[2] In addition, estrogen may possibly affect organ maturation, such as lung maturation, whereas the lack of estrogen may lead to prolonged or delayed labor as seen in estrogen deficiency states such as anencephaly, steroid sulfatase deficiency and aromatase deficiency, which also can lead to masculinization of the female fetus.[2] Exogenous estrogen treatment of pregnant women, i.e. diethylstilbestrol, can lead to cancer and abnormal histology and development of the reproductive tract in affected offspring.

Progesterone has been proposed to lead to uterine quiescence and the prevention of uterine contractions and labor at least in some animal species.[2] Progesterone has no known physiologic role in the fetus, however it has been proposed to affect the immune system.[27] Some have suggested that progesterone leads to an alteration of helper and suppressor T-cells which may result in maternal immunodeficiency and which can decrease the chance of fetal rejection; this may explain the increased appearance of autoimmune diseases in pregnancy.[28]

REFERENCES

1. Brown JB 1956 Urinary excretion of oestrogen during pregnancy, lactation and the re-establishment of menstruation. Lancet 1956: 704–707
2. Carr BR 1995 The maternal-fetal-placental unit. In: Becker KL (ed) Principles and practice of endocrinology and metabolism, 2nd edn. Lippincott, Philadelphia, ch 106, pp 987–1000
3. Siiteri PK, MacDonald PC 1963 The utilization of circulating dehydroisoandrosterone sulfate for estrogen synthesis during human pregnancy. Steroids 2: 713–730
4. Carr BR, Simpson ER 1984 Cholesterol synthesis by human fetal hepatocytes: effect of hormones. Journal of Clinical Endocrinology and Metabolism 58: 1111–1116
5. Carr BR, Simpson ER 1981 Lipoprotein utilization and cholesterol synthesis by the human fetal adrenal gland. Endocrine Reviews 2: 306–326
6. Pasqualini JR, Kincl FA 1985 Hormones and the fetus, vol I. Pergamon Press, Oxford, pp 348–351
7. Pulkkinen MO 1961 Arylsulfatase and the hydrolysis of some steroid sulfates in developing organisms and placenta. Acta Physiologica Scandinavica 52 (Suppl.) 180: 1–92
8. Levitz M, Condon GP, Dancis J 1961 Sulfurylation of estrogens by the human fetus. Endocrinology 68: 832–833
9. Pasqualini JR, Kincl FA 1985 Hormones and the fetus, vol I. Pergamon Press, Oxford, pp 210–211
10. Ryan KJ, Engel LL 1953 The interconversion of estrone and estradiol by human tissue slices. Endocrinology 52: 287–291
11. Strickler RC, Tobias B 1980 Estradiol 17β-dehydrogenase and 20α-hydroxy-steroid dehydrogenase from human placental cytosol: one enzyme with two activities? Steroids 36: 243–253
12. Pasqualini JR, Kincl FA 1985 Hormones and the fetus, vol I. Pergamon Press, Oxford, p 135
13. Geroge FW, Wilson JD 1978 Conversion of androgen to estrogen by the human fetal ovary. Journal of Clinical Endocrinology and Metabolism 47: 550–555
14. Pasqualini JR, Kincl FA 1985 Hormones and the fetus, vol I. Pergamon Press, Oxford, pp 205–209
15. Shutt DA, Smith ID, Shearman RP 1974 Oestrone, oestradiol-17β and oestriol levels in human foetal plasma during gestation and at term. Journal of Endocrinology 60: 333–341
16. Tulchinsky D 1973 Placental secretion of unconjugated estrone, estradiol and estriol into the maternal and the fetal circulation. Journal of Clinical Endocrinology and Metabolism 36: 1079–1087
17. Laatikainen T, Peltonen J 1975 Foetal and maternal plasma levels of steroid sulphates in human pregnancy at term. Acta Endocrinologica (Copenhagen) 79: 577–588
18. Whittle MJ, Anderson D, Lowensohn RI et al 1979 Estriol in pregnancy VI. Experience with unconjugated plasma estriol assays and antepartum fetal heart rate testing in diabetic pregnancies. American Journal of Obstetrics and Gynecology 135: 764–772
19. Forest MG 1990 Pituitary gonadotropin and sex steroid secretion during the first two years of life. In: Grumbach MM, Sizonenka PG, Auberet MI (eds) Control of the onset of puberty. William & Wilkins, Baltimore, pp 451–477
20. Parker CR, Illingworth DR, Bissonnette JL, Carr BR 1986 Endocrine changes during pregnancy in a patient with homozygous familial hypobeta lipoproteinemia. New England Journal of Medicine 314: 557–560
21. Scommegna A, Burd L, Bieniarz J 1972 Progesterone and pregnenolone sulfate in pregnancy plasma. American Journal of Obstetrics and Gynecology 13: 60–65
22. Escargena L, Clark H, Gurpide E 1978 Contribution of maternal circulation to blood-borne progesterone in the fetus. American Journal of Obstetrics and Gynecology 130: 462
23. Pasqualini JF, Kincl FA 1985 Hormones and the fetus, vol I. Pergamon Press, Oxford, pp 203–204
24. Tulchinsky D, Okada D 1975 Hormones in human pregnancy IV. Plasma progesterone. American Journal of Obstetrics and Gynecology 121: 293–299
25. Runnebaum B, Stober I, Zander J 1975 Progesterone, 20α-dihydroprogesterone and 20β-dihydroprogesterone in mother and child at birth. Acta Endocrinologica (Copenhagen) 80: 569–576
26. Hagemenas FC, Kittinger GW 1973 The influence of fetal sex on the levels of plasma progesterone in the human fetus. Journal of Clinical Endocrinology and Metabolism 36: 389–391
27. Siiteri PK, Febres F, Clemens LE et al 1977 Progesterone and maintenance of pregnancy: is progesterone nature's immunosuppressant? Annals of the New York Academy of Science 286: 384–389
28. Sridama V, Pacini F, Yang J-L et al 1982 Decreased levels of helper T cells: possible cause of immunodeficiency in pregnancy. Steroids 307: 352–355

SECTION 4

Pharmacology

CONTENTS

25. Pharmacokinetics of estrogens and progestogens

Johann W. Faigle Lotte Schenkel

Introduction

Pharmacokinetics, as first defined by Dost[1] in 1953, simply means the time course of circulating drug concentrations. Any concentration time course is determined by the processes of drug absorption, distribution and elimination. The aim of a pharmacokinetic investigation is to describe these processes in a quantitative manner. Although the pharmacokinetic discipline does not primarily deal with the biological activities of a drug, it is an indispensable complement to pharmacology.

In drug therapy it is essential to know the pharmacokinetic processes, because they modulate and influence the pharmacodynamic outcome. For instance, if a systemically active substance is intensely metabolized during its first passage through the gut wall and liver, it may not show adequate efficacy after oral administration. Safety aspects can also be addressed by pharmacokinetics, in that retention or accumulation of a drug in the organism can be detected or predicted long before possible adverse effects arise. Therefore, pharmacokinetic information is important from both a clinical and a drug regulatory point of view.

Knowing the time course of concentrations in blood, organs and excretory products, it is possible to optimize the dosage regimen of a drug. Generally, one has to assume that the pharmacological and clinical effects correlate less well with the amount of drug administered than with the concentration achieved at the site of action. In most cases, however, the true site of action is inaccessible to drug analysis. Measurement in blood, plasma or serum is then an alternative, because the circulating drug levels run roughly parallel with the levels in the organ of interest. The absolute concentrations may differ between the two body compartments, but the concentration ratio will be largely stable, especially at steady state.

Numerous technical terms are established now in pharmacokinetics, but quite a few of them are only interesting for the specialists in the field. Terms or parameters required to describe those processes which are essential in the clinical pharmacology of steroid hormones are summarized in Table 25.1. They include well known expressions like bioavailability (BAV, % of dose reaching systemic circulation), maximum concentration (Cmax), area under the concentration–time curve (AUC) and elimination half-life ($T_{1/2}$). When we consider the kinetics of steroid

Table 25.1 Basic parameters required to describe pharmacokinetic processes.

Process	Parameter	Brief term
Absorption (exogenous hormones)	Bioavailability Maximum concentration Time to reach maximum concentration	BAV Cmax Tmax
Production (endogenous hormones)	Blood production rate	BPR
Distribution	Volume of distribution Binding to serum proteins	V % bound
Elimination	Half-life of elimination Metabolic clearance rate	$T^1/_2$ MCR

hormones stemming from endogenous sources, however, we need further descriptors such as blood production rate (BPR, total amount of hormone entering circulation).[2]

Pharmacokinetic data are usually presented as an average of results from a studied population. Mean values are indeed important to characterize a drug in a general sense. On the other hand, information on the pharmacokinetic variability between subjects is also needed, because the extremes of a range may be associated with treatment failures or unwanted side effects. It should be kept in mind that the inter-subject variability of a kinetic parameter may be tenfold, even under well controlled study conditions.[2]

Pharmacokinetic investigations are based on the measurement of drugs or their metabolites in body fluids, but the raw data obtained can be evaluated by different approaches. They extend from a simple description of the processes involved to sophisticated methods like compartment modeling and iterative curve fitting. The latter approaches require specially designed studies with long observation periods and large numbers of biological samples. Such studies are not available for most of the steroids to be considered in this chapter. Therefore, we wish to follow a pragmatic approach which combines descriptive elements with some basic kinetic parameters, as outlined in Table 25.1

In the present class of substances, serious analytical problems may arise. Concentrations in body fluids are generally low for both endogenous and exogenous steroids. In plasma or serum, for instance, concentrations lie in the range of picograms or nanograms per milliliter (pg/ml; ng/ml). Only a few technologies are actually suitable for that range, variations on radioimmunoassay (RIA) being the most important ones.[3] Although an RIA may be sufficiently sensitive for the desired steroid, it may lack specificity in that it cross-reacts with related compounds or metabolites. Newer methods are more reliable than older methods in this respect. Thus, we shall refer to more recent studies, where possible.

This chapter will comprise three main areas. The first one will deal with the kinetics of endogenous and exogenous estrogens in women. The influence of variables, such as ovarian function for endogenous estrogens, and route of administration for exogenous estrogens, will also be discussed. Metabolic transformations will be mentioned, as far as they are decisive for the understanding of the pharmacokinetics. The second area will comprise the same topics for endogenous and exogenous progestogens. In the last area, factors which may influence the kinetics of estrogens and progestogens will be included. Here we shall refer to genetic, racial and environmental factors, as well as to interactions with xenobiotics such as drugs, alcohol or tobacco.

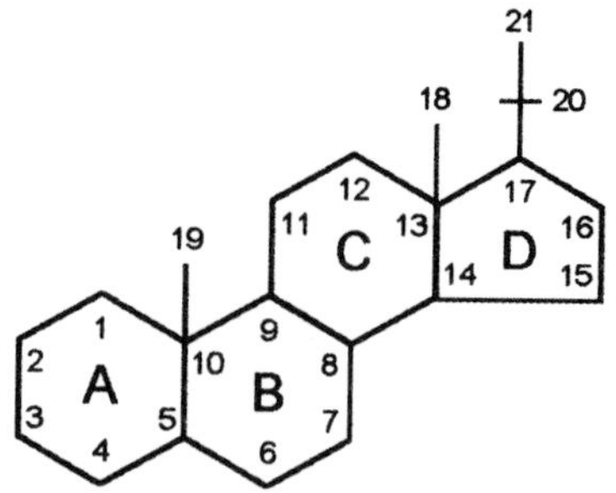

Fig. 25.1 Basic skeleton of estrogen and progestogen molecules,[4] including designation of rings and numbering of positions of C atoms. (Side chains containing C atoms 19, 20 & 21 are absent in some of the steroids.)

To describe the kinetics of steroid hormones and their biologically active metabolites in a reasonable way, some reference has to be made to chemical structures. For instance, it is essential to specify those parts of a molecule where side chains are attached, or where metabolic reactions take place. In this chapter, we adhere to the standard designation of rings and positions in the basic skeleton of estrogens and progestogens,[4] as shown in Figure 25.1.

As far as the pharmaceutical estrogens and progestogens are concerned, we shall focus on commercially available products, disregarding experimental and investigational drugs. However, we do not intend to list the proprietary names of all the products. Naming is rather complex and may change from one country to another. Readers interested in proprietary names are referred to national or international compendia, such as Martindale's Extra Pharmacopoeia, The Merck Index, or Physicians' Desk Reference.[5–7]

PHYSIOLOGICAL ESTROGENS AND MAIN PHARMACEUTICAL PRODUCTS

Kinetics of physiological estrogens

The major physiological estrogens present in the female organism are 17β-estradiol (abbreviated E_2), estrone (E_1) and estriol (E_3). They exert their activities by binding to specific estrogen receptors in the target cells. The receptor affinity of E_2 is higher than that of E_1, and is much higher than that of E_3.[8,9]

The essential pathways of formation and interconversion of physiological estrogens are described in detail in chapters 4, 7 and 8. In young women, E_2 and E_1 are secreted by the ovaries, the rate of secretion being dependent on the cycle phase. Small amounts of E_1 are independently produced from androstenedione which stems from the adrenal glands and ovaries.[8–12] Metabolic oxidation of E_2 at position C17 results in E_1, and metabolic reduction leads back to E_2 again. E_1 is also reversibly interlinked with a product of conjugation, estrone 3-sulfate (E_1S). Owing to its high physiological concentrations, E_1S serves as a reservoir for E_1 and E_2 in the body.[13,14] The least potent estrogen, E_3, is formed by irreversible metabolism of E_1 at C-16 and C-17.[15]

The conversion of androstenedione to E_1 is mediated by an aromatase primarily present in adipose tissue, liver, spleen and neural tissue.[11] The reversible equilibrium between E_2, E_1 and E_1S is regulated by three enzyme systems, i.e. 17β-hydroxysteroid dehydrogenase, sulfortransferase and aryl sulfatase. These enzymes are located in the liver and many other sites such as the endometrium, breast and adipose tissue. Extent and direction of the latter reactions are concentration dependent. Hydroxylation of E_1 and E_2 at C-2 or C-4 leading to catechol estrogens is catalysed by an isoenzyme of the hepatic cytochrome P450 complex.[16,17]

During reproductive life, the blood production rate of E_2 averages from 100–600 µg per day, depending on the phase of the cycle. The corresponding figures for E_1 are 100–500 µg per day. Both estrogens originate mostly from ovarian secretion.[18–21] After menopause, ovarian secretion ceases completely. The residual amounts of E_2 and E_1 are then only in the range 15 µg and 45 µg per day, respectively. They originate mainly from aromatization of androstenedione. Because this process does also occur in adipose tissue, obese women may produce twice as much E_2 as slender women.[8]

The differences in estrogen production are reflected by the plasma or serum levels of physiological E_2 and E_1 in women before and after menopause (Fig. 25.2).[8,10,19,21–23] The concentration ratio E_2:E_1 is ≥1 in premenopausal women. However, concentrations drop drastically at the end of fertile life. In this phase, E_2 is a conversion product of E_1 and, therefore, E_1 is now predominant.

The processes of distribution and elimination of physiological estrogens can be described by pharmacokinetic methods. The parameters obtained are listed in Table 25.2. The most potent estrogen, E_2, is rapidly cleared from the circulation; the mean half-life being 1.7 hours. The half-lives reported for E_1 and E_1S are about four times longer.[24,25] Judged from its large volume of distribution, E_2 is widely distributed in organs and tissues. The metabolic clearance rate of E_1 is somewhat higher than that of E_2, and both are about ten times that of E_1S. Metabolic clearance rates are similar before and after menopause which implies that they are independent of ovarian function.[12,21,23,26,27]

Kinetics of exogenous estrogens: E_2 and E_2 esters

Oral administration of E_2 and E_2 valerate

The main commercial products available for oral administration contain micronized E_2 (0.5, 1.0 and

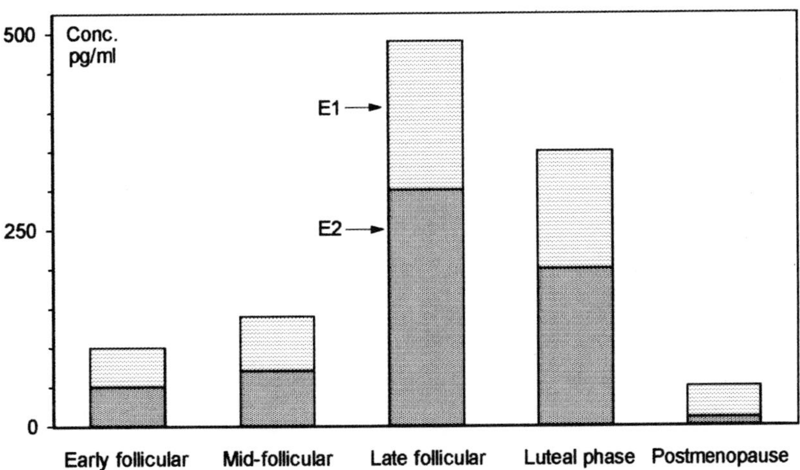

Fig. 25.2 Concentrations of physiological E_2 and E_1 in plasma or serum of premenopausal and postmenopausal women. Approximate mean values.[10,19,21–23]

Table 25.2 Pharmacokinetic parameters of physiological estrogens in women (mean or approximate values).[12,21,23–27]

Parameter	E_2	E_1	E_1S
Elimination half-life (hours)	1.7	~7	5–9
Distribution volume (liter)	73	–*	–*
Metabolic clearance rate (liter/day)	1100–1200	1600–1900	150

*No data available.

2.0 mg per tablet), or an esterified form, E_2 valerate (1 and 2 mg per tablet).[18,28–30]

Micronized E_2 and its esters are readily absorbed from the gastrointestinal tract, but a high fraction of the dose is metabolized during the first passage through the intestinal mucosa and liver. First pass metabolism of E_2 involves extensive oxidation to E_1, partly followed by conjugation to E_1S. Esters like E_2 valerate are first hydrolysed and, subsequently, the resulting free E_2 molecule undergoes oxidation and conjugation as above. Thus, the estrogen concentrations in blood produced by oral E_2 are comparable to those produced by an equivalent dose of E_2 valerate.[29]

Owing to the first pass metabolism, only a small fraction of the dose becomes bioavailable as unchanged E_2 in the circulation. This fraction is barely 5% for both oral E_2 and E_2 valerate.[24,31] The principal metabolites, E_1 and E_1S, enter the bloodstream in larger amounts. Therefore, oral administration of E_2 to postmenopausal women results in low plasma concentrations of E_2 and higher ones of E_1, the average ratio lying between 1:3 and 1:6. This concentration pattern differs basically from the physiological pattern observed in premenopausal women in whom the ratio of E_2:E_1 is ≥ 1 (see above).

The aim of hormone replacement therapy (HRT) in postmenopausal women is to raise plasma levels of E_2 back to the premenopausal range. Oral administration of E_2 or E_2 valerate in daily doses of 2 mg, for instance, have been reported to produce mean levels of 60–65 pg/ml.[9,19] These E_2 levels do indeed approach the range aimed at (Figs. 25.2 & 25.3). The accompanying levels of E_1, however, reach unphysiologically high values of up to 35 pg/ml.

Transdermal administration of E_2

There are two established pharmaceutical principles which allow transfer of efficacious amounts of E_2 through the skin, i.e. application of E_2 incorporated in a gel, and application of a transdermal therapeutic

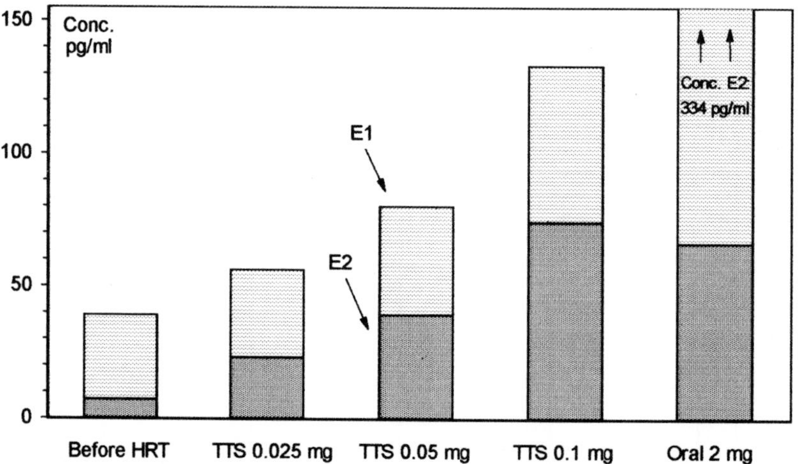

Fig. 25.3 Mean concentrations of E_2 and E_1 in plasma of postmenopausal women following administration of E_2 by the transdermal and oral route. Transdermal therapeutic systems (TTS) releasing 0.025, 0.05 and 0.1 mg E_2 per day are compared to micronized oral E_2 in daily doses of 2 mg.[32,33]

system (TTS) of E_2. The gel formulation contains 0.6 mg E_2 per g of gel, the recommended daily dose being 2.5–5 g of gel, or 1.5–3 mg of E_2. The original TTS is a self-adhesive reservoir patch designed to release E_2 in a controlled manner during 3–4 days. The three patch sizes available have average release rates of 0.025 mg, 0.05 mg and 0.1 mg of E_2 per day.[7,32]

E_2 is the most potent among the physiological estrogens, but it is not optimally suited for oral administration, as pointed out earlier. Because of the first pass metabolism, high doses are required to reach effective plasma levels. When E_2 is administered transdermally — or by any other parenteral route — the sites of first pass metabolism are fully circumvented. Therefore, the daily E_2 doses needed for HRT in postmenopausal women are many times lower for the transdermal than for the oral route of administration.

In Figure 25.3, the mean plasma concentrations achieved by patches (TTS in doses of 0.025, 0.05 and 0.1 mg E_2 per day) are compared with those achieved by oral micronized E_2 (in daily doses of 2 mg).[32,33] All treatments show a distinct increase of E_2 concentrations over the pretreatment base values of postmenopausal women. With TTS, this increase is linearly related to the daily dose. A transdermal dose of 0.1 mg corresponds to an oral dose of 2 mg in terms of E_2 levels in plasma. The levels of the second estrogen, E_1, increase only moderately during TTS application. With the oral route of E_2 administration, in contrast, E_1 levels increase several fold.

Figure 25.4 demonstrates that E_2 concentrations in plasma can be kept fairly constant, when a TTS is applied to skin, is left there for three to four days, and is then replaced by a new one. The example relates to the medium patch size releasing 0.05 mg of E_2 per day.[32] Thus, the TTS is an easy to use and safe product for HRT in postmenopausal women. A more recently described transdermal matrix patch system delivers 0.05 or 0.1 mg of E_2 daily during seven days in a slightly more constant manner than the twice weekly systems.[34]

Transdermal administration of E_2 is also possible with the gel formulation. A dose of 5 g of the gel (or 3 mg E_2), applied to 300–500 cm^2 of skin, results in E_2 plasma concentrations of 225–300 pg/ml after 9 hours, and 110–190 pg/ml after 24 hours.[8] Application of the gel is nonocclusive, and this is one of the reasons why the bioavailability of E_2 is low and greatly variable.

Vaginal administration of E_2

Several products for vaginal administration of E_2 are available. They include a vaginal cream formulation containing 0.1 mg E_2 per gram (recommended daily dose 1–4 g of cream), a vaginal ring containing 2 mg E_2 (delivery rate 7.5 µg/day for three months) and a vaginal tablet containing 25 µg E_2 (for once daily use).[30]

Vaginal preparations were originally developed for topical treatment of an atrophic vagina. It was assumed that only small amounts of E_2 would be absorbed and that the undesirable effects of systemic treatment, such as endometrial stimulation, would not occur. However, estrogens do readily penetrate the

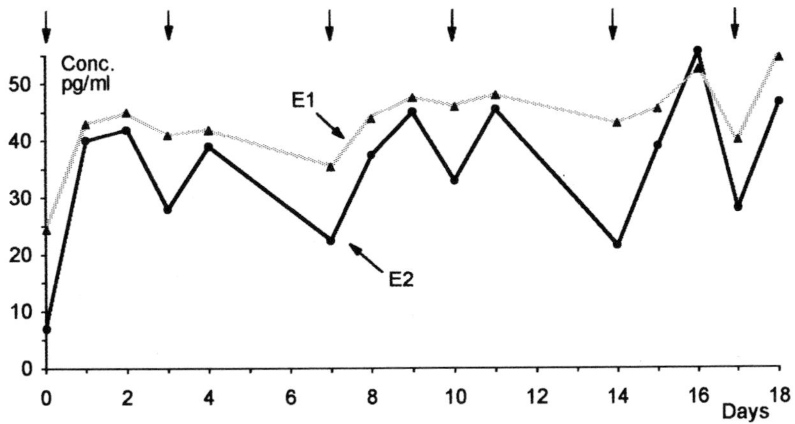

Fig. 25.4 Time course of concentrations of E_2 and E_1 in plasma of postmenopausal women during repeated use of transdermal therapeutic systems (TTS). Release rate 0.05 mg E_2 per day. Replacement of TTS every three or four days, as indicated by the arrows at the top of the diagram.[32,33]

vaginal mucosa and, depending on the dose and the structure of the vaginal wall, an increase of plasma estrogen levels can be observed.

Application of vaginal cream induces a massive but transient rise of plasma E_2, and a much smaller rise of plasma E_1. At 3 hours after a dose of 1 mg E_2, for instance, concentrations of E_2 and E_1 amounted to about 800 pg/ml and 150 pg/ml, respectively.[8] The high E_2:E_1 ratio is again typical for parenteral administration of E_2; it is in contrast to the oral route, where E_2 concentrations in plasma are always inferior to E_1.

With the high degree of E_2 absorption from an atrophic vagina, it was essential to develop a controlled type of delivery system which would ensure a more accurate dosing than vaginal cream. Some products of this kind are now available in Europe: the vaginal ring mentioned before releases E_2 at a low rate 7.5 μg/day only. It is effective in the treatment of atrophic vaginitis in postmenopausal women.[35,36] Even with this low dose, a transient initial increase of plasma E_2 to about 50 pg/ml, and a more persisting increase of E_1S were observed. The third product mentioned, i.e. vaginal tablets containing 25 μg E_2, resulted also in an increment of plasma estrogen. The levels of E_2 rose maximally by about 30 pg/ml, while those of E_1 remained virtually unchanged.[37,38]

Intramuscular injection of E_2 valerate

E_2 valerate is commercially available as a depot formulation for i.m. injection (10 mg/ml in oil). The recommended dose is 10 mg of E_2 valerate every two weeks.[30]

Following i.m. injection of 5 mg E_2 valerate, E_2 appears rather slowly in plasma and reaches a very high Cmax of 600 pg/ml at day 2. At day 4 and day 6 levels are still in the range of 300 pg/ml and 150 pg/ml, respectively, indicating continued release of the ester from the depot. Baseline levels are attained 8–10 days after injection. Levels of E_1 show a similar pattern, but are generally lower than those of E_2.[39,40]

Kinetics of exogenous estrogens: conjugated equine estrogens (CEE)

Oral administration of CEE

The main products for oral use are tablet formulations containing 0.625 and 1.25 mg of CEE. In some countries, tablet strengths of 0.3, 0.9 and 2.5 mg are marketed in addition. The usual daily dose in HRT is 0.625 mg.[7,30]

The term CEE stands for a mixture of substances isolated from the urine of pregnant mares. The mixture contains the sodium sulfate esters of at least 10 estrogens, including E_1, E_2 and some specific equine estrogens. These equine steroids are characterized by one or two double bonds in ring B, but otherwise their structures resemble those of E_1 and E_2. Figure 25.5 shows the metabolic reactions of four essential equine estrogens in the human body. Equilin and equilenin undergo reversible reduction at position 17, in analogy to the interconversion between E_1 and E_2.

Table 25.3 summarizes the composition of CEE, and the relative estrogenic potencies of the components in unconjugated form.[39,41,42] Taking both the fractions and potencies into account, E_1 and equilin constitute the essential estrogens of CEE. When the mixture is administered orally, only a small part of the dose is absorbed as intact sulfates. Most is hydrolysed in the gut and is resulfated after absorption. The circulating sulfates are in equilibrium with the unconjugated substances, as described above for the physiological female estrogens.[43,44]

The pharmacokinetics of CEE in postmenopausal women are complex, as a result of the large number of estrogens, and of their metabolic reactions and interconversions.[45,46] Some kinetic characteristics are known for equilin and its main metabolite 17β-dihydroequilin: their mean MCRs are in the range of 4000 and 2000 L/day, respectively; the values of their sulfate esters amount to 280 and 620 L/day only. Thus, the clearances of these equine steroids are about twice as high as those of the corresponding endogenous estrogens (Table 25.2).

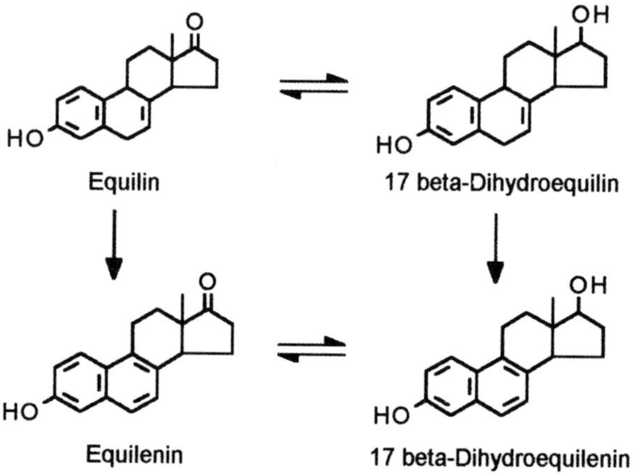

HO O Equilin ⇌ HO OH 17 beta-Dihydroequilin

HO O Equilenin ⇌ HO OH 17 beta-Dihydroequilenin

Fig. 25.5 Structures and metabolic conversions of four essential equine estrogens.[46]

Table 25.3 Composition of the mixture of conjugated equine estrogens and relative binding affinities of the unconjugated estrogens to estrogen receptor.[39,41,42]

Conjugated estrogen (sodium sulfate ester)	Composition* (conjugated form)	RBA** (unconjugated form)
Estrone (E_1)	50–57.5	11
Equilin	21.5–27.5	40
17 alpha-dihydroequilin	13.5–19.5	31
Estradiol (E_2)	2.5–9.5	100
Equilenin	~2.4	7
17 beta-dihydroequilenin	0.5–4.0	47
17 alpha-dihydroequilin	~1.3	18
17 beta-dihydroequilenin	~0.5	46

*In weight percent (total CEE mixture = 100%); **relative binding affinity to estrogen receptor *in vitro* (affinity of E_2 = 100%)

The plasma concentrations produced by oral doses of CEE are documented for a few of the individual estrogens only. Single dose data for E_1 and equilin are plotted in the left half of Figure 25.6, and multiple dose data for E_1 and E_2 are plotted in the right half. All data refer to postmenopausal women.[32,42] Following a single oral dose of 1.25 mg CEE, plasma E_1 reaches a Cmax of about 130 pg/ml at about 10 hours. Concentrations of equilin are generally lower, Cmax barely exceeding 50 pg/ml. Following repeated daily doses of 1.25 mg, mean levels of E_1 and E_2 amount to 150 and 30 pg/ml, respectively. The value of E_2 approaches that of a TTS delivering 0.05 mg E_2 daily (Fig. 25.3). However, oral CEE results in the same unphysiologically high E_1:E_2 ratio as oral dosage forms of E_2 do.

Vaginal administration of CEE

A vaginal cream containing 0.625 mg CEE per gram is available for the topical treatment of atrophic vaginitis.[7] Dosage recommendations were initially 2–4 g of cream per day which corresponds to 1.25–2.5 mg of CEE. Now it is recommended to use vaginal CEE cyclically, and not for prolonged periods, in amounts of 1–4 g of cream per application.

In an early study[47] it was found that a daily CEE dose of 1.25 mg resulted in plasma levels of E_1 and E_2 well above the premenopausal midcycle ovulatory range. E_1 levels were similar to those achieved by oral doses of 1.25 mg CEE (Fig. 25.6). The levels of E_2, on the other hand, appeared to be higher after vaginal than after oral administration.

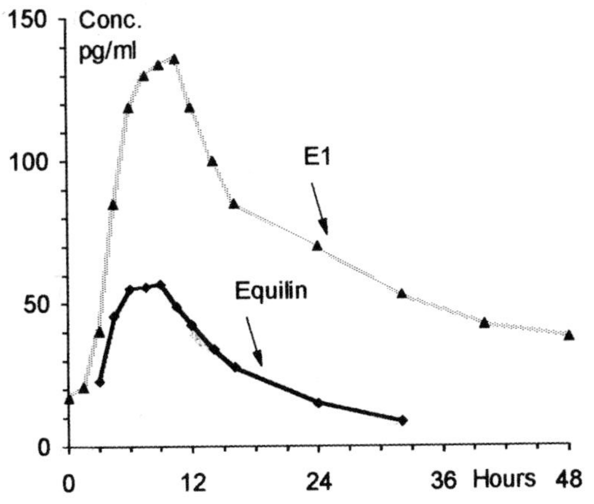

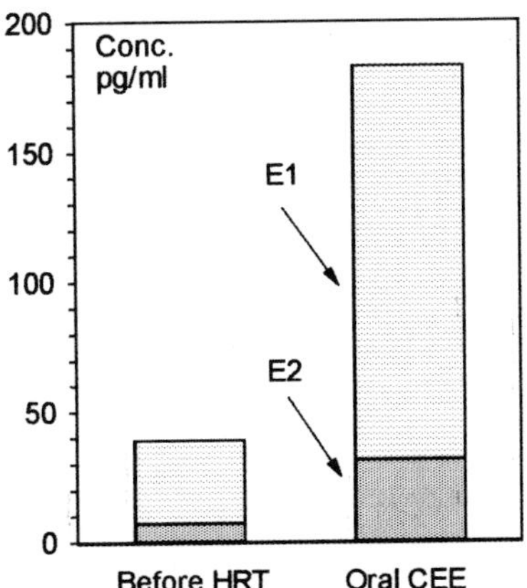

Fig. 25.6 Left panel: time course of concentrations of E_1 and equilin in plasma of postmenopausal women following single oral administration of 1.25 mg CEE. Right panel: mean concentrations of E_1 and E_2 during repeated oral administration of 1.25 mg CEE daily.[32,42]

In a later study, daily doses of 0.3, 0.625, 1.25 and 2.5 mg CEE were administered as vaginal cream for four weeks each.[48] They produced a dose-related increase of both E_1 and E_2 in plasma. Gonadotropins were reduced in a stepwise, dose dependent way, and the effects on the vaginal epithelium were significant even at the lowest dose of 0.3 mg of CEE or 0.5 g of cream per day.

Kinetics of exogenous estrogens: E_1, E_1S, E_3 and ethinyl estradiol (EE)

Oral administration of E_1S, E_3 and EE

A synthetic piperazine salt of E_1S (estropipate) is available as a tablet formulation for oral use. Tablets contain 0.625, 1.25, 2.5 or 5 mg, expressed in equivalents of E_1S.[7]

Absorption takes place as described above for oral CEE. The sulfate, E_1S, is first hydrolysed in the gut, free E_1 is absorbed and then largely resulfated in the gut wall or liver. Repeated estropipate doses of 2.5 mg daily result in mean plasma concentrations of 280 pg/ml of E_1 and 40 pg/ml of E_2. Again, the ratio E_1:E_2 is unphysiologically high. It is interesting to note that equimolar oral doses of E_1 and E_2 derivatives, e.g. estropipate and E_2 valerate, produce the same E_1:E_2 concentration profile in plasma.[28,49]

Another oral product contains E_3, in an amount of 1 mg per tablet. The recommended initial dose is 4–8 mg daily, the maintenance dose is 1–2 mg daily.[30] E_3 is a weak estrogen and is not converted to either of the more potent estrogens, E_2 or E_1. When administered orally in a dose of 8 mg, E_3 reaches a Cmax in plasma of 75 pg/ml after 2 hours. The steady state level is reported to be 130 pg/ml.[39] The bioavailability of oral E_3 is low. The steroid is extensively sulfated during absorption, and the plasma levels of the sulfate are 500 times those of unconjugated E_3.

A synthetic compound, 17α-ethinylestradiol (EE), is contained as an estrogen component in numerous oral contraceptives. Bioavailability of oral EE averages 40–50%, and is thus about ten times higher than that of oral E_2.[50] This is attributable to the ethinyl group at C-17 which makes metabolic oxidation of the hydroxyl function at C-17 impossible. That kind of oxidation occurs when E_2 is converted to E_1 during the first passage through gut wall and liver (see above). Following an i.v. dose, the elimination half-life of EE is 7–9 hours; the MCR averages 1345 L/day. Oral doses of 30 µg of EE result in mean plasma Cmax values of between 100 and 200 pg/ml after 1–2 hours, indicating rapid absorption. The interindividual variation of kinetic parameters is large, however.[51,52]

Mestranol is a biologically inactive prodrug of EE which carries an O-methyl group at position 3 of the molecule. Following oral administration, mestranol is absorbed as such and is activated by enzymatic demethylation in the liver. The efficiency of this conversion to EE is 70%. In a contraceptive pill, therefore, 50 µg of mestranol should be equivalent to 35 µg of EE. The plasma concentrations of EE resulting from these two dosages are indeed almost identical.[50]

Vaginal administration of E_3

Vaginal creams containing E_3 are available, a typical concentration being 1 mg E_3 per gram of cream.[30] The recommended dosage is 0.5 mg E_3 daily for the first two to three weeks, followed by a twice weekly regimen.

The bioavailability of vaginal E_3 is much higher than that of oral E_3: a vaginal dose of 0.5 mg produces about the same plasma concentrations as an oral dose of 10 mg.[39] Following 0.5 mg E_3 vaginally, plasma levels reach a peak of 100–150 pg/ml within 2 hours, with a subsequent decrease to about 50 pg/ml at 12 hours. No change in E_2 or E_1 concentrations occurs. This study demonstrates that E_3, like other estrogens, is readily absorbed from the vagina.

PROGESTERONE AND MAIN SYNTHETIC PROGESTOGENS

Chemical characteristics of progestogens

Pharmaceutic products containing natural progesterone are commercially available, but their clinical use is limited by the rapid inactivation of progesterone in the gastrointestinal tract and liver. Therefore, attempts have been made to synthesize steroid hormones which mimic the activities of progesterone, but are more resistant to metabolic inactivation. Stability can be improved, for instance, by attaching additional substituents to metabolically sensitive sites of a molecule.

The structures of the major synthetic progestogens used today for oral contraception and for HRT are illustrated in chapter 4. Four of the synthetic progestogens, i.e. medroxyprogesterone acetate, cyproterone acetate, medrogestone and dydrogesterone, are structurally related to natural progesterone. The remaining compounds, i.e. norethindrone and its acetate, levonorgestrel, desogestrel, gestodene and norgestimate, are classified as 17-ethinyl derivatives of 19-nortestosterone.[6]

Progestational activity depends on the presence of a 3-keto group in ring A of the steroid skeleton. Most of the progestogens used today do indeed carry such a group in their original molecules. However, the 3-keto group is initially missing in the case of desogestrel and norgestimate. They are prodrugs which undergo metabolic conversion to active 3-keto derivatives in the body.

Kinetics of physiological progesterone

The major amount of physiological progesterone is produced by the corpus luteum during the luteal phase of the female menstrual cycle. A small fraction of progesterone, secreted by the adrenal gland, is negligible for the biological actions of the hormone. Clearance of progesterone from the organism is governed by several metabolic reactions. The major ones are reduction of the C=O and C=C double bonds, and hydroxylations at different C atoms of the molecule. For details see chapters 4 and 8.

Two of the reactions are of interest for this chapter, because they lead to metabolites which possess biological activities of their own. One of these metabolites is 20α-dihydroprogesterone (20-DHP). Qualitatively, it shows the same progestational activities as the parent substance, but is only half as effective as progesterone. The second metabolite is 11-deoxycorticosterone (DOC) which may exert mineralocorticoid effects.[3,39,53]

Some pharmacokinetic characteristics of progesterone, derived from the physiologic plasma concentrations in premenopausal women,[27,54] are listed in Table 25.4. The production rate of progesterone is as high as 15–50 mg daily in the luteal phase of the menstrual cycle. It falls to 5% of this value in the follicular phase, when the adrenal gland is the only source of progesterone. The same is true for ovariectomized and postmenopausal women. The mean MCR lies between 2100–2500 L per day, with no obvious influence of ovarian function. About half of the metabolic clearance occurs in liver and the rest in extrahepatic tissues. The elimination half-life of progesterone is in the range of 30 minutes, which is in agreement with its high MCR.[55,56]

As the MCR is virtually constant, the plasma level pattern of progesterone reflects exactly the rate of production (Table 25.4). In cycling women, luteal secretion may bring the levels up to 20 ng/ml, while adrenal production suffices for barely 1 ng/ml. The plasma concentrations of 20-DHP and DOC follow the same time course, but amount to only a few percent of those of the parent substance.[53,57]

Kinetics of pharmaceutic progestogens: luteal supplementation and HRT

Oral administration of progesterone

The main commercial product of progesterone is a tablet formulation containing 100 mg progesterone in micronized form.[30] The recommended daily dose is 300 mg.

Following oral administration, progesterone undergoes marked first pass metabolism in the gut wall and liver. Thus only a quarter of an oral dose, or even less, reaches the general circulation as unchanged progesterone.[53,58,59] Mean plasma levels observed in women following single doses of micronized progesterone are plotted in Figure 25.7. The left panel shows the concentration–time course of unchanged progesterone within 24 hours of administration of a 200 mg dose.[39] A peak level of 21 ng/ml is reached after two hours already, indicating rapid absorption from the gastrointestinal tract. Concentrations are almost at baseline again after 12 hours and, therefore, a twice daily intake of oral progesterone is recommended in HRT.[30] The Cmax produced by a 200 mg dose of progesterone lies well within the range of luteal phase values.

The active metabolites reach much lower maximal plasma concentrations than unchanged progesterone

Table 25.4 Pharmacokinetic parameters of physiological progesterone in normal premenopausal women and after ovariectomy (mean or approximative values).[27,54]

Parameter	Follicular phase	Luteal phase	After ovariectomy
Production rate (mg/day)*	0.8–2.5	15–50	0.8
Metabolic clearance rate (liter/day)	2510	2510	2100
Plasma concentration (ng/ml)	0.3–1	6–20	0.4

*Calculated for plasma.

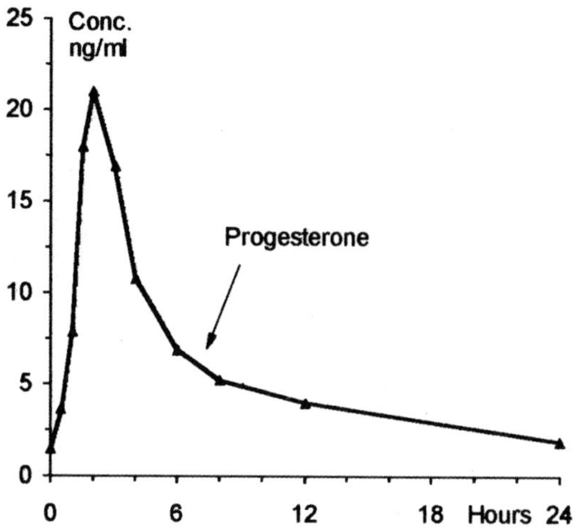

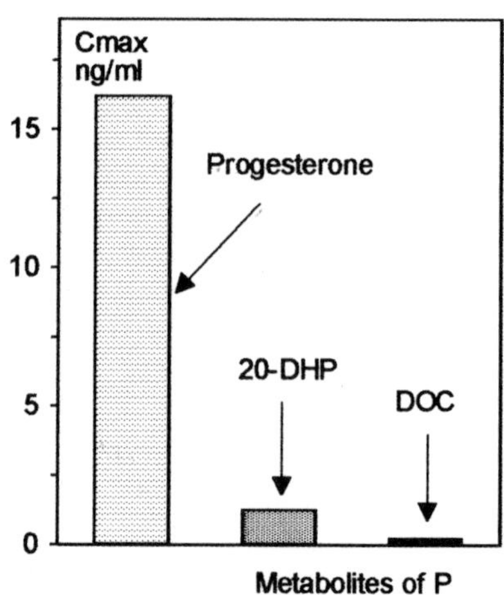

Fig. 25.7 Left panel: time course of mean plasma concentrations of unchanged progesterone in women following single oral doses of 200 mg progesterone.[39] Right panel: comparison of mean Cmax values of progesterone and its active metabolites, 20-DHP and DOC, following single oral doses of 100 mg progesterone.[53]

does. This is evident from the Cmax values found in an independent study with single oral doses of 100 mg progesterone (right panel of Fig. 25.7). Compared to Cmax of progesterone, the values of 20-DHP and DOC correspond to 8% and 1.5%, respectively.[53] Although the plasma levels of DOC seem to be low, it has been hypothesized that they may have adverse effects, as DOC is a potent mineralocorticoid. Its plasma concentration is actually higher after oral than after parenteral dosing of progesterone, indicating that DOC stems at least in part from first pass metabolism.

In a recent paper,[58] the plasma concentrations resulting from oral progesterone have been reported to be several times lower than those shown in Figure 25.7. The authors of the new study explain this discrepancy with the use of insufficiently specific assays in the earlier trials. It will be up to further investigations to obtain an unequivocal answer.

Oral and intramuscular administration of synthetic derivatives of progesterone

The following synthetic derivatives of progesterone are contained in commercial products used for luteal supplementation or HRT.[7,30] Medroxyprogesterone acetate (MPA): usual oral dosage form 5–10 mg daily; intramuscular dosage form 150 mg every three months. Cyproterone acetate (CPA): oral dosage form 10–50 mg daily. Medrogestone: oral dosage form (single substance) 5–10 mg daily; oral dosage form (combined with conjugated estrogens) 5 mg daily. Dydrogesterone: oral dosage form 10–20 mg daily. Low-dose CPA (2 mg) combined with EE (35 µg) is also used for fertility control.

It should be kept in mind that natural progesterone has a short elimination half-life of 30 minutes only. The synthetic progestogens, on the other hand, have been designed for prolonged half-lives.

The half-lives of MPA and CPA range from 2–3 days.[39,60,61] In contrast to progesterone, both MPA and CPA are completely bioavailable. These synthetic progestogens are highly effective after oral administration. Following repeated daily doses of MPA or CPA, plasma levels reach a steady state within a few days. For instance, a low dose of CPA (2 mg plus 50 µg EE), as used for contraception, produces peak levels of 15 ng/ml and 24 ng/ml, respectively, after single and repeated oral administration.[62] Intramuscular injection of 150 mg of MPA results in long lasting plasma concentrations, decreasing from 3 ng/ml to 1 ng/ml during 90 days.[40]

The pharmacokinetics of dydrogesterone and medrogestone are not well documented. Absorption of oral doses is rapid, Cmax in plasma being reached after 1–2 hours.[30] The elimination half-life of medrogestone is only 4–5 hours, and that of dydrogesterone must be short, too, because 85% of a dose is excreted again in 24 hours. Fast elimination may be explained by the fact that medrogestone carries only a small additional substituent at position 17, while dydrogesterone carries none.

Oral and transdermal administration of norethisterone and its acetate ester

Norethindrone (NET) and norethindrone acetate (NETA) are used for luteal supplementation in oral daily doses of 5 mg and 2.5 mg, respectively. For HRT, the recommended oral doses are lower, e.g. ≤1 mg of NET per day. For the latter indication, a combined transdermal system is also available, with a nominal release rate of 0.25 mg NETA and 50 µg E_2 per day.[7,30] (For the use of NET/NETA in oral contraception see chapters 44–46.)

NET is rapidly absorbed from the gastrointestinal tract, but its bioavailability is incomplete. Owing to first pass metabolism, only about 65% of an oral dose reaches the general circulation as unchanged NET. A 5 mg dose of NET results in a plasma Cmax of 30ng/ml. Elimination follows a half-life of 8 hours. These values represent the means of several studies.[39,60] NETA is actually a prodrug of NET. Efficient cleavage of the acetate ester bond of NETA is mediated by esterases present in body fluids and tissues. Following oral or transdermal administration, the acetyl group of NETA is readily split off during its passage through the intestinal wall or skin, and NET is released into the circulation.

When the combined transdermal system is applied to skin, it releases NETA and E_2 continuously during 3–4 days. The plasma levels of NET increase during two days after the first application. Then they remain constant at an average of 0.7–0.8 ng/ml for the entire treatment period, provided the system is replaced twice weekly. The concentrations of E_2 resemble those produced by a system containing solely the estrogen component (Fig. 25.4). For HRT in postmenopausal women, E_2 systems and E_2/NETA systems can be used cyclically or continuously. Treatment conventionally begins with E_2 and is switched to E_2/NETA in the middle of each 4 week period, to simulate the menstrual cycle.[30,63] More recently, continuous combined regimens are being explored.

Kinetics of exogenous progestogens: contraception

General data on progestogens used for contraception

Most oral contraceptives contain nowadays one of the 19-nortestosterone derivatives carrying an ethinyl group at C-17. A first series of such derivatives comprises well-known steroids like NET, NETA and levonorgestrel (LNG). A second series is represented by products of more recent development, e.g. desogestrel (DSG), gestodene (GSD) and norgestimate (NGM).[39,60,64] The newer progestogens are claimed to act more selectively than the older ones, and to have less unwanted side-effects.

There is a vast variety of contraceptive dosage forms on the market. They consist of a progestogen which is normally combined with EE as an estrogenic component. Typical combinations and dose strengths of oral products are summarized in Table 25.5. In some products for oral intake, the progestogen dose is not constant during a treatment cycle, but changes in two or three phases of the cycle. The more recently introduced products contain generally lower doses of both the progestogen and the estrogen.

Many attempts have been made to develop long-acting contraceptives for implantation or injection, but the number of commercial products is still rather modest.[40,65] One of the available products (Norplant®) contains a total amount of 216 mg of LNG, incorporated in six silastic capsules which are simultaneously implanted under the skin. This system

Table 25.5 Amounts of active substances contained in contraceptive dosage forms for oral use. Usual daily doses of progestogens are given in mg, those of the estrogen (EE) in µg.[7,64]

Progestogen generic name	Abbreviation	Progestogen dose (mg)	Estrogen (EE) dose (µg)
Norethindrone	NET	0.35–10	35–50
Norethindrone	NET	0.35	None
Norethindrone acetate	NETA	1.0–1.5	20–50
Norgestrel		0.3–0.5	30–50
Levonorgestrel	LNG	0.05–0.15	30–40
Desogestrel	DSG	0.15	20–30
Gestodene	GSD	0.05–0.15	30–40
Norgestimate	NGM	0.25	35

has been designed to release LNG continuously at a relatively constant rate during a period of at least five years.[7]

Oral administration of NET, NETA and LNG

The general kinetic features of NET and its acetyl ester NETA have already been described in the context of HRT and luteal supplementation (see above). Some numerical kinetic parameters are listed in Table 25.6, together with those of LNG.[60,64,66]

The daily oral dose of NET in contraceptives is 1 mg at most. Single doses of that strength produce maximum plasma concentrations of about 6 ng/ml, mostly within two hours of administration. Concentrations fall below 1 ng/ml after 24 hours. Steady state levels are reached after about two days of repeated treatment. First pass metabolism reduces the bioavailability of both NET and NETA considerably.

Norgestrel is a racemic compound consisting of the hormonally active levorotatory enantiomer (LNG) and an inactive dextrorotatory enantiomer.[67] The latter is considered as isomeric ballast. Therefore, only a few of the oral contraceptives used today contain racemic norgestrel; most of them contain half of the dose as LNG (Table 25.5). Regarding the pharmacokinetics, LNG is well documented, while only little is known about norgestrel.

Orally administered LNG does not undergo any first pass metabolism and is completely bioavailable, as opposed to NET (Table 25.6). Following single doses of 0.15 mg LNG (plus 30 μg EE), plasma levels of LNG reach a peak of 3–4 ng/ml, and drop to values of <1 ng/ml at the time of the next daily dose.[60,66] Absorption is rapid, as indicated by a mean Tmax of 1–2 hours. There is a linear relationship between plasma concentrations and dose-height. Steady state levels are attained after a few days of repeated treatment, but they are about three times higher than anticipated from the single dose data. This is largely attributable to an interaction with EE, as will be discussed later.

Implantation of long-acting LNG systems

When the silastic capsules mentioned above are inserted under the skin, they release LNG at a rate of 50–80 μg per day during the first year. From the second to the fifth year of use, the release rate averages 30–35 μg per day.[7,40] Mean plasma concentrations of LNG rise to 1.6 ng/ml within 24 hours after implantation of the capsules. The levels fall rapidly during the first month to about 0.4 ng/ml, but afterwards they decline only slightly to values of 0.33 ng/ml at 12 months and 0.26 ng/ml at 60 months. The initial fall is partially attributable to a feedback mechanism: LNG is tightly bound to sex hormone-binding globulin (SHBG), but SHBG is suppressed by the presence of LNG. As a consequence, the plasma concentration of LNG decreases.

Oral administration of GSD, DSG and NGM

The kinetic parameters of three newer progestogens, GSD, DSG and NGM, are summarized in Table 25.7. Only GSD carries a 3-keto group in its molecule, and is thus active in its unchanged form. DSG and NGM can be considered as prodrugs which are activated in the body by metabolic reactions.

Following ingestion of GSD, no first pass metabolism occurs. This progestogen is fully bioavailable. A single dose of 0.075 mg GSD (plus 30 μg EE) results in peak plasma concentrations of 3–4 ng/ml within 1 hour; they decrease to about one tenth after 24 hours (Fig. 25.8, left panel). Peak levels at steady state are in the range of 10 ng/ml.[39,60,68] During multiple intake, the initial elimination half-life of 12 hours rises to 18 hours, probably because GSD inhibits its own metabolism to some extent.

The next substance of this series, DSG, is efficiently metabolized to 3-keto-DSG during its first passage through the gut wall and liver (Fig. 25.9). About 75% of an oral dose is available in the circulation as 3-keto-DSG in which the progestational activity resides. All kinetic data refer to the metabolite, therefore.[39,60,69]

Table 25.6 Pharmacokinetic parameters of a first group of synthetic progestogens: NET, NETA and LNG (approximate mean values).[60,64,66]

Parameter	NET	NETA	LNG
Bioavailability (% of oral dose)	65	~50*	100
Elimination half-life (hours)	8	8*	16
Distribution volume (liter)	240	240*	120
Metabolic clearance rate (liter/day)	530	530*	145

*Data relate to NET which is the major active metabolite of NETA.

Table 25.7 Pharmacokinetic parameters of a second group of synthetic progestogens: GSD, DSG and NGM (approximate mean values).[60,64,68,69]

Parameter	GSD	DSG	NGM
Bioavailability (% of oral dose)	100	75*	_***
Elimination half-life (hours)	12	12*	16**
Distribution volume (liter)	32	110*	_***
Metabolic clearance rate (liter/day)	70	190*	_***

*Data refer to the major active metabolite, 3-keto-DSG; **half-life of an active metabolite, deacetyl-NGM; ***No data available.

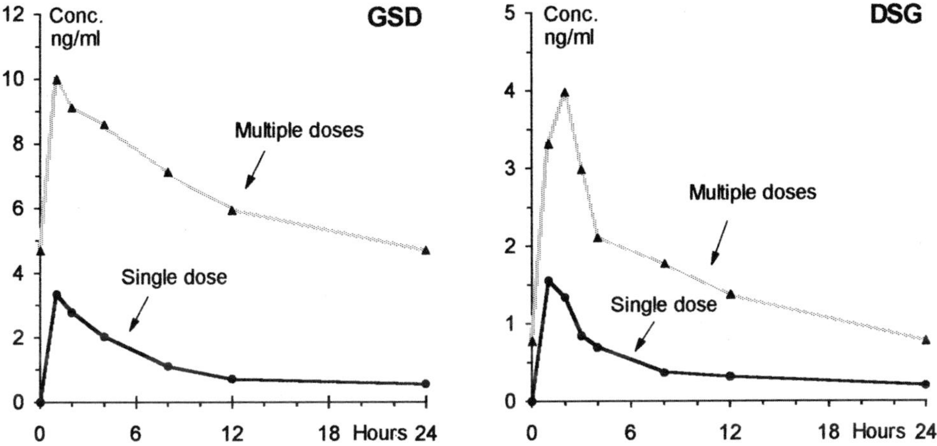

Fig. 25.8 Plasma concentrations observed following single and repeated doses of GSD (left panel) and DSG (right panel; note the expanded ordinate scale). Doses: 0.075 mg GSD or 0.15 mg DSG, always combined with 30 mg EE. The data of DSG stand for its active metabolite, 3-keto-DSG.[60]

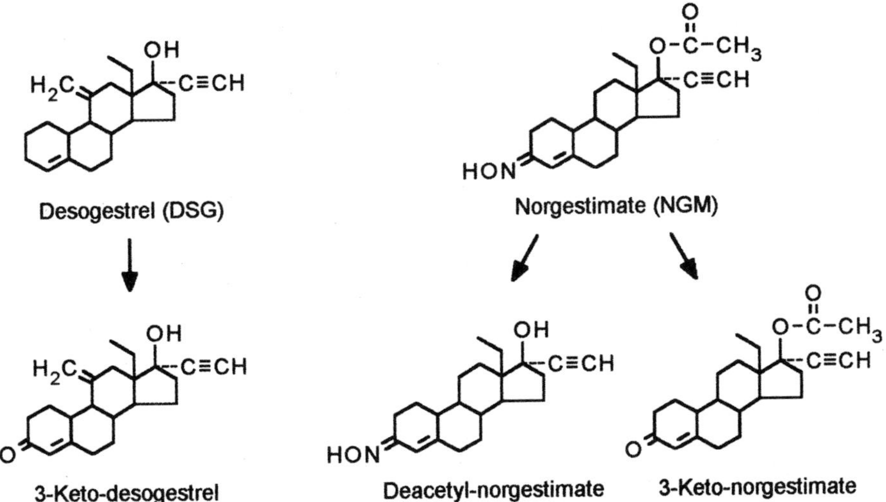

Fig. 25.9 Formation of active metabolites by enzymatic oxidation of DSG (left side) and hydrolysis of NGM (right side).[39,60]

DSG is rapidly absorbed from the gastrointestinal tract, as indicated by a Tmax in plasma of 1–2 hours. Cmax amounts to about 1.5 ng/ml after a single dose of 0.15 mg DSG (combined with 30 μg EE), and rises to 4 ng/ml at steady state (Fig. 25.8, right panel).

The two progestogens GSD and DSG resemble each other in their bioavailabilities and elimination half-lives (Table 25.7). Nevertheless, the plasma concentrations of GSD exceed by far those of 3-keto-DSG, when the differences in dose-heights are taken into account (Fig. 25.8). The high levels of GSD are presumably attributable to the strong association of GSD with circulating SHBG. The distribution volumes in Table 25.7 suggest that GSD is indeed less widely distributed in the organism than 3-keto-DSG.

The pharmacokinetic pattern of NGM is rather complex and is not well investigated. It is known that at least two active metabolites contribute to the progestogenic effects of NGM. The structures of these metabolites, i.e. deacetyl-NGM and 3-keto-NGM, are included in Figure 25.9. Deactyl-NGM reaches a plasma Cmax of about 3.5 ng/ml following single oral doses of 0.36 mg NGM (plus 70 μg EE); the steady state concentration during multiple dosing averages 4.5 ng/ml.[60,70] The elimination rate of deacetyl-NGM is in the same range as that of other progestogens of this series (Table 25.7). The second metabolite, 3-keto-NGM; seems to reach sizeable plasma levels, too, but accurate data are missing. The concentrations of unchanged NGM do not exceed 0.1 ng/ml.

VARIABILITY OF PHARMACOKINETIC PARAMETERS OF ESTROGENS AND PROGESTOGENS

Overview of processes controlling the kinetics of steroid hormones

When drug molecules are absorbed following oral administration, they traverse the gastrointestinal tract, the liver, the heart, the lungs, and pass back to the heart, before they reach the general circulation. The molecules then distribute reversibly between the bloodstream and organs and tissues. Eventually they are eliminated from the body by hepatic or renal mechanisms. A simplified diagram of the essential organs and processes is given in Figure 25.10.

Drug concentrations in the blood or at the site of action are the result of an interplay of many independent events. Extent and rate of each individual process are determined by two principles: the physicochemical properties of the drug, and the functions of the biological system. The latter functions are in no way constant in a population, or even in an individual person. For a given drug substance, therefore, the pharmacokinetics will vary inter- and intra-individually. Some of the functions or processes may give rise to clinically relevant variations, some others not. In the following we wish to discuss those processes which may become critical for estrogens and progestogens.

Absorption of estrogens and progestogens from the gastrointestinal tract is normally unproblematic. Dosage forms are designed for rapid release; the steroid is incorporated in micronized form, should low water solubility be a problem. The active substances are absorbed in the upper part of the intestine, and concomitant administration of antacids has no effect on bioavailability.[71–73]

First pass metabolism is theoretically possible everywhere on the drug's pathway from the gut lumen to the general circulation. For steroid hormones, however, only the intestinal wall and liver are important (Fig. 25.10). Sensitive substances, such as E_2 and progesterone, are indeed largely metabolized during their first passage through these tissues. As the fraction of dose lost is not constant, steroids

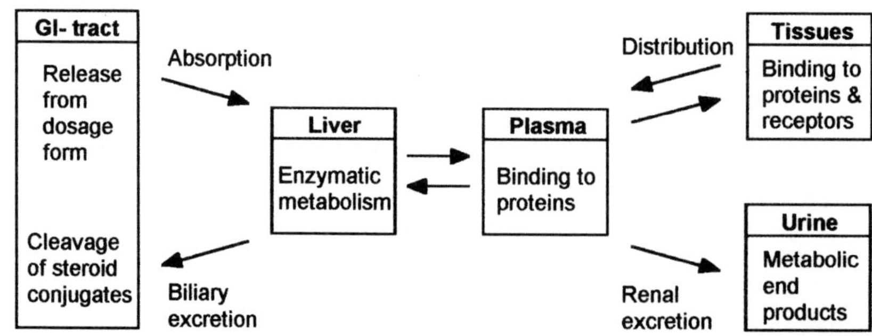

Fig. 25.10 Scheme of major processes determining the pharmacokinetics of a steroid hormone following oral administration.

undergoing first pass metabolism tend to show a higher degree of kinetic variability than steroids which escape this kind of breakdown. It should be mentioned here that first pass metabolism may also occur in the skin or mucosa, when a steroid is administered by the transdermal or vaginal route.

An estrogen or progestogen spreads between blood and tissues by passive diffusion. The pattern of distribution is largely controlled by the binding of the substance to transport proteins and tissue receptors. Binding is reversible so that each change of concentration in one compartment is followed by a re-equilibration of substance. Some lipophilic steroids are taken up by body fat. In the blood compartment, steroids are preferentially associated with two proteins, i.e. albumin and sex hormone-binding globulin (SHBG; see ch. 8). Consequently, steroid kinetics may be influenced by the amount of adipose tissue or the concentration of SHBG.[71] Such distribution processes may also contribute to the kinetic variability.

Because of their low solubility in aqueous media, estrogens and progestogens are not apt for direct excretion by the kidneys. Metabolic reactions in the liver make the steroids water soluble. The end products of this process, such as glucuronides, are then largely removed by the renal route. Therefore, impaired kidney function may increase the levels of circulating steroid metabolites, but the levels of the unchanged steroids will not be greatly influenced.

The rates of the metabolic reactions in the liver are actually a major determinant of the kinetics of estrogens and progestogens. These reactions are catalysed by drug-metabolizing enzymes, including oxidases, reductases and transferases (see ch. 4 and 8). Activities of such enzymes differ considerably from one person to another. For example, factors of interindividual variation were found to range from 3–11, when the metabolic clearance of a series of chemically different drugs was investigated in normal subjects.[74] Most of this high degree of variation is genetically controlled. Variability is therefore always larger between subjects than within a subject, although factors like drug intake, special diets and pathologic conditions may also influence enzyme activities.

Enterohepatic recirculation of active substances is a specific feature of estrogen kinetics. Active estrogen molecules contain hydroxyl groups in positions 3 and 17, which undergo conjugation in the intestinal wall or liver. The resulting sulfates and glucuronides of the otherwise unchanged estrogen are partly excreted into the bile, and are transported to the duodenum (Fig. 25.10). The conjugates are cleaved by the natural gut flora in the lower parts of the intestine, and the released estrogen is absorbed again. This process may prolong the residence time of an estrogen in the circulation. On the other hand, it is a further source of variability.

Plasma concentrations of the endogenous hormones E_2, E_1, E_3 and progesterone depend primarily on their physiologic production rates. That aspect has been discussed above already. The subsequent sections will focus on exogenous estrogens and progestogens, and on the processes which are responsible for pharmacokinetic variability. This will particularly include hepatic metabolism, but attention will also be paid to less critical phenomena, such as first pass effect, enterohepatic recirculation and tissue distribution.

Factors which influence the kinetics of estrogens

Genetic and environmental factors

The plasma levels of exogenous estrogens show a similar degree of interindividual variability as shown by the levels of other synthetic drugs.[74] Following single oral doses of EE, for instance, the plasma AUC of EE varied 9-fold across a group of healthy women, even when external factors were strictly controlled. The variability observed after oral E_2 is in the same order of magnitude.[24,51,52] Part of this effect is attributable to the gastrointestinal first pass metabolism, because kinetic variability is 2–3 times lower when E_2 is administered by the intravenous route. Even after allowing for the variability of first pass metabolism, a variation factor of 3–4 is still left which must be largely assigned to the hepatic clearance of estrogens from the general circulation.

Circulating estrogens are cleared by two main processes, i.e. conjugation of hydroxyl groups and hydroxylation at C-2 and C-4. Conjugation is catalysed by glucuronyltransferases and by sulfotransferases, whereas hydroxylation is catalysed by isoenzymes of the cytochrome P450 complex, mainly CYP3A4 and CYP1A2. The activities of these enzymes may differ several times between subjects, but age has little or no influence.[17,50,75,76] Basal activities of such enzymes are genetically controlled, as shown by studies in twins.[74]

Genetic factors are frequently associated with ethnic or geographic differences in drug kinetics. Studies with EE in women from the US, Nigeria and some southeast Asian countries have shown that mean plasma levels of EE vary almost 4-fold between these populations. Oxidative metabolism prevails in the US women, and conjugations in all other populations. Nevertheless, it is still speculative whether this difference is attributable to genetic, dietary or other factors.[50] Dietary factors seem to have some influence on 2-hydroxylation of estrogens: high protein and low fat diets enhance this process, while high carbohydrate diets decrease it. Whether metabolism of steroids generally differs between vegetarians and nonvegetarians is still controversial.[71] The high fiber content in vegetarian diets leads possibly to decreased plasma concentrations of natural E_2, owing to a reduced enterohepatic recirculation.

Cigarette smoking has been reported to influence the kinetics of exogenous estrogens in women receiving oral HRT.[77,78] During treatment with high oral doses of E_2 (4 mg/day), for instance, the plasma levels of E_2 and E_1 in smokers were 50% lower than those in nonsmokers. Smoking induces the hepatic cytochrome P450 isoenzyme responsible for 2-hydroxylation of natural estrogens which is accompanied by a loss of activity. It is assumed that this kind of hydroxylation occurs during the first passage through the liver. After transdermal administration of E_2 — when no hepatic first pass metabolism can occur — the estrogen levels in plasma do not actually differ between smokers and nonsmokers.[78,79] Such a first pass mechanism would also explain why smoking has no significant influence on the production rate and metabolic clearance rate of endogenous estrogens in pre- and postmenopausal women.[80–82]

Considering the pharmacokinetics of EE in women taking oral contraceptives, smoking has no significant effect, although EE is also inactivated by 2-hydroxylation. The specific P450 isoenzyme catalysing the 2-hydroxylation of synthetic estrogens, such as EE, is not inducible by tobacco smoke. Accordingly, cigarette smoking does not seem to increase the failure rate of oral contraceptives.[79,83,84]

Little is known about a possible influence of alcohol on the pharmacokinetics of estrogens. In particular, there are no reports as regards the kinetics of exogenous estrogens used for HRT or contraception. According to a recent study in premenopausal women, chronic alcohol ingestion has no effect on endogenous plasma estrogens in the follicular, midcycle or luteal phases of the menstrual cycle.[85] The women investigated included light, moderate and heavy drinkers, but none had signs of chronic liver disease.

We conclude that genetic factors are responsible for a considerable part of the interindividual variability of estrogen pharmacokinetics. Dietary habits or other environmental factors may have an additional effect. However, there is no simple means to determine the kinetic or metabolic status of an individual woman before prescribing an estrogen-containing drug. Not knowing this status, selection of the optimal product and adjustment of dose have to rely on therapeutic or clinical effects. For estrogen replacement in postmenopausal women, products for transdermal use are superior to oral dosage forms. By avoiding first pass metabolism, transdermal therapy reduces the variability of estrogen kinetics.

Effects of drugs on estrogen kinetics

The problem of pharmacokinetic interactions between drugs and estrogens has been addressed in numerous clinical studies. Yet, our knowledge about drug interactions with E_2 and E_1 is scanty, because investigators were mainly interested in interactions with EE in oral contraceptives. This is easy to understand, when the potential consequences are considered: in postmenopausal women receiving HRT, intermittent impairment of the kinetics of E_2 or E_1 by a second drug may result in discomfort but not in serious side-effects. In women taking contraceptive steroids, however, any suppression of plasma levels by a second drug increases the risk of breakthrough bleeding and unexpected pregnancy. Although a clinically important decrease of contraceptive efficacy is a rare event, the absolute number of women affected is still high, considering the widespread use of oral contraceptives.[71,86]

There are two major mechanisms by which other drugs can lower the plasma concentrations of EE. Firstly, inducers of hepatic enzymes may enhance the metabolic inactivation of EE. Secondly, oral antibiotics may interfere with the enterohepatic recycling of EE by decimating the gut flora responsible for the cleavage of estrogen conjugates secreted into the intestine by way of bile.

Inducers of hepatic enzymes include several anticonvulsant drugs, such as phenobarbital, primidone, phenytoin and carbamazepine. The antibiotic rifampicin is a further potent inducer. Upon repeated administration of any of these drugs, activities of CYP3A4 and other isoforms of cytochrome P450 are raised. As a consequence, 2-hydroxylation of EE is enhanced. Figure 25.11 illustrates how repeated therapeutic doses of inducing agents lower the plasma concentrations of EE in premenopausal women.[83] Under the influence of phenytoin, carbamazepine and rifampicin, the plasma AUC of EE falls to 50–60% of the control value. Valproic acid is a non-inducing anticonvulsant and has virtually no effect.

Higher doses of contraceptive steroids have been recommended to ensure contraceptive efficacy in women taking anticonvulsants with the potential to induce metabolising enzymes in the liver. In the case of rifampicin, some specialists feel that the additional use of mechanical contraceptives should suffice, while others consider the simultaneous use of rifampicin and oral contraceptives as being contraindicated.[83,86,87]

A few drugs have the opposite effect on estrogen kinetics. Paracetamol and vitamin C are examples of drugs undergoing extensive sulfation during absorption through the gut wall. Thus, the sulfate pool may temporarily be exhausted. When such a drug is ingested together with contraceptive steroids, the sulfation of EE in the gut wall may be impaired. As a consequence, the circulating levels of EE will rise. This interaction can easily be avoided by taking the drugs at least two hours apart.[86,88]

The metabolic processes leading to enterohepatic recirculation of estrogens are outlined in Figure 25.12, taking EE and its 3-sulfate as an example. Other estrogens or conjugates, e.g. glucuronides, undergo the same kind of recycling. Only a fraction of an estrogen dose is entering such a cycle, because of competing metabolic pathways.[83,86] If hydrolysis of a conjugate in the gut is inhibited, less of the free estrogen will be reabsorbed, and more of the conjugate will be excreted in the feces.

Broad spectrum antibiotics, like ampicillin and tetracycline, are known to kill intestinal bacteria which hydrolyse estrogen conjugates. Several studies have shown, however, that these antibiotics do not

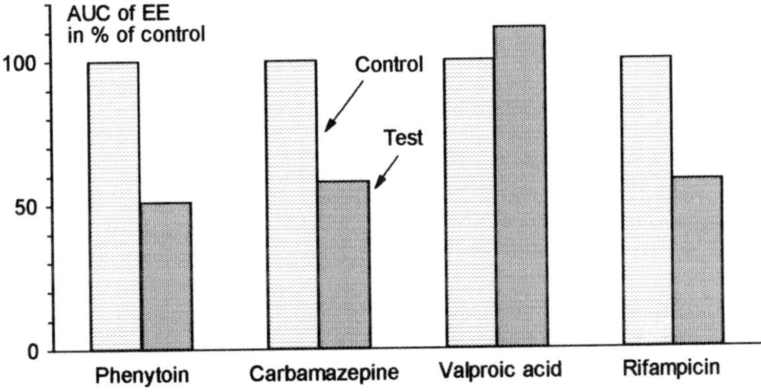

Fig. 25.11 Influence of enzyme inducers (phenytoin, carbamazepine, rifampicin) and of a noninducing agent (valproic acid) on the concentrations of EE in plasma of premenopausal women. The left column of each pair represents the AUC of EE observed without second drug (control value = 100%); the right bar represents the AUC observed during repeated administration of the second drug (test value in % of control).[83]

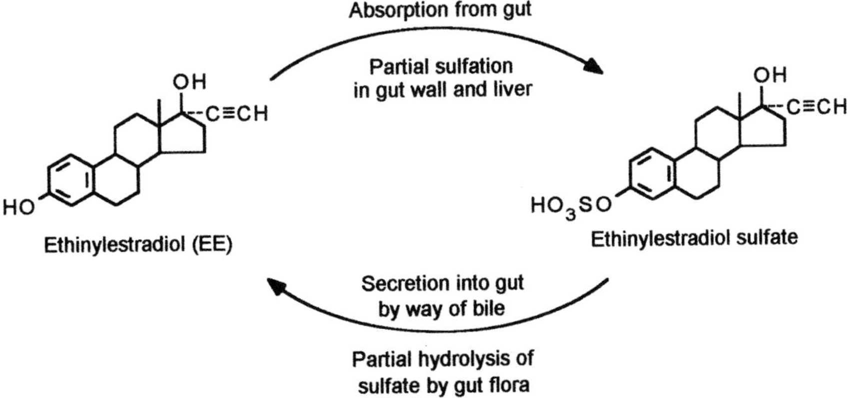

Fig. 25.12 Scheme of enterohepatic circulation of estrogens, exemplified with EE and its 3-sulfate. The same kind of cycle occurs with the glucuronide

systematically lower EE plasma levels in women taking oral contraceptives.[83,86] On the other hand, contraceptive failures have been reported to occur with such drug combinations. It is assumed that a minority of women may be at risk, in whom the pill produces generally low EE levels, e.g. by genetic reasons. Alternative contraceptive precautions are therefore recommended. Cholestyramine is another drug supposed to lower EE concentrations in plasma. It is an anion exchange resin which binds bile acid conjugates and impairs their enterohepatic circulation. In the same way it reduces reabsorption of estrogens.[89]

Factors which influence the kinetics of progestogens

Genetic and environmental factors

Progestogens are cleared from the circulation by hepatic metabolism mainly. Reduction of the double bonds at positions 3 and 5 is a major reaction leading to inactive metabolites. The exact nature of the reductases involved remains to be identified. Oxidative attack is catalysed by a cytochrome P450 isoenzyme (CYP3A4); it occurs at C-6 and, in the case of ethinyl-substituted steroids, also at the ethinyl group. Direct conjugation is possible at the hydroxyl group in position 17, but it is a minor reaction only.[16,17,60,90] Therefore, progestogens do not undergo enterohepatic circulation to any substantial degree which is quite in contrast to the estrogens (Fig. 25.12).

One has to assume that much of the interindividual variability of the progestogen kinetics is again attributable to the activities of the drug metabolizing enzymes, and thus to genetic factors. This is supported by the fact that variability between subjects exceeds variability within a subject.[86,91] Experimental data on kinetic variability are still scarce, however. Little is known about natural progesterone and its synthetic derivatives, like MPA and CYP. Progestogens related to 19-nortestosterone, being components of oral contraceptives, are better documented.

The interindividual variability of plasma levels of the 19-nortestosterone derivatives lies in the same region as that of EE. This is evident from a paper in which the coefficients of variation of plasma AUCs following single oral doses have been compared.[92] For NET, LNG, GSD and DSG, these coefficients range from 31%–47%, and for EE it is 37%. One would expect that the two progestogens undergoing first pass metabolism (NET; DSG) show larger coefficients of variation than the others do (LNG; GSD). Because there is in fact no systematic difference, first pass metabolism does not seem to add much to the kinetic variability of these progestogens.

Factors other than genetic must also play a role in both the inter- and intra-individual variability. It is known, for instance, that intake of a meal may decrease the serum levels of progesterone by one third, probably by increasing hepatic blood flow and clearance of progesterone. However, cigarette smoking has no effect on the production and metabolism of natural progesterone in cycling women.[82,90] Apart from such anecdotal reports, however, virtually nothing has been published on environmental factors like diet, tobacco smoking and alcohol ingestion. Information on ethnic differences is also not available for this class of steroids.

Effects of drugs on progestogen kinetics and interactions with estrogens

Most of our present knowledge about kinetic interactions between progestogens and other drugs arises from studies with oral contraceptives. Induction of hepatic enzymes of the cytochrome P450 complex is an important mechanism of such interactions. Upon repeated administration of an enzyme inducer, the metabolic clearance of the estrogenic component of oral contraceptives is enhanced, as outlined previously.

The effect of three anticonvulsants and one antibiotic on the plasma levels of progestogens is virtually identical to that demonstrated for EE in Fig. 25.11. During concomitant administration of phenytoin and carbamazepine, the plasma AUCs of LNG decrease to about 60% of the control values.[83] A non-inducing anticonvulsant, valproic acid, has no influence. The antibiotic rifampicin lowers the AUC of NET also to 60% of controls. Measures to avoid contraceptive failures in such cases have been mentioned already.

Enterohepatic circulation is important for estrogens, but is unimportant for progestogens. Any disturbance of the gut flora by broadspectrum antibiotics will not impair the kinetics of progestogens. Estrogens undergo significant sulfation during absorption through the gut wall, but progestogens do not. Plasma concentrations of LNG are unaltered by concurrent administration of paracetamol, which is a drug competing with steroid sulfation.[93]

An interesting though very complex area of kinetic interactions is that between estrogens and progestogens. This applies particularly to steroids carrying an ethinyl group in position 17, including EE, NET, LNG, DSG and GSD. Such interactions may be caused by two independent mechanisms, namely changes in SHBG binding capacity and inhibition of cytochrome P450 isoenzymes.

Exogenous estrogens enhance the production of SHBG. Therefore, the plasma levels of SHBG will increase during intake of an oral contraceptive containing EE. On the other hand, the SHBG levels may be lowered by the progestogenic component, because some of the progestogens have a pronounced antiestrogenic activity. As a net result, combinations of LNG+EE show virtually no effect on plasma SHBG, while GSD+EE or DSG+EE lead to a doubling of concentrations. The combination of NET+EE holds an intermediate position.[64,66,94,95] Progestogens are bound to SHBG and their plasma concentrations will correspondingly rise, when the amount of SHBG goes up.

The inhibition of cytochrome P450 seems to be a secondary effect of metabolic oxidation of the ethinyl group attached to position 17 of EE and of several progestogens. Reactive intermediates resulting from this oxidation bind irreversibly to the catalysing P450 enzyme, thus reducing its activity. As a consequence, the hepatic clearance of EE and of progestogens may be reduced during repeated administration of oral contraceptives.[16,17,90]

The list in Table 25.8 is an attempt to arrange the individual factors and influences of both kinds of interaction in a systematic way. GSD is the most extreme among the progestogens, inasmuch as it strongly inhibits P450, does not suppress SHBG production and shows the highest degree of binding to SHBG. The combined result of these three factors is a plasma concentration of GSD at steady state which is considerably higher than to be expected from the single dose kinetics (Fig. 25.8).

To sum up, the pharmacokinetic variability caused by genetic and environmental factors may be aggravated by interactions. However, there is no apparent relationship between the plasma concentrations of a progestogen and the pharmacological effects of the oral contraceptive containing it. The concentration range achieved is presumably near the upper end-point of the concentration-response curve of a progestogen. Thus, even the low dose formulations used today seem to produce adequate plasma levels in the vast majority of cases.

Conclusion

Endogenous female sex hormones, especially E_2 and progesterone, have short plasma half-lives. The residence time of E_2 is prolonged by reversible conversion to E_1, and by enterohepatic recirculation of estrogen conjugates excreted in the bile.

Natural hormones have to be administered in large oral doses to obtain effective plasma concentrations. Doses can considerably be reduced with parenteral administration, because first pass metabolism in the gut and liver is avoided. Continuous delivery of E_2 from a transdermal patch results in a physiologic pattern of plasma levels with low daily doses.

Synthetic estrogens and progestogens have been designed to prevent their rapid metabolic breakdown during both absorption and circulation. Elimination half-lives are indeed several times those of their natural counterparts. For synthetic steroids with a high degree of metabolic resistance, only low oral doses are required.

Plasma levels of estrogens and progestogens show a wide range of variability between subjects, a substantial part of which being attributable to genetic factors. For kinetic differences observed between populations, specific diets may be more important than ethnic factors. Moderate tobacco smoking and alcohol intake have no critical influence on the kinetics.

Some anticonvulsants and antibiotics are known to impair the efficacy of oral contraceptives by enhancing the elimination of estrogens and progestogens. When such drugs are administered concomitantly, oral contraceptives should be used in higher doses, or alternative contraceptive measures considered.

Table 25.8 Factors which influence the kinetic interactions between estrogens and progestogens during continued intake of oral contraceptives.[16,60,94]

Steroid	Effect on SHBG production	Binding to SHBG	Effect on cytochrome P450
EE	Strong stimulation	None	Weak inhibition
NET	Moderate suppression	36%	Weak inhibition
LNG	Strong suppression	48%	Weak inhibition
DSG*	Weak suppression	32%	Moderate inhibition
GSD	Weak suppression	76%	Strong inhibition

*Data refer to 3-keto-DSG, the active main metabolite of DSG.

REFERENCES

1. Dost FH 1953 Der Blutspiegel; Kinetik der Konzentrationsabläufe in der Körperflüssigkeit. Thieme Verlag, Leipzig
2. Hvidberg EF 1990 Why do we need pharmacokinetic studies? American Journal of Obstetrics and Gynecology 163: 316–318
3. Pazzagli M, Serio M 1987 Immunochemical methods for adrenal and gonadal steroids. In: Patrono C, Peskar BA (eds) Radioimmunoassay in basic and clinical pharmacology. Handbook of Experimental Pharmacology vol 82. Springer, Berlin, pp 363–400
4. Moss GP 1991 The nomenclature of steroids. IUPAC-IUB Joint Commission on Biochemical Nomenclature (JBCN). Recommendations 1989. In: Hill RA, Kirk DN, Makin HLJ, et al (eds) Dictionary of steroids. Chemical data, structures and bibliographies. Chapman & Hall, London, pp XXX–LIX
5. Martindale 1996 The extra pharmacopoeia, 31st edn. Reynolds JEF, Parfitt K, Parsons AV, Sweetman SC (eds). Royal Pharmaceutical Society, London
6. The Merck Index 1996 An encyclopedia of chemicals, drugs, and biologicals, 12th edn. Budavari S, O'Neil MJ, Smith A, Heckelman PE, Kinneary JF (eds) Merck Whitehouse Station, New Jersey
7. Physicians' Desk Reference, 52nd edn. 1998 Medical Economics Company, Montvale, New Jersey
8. Nichols KC, Schenkel L, Benson H 1984 17β-estradiol for postmenopausal estrogen replacement therapy. Obstetrics and Gynecological Survey 39: 230–245
9. O'Connell MB 1995 Pharmacokinetic and pharmacologic variation between different estrogen products. Journal of Clinical Pharmacology 35: 18S–24S
10. Adlerkreutz H, Gorbach SL, Goldin BR, Woods MN, Dwyer JT, Hämäläinen E 1994 Estrogen metabolism and excretion in oriental and caucasian women. Journal of the National Cancer Institute 86: 1076–1082
11. Gavaler JS 1988 Effects of moderate consumption of alcoholic beverages on endocrine function in postmenopausal women. Bases for hypotheses. Recent Developments in Alcoholism 6: 229–251
12. Longcope C, Baker S 1993 Androgen and estrogen dynamics: relationships with age, weight, and menopausal status. Journal of Clinical Endocrinology and Metabolism 76: 601–604
13. Hawkins RA, Oakey RE 1974 Estimation of oestrone sulphate, oestradiol-17β and oestrone in peripheral plasma: concentrations during the menstrual cycle and in men. Journal of Endocrinology 60: 3–17
14. Roberts KD, Rochefort JG, Bleau G, Chapdelaine A 1980 Plasma estrone sulfate levels in postmenopausal women. Steroids 35: 179–187
15. Guerami A, MacDonald PC, Casey ML 1984 Variation in the fractional conversion of plasma estrone to estriol among women and men. Journal of Clinical Endocrinology and Metabolism 58: 1148–1152
16. Guengerich FP 1990 Inhibition of oral contraceptive steroid-metabolizing enzymes by steroids and drugs. American Journal of Obstetrics and Gynecology 163: 2159–2163
17. Guengerich FP 1992 Oxidation of estrogens and other steroids by cytochrome P-450 enzymes: relevance to tumorigenesis. In: Li JJ, Nandi S, Li SA (eds) Hormonal carcinogenesis (Proceedings of the First International Symposium). Springer, New York, pp 104–109
18. Anderson F 1993 Kinetics and pharmacology of estrogens in pre- and postmenopausal women. International Journal of Fertility 38 (Suppl 1): 55–64
19. Balfour JA, Heel RC 1990 Transdermal estradiol. A review of its pharmacodynamic and pharmacokinetic properties, and therapeutic efficacy in the treatment of menopausal complaints. Drugs 40: 561–582
20. Longcope C, Jaffee W, Griffing G 1981 Production rates of androgens and oestrogens in post-menopausal women. Maturitas 3: 215–223
21. Nordin BEC, Crilly RG, Marshall DH, Barkworth SA 1981 Oestrogens, the menopause and the adrenopause. Journal of Endocrinology 89: 131P–143P
22. Cauley JA, Gutai JP, Kuller LH, Powell JG 1991 Reliability and interrelations among serum sex hormones in postmenopausal women. American Journal of Epidemiology 133: 50–57
23. Ridgway EC, Maloof F, Longcope C 1982 Androgen and oestrogen dynamics in hyperthyroidism. Journal of Endocrinology 95: 105–115
24. Kuhnz W, Gansau C, Mahler M 1993 Pharmacokinetics of estradiol, free and total estrone, in young women following single intravenous and oral administration of 17β-estradiol. Arzneimittelforschung 43: 966–973
25. Ruder HJ, Loriaux L, Lipsett MB 1972 Estrone sulfate: production rate and metabolism in man. Journal of Clinical Investigation 51: 1020–1033
26. Hembree WC, Bardin CW, Lipsett MB 1969 A study of estrogen metabolic clearance. Rates and transfer factors. Journal of Clinical Investigation 48: 1809–1819
27. Little B, Billiar RB, Longcope C, Jassani M 1979 Uterine metabolism of gonadal steroids during the menstrual cycle. American Journal of Obstetrics and Gynecology 135: 957–964
28. Aedo AR, Landgren BM, Diczfalusy E 1990 Pharmacokinetics and biotransformation of orally administered oestrone sulphate and oestradiol valerate in postmenopausal women. Maturitas 12: 333–343
29. Svensson LO, Hedman Johnson S, Olsson SE 1994 Plasma concentrations of medroxyprogesterone acetate, estradiol and estrone following oral administration of Klimaxil®, Trisequence®/Provera® and Divina®. A randomized, single-blind, triple cross-over bioavailability study in menopausal women. Maturitas 18: 229–238
30. Arzneimittel-Kompendium der Schweiz 1998. Morant J, Ruppanner H (eds) Documed, Basel
31. Düsterberg B, Schmidt-Gollwitzer M, Hümpel M 1985 Pharmacokinetics and biotransformation of estradiol valerate in ovariectomized women. Hormone Research 21: 145–154
32. Powers MS, Schenkel L, Darley PE, Good WR, Balestra JC, Place VA 1985 Pharmacokinetics and pharmacodynamics of transdermal dosage forms of 17β-estradiol: comparison with conventional oral estrogens used for hormone replacement. American Journal of Obstetrics and Gynecology 152: 1099–1106
33. Bercovici JP, Schenkel L 1987 Estraderm TTS® et ménopause. L'estrogénothérapie transcutanée réactualisée. Contraception-fertilité-sexualité 15: 1095–1103

34. Gordon SF 1995 Clinical experience with a seven-day estradiol transdermal system for estrogen replacement therapy. American Journal of Obstetrics and Gynecology 173: 998–1004
35. Birgerson L, Gabrielsson J 1993 Pharmacokinetics of estradiol released by an E_2 vaginal ring. In: Notelovitz M (ed) Proceedings of the First International Workshop on Estring. International Congress and Symposium Series No. 203. Royal Society of Medicine Services, London, pp 25–32
36. Schmidt G, Andersson SB, Nordle Ö, Johansson CJ, Gunnarsson PO 1994 Release of 17-beta-oestradiol from a vaginal ring in postmenopausal women: pharmacokinetic evaluation. Gynecologic and Obstetric Investigation 38: 253–260
37. Nilsson K, Heimer G 1992 Low-dose oestradiol in the treatment of urogenital oestrogen deficiency — a pharmacokinetic and pharmacodynamic study. Maturitas 15: 121–127
38. Nilsson K, Heimer G 1995 Low-dose 17β-oestradiol during maintenance therapy — a pharmacokinetic and pharmacodynamic study. Maturitas 21: 33–38
39. Kuhl H 1990 Pharmacokinetics of oestrogens and progestogens. Maturitas 12: 171–197
40. Primiero FM, Benagiano G 1994 Long-acting contraceptives. In: Goldzieher JW, Fotherby K (eds) Pharmacology of the contraceptive steroids. Raven Press, New York, pp 153–183
41. Johnson RN, Masserano RP, Kho BT, Adams WP 1978 Steady-state urinary excretion method for determining bioequivalence of conjugated estrogen products. Journal of Pharmaceutical Sciences 67: 1218–1224
42. Troy SM, Hicks DR, Parker VN, Jusko WJ, Rofsky HE, Porter RJ 1994 Differences in pharmacokinetics and comparative bioavailability between Premarin® and Estratab® in healthy postmenopausal women. Current Therapeutic Research 55: 359–372
43. Bhavnani BR, Woolever CA, Wallace D, Pan CC 1989 Metabolism of [^{3}H]equilin [^{35}S]sulfate and [^{3}H]equilin sulfate after oral and intravenous administration in normal postmenopausal women and men. Journal of Clinical Endocrinology and Metabolism 68: 757–765
44. Ansbacher R 1993 Bioequivalence of conjugated estrogen products. Clinical Pharmacokinetics 24: 271–274
45. Bhavnani BR, Cecutti A 1993 Metabolic clearance rate of equiline sulfate and its conversion to plasma equilin, conjugated and unconjugated equilenin, 17β-dihydroequilin, and 17β-dihydroequilenin in normal postmenopausal women and men under steady state conditions. Journal of Clinical Endocrinology and Metabolism 77: 1269–1274
46. Bhavnani BR, Cecutti A 1994 Pharmacokinetics of 17β-dihydroequilin sulfate and 17β-dihydroequilin in normal postmenopausal women. Journal of Clinical Endocrinology and Metabolism 78: 197–204
47. Whitehead MI, Minardi J, Kitchin Y, Sharples MJ 1978 Systemic absorption of estrogen from Premarin vaginal cream. In: Cooke ID (ed) The role of estrogen/progestogen in the management of the menopause. MTP Press, Lancaster, pp 63–71
48. Mandel FP, Geola FL, Meldrum DR et al 1983 Biological effects of various doses of vaginally administered conjugated equine estrogens in postmenopausal women. Journal of Clinical Endocrinology and Metabolism 57: 133–139
49. Aedo AR, Sundén M, Landgren BM, Diczfalusy E 1989 Effect of orally administered oestrogens on circulating oestrogen profiles in post-menopausal women. Maturitas 11: 159–168
50. Goldzieher JW 1994 Pharmacokinetics and metabolism of ethinyl estrogens. In: Goldzieher JW, Fotherby K (eds) Pharmacology of the contraceptive steroids. Raven Press, New York, pp 127–151
51. Goldzieher JW 1990 Selected aspects of the pharmacokinetics and metabolism of ethinyl estrogens and their clinical implications. American Journal of Obstetrics and Gynecology 163: 318–322
52. Goldzieher JW, Brody SA 1990 Pharmacokinetics of ethinyl estradiol and mestranol. American Journal of Obstetrics and Gynecology 163: 2114–2119
53. Ottoson UB, Carlstrom K, Damber JE, von Schoultz B 1984 Serum levels of progesterone and some of its metabolites including deoxycorticosterone after oral and parenteral administration. British Journal of Obstetrics and Gynaecology 91: 1111–1119
54. Lin TJ, Billiar RB, Little B 1972 Metabolic clearance rate of progesterone in the menstrual cycle. Journal of Clinical Endocrinology and Metabolism 35: 879–886
55. Little B, Billiar RB, Rahman SS, Johnson WA, Takaoka Y, White RJ 1975 In vivo aspects of progesterone distribution and metabolism. American Journal of Obstetrics and Gynecology 123: 527–534
56. Thijssen JHH, Zander J 1966 Progesterone-4-^{14}C and its metabolites in the blood after intravenous injection into women. Acta Endocrinologica 51: 563–567
57. Diczfalusi E 1978 Circulating steroids and the menstrual cycle. In: Vokaer R, de Maubeuge R (eds) Sexual endocrinology. Masson, New York, pp 245–264
58. Nahoul K, Dehennin L, Jondet M, Roger M 1993 Profiles of plasma estrogens, progesterone and their metabolites after oral or vaginal administration of estradiol or progesterone. Maturitas 16: 185–202
59. Whitehead MI, Townsend PT, Gill DK, Collins WP, Campbell S 1980 Absorption and metabolism of oral progesterone. British Medical Journal 280: 825–827
60. Fotherby K 1994 Pharmacokinetics and metabolism of progestins in humans. In: Goldzieher JW, Fotherby K (eds) Pharmacology of the contraceptive steroids. Raven Press, New York, pp 99–126
61. Huber J, Zeilinger R, Schmidt J, Täuber U, Kuhnz W, Spona J 1988 Pharmacokinetics of cyproterone acetate and its main metabolite 15β-hydroxycyproterone acetate in young healthy women. International Journal of Clinical Pharmacology, Therapy and Toxicology 26: 555–561
62. Kuhnz W, Staks T, Jütting G 1993 Pharmacokinetics of cyproterone acetate and ethinylestradiol in 15 women who received a combination oral contraceptive during three treatment cycles. Contraception 48: 557–575
63. Wiseman LR, McTavish D 1994 Transdermal estradiol/norethisterone. A review of its pharmacological properties and clinical use in postmenopausal women. Drugs and Aging 4: 238–256
64. Fotherby K, Caldwell ADS 1994 New progestogens in oral contraception. Contraception 49: 1–32
65. Garza-Flores J 1994 Pharmacokinetics of once-a-month injectable contraceptives. Contraception 49: 347–359

66. Kuhnz W 1990 Pharmacokinetics of the contraceptive steroids levonorgestrel and gestodene after single and multiple oral administration to women. American Journal of Obstetrics and Gynecology 163: 2120–2127
67. Stanczyk FZ, Roy S 1990 Metabolism of levonorgestrel, norethindrone, and structurally related contraceptive steroids. Contraception 42: 67–96
68. Kuhnz W, Schütt B, Power J, Back DJ 1992 Pharmacokinetics and serum protein binding of gestodene and 3-keto-desogestrel in women after single oral administration of two different contraceptive formulations. Arzneimittelforschung 42: 1139–1141
69. Kuhnz W, Al-Yacoub G, Power J, Ormesher SE, Back DJ, Jütting G 1992 Pharmacokinetics and serum protein binding of 3-keto-desogestrel in women during three cycles of treatment with a low-dose combination oral contraceptive. Arzneimittelforschung 42: 1142–1146
70. McGuire JL, Phillips A, Hahn DW, Tolman EL, Flor S, Kafrissen ME 1990 Pharmacologic and pharmacokinetic characteristics of norgestimate and its metabolites. American Journal of Obstetrics and Gynecology 163: 2127–2131
71. Fotherby K 1990 Interactions with oral contraceptives. American Journal of Obstetrics and Gynecology 163: 2153–2159
72. Hanker JP 1990 Gastrointestinal disease and oral contraception. American Journal of Obstetrics and Gynecology 163: 2204–2207
73. Orme ML'E, Back DJ 1990 Factors affecting the enterohepatic circulation of oral contraceptive steroids. American Journal of Obstetrics and Gynecology 163: 2146–2152
74. Vesell ES, Penno MB 1983 Assessment of methods to identify sources of interindividual pharmacokinetic variations Clinical Pharmacokinetics 8: 378–409
75. Kerlan V, Dreano Y, Bercovici JP, Beaune PH, Floch HH, Berthou F 1992 Nature of cytochromes P450 involved in the 2-/4-hydroxylations of estradiol in human liver microsomes. Biochemical Pharmacology 44: 1745–1756
76. Martucci CP, Fishman J 1993 P450 enzymes of estrogen metabolism. Pharmacology and Therapeutics 57: 237–257
77. Jensen J, Christiansen C, Rødbro P 1985 Cigarette smoking, serum estrogens, and bone loss during hormone-replacement therapy early after menopause. New England Journal of Medicine 313: 973–975
78. Jensen J, Christiansen C 1988 Effects of smoking on serum lipoproteins and bone mineral content during postmenopausal hormone replacement therapy. American Journal of Obstetrics and Gynecology 159: 820–825
79. Michnovicz J 1987 Environmental modulation of oestrogen metabolism in humans. International Clinical Nutrition Review 7: 169–173
80. Cassidenti DL, Vijod AG, Vijod MA, Stanczyk FZ, Lobo RA 1990 Short-term effects of smoking on the pharmacokinetic profiles of micronized estradiol in postmenopausal women. American Journal of Obstetrics and Gynecology 163: 1953–1960
81. Longcope C, Johnston CC 1988 Androgen and estrogen dynamics in pre- and postmenopausal women: a comparison between smokers and nonsmokers. Journal of Clinical Endocrinology and Metabolism 67: 379–383
82. Thomas EJ, Edridge W, Weddell A, McGill A, McGarrigle HHG 1993 The impact of cigarette smoking on the plasma concentrations of gonadotrophins, ovarian steroids and androgens and upon the metabolism of oestrogens in the human female. Human Reproduction 8: 1187–1193
83. Back DJ, Orme ML'E 1994 Drug interactions. In: Goldzieher JW, Fotherby K (eds) Pharmacology of the contraceptive steroids Raven Press, New York, pp 407–425
84. Miller LG 1990 Cigarettes and drug therapy: pharmacokinetic and pharmacodynamic considerations. Clinical Pharmacology 9: 125–135
85. Dorgan JF, Reichman ME, Judd JT et al 1994 The relation of reported alcohol ingestion to plasma levels of estrogens and androgens in premenopausal women (Maryland, United States). Cancer Causes and Control 5: 53–60
86. Shenfield GM 1993 Oral contraceptives. Are drug interactions of clinical significance? Drug Safety 9: 21–37
87. Szoka PR, Edgren RA 1988 Drug interactions with oral contraceptives: compilation and analysis of an adverse experience report database. Fertility and Sterility 49 (Suppl): 31S–38S
88. Orme M, Back DJ 1991 Oral contraceptive steroids — pharmacological issues of interest to the prescribing physician. Advances in Contraception 7: 325–331
89. Bolt HM 1994 Interactions between clinically used drugs and oral contraceptives. Environmental Health Perspectives 102 (Suppl 9): 35–38
90. Jung-Hoffmann C, Kuhl H 1990 Pharmacokinetics and pharmacodynamics of oral contraceptive steroids: factors influencing steroid metabolism. American Journal of Obstetrics and Gynecology 163: 2183–2197
91. Fotherby K 1990 Pharmacokinetics of gestagens: some problems. American Journal of Obstetrics and Gynecology 163: 323–328
92. Bergink W, Assendorp R, Kloosterboer L, van Lier W, Voortman G, Qvist I 1990 Serum pharmacokinetics of orally administered desogestrel and binding of contraceptive progestogens to sex hormone-binding globulin. American Journal of Obstetrics and Gynecology 163: 2132–2137
93. Back DJ, Orme ML'E 1990 Pharmacokinetic drug interactions with oral contraceptives. Clinical Pharmacokinetics 18: 472–484
94. Fotherby K 1990 Potency and pharmacokinetics of gestagens. Contraception 41: 533–550
95. Shenfield GM, Griffin JM 1991 Clinical pharmacokinetics of contraceptive steroids. An update. Clinical Pharmacokinetics 20: 15–37

26. Pharmacodynamic effects of estrogens and progestogens

Joseph W. Goldzieher

Introduction

In addition to dose and potency, many factors affect the response to administered estrogens and progestogens. These include:

1. Specific characteristics of the compound
2. Route of administration (oral, intramuscular, intravenous, vaginal, percutaneous, subcutaneous [implants] and intrauterine)
3. Time of administration in the menstrual cycle
4. Pharmacokinetic characteristics achieved (C_{max}, AUC, duration of significant blood levels)
5. Inter- and intra-individual variability of these parameters
6. Subject's age, weight, ethnicity
7. Methods of determining the response parameter, especially if it is subjective.

Estrogens

There are several classes of estrogens. The 'biologic' compounds of interest are estrone and estradiol (E_2), as well as conjugates such as estrone sulfate and conjugated equine estrogens (CEE) — a preparation which consists of estrone sulfate plus a variety of equine estrogen conjugates of different potencies. The common synthetic estrogens include ethynyl estradiol (EE) and its methyl ether, mestranol (which must be demethylated to become biologically active). Because of this, 50 µg of mestranol, for example, is bioequivalent to 35 µg of ethynyl estradiol.[1] There are also quinestrol and diethylstilbestrol (DES); other synthetic estrogens are currently being developed. The triphenyl compounds such as clomiphene have estrogenic effects, and a phytoestrogen from soybeans, genistein, is being researched intensively because of its unusual spectrum of estrogenic properties.

The common effects of estrogens are receptor-mediated, but nonreceptor effects such as acute vasodilatation induced in minutes from sublingual administration of E_2,[2] and actions on the arterial endothelium and subendothelial cells are also extremely important.[3] It must be kept in mind that different organs or tissues have different thresholds of response and different dose-response curves. Thus, an estrogen dose which fully matures the vaginal epithelium (the most estrogen-sensitive tissue of all) will have only a modest effect on the endometrium and little if any effect on bone. How the physiologic secretion of estrogen manages to keep all estrogen-sensitive tissues optimally exposed is truly remarkable, and is the challenge that is faced by therapeutic attempts at estrogen replacement (ERT).

The formulations for clinical use have individual properties. Estradiol administered orally in milligram quantities must be micronized to be absorbed by the gastrointestinal tract. Commercial formulations of CEE have a slow-release characteristic not shared by synthetic sodium estrone sulfate. This is not a problem with the ethynyl estrogens, which are active in microgram quantities. All oral estrogens undergo enterohepatic recirculation (the first pass effect). Thus, the liver is exposed to high concentrations of estrogen and this is reflected, for example, in the rate of synthesis of proteins such as sex hormone-binding globulin (SHBG), cortisol-binding globulin (CBG) and others. These responses can be used to make comparisons of oral potencies of estrogenic compounds.[4] The first pass effect, for any compound, is known to introduce considerable inter-individual variability in blood levels (Fig. 26.1); this consequently widens the range of clinical responses and makes comparisons between compounds and doses more difficult. There is also an increase in intra-individual variability (Table 26.1) so that a minimally effective dose on one day may not be sufficient for a particular purpose (e.g. endometrial maintenance) at another time. These difficulties offset to some extent the convenience of oral administration and favor the percutaneous or transvaginal (tablet, cream) routes,[5]

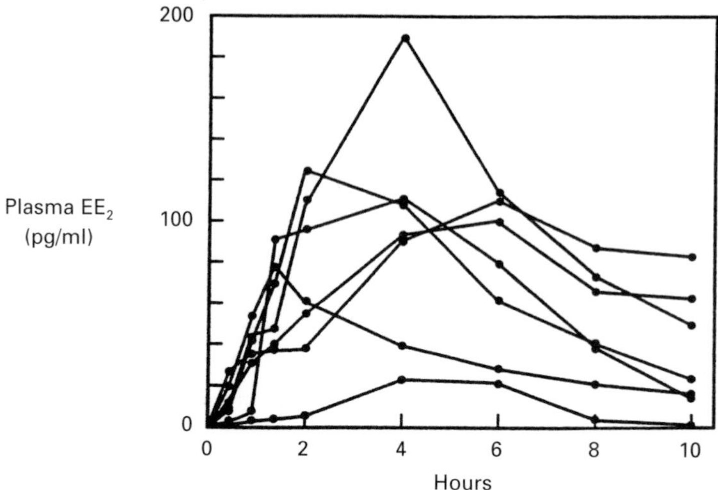

Fig. 26.1 Plasma ethynyl estradiol levels in seven individuals given a single oral dose of 50 μg. Note the large inter-individual variability.

Table 26.1 Representative plasma ethynyl estradiol AUC_{0-24} values for triplicate studies, a month apart, in 10 individuals given a single COC tablet containing 35 μg ethynyl estradiol or 50 μg mestranol (as well as norethindrone).

Subject no.	Trial no. 1	2	3
35 μg ethynyl estradiol			
2	1002	431	855
9	252	499	569
12	1892	637	1390
13	1563	539	934
20	657	1594	2122
50 μg mestranol			
104	215	1230	658
106	1355	854	1080
3	768	963	696
16	1033	839	818
25	433	289	331

which bypass the gastrointestinal tract, produce smoother and higher blood levels and avoid side-effects such as nausea and increased hepatic synthesis of certain proteins and lipids, especially triglyceride.

Variability in the effect of estrogens may also be due to body weight or age: elderly women being re-exposed to estrogens by initiation of ERT must be started with very small, intermittent dosages; adolescents are more likely to have nausea and other side effects from estrogens in oral contraceptives; and women of low body weight, as in Sri Lanka, do better with very low dose OCs. Further, ethnicity also has an impact.[6] In studies with radiolabeled ethinyl estradiol, significant differences were noted both in the type of urinary conjugates and in the free estrogen metabolites themselves in women from Nigeria, Sri Lanka and the USA (Fig. 26.2).[6] The basis of these hepatic (and possibly renal) differences is not known.

The pharmacodynamic effects of estrogens, from the receptor level on up, are affected by the concomitant administration of progestogens in complex ways; only interactions at the organ and tissue level will be described.

Progestogens

Although both the C_{21}-acetoxy and the 19-nor steroids are powerful progestogens, their biologic profiles[7] and

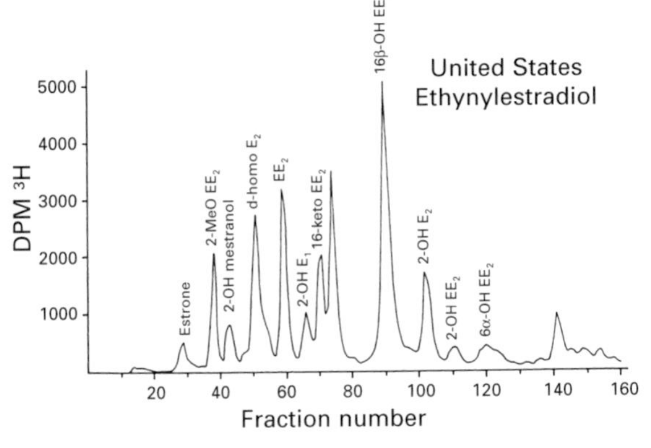

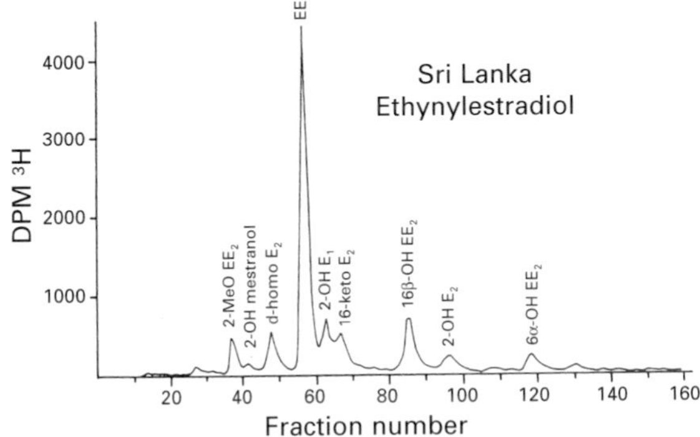

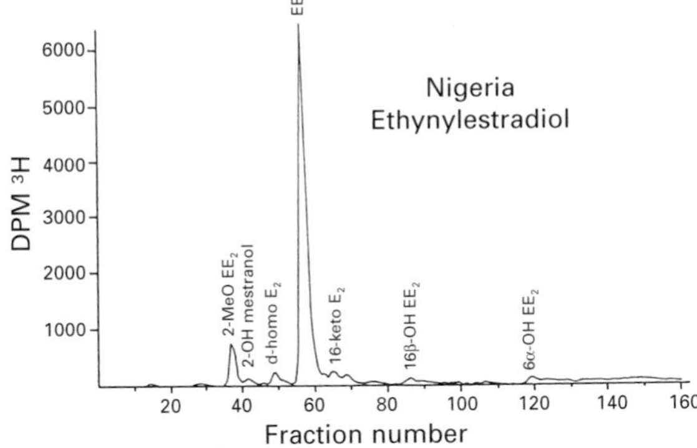

Fig. 26.2 Deconjugated urinary metabolites of ethynyl estradiol, as separated by high pressure liquid chromatography, from women given a single dose of radiolabeled ethynyl estradiol. The Nigerian sample shows chiefly unaltered ethynyl estradiol, with traces of oxidative metabolites. Higher oxidative activity is seen in the Sri Lankan sample although ethynyl estradiol is still preponderant. In the USA sample, the oxidative metabolites far exceed the starting material.[6]

hence their pharmacodynamic effects differ substantially. The former group (medroxyprogesterone, megestrol, medrogestone, chlormadinone) simulate the profile of progesterone more closely, especially in their effect on the hypothalamopituitary system and on carbohydrate and lipid metabolism. The 19-nor steroids consist of two groups: those related to 19-nortestosterone (norethindrone, norethynodrel, ethynodiol) and those which have an 18-ethyl instead of an 18-methyl group and are classed as gonanes. The parent and reference compound in this latter group is levonorgestrel. More recently developed, closely related compounds are gestodene, desogestrel (which is an inactive prodrug of 3-ketodesogestrel) and norgestimate (which is a prodrug of levonorgestrel). Hybrid compounds of the C_{21}-acetoxy 19-nor type are under investigation. Interestingly, the 19-nortestosterone derivatives are subject to the first pass effect, with consequent impact on bioavailability and pharmacokinetic variability, whereas the gonanes are 100% bioavailable. The reason for this is not known.

Compared to the C_{21}-acetoxy steroids, the 19-norsteroids are not only much more potent, but they have selectively greater activity in suppressing gonadotropin secretion; additionally, in animal assays some of them have definite androgenic activity. Whether or not this is clinically significant will be discussed below. Further, the 19-nortestosterone derivatives and levonorgestrel have an impact on laboratory parameters of carbohydrate and lipid metabolism. The newer gonane progestogens (gestodene, desogestrel) appear to have less impact on these metabolic areas.

The synthetic progestogens are orally active, in contrast to progesterone, which is very poorly absorbed even in micronized form: this is one reason why there was commercial interest in synthesizing new progestogens. They can also be absorbed transvaginally in tablet form (South American investigators have demonstrated the efficacy of combination oral contraceptives used intravaginally;[8] intramuscularly as esters (as in the one and two month injectable contraceptives)[9] or in microcrystalline aqueous suspension as depot medroxyprogesterone (DMPA). Intra-uterine administration is effective in levonorgestrel-containing IUDs. Subcutaneous silicone implants (Norplant®) and biodegradable rods and other formulations are used for long-range contraception.[10]

SYSTEMIC EFFECTS OF ESTROGENS AND PROGESTOGENS

Subjective effects

Symptoms such as nausea, headache, bloating, mood changes, etc. are common complaints after the administration (primarily oral) of estrogens and progestogens. They may vary by compound: biologic estrogens provoke much less nausea than ethynyl estrogens or DES, for example. However, the origin of these symptoms is unclear and they are difficult to quantitate. Figure 26.3 shows the very large range of the frequency of nausea (and, for comparison, the incidence of an objective symptom, breakthrough bleeding) in a multicenter study where large numbers of subjects and cycles were collected. The reasons for such variability are unclear, but it is well known that methods of data collection and consumer/provider interactions influence such results heavily. Users' prior knowledge about the side effects of the administered medication are also critical. In a double blind, randomized, placebo-controlled study of the effect of oral progesterone on the symptoms of premenstrual tension syndrome, all subjects were required to read the FDA-approved patient information insert.[11] Upon completion of the study the data were uncoded, and 62% of the placebo subjects had reported side effects such as those listed in the information insert. Given experiences such as these, it is evident that comparisons of different estrogens or different kinds of oral contraceptives are fraught with difficulties of interpretation.

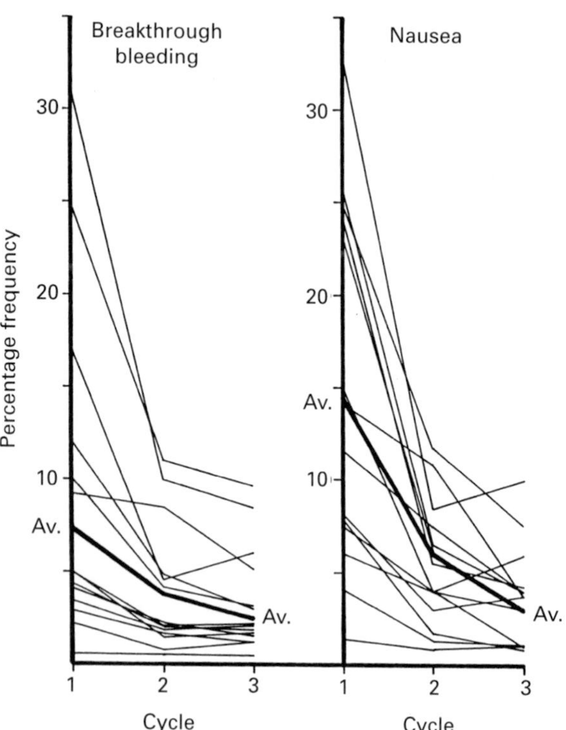

Fig. 26.3 Frequency of an objective side-effect (breakthrough bleeding) and a subjective side-effect (nausea) in 14 USA localities (> 200 patients each) engaged in a multicenter phase III trial of a high dose COC (Goldzieher, unpublished).

Hypothalamopituitary system

Significant changes occur in the hypothalamopituitary-ovarian system during the perimenopausal transition.[12] Subtle changes can be seen in FSH levels even when comparing women in their 20s, 30s and 40s.[13] Eventually, of course, there is a permanent, large elevation of plasma and urinary FSH (and to a lesser extent, LH) levels. The institution of ERT with biologic estrogens such as E_2 and CEE at the usual doses does not normalize FSH, and suppression of the elevated level of this hormone should not be used to determine the adequacy of replacement regimens. Substantial levels of CEE — 1.25–3.75 mg/day as used in young post-oophorectomy women — just begin to have some impact on plasma FSH.

On the other hand, the ethynyl estrogens have a more powerful suppressive effect, and 0.02 mg ethinyl estradiol daily, a commonly used ERT regimen, will reduce FSH levels to normal or below. The high potency of ethynyl estrogens vs. biologic estrogens in inhibiting gonadotropin secretion is at the heart of their effectiveness in combined oral contraceptives.[14] Biologic estrogens, when added to contraceptive progestogens used for contraception, add little to their ovulation-inhibitory activity and such mixtures are not much more efficacious than progestogen-only (POP) pills (however, cycle control is improved). Indeed, our early studies of ethynyl estrogens (reviewed by Gual et al[15]) showed that ethynyl estrogens inhibited gonadotropin secretion so well that they could be used by themselves for oral contraception, and in 1961 appropriate clinical trials were undertaken; the result was a type of oral contraceptive designated as 'sequential'[16] (where mestranol alone was used for 15 days, followed by the same dose of estrogen with 10 days of progestogen (to mature the endometrium). However, it required 75–80 μg of mestranol to ensure consistent ovulation inhibition, and when efforts were made to diminish side-effects by lowering the hormone dosage, the sequentials fell by the wayside.

The synergistic effect of ethynyl estrogens and 19-nor progestogens on gonadotropin secretion probably occurs both at the hypothalamic and pituitary gonadotrope levels. An example of this synergistic effect is shown in Figure 26.4. This phenomenon has made possible the progressive lowering of the dosage of

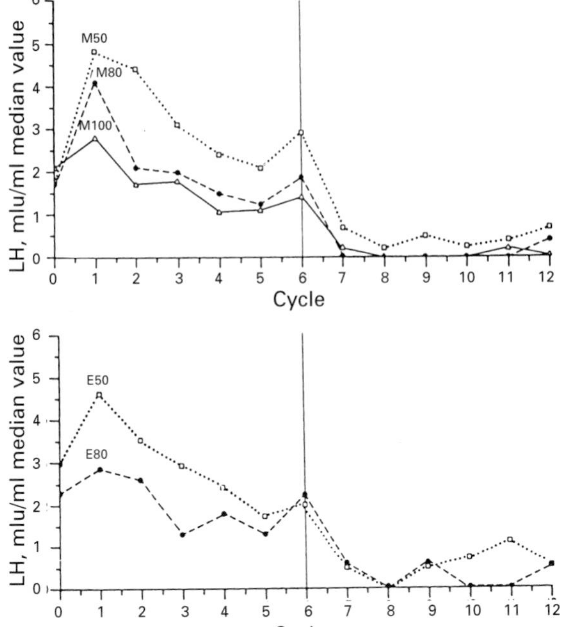

Fig. 26.4 Median values for plasma LH levels in groups of subjects receiving cyclic ethynyl estrogen for six cycles, followed by six cycles during which a progestogen was added, to make a COC. (**A**) Administration of mestranol at 50, 80 and 100 µg per day; (**B**) Administration of ethynyl estradiol at 50 and 80 µg per day.[6]

estrogen and progestogen to the levels in current 'low-dose' oral contraceptives without impairing contraceptive efficacy. The multiphasic formulations probably have the least gonadotropin-suppressive effect.

Suppression wears off quickly and is gone by the end of the 7-days-off-pills interval, although sophisticated tests with gonadotropin-releasing hormone sometimes show residual, clinically insignificant effects.[17,18] In perimenopausal and postmenopausal women on oral contraceptives it may take two weeks for gonadotropins to rebound fully.[13] In any event, in reproductive-age women ovulation and fertility are restored almost immediately, even with the high-dose formulations no longer in use.[19]

Progestogen-only oral contraceptives ablate the preovulatory surge in gonadotropins, but do not affect the average level. Consequently, the effect on the ovary is quite variable,[20] ranging from complete inhibition of follicular activity to inadequate luteal phases to normal progesterone levels (in which case the other contraceptive mechanisms of progestogen-only administration are the limiting factor). The same ablation of the preovulatory gonadotropin surge is seen in the case of injected DMPA and progestogen implants. The estrogen levels during use of both these modalities range round the early follicular phase level. The gonadotropic effects of the combined estrogen-progestogen (one and two month) injectables have not been studied in detail.

Inhibition of ovarian secretory activity is also reflected in the plasma level of androgens, as the ovary is a major producer of androstenedione. Decreased follicular and stromal activity are reflected in lower androstenedione and testosterone levels; this is the basis for the use of COCs (preferably at higher dose levels) in the treatment of seborrhea, hirsutism and acne.

The return of the hypothalamopituitary gonadotropic system to normalcy after discontinuation of COCs is prompt, and fertility normalizes within one or two cycles. After removal of subcutaneous implants the return to fertility is of course equally prompt. Normalization after various injectables depends on their nature. With DMPA, fertility is essentially restored to normal within one year after the last injection, and certainly after two.[19]

The effect of these various contraceptive formulations and delivery systems on other pituitary activity (i.e. growth hormone and prolactin) have been examined[21] but have not revealed any changes of clinical consequence.

Vagina

The vaginal epithelium is said to be the most estrogen-sensitive tissue in the body, and (as used in rodents) formed the basis of early estrogen bioassays. The response is altered by the concomitant administration of progestogens ('mucification') and inhibited by androgens and some other steroids. Human vaginal epithelium is restored quickly to normalcy by ERT in estrogen-deficient women; the deeper tissues of the vaginal wall may take several months to recover elasticity and lubricity. Improvement of dyspareunia should follow. Susceptibility to surface invasion by bacteria and fungi is diminished as the epithelium is restored and the pH returns to its normal acidity by the resurgence of Döderlein bacilli.

Vaginal creams or tablets containing estrogen are an effective delivery system and the creams are particularly useful in the case of atrophic vaginitis. Estrogen absorption into the systemic circulation occurs readily; however, absorption decreases somewhat as the epithelium and the other vaginal wall tissues thicken and normalize. Nevertheless, this remains a convenient and effective delivery system.

Susceptibility of the vagina to the common infections in the course of contraceptive steroid use has been investigated, and the findings are inconsistent. In any event, the effectiveness of the antibiotics used to manage these problems is unaltered.

Cervix

The effect of the estrogens and progesterone on the cervix during the normal cycle has been described elsewhere. In hypogonad women, the cervical epithelium is restored by estrogen and mucus production resumes. The normal effects of progesterone are exaggerated by exogenous progestogens, whether locally delivered (as by vaginal rings, intracervical or intra-uterine devices), or by oral, subcutaneous or parenteral administration. The cervical mucus diminishes, thickens and its cell content and molecular structure change.[22] Sperm motility and penetrability are inhibited. The effect of oral administration on cervical mucus takes effect within a couple of hours, peaks in 3–4 hours (others have found it to peak at 5–10 hours), and remains high for 16–19 hours. These antifertility effects are clearly the first line of defense for the POPs, whose dosage is too low to have a consistent gonadotropin-inhibiting, antiovulatory effect. The morphology of the cervix exposed to high-dose COCs has been described.[23] Squamous metaplasia, glandular hypersecretion and some stromal edema occur. The effect of COCs on the incidence of cervical carcinoma is controversial due to numerous confounding factors (see ch. 67).

Endometrium

The stimulatory effect of estrogens on the endometrium is well known, and its histology has been extensively studied. The tendency of endometrium under continuous estrogen stimulation to undergo hypertrophy, hyperplasia, metaplasia and in some instances to progress to a histological malignancy is documented. (The relation of ERT to endometrial cancer is discussed in ch. 67.) Assessment of the endometrium by biopsy has been greatly augmented, and in many instances replaced, by transvaginal ultrasonography. An endometrial thickness of <4 mm indicates atrophy, and with a thickness of <8 mm, pathology is unlikely.[24] This technique has shown that some endometria are very sensitive, while others are very slow to respond to ERT. If progestogen is administered in the case of an atrophic endometrium and then withdrawn, no bleeding will occur; however bleeding will occur within 10 days of progestogen administration if the endometrium is proliferative. The duration and intensity of bleeding correlate to some extent with endometrial thickness and shedding. In some instances of ERT management, it may be impossible or unacceptable to perform indicated endometrial biopsies; in these circumstances ultrasound may be extremely useful. This is also true for women who develop adverse reactions to oral progestogens (given to protect the endometrium during ERT) and reject this treatment or wish it to be administered as infrequently as possible.

The effect of progestogens on the endometrium has been well summarized by Song and Fraser.[25] The various bleeding patterns provoked by POPs are probably a reflection of the variety of endometrial patterns produced. Various progestogens seem to produce different histological effects.[26] However, the correlation of bleeding with endometrial morphology is still a mystery.[27] The pattern of glands and stroma may range from mixed to atrophic, and significant changes in the endometrial circulatory system[20,25] are observed by standard and immunohistochemical techniques. Similar findings with Norplant suggest that long-term progestogen administration acts differentially on the different types of endometrial blood vessels, reducing arterioles and increasing capillaries and small veins. Intra-uterine progestogens and DMPA produce wholly suppressed endometria (as reflected by the development of almost universal amenorrhea with prolonged use of DMPA).

The early high dose COCs produced glandular involution and intense stromal edema and hyperplasia. Such changes are greatly reduced in modern COCs, where endometrial development is inhibited and the tissue thinned. The glands are poorly developed and show decreased mitotic activity and pseudostratification. Stroma shows various degrees of edema and occasionally, some pseudodecidual changes. The spiral arterioles are poorly developed but the venules may be ectatic; endothelial cells are also affected and leukocytes and macrophages show important effects. Eventually, with prolonged use, the endometrium becomes atrophic with poor gland elements and an edematous, fibroblastic stroma. It is generally believed that these histologically abnormal endometria represent one of the mechanisms of contraceptive efficacy. However, when one recalls the ease with which women on POPs conceive, and also the significant number of pregnancies attributed to poor compliance with COCs as well, it is evident that the influence of these morphological changes is limited.

Return to normalcy of the endometrium is prompt whether old high dose or current types of COCs were used. Duration of use is not a factor. Even with the former preparations, two-thirds of endometria are normal after a single cycle of discontinuation,[28,29] and this is consistent with the rapid return of fertility after discontinuation of COCs. This is equally true after removal of subcutaneous implants. Histological normalization of the endometrium after the use of injectable or biodegradable implant contraceptives obviously depends on their duration of action.

A decrease in the incidence of fibroids in COC users has been reported (Table 26.2), in contrast to early observations with very high-estrogen COCs, which produced some stimulation of fibroid cells. High dose oral contraceptives as well as DMPA were used several decades ago for the treatment of endometriosis (q.v.) and recent studies show a lower incidence of endometriosis in COC users than nonusers.[30]

Continuous use of ERT, unassociated with exposure to progestogens, increases the risk of a relatively benign form of endometrial carcinoma; this risk is eliminated by progestagen use. It is now well established that COC use decreases the relative risk of endometrial cancer, even with as brief an exposure as 1–2 years of a high dose COC. Epidemiologic studies with low dose formulations are awaited. Long-term studies of Depo-provera by the WHO also show a major decrease in relative risk of endometrial cancer. This subject is discussed in chapter 67.

Fallopian tubes

Data on the effect of contraceptive progestogens or COCs on tubal motility and environment are scanty (see McCann and Potter[20] for review). The negative effects of progestogens on spermatozoal function[31] may occur in the tubal environment as well as in the uterus.

Emergency contraception: postcoital use of estrogens and progestogens

The administration of high doses of estrogens (DES, CEE or ethinyl estrogens) or estrogen-progestogen combinations (e.g. the Yuzpe regimen of two tablets of ethinyl estradiol 50 µg/levonorgestrel, taken twice at a 12 hour interval within 72 hours of unprotected intercourse) is highly effective,[32] reducing the expected risk of pregnancy by 75% or more. Danazol, another type of steroid, is considerably less effective. Regimens using an antiprogestogen such as mifepristone are at least as effective as the Yuzpe regimen, and have far fewer side-effects. Details as to appropriate dosage are still under development. The mechanism by which such regimens prevent implantation is not clear, but is likely to involve both tubal and intrauterine environmental changes.

Table 26.2 Effect of continued use of high-dose COCs on uterine myomata (fibroids)

Duration of COC use (years)	Relative risk of myomata
2–4	0.8
4–8	0.79
8–10	0.73
10 or more	0.54

Modified from: Ross et al 1986 Risk factors for uterine fibroids: reduced risk associated with oral contraceptives British Medical Journal 293: 359

Breast

Concern about the relationship of breast cancer to estrogens is one of the major obstacles to the widespread use of ERT. Recently the dogma surrounding this issue has been reviewed and called into question;[33] even the prohibition of estrogen use in breast cancer survivors may be unfounded.[34] Interestingly, the simultaneous use of estrogen and tamoxifen (an estrogen agonist/antagonist used in breast cancer recurrence prophylaxis) appears not to offset the effect of tamoxifen.[34] The issue of breast cancer is discussed in detail elsewhere.

As early as 1970[35] it was noted that users of high-dose COCs had a significant reduction in fibrocystic disease and fibroadenomas of the breast, with a substantial decrease in the number of breast biopsies as a result. The incidence decreased by 30% after a year's use and by 65% after two or more years of use. The decreased risk appeared related to the progestogen dosage, duration of use and current use[36] although one study[37] among many did not confirm these findings. In a cohort study of premenopausal women with benign breast disease[38] the use of 19-nortestosterone derivatives was found to be significantly associated with a lower risk of breast cancer.

The effect of hormonal contraceptives on lactation is an important one, especially in the developing world, where infant nutrition and maternal fertility are major concerns. Studies with radioactively labeled steroids as well as orally administered estradiol[39] have shown that minuscule quantities of contraceptive steroids or their metabolites appear in milk[40] and it is generally agreed that this exposure is clinically insignificant. There is a very large literature on the effect of contraceptive steroids on quality and quantity of breast milk, but relatively few controlled studies on neonatal health (for a review see Erwin[41]). High dose COCs no longer in use had a definite negative impact on lactation, especially when started before lactation was fully established. However, careful review of studies with lower dose COCs show no adverse effect on the newborn, despite change in some of the characteristics of milk production.[40] This is especially true if onset of use is delayed briefly, until full lactation has set in. The alternatives are the immediate institution of progestogen-only pills[42] or the use of DMPA, which actually has some positive effects on lactation. Many family planning experts emphasize that prompt initiation of hormonal contraception is mandatory, in spite of conservative recommendations by various regulatory bodies;[42] the risk of unintended pregnancy far outweighs any risk to newborn or mother.

Urinary tract

The effect of sex hormones on the female urinary tract during menses, in pregnancy and after menopause has been well reviewed by Miodrag et al.[43] Tissues of the lower urinary tract are estrogen-sensitive. Urge and stress incontinence increase with age and estrogen deficiency plays a role. Estrogens may aid continence by increasing urethral resistance, raising the sensory threshold of the bladder, and increasing I-adrenergic receptor sensitivity in the urethral smooth muscle.[44] Atrophic vaginitis may be related to recurrent urinary tract infections, and treatment of the vaginitis with estrogen, with restoration of normal bacterial flora, appears to be helpful. The effects of ERT on urinary symptomatology, urge and stress incontinence are inconclusive, especially with regard to the latter problem;[45] however, the tendency to use small estrogen doses or weak estrogens such as estriol may account for some of the negative reports.

Concern has been expressed regarding the impact of COCs on diabetic nephropathy, because of the alterations of laboratory parameters of carbohydrate and lipid metabolism by certain formulations. Careful studies, however, have shown no effect on either renal or retinal vasculature in insulin-dependent diabetics.[46]

Thyroid

The effects of pregnancy and estrogen therapy on the laboratory parameters of thyroid function are well known. These alterations are due to increased plasma levels of thyroxine-binding globulin (TBG) consequent upon increased hepatic synthesis. The changes are estrogen-dose related; progestogens themselves have no effect. Thyroidal iodine metabolism and thyroid function are unaffected, and there is no change in the incidence of thyroid disorders in users of oral contraceptives.[47]

Adrenal cortex

There is considerable evidence for direct effects of COCs on the steroidogenic pathways in the adrenals and on the regulatory mechanisms of the pituitary-adrenal axis.[48] These effects depend on the relative amounts of estrogens and progestogens and their potency, for the two components have different effects, and interactions as well. Estrogens may augment ACTH release by down-regulating pituitary glucocorticoid receptors and also potentiate adrenal responsiveness, while progestogens with glucocorticoid activity tend to decrease ACTH release. High doses of estrogens may interfere with interpretation of dexamethasone suppression tests and urinary free cortisol levels.

Most importantly, hepatic transcortin (CBG) synthesis is stimulated by estrogens, thus raising the level of total plasma cortisol. The effects on free (biologically active) cortisol are controversial, but there is no clinical evidence of hypercortisolism from the use of estrogens or COCs. Similarly, estrogens increase the level of aldosterone-binding globulin, but no change in aldosterone levels has been detected in users of COCs. Some progestogens, such as gestodene, are aldosterone receptor antagonists, as is progesterone itself.

COCs containing 19-nortestosterone derivatives or levonorgestrel reduce circulating levels of DHEA sulfate, pregnenolone and 17-hydroxypregnenolone, either by the decrease in ACTH stimulation or by a direct effect on cytochrome P450.[49] Plasma androstenedione and testosterone may also be decreased especially in women with hyperandrogenic hirsutism and/or low SHBG levels.

Immune system

Despite many studies on the effect of estrogens and progestogens on humoral and cell-mediated immunity,[51] it is impossible to draw a coherent picture of the properties of these steroids. Interestingly, the immunomodulating effects do not parallel estrogenic or progestational activities.

Investigations of susceptibility to infections of viral, bacterial or fungal origin in COC users have been beset by a variety of problems which confound the results of epidemiologic studies; in general, no consistent effects have been observed.

Certain autoimmune disorders appear to be influenced by estrogen, for example systemic lupus erythematosus; switching to a progestogen-only contraceptive avoids recrudescence of the disorder.[52] The impact of COCs on rheumatoid arthritis is problematic: European studies show a protective effect, whereas studies in the USA do not confirm these findings.[51]

Cardiovascular system: atherogenesis

The role of estrogen deficiency and ERT in postmenopausal women is discussed in chapter 55. Most attention has been focussed on the lipoprotein profile. However, the non-receptor-mediated coronary vasodilator effect of estrogens as shown in women with coronary stenosis is also important.[53] Experiments in estrogen-deprived cynomolgus monkeys[54] showed coronary artery vasoconstriction following acetylcholine infusion, whereas animals with physiologic estrogen replacement responded with vasodilatation instead. Vasomotion could be restored to normal in the estrogen-deprived monkeys within 20 minutes of intravenous estradiol administration, in parallel to the clinical study of Collins et al.[53] Medroxyprogesterone acetate reduced this vasodilator effect by half, but norethindrone did not. Endothelium-dependent vasoconstriction may promote atherogenesis, especially in conjunction with the adverse effects of nitric oxide depletion which increases LDL uptake in coronary artery cell metabolism.

There are other direct protective effects on the arterial wall itself that are seen with COC administration, such as decreased degradation of LDL into plaque.[54,55] In monkeys exposed to an atherogenic diet, severe (atherogenic) social stress and high dose oral contraceptives,[55] the estrogen in the COC protected against the adverse lipoprotein profile caused by the progestogen, actually yielding substantially *less* coronary atherogenesis (as shown at autopsy) than in the control animals not given the COC. Clinical correlates are the absence of any increase in atherogenesis in long-term prospective studies of COC users,[56] and a lower incidence of diffuse coronary atheromatosis (by angiography) in young women sustaining their first myocardial infarction, as compared to never-users of COCs.[57]

It therefore turns out that COCs, like ERT, are probably protective against atherogenic cardiovascular disease, contrary to early epidemiologic studies, which were confounded by the adverse effects of cigarette smoking and various other errors.[58] There remains the allegation that coagulation disorders are the mechanism responsible for thrombotic strokes and deep vein thrombosis in high dose COC users. An increased risk of stroke was never observed in large prospective studies in the USA.[58,59] and all studies of deep vein thrombosis are confounded by the high incidence of false positive clinical diagnoses: when checked by ultrasonography over 80% of such diagnoses were wrong in women known by their clinician to be COC users.[60]

In late 1995 several epidemiological papers reported an increased risk of venous thrombosis in users of COCs containing gestodene or desogestrel, as compared to 'second-generation' COCs containing levonorgestrel. This implausible finding (there is no biological reason why any progestogen should be thrombogenic (consider pregnancy!), let alone why one progestogen should be more thrombogenic than another), has generated a huge controversy, aggravated in no small degree by the inappropriate way regulatory agencies made these results public. At the time of writing, the confounding factors unavoidable in such studies seem to be the most plausible explanation. In any event, the difficulties in the assessment of an association of contraceptive steroids and venous thrombosis are being addressed seriously by the epidemiologic community for the first time since the initial (1961) report of such an occurrence.

Nervous system

The steroid hormones are intimately involved, at many neurobiological levels, with the function of the central and autonomic nervous systems.[61,62] The actions of estrogen in particular have been subjected to intensive investigation.[63] Locally-synthesized catechol estrogens (despite their extremely short half-life) as well as 5α-pregnanolone and related progestogens have sparked considerable interest. In very large doses, certain progestogens even have an anesthetic effect. Cognitive function, mood, feelings of well-being, even the dementia of Alzheimer's disease[64] are affected by levels of these steroid hormones. In general, estrogens can be seen to have 'activating' effects on mood and activity, while progestogens exert an 'inhibitory' effect; these changes are noted both during the menstrual cycle and with ERT. However, the symptomatic changes induced by estrogen and progestogen replacement therapy are very variable and difficult to verify and quantitate, as are the effects of these steroids on conditions such as premenstrual tension.[11]

Meningiomas possess both estrogen and progesterone receptors;[50] use of the progesterone antagonist, mifepristone, is under investigation as chemotherapy.

Conclusion

The pharmacodynamics of estrogens and progestogens is a classical example of the complexity of human pharmacology and the need to study the action of drugs under a wide variety of circumstances and in many individuals. It is easy to make lists of subjective and objective effects observed during use of a particular drug, but much more difficult to provide a biologically plausible explanation for the observations. In the absence of such investigations, much constraint may be imposed on their use on the basis of 'prudence' — often a pseudonym for maintaining the status quo. Continuing research on pharmacodynamics at the subcellular level will not only clarify mechanisms but also provide unanticipated applications to problems of human health.

REFERENCES

1. Brody SA, Turkes A, Goldzieher JW 1989 Pharmacokinetics of three bioequivalent norethindrone/mestranol 50 mcg and three norethindrone/ethinyl estradiol 35 mcg OC formulations: are low-dose pills really lower? Contraception 40: 269–284
2. Rosano GMC, Sarrel PM, Poole-Wilson PA et al 1993 Beneficial effect of estrogen on exercise-induced myocardial ischemia in women with coronary artery disease. Lancet 342: 133–136
3. Clarkson TB, Prichard RW, Morgan TM et al 1994 Remodeling of coronary arteries in human and nonhuman primates. Journal of the American Medical Association 289–294
4. Judd HL 1987 Effects of estrogen replacement on hepatic function. In: Mishell DR Jr (ed) Menopause, physiology and pharmacology. Year Book Medical Publishers, Chicago, pp 237–253
5. Nahoul K, Dehennin L, Jondet M et al 1993 Profiles of plasma estrogens, progesterone and their metabolites after oral or vaginal administration of estrogen or progesterone. Maturitas 16: 185–193
6. Goldzieher JW 1994 Pharmacology of ethynyl estrogens in various countries. In: Snow R, Hall P (ed) Steroid contraceptives and women's response. Plenum Press, New York, pp 85–90
7. Edgren RE 1994 Issues in animal pharmacology. In: Goldzieher JW, Fotherby K (eds) Pharmacology of the contraceptive steroids. Raven Press, New York, pp 81–98
8. Coutinho EM, Mascarenhas I, Mateo de Acosta O et al 1993 Comparative study on the efficacy, acceptability and side effects of a contraceptive pill administered by the oral and the vaginal route: an international multicenter clinical trial. Clinical Pharmacology and Therapeutics 54: 540–545
9. WHO task force on long-acting systemic agents for fertility control 1988: a multicentered phase III comparative study of two hormonal contraceptive preparations given once-a-month by intramuscular injection. I. Contraceptive efficacy and side effects. Contraception 37: 1–20
10. Primiero FM, Benagiano G 1994 Long-acting contraceptives. In: Goldzieher JW, Fotherby K (eds) Pharmacology of the contraceptive steroids. Raven Press, New York, pp 153–184
11. Shangold MM, Tomai TP, Cook JD et al 1991 Factors associated with withdrawal bleeding after administration of oral micronised progesterone in women with secondary amenorrhea. Fertility and Sterility 56: 1040–1047
12. MacNaughton J, Bangah M, McCloud P et al 1992 Age related changes in follicle stimulating hormone, luteinizing hormone, estradiol and immunoreactive inhibin in women of reproductive age. Clinical Endocrinology 36: 339–345
13. Castracane VD, Gimpel T, Goldzieher JW 1995 When is it safe to switch from oral contraceptives to hormonal replacement therapy? Contraception 52: 371–376
14. Goldzieher JW 1994 The hypothalamo-pituitary-ovarian system. In: Goldzieher JW, Fotherby K (eds) Pharmacology of the contraceptive steroids. Raven Press, New York, pp 185–194
15. Goldzieher JW, de la Pena A, Chenault CB et al 1975 Comparative studies of the ethynyl estrogens used in oral contraceptives II. Antiovulatory activity. American Journal of Obstetrics and Gynecology 122: 619–624
16. Goldzieher JW, Martinez-Manautou J, Livingston NB Jr et al 1963 The use of sequential estrogen and progestin to inhibit fertility. A preliminary report. Western Journal of Surgery, Obstetrics and Gynecology 71: 187–190
17. Mishell DR Jr, Kletzky OA, Brenner PF et al 1977 The effect of contraceptive steroids on hypothalamopituitary function. American Journal of Obstetrics and Gynecology 128: 60–74
18. Scott JA, Brenner PF, Kletzky OA et al 1978 Factors affecting gonadotropin function in users of oral contraceptive steroids. American Journal of Obstetrics and Gynecology 130: 817–821
19. Anon 1984 After contraception: dispelling rumors about later childbearing. Population Reports, Sept, Series J, no. 28 Hampton House
20. McCann MF, Potter LS 1994 Progestin-only contraception: a comprehensive review. Contraception 50: Suppl. 1
21. Pituitary adenoma study group 1983 Pituitary adenomas and oral contraceptives: a multicenter case-control study. Fertility and Sterility 39: 753–760
22. Chretien FC, Sureau C, Neau C et al 1980 Experimental study of cervical blockade induced by continuous low-dose oral progestogens. Contraception 22: 445–456
23. Maqueo M, Azuela JC, Calderon JJ et al 1966 Morphology of the cervix in women treated with synthetic progestins. American Journal of Obstetrics and Gynecology 96: 994–998
24. Meuwissen JHJM, Brolmann HAM 1993 Vaginosonography of the endometrium. In: Berg G, Hammar M (eds) The modern management of the menopause. Parthenon Publishing Group, New York, pp 207–216
25. Song JU, Fraser IS 1995 Effects of progestogens on human endometrium. Obstetric and Gynecology Survey 50: 385–394
26. Johannisson E, Brosens I 1994 The lower reproductive tract. In: Goldzieher JW, Fotherby K (eds) Pharmacology of the contraceptive steroids. Raven Press, New York, pp 211–232
27. Alexander NJ, d'Arcangues C 1992 Steroid hormones and uterine bleeding. American Association for the Advancement of Science Press, Washington DC, xii–xv

28. Maqueo MM, Rice-Wray E, Goldzieher JW et al 1990 Endometrial regeneration in patients discontinuing oral contraceptives. Fertility and Sterility 21: 224–229
29. Maqueo MM, Gorodovsky J, Rice-Wray E et al 1970 Endometrial changes in women taking hormonal contraceptives for periods up to ten years. Contraception 1: 115–129
30. Kirshon B, Poindexter AN 1988 Contraception: a risk factor for endometriosis. Obstetrics and Gynecology 71: 829–831
31. Hyne RV, Murdoch RN, Boettcher B 1978 The metabolism and motility of human spermatozoa in the presence of steroid hormones and synthetic progestogens. Journal of Reproduction and Fertility 53: 315–322
32. Trussell J, Stewart F 1992 The effectiveness of postcoital hormonal contraception. Family Planning Perspectives 24: 262–264
33. Lobo RA 1993 Oestrogen replacement after treatment for breast cancer? Lancet 341: 1313–1314
34. Cobleigh MA, Berris RF, Bush T et al: 1994 Estrogen replacement therapy in breast cancer survivors: a time for change. Journal of the American Medical Association 272: 540–545
35. Ory H, Cole P, MacMahon B et al 1976 Oral contraceptives and reduced risk of benign breast diseases. New England Journal of Medicine 294: 419–422
36. Brinton LA, Vessey MR, Flavel R et al 1981 Risk factors for benign breast disease. American Journal of Epidemiology 113: 203–214
37. Rohan TE, L'Abbe KA, Cook MG 1992 Oral contraceptives and risk of benign proliferative epithelial disorders of the breast. International Journal of Cancer 50: 891–894
38. Plu-Bureau G, Le MG, Sitruk-Ware R et al 1994 Progestogen use and decreased risk of breast cancer in a cohort study of premenopausal women with benign breast disease. British Journal of Cancer 70: 270–288
39. Nilsson S, Nygren KG 1979 Transfer of contraceptive steroids to human milk. Research in Reproduction 11: 1–2
40. WHO 1994 Task force for epidemiological research on reproductive health. Progestogen-only contraceptives during lactation. Contraception 50: 35–40
41. Erwin PC 1994 To use or not use combined hormonal oral contraceptives during lactation. Family Planning Perspectives 26: 26–30
42. Fraser I 1991 A review of the use of progestogen-only minipills for contraception during lactation. Reproduction and Fertility Developments 3: 245–254
43. Miodrag A, Castleden CM, Vallance TR 1988 Sex hormones and the female urinary tract. Drugs 36: 491–504
44. Cardozo J, Kelleher C 1993 Estrogen deficiency and urinary incontinence. In: Berg G, Hamma M (eds) The modern management of the menopause. Parthenon Publishing Group, New York, pp 187–200
45. Sultana CJ, Walters MD 1994 Estrogen and urinary incontinence in women. Maturitas 20: 129–138
46. Garg SK, Chase HP, Marshall G et al 1994 Oral contraceptives and renal and retinal complications in young women with insulin-dependent diabetes mellitus. Journal of the American Medical Association 271: 1099–1102
47. Goldzieher JW 1994 The thyroid gland. In: Goldzieher JW, Fotherby K (eds) Pharmacology of the contraceptive steroids, Raven Press, New York, pp 243–247
48. Petak SM, Steinberger E 1994 The adrenal gland. In: Goldzieher JW, Fortherby K (eds) Pharmacology of the contraceptive steroids. Raven Press, New York, pp 233–242
49. Fern M, Rose DP, Fern EB 1978 Effect of oral contraceptives on plasma androgenic steroids and their precursors. Obstetrics and Gynecology 51: 541–544
50. Poison M 1984 Steroid receptors in human meningiomas. Clinical Neuropharmacology 7: 320–324
51. Schuurs AHWM, Geurts TBP, Goorissen EM et al 1994 Immunologic effects of estrogens, progestins, and estrogen-progestin combinations. In: Goldzieher JW, Fotherby K (eds) Pharmacology of the contraceptive steroids. Raven Press, New York, pp 379–400
52. Jungers P, Dougados M, Pelissier C et al 1982 Influence of oral contraceptive therapy on the activity of systemic lupus erythematosus. Arthritis and Rheumatology 25: 618–623
53. Collins P, Rosano GM, Jiang C et al 1993 Cardiovascular protection by oestrogen — a calcium antagonist effect? Lancet 341: 1264–1265
54. Williams JK, Honore EK, Washburn SA et al 1994 Effects of hormone replacement therapy on reactivity of atherosclerotic coronary arteries in cynomolgus monkeys. Journal of the American College of Cardiology 24: 1757–1761
55. Wagner JD, Adams MR, Schwenke DC et al 1993 Oral contraceptive treatment decreases arterial low density lipoprotein degradation in female cynomolgus monkeys. Circulation Research 72: 1300–1307
56. Colditz GA, and the Nurses' Health Study Research Group 1994 Oral contraceptive use and mortality during 12 years of follow up: the Nurses' Health Study. Annals of Internal Medicine 120: 821–826
57. Engel HJ 1991 Angiographic findings after myocardial infarctions of young women: role of oral contraceptives. Advances in Contraception 7 (Suppl 3): 235–241
58. Realini JP, Goldzieher JW 1985 Oral contraceptives and cardiovascular disease: a critique of the epidemiologic studies. American Journal of Obstetrics and Gynecology 152: 729–748
59. Grimes DA 1992 The safety of oral contraceptives: epidemiologic insights from the first 30 years. American Journal of Obstetrics and Gynecology 166: 1950–1954
60. Barnes RW, Krapf T, Joak JC 1978 Erroneous clinical diagnosis of leg vein thrombosis in women on oral contraceptives. Obstetrics and Gynecology 51: 556–558
61. Smith LH Jr, Fitz JG 1984 Oral contraceptives and benign tumors of the liver. Western Journal of Medicine 140: 260–267
62. McEwen HS 1993 Ovarian steroids have diverse effects on brain structure and function. In: Berg G, Hammer M (eds) The modern management of the menopause. Parthenon Publishing Group, New York, pp 269–278
63. Smith SS 1993 Activating effects of estradiol on brain activity. In: Berg G, Hammar M (eds) The modern management of the menopause. Pathenon Publishing Group, New York, pp 279–294
64. Ohkura T, Isse K, Akazawa K et al 1993 An open trial of estrogen therapy for dementia of the Alzheimer type in women. In: Berg G, Hammar M (eds) The modern management of the menopause. Parthenon Publishing Group, New York, pp 315–336

27. The pharmacology of antiestrogens and antiprogestogens

G. C. Davies

Introduction

Antihormones are efficacious agents in a number of therapeutic indications, including hormone dependent tumors, sex steroid dependent gynecological conditions, infertility and contraception. More recently, the selective estrogen receptor modulator (SERM)[1] properties of certain phytoestrogens and synthetic antiestrogens have been investigated; these agents attempt to harness the beneficial properties of estrogen without the incumbent proliferative effects on the uterus and breast.

ANTIESTROGENS

These molecules have a spectrum of activity ranging from 'pure' antagonism to tissue selective agonist/antagonist activity.

Mechanism of action at receptor

Animal studies have demonstrated that estrogen increases the rate of cell proliferation by a reduction in the length of the G1 phase and recruiting noncycling cells into the cell cycle.[2] The mitogenic effects of estrogen appear to be dependent on the additional presence of peptide growth factors.[3]

The estrogen receptor (ER) protein consists of several domains: a ligand-binding domain at the C terminus, a DNA-binding domain in the centre, responsible for recognizing the DNA palindromic sequence of the target gene, and two domains with transactivation functions: TAF 1 in the N terminal domain and TAF 2 in the ligand-binding domain.[4] The TAF domains are responsible for stimulation of transcription. In the resting state, the ER is in the form of a large macromolecular complex consisting of receptor, heat shock proteins (HSP) and immunophilins.[5] Following binding of estrogen, the receptor undergoes a conformational change with dissociation of the HSPs, dimerization, nuclear translocation and interaction with DNA sequences in the regulatory regions of the target genes.[6] Transcriptional initiation by RNA polymerase II follows, ultimately resulting in a physiological response. The response may be influenced by repressor proteins (SSN6, TUP 1) and growth promoting signals (epidermal growth factor, insulin like growth factor, transforming growth factor).

In vitro antiestrogens appear to induce conformational changes in the ER sufficient to enable interaction with target gene DNA.[7] McDonnell and coworkers[7] have proposed that it is the degree of conformational change, subsequent presentation of TAF domains to the transcription apparatus and the cell type that determines the selectivity of individual antiestrogens. A classification of antiestrogens has been proposed based on the response of an ER model to the 'pure' antiestrogen ICI 182,270, tamoxifen, clomiphene, raloxifene and nafoxidine. Under the proposed classification, a type 1 antiestrogen is one that inhibits the binding of the estrogen receptor ligand complex (ERLC) to DNA; such a ligand is yet to be described. A type II antiestrogen as typified by ICI 182,270 produces an ERLC closest in conformation to the inactive receptor. A type III antiestrogen is characterized and approaches the change which occurs following binding of the ER with estrogen. In this situation, however, the TAF are presented in such a way that the agents demonstrate transcriptional activity in a number of ER sensitive genes such as bone but demonstrate diminished or no activity in a uterus or breast. The type IV antiestrogen ERLC undergoes the conformational changes which are closest to those that occur following the binding of estrogen. These agents, characterized by tamoxifen, demonstrate transcriptional activity in an increasing number if ER responsive genes. The classification is not exhaustive and with the advent of new antiestrogens or receptor subtypes further subclassification may be necessary.

In vitro studies have also suggested the existence of primary and secondary binding sites in the estrogen receptor. The primary site has a common high binding affinity for estrogen and type IV antiestrogens.[8] At all concentrations, estradiol interacts solely with the primary site, leading to characteristic conformation change of the ERLC and transcription activation. *In vitro* studies suggest that at low concentrations the type IV antiestrogens preferentially bind with the primary site resulting in a conformational change characteristic for that antiestrogen. If the primary site is occupied with estrogen it may be postulated that at concentrations suboptimal for competitive antagonism, the secondary site occupation by the antiestrogen results in a conformational change which is a hybrid of the two individual conformational changes. The resultant transcriptional activity of the hybrid conformation is organotypic and dependent on the TAF domain presentation. This may help explain the enigmatic actions of tamoxifen in the uterus in the presence of estrogen.[9] The lack of agonist activity of the type II antiestrogens may be explained by a greater affinity for its secondary site leading to transcriptional block.[8]

Ligand independent estrogen receptor-mediated transcriptional activity has been demonstrated in the presence of epidermal growth factors.[10] Evidence suggests that the link between the TAF domains and the apparatus of transcription is through a number of cofactors which include cAMP, epidermal growth factors and transforming growth factor α.[11] Activation of these factors may be sufficient to 'bridge the conformational gap' between the antagonist conformation of the TAF domains and the RNA polymerase complex leading to an agonist profile. Ligand-independent ER transcriptional activity occurs in a variety of tissues and may be modulated by receptor ligands.[12] Under the selective antagonistic pressure of tamoxifen, a cell line with an activated pathway may account for the development of tumor resistance to or stimulation by tamoxifen.[11]

Net changes in cellular growth may be achieved by apoptosis (cell death) as well as progression through the cell cycle. Some antiestrogens appear to have cytotoxic effects which are independent of ER requirements.[13]

Phytoestrogens

Phytoestrogens are plant-derived chemicals with estrogenic activity. The isoflavones and coumestans to date have demonstrated the greatest potency. Animal studies suggest that the isoflavones, genistein and daidzein, constituents of a soy-based diet, have the potential to demonstrate beneficial estrogen agonist effects and antiestrogenic activity in breast and prostatic carcinoma.[14] Ginseng is a traditional Chinese medicine and is consumed by over five million people in North America for its proposed beneficial properties. The term ginseng, however, is misleading as it refers to seng, the fleshy underground portion of more than 25 different plant species which to date have complicated accurate assessment of 'ginseng's' profile.[15] Estrogenic[16] and androgenic[17] and antiestrogenic properties have been described.

The mechanisms by which certain phytoestrogens display both estrogenic and antiestrogenic activity is yet to be fully established. One source of antiestrogenic activity is via the enzyme 17β-hydroxysteroid oxidoreductase type 1 (17β-HSOR) inhibition.[19] This enzyme catalyses the reversible conversion of endogenous estrone to estradiol. The inhibition of 17β-HSOR is dependent on the structure of the phytoestrogen; inhibitory activity is high in coumestrol and genistein compared to coumerin and quercetin.

Phytoestrogens also possess significant intrinsic estrogenic activity (Table 27.1). It is difficult to postulate that 17β-HSOR inhibition alone is sufficient to explain the beneficial impact diets rich in these molecules have on estrogenic tumors unless the molecule itself is acting as an estrogen with a spectrum of estrogenic and antiestrogenic effects. The phytoestrogen, enterolactone, has demonstrated mild to moderate aromatase inhibitory properties and may, by reducing endogenous estrogen, act as a chemoprotective agent.[20]

Genistein binds to the estrogen receptor *in vitro*, however its inhibitory effect on tumor growth appears to be estrogen receptor independent.[21] There are

Table 27.1 Relative estrogenicity and food content of selected phytoestrogens.[18,19]

Molecule	Source	Food content mg/kg	Emax*
Genistein	Soy flour	1122.6	72
Daidzein	Soy flour	654.7	
Biochanin A	Clover sprouts (freeze dried)	88.1	64
Coumestrol	Clover sprouts (freeze dried)	5661.4	78

*The maximal estrogenic effect at a concentration of 1 μM taken as the capability to enhance proliferation of MCF-7 breast cancer cells in culture as a percentage of 17β estradiol.

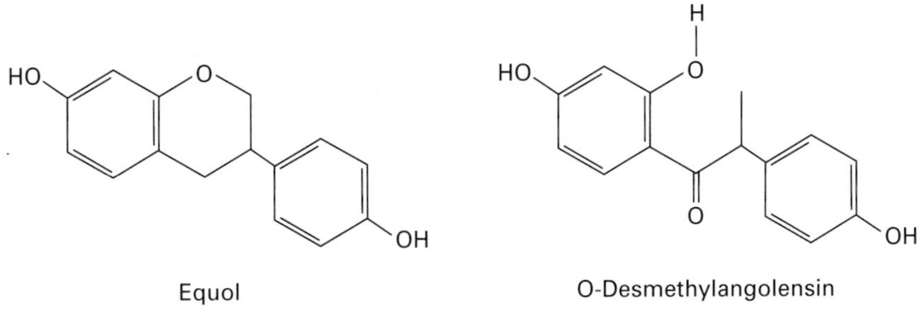

Fig. 27.1 Isoflavonoid metabolites, equol and O-desmethylangolensin.

several potential anticarcinogenic sites at which genistein may act. The protective effects of genistein may be initiated as early as the neonatal period, where administration has been shown to reduce carcinogen induced mammary cancer in rats.[22] Possible sites of action include protein tyrosine kinase (PTK) inhibition. Cellular PTKs are responsible for phosphorylation of mutated proteins encoded from oncogenes resulting in growth factor stimulated signal transduction. Hydrophobic rather than ionic substituents at C2 are necessary to maintain an inhibitory effect, suggestive that genistein must enter cells to have an effect.[23] Genistein has also demonstrated *in vitro* inhibition of topoisomerase II, an enzyme involved in cellular replication.[24] The chemopreventative action of genistein may in part be due to its ability to promote terminal differentiation in human tumor cells.[24] Genistein may also inhibit tumor promotion by having an antioxidant effect on mutagenic oxygen radicals.[21]

Postmenopausal women with hot flashes have been shown to benefit from the estrogenic effects of a diet supplemented with soya flour.[25] A significant reduction in the number of hot flashes has been demonstrated. An increase in the vaginal maturation index has been demonstrated by Wilcox et al[25] but not by Murkies et al.[26] An increase in urinary hydroxyproline demonstrated in the control group over 12 weeks was not matched by the soy group, suggesting an inhibitory effect on bone turnover.[26]

Little is known about the metabolism of phytoestrogens in humans. Isoflavonoids are present in plants as glycosides. The estrogen active aglycones are rapidly released by acid hydrolysis. Following ingestion, the isoflavones undergo intestinal metabolism leading to absorption and excretion of genistein and diadzein and their intestinal estrogenic metabolites, equol and O-desmethylangolensin. There is a high degree of variability in metabolism, either due to differential metabolic capacity and/or differentially active metabolic pathways. Peak equol excretion levels vary by a factor of up to 1527.[27]

Individual phytoestrogens are under investigation but little is yet known of potential development, reproductive and carcinogenic effects. The effects of interactions with other phytoestrogens or chemically active/inert substances from within the foodstuff have yet to be elucidated.

Nonsteroidal antiestrogens

This heterogenic group contains agents synthesized from a number of different chemical entities (Table 27.2).

Triphenylethylene derivatives:

Fertility agents. Clomiphene was first synthesized in the 1950s, along with tamoxifen and nafoxidine. It

Table 27.2 The nonsteroidal antiestrogens.

Structure	Antiestrogen	Indication
Triphenylethylene	Clomiphene	Ovulation induction
	Tamoxifen	Breast carcinoma
	Droloxifene*	Breast carcinoma Osteoporosis
	Idoxifene*	Breast carcinoma
	Toremphene*	Breast carcinoma
	Nitromifene*	Breast carcinoma
Naphthalenes	Nafoxidene	Breast carcinoma
	Trioxifene	Breast carcinoma
Indoles	Zindoxifene*	Breast carcinoma
	ZK 119010*	Breast carcinoma
Benzothiaphenes	Raloxifene*	Osteoporosis
	T-588*	Alzheimer's disease
Benzopyran	Centchroman*	Osteoporosis
Benzofuroquinolone	KCA 098*	Osteoporosis

*Drug under development with suggested indications.

is a racemic mixture of zuclomiphene (cis isomer) and enclomiphene (trans isomer). The pharmacokinetic properties of tamoxifen and clomiphene are very similar. Clomiphene undergoes hydroxylation and conjugation in the liver; the metabolite trans 4-hydroxy clomiphene has potent antiestrogenic activity. The half life of clomiphene is between 5–7 days due to high affinity binding to sex steroids, enterohepatic circulation and accumulation in fatty tissues. Clomiphene and its metabolites are cleared from the circulation within three weeks and excreted in the feces.

Clomiphene is an important agent in the treatment of anovulatory women. The usual treatment regimen is 50 mg daily for five days commenced within five days of the onset of menstruation. Tamoxifen given in a similar cyclical fashion can also induce ovulation.[28] The mechanisms of action are similar: a reduced amount of estrogen available to the hypothalamus leads to an increase in the secretion of gonadotropin releasing hormone and the secretion of pituitary gonadotropins. Prolonged treatment with clomiphene at doses of 100–200 mg and tamoxifen at 20 mg can lead to ovarian hyperstimulation syndrome.[29] An association between prolonged clomiphene therapy for ovulation induction and risk of borderline or invasive ovarian tumor has been suggested.[30]

Both clomiphene and tamoxifen administration have been used in an attempt to improve sperm quality in normogonadotropic men with oligospermia. Tamoxifen, with less intrinsic estrogenic activity than clomiphene, has demonstrated some benefit in the improvement of sperm density.[31]

Breast chemotherapeutics: tamoxifen. Breast cancer is the most frequent cancer in women and the leading cause of cancer death. The current benchmark in the adjuvant treatment of primary breast carcinoma and endocrine therapy of advanced breast carcinoma is the triphenylethylene, tamoxifen. Tamoxifen was synthesized in 1966 and initially developed as an infertility agent; it was subsequently found to stimulate ovulation and its efficacy in breast carcinoma was first described in 1971.[32] Currently, tamoxifen is the most widely prescribed antineoplastic for the treatment of breast carcinoma in the United States and Great Britain.

Following oral administration of the standard 20 mg dose of tamoxifen, steady state concentration is reached after approximately four weeks' treatment. There is a wide therapeutic range of drug concentrations. Tamoxifen undergoes extensive hydroxylation and conjugation in the liver. The principal metabolites are N-desmethyltamoxifen, which reaches steady state by eight weeks, and 4-hydroxytamoxifen. These metabolites bind to the ER, N-desmethyltamoxifen at approximately the same affinity as tamoxifen and 4-hydroxytamoxifen at 25–30 times the affinity of tamoxifen, approximately equal to estradiol.[33]

The majority of tamoxifen is excreted in the bile with a minimal amount excreted unchanged in the urine. Tamoxifen and its major metabolite, N-desmethyltamoxifen, have long half lives—7 and 14 days respectively—due to extensive plasma binding and enterohepatic recirculation. Tamoxifen and N-desmethyltamoxifen may remain in the serum for up to six weeks following cessation of treatment.

The endocrine effects of tamoxifen are dependent in many systems on the presence or absence of endogenous estrogen (Table 27.3).

Tamoxifen prolongs disease-free interval and overall survival in 50–80% of postmenopausal women positive for ER and PR and 20–40% of premenopausal

Table 27.3 The endocrine effects of long-term tamoxifen therapy in the pre and postmenopause.

	Premenopause	Postmenopause
Estrogen and progesterone	↑ 1–3×[34]	→[35]
Gonadotrophins	→ or ↑[36]	↓[35]
Thyroid-binding globulin	↑[37]	↑[37]
Sex hormone-binding globulin	↑[38]	↑[38]
Prolactin	↓ or →[36]	↓ or →[36]
Ovulation	→[34]	Not applicable
Amenorrhea	16–39%[39]	Not applicable
Vaginal cornification	↓[40]	↑[41]

(↑ = increases; → = unchanged; ↓ = decreases.)

women when used as an adjuvant to primary surgery in breast carcinoma. Efficacy is also demonstrated in over 50% of patients with metastatic disease in ER positive tumors.[42] The report from the National Surgical Adjuvant Breast and Bowel Project suggests that treatment beyond five years confers no improvement in survival.[43]

Breast tumors may become resistent or stimulated following prolonged tamoxifen administration.[44] The most likely cause for resistance is the selection of proliferating colonies of resistant cells[11] due to activation of dormant signal pathways or point mutations in the estrogen receptor. There are several experimental conditions which would support these theories: long-term treatment with 'pure' antiestrogens led to proliferating tumor colonies sensitive to tamoxifen;[45] estrogen can act as an antagonist in tamoxifen-resistant breast cells;[44] a mutation of a sole pair of amino acids in the TAF2 region was sufficient to convert tamoxifen and the 'pure' antiestrogen ICI 164,384 from antagonists to agonists.[46]

The ability of tamoxifen to demonstrate inhibitory activity in 10–15% of ER negative tumors suggests an ER independent activity;[47] such activity may involve the inhibition of the tumor promoting factors, PKC and calmodulin, enhancing immunogenic activity towards the tumor and inhibition of tumor angiogenesis.[48]

In postmenopausal women, tamoxifen at a dosage of 20 mg per day offers some protection from osteoporosis, but to a lesser degree than estrogen or the bisphosphonates.[49] Tamoxifen reduces low density lipoprotein cholesterol (LDL) and cholesterol, high density lipoprotein cholesterol (HDL) remains unchanged. Cardioprotective properties of tamoxifen have been suggested by a halving of deaths due to myocardial infarction in the Scottish adjuvant trial and a 25% reduction in cardiovascular deaths in the early Breast Cancer Trialist's Collaborative Group.[42,50]

About 40 side effects have been attributed to tamoxifen. The most common are hot flashes, vaginal changes and irregular menses. A doubling of menopausal symptoms in tamoxifen users compared to placebo (48.5:21.2 %) has been reported in addition to depression (1%) and nonspecific CNS symptoms.[51]

The most concerning complications of tamoxifen use are carcinoma, thromboembolism and bone loss in premenopausal women.[52] Initial concerns over ocular effects seem to be limited to doses of tamoxifen greater than 180 mg per day.[53]

There appears to be an increased incidence of venous thromboembolism associated with tamoxifen. Fisher[54] describes a higher rate of deep vein thrombosis (0.4:0.1%), pulmonary embolus (0.4:0.1%) and death due to thromboembolic causes (0.2:0.0%) compared to controls. In a risk/benefit analysis of entering a tamoxifen trial a 3.5 (range 0–7) increased risk of thromboembolic death has been described.[55] The mechanism for this phenomenon is unclear, however the finding of a reduction in antithrombin III activity in 42%[56] of women taking tamoxifen has not been verified in subsequent studies.[57]

Studies have linked the use of tamoxifen to endometrial carcinoma, the largest data set is derived from the National Surgical Adjuvant Breast and Bowel Project (NASBP) B-14.[58] The patients were followed up for an average of 8 years. Including all originally reported endometrial cancers an annual hazard rate of 0.2/1000 in the placebo group and 1.6/1000 in the patients randomized to tamoxifen was reported. A relative risk of 7.5. The incidence of endometrial carcinoma appears to remain constant over time, 36% of the women who developed endometrial carcinoma received tamoxifen for less than 2 years.

The NASBP failed to show any significant increase in any other carcinoma. A joint analysis of the incidence of endometrial and gastrointestinal cancers has been performed on pooled data from three major Scandinavian studies evaluating adjuvant tamoxifen treatment. A six fold increase in endometrial carcinoma and a three fold increase in gastrointestinal tumors were described. The majority of the GI tumors were colorectal and stomach cancers.[59] The link between tamoxifen and GI tumors, however, remains tenuous with inconsistencies in dose, duration and demographic risk factors.[60]

Chemotherapeutics under development. There are many agents under development in the nonsteroidal antiestrogen group designed to improve on the estrogen agonist/antagonist profile of tamoxifen, and many are currently undergoing clinical trial for the treatment of breast cancer.

Droloxifene (3-hydroxy tamoxifen) has a number of advantages over tamoxifen including a 20–60 fold higher affinity for the ER.[61] Droloxifene requires no further metabolism to achieve activity, it has a half life of 1.5 days and is rapidly eliminated in the feces. Droloxifene appears to have less impact on SHBG and gonadotropins compared to tamoxifen in postmenopausal women.[62]

Idoxifene demonstrates superior binding affinity for the ER, improved antitumor activity and less uterotrophic effects than tamoxifen in rat and mouse models.[63]

Toremifene has ER dependent activity and apoptotic activity.[64] The drug is well absorbed and strongly binds to plasma proteins.

Naphthalene derivatives

Nafoxidene[65] and trioxifene[66] have been tested in phase I and II breast cancer trials with similar objective results as tamoxifen but an unacceptable side effect profile.

Indole derivatives

Zindoxifene the first member of this group to be assessed demonstrated marginal therapeutic activity in advanced breast cancer. ZK 119010 is less estrogenic than zindoxifene in rats and mice and may be of value in breast carcinoma.[67]

Selective estrogen receptor modulators (SERM)

Several antiestrogens have demonstrated SERM properties. These molecules have a selective estrogenic action with minimal uterotropic activity and a beneficial or neutral profile in breast tissue. The SERM properties of antiestrogens currently under development as breast chemotherapeutics have yet to be fully evaluated.

Raloxifene. Raloxifene has beneficial effects on markers of bone turnover and on lipids and no demonstrable effect on endometrial histology.[68] It is currently undergoing phase III studies for the prevention and treatment of osteoporosis. One mechanism by which raloxifene appears to prevent osteoporosis is by inhibition of IL-6 stimulated differentiation of osteoclasts with a limited effect on fully differentiated osteoclasts.[69]

Centachroman. The benzopyran centachroman was originally developed as a postcoital contraceptive with antiestrogenic and mild estrogenic properties,[70] it also appears to have an osteoclastic inhibitory activity and may demonstrate other SERM properties.[71]

Ipriflavone. Phytoestrogens are a potentiall source of SERMs. Ipriflavone is a synthetic flavonoid derivative devoid of estrogenic activity in animals and humans but it enhances the uterotropic effects of estrogen in the rat uterus.[72] Ipriflavone reduces bone turnover in postmenopausal women the mechanism of action has not yet been fully elucidated.

Steroidal antiestrogens

The partial estrogenic action of the nonsteroidal antiestrogens has been implicated in the resistance that develops in ER positive breast tumors. The steroidal antiestrogens are devoid of estrogenic activity. These 'pure' agents are being developed as both first and second line treatments for breast carcinoma and include ICI 164384, ICI 182780, RU 586668, EMI 139 and ME 170.

Preclinical *in vivo* studies with ICI 164384 demonstrated inhibitory properties at doses too high for human development.[73] ICI 182780 is more potent than ICI 164384 and demonstrates a four to five fold improvement in binding affinity to the ER coupled with a five fold increase in inhibition of MCF-7 cells.[74] ICI 164384 and ICI 182780 have twice the ability to inhibit MCF-7 cells as tamoxifen.[73,74]

Progress with ICI 182780 has been delayed by its low oral bioavailability, however oil-based formulations demonstrating long-acting antiestrogenic activity are under development.[75] An antiuterotropic effect of ICI 182780 in monkeys appears to be devoid of an associated increase in gonadotropins.[75] This agent also failed to induce any loss in bone mineral density in rats compared to OVEX controls.[76] Administration of ICI 182780 during the follicular phase of the menstrual cycle in women prior to hysterectomy produced a significant increase in plasma estradiol compared to controls but no increase in endometrial thickness or gonadotropin levels.[77] There may therefore be a role for these molecules in estrogen-dependent gynecological disease.

The method of action of these agents, apart from inducing an ER conformational change hostile to transcription activity, may include increased turnover of the receptor as a consequence of impaired dimerization[78] and inhibition of 17 β-hydroxysteroid dehydrogenase, the enzyme responsible for the conversion of estrone to estradiol.[79]

Pathway inhibitors

The peripheral aromatization of circulating androstenedione is the mechanism proposed for the majority of estrogen production in the postmenopausal woman, with approximatedly two thirds of androstenedione originating from the adrenal and one third from the ovary.

Aminoglutethimide

Aminoglutethimide, originally developed as an anticonvulsant, was the first agent to be utilized in this fashion. Aminoglutethimide competitively inhibits two enzyme systems: desmolase catlyses the conversion of cholesterol to pregnenolone in the adrenal gland and aromatase converts androstenedione and testosterone to estrone and estradiol respectively in the periphery (Fig. 27.2). The observation of estrogen levels at

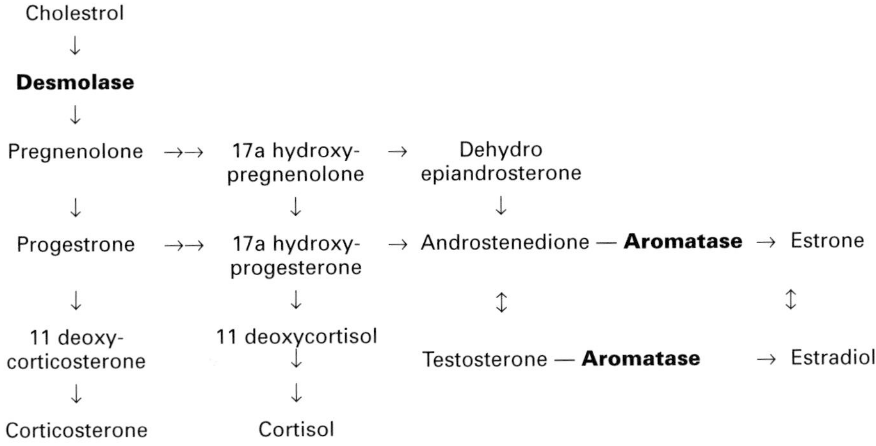

Fig. 27.2 Pathway of non-gonadal sex steroid production (target enzymes in bold).

40–60% of control despite efficient inhibition of aromatization with aminoglutethimide suggests the presence of alternative production pathways.[80]

New selective aromatase inhibitors are under development with improved selectivity and side effect profiles. This group may be subdivided into competitive inhibitors, including both steroidal and nonsteroidal agents, and mechanism-based (suicide) inhibitors.

Steroidal competitive inhibitors have potential unwanted agonist or antagonist activity at the estrogen, progesterone, androgen or glucocorticoid receptor. In contrast, the nonsteroidal competitive inhibitors can have unwanted effects due to lack of specificity on the cytochrome aromatases. The mechanism-based inhibitors are converted to reactive alkylating agents by the aromatase and form covalent bonds close to the binding site, irreversibly inactivating the enzyme. The effects of these agents are long-lasting and specific for their substrate enzyme.

Rogletimide

Rogletimide (pyridoglutethimide) is an analogue of aminoglutethimide which lacks desmolase activity but has half the potency of aminoglutethimide.[81]

Formestane

Formestane, 4-hydroxyandrostenedione (4-OHA), a derivative of androstenedione, is the first steroidal, mechanism-based aromatase inhibitor investigated in humans. *In vitro* it is 60 times more potent than aminoglutethimide.[82]

Fadrozole

Fadrozole is a nonsteroidal competitive inhibitor, 500 fold more potent than aminoglutethimide. Fadrozole lacks complete specificity and small changes in plasma electrolyte and aldosterone levels with associated blunting of aldosterone and cortisol response to ACTH have been reported.[83]

Letrozole

Letrozole has similar potency and method of action as fadrozole but improved specificity. In phase I studies there was no evidence of changes in aldosterone and cortisol[84] and good efficacy in advanced breast carcinoma.

Exemestane

Exemestane is a mechanism-based aromatase inhibitor. Preclinical and phase I studies have demonstrated a high level of specificity and efficacy. The most common side effect is headache.[85]

Arimidex, virazole

Arimidex and virazole are nonsteroidal competitive inhibitors of aromatase, which appear to have no effects on key enzymes that regulate cortisol and aldosterone biosynthesis. The (+) enantiomer of virazole, R83842, is highly selective and over 1000 fold more potent than aminogluetethimide *in vitro*.[86]

The mismatch between the extent to which individual aromatase inhibitors inhibit aromatase and the response rate demonstrated suggests alternative pathways of estrogen production. These pathways may be susceptible to secondary effects of those aromatase inhibitors demonstrating higher efficacy.

COMBINED ANTIESTROGEN-ANTIPROGESTOGENS

Steroids

Danazol

Danazol is a synthetic derivative of 17 α-ethinyl testosterone with mild antiestrogenic and antiprogestogenic effects, which is administered orally in a dose range between 200–800 mg daily. The hepatic activity of danazol results in a lowering of SHBG and HDL-C levels.[87] The reduction in SHBG concentration in addition to the binding of danazol to SHBG results in a doubling of free testosterone concentrations. Danazol is metabolized to over 60 metabolites, including ethinyl testosterone with progestogenic and weak androgenic effects. Recent studies have demonstrated no effect on serum estrogen concentration or gonadotropin concentration/pulsatility.[88] The *in vitro* administration of danazol to monocytes reduces the ER levels.[89] This may be one of a range of activities, including inhibition of enzyme activities in steroidogenesis[90] and binding to steroid hormone receptors in target organs, responsible for danazol's efficacy in sex steroid-activated diseases.

Gestrinone

Gestrinone is a synthetic 19-nonsteroid with androgenic, antiestrogenic and antiprogestogenic properties. In addition to moderate antigonadotropic activity, gestrinone demonstrates similar endocrine effects, side effect profile and efficacy as danazol.

ANTIPROGESTOGENS

Mechanisms of action at receptor

As is the case with the ER, the progesterone receptor (PR) is a latent transcription factor with the capacity to interact with the recognition sequences of target genes. The progesterone receptor, its activation and inhibition are discussed in chapters 11 and 12.

Mifepristone

Mifepristone (RU 38486) was initially developed as an antiglucocorticoid but became the first steroid to be utilized as an antiprogestogen for termination of pregnancy and emergency contraception. Mifepristone binds competitively to the PR with a binding affinity twice that of progesterone but possesses mild antiglucocortoid and antiandrogenic properties.

Approximately 98% of mifepristone is bound to plasma proteins with a high affinity to α1 acid glycoprotein (AAG) and to a lesser extent albumin. Clearance and distribution is time and dose-dependent and inversely related to AAG concentration. The half-life is approximately 24 hours. Mifepristone is metabolized to hydroxylated, mono and dimethylated compounds. The principal route of excretion is biliary (90%) with enterohepatic recirculation. Mifepristone is generally well tolerated, however prolonged administration leads to increased plasma levels of ACTH and cortisol.[91]

Antiprogestogens demonstrate potent PR-mediated antiproliferative effects in human breast cancer cells. Evidence is accumulating that antiprogestogens either alone or in combination with an antiestrogen are of benefit as adjuvant endocrine therapy in PR-positive breast cancer.[92] Progesterone receptors are present in the meninges, and mifepristone has demonstrated efficacy in the management of meningiomas.[93] Analogues of mifepristone are being developed to increase the potency and reduce the antiglucocorticoid activity and side effect profile.

Antiprogestogens under development

Table 27.4 gives the receptor binding profiles of antiprogestogens.

Onapristone (ZK 98299) showed lowered binding affinity to plasma proteins, reduced half life (6 hrs) and glucocorticoid activity compared to mifepristone. However it also demonstrated reduced PR binding.

The newer agents Org 31710 and Org 31806 demonstrate similar PR binding affinities as mifepristone with the benefit of a reduced GR and AR binding affinity.

Org 33628 possesses a high PR binding affinity in conjunction with a low GR, AR and MR binding affinity and is currently the most powerful orally administered antiprogestogen.[94] Org 33628 demonstrates strong abortifacient and antitumor properties and unlike other antiprogestogens is also a potent inhibitor of ovulation.

Conclusion

The antihormones are a key focus area for the health care industry due to their potential efficacy in a multitude of disease states. Antihormones may have an important role in reducing the morbidity and mortality associated with an increasing aged population and sex hormone-dependent diseases.

Table 27.4 Relative binding affinities (%) of antiprogestogens to the cytosolic progesterone (Prc), estrogen (Erc) and androgen (Arc) receptor of MCF-7 cells, IM-9 nuclear glucocorticoid receptor (Grn) and rat cytosolic mineralocorticoid receptor (Mrc). (DHT: dihydrotestosterone; nc: no competition; nd: not determined.)[24]

Absolutes: 100% affinity	ORG 2058 Prc	Estradiol Erc	DHT Arc	Dexamethasone Grn	Aldosterone Mrc
RU 38486	35	nc	4.7	366	nd
ZK 98299	4.1	nd	nd	21	nc
Org 31710	31	nc	2.3	11.2	18.6
Org 31806	32	nc	2.4	5.2	3.5
Org 33628	77	nc	3.7	16	3.3

REFERENCES

1. Bryant HU, Glasebrook AL, Yang NN, Sato M 1995 A pharmacological review of raloxifene. Journal of Bone and Mineral Metabolism 13: 75–83
2. Sutherland RL, Reddel RR, Green MD 1983 Effects of estrogen on cell proliferation and cell cycle kinetics. A hypothesis on the cell cycle effects of antiestrogens. Eur J Cancer Clin Oncol 19: 307–318
3. Stewart AJ, Johnson MD, May FEB, Westley BR 1990 Role of insulin like growth factors and the type I insulin like growth factor receptor in the estrogen stimulated proliferation of human breast cancer cells. J Biol Chem 265: 21172–21178
4. Tzukerman MT, Esty A, Santiso-Mere D et al 1994 Human estrogen receptor transactivational capacity is determined by both cellular and promotor context and mediated by two functionally distinct intramolecular regions. Mol Endocrinol 8: 21–30
5. Smith D, Toft D 1993 Steroid receptors and their associated proteins. Mol Endocrinol 7: 4–11
6. Beekman JM, Allan GF, Tsai MJ, O'Malley BW 1993 Transcriptional activation by the estrogen receptor requires a conformational change in the ligand binding domain. Mol Endocrinol 7: 1266–1274
7. McDonnell DP, Clem DL, Hermann T, Goldman ME, Pyke JW 1995 Analysis of estrogen receptor function in vitro reveals three distinct classes of antiestrogens. Mol Endo 9: 659–669
8. Heddon A, Muller V, Jensen EV 1995 A new interpretation of antiestrogen action. Ann New York Acad Sci 761: 109–120
9. Branham WS, Sheehan DM, Zehr DR, Medlock KL, Nelson CJ, Ridlon E 1988 Inhibition of rat uterine gland genesis by tamoxifen. Endocrinology 117: 2238–2248
10. Ignar-Trowbridge DM, Nelson KG, Bidwell MC, Curtis SW, Washburn TF, McLachlan JA, Korach KS 1992 Coupling of dual signal pathways: epidermal growth factor action involves the estrogen receptor. Proc Natl Acad Sci USA 89: 4658–4662
11. Nordeen SK, Bona BJ, Beck CA, Edwards DP, Borror KC, DeFranco DB 1995 The two faces of a steroid antagonist: when an antagonist isn't. Steroids 60: 97–104
12. Smith CL, Conneely OM, O'Malley BW, 1993 Modulation of the ligand independent activation of the human estrogen receptor by hormone and anti-hormone. Proc Natl Acad Sci USA 90: 6120–6124
13. Hwang PL, Shoon MY, Low YL, Lin L, Ng HL 1995 Inhibitors of protein and RNA synthesis block the cytotoxic effects of non-steroidal antiestrogens. Biochemica et Biophysica Acta 1266: 215–222
14. Barnes S, Grubbs C, Setchel KDR 1990 Soybeans inhibit mammary tumors in models of breast cancer. In: Pariza M, Ed. Mutagens and Carcinogens in the Diet. New York: Wiley-Liss 239–253
15. Awang DVC 1991 Maternal use of Ginseng and neonatal androgenization (letter comment). JAMA 265: 1828
16. Hopkins MP, Androff L, Benninghoff AS 1988 Ginseng face cream and unexplained vaginal bleeding. Am J Obstet Gynecol 159: 1121–1122
17. Bespalov VG, Alexsandrov, Davydov VV et al 1993 Inhibition of the mammary gland carcinogenesis by tincture from biomass of cultivated tissue of ginseng. Byull Eksp Biol Med 115: 459–461
18. Franke A, Custer L, Cerna C, Narala K 1995 Rapid HPLC analysis of dietary phytoestrogens from legumes and from human urine. Proc Soc Exp Biol Med 208: 18–26
19. Makela TS, Poutanen J, Lehtimaki M, Kostian ML, Santti R, Vihko R 1995 Estrogen specific 17β-hydroxysteroid oxidoreductase type 1 as a possible target for the action of phytoestrogens. Proc Soc Exp Biol Med 208: 51–59
20. Adlercreutz H, Bannwart C, Wahala K et al 1993 Inhibition of human aromatase by mammalian lignans and isoflavonoid phytoestrogens. J Steroid Biochem Mol Bio 44: 147–153
21. Barnes S, Peterson TG 1995 Biochemical targets of the isoflavone Genistein in tumor cell lines. Proc Soc Exp Biol Med 208: 103–108
22. Lamartiniere CA, Moore J, Holland M, Barnes S 1995 Neonatal genistein chemoprevents mammary cancer. Proc Soc Exp Biol Med 208: 120–123
23. Ogawara H, Akiyama T, Ishida J, Watanabe S, Ito N, Kobori M, Seoda Y 1989 Inhibition of tyrosine protein kinase activity by synthetic isoflavones and flavones. J Antibiotics 42: 340–343
24. Constantinou A, Kigucji K, Huberman E 1990 Induction of differentiation and DNA strand breakage in human HL-60 and K562 leukemia cells by genistein. Cancer Res 50: 2618–2624
25. Wilcox G, Wahlqvist ML, Burger HG, Medley G 1990 Oestrogenic effects of plant foods in postmenopausal women. BMJ 301: 905–906

26. Murkies AL, Lombard C, Strauss BJG, Wilcox G, Burger HG, Morton MS 1995 Dietary flour supplementation decreases post-menopausal hot flushes: effect of soy and wheat. Maturitas 21: 189–195
27. Kelly GE, Joannou GE, Reeder AY, Nelson C, Waring MA 1995 The variable metabolic response to dietary isoflavones in humans. Proc Soc Exp Biol Med 208: 40–43
28. Gerhard I, Runnebaum B 1979 Comparison between tamoxifen and clomiphene therapy in women with anovulation. Arch Gynecol 277: 279–288
29. Jolles CJ, Smotkin D, Ford KL, Jones KP 1990 Cystic ovarian necrosis complicating tamoxifen therapy for breast cancer in premenopausal woman. J Reprod Med Obstet Gynecol 35: 299–300
30. Rossing MA, Daling JR, Weiss NS, Moore DE, Self SG 1994 Ovarian tumors in a cohort of infertile women. N Engl J Med 331: 771–776
31. Schill WB, Landthaler M 1981 Erfahrung mit dem antioestrogen Tamoxifen zur therapie des oligoospermie. Hautartz 32: 306–308
32. Cole MP, Jones CTA, Todd IDH 1971 A new antiestrogenic agent in late breast cancer. An early clinical appraisal of ICI 46,474. Br J Cancer 25: 270–275
33. Fabian C, Tilzer L, Stenson L 1981 Comparative binding affinities of tamoxifen, 4-hydroxytamoxifen and desmethyltamoxifen for estrogen receptors isolated from human breast carcinoma: correlation with blood levels in patients with metastatic breast carcinoma. Biopharm Drug Dispos 2: 381–390
34. Jordan VC, Fritz NF, Langan-Fahey S et al 1991 Alteration of endocrine parameters in premenopausal women with breast carcinoma during long term adjuvant therapy with tamoxifen as the single agent. J Natl Cancer Inst 83: 1488–1491
35. Boccardo F, Guarneri D, Rubagotti A et al 1984 Endocrine effects of tamoxifen in post menopausal breast cancer patients. Tumori 70: 61–68
36. Groom GV, Griffiths K 1976 Effects of the anti-oestrogen tamoxifen on plasma levels of luteinizing hormone, follicle stimulating hormone, prolactin, oestradiol and progesterone in normal pre-menopausal women. J Endocrinol 70: 421–428
37. Jensen IW 1985 Oestrogen like effects of tamoxifen on thyroid binding globulin. Lancet 2: 1020–1021
38. Sakai F, Cheix F, Clavel M et al 1978 Increases in steroid binding globulins induced by tamoxifen in patients with carcinoma of the breast. J Endocrinol 76: 219–226
39. Planting AST, Alexieva-Figusch J, Blonk-vd Wijst J et al 1985 Tamoxifen therapy in premenopausal women with metastatic breast cancer. Cancer Treat Rep 69: 363–368
40. Tajima C 1984 Luteotropic effects of tamoxifen in infertile women. Fertil Steril 42: 223–227
41. Boccardo F, Bruzzi P, Rubagotti A et al 1981 Estrogen like action of tamoxifen on vaginal epithelium in breast cancer patients. Oncology 38: 281–285
42. Early breast cancer trialists collaborative Group. Systemic treatment of early breast cancer by hormonal, systemic or immune therapy: 133 randomized trials involving 31,000 recurrences and 24,000 deaths among 75,000 women. Lancet 339: 1–14, 71–85
43. Bulbrook RD 1996 Long term adjuvant therapy for primary breast cancer. More than five years of tamoxifen is no longer justified. BMJ 312: 389–390
44. Osborne CK, Fuqua SAW 1994 Mechanisms of tamoxifen resistance. Breast Cancer Res Treat 32: 49–55
45. Lykkesfeldt AE, Larsen SS, Briand P 1995 Human breast cancer cell lines resistant to pure antiestrogens are sensitive to tamoxifen treatment. Int J Cancer 61: 529–534
46. Mahfoudi A, Roulet E, Dauvois S, Parker M, Wahli W 1995 Specific mutations in the estrogen receptor change the properties of antiestrogens to full agonists. Proc Natl Acad Sci 92: 4206–4210
47. Vignon F, Bouton MM, Rochefort H 1987 Antiestrogens inhibit the mitogenic effect of growth factors on breast cancer cells in the total absence of estrogens. Biochem Res Comm 146: 1502–1508
48. Jaiyesimi IA, Buzdar AU, Decker DA, Hortobagyi GN 1995 Use of tamoxifen for breast cancer twenty eight years later. J Clin Oncol 13: 513–529
49. Grey AB, Stapleton JP, Evans MC, Tatnell MA, Ames RW, Reid IR 1995 The effect of the antiestrogen tamoxifen on bone mineral density in normal late postmenopausal women. Am J Med 99: 636–642
50. McDonald CC, Stewart HJ 1991 Fatal myocardial infarction in the Scottish adjuvant tamoxifen trial. The Scottish Breast Cancer Committee. BMJ 303: 435–437
51. Love RR, Cameron L, Connell BL 1991 Symptoms associated with tamoxifen treatment in postmenopausal women. Arch Intern Med 151: 1842–1847
52. Powles TJ, Hickish T, Kanis JA, Tidy A, Ashley S 1996 Effect of tamoxifen on bone mineral density measured by dual energy X ray absorptiometry in healthy premenopausal and postmenopausal women. J Clin Oncol 31: 251–257
53. Kaiser-Kupfer M, Kupfer C, Rodriguez MM 1981 Tamoxifen retinopathy. A clinicopathologic report. Ophthalmology 88: 89–93
54. Fisher B 1992 NSABP Protocol P1. A clinical trial to determine the worth of tamoxifen for preventing breast cancer. National Surgical Adjuvant Breast and Bowel Project January 24
55. Nease RF, Ross JM 1995 The decision to enter a randomized trial of tamoxifen for the prevention of breast cancer in healthy women; An analysis of the tradeoffs. Am J Med 99: 180–189
56. Enck RE, Rios CN 1984 Tamoxifen treatment of metastatic breast cancer and antithrombin III levels. Cancer 53: 2607–2609
57. Auger MJ, Mackie MJ 1988 Effects of tamoxifen on blood coagulation. Cancer 61: 1316–1319
58. Fisher B, Costantino JP, Redmond CK, Fisher ER, Wickerham DL, Cronin WM 1994 Endometrial cancer in tamoxifen treated breast cancer patients: findings from the National Surgical Adjuvant Breast and Bowel (NSABP) B-14, J Natl Cancer Inst 86: 527–537
59. Rutqvist LE, Johansson H, Signomklao T, Johansson U, Fomander T, Wilking N 1995 Adjuvant tamoxifen therapy for early stage breast cancer and secondary primary malignancies. Stockholm Breast Cancer Study Group. J Natl Cancer Inst 87: 627–629
60. Jordan VC 1995 Tamoxifen and tumorigenicity: a predictable concern. J Natl Cancer Inst 87: 645–651
61. Rauschning W, Pritchard KI 1994 Droloxifene, a new antiestrogen; its role in metastatic breast cancer. Breast Cancer Res Treat 31: 83–94

62. Geisler J, Ekse D, Hosch S, Lonning PE 1995 Influence of droloxifene (3-hydroxytamoxifen), 40 mg daily, on plasma gonadotrophins, sex hormone binding globulin and estrogen levels in post menopausal breast cancer patients. J Steroid Biochem Molec Biol 55: 193–195
63. Coombes RC, Haynes BP, Dowsett M et al 1995 Idoxifene: report of a phase I study in patients with metastatic breast cancer. Cancer Res 55: 1070–1074
64. Anttila M, Laakso S, Nylanden P, Sotoniemi EA 1995 Pharmacokinetics of the novel antiestrogenic agent toremifene in subjects with altered liver and kidney function. Clin Pharmacol Ther 57: 628–635
65. Bloom HJG, Boesen E 1974 Antiestrogens in treatment of breast cancer. Value of nafoxidine in 52 advanced cases. Br Med J 2: 7–10
66. Lee RW, Buzdar AU, Blumenschein GR, Hortobagyi GN 1986 Trioxifene mesylate in the treatment of advanced breast cancer. Cancer 57: 40–43
67. Nishino Y, Schneider MR, Michna H, von Angerer 1991 Pharmacological characterization of a novel oestrogen antagonist, ZK 119010, in rats and mice. J Endocrin 130: 409–414
68. Draper MW, Flowers DE, Huster WJ, Neild JA 1993 Effects of raloxifene (LY 139481 HCL) on biochemical markers of bone and lipid metabolism in healthy post menopausal women. In: Christiansen C, Riis B, editors. Proceedings. Fourth International Symposium on Osteoporosis and Consensus Development Conference. Aalborg, Denmark: Handelstrykkeriet Aalborg ApS 119–121
69. Sato M, Rippy MK, Bryant HU Comparative analysis of raloxifene, tamoxifen, nafoxidine or estrogen effects on reproductive and non reproductive tissues in ovaiectomized rats and on rat osteoclasts. J Pharmacol Exp Ther. In press
70 Kamboj VP, Setty BS, Chandra H, Roy SK, Kar AB 1977 Biological profile of centchroman – a new post coital contraceptive. Indian J Exp Biol 15: 1144–1150
71. Hall TJ, Nyugen H, Schaueblin M, Fornier B 1995 The bone specific estrogen centchroman inhibits osteoclastic bone resorption in vitro. Biochem Biophys Res Comm 216: 662–668
72. Reginster JYL 1993 Ipriflavone: pharmacological properties and usefulness in postmenopausal osteoporosis. Bone and Mineral 23: 223–232
73. Wakeling AE, Bowler J 1988 Novel antiestrogens without partial agonist activity. J Steroid Biochem 31: 645–653
74. Wakeling AE, Dukes M, Bowler J 1991 A potent specific pure antiestrogen with clinical potential. Cancer Res 51: 3867–3873
75. Dukes M, Miller D, Wakeling AE, Waterson JC 1992 Antiuterotrophic effects of a pure antiestrogen ICI 182780: magnetic resonance imaging of the uterus in ovariectomized monkeys. J Endocrinol 135: 239–247
76. Wakeling AE 1993 The future of new pure antiestrogens in clinical breast cancer. Breast Cancer Res Treat 25: 1–9
77. Thomas EJ, Walton PL, Thomas NM, Dowsett M 1994 The effects of ICI 182,780, a pure anti-oestrogen, on the hypothalamic-pituitary-gonadal axis and on endometrial proliferation in pre-menopausal women. Hum Repro 9: 1991–1996
78. Parker MG 1993 Action of "pure" antiestrogens in inhibiting estrogen receptor action. Breast Cancer Res Treat 26: 131–137
79. Labrie C, Martel C, Dufour JM, Levesque C, Merand Y, Labrie F 1992 Novel compounds inhibit estrogen formation and action. Cancer Res 52: 610–615
80. Lonning PE, Dowsett M, Powles TJ 1990 Postmenopausal estrogen synthesis and metabolism: alterations caused by aromatase inhibitors used for the treatment of breast cancer. J Steroid Biochem 35: 355–366
81. Fox KR, Glick JH, MacDonald JS et al 1993 Randomized phase II trial of Rogletimide in advanced breast cancer; A preliminary report. Breast Cancer Treat 27: 152
82. Dowsett M, Coombes RC 1994 Second generation aromatase inhibitor-4-hydroxyandrostenedione. Breast Cancer Res Treat 30: 81–87
83. Santen RJ, Demers LM, Lynch J et al 1991 Specificity of low dose fadrozole hydrochloride (CGS 16949A) as an aromatase inhibitor. J Clin Endocrinol Metab 73: 99–106
84. Iveson TJ, Smith IE, Ahern J et al 1993 Phase I study of the oral non steroidal aromatase inhibitor CGS 20267 in postmenopausal patients with advanced breast cancer. Cancer Res 53: 266–270
85. di Salle E, Ornati G, Giudici D et al 1992 Exemestane (FCE 24304) a new steroidal aromatase inhibitor. J Steroid Biochem Mol Biol 43: 137–143
86. Goss PE, Gwyn KMEH 1994 Current perspectives on aromatase inhibitors in breast cancer. J Clin Onc 12: 2460–2470
87. Allen JK, Fraser IS 1981 Cholesterol, high density lipoproteins and danazol. J Clin Endocrinol Metab 53: 149–151
88. Sakata M, Ohtsuka S, Kurachi H, Miyake A, Terakawa N, Tanizawa 1994 The hypothalamic-pituitary-ovarian axis in patients with endometriosis is suppressed by leuprolide acetate but not by danazol. Fertil Steril 61: 432–437
89. Fujimoto J, Hori M, Itoh T, Ichigo S, Nishigaki M, Tamaya T 1995 Danazol decreases transcription of estrogen receptor gene in human monocytes. Gen Pharmac 26: 507–516
90. Barbieri RL, Ryan KJ 1981 Danazol endocrine pharmacology and therapeutic application. Am J Obstet Gynecol 141: 453–465
91. Brogden RN, Goa KL, Faulds D 1993 Mifepristone: a review of its pharmacodynamic and pharmacokinetic properties and therapeutic potential. Drugs 45: 384–409
92. Horwitz KB 1992 The molecular biology of RU486. Is there a role for antiprogestins in the treatment of breast cancer. Endocrine Rev 13: 146–163
93. Grunberg SM, Weiss MH, Spitz IM et al 1991 Treatment of unresectable meningiomas with the antiprogesterone agent, mifepristone. J Neurosurg 74: 861–866
94. Kloosterboer HJ, Deckers GH, De-Gooyer ME, Dijkema R, Orlemans EOM, Schoonen W GEJ 1995 Pharmacological properties of a new selective antiprogestogen: Org 33628. Ann New York Acad Sci 761: 192–201

SECTION 5

Laboratory Assessment

CONTENTS

28. Assays for estrogens and progestogens

W.P. Collins

Introduction

Methods for measuring estrogenic or progestogenic activity, or the concentration of individual estrogens or progestogens, are still evolving. Bioassays were used initially to identify the principal estrogens and progestogens from ovarian fluids and tissues.[1] Subsequently chemical methods were developed to measure the steroid moiety of the main metabolites in urine.[2–4] The advent of competitive protein-binding assay[5] (particularly immunoassay) enabled the measurement of physiologically important steroids in peripheral blood[6] and saliva,[7] and related steroid glucuronides in urine.[8] Gas-liquid chromatography followed by mass spectrometry is widely regarded as the best reference method for quantitative steroid analysis.[9] Recently, genetic engineering techniques have been used to produce novel cellular assays of estrogenic activity.[10]

The advances in assay principles, design, format and equipment have been impressive, and even more exciting prospects are on the horizon with the development of nanotechnology (i.e. the systematic assembly of tests from individual molecules).[11] There is a notion, however, that most developments of clinical tests for estrogens or progestogens are more concerned with reducing the assay time and cost than with improving the accuracy and usefulness of the results under different circumstances. Accordingly, there is still a need for more information about the physiological and pathological changes that can occur in the production, transformation, protein binding and excretion of estrogens and progestogens. The role of non-protein bound (i.e. apparent free) or weakly protein bound steroids in peripheral blood is particularly intriguing.[12] There is also increasing evidence that the activity of endogenous estrogens (particularly in postmenopausal women) is affected by the uptake of estrogen mimetics in food[13] and water.[14]

The development of assays for the assessment of estrogenic and progestogenic status in women is reviewed in this chapter. Selected references are quoted to illustrate various trends and to provide a source of more detailed information. The ultimate technical objectives appear to be the production of self-contained procedures for the measurement of specific estrogens or progestogens (from endogenous or exogenous sources), or for the determination of indices that reflect estrogenic or progestogenic activity. There has been a long-term need for some of the tests to be performed at frequent intervals in sites outside of the laboratory.[15] Consequently, the research effort has been applied systematically to the measurement of biochemical markers in urine, peripheral blood and saliva. Recent developments should fulfil the technical desiderata, but prospective clinical trials will be required to evaluate and subsequently improve the assays for defined clinical purposes.

BIOASSAY

The original bioassays for estrogenic or progestogenic activities were based upon responses in the genital organs (oviducts, uterus, cervix and vagina) of experimental animals.[16,17] Estradiol (with a phenolic A ring) and progesterone (with a 3-oxo, 4 ene group) were found to be the most active of the estrogens or progestogens respectively. The presence of enzymes (e.g. 17β-hydroxysteroid dehydrogenase and 20α-hydroxysteroid reductase) in responsive tissues could have accounted for some of the observed activities of closely related steroids (e.g. estrone and 20α-dihydroprogesterone).

The most noticeable extragonadal effects of estrogens are on the skeleton and on the cardiovascular, endocrine and immune systems.[18] Some of the responses could be the result of changes in intra-organ blood flow. There is good evidence that the administration of estradiol to postmenopausal women can enhance blood flow in the uterine[19] and carotid[20] arteries. This action could result from the formation of catecholestrogens (e.g. 2-hydroxyestrone), which inhibit catechol methyl transferase activity, and thereby modulate the effects of catecholamines.[21] A multitude of biochemical indices (e.g. electrolytes, lipids, carbohydrates, proteins and nucleic acids) are modified by the presence of estrogens. Changes in the concentration of individual analytes in selected body fluids or tissues have been used to reflect estrogenic status and potential fertility.[22]

Recently, cellular based bioassays have been developed to test for estrogenic activity in new drugs and in samples of food or drink. The assays include the use of a breast cancer cell line (MCF 7) in a proliferation assay,[23] in an epithelial cell line which is only responsive to estrogenic compounds in terms of producing alkaline phosphatase,[24] in fish hepatocytes that produce vitellogenin,[25] and in cultured mammalian cells transformed by the introduction of the estrogen receptor gene.[10]

Protein binding assays

The concentrations and activities of putative estrogenic and progestogenic substances in peripheral blood are regulated by groups of circulating transport proteins.[12] Similarly, the main estrogenic and progestogenic effects at gonadal sites appear to be mediated through receptor proteins.[26] Crude preparations of the uterine receptor for estradiol and the main circulating protein for progesterone (corticosteroid-binding globulin), were used to develop the first protein binding assays.[27,28] These assays were quickly superseded by radioimmunoassays for the principal endogenous estrogens and progestogens,[29] due to the superior avidity, specificity, stability and availability of antibodies.

Immunoassay

Immunoassay is a technique based on the reaction between an antigen and an antibody for measuring the concentration of either reactant in solution. The development of immunoassays for steroids has generally followed the establishment of methods for the measurement of proteins, and alternative procedures have been described.[30,31] The description and classification of each immunoassay is complicated because the terminology can change when the technique is viewed from different perspectives. Immunoassays for estrogens or progestogens may involve a procedure for extracting the analyte from the biological fluid (i.e. extraction as opposed to direct assay). Some of the variables that contribute to the analytical performance and classification of an immunoassay are:

1. The underlying principle
2. The reference preparation and matrix
3. The binding characteristics of the antibodies
4. The technique for distinguishing between bound and free fractions of the labelled reagent
5. The type of label to monitor the binding reaction
6. The end-point reaction and measurement.

Extraction or direct assay

An extraction procedure can be used to isolate the total amount (i.e. protein-bound and apparent free fractions) of a particular estrogen or progestogen from a biological fluid or tissue prior to immunoassay. Traditionally, steroids have been extracted with an organic solvent (e.g. diethyl ether), which is subsequently evaporated. The extract is redissolved in buffer before analysis. Alternatively, direct immunoassays have been developed to approximate the total amount of a particular biologically active compound or a metabolite in the original matrix (e.g. serum, urine or saliva).

Competitive or noncompetitive assay

There are two basic types of immunoassay, which are usually referred to as competitive and non-competitive. The principles are illustrated in Figure 28.1. The first type is the conventional competitive binding assay with limited, constant amounts of reagents. In this example a specific (capture) antibody is coated onto a solid phase, and a labeled antigen is allowed to compete with the analyte for antibody binding sites. After the binding reaction the amount of labeled antigen associated with the solid phase (i.e. the number of antibody binding sites not occupied by the analyte) is inversely related to the amount of analyte. Accordingly, the level of nonspecific binding has a disproportionate effect on the measurement of higher amounts of analyte. A well optimized assay should measure the amount of estrogen or progestogen over two to three orders of magnitude with good precision (e.g. $<10\%$ coefficient of variation). The detection limit is dependent upon the practical errors (i.e. pipetting the sample, antibodies and antigen, and measuring the signal) and the affinity binding of the antibodies.

The second type is the noncompetitive binding, excess reagent assay (also known as the immunometricassay), which was developed initially for the

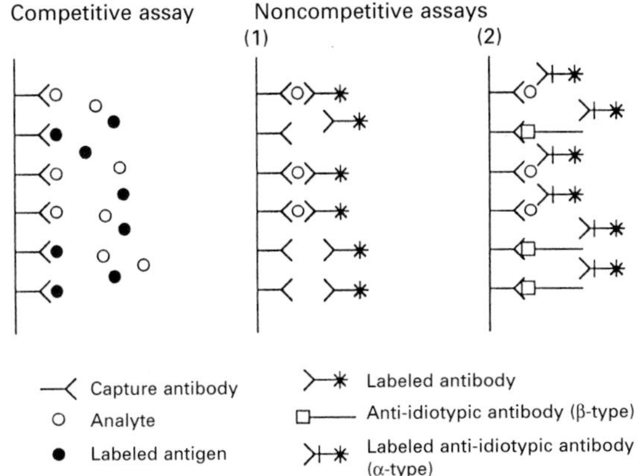

Fig. 28.1 Examples illustrating the principles of competitive and noncompetitive immunoassay. See text.

measurement of proteins with at least two epitopes (antigen binding sites). In this system (see Fig. 28.1, example 1, noncompetitive assay) an excess amount of capture antibody is attached directly, or indirectly, to a solid phase. A second, labelled antibody against a different epitope is added in excess at the start of the primary binding reaction (a one step procedure) or following phase separation (a two step procedure). After the binding reactions, the amount of labeled antibody associated with occupied binding sites of the capture antibody is directly related to the amount of analyte. The level of the nonspecific binding has a larger effect on the measurement of lower amounts of analyte. A good noncompetitive assay should measure the amount of analyte over four to five orders of magnitude with good precision (e.g. <5% coefficient of variation). The detection limit is dependent upon the sampling error, the nonspecific binding and the binding affinity of the antibodies.

Noncompetitive immunoassay has proved difficult to apply to estrogens or progestogens. Accordingly, alternative approaches have been devised to measure the number of binding sites on the capture antibody that have been occupied by analyte. An example using anti-idiotypic antibodies is illustrated in Figure 28.1, example 2, noncompetitive assay. A specific antibody is used to capture the analyte. An antibody against the binding site of the capture antibody (i.e. an anti-idiotypic antibody β type) is used to block the sites not occupied by analyte. A second (labeled) anti-idiotypic antibody (α type), which binds close to the binding site in the presence of analyte (but not in the presence of β-type anti-idiotypic antibody), is added to determine the number of occupied binding sites and hence the end-point of the assay.

Reference preparation and matrix

The form and purity of the authentic material and the composition of the surrounding matrix will affect the type and analytical performance of immunoassays for estrogens and progestogens. Reference preparations are used:

1. As solid phase antigens
2. For the production of immunogens and hence antibodies,
3. For the assay of extracted analytes
4. For the direct assay of total or weakly protein-bound and free analytes.

Most steroids are readily available in sufficient quantities to allow recrystallization before use. These materials fulfil the requirements for the first three uses. The development of universal matrices for the direct assay of different estrogenic and progestogenic fractions in peripheral blood or saliva is more difficult in theory and in practice. The direct assay of steroid glucuronides in diluted urine is relatively simple and noncontroversial.

Characteristics of antibodies

Antibodies constitute the most important reagents in immunoassays for estrogens and progestogens. Free steroid molecules (haptens) are too small to produce an immune response. There are, however, many chemical methods for linking steroids to larger carrier molecules (usually proteins) for the production of antibodies that are mainly directed against the characteristic functional groups of the hapten. The antibodies can be:

1. Poly or monoclonal
2. Mono, di or polyvalent
3. Mono or bispecific,
4. Antiallotypic or anti-idiotypic, and
5. Labeled or linked to a solid phase in a variety of ways.

Monoclonal antibodies are preferred in competitive binding immunoassays to ensure that the labeled or solid phase antigen and the analyte compete for the same binding site. They are essential in noncompetitive binding assays because of their well defined epitope specificity and purity. Most naturally occurring antibodies are divalent and all are monospecific. Recently, novel antibodies have been produced by hybrid-hybridomas and by the manipulation of antibody producing genes. The products may be labeled or linked to a solid phase by passive adsorption or covalent linkage.

Separation and nonseparation assays

Competitive and noncompetitive assays can be subdivided into separation (also known as heterogeneous) and nonseparation (also known as homogeneous) systems. A separation assay involves a step to isolate the antibody-bound or free fraction, in order to quantify the amount of label present. Conversely, the signal is measured in the presence of all reactants in a nonseparation assay — although a physical separation may occur in the assay tube (e.g. hemagglutination tests). The nonseparation assays are usually based on the finding that the antibodies can modulate the signal from either the bound or free fractions of analyte. Alternatively, the technique may involve fluorescence or chemical energy transfer from a labeled antigen to a labeled antibody.

Solid phases and labels

Traditionally, liquid-phase systems were preferred for the measurement of estrogens and progestogens. The antibody-bound fraction was either precipitated (e.g. with a second antibody) or the free analyte was absorbed with Dextran-coated charcoal (a solid phase reagent). Currently, solid phase systems are more popular because they permit simplification of the assay format and reduction of background binding. Some options in the choice of solid-support are: tubes, beads, particles, microtiter plates or strips, dipsticks, cards, pegs, electrodes, slides or fibers. The profusion of labels to monitor the antibody/antigen binding reaction can be categorized as particles, radionuclides, enzymes, substrates, cofactors, preluminescent derivatives or electronically active compounds.

End-points

Different labels can produce a variety of end-points. The ones used most frequently are listed in Table 28.1. The amount of label (in the antibody-bound or free fractions) at the end of an immunoassay may be measured in total or as a concentration. Alternatively, the end point may be a reaction rate.

Data processing and statistical analysis

Appropriate algorithms have been developed to fit the dose–response curves from competitive and noncompetitive assays, using four and five parameters respectively. Indices of the reliability of an assay include sensitivity (also known as the detection limit), within and between assay variation (also known as intra- and inter-assay variation) and precision and bias profiles.[33,33]

Body fluids

Analytes have been measured by immunoassay most frequently in peripheral venous or capillary plasma or serum; early morning, midmorning, early evening, daily or 24-hour urine collections; and saliva. Some characteristics of the three fluids are listed in Table 28.2. Methods have also been developed for the measurement of analytes in other body compartments, e.g. cervicovaginal fluid, milk or amniotic fluid.

Weakly protein-bound or free analytes

Most immunoassays for haptens involve the measurement of the total analyte in peripheral venous plasma or serum. There is a considerable amount of theoretical and experimental evidence, however, which is consistent with the hypothesis that the apparent free or weakly protein-bound fractions are associated with

Table 28.1 Labels and end-points used in immunoassay.

Labels	End-points
Particles	visual, turbidimetric, colorimetric, size analysis
Radionuclides	radioluminometric
Enzymes substrates cofactors	visual, turbidimetric colorimetric, fluorimetric, bioluminometric, potentiometric
Preluminescent compounds	fluorimetric chemiluminometric

Table 28.2 Some advantages and limitations to the use of alternative body fluids for the analysis of estrogens and progestogens.

Fluid	Characteristics
Urine	Noninvasive technique Contains high concentration of metabolites Uncertain relationship between concentration of analyte and fluid intake Use of early morning urine limits frequency of sampling pH and osmolarity may affect assay result
Peripheral or capillary venous blood	Invasive technique Requires the separation of erythrocytes Contains biologically active compounds Requires frequent sampling Contains endogenous binding proteins
Saliva	Sampling procedure can be invasive Contains particulate matter Low concentrations of estrogens and progestogens can reflect biologically active components pH, enzymes and endogenous binding proteins can affect assay result

the main biological activity of hormones and drugs. Consequently, methods have been devised for the measurement of free thyroid hormones, which either involve:

1. The back titration of exogenous antibody with labeled antigen
2. The competitive binding of a labeled analog of the antigen to a solid phase antibody
3. The use of a solid phase antigen and a labeled antibody.[34]

To date, there have been no reports of attempts to apply these approaches to the measurement of the relatively low levels of apparent free estrogens or progestogens.

Location and requirements

Immunoassays are usually performed in a laboratory — either by staff providing a centralized routine service or by research workers. The methodological requirements are for:

1. High sensitivity
2. The ability to process large numbers of samples and analytes
3. Rapid inexpensive assays with good quality control.

There is also a trend towards the development of tests for extra-laboratory use, such as in the clinic or ward (for point of contact testing) and the home (for self-testing). The requirements are for simple, quick, reliable, inexpensive tests (e.g. in the form of tube tests, pads, dipsticks or biosensors).

ESTROGENS

The development of methods for the estimation of individual endogenous estrogens (including estrone and estriol), pharmaceutical estrogen mimetics, and phytoestrogens (plant estrogens) in different biological samples has been reviewed.[35] Assays have also been reported for the measurement of xenoestrogens (i.e. industrial chemicals that have been released into the environment and mimic the activity of endogenous estrogens).[36]

Endogenous compounds

Approximate dates for the introduction of new assays, or important technical refinements for the measurement of estrogens in urine or estradiol in peripheral plasma or saliva are shown in Figure 28.2. The main trends appear to be towards the development of one step self-tests for estrone-3-glucuronide (EG) in urine and automated laboratory assays for estradiol in plasma or serum. The development of multi-analyte assays[37] is probably a desirable long-term objective for both approaches. Some details about the concentration of EG in early morning urine and estradiol in peripheral serum and saliva are given in Table 28.3.

Urinary estrone glucuronide

Urinary EG is an early, quantitively important metabolite of plasma estradiol.[15] Initially, reagents were prepared to measure the concentration of EG by

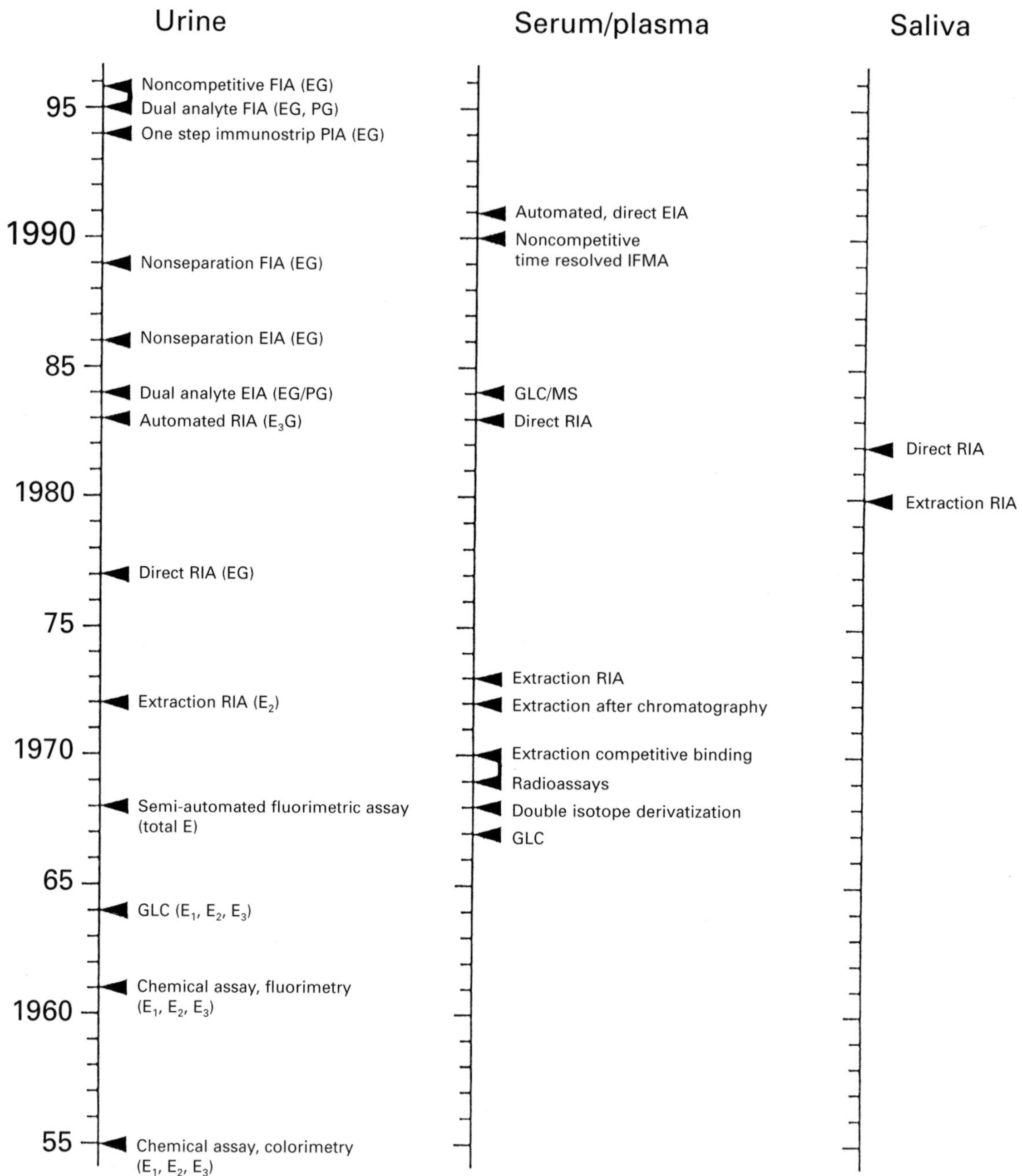

Fig. 28.2 Approximate dates for the introduction of new techniques (or important developments in immunoassay) for the measurement of estrogens in urine or estradiol in serum/plasma or saliva.[1,35,44]

direct, competitive radioimmunoassay. Reference preparations were prepared in assay buffer, and a tritiated antigen was synthesized.[8] The positions that have been used to link EG to a carrier molecule to form immunogens and the positions of functional groups on related steroid glucuronides or sulphates are shown in Figure 28.3. To date, antibodies to EG have been raised against immunogens in which a protein has been linked to the carboxyl group of the glucuronyl moiety (e.g. estrone-3-glucuronyl-6-bovine serum albumin).

Table 28.3 Immunochemical indices of estrogenic status during the follicular phase of the ovarian cycle.

Analyte	Fluid	Concentration		
		SI units	Median*	CF**
Estrone glucuronide	EMU	nmol/l	51	×0.446
Estradiol	Serum	pmol/l	325	×0.272
Estradiol	Saliva	pmol/l	6	×0.272

EMU: early morning urine; *day 1 of menses to day of urinary LH peak, data from author's laboratory; **conversion factor SI units to mass units

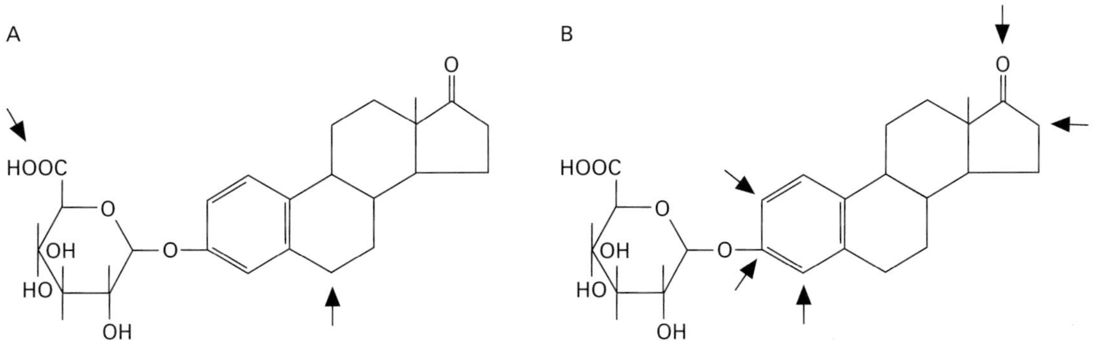

A

HOOC

O

OH

HO

O

OH

O

B

HOOC

O

OH

HO

O

OH

O

Fig. 28.3 (**A**) Principal sites of linkage between estrone glucuronide and a carrier molecule to form immunogens. (**B**) Positions of functional groups on related molecules.

There is, however, a paradigm of raising antibodies to an estrogen glucuronide by linking the hapten at carbon 6 of the steroid molecule to bovine serum albumin.[38] Similarly, antibodies to estrone-3-sulphate have been raised in a rabbit immunized with estrone-3-sulphate 6α hemisuccinyl-bovine serum albumin.[39] Monoclonal antibodies have been raised to estrone-3-glucuronide-6-bovine serum albumin. The best antibodies have <5% cross reactivity (CR) with unconjugated estrone and 2-hydroxyestrone-3-glucuronide, and <0.01% CR with unconjugated estradiol or estriol, and estrone-3-sulphate.

Self-contained assays

A nonseparation enzyme immunoassay for urinary EG has been described.[40,41] Lysozyme is used as the label and micrococcus as the substrate. The reagents are spatially distributed in an immunotube. The reactions are initiated sequentially by the addition of water and sample. Timed specimens of urine are collected for analysis. Each urine sample is diluted with tap water in a graduated jug to a final volume which corresponds to a secretion rate of 100 or 125 mL of urine/hour. A portion of the diluted urine is heated for 10 minutes in a water bath at 80°C to destroy endogenous lysozyme or bacteria. The test takes approximately 30 minutes to complete and has been evaluated for home use.

A method for the measurement of EG in early morning urine based upon nonseparation x time-resolved fluorescence has been developed.[42,43] The reference preparations are prepared in diluted male urine. A europium chelate, which is fluorescent in aqueous solution, is linked to EG to form the labeled antigen. The antibodies, labeled antigen and urine are incubated for 10 minutes at room temperature and fluorescence from the unbound fraction is measured. Background fluorescence is allowed to decay for 400 μsec after a pulse of light before the signal from the unbound labeled antigen is integrated over 600 μsec. The cycle is then repeated each millisecond for one second. The assay procedure has been shown to offer some correction for changes in urine production which may affect EG excretion (an unknown endogenous fluorescence quenching agent is apparently secreted in parallel with EG).

Noncompetitive immunoassay

A noncompetitive time-resolved fluoroimmunoassay has been reported for EG.[44] Two types of monoclonal anti-idiotypic antibodies are used that recognize different epitopes within the hypervariable region of the primary antibody. The principle of the assay is illustrated in Figure 28.1 (noncompetitive assays 2). This assay has vastly increased sensitivity compared with a competitive method using the same primary antibody, but requires the use of three (rather than two) reagents. The high sensitivity (0.4 nmol/L) and working range of the assay (up to 10 nmol/L) were appropriate for the direct assay of diluted urine during the menstrual cycle, but might be of particular value for the study of prepubertal and postmenopausal women. The β-type anti-idiotypic antibody has been labeled with a europium chelate and used in a conventional competitive immunoassay for studies of women during reproductive life.

Plasma/serum estradiol

There is a consensus that the concentration of total unconjugated estradiol in the peripheral circulation is the best hormonal index of estrogen status, particularly in terms of endogenous production in the premenopausal woman. Recommendations for the provision of a laboratory service for the measurement of estradiol have been published.[45] There is some evidence that the amount of apparent free and weakly protein-bound estradiol represents the potentially active fraction in growth responsive tissues.[35]

Total unconjugated estradiol

The first immunoassays for plasma or serum estradiol involved the use of a tritiated antigen and polyclonal antibodies to estradiol 17β-hemisuccinate-bovine serum albumin. The cross reactivity of this antiserum with estrone, estradiol 17β-sulphate and estradiol 17β-glucuronide necessitated the use of an extraction step and the chromatographic separation of unconjugated estradiol from related phenolic steroids. The purified extracts were dried and redissolved in assay buffer. The reference preparation was prepared in the same matrix.

More specific polyclonal antisera were produced from alternative immunogens. The principal sites of estradiol metabolism in nonpregnant women (so producing potentially cross reacting compounds) and the positions of chemical linkage to carrier molecules to form immunogens are shown in Figure 28.4. Estradiol-6-carboxymethyl-oxime-bovine serum albumin produced the best antisera (polyclonal and monoclonal) for use in immunoassay. This development reduced the need for a chromatographic step before the antibody binding reaction in the assay procedure.

Iodine-125 (which does not require scintillation fluid to produce an end-point) was used subsequently to label various derivatives of estradiol. Representations of the structure of 2,4,6,7-tritiated estradiol and estradiol-6-carboxymethyl oxime-diiodohistamine are shown with the authentic steroid and a relevant part of the corresponding immunogen in Figure 28.5. The structure of the tritiated derivative is similar to estradiol (only differing by four protons), whereas the iodinated derivative resembles a larger portion of the immunogen. The relative affinities of these compounds is dependent upon the characteristics of the antibodies.

The use of iodinated labeled antigens (together with agents to block binding to endogenous circulating proteins) facilitated the development of direct (nonextraction) immunoassays (some of which now involve the use of nonisotopic labels). These assays are undoubtedly simpler and are widely used in clinical laboratories. Nevertheless doubts have been raised

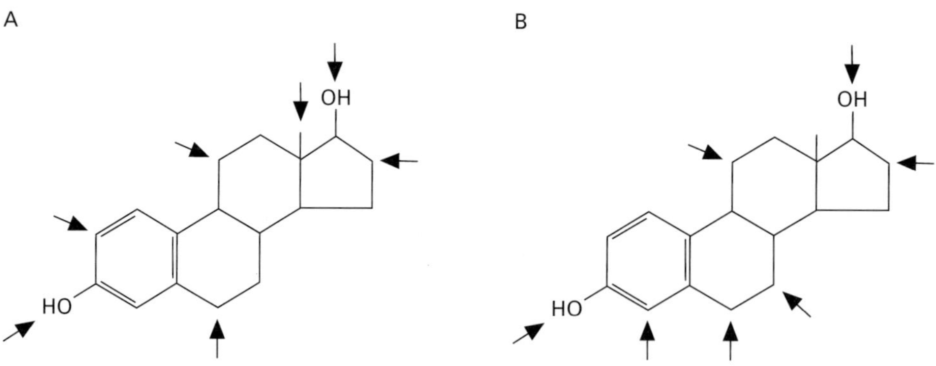

Fig. 28.4 **A** Principal sites of estradiol metabolism in women. **B** Positions of chemical linkage to carrier molecules to form immunogens.

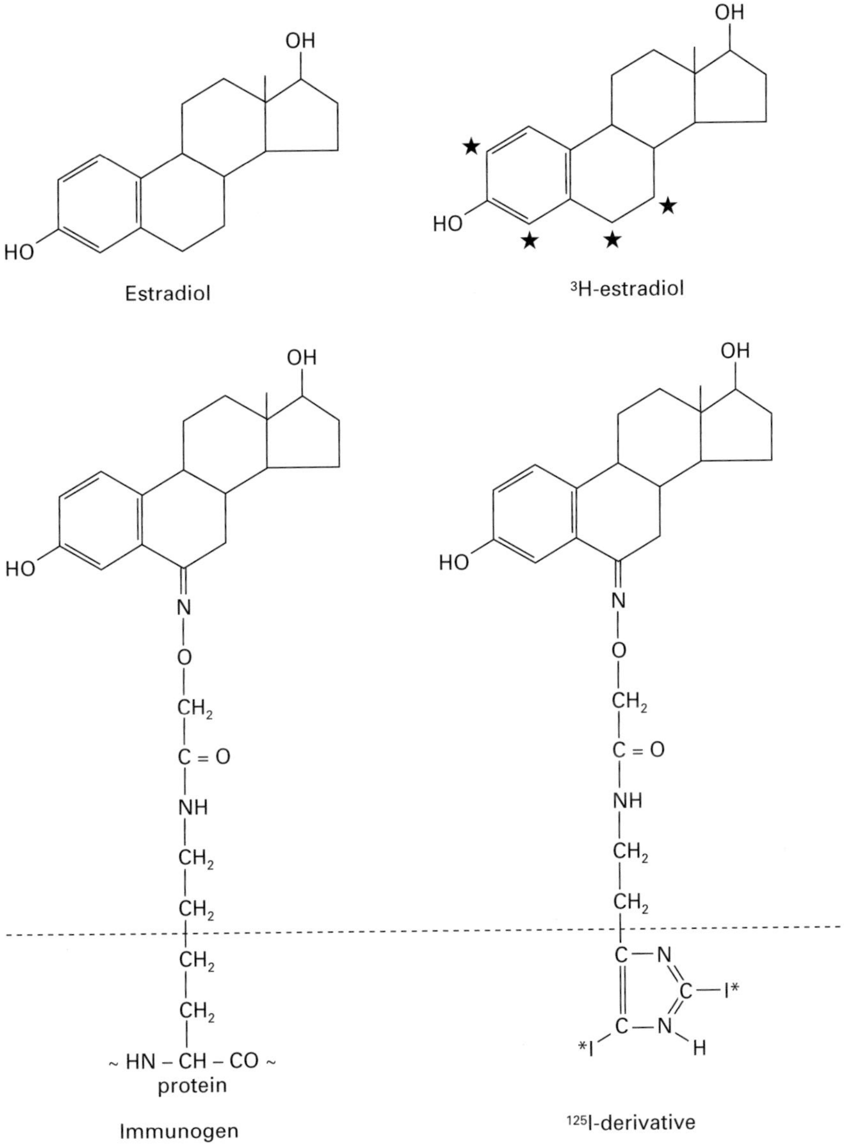

Fig. 28.5 Molecular structure of the principal immunogen for raising antibodies to estradiol and examples of labeled antigens.

about the reliability of some test results.[46] The labeled antigens bind to some extent to plasma proteins and a two step procedure for the assay of estradiol has been shown to be more reliable.[47]

Noncompetitive immunoassay

A direct, noncompetitive assay using time-resolved fluorescence as the end-point has been reported.[48] This development, which involved the sequential incubation of reagents, initially produced a similar sensitivity (around 50 pmol/L) to a conventional competitive assay using the same primary antibody, but a wider working range (from 50 pmol/L – > 50 000 pmol/L). The within assay batch precision was < 10%. The assay bias was negligible at all dose levels. Similar results were obtained with a europium label[49] or an enzyme label in a single stage assay.[50] The β-type anti-idiotypic antibody has been labeled with a europium chelate and used in a competitive immunoassay.[49]

Apparent free/weakly protein-bound estradiol

Indirect procedures involving the use of tritiated estradiol and equilibrium dialysis, steady state gel filtration or ultracentrifugation have been used to estimate the level of apparent free estradiol in the peripheral circulation.[35] Values of 0.5–2.0% of the total level of estradiol have been reported. To date, there is no convincing evidence to justify the use of these methods in clinical practice. The development of a reliable method to measure the amount of estradiol which is weakly bound to proteins remains a challenge.

Catechol estrogens

The catechol estrogens contain an additional hydroxyl group at C-2 or C-4. These compounds are regarded as metabolites of estrone or estradiol that may link the endocrine and neuroendocrine systems by competing with catecholamines for the enzyme catechol-O-methyl transferase.[21] The corresponding monomethyl ethers of the catechol estrogens are relatively stable compounds. Under certain conditions, however, catechol estrogens can be oxidized to quinones, which can form DNA adducts and possibly cause gene mutations.[51]

Extraction immunoassays using tritiated antigens have been reported for the measurement of 2-hydroxyestrone and 2-methoxyestrone in acid hydrolysed urine.[35] Antisera to both metabolites were raised by linking the authentic compounds through C-17 to bovine serum albumin. The concentration of the methylated form was found to be about ten fold higher than the unconjugated estrogen. The pattern of daily levels throughout the menstrual cycle was similar to that reported for EG in urine.[52] The concentration of 2-hydroxyestrone in peripheral plasma remains controversial.[35]

Salivary estradiol

The concentration of estradiol in saliva is independent of the flow rate of the fluid and probably reflects the apparent free concentration in plasma or serum[53] (see Table 28.3 for mean concentration in premenopausal women). Accordingly, well matched antibodies and labeled antigens with a high specific activity (i.e. the signal to mass ratio) are required to achieve the sensitivity needed for direct (nonextraction) assays. Appropriate methods involving the use of antibodies to estradiol-6-carboxymethyl oxime-bovine serum albumin and radioactive, enzymatic or chemiluminescent labels have been reported.[35] Reference preparations of authentic estradiol are usually prepared in pooled saliva samples from men. The results from a multicenter evaluation of assays for estradiol in saliva that included the provision of common samples for quality assessment were encouraging.[54]

Extracted or synthetic drugs

A mixture of estrogens from pregnant mares' urine (predominantly estrone, equilin, equilenin and the corresponding 3-sulphate derivatives, Premarin) or ethinyl estradiol (a synthetic estrogen), can be used for estrogen replacement therapy in women. Ethinyl estradiol (or its 3-methyl ether derivative, mestranol) is used for the estrogen component of oral contraceptive formulations.

Plasma or serum equilin

An extraction radioimmunoassay for equilin has been reported using an antiserum to equilin-3-hemisuccinate-bovine serum albumin and the corresponding ^{125}I-iodohistamine derivative as the labeled antigen. There was minimal cross reactivity with estrone, equilenin, estradiol or ring-β diunsaturated steroids. The method was suitable for measuring equilin in peripheral plasma from postmenopausal women taking the preparation of equine estrogens (Premarin).[55]

Plasma or serum ethinyl estradiol

An extraction radioimmunoassay for 17α-ethinyl estradiol has been reported using an antiserum to ethinyl estradiol-3-hemisuccinate-bovine serum albumin.[56] Tritiated ethinyl estradiol was used to monitor extraction losses and higher amounts constituted the labeled antigen in the antibody binding reaction. The cross-reactivity with related naturally occurring, unconjugated estrogens was $<3\%$. Antisera with good specificity (even to conjugated estrogens) have been raised to ethinyl estradiol-6-thioproprionate-bovine serum albumin.[57] The same approach produced good antisera to 17α-ethinyl estradiol-3-methyl ether (mestranol). Importantly, antibodies for natural estradiol-17β do not cross react with ethinyl estradiol or mestranol.

Phytoestrogens

Two groups of compounds with diphenolic structures (the lignans and the isoflavonic phytoestrogens) have been identified in human urine and other biological fluids. A method involving gas-liquid chromatography/mass spectroscopy (using selection monitoring and deuterated internal standards) has been reported[13] for measuring the lignans enterolactone and enterodiol and the isoflavonic phytoestrogen metabolites daizein, equol and O-desmethylangolensin. The appropriate conjugated derivatives were extracted from urine (2.5–10.0 ml), purified by ion-exchange chromatography and hydrolysed enzymatically. The products were re-extracted and the trimethyl silyl ether derivatives were formed for analysis. The method has been used to study the urinary excretion of lignans and isoflavonoid phytoestrogens in women (and men) consuming a traditional Japanese diet.[58]

Xenoestrogens

A variety of phenolic compounds (used in the manufacture of various pesticides, plasticisers, food additives, detergents or antioxidants) have been shown to possess estrogenic activity.[14,25] An attempt to separate the xenoestrogens in human peripheral plasma from the endogenous estrogens and phytoestrogens has been reported. The initial aim was to assess estrogenic activity in the purified fractions using a cell proliferation bioassay or by measuring the induced formation of a progesterone receptor protein.[36]

PROGESTOGENS

The development of methods for the estimation of individual endogenous progestogens (or their inactive metabolites) in various body fluids and of synthetic progestogens in the peripheral circulation has been reviewed in detail.[59] Recommendations for the provision of a laboratory service for the measurement of plasma or serum progesterone have been published.[60]

Endogenous compounds

Approximate dates for the introduction of new assays and other important technical developments for the measurement of the main progestogen metabolites in urine or progesterone in peripheral plasma or saliva are shown in Figure 28.6. There has always been the tendency to measure total pregnanediol — mainly pregnanediol-3α, 20α-diol (after hydrolysis) or the main conjugate 5β-pregnanediol-20α-ol-3α-glucuronide (PG) in urine, and progesterone in peripheral plasma or saliva. The relatively high levels of these compounds compared to the estrogens has facilitated the development of methods for their measurement. Some details about the concentration of PG in EMU and progesterone in peripheral serum and saliva are given in Table 28.4.

Urinary pregnanediol glucuronide

Urinary PG is a quantitatively important metabolite of plasma progesterone.[15] The concentration can be measured in diluted urine by direct immunoassay using a tritiated antigen.[8] The position that has been used to link PG to a carrier molecule to form an immunogen, and the positions of functional groups on related steroid glucuronides or sulfates, are shown in Figure 28.7. Polyclonal and monoclonal antibodies have been raised for use in immunoassay with a variety of labelled antigens.[15] The best antibodies have <5% cross reactivity (CR) with unconjugated 5β-pregnanediol, and <2% with 5β-pregnanetriol-3α-glucuronide (a metabolite of 17-hydroxyprogesterone). The reference preparations are usually prepared in assay buffer (for radioimmunoassay) or diluted male urine (for nonisotopic immunoassay).

A separation enzyme immunoassay involving immunoconcentration for urinary PG has been marketed as a self-test (SAFEPLAN™, Quidel, San Diego, California, USA) with the aim of helping women to locate the start of the infertile (luteal) phase of the menstrual cycle.

Self-contained immunoassay

A nonseparation enzyme immunoassay for urinary PG has been evaluated for use in the clinic or home.[40,41] The test procedure is similar to that described for estrone glucuronide, but the reactions take only 10 minutes to complete. The use of immunotubes and an electronic device to measure EG and PG in daily samples of urine constitutes the Home Ovarian Monitor (St Michael Research Foundation, University of Melbourne, Australia) which was launched in 1987.

Plasma/serum progesterone

Immunoassays have been developed for the measurement of progesterone, 17-hydroxprogesterone[61] or 20α-dihydroprogesterone[62] in the peripheral circulation. The concentration of progesterone appears to be the most informative hormonal index of corpus luteum function. There is also the possibility that the apparent free and weakly protein-bound progesterone represents the potentially active fraction in responsive tissues.

The first immunoassays for plasma or serum progesterone involved the use of progesterone labeled

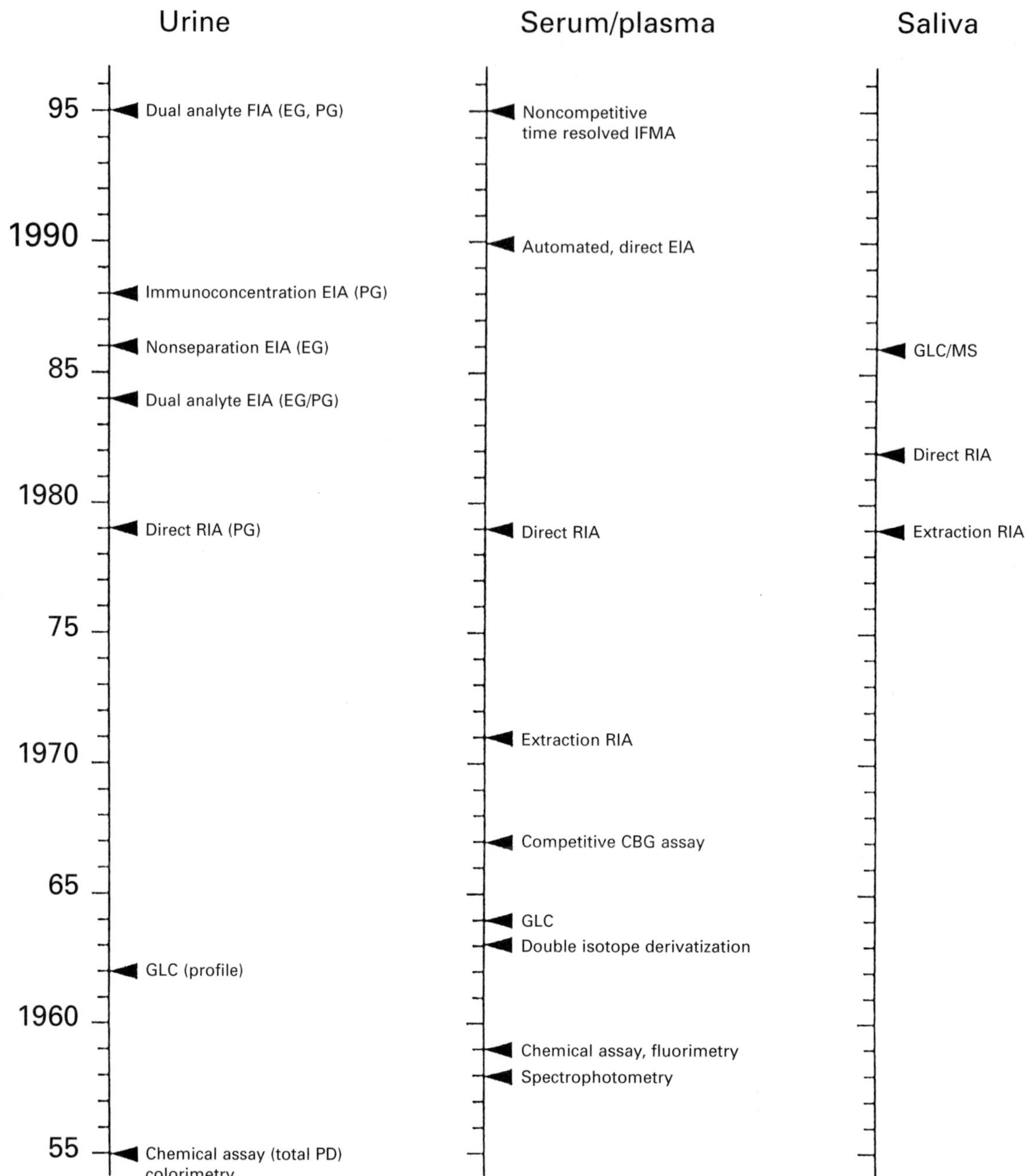

Fig. 28.6 Approximate dates for the introduction of new techniques (or important developments in immunoassay) for the measurement of progesterone metabolites in urine or progesterone in serum/plasma or saliva.[1,59,64]

with tritium in the 1, 2, 6 and 7 positions, and polyclonal antibodies to 11-desoxycortisol-21-hemisuccinate-human serum albumin or progesterone-3-carboxymethyl oxime-bovine serum albumin. The cross reactivities of these antisera with related steroids necessitated the use of an extraction step (with hexane or diethyl ether) and the chromatographic separation of progesterone from related neutral steroids. The

Table 28.4 Immunochemical indices of progestogenic status during the luteal phase of the ovarian cycle.

Analyte	Fluid	Concentration		
		SI units	Median*	CF**
Pregnanediol glucuronide	EMU	µmol/l	9.4	×0.496
Progesterone	Serum	nmol/l	17.2	×0.315
Progesterone	Saliva	pmol/l	223.6	×0.315

EMU: early morning urine; *day of urinary LH peak plus 1, to day 1 or next menses minus 1, data from author's laboratory; **conversion factor SI units to mass units

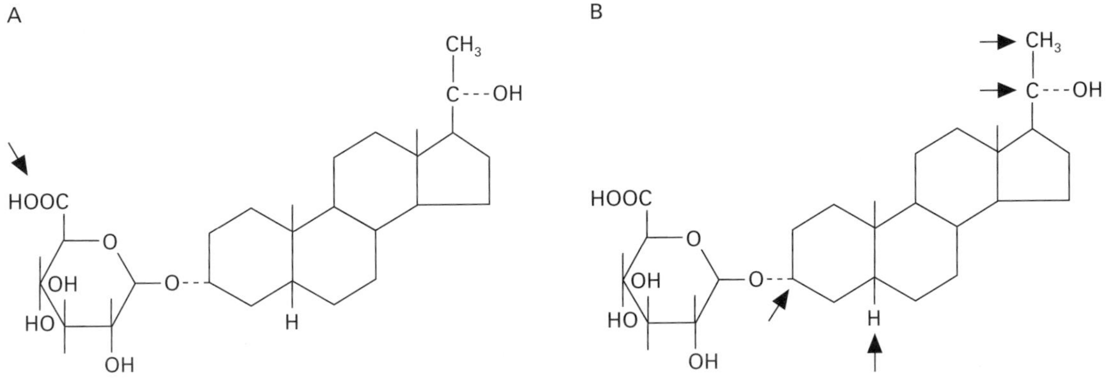

Fig. 28.7 (**A**) Principal site of linkage between pregnanediol glucuronide and a carrier molecule to form an immunogen. (**B**) Positions of functional groups or stereochemical changes in related molecules.

purified extracts were dried and redissolved in assay buffer. The reference preparation was prepared in the same matrix.

More specific polyclonal antisera were produced from other immunogens. The principal sites of progesterone metabolism in nonpregnant women (so producing potentially cross-reacting compounds) and the positions of chemical linkage to carrier molecules to form immunogens are shown in Figure 28.8. A detailed analysis of the relative concentrations of metabolites in peripheral plasma from nonpregnant women suggests that more specific antisera would be

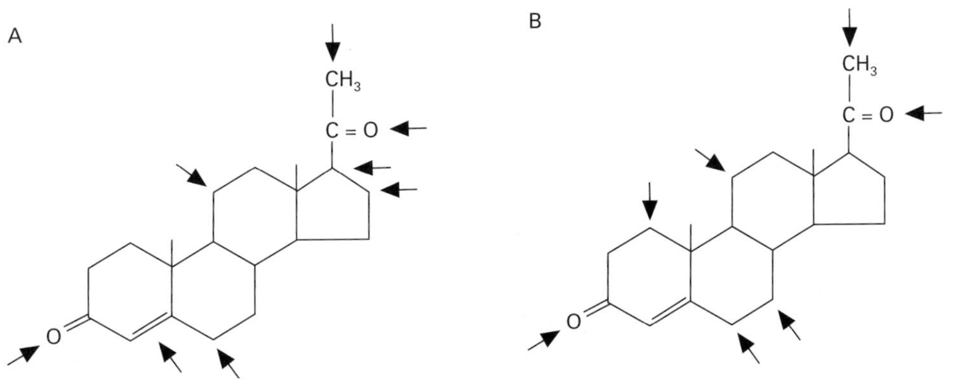

Fig. 28.8 (**A**) Principal sites of progesterone metabolism in women. (**B**) Positions of chemical linkage to carrier molecules to form immunogens.

produced if the linkage was applied to the 11α position on the progesterone molecule. The use of progesterone-11α-hemisuccinate-bovine thyroglobulin has produced good antisera (polyclonal and monoclonal) for use in immunoassay. This development reduced the need for a chromatographic step in assays designed to assess corpus luteum function.

Various derivatives of progesterone labeled with iodine-125 have been synthesized and tested in direct immunoassays (e.g. 11α-hydroxyprogesterone-11α-(4-hydroxyphenol) proprionate, progesterone-11α-succinyl iodohistamine). These assays are easy to use and produce reliable results during the luteal phase of the ovarian cycle.[63]

Noncompetitive immunoassay

A direct, noncompetitive assay using time-resolved fluorescence as the end-point has been reported for the measurement of plasma progesterone using primary (labeled) antibodies to progesterone-7α-carboxy-methyl-thioether bovine serum albumin.[64] The detection limit was 0.32 nmol/L and the working range extended to 7000 nmol/L. There was no apparent bias in the results (compared with a direct RIA) for samples taken from healthy women or patients undergoing treatment for infertility by *in vitro* fertilization and embryo transfer.

Apparent free/weakly protein-bound progesterone

The results of studies involving equilibrium dialysis and ultrafiltration have shown that a large percentage (>98%) of the progesterone in plasma is bound to various protein fractions — serum albumin, α_1-glycoprotein or corticosteroid binding globulin.[59] By analogy with plasma cortisol, the apparent free or weakly bound fraction is thought to be the biologically active material.

Salivary progesterone

The original assays for salivary progesterone involved solvent extraction (2–10 ml of saliva), the use of a tritiated antigen and antisera to progesterone-11α-hemisuccinate-bovine serum albumin.[65] The synthesis of radio-iodinated progesterone-11α-glucuronide tyramine enabled the development of a direct assay.[66] The standards were prepared in pooled male saliva. Although occasional anomalously high results have been reported, the method produces useful serial data for the assessment of ovarian function.

A gas-liquid chromatographic/mass spectrometric method has been developed for the measurement of progesterone in saliva. The procedure involved the use of 7,7-$^2H_2$ progesterone as an internal standard.[67] Progesterone was extracted by immunoadsorption and the 3-enol heptafluorobutyrate derivative was formed. The derivative was purified by gas-liquid chromatography using a capillary column, and the amount of progesterone was determined by selected ion monitoring. The sensitivity of the method was 10 pg per aliquot. There was a good correlation with values obtained by the radioimmunoassay of progesterone in saliva from adolescent girls.

Synthetic drugs

Extraction radioimmunoassays have been reported for the measurement of the synthetic progestogens based on 19-nortestosterone (norethindrone and D-norgestrel), the C-21 progestogens (medroxprogesterone acetate and cyproterone acetate) and an antiprogestogen (mifepristone). Immunoassays have also been reported for the measurement of norethisterone in saliva and D-norgestrol in milk. The procedures have been reviewed.[59] Methods for the measurement of norethindrone and medroxyprogesterone acetate have been validated by the concomitant use of gas-liquid chromatography/mass spectrometry.

TECHNICAL DEVELOPMENTS

There have been notable recent developments in the immunoassay of estrogens and progestogens, and in the production of novel binding reagents for individual compounds and specific molecular groupings.

Automated systems

Methods for the direct, separation enzyme immunoassay of estradiol and progesterone in peripheral plasma or serum have been automated. For example, the BAYER IMMUNO 1™ system (Bayer Corporation, Business Group Diagnostics, Tarrytown, New York, USA) involves the use of an alkaline phosphatase label and a spectrophotometric end-point. The antibodies are linked to solid particles and a magnet is used to separate the bound labeled antigen. The IMMUNOLITE™ system (Diagnostics Products Corporation, Los Angeles, California, USA) involves the use of an alkaline phosphatase label and a chemiluminescence end-point. The respective antibodies are linked to polystyrene beads and the unbound label is removed by washing. The tests take from 40–60 minutes to complete. Preliminary data show that the sensitivity for both analytes is adequate for routine purposes and the within and between assay precision is good.[68-70] There were close correlations between the values derived by automated assay and those obtained by established manual direct radioimmunoassays.

Point of contact and self-tests

Simple one step tests for urinary hCG and LH based on immuno-chromatography have been marketed by Unipath Ltd, Bedford, UK. The devices for home use (Clearblue One Step and Clearplan One Step) contain a wick to be held in a stream of urine. A predetermined amount of the absorbed sample is transferred automatically to an immunostrip which contains dried reagents for a noncompetitive binding particle immunoassay. One of the antibodies is labeled with latex spheres loaded with blue dye. The sample and reagent travel along the strip by capillary action. After the binding reaction, the components containing the labeled reagent are held in a window by capture antibodies. A second window contains a reagent to show that the test has worked and (in the case of LH) indicates when the value for the unknown sample has passed a predetermined level. Each test takes less than two minutes to produce a result.

The test strips have been modified to measure the concentrations of estrone glucuronide and LH simultaneously in the same sample.[71] The estrone glucuronide is measured by a direct competitive binding particle immunoassay. A limited amount of antibody labeled with the colored latex spheres reacts with the analyte. The labeled antibody with unoccupied binding sites is captured by immobilized immunogen at a separate location in the detection zone. An electronic instrument measures the end-point and processes the signal. The tests and instrument comprise the Personal Contraceptive System (Unipath Ltd, Bedford, UK), which is designed to locate the time of potential fertility during each menstrual cycle. The same procedure with appropriate reagents could be used to measure the concentration of pregnanediol glucuronide in urine.

Conclusion

There have been remarkable advances in the development of tests to measure the concentration of individual estrogens or progestogens, or total estrogenic or progestogenic activity. Nevertheless, the ultimate aim of producing simple protein binding tests for use in the home or at the point of patient contact remains to be achieved. The availability of such tests, used in conjunction with techniques for diagnostic imaging, would provide immediate complementary information for clinical or research purposes. The main problems to be overcome are the wide variations in the concentration of the principal endogenous estrogens and progestogens (over four orders of magnitude throughout life including pregnancy), corresponding changes in the proportion of related compounds (hence potentially interfering with specific assays), and the changing presence of endogenous binding proteins in various biological fluids.

Technical strategies to improve assay simplification, specificity and clinical usefulness have included the development of new assay formats (including polymerized bilayer assemblies) and the use of new labels and techniques for signal amplification.[72] The use of new approaches for the production of more specific antibodies or binding peptides[73] with a high affinity for individual estrogens or progestogens would enhance the development of single or multi-analyte assays. Similarly the availability of antibodies or peptide fragments that mimic the hapten binding characteristics of estrogen or progestogen receptors could lead to the development of simple tests for total estrogenic or progestogenic activities. Alternative methods of measuring more than one analyte in the same sample have included the use of different labels[74] or the spatial distribution of reagents.[75,76]

The pioneering work of Brown et al on the application of self-contained enzyme immunoassays for urinary EG and PG demonstrated that home tests could be used to monitor ovulation induction[77] and to locate the period of potential fertility during successive normal menstrual cycles.[78] The production of simpler one step tests (with a urine sampling member) based on particle labeled immunochromatography[71] has provided a paradigm for the development of simple multi-analyte tests for combinations of estrogens and/or progestogens (or their metabolites). Modifications to the basic immunochromatography format which may improve the competitive immunoassay of some haptens (drugs) have been suggested.[79] Alternative approaches to the development of non-competitive immunoassays for haptens have also been reported. For example, Piran et al.[80] have produced an assay for tri-iodothyronine based upon a solid-support for one of the reagents producing steric hindrance to one of the binding reactions. Self et al have achieved the ultimate objective of a conventional two site assay for digoxin after raising an antibody against the occupied binding site of the captive antibody.[81] Both approaches to the development of noncompetitive assays might be used eventually for the assay of estrogens or progestogens (or their metabolites) in conjunction with a dipstick or biosensor.

There has been a tendency to apply the new technologies to the measurement of metabolites in urine. This approach appears to be the most practicable for the longitudinal multi-analyte assessment of endogenous estrogen and progestogen production and metabolism. The analysis of random samples of peripheral venous blood, however, would appear to be more suitable for the assessment of estrogenic or progestogenic status at the target tissues of postmenopausal women — particularly if the weakly protein-bound and apparent free fractions could be isolated (e.g. by using antibodies to sex hormone-binding globulin and corticosteroid-binding globulin to remove the strongly bound fractions). Stabilized forms of the estrogen and progestogen receptors, or antibody fragments with similar binding characteristics, could be used to measure total estrogenic and progestogenic activities. The development of efficient, simple devices for sampling saliva[82] might encourage the development of alternative tests for the serial determination of biologically active estrogens and progestogens in a readily accessible body fluid. There is also a need for the production of simple tests that provide a measure of hormonal concentration or activity together with a biochemical index of a resultant biochemical action.

The awareness of the necessity to monitor the production and activity of endogenous estrogens and the intake and influence of exogenous estrogen mimetics will undoubtedly stimulate the production of a new generation of protein binding tests.

REFERENCES

1. Loraine JA 1958 Clinical applications of hormone assay. Churchill Livingstone, Edinburgh
2. Brown JB 1955 A chemical method for the determination of oestriol, oestrone and oestradiol in human urine. Biochemical Journal 60: 185–193
3. Brown JB, Macleod SC, Macnaughton C, Smith MA, Smyth B 1968 A rapid method for estimating estrogens in urine using a semi-automated extractor. Journal of Endocrinology 42: 5–15
4. Klopper A 1968 Determination of pregnanediol in urine by spectrophotometry or gas-liquid chromatography. In: Dorfman RI (ed) Methods of hormone research. Academic Press, New York, pp 273–280
5. Murphy BEP 1967 Some studies of the protein binding of steroids and their application to the routine micro and ultramicro measurement of various steroids in body fluids by competitive protein-binding radioassay. Journal of Endocrinology 27: 973–990
6. Abraham GE, Garza R. Radioimmunoassay of steroids. In: Abraham GE (ed) Handbook of radioimmunoassay. Marcel Dekker, New York, pp 591–656
7. Vining RF, McGinley RA 1986 Hormones in saliva. CRC Critical Reviews in Clinical Laboratory Science 23: 95–146
8. Samarajeewa P, Baker TS, Coulson WF 1983 The urinary assay of steroid glucuronides: their value and methodology. In: Hunter WM, Corrie JET (eds) Immunoassays for clinical chemistry. Churchill Livingstone, Edinburgh, pp 414–421
9. Makin HLJ, Honour JW, Shackleton CHL 1995 General methods of steroid analysis. Part 1. Extraction, purification and measurement of steroids by high-performance liquid chromatography, gas-liquid chromatography and mass spectrometry. In: Makin HLJ, Gower DB, Kirk DN (eds) Steroid analysis. Blackie Academic and Professional, London, pp 114–184
10. Miksicek RJ 1994 Interaction of naturally occurring nonsteroidal estrogens with expressed recombinant human estrogen receptor. Journal of Steroid Biochemistry and Molecular Biology 49: 153–160
11. Kaehler T 1994 Nanotechnology: basic concepts and definitions. Clinical Chemistry 40: 1797–1799
12. Tait JF, Tait SAS 1991 The effect of plasma protein binding on the metabolism of steroid hormones. Journal of Endocrinology 131: 339–357
13. Adlercreutz H, Fotsis T, Bannwart C, Wahalak K, Makela T, Brunow G, Hase T 1986 Determination of urinary lignans and phytoestrogen metabolities, potential antiestrogens and anticarcinogens, in urine of women on various habitual diets. Journal of Steroid Biochemistry 25: 791–797
14. White R, Jobling S, Hoare SA, Sumpter JP, Parker MG 1994 Environmentally persistent alkyphenolic compounds are estrogenic. Endocrinology 135: 175–182
15. Collins WP 1992 Immunochemical tests of potential fertility. Biochemical Society Transcripts 20: 234–237
16. Emmens CW 1962 Estrogens. In: Dorfman RI (ed) Methods in hormone research, vol 2. Academic Press, New York, pp 59–111
17. Miyake T 1962 Progestational substances. In: Dorfman RI (ed) Methods in hormone research, vol 2. Academic Press, New York, pp 127–178
18. Lobo RA 1994 Treatment of the postmenopausal woman: basic and clinical aspects. Raven Press, New York
19. Bourne T, Hillard T, Crook D, Campbell S 1990 Evidence for a rapid effect of oestrogens on the arterial status of postmenopausal women. Lancet 335: 1470–1471
20. Gangar K, Vyas S, Whitehead MI, Crook D, Meire H, Campbell S 1992 Pulsatility index in the internal carotid artery is influenced by transdermal oestradiol and time since menopause. Lancet 338: 839–842
21. Ball P, Knuppen R 1990 Formation, metabolism and physiologic importance of catecholestrogens. American Journal of Obstetrics and Gynecology 163: 2163–2170
22. Albertson BA, Zinaman MJ 1987 The prediction of ovulation and monitoring of the fertile period. Advances in Contraception 3: 263–290

23. Soto AM, Sonnenschein C, Chung KL, Fernandez MF, Olea N, Olea-Serrano MF 1995 The E-SCREEN assay as a tool to identify estrogens: an update on estrogenic environmental pollutants. Environmental Health Perspectives 103: 113–122
24. Littlefield BA, Gurpide E, Markiewicz L, McKinley B, Hockberg RB 1990 A simple and sensitive microtitre plate estrogen bioassay based on stimulation of alkaline phosphatase in Ishikawa cells: estrogenic action of Δ^5 adrenal steroids. Endocrinology 127: 2757–2762
25. Jobling S, Sumpter JP 1993 Detergent components in sewage effluent are weakly estrogenic to fish — an in vitro study using rainbow trout (*Oncorhynchus mykiss*) hepatocytes. Aquatic Toxicology 27: 361–372
26. Parker MG 1993 Steroid and related receptors. Current Opinion in Cell Biology 5: 499–504
27. Korenman SG 1968 Radio-ligand binding assay of specific estrogens using a soluble uterine macromolecule. Journal of Clinical Endocrinology and Metabolism 28: 127–130
28. Johansson EDB 1969 Progesterone levels in peripheral plasma during the luteal phase of the normal human menstrual cycle measured by a rapid competitive protein binding technique. Acta Endocrinologica 61: 592–606
29. Collins WP, Hennam JF, Tyler JPP, Barnard GJR 1975 Factors affecting the radioimmunoassay of gonadal steroids. In: Pasternak CA (ed) Radioimmunoassay in clinical biochemistry. Heydon, London, pp 153–169
30. Collins WP 1985 Alternative immunoassays. John Wiley & Sons, Chichester
31. Collins WP 1988 Complementary immunoassays. John Wiley & Sons, Chichester
32. Jeffcoate SL 1981 Efficiency and effectiveness in the endocrine laboratory. Academic Press, London
33. Dudley RA, Edwards P, Ekins RP, Finney DJ, McKenzie IGM, Raab GM, Rodbard D, Rogers RPC 1985 Guidelines for immunoassay data processing. Clinical Chemistry 31: 1264–1271
34. Ekins R 1992 The free hormone hypothesis and measurement of free hormones. Clinical Chemistry 38: 1289–1293
35. Oakey RE, Holder G 1995 The measurement of estrogens. In: Makin HLJ, Gower DB, Kirk DN (eds) Steroid analysis. Blackie Academic and Professional, London, pp 427–467
36. Sonnenschein C, Soto AM, Fernandez MF, Olea N, Olea-Serrano FM, Ruiz-Lopez MD 1995 Development of a marker of estrogen exposure in human serum. Clinical Chemistry 41: 1888–1895
37. Kricka LJ 1992 Multianalyte testing. Clinical Chemistry 38: 327–328
38. Honjo H, Otsubo K, Yasuda J, Kitawaki J, Okada H, Ohkubo T, Nambara T 1984 Conjugated estrogen during the menstrual cycle measured by direct radioimmunoassay with an antiserum prepared against oestradiol-17-glucosiduronate -[C-6]- BSA conjugate. Acta Endocrinologica 106: 374–380
39. Nambara T, Shimada K, Ohta H 1980 Preparation of specific antiserum to estrone sulphate. Journal of Steroid Biochemistry 13: 1075–1079
40. Brown JB, Blackwell LF, Cox RI, Holmes JM, Smith MA 1988 Chemical and homogeneous enzyme immunoassay methods for the measurement of estrogens and pregnanediol and their glucuronides in urine. Progress in Biological and Clinical Research 285: 119–138
41. Brown JB, Blackwell LF, Holmes J, Smyth K. 1989 New assays for identifying the fertile period. International Journal of Gynecology and Obstetrics (Suppl 1): 111–122
42. Barnard G, Kohen F, Mikola H, Lovgren T 1989 Measurement of estrone-3-glucuronide in urine by rapid, homogenous time-resolved fluoroimmunoassay. Clinical Chemistry 35: 455–459
43. Barnard G, O'Reilly CP, Dennis K, Collins WP 1989 A nonseparation, time-resolved fluoroimmunoassay to monitor ovarian function and predict potential fertility in women. Fertility and Sterility 52: 60–65
44. Barnard G, Amir-Zaltsman Y, Lichter S, Gayer B, Kohen F 1995 The measurement of oestrone-3-glucuronide in urine by noncompetitive idiometric assay. Journal of Steroid Biochemistry and Molecular Biology 55: 107–114
45. Ratcliffe WA, Carter GD, Dowsett M, Hillier SG, Middle JG, Reed MJ 1988 Oestradiol assays: applications and guidelines for the provision of a clinical biochemistry service. Annals of Clinical Biochemistry 25: 466–483
46. Tietz NW 1994 Accuracy in clinical chemistry — does anybody care? Clinical Chemistry 40: 859–861
47. Micallef JV, Hayes MM, Latef A, Ahsan R, Sufi SB 1995 Serum binding of steroid tracers and its possible effects on direct steroid immunoassay. Annals of Clinical Biochemistry 32: 566–574
48. Barnard G, Kohen F 1990 Idiometric assay: noncompetitive immunoassay for small molecules typified by the measurement of estradiol in serum. Clinical Chemistry 36: 1945–1950
49. Altamirano-Bustamante A, Barnard G, Kohen F 1991 Direct time-resolved fluorescence immunoassay for serum oestradiol based on the idiotypic anti-idiotypic approach. Journal of Immunological Methodology 138: 95–101
50. Mares A, De Boever J, Osher J, Quirogo S, Barnard G, Kohen F 1995 A direct noncompetitive idiometric enzyme immunoassay for serum oestradiol. Journal of Immunological Methodology 181: 83–90
51. Liehr JG 1990 Genotoxic effects of estrogens. Mutation Research 238: 269–276
52. Berg FD, Kuss E 1991 Urinary excretion of catecholestrogens, 2-methoxy-estrogens and 'classical estrogens' throughout the normal menstrual cycle. Archives of Gynecology and Obstetrics 249: 201–207
53. Vining RF, McGinley RA, Symons RG 1983 Hormones in saliva: mode of entry and consequent implications for clinical interpretation. Clinical Chemistry 29: 1752–1756
54. Sufi SB, Donaldson A, Gandy SC, Jeffcoate SL, Chearskul S, Goh H, Hazra D, Romero C, Wang HZ 1985 Multicentre evaluation of assays for estradiol and progesterone in saliva. Clinical Chemistry 31: 101–103
55. Morgan MRA, Whittaker PG, Fuller BP, Dean PGD 1980 A radioimmunoassay for equilin in postmenopausal plasma: plasma levels of equilin determined after oral administration of conjugated equine oestrogens (Premarin). Journal of Steroid Biochemistry 13: 551–555

56. Akpoviroro J, Fotherby K 1980 Assay of ethinyl estradiol in human serum and its binding to plasma proteins. Journal of Steroid Biochemistry 13: 773–779
57. Rao PN, de la Prena A, Goldzieher JW 1974 Antisera for radioimmunoassay of 17α-ethinylestradiol and mestranol. Steroids 24: 803–808
58. Adlercreutz H, Honjo H, Higashi A, Fotsis T, Hamalainen E, Hasegawa T, Okada H 1991 Urinary excretion of lignans and isoflavonoid phytoestrogens in Japanese men and women consuming a traditional Japanese diet. American Journal of Clinical Nutrition 54: 1093–1100
59. Read GF, Barnard G, Collins WP 1995 Analysis of progestogens. In: Makin HLJ, Gower DB, Kirk DN (eds) Steroid analysis. Blackie Academic and Professional, London, pp 369–426
60. Wood P, Groom G, Moore A, Ratcliffe W, Selby C 1985 Progesterone assays: guidelines for the provision of a clinical biochemistry service. Annals of Clinical Biochemistry 22: 1–24
61. Youssefnejadian E, Florensa E, Collins WP, Sommerville IF 1972 Radioimmunoassay of 17-hydroxyprogesterone. Steroids 20: 773–781
62. Florensa E, Sommerville IF 1973 Radioimmunoassay of plasma 20α-dihydroprogesterone. Steroids 7(10): 451–465
63. Ratcliffe WA, Corrie JET, Dalziel A, McPherson JS 1982 Direct ^{125}I-radioligand assays for serum progesterone compared with assays involving extraction of serum. Clinical Chemistry 28: 1314–1318
64. Barnard G, Osher J, Lichter S, Gayer B, De Boever J, Limor R, Ayalon D, Kohen F 1995 The measurement of progesterone in serum by noncompetitive idiometric assay. Steroids 60: 824–829
65. Walker RF, Read GF, Riad-Fahmy D 1979 Radioimmunoassay of progesterone in saliva: application to the assessment of ovarian function. Clinical Chemistry 25: 2030–2033
66. Corrie JET 1984 A direct radioimmunoassay for salivary progesterone using a radiolebelled tracer. In: Read GF, Riad-Fahmy D, Walker RF, Griffiths K (eds) Ninth Tenovus Workshop: Immunoassays of steroids in saliva. Alpha Omego Publishing, Cardiff, pp 127–133
67. Leith HM, Truran PL, Gaskell SJ 1986 Quantification of progesterone in human saliva. Biomedical and Environmental Mass Spectrometry 13: 257–261
68. Lévesque A, Letellier M, Dillon PW, Grant A 1997 Analytical performance of Bayer Immuno 1™ estradiol and progesterone assays. Clinical Chemistry 43: 1601–1609
69. Lei J-D, El Shami AS, Young KK 1994 An automated chemiluminescent immunoassay for estradiol on the Immulite system. Clinical Chemistry 40: 1035
70. Wilson H, El Shami AS, Lei J-D 1994 An automated chemiluminescent immunoassay for progesterone on the Immulite system. Clinical Chemistry 40: 1035
71. May K 1996 The Unipath Personal Contraceptive System. In: Bonnar J (ed) Natural contraception through personal hormone monitoring. Parthenon Publishing, New York, pp 35–44
72. Kricka LJ 1994 Selected strategies for improving sensitivity and reliability of immunoassay. Clinical Chemistry 40: 347–357
73. Pluckthun A 1994 Antibodies from *Escherichia coli*. In: Rosenberg M, Moore GP (eds) The pharmacology of monoclonal antibodies. Handbook of pharmacology, vol. 113. Springer Verlag, pp 269–315
74. Barnard G, Beazley C, Kohen F 1994 Monitoring ovarian function by a simultaneous time-resolved fluorescence immunoassay of three urinary metabolites. Journal of Endocrinology 140: 42
75. Ekins R, Chu FW 1991 Multianalyte microspot immunoassay — microanalytical 'compact disk' of the future. Clinical Chemistry 37: 1955–1967
76. Kakabakos SE, Christopoulos TK, Diamandis EP 1992 Multianalyte immunoassay based on spatially distinct fluorescent areas quantified by laser-excited solid phase time-resolved fluorimetry. Clinical Chemistry 38: 338–342
77. Thornton SJ, Pepperell RJ, Brown JB 1990 Home monitoring of gonadotropin ovulation induction using the ovarian monitor. Fertility and Sterility 54: 1076–1082
78. Brown JB, Holmes J, Barker G 1991 Use of the home ovarian monitor in pregnancy avoidance. American Journal of Obstetrics and Gynecology 165: 2008–2011
79. Klimov AD, Tsai S-CJ, Towt J, Salamone SJ 1995 Improved immunochromatographic format for competitive-type assays. Clinical Chemistry 41: 1360
80. Piran U, Riordan WJ, Livshin LA 1995 New noncompetitive immunoassays of small analytes. Clinical Chemistry 41: 986–990
81. Self CH, Desse JL, Winger LA 1994 High-performance assays of small molecules: enhanced sensitivity, rapidity and convenience demonstrated with noncompetitive immunometric anti-immune complex assay system for digoxin. Clinical Chemistry 40: 2035–2041
82. Wade SE 1992 An oral-diffusion-sink device for extended sampling of multiple steroid hormones from saliva. Clinical Chemistry 38: 1878–1882

29. Imaging of the reproductive tract

Philippa A. Ramsay Ian S. Fraser

Introduction

The pelvic organs in a woman of reproductive age are constantly responding to the changing hormonal milieu of the menstrual cycle. In clinical practice, we often need to observe these changes and to document departures from normal. We need imaging modalities that can be used repeatedly to document the progress or resolution of a lesion, without perturbing the menstrual cycle we are studying.

Ultrasound has become the imaging modality of choice for examining the ovaries and their developing follicles, as well as the endometrium. The transvaginal transducer has allowed high frequency, high resolution imaging, and other developments such as color Doppler imaging and sonohysterography have further expanded its scope. But ultrasound has its limitations, so hysterosalpingography (HSG), computerized tomography (CT) and magnetic resonance imaging (MRI) have a place in certain clinical situations (Fig. 29.1), and when a definite histological diagnosis is required direct visualization and biopsy via colposcopy, hysteroscopy, laparoscopy or other endoscopic or open operation is then usually optimal.

The size and structure of the uterus, tubes and ovaries changes with reproductive age and the phase of the menstrual cycle. Therefore, a clinical history, an understanding of the normal physiological events, and sometimes serial examinations can be needed to come to an accurate understanding of the pathology.

IMAGING MODALITIES

Ultrasound

Ultrasound waves are created by the piezoelectric effect on a crystal within an ultrasound transducer. The ultrasound waves are transmitted through the skin or mucosa and are then attenuated and reflected by the deeper tissues. The reflected waves are detected by the transducer, and their amplitude and time delay are interpreted into a grey-scale image of intensity and depth. Different tissues have different absorption coefficients, so the returning waves reflect this. Ultrasound imaging is in real-time, so the peristalsis of bowel, the wave motion of endometrium and the pulsation of arteries are all clearly seen, as is fetal heart motion in a pregnant patient. With the transabdominal approach, the pelvic organs are often obscured by swirling loops of bowel unless the patient has a full bladder. The bladder serves to displace the bowel superiorly, as well as provide a clear reflection-free window to the uterus and ovaries (Fig. 29.1A). Higher frequency transducers give the best spatial resolution but at the expense of penetration. Therefore, it is difficult to get good resolution at depth. In gynecology this problem has been circumvented by the development of the transvaginal transducer, which is long and narrow. It is usually placed in the anterior vaginal fornix, only 1–2 cm from the uterus and ovaries, so very high resolution images can be achieved.

Sonohysterography can be used to further differentiate small endometrial lesions. Saline, or a contrast agent, is introduced into the endometrial cavity by way of a small trans-cervical catheter to distend the cavity slightly and provide a contrast with the endometrial lining (Fig. 29.2). This technique is also helpful in providing information on the myometrium underlying endometrial lesions.

Color Doppler imaging is available on some machines. It consists of an extra beam of ultrasound that is aimed at blood vessels or tissue to detect blood flow within. Because of the Doppler effect on the moving blood cells, the reflected waves have a different frequency, which can be perceived by the transducer and demonstrated as red or blue, according to the direction of flow. This facility is used commonly to assess vascularity and vascular – pulsatility and particularly to detect neovascularization and increased flow in neoplastic tissues.

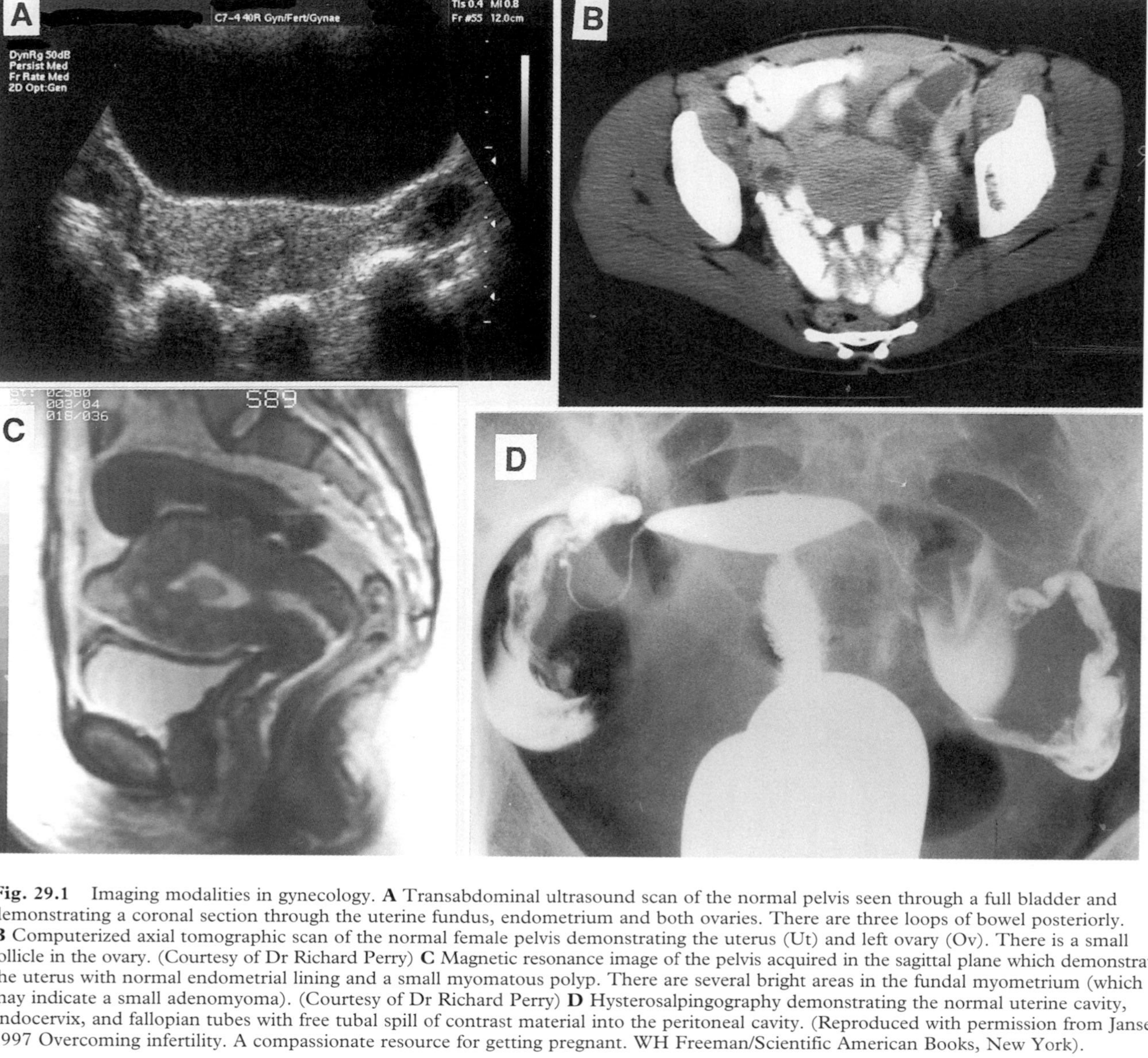

Fig. 29.1 Imaging modalities in gynecology. **A** Transabdominal ultrasound scan of the normal pelvis seen through a full bladder and demonstrating a coronal section through the uterine fundus, endometrium and both ovaries. There are three loops of bowel posteriorly. **B** Computerized axial tomographic scan of the normal female pelvis demonstrating the uterus (Ut) and left ovary (Ov). There is a small follicle in the ovary. (Courtesy of Dr Richard Perry) **C** Magnetic resonance image of the pelvis acquired in the sagittal plane which demonstrates the uterus with normal endometrial lining and a small myomatous polyp. There are several bright areas in the fundal myometrium (which may indicate a small adenomyoma). (Courtesy of Dr Richard Perry) **D** Hysterosalpingography demonstrating the normal uterine cavity, endocervix, and fallopian tubes with free tubal spill of contrast material into the peritoneal cavity. (Reproduced with permission from Jansen, 1997 Overcoming infertility. A compassionate resource for getting pregnant. WH Freeman/Scientific American Books, New York).

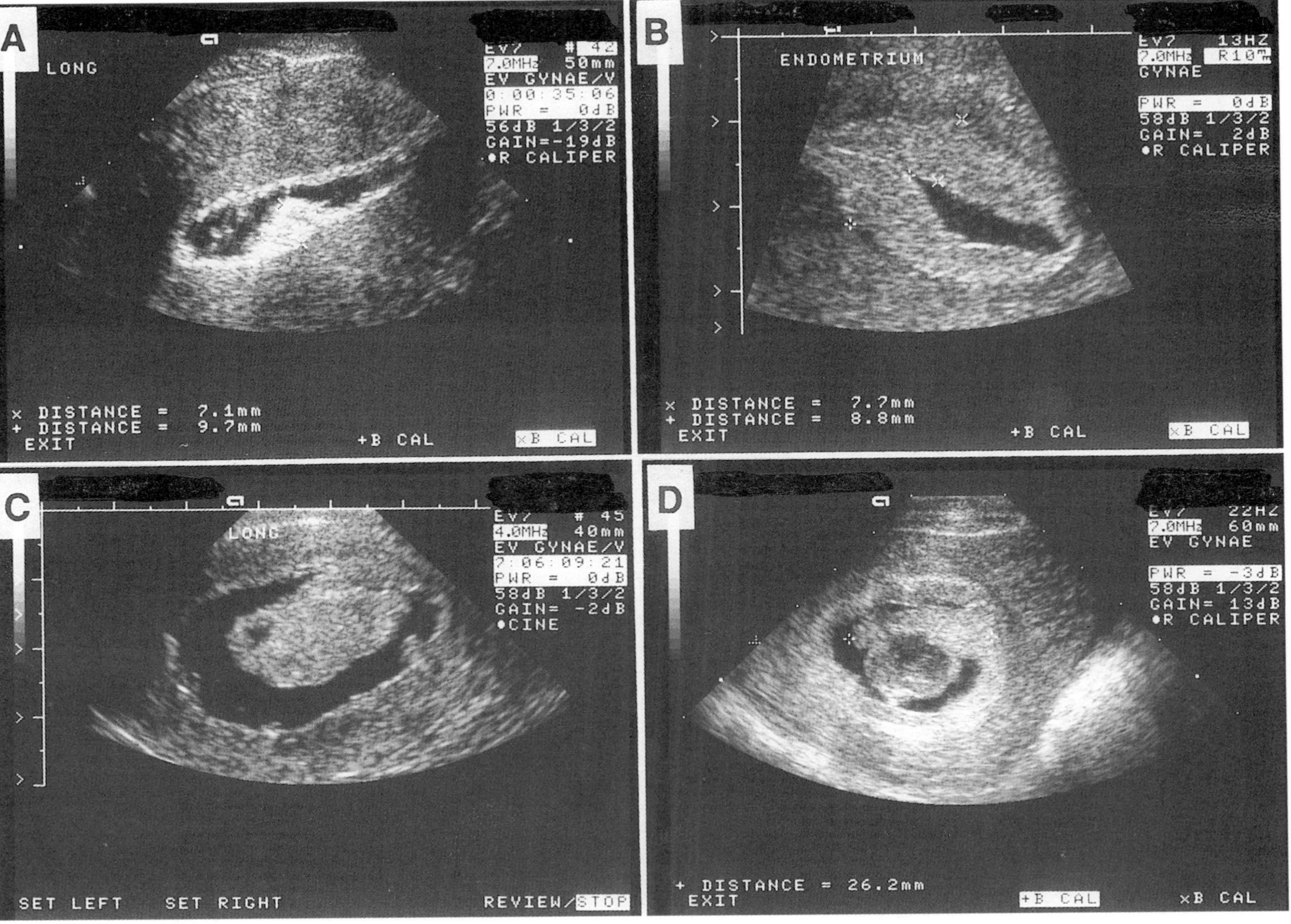

Fig. 29.2 Sonohysterography of the endometrium. **A** A small polyp arising from the posterior endometrial layer. **B** No obvious polyp but thick hyperplastic endometrium along anterior and posterior walls. **C** A large polyp arising from thin atrophic endometrium. **D** A large polyp arising from thick hyperplastic endometrium.

Gynecological applications

Ultrasound has extensive applications in gynecology, from the investigation of symptoms like pelvic pain or abnormal bleeding, to the monitoring of follicle stimulation, hormone replacement therapy or an asymptomatic ovarian cyst. It is usually the first line imaging modality, and will often avoid further investigation.

Hysterosalpingography

Hysterosalpingography is a well-established technique that displays the cervical canal, the uterine cavity and the Fallopian tubes by x-ray examination (Fig. 29.1B). To outline these soft tissues, contrast must be injected after insertion of a speculum and cannulation of the cervix with a balloon or suction-cup catheter. A plain x-ray is taken beforehand, and fluoroscopic guidance is used during the procedure. The most common indication is to determine tubal patency in a woman presenting with infertility. If tubal patency cannot be established, some would proceed to fluoroscopically guided fallopian tube catheterization and selective salpingography.[1] The main complication of both of these procedures are pain, and a small risk of pelvic infection, particularly if there has been a past history of pelvic inflammatory disease or distally blocked tubes.

Computerized tomography

Computerized tomography, or CT, scan images are constructed from multiple x-ray images which are taken from different angles while the x-ray tube is rotating around the patient who lies supine. The different tissues of the body attenuate the x-rays to different degrees. The intensity of x-rays emerging from the patient is measured with an array of detectors and a computer image of the values is reconstructed after assessment of multiple views of each slice of tissue (Fig. 29.1C). This results in multiple images of transaxial slices of the body. The resolution depends in part on the thickness of each slice, as partial volume averaging artefacts make it difficult to assess the density of small structures. Intravenous injections of contrast agent may be required to delineate vascular structures or the bladder. Oral contrast is regularly used to highlight the bowel.

Gynecological applications

The spatial resolution of CT is not as good as ultrasound. Nevertheless, CT has a role in clinical situations where ultrasound is limited. It is excellent for the evaluation of complex adnexal masses, where differentiation from bowel has been difficult with ultrasound. It is often valuable in the assessment of a mass in a grossly obese patient, where ultrasound images are poor because of excessive wave attenuation.

Magnetic resonance imaging

Magnetic resonance imaging (MRI) relies on electromagnetic coils to cause a magnetic field across the body. A radiofrequency pulse is then applied. This distorts the hydrogen atoms in the tissues, and as they realign they give off a magnetic resonance signal. This signal differs according to the chemical bonds around the hydrogen atoms. Thus, different signals emanate from different tissues. In 'T1-weighted' images fat produces a strong signal and looks white, whereas muscle and fluid appear dark. In 'T2-weighted' images fat looks dark, fluid looks light, endometrium looks white and myometrium is intermediate. The spatial resolution of MRI is excellent and images can be acquired in any plane (Fig. 29.1D).

Gynecological applications

MRI is particularly good at imaging adnexal masses and the myometrium. Many authorities feel that it is better than ultrasound.[2] MRI cannot be used in most centers for these indications alone because of its cost and limited availability.

Reproductive diagnostic endoscopy

Endoscopy remains an essential component of pelvic imaging, and is complementary to the less invasive ultrasound and radiology investigations summarized above. Endoscopic imaging is discussed in detail below.

IMAGING THE UTERUS

The size of the adult uterus depends on parity and menopausal status. The normal length varies from 7 cm in nullipara to 9 cm in multiparous women,[3] and in postmenopausal women the uterus reduces in size proportionate to the number of years since menopause.[4] Normal myometrium is homogeneously echodense with a moderately fine echotexture. The uterine walls are approximately 1.5–2 cm in thickness, and they curve around in the 'pear' shape of a normal uterus. Müllerian anomalies such as a bicornuate or subseptate uterine shape can be detected by careful assessment of the outer contour of the uterus and comparison with the endometrial cavity contour.

The newborn and prepubescent uterus

In the neonatal period the cervix is longer than the uterine corpus and the organ is tubular in shape. Removed from the influence of maternal hormones, it involutes in the first year of life, and its size stays relatively unchanged, at about 3 cm in length, until slow steady growth ensues between 7–10 years of age.[5] This growth results in a corpus:cervix ratio of approximately 2:1 — an adult configuration and an adult size.

The adult uterus and the menstrual cycle

The most apparent changes in the uterus through the menstrual cycle are in the endometrium (Fig. 29.3 and see ref. 5a). Under the influence of endogenous estrogen and progesterone, the endometrium undergoes impressive but predictable histological change, and these changes affect the thickness and density of the endometrium enough to be clearly perceptible with ultrasound.

The proliferative phase

After menstruation the functional layer of the endometrium responds to the estrogen secreted by the ovary. The glands proliferate, lengthen and become tortuous; the stroma accumulates glycogen and the endometrium becomes thicker. The double layer, midsagittal endometrial thickness of this proliferative endometrium increases from 1 mm to 18 mm. One thin echogenic line is seen from menstruation to about seven days before ovulation (Fig. 29.3A), then, towards the late proliferative phase, a change from one to three echogenic lines is observed. The outer lines represent the myometrial–endometrial interface, and the central line represents the apposition of the anterior and posterior endometrial layers. The endometrial tissue in between is thick and hypoechoic.[6] These changes reflect the increasing serum concentration of estradiol.

The secretory phase

In the secretory phase the endometrial glands become more tortuous and produce a mucoid secretion which is rich in glycogen. Histologically, this is initially seen as subnuclear vacuolation but the collection soon fills the whole cell and appears in the glands themselves. On ultrasound examination from days one to six after ovulation an increasing blurring of the three lines becomes apparent as the previously hypoechoic layers become echogenic.[6] By seven days after ovulation through to menstruation the endometrium remains thick and echogenic, corresponding to the predecidual reaction on histology (Fig. 29.3B). The cells are full of glycogen, ready to nourish the blastocyst in case fertilization has occurred, whence it would go on to a fully developed decidual reaction. If pregnancy does not ensue, the growth of the endometrium plateaus[6] and without progesterone support from an ongoing corpus luteum of pregnancy the functional layers of the endometrium break down and slough off with menstruation.

The menstrual phase

During menstruation, blood, blood-clot and endometrial fragments can be seen in the endometrial cavity. The blood is echolucent or faintly echogenic, and the clots and endometrial debris are echogenic. The interface between the basal layer of endometrium and myometrium is poorly defined and irregular. Finally the cavity is empty of debris, but a thin layer of echolucent fluid, presumably blood, remains. Then regeneration begins in the proliferative phase of the next cycle.

The postmenopausal uterus

Uterine involution at the time of menopause results in reduction of the size of both the cervix and uterine body. This occurs steadily with the uterine length ultimately decreasing to approximately 5 cm.[4]

In postmenopausal women the ovaries are quiescent and the endometrium should be thin and atrophic, with no cyclic changes. The mean endometrial thickness is 2.3 ± 1.8 mm (range 0–10 mm).[7] However, the peripheral conversion of androstenedione to estrogen by fat cells causes a background level of estrogen even in postmenopausal women, which can sometimes cause endometrial thickening. Thus fatter women tend to have thicker postmenopausal endometrium, even within the normal range.[7] Once the endometrial thickness is greater than 5 mm, the risk of endometrial hyperplasia or carcinoma increases proportionately with the thickness.[8] The endometrium in postmenopausal women is homogeneously echodense, with the two layers not separately discernible unless there is fluid in the cavity. A small amount of endometrial fluid is commonly seen with high resolution ultrasound. As long as the endometrium around it is thin and regular,

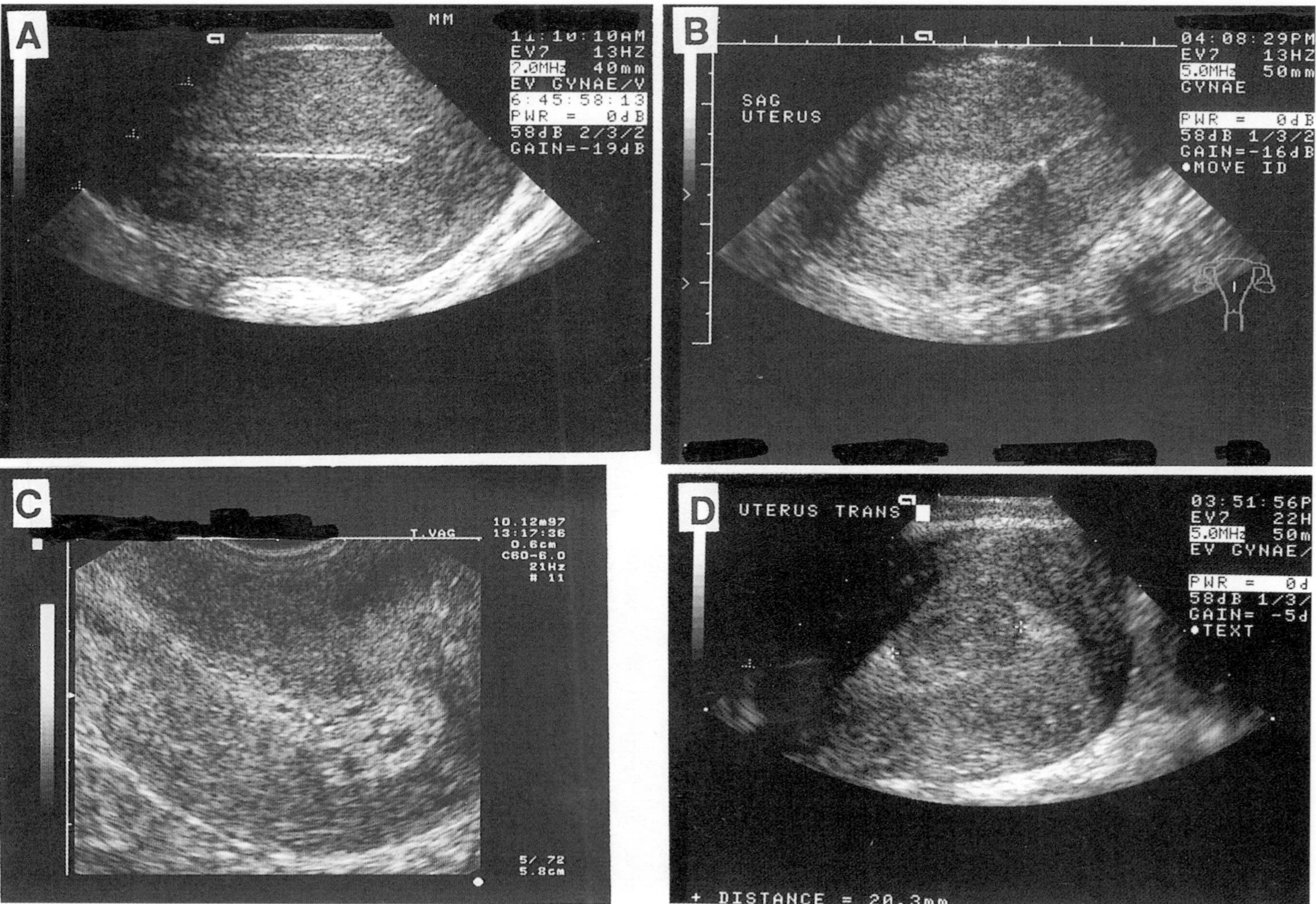

Fig. 29.3 Transvaginal ultrasound scans of the endometrium. **A** Normal early proliferative endometrium with a thin bright central line. **B** Normal secretory endometrium greatly thickened in the fundal region. **C** Tamoxifen-exposed and thickened endometrium, containing several small cystic areas. **D** Secretory endometrium distorted by a 20 mm submucous fibroid (delineated by the two electronic markers).

and there are no symptoms, it is thought to be a normal finding.

The effect of drugs on the endometrium

The combined oral contraceptive usually causes 'pseudosecretory' endometrium, which is thin, regular in outline and highly echogenic. It varies little throughout the month until the time of the withdrawal bleed when it has an appearance similar to natural cycle menstruation. Some estrogen/progestogen combinations can cause the endometrium to look 'early proliferative', 'secretory' or atrophic, depending on the contribution of endogenous hormones.

Tamoxifen is an estrogen antagonist that has some agonistic properties. It is used to inhibit breast cancer recurrence, but paradoxically it can stimulate endometrial growth and has been implicated in the development of endometrial polyps, endometrial hyperplasia and adenocarcinoma.[9] The endometrium looks thick and echogenic, with multiple small cystic spaces throughout (Fig. 29.2C) possibly due to changes in the subendometrial myometrial layer.[10] Annual vaginal sonography and endometrial biopsy have been suggested for surveillance in women on tamoxifen.[11]

Benign conditions of the endometrium

Cystic, adenomatous and atypical hyperplasia are all thought to be precursors of endometrial cancer. They typically cause endometrial thickening, and sometimes a change to hyperechoic endometrium with multiple small cystic spaces within. Endometrial polyps appear as well circumscribed echogenic masses in the endometrial cavity. They are best demonstrated when surrounded by fluid — either menstrual blood or fluid purposefully introduced by way of sonohysterography (Fig. 29.2). Otherwise, as they are not responsive to cyclic hormonal changes, they can be better demonstrated when the surrounding endometrium is thin, in the early proliferative phase. Endometrial atrophy causes a thin, faint appearance on ultrasound examination. This is so reliable that in women with postmenopausal bleeding and an endometrial thickness of less than 5 mm, curettage can be avoided, as it will probably just yield scant, if any tissue, with endometrial atrophy the only finding on histopathology.[8]

Malignant conditions of the endometrium

Unfortunately, the resolution of ultrasound does not approach that of a microscope, so histological diagnosis of cancer cannot be achieved with ultrasound examination alone. It is suspected in a postmenopausal woman who is not on hormone replacement therapy when the endometrium is greater than 5 mm in thickness, or when it is greater than 9 mm in thickness on combined HRT. The sonographic appearance can be indistinguishable from that of secretory endometrium, decidua, or endometrial hyperplasia, unless it is advanced and invades the myometrium.

An appearance which is normal in reproductive life might be abnormal after the menopause. For example, normal premenstrual endometrium in a young woman can look similar to hyperplastic endometrium in an older woman. It is therefore impossible to determine whether an image is normal or abnormal without knowing the patient's age, menstrual history and recent medications.

Benign conditions of the myometrium

The most common myometrial lesion is the myoma (fibroid). These lesions are usually clearly seen with transvaginal ultrasound as well circumscribed, encapsulated, rounded masses of myometrium. Their echotexture is similar to the surrounding myometrium, but often slightly hypoechoic, with good posterior acoustic enhancement. Fibroids are often multiple, and they can be submucosal, subserous or intramural. The submucosal fibroids (Fig. 29.3D) often cause irregular bleeding, menorrhagia or infertility in the reproductive age-group.

Adenomyosis is a difficult diagnosis to make with ultrasound. Focal adenomyosis can be indistinguishable from a fibroid with ultrasound alone. In clear examples adenomyosis produces a nonencapsulated rounded mass of irregular echotexture, predominantly in the posterior wall of the uterus with an elevation of serum CA125 antigen.[11a] In the past, MRI has been considered to be the imaging modality of choice for this condition, however recent evidence has demonstrated a similar sensitivity and specifity for MRI and transvaginal ultrasound.[12]

IMAGING OF THE VAGINA

The vagina can be imaged with a transabdominal ultrasound transducer angled caudally through the full bladder. The vaginal walls are usually 3 mm in thickness and due to their fibromuscular nature these walls are hypoechoic. Apposition of the epithelial mucosal layers results in a bright specular reflection in the midsagittal plane.

Its absence might be noted in women with untreated vaginal atresia. Its length cannot be reliably measured with ultrasound as it is so dependent on the extent of bladder filling. Transperineal ultrasound has been successfully utilised to demonstrate solid tissue septums and to plan appropriate surgery.[13] Paradoxically, transvaginal ultrasound often fails to demonstrate the vaginal wall, because the wall is closer than the focal zone of the transducer.

IMAGING OF THE FALLOPIAN TUBES

Hysterosalpingography (HSG) and occasionally fluoroscopically guided fallopian tube catheterization and selective salpingography are used to establish tubal patency in women presenting with infertility. These techniques can demonstrate whether there is a proximal or distal obstruction, as well as the presence of hydrosalpinges. HSG also demonstrates Müllerian anomalies of the uterus and indentations of the cavity due to submucous fibroids.

The fallopian tubes are difficult to demonstrate with ultrasound as they are long and narrow and they often adopt a serpiginous course surrounded by swirling loops of bowel. If there is fluid in the lumen or in the pelvis around them they are more easily demonstrated though in one targeted study even a single tube could be identified in only 15% of patients.[14] The interstitial segment of the fallopian tube can be demonstrated, passing through the wall of the uterus and the tubal ostia can be cannulated for the purposes of sonosalpingography or tubal embryo transfer.

Sonohysterography is gaining in popularity. Various different methods of proving tubal patency have been described, including watching for distension of the tube in the adnexa, using color Doppler imaging to show rapid flow through the tubal isthmus and demonstrating the accumulation of instilled fluid in the pouch of Douglas (cul de sac). This technique is excellent for examining the uterine cavity, but its role in the diagnosis of tubal patency is uncertain. Sonohysterography with an ultrasonic contrast liquid (sometimes known as hystero-contrast-sonography or HyCoSy), might be more effective, but there are as yet no good studies comparing it to HSG or laparoscopy and dye.

IMAGING OF THE OVARIES

Transvaginal ultrasound allows close examination of the ovaries, but the technique requires good equipment and a skilled operator. The ovaries are seen as small elliptical organs with a coarse echotexture which is slightly less echodense than that of myometrium. They usually contain a few follicles that vary in size from 2–30 mm and are usually spherical and filled with echolucent fluid. Ovarian cysts and masses are easily demonstrated, measured and characterized.

The newborn and prepubescent ovary

In the newborn infant it can be difficult to identify the ovaries because they are small, usually without follicles, and the bladder is not reliably full. The transvaginal approach is obviously inappropriate but the transperineal approach can sometimes be used. The mean ovarian volume is 1.06 cm^3 (range 0.7–3.6 cm^3) among girls up to three months old; 1.05 cm^3 (range 0.2–2.7 cm^3) among girls 4–12 months old and 0.67 cm^3 (range 0.1–1.7 cm^3) among girls 13–24 months old.[15] The ovaries grow slowly but continuously throughout childhood increasing from a mean ovarian volume of 0.51 cm^3 at the age of three, to a mean ovarian volume of 2.77 cm^3 at the age of 18 years.[16]

Small ovarian cysts can be present in the normal newborn, but they are occasionally larger than 9 mm in diameter.[15] These cysts sometimes develop *in utero* under the influence of maternal estrogen. Most are simple, with no solid elements, and if so they are usually benign and resolve with time.[17] Occasionally, dermoid cysts present in this age group. Failure to demonstrate one or both ovaries at this age is common and does not imply that there is ovarian dysgenesis.

The adult ovary and the ovarian cycle

After puberty ovarian follicles develop regularly, and measurement of ovarian volumes becomes difficult. This could explain the contradiction between one report that the ovarian volume remains the same throughout the menstrual cycle in both ovaries,[18] and another which documented an increase in the stromal volume throughout the follicular phase of the ovulating ovary, with no change in the contralateral ovary.[19]

The follicular phase

Ovarian follicles develop under the influence of follicle stimulating hormone. Once they reach 2 mm in diameter these 'recruited' follicles become evident on transvaginal ultrasound.[20] The diameter of the dominant follicle increases at a rate of 2.5 mm per day until it reaches about 20 mm in size. Then the growth rate slows to 1.3 mm/day.[21] The oocyte and surrounding cumulus oophorus protrude into the follicular antrum and have been described as a small papillary projection from the wall of the follicular antrum on transabdominal ultrasound. However using a high resolution transvaginal transducer others have failed to visualize the cumulus oophorus, and failed to accurately predict the time of ovulation.[22] As well as the dominant follicle, several other follicles may also continue to grow, particularly in the dominant ovary, and in 5% of cycles there are two dominant follicles.[23,24] The side of ovulation in successive cycles is not affected by the side of ovulation in the preceding cycle.[25]

Ovulation

By the time it reaches approximately 21 mm in diameter (range 16–33 mm) the follicle is ready to ovulate.[26] The follicle wall ruptures and the egg is released. The ultrasonically recognizable events are sudden disappearance or slow collapse of the dominant follicle, the appearance of peri-adnexal fluid, and the subsequent development of a corpus luteum.[27]

If ovulation does not occur and the follicle does not involute it may continue to grow and become a follicular cyst. These are typically simple, with sharply marginated thin walls and echolucent fluid within. They may grow to become very large but are typically 3–4 cm in diameter, and usually regress if left alone (Fig. 29.4B). Occasionally, hemorrhage can occur into the cyst.

The luteal phase

On transvaginal ultrasound the corpus luteum might be barely visible or it may be seen as a solid dimple on the surface of the ovary, about 18 mm in diameter (Fig. 29.4A). Its thick, echogenic walls often have a crenated appearance, with a hypoechoic hollow centrally. There is much neovascularization in and around the corpus luteum which is well documented with color Doppler imaging.[28] Occasionally, after ovulation the follicle immediately fills up with blood, when it is called a hemorrhagic corpus luteum. The blood is seen as homogeneously echodense fluid, with a trabecular network of echoes (Fig. 29.4C) or, occasionally, gravity-dependent particles or clot (Fig. 29.4D).[29] They can expand to be 5–6 cm in diameter and the ultrasound appearances can easily mimic (and indeed can coexist with) an endometrioma (Fig. 29.4E). If there is no hemorrhage, the corpus luteum can fill with serous fluid and become a luteal cyst. Luteal cysts are thought to have thicker walls than follicular cysts, but in practice it can be impossible to differentiate between them unless there has been ultrasound or hormonal documentation of ovulation. Luteal cysts are more likely to cause pain but the management of these functional cysts is conservative as most regress spontaneously. Aspiration under ultrasound guidance or laparoscopic surgery is warranted in those uncommon cases where the symptoms are too severe for the patient to wait for spontaneous resolution.

Because the ultrasonographic appearance of the postovulatory ovary is so varied, much diagnostic difficulty can be avoided by scanning before ovulation.

The postmenopausal ovary

During the perimenopausal years it is common to have small simple cysts on the ovaries. By three years after the last menstrual period the ovaries are usually quiescent and no follicle development is evident. The ovaries become small and homogeneous in echotexture, and can be difficult to find because of overlying bowel and the lack of distinguishing follicles.

The effect of drugs

The combined oral contraceptive and certain progestogen-only contraceptives suppress ovulation in most women, but some development of follicles will usually still be evident with ultrasound. Hormone replacement therapy and tamoxifen have little if any effect on imaging of the ovary.

Benign and malignant conditions of the ovary

Polycystic ovaries

Polycystic ovaries contain multiple small cystic structures that represent immature and atretic follicles. They are peripherally located around the central ovarian stroma, which is echogenic due to hypertrophy (in a typical 'necklace' pattern; Fig. 29.4F). The follicles measure 3–10 mm in diameter and there are at least 5–10 and sometimes as many as 30. They are usually bilateral and the ovaries are usually enlarged but do not usually demonstrate signs of ovulation, such as a corpus luteum or a dominant follicle.[30]

Multicystic ovaries

Follicular development is not always sustained and ovulation does not always follow. Particularly in young teenagers, one follicle can take another's place without ovulation, giving menstrual cycles that are long and irregular. The variable persistence of differently-sized follicles, some functional, some atretic and some large

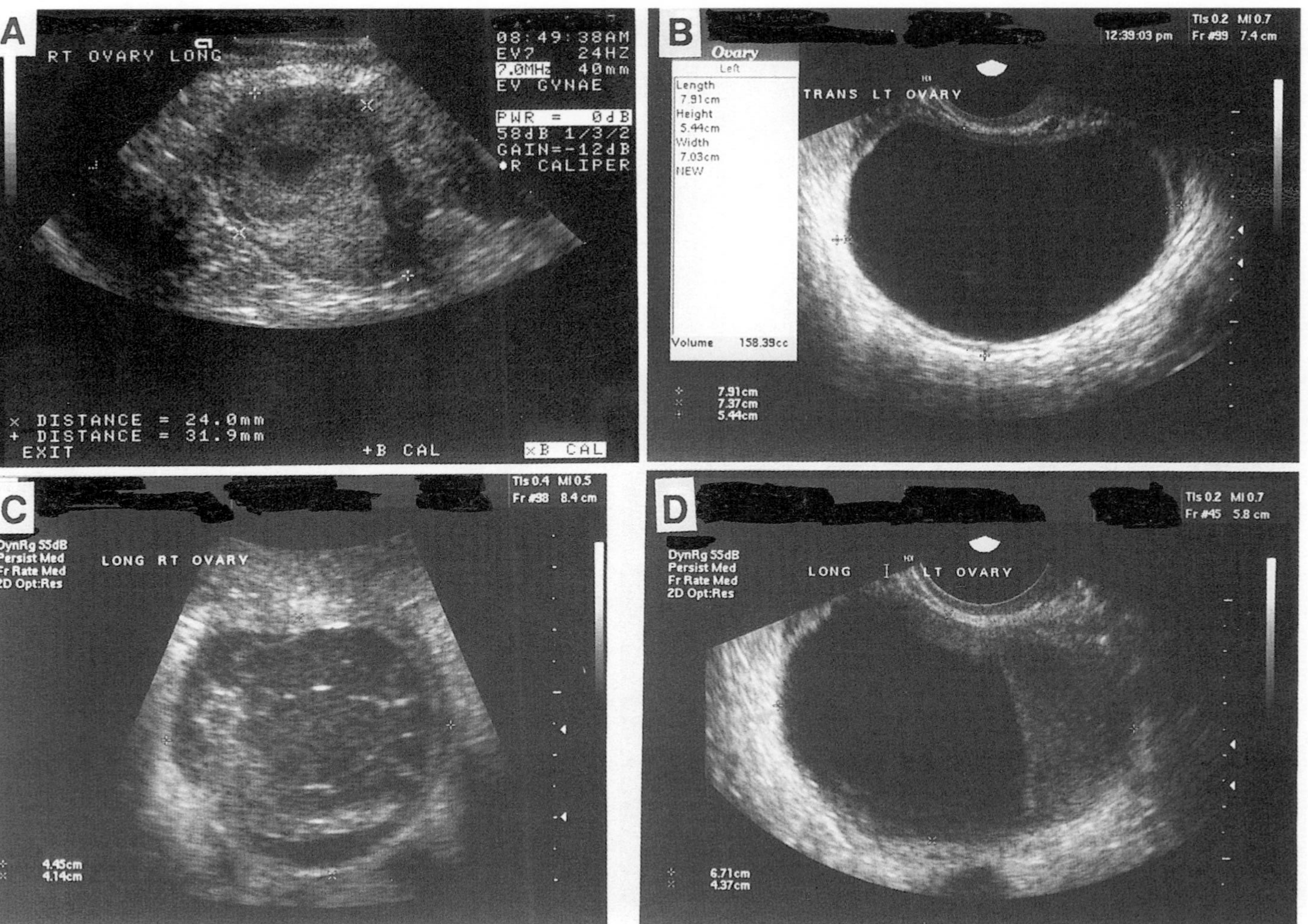
A
RT OVARY LONG
08:49:38AM
EV7 24HZ
7.0MHz 40mm
EV GYNAE
PWR = 0dB
58dB 1/3/2
GAIN=-12dB
●R CALIPER
× DISTANCE = 24.0mm
+ DISTANCE = 31.9mm
EXIT
+B CAL
×B CAL
B
Tls 0.2 MI 0.7
12:39:03 pm
Fr #99 7.4 cm
Ovary
Left
Length
7.91cm
Height
5.44cm
Width
7.03cm
NEW
Volume 158.39cc
TRANS LT OVARY
7.91cm
7.37cm
5.44cm
C
Tls 0.4 MI 0.5
Fr #98 8.4 cm
DynRg 55dB
Persist Med
Fr Rate Med
2D Opt:Res
LONG RT OVARY
4.45cm
4.14cm
D
Tls 0.2 MI 0.7
Fr #45 5.8 cm
DynRg 55dB
Persist Med
Fr Rate Med
2D Opt:Res
LONG LT OVARY
6.71cm
4.37cm

Fig. 29.4 A–D

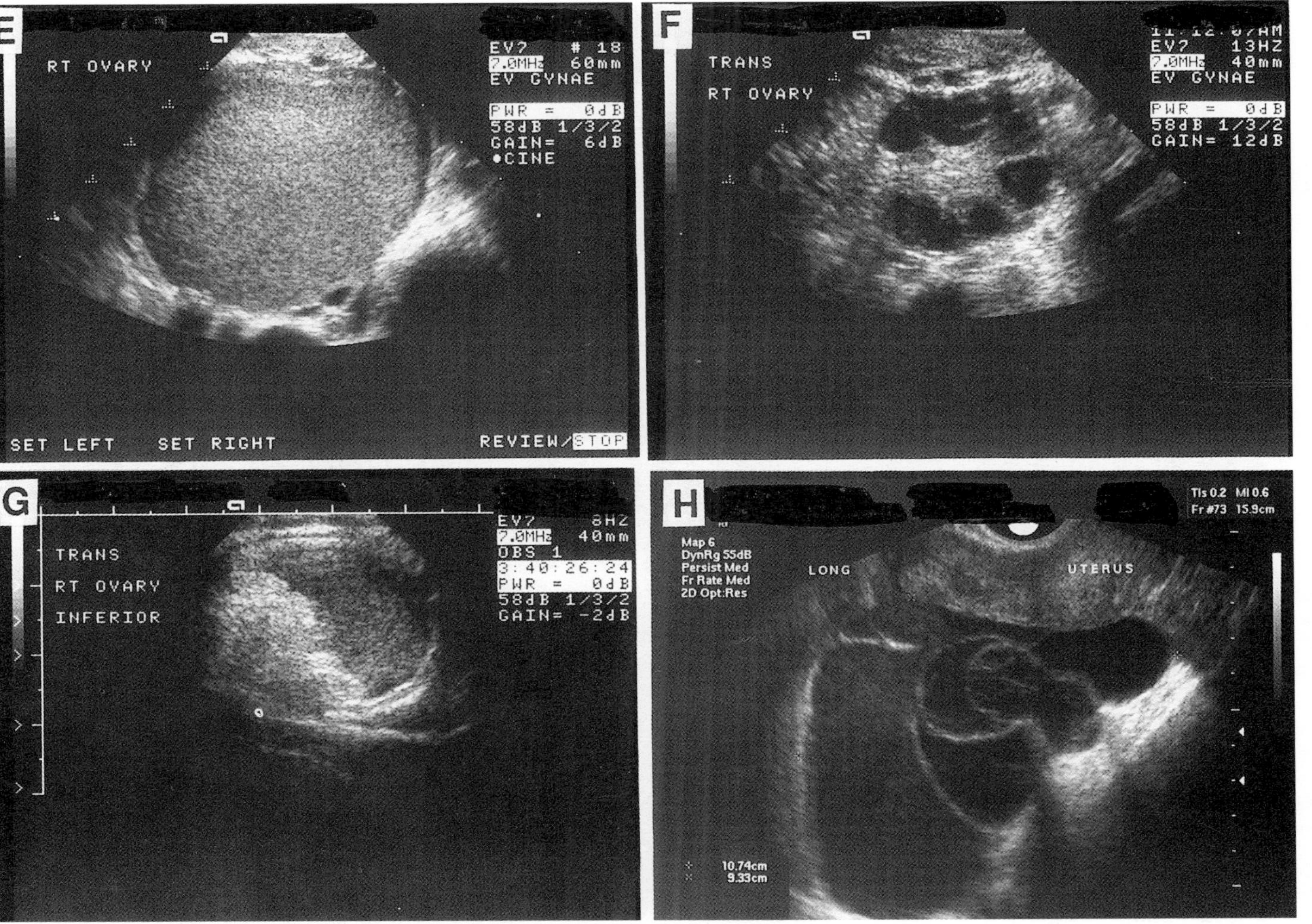

Fig. 29.4 Transvaginal ultrasound scans of the ovary demonstrating a range of physiological and pathological conditions. **A** A normal ovary (delineated by the electronic markers) with a cystic corpus luteum at the upper pole. **B** A functional ovarian cyst measuring 7 cm in diameter, with little identifiable normal ovarian tissue around it. **C** A hemorrhagic ovarian cyst measuring 4 cm in diameter (possible luteal or endometriotic). **D** A hemorrhagic cyst demonstrating a vertical fluid/fluid level to the right of the midline. **E** An endometrioma (6 cm) with homogeneously echogenic fluid within. **F** Coronal view of a polycystic ovary with multiple small follicular structures peripherally placed around echogenic cortex. **G** An ovarian dermoid cyst (4 cm) with highly echogenic sebaceous material within. **H** A large multi-septated serous cystadenoma of the ovary (10.7 cm), lying posterior to the uterus.

and cystic is the cause of the ovarian appearance sometimes called 'multicystic ovaries'.[31] This picture can also be seen leading up to the menopause, when there are few follicles left and FSH levels are high. The follicular phase can be extremely short and ovulation is disordered. Thus multicystic ovaries can be a normal phenomenon at both the beginning and end of the reproductive years.[32] They may also be seen in women with anovulatory dysfunctional uterine bleeding.

Ovarian endometriomata

When peritoneal endometriosis consists only of small deposits of functioning endometrioid tissue it cannot be resolved with ultrasound, CT or MRI, and laparoscopic visualization is necessary. But if the endometriosis affects the ovaries, the resulting cystic masses can be well seen.[33] The typical ultrasound appearance is of a well-circumscribed thin or thick-walled cyst which contains homogenously echogenic fluid (Fig. 29.4E). The fluid is altered blood which has been released from the ectopic endometrial tissue but is unable to escape. The walls are regular with no papillary projections, but internal septations may be present. Occasionally there is a fluid–fluid level. MRI is also excellent at imaging endometriomata[34] and other types of adnexal masses.[35]

Germ cell tumors — ovarian dermoid cysts

Dermoid cysts, or teratomas, contain a mixture of tissues because of the totipotent nature of the germ cells from that they arise. They typically contain apocrine glands produce sebum as well as hair and, occasionally, rudimentary tooth formation. Malignant change is rare. Because of the variable components, the ultrasound appearance is also variable, from the pathognomonic appearance of a cyst containing hyperechoic sebaceous fluid and a calcified tooth, to a confusing appearance of a complex cyst with multiple loculations and papillary projections that resembles malignancy (Fig. 29.4G). If the diagnosis is not obvious with ultrasound, but a dermoid cyst is suspected, CT and MRI are useful: both modalities are sensitive to the presence of fat in the lesion.[36]

Sex cord–stromal tumors

Thecomas and fibromas represent two extremes of a group of tumors that consist of varying proportions of stromal and thecal elements. They are virtually all benign but are of interest because tumours containing thecal elements can secrete estrogen, and occasionally androgens, and thus cause systemic effects, the most common of which is endometrial hyperplasia. Fibromas are occasionally associated with Meigs' syndrome — the development of ascites and a pleural effusion.

On ultrasound examination a fibrothecoma presents as an ovarian mass that is homogeneously hypoechoic, with posterior acoustic shadowing, as opposed to posterior acoustic enhancement, which is usually seen behind hypoechoic fluid-filled structures. Some fibromas have areas of calcification that would cause posterior acoustic shadowing.

Granulosa cell tumors also secrete estrogen and they usually present with abnormal bleeding in the reproductive years or postmenopausally (See Chapter 58). The ultrasonographic appearances are variable.

Epithelial tumors

The sonographic features of serous and mucinous cystadenomas and cystadenocarcinomas are not characteristic enough to come close to an accurate histological diagnosis. The main role of ultrasound is to identify the ovarian mass, recognize its malignant potential and allow appropriate surgical planning. The normal ovarian tissue is often obliterated, or might be demonstrable in the wall of the tumor. These ovarian tumors are seen as adnexal masses which are predominantly cystic (Fig. 29.4H). They can be unilocular or multilocular, but they are usually complex, with some solid component, septa and perhaps papillary projections. Many different scoring systems have been proposed to objectively assess these lesions. The signs that suggest malignancy include: size >5 cm in diameter, multilocularity, thick walls, papillary projections and the presence of ascites.[37,38] Particularly in an older woman, these features suggest malignancy. Color Doppler imaging should show neovascularization, with low resistance flow as measured by the resistance and pulsatility indices, but the false positive rates of these findings is high, so color Doppler imaging is seen as an adjunct to the gray-scale images.[39] MRI also has a major role in the characterization of adnexal masses.[35]

DIAGNOSTIC REPRODUCTIVE ENDOSCOPY

Systematic and careful diagnostic endoscopy using high quality endoscopic technology remains a very important part of modern pelvic imaging. The uses of endoscopy, ultrasound and radiology techniques are frequently complementary, and the modern gynecologist needs to have a clear understanding of the role of each in evaluating normal and abnormal pelvic anatomy and function. Until recently, conventional diagnostic laparoscopy and hysteroscopy have usually required general anesthesia and moderate-sized endoscopes. Modern technology has allowed the development of minihysteroscopes and minilaparoscopes, both of which can be used effectively under local anesthesia (or in the case of hysteroscopy, with no analgesia) on outpatients. Extensive recent data have shown office hysteroscopy to be substantially superior to diagnostic curettage for the exclusion of intrauterine pathology[40] and marginally superior to transvaginal ultrasound scanning.[41,42] The technology of this equipment is continuing to advance rapidly, but important basic training and skills will always be required for appropriate application of the technology.

Endoscopes are now available to effectively image the lumen of the fallopian tube (falloposcopy and salpingoscopy), as well as the inside of ovarian cysts (ovarioscopy), although it seems likely that technologies such as these will generally be limited to highly specialized centers for the foreseeable future.

This field is much too large to be covered adequately in this short chapter, and the reader is referred to the following excellent review volumes for further information.[43–45]

MINIHYSTEROSCOPY

This is still regarded as the 'gold standard' for evaluation of the uterine cavity and the endometrial surface,[41,42,46,47] although newer ultrasound techniques such as sonohysterography are providing increasingly useful complementary diagnostic information.[48] Both of these approaches to imaging require skilled operators for optimum use and there is increasing debate as to which evaluation should be carried out first. Most ultrasound techniques are less invasive and cheaper, are less precise in evaluating the endometrial surface, but do provide information about endometrial thickness and echogenicity and about the underlying myometrium.

Outpatient diagnostic hysteroscopy is usually carried out with narrow rigid telescopes with an outer sheath diameter of 2.5–5.0 mm and a 25° objective lens to allow inspection of the cavity walls and tubal ostia. Uterine distension is nowadays achieved in most centres using normal saline under pressure of 50–150 mmHg. This fluid medium is technically easier to use than carbon dioxide, allows a more natural view of soft and mobile surface structures and can give a clearer view in the presence of intracavitary blood. The most recent developments in technology have resulted in the availability of very narrow semi-rigid endoscopes with an outer sheath diameter of less than 2 mm. These can usually be used without any analgesia and even without a cervical tenaculum, but the clarity of vision is not quite as good as with the wider diameter endoscopes. Nevertheless, vision is adequate for routine diagnostic purposes, and can be combined with directed biopsy.

Hysteroscopy is valuable for the diagnosis and evaluation of cervical and endometrial polyps, submucous and intracavitary myomata, uterine septa, intrauterine and cervical adhesions, abnormalities of the tubal ostia, endometritis, areas of endometrial hyperplasia, severe adenomyosis and endometrial carcinoma. Therefore, hysteroscopy is a valuable routine investigation for abnormalities of vaginal bleeding, infertility and recurrent miscarriage.

MINILAPAROSCOPY

Diagnostic laparoscopy has progressed considerably since the 1960s when it was popularized by Steptoe, Palmer and Frangenheim. It is now being increasingly undertaken as an 'office' procedure using local analgesia and mild sedation with endoscopes that are just 1–2 mm diameter, and with outer sheaths of only 2–3 mm diameter, although many surgeons gain initial experience with these procedures in the operating room.[49–51] Although the clarity of vision is less than that provided by the conventional 5–8 mm operative laparoscopes, it is satisfactory for many diagnostic purposes. In most cases abdominal distension is achieved with carbon dioxide, but some investigators are inspecting the ovaries and tubes through saline or Hartman's solution.

The diagnostic information provided by laparoscopy is an important adjunct to that provided by ultrasound. Laparoscopy generally permits more reliable assessment of pelvic adhesions, mobility of pelvic organs, surface appearance of pelvic structures (including endometriosis) and tubal patency than vaginal ultrasound, although ultrasound provides better information on the structure of ovarian and uterine lesions. Laparoscopy also allows the opportunity for inspection of the upper part of the abdominal cavity.

Laparoscopy is not entirely without risk, even in the most skilled hands, and occasional serious complications such as bowel or vascular injury can occur.

Other types of pelvic endoscopy

These have been well reviewed by Brosens and Wamsteker.[44] Evaluation of the fallopian tubal lumen with flexible fiberscopes can be undertaken by salpingoscopy, with cannulation of the fimbrial ostium and ampulla under direct vision at laparoscopy, or by falloposcopy with transuterine cannulation of the uterine ostium and interstitial portion of the tube. Salpingoscopy allows inspection of the ampullary portion of the tube as far as the isthmic-ampullary junction, whereas the narrower fiberscope of the falloposcope allows inspection of the full length of the tubal lumen. Due to the small number of fibers in these tiny scopes the image tends to lack clarity, but with practice intratubal pathology can be accurately evaluated.

Ovarioscopy with a double lumen sheath allows irrigation and inspection of the interior of an ovarian cyst without spillage of cyst contents. This can be helpful in identifying active areas of endometriosis within an endometrioma, which can then be ablated by laser or electrocautery, or in identifying suspicious areas inside other types of cyst for directed biopsy.

Other pelvic organs that can be inspected endoscopically include the uterine cervix (colposcopy), urinary tract (urethroscopy, cystoscopy, ureteroscopy) and bowel (proctoscopy, sigmoidoscopy, colonoscopy). Detailed discussion of these techniques is beyond the scope of this chapter.

Conclusion

Precise imaging of the pelvic organs is an increasingly important approach to the diagnosis, assessment and treatment of conditions that are influenced by estrogens and progestogens. Continued refinement of a range of imaging techniques is likely over the next few years.

REFERENCES

1. Thurmond AS 1994 Pregnancies after selective salpingography and tubal recanalization. Radiology 190: 11–13
2. Outwater E, Mitchell DG, Wilson KM 1998 CT and MRI of the myometrium. In: Anderson JA (ed) Gynaecological imaging with clinical and pathological correlates. Churchill Livingstone, London, ch 16
3. Platt JF, Bree FL, Davidson D 1990 Ultrasound of the normal non-gravid uterus: correlation with gross and histopathology. Journal of Clinical Ultrasound 18: 15–19
4. Merz E, Miric-Tesanic D, Bahlman F, Weber G, Wellek S 1996 Sonographic size of uterus and ovaries in pre- and postmenopausal women. Ultrasound Obstet Gynecol Jan 7(1): 38–42
5. Orsini LF, Salardi S, Pilu G, Bovicelli L, Cacciari E 1984 Pelvic organs in premenarcheal girls: real-time ultrasonography. Radiology 153: 113–116

5a. Ramsey PA, Jansen RPS 1998 Ultrasonography of the normal female pelvis. In: Anderson JA (ed) Gynecologic imaging with clinical and pathological correlate. Churchill Livingstone, London

6. Bakos O, Lundkvist O, Bergh T 1993 Transvaginal sonographic evaluation of endometrial growth and texture in spontaneous ovulatory cycles — a descriptive study. Human Reproduction 8: 799–806
7. Andolf E, Dahlander K, Aspenberg P 1993 Ultrasonic thickness of the endometrium correlated to body weight in asymptomatic postmenopausal women. Obstetrics and Gynecology 82: 936–940
8. Ferrazzi E, Torri V, Trio D, Zannoni E, Filiberto S, Dordoni D 1996 Sonographic endometrial thickness: a useful test to predict atrophy in patients with postmenopausal bleeding. An Italian multicentre study. Ultrasound in Obstetrics and Gynecology 7: 315–321
9. Cohen I, Altaras MM, Shapira J, Tepper R, Beyth Y 1994 Postmenopausal tamoxifen treatment and endometrial pathology. Obstetrics and Gynecology Survey 49: 823–829
10. Goldstein SR 1994 Unusual ultrasonographic appearance of the uterus in patients receiving tamoxifen. American Journal of Obstetrics and Gynecology 170: 447–451
11. Schwartz PE 1994 Gynaecological surveillance of women on tamoxifen. Connecticut Medicine 58: 515–521

11a. Ota H, Maki M, Shidara Y, Kodama H, Takaheshi H, Hayakawa M et al 1992 Effect of donazol at the immunological level in patients with adenomyosis, with special reference to autoantibodies: a multi-center cooperative study. American Journal of Obstetrics and Gynecology 167: 481–486

12. Reinhold C, McCarthy S, Bret PM, Mehgio B, Atri M, Zakarian R, Glaude Y, Liang L, Seymour RJ 1996 Diffuse adenomyosis: comparison of endovaginal US and MR imaging with histopathological correlation. Radiology 199: 151–158
13. Scanlan KA, Pozniak MA, Fagerholm M, Shapiro S 1990 Value of transperineal sonography in the assessment of vaginal atresia. American Journal of Radiology 154: 545–548
14. Rottem S, Thaler I, Goldstein SR, Timor-Trisch IE, Brandes JM 1990 Transvaginal sonographic technique: targeted organ scanning without resorting to 'planes'. Journal of Clinical Ultrasound 18: 243
15. Cohen HL, Shapiro MA, Mandel FS, Shapiro ML 1993 Normal ovaries in neonates and infants: a sonographic study of 77 patients 1 day to 24 months old. American Journal of Roentgenology 160: 583–586
16. Bridges NA, Cooke A, Healt MJ, Hindmarsh PC, Brook CG 1993 Standards for ovarian volume in childhood and puberty. Fertility and Sterility 60: 456–460
17. Muller-Leisse C, Bick U, Paulussen K, Troger J, Zachariou Z, Holzgreve W, Schumacher R, Horvitz A 1992 Ovarian cysts in the fetus and neonate — changes in sonographic pattern in the follow-up and their management. Pediatric Radiology 22: 395–400
18. Cohen HK, Tice HM, Handel FS 1990 Ovarian volumes measured by US: bigger than we think. Radiology 177: 189–192

19. Meroo LT, Andrino R, Barco MJ, de la Fuente F 1990 Cyclic changes of the functional ovarian compartments: echographic assessment. Acta Obstetrica Gynecologica Scandinavica 69: 327–332
20. Pache TD, Wladimiroff JW, deJong FH, Hop WC, Fauser BCJ 1990 Growth patterns of non-dominant ovarian follicles during the normal menstrual cycle. Fertility and Sterility 54: 638–642
21. Rossavik IK, Gibbons WE 1985 Variability of ovarian follicular growth in natural menstrual cycles. Fertility and Sterility 44: 195–199
22. Zandt-Stastry D, Thorsen MK, Middleston WB, Aiman J, Zion A, McAsey M, Harns L 1989 Inability of sonography to detect imminent ovulation. American Journal of Radiology 152: 91–95
23. O'Herlihy C, DeCrespigny L, Lopata A, Johnston I, Hoult I, Robinson H 1990 Preovulatory follicular size: a comparison of ultrasound and laparoscopic measurements. Fertility and Sterility 34: 24–26
24. Marinho AO, Sallam HN, Goessens LKV, Collins WP, Rodeck CH, Campbell S 1982 Real-time pelvic ultrasonography during the periovulatory period of patients attending an artificial insemination clinic. Fertility and Sterility 37: 633–638
25. Check JH, Dietterich C, Houck MA 1991 Ipsilateral versus contralateral ovary selection of dominant follicle in succeeding cycles. Obstetrics and Gynecology 77: 968–970
26. Hamilton CJCM, Evers JLH, Tan FES, Hoogland HJ 1987 The reliability of ovulation prediction by a single ultrasonographic follicle measurement. Human Reproduction 2: 103–107
27. Hanna MD, Chizen DR, Pierson RA 1994 Characteristics of follicular evacuation during human ovulation. Ultrasound in Obstetrics and Gynecology 4: 488–493
28. Ttinkanen H 1994 The role of vascularisation of the corpus luteum in the short luteal phase studied by doppler ultrasound. Acta Obstetrica Gynecologica Scandinavica 73: 321–323
29. Okai T, Kobayashi K, Ryo E, Kagawa H, Koxuma S, Taketani Y 1994 Transvaginal sonographic appearance of hemorrhagic functional ovarian cyst and their spontaneous regression. International Journal of Gynaecology and Obstetrics 44: 47–52
30. Pache TD, Wladimiroff JW, Hop WCJ et al 1992 How to discriminate between normal and polycystic ovaries: transvaginal US study. Radiology 183: 421
31. Venturoli S, Porcu E, Fabbri R, Maguini O, Paradisi R, Pallotti G, Gammi L, Flamigni C 1987 Postmenarchal evolution of endocrine pattern and ovarian aspects in adolescents with menstrual irregularities. Fertility and Sterility 48: 78–85
32. Haber HP, Mayer EI 1994 Ultrasound evaluation of uterine and ovarian size from birth to puberty. Pediatric Radiology 24: 11–13
33. Kupfer MC, Schwimer SR, Lebovic J 1992 Transvaginal sonographic appearance of endometriomata: spectrum of findings. Journal of Ultrasound in Medicine 11: 129–133
34. Zawin M, McCarthy S, Scorett L et al 1989 Endometriosis appearance and detection at MR imaging. Radiology 171: 693
35. Yamashita Y, Torashima M, Hatanaka Y, Harada M, Higashida Y, Takahashi M et al 1995 Adnexal masses: accuracy of characterization with transvaginal US and precontrast and postcontrast MR imaging. Radiology 1994: 557–565
36. Thurmond AS, Jones MK, Cohen DJ 1996 Gynecologic, obstetric and breast radiology. A text/atlas of imaging in women. Blackwell Science, Cambridge, Massachusetts, USA, pp 296–297
37. Sassone AM, Timor-Tritsch IE, Artner A, Westhoff C, Warren WB 1991 Transvaginal sonographic characterization of ovarian disease: evaluation of a new scoring system to predict ovarian malignancy. Obstetrics and Gynecology 78: 70–76
38. Ferrazzi E, Zanetta G, Dordoni D, Berlandi N, Mezzopane R, Lissoni G 1997 Transvaginal ultrasonographic characterization of ovarian masses: comparison of live scoring systems in a multicenter study. Ultrasound in Obstetrics and Gynecology 10: 192–197
39. Timor-Tritsch LE, Lerner JP, Monteagudo A, Santos R 1993 Transvaginal ultrasonographic characterization of ovarian masses by means of color flow-directed Doppler measurements and a morphologic scoring system. American Journal of Obstetrics and Gynecology 168: 909–913
40. Goldrath MH, Sherman AI 1985 Office hysteroscopy and suction curettage: can we eliminate the hospital diagnostic dilation and curettage? American Journal of Obstetrics and Gynecology 155: 202–229
41. Emanuel MH, Verdel MJ, Wamsteker K, Lammes FB 1995 A prospective comparison of transvaginal ultrasonography and diagnostic hysteroscopy in the evaluation of patients with abnormal uterine bleeding. American Journal of Obstetrics and Gynecology 172: 547–552
42. Towbin NA, Gviazda IM, March CM 1996 Office hysteroscopy versus transvaginal ultrasonography in the evaluation of patients with excessive uterine bleeding. American Journal of Obstetrics and Gynecology 174: 1678–1682
43. Hamou JE 1991 Hysteroscopy and microhysteroscopy. Appleton and Lange, Norwalk
44. Brosens I, Wamsteker K (eds) 1997 Diagnostic imaging and endoscopy in gynaecology. WB Saunders, London
45. Kadar N 1995 Atlas of laparoscopic pelvic surgery. Blackwell Science, Cambridge, Ma
46. Nagele F, O'Connor H, Davies A, Badawy A, Mohamed H, Magos A 1996 2500 outpatient diagnostic hysteroscopies. Obstetrics and Gynecology 88: 87–92
47. Fraser IS 1993 Personal techniques and results for outpatient diagnostic hysteroscopy. Gynaecological Endoscopy 2: 29–34
48. Laughead MK, Stones LM 1997 Clinical utility of saline solution infusion in a primary care obstetric-gynecologic practice. American Journal of Obstetrics and Gynecology 176: 1313–1318
49. Molloy D 1995 The diagnostic accuracy of a microlaparoscopy. Journal of the American Association of Gynecologic Laparoscopists 2: 203–206
50. Palter SF, Olive DL 1996 Office microlaparoscopy under local anesthesia for chronic pelvic pain. Journal of the American Association of Gynecologic Laparoscopists 3: 359–364
51. van der Wat J 1997 Microendoscopy in the operating room. Gynaecological Endoscopy 6: 265–268

SECTION 6

Therapeutics

CONTENTS

Cancer of Reproductive Organs

Metabolic actions and long term side-effects of therapeutic steroids used for contraception, hormone replacement and gynecologic disease

30. Primary and secondary amenorrhea

Rogerio A. Lobo

Introduction

Amenorrhea is defined as the absence of menses and can be primary or secondary. In primary amenorrhea menses have never occurred; and in secondary amenorrhea absence of menstruation occurs after some pattern of bleeding has been established. Alterations in the endogenous secretion of estrogen, and also of progesterone, lead to amenorrhea. Uterine bleeding is dependent on the appropriate priming of the endometrium with estrogen, followed by progesterone. Apart from structural abnormalities of the mullerian tract, we will see that the majority of cases of amenorrhea are due to alterations in the secretion of estrogen. Primary amenorrhea will be discussed first, followed by the evaluation of secondary amenorrhea. A practical approach to the differential diagnosis will be stressed. Finally, the possible treatment of these disorders with estrogen and/or progestogens will be presented.

PRIMARY AMENORRHEA

Primary amenorrhea is somewhat arbitrarily diagnosed when uterine bleeding has not occurred by age 16½ years.[1] Other authors have used the aged of 16 or 17 years. It is important under these circumstances to know whether other signs of puberty exist. Puberty usually begins with breast budding (thelarche) followed closely by pubic hair development and a growth spurt. The latter can overlap or even precede the other signs. The mean age ± SD of obvious clinical signs of thelarche, pubic hair appearance and menarche in the US are 10.8 ± 1.1, 11.0 ± 1.2 and 12.9 ± 1.2 years. The normal interval between thelarche and menarche is 2.3 years. The range is 1.5–5 years. If thelarche has not occurred by age 14, it is likely that primary amenorrhea will follow (no bleeding by age 16½), and an evaluation for delayed onset of puberty is warranted.

Because the breast is extremely sensitive to estrogen, and development is usually the first obvious sign of puberty, the presence or absence of breast growth is a major criterion in the diagnostic evaluation of primary amenorrhea. The other important variable is the presence of an end-organ or uterus. Thus a differential diagnosis can be established by physical examination based on the findings of the presence or absence of the breast and the uterus.[2] Clearly, before an examination occurs, important historical clues need to be sought such as a history of abnormal growth and development, systemic illnesses, operations, family history, etc. Table 30.1 lists the etiologies based on the physical findings (breast and uterus).

Uterus present, breast absent

If on examination, or by ultrasound, a uterus is present yet there is no breast development, it may be assumed that the estrogen status is low. It must be recognized that an infantile uterus is sometimes so small that it is missed on abdominal scanning. Therefore either ovarian failure is present (usually due to genetic factors) or there is an inhibition of the hypothalamic-pituitary axis. The measurement of FSH distinguishes between these two. If FSH is elevated, a karyotype is indicated to rule in or out gonadal dysgenesis. Features of Turner's syndrome (webbed neck, etc.), if present, will be helpful but need not be present. Genetic abnormalities are the most common cause of primary amenorrhea, making up 30% of all cases.[2,3]

Either the absence of an X chromosome or a defect on X will lead to ovarian failure and amenorrhea. Mosaicism is also common. In general, height is affected by a defect in Xp for most women. Xq abnormalities usually result in individuals who have normal height. A portion of the Y chromosome may also appear in the karyotype, either as a whole or as a fragment. The latter might only be detectable with a

Table 30.1 Differential diagnosis of primary amenorrhea.

1. **Uterus present, breast absent** *Elevated FSH* Gonadal dysgenesis — karyotype (rule out Y) 17α-hydroxylase deficiency *Normal/low FSH* — CNS imaging Hypothalamic (GnRH deficiency) Pituitary causes 2. **Uterus absent, breast present** *Testosterone* (Male range) Androgen insensitivity — 46XY (confirmatory) (Female range) Congenital absence of uterus	3. **Uterus absent, breast absent** Agonadism 17,20-desmolase deficiency 17α-hydroxylase deficiency (46,XY) 4. **Uterus present, breast present** *PRL, estradiol/progesterone challenge* Work up as in secondary amenorrhea

Y-specific probe. Nevertheless, if Y is either detected or any signs of masculinization exist (even if no Y is detected), gonadectomy should be performed by laparoscopy because of the high risk of neoplasms. In no other condition in this category is removal of the streak gonad or diagnostic laparoscopy necessary.

The only other diagnosis in this category is 17α-hydroxylase deficiency.[4,5,6] This rare diagnosis is associated with hypertension and hypokalemia. The phenotype is similar (eunuchoid) in these individuals, whether the karyotype is 46,XX or 46,XY. In 46,XY individuals, who present as phenotypic females with primary amenorrhea, a uterus is not usually present. In 46,XX, the ovaries are usually multicystic and the gonadotropins are elevated, resulting in the stimulation of steroidogenesis through progesterone to form deoxycorticosterone (DOC). The diagnosis is confirmed by the finding of a luteal phase level of progesterone (>3 ng/mL; >9 nmol/L) and very low levels of 17 OH progesterone (<0.2 ng/mL; <0.6 nmol/L) because of the block in steroidogenesis.

If serum FSH is low, then a defect in the hypothalamic-pituitary axis can be assumed. In this category, either constitutional delay of puberty or a pathological deficiency in GnRH secretion should be entertained. Isolated deficiency of GnRH secretion might be present (hypogonadotropic hypogonadism) and this can be associated with anosmia in Kallmann's syndrome.[7,8,9]

It is important to image the hypothalamic-pituitary areas whenever a defect in gonadotropin secretion is suspected. An MRI is usually preferred over a CT scan, although a CT scan with contrast is more precise than plain X-rays. A plain cone-view X-ray might be all that is needed, as CNS lesions outside the hypothalamic-pituitary area are usually large and easy to diagnose. If no lesion is visible, most of the defects are hypothalamic in origin. However, in order to differentiate between these and the more rare pituitary causes, a GnRH stimulation test may be helpful. GnRH 100 µg is given as a bolus to elicit a rise in LH. It is usually necessary to prime the pituitary if there is no response by administering the same dose of GnRH intramuscularly for at least five days.

Uterus absent, breast present

Here, estrogen or steroid action on the breast is adequate, suggesting normal gonadal development. Absence of the uterus suggests a mullerian abnormality. The two possibilities can be differentiated using measurements of serum testosterone.[2] In the first, *androgen insensitivity syndrome*, testosterone is in the normal male range (200–1000 ng/dL) and the diagnosis can be confirmed by a karyotype (showing 46,XY). In the second case, serum testosterone is in the female range and the defect is that of congenital absence of the uterus and vagina (Mayer-Rokitansky-Kuster-Hauser syndrome).

Androgen insensitivity (complete)

Formerly called *testicular feminization syndrome*, the defect is one of androgen action: either a receptor or postreceptor defect. An individual with the androgen insensitivity syndrome has a 46,XY karyotype, testes and a female phenotype.[10] In the complete form, the clinical features include a total absence of axillary and pubic hair, normal breast development and a blind vaginal pouch. A family history is an important part of the patient's evaluation as this syndrome — which is either X-linked recessive or X-linked dominant with incomplete penetrance — can be found in several members of a family.

The uterus and oviducts are absent, and the testes secrete normal amounts of müllerian-inhibiting substance (MIS), which exerts its action even in the absence of receptors. Because the testes also produce normal male levels of testosterone and estradiol, the serum levels of gonadotropins remain normal. Normal breast development occurs, even with low levels of estradiol (30 pg/mL; 100 pmol/L), because of the lack of any androgen opposition. The small amounts of estrogen secreted by the adrenals and testes are enhanced by peripheral conversion of androstenedione to estrone. When unopposed by androgens, they promote either normal breast development or enlarged breasts.

Any phenotypic female with a Y chromosome should have the gonads removed because of the high incidence of malignancy. For women over the age of 30 with the androgen insensitivity syndrome, the incidence of malignant gonadal neoplasia is 22%. The malignant gonadal neoplasias are usually dysgerminomas or gonadoblastomas. Because malignant tumors have not been reported in prepubertal patients with this syndrome, the testes should not be removed until full breast development and epiphyseal closure have occurred; this allows endogenous testicular steroid secretion to exert its effects on these areas. After sexual maturity is achieved, the testes should be removed and estrogen replacement given to prevent osteoporosis and other sequelae of steroid deficiency. If necessary, progressive vaginal dilation based on the original principal of Frank[11] or skin graft or other types of vaginoplasty[12] should be performed when the patient wishes to become sexually active.

Uterovaginal agenesis

Complete uterine agenesis is the second most common cause of primary amenorrhea. Because they have ovaries, these individuals demonstrate normal secondary sex characteristics and often experience cyclic breast and mood alterations compatible with ovulation.

Since most patients with congenital absence of the uterus have normal ovarian function, hormone replacement is unnecessary. If the vagina is also absent (Mayer-Rokitansky-Kuster-Hauser syndrome), either vaginal dilation with progressively larger dilators or vaginoplasty will correct the defect. Using a surrogate mother, a patient with this disorder can now have her own genetic children.

Patients with congenital agenesis of the uterus alone or in association with vaginal agenesis have been found to have associated abnormalities such as urinary tract anomalies. Major defects (e.g. absence of a kidney) have been reported in approximately 15% of patients, and minor defects (e.g. double collecting system) in as many as 40% of patients. A 5% incidence of anomalies of the bony structures has also been reported in association with anomalies of the mullerian oviducts. Among the most common bony anomalies is the congenital fusion of the cervical vertebrae, which may present a problem when administering anesthesia because the rigidity of the neck renders intubation very difficult.

Uterus absent, breast absent

This is the rarest category. Here a karyotype is useful and is usually 46,XY. Typically, serum gonadotropin levels are elevated and testosterone is low (female range).

Agonadism

Individuals with agonadism have no breast development, uterine agenesis and no gonads. Federman[13] described this disorder, which presents with female or ambiguous external genitalia, and results from congenital anorchia (the loss of male gonads *in utero*). As there is no mullerian development, this occurs at a stage later than the production of anti-mullerian hormone by the testes.

17,20-desmolase deficiency

Patients with a complete deficiency of 17,20-desmolase lack the enzyme necessary to convert 17α-hydroxypregnenolone to dehydroepiandrosterone (Δ^5) and 17α-hydroxyprogesterone to androstenedione (Δ^4)[14]. With both of these pathways blocked, patients fail to synthesize any sex steroids, but are capable of producing cortisol and DOC. These individuals are phenotypically female, but with a 46,XY karyotype, and have intra-abdominal testes, which require surgical removal.[14]

Uterus present, breast present

Up to one third of patients with primary amenorrhea are in this category.[2] Since the uterus is present and breast development has occurred, the defect is one that occurred after estrogen stimulation of breast development and the full integration of the hypothalamic-pituitary-ovarian axis. Hyperprolactinemia may be responsible and has been found in 25% of patients in this category. Therefore prolactin (PRL) should be measured. Other patients should be evaluated in the same manner as for patients with secondary amenorrhea, beginning with measurements of serum estradiol (and/or a progestogen challenge). This situation can occur with the development of any cause of secondary amenorrhea in the interval between breast development and menarche (e.g. hypothalamic amenorrhea or polycystic ovarian disease).

SECONDARY AMENORRHEA

Our evaluation of this diagnosis presupposes that there are no other confounding factors influencing the reproductive axis. Thus PRL abnormalities are dealt with separately as are androgen abnormalities. In all other patients it is necessary to know what the current estrogen status is, as the first step in the evaluation.

Estrogen status is generally assessed by measurement of serum E_2-levels (levels <35 pg/mL; <100 pMol/L) generally imply a degree of hypoestrogenism that is insufficient to proliferate the endometrium). In the past, a progesterone withdrawal test was used. Here either i.m. progesterone (100–200 mg) or oral progestogen was administered with the anticipation of withdrawal bleeding within two weeks.[15] Since this test is less reliable, serum E_2 is favored. Note that the threshold level of serum E_2 varies from lab to lab. Serum E_2 <35 pg/mL (<100 pMol/L) represents a level that is generally below the normal follicular phase range.

A cause of secondary amenorrhea that needs to be considered early is a uterine defect, e.g. intrauterine adhesions (Asherman's syndrome), and/or severe cervical stenosis. This can occur as frequently as 7% in selected clinics[16,17] and may be suggested by a history of instrumentation, infection or other traumatic injury. If suspected, a diagnostic test (hysterosalpingogram, sonohysterography or hysteroscopy) should be considered initially.

If a uterine cause can be eliminated, the differential diagnosis is then based on whether E_2 is normal or low (Fig. 30.1).

Serum E_2 is normal (>35 pg/mL; >100 pMol/L)

If the serum E_2 is normal with a normal uterus, amenorrhea is due to anovulation. That is, even though the ovary has an adequate amount of basal GnRH and LH-FSH secretion to allow some E_2 production, the degree is insufficient for normal follicular activity and ovulation. This is often due to a lack of normal *pulsatile* secretion. Most of these causes are due to hypothalamic functional abnormalities. Hypothalamic amenorrhea, in turn, can be due to changes in body weight (and diet), exercise, stress, drug exposure, etc.[18–23] In general, these causes disrupt the final common pathway of GnRH pulsatile secretion due to abnormal signaling from neurotransmitters (opioids, catecholamines, serotonin, etc.). These interactions are discussed in chapter 7.

The other major cause of anovulation with normal estrogen status is due to the finding of polycystic ovarian syndrome (PCOS). This is discussed in detail in chapter 34. Indeed, here, estrogen status is moderately increased. Regarding the diagnosis of PCOS, even if obvious androgen excess *per se* is not present, clinical findings of anovulation and polycystic ovaries on ultrasound usually point to the diagnosis. However, because of clinical heterogeneity, not all findings need to be present. For example, only 70–75% of women with this diagnosis will have clear cut elevations in serum LH. Therefore, this confirmatory measurement is not necessary to make the diagnosis. Many investigators now accept a diagnosis of PCOS when typical 'polycystic' changes are present on ultrasound in combination with one or more relevant symptoms.

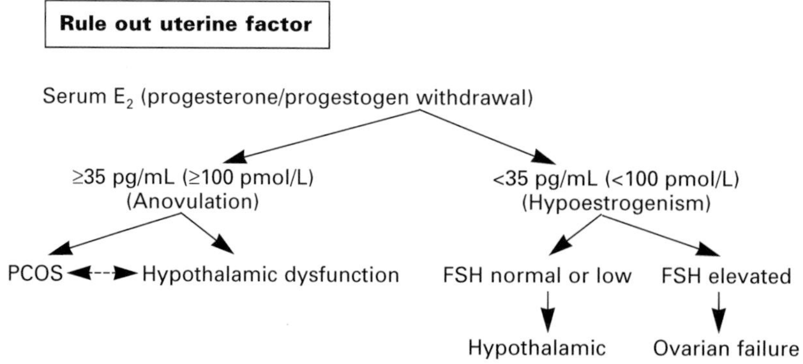

Fig. 30.1 Secondary amenorrhea (absent PRL and androgen abnormalities).

Serum E_2 is <35 pg/mL (<100 pMol/L)

Here, one simple diagnostic test is valuable in distinguishing why E_2 is low. Elevations of serum FSH point to premature ovarian failure if the women is less than 40 years old. If she is older than 40, her amenorrhea constitutes natural menopause.

If FSH levels are normal or low, a more severe form of hypothalamic amenorrhea is present (complete shut down of the axis). In this setting, unless there is a definitive history of drug use, etc., CNS imaging may be important to rule out rare neoplastic processes. If this is ruled out by CT scan or MRI, a functional or benign cause may be anticipated, sometimes with complete spontaneous recovery. Nevertheless, although rare, subtle defects in the ACTH-cortisol system can exist and therefore should be tested for, or taken into consideration if these patients require surgery or undergo medical stress (severe infections, etc.).

Premature ovarian failure is like the perimenopause in that the status may wax and wane.[24,25] Thus FSH levels may fluctuate above and below a diagnostic value of 40 mIU/mL. Once the diagnosis is established, other contributing causes should be evaluated, such as chromosomal or autoimmune disease.[26] Screening tests such as antinuclear antibodies, antiovarian antibodies, antimicrosomal antibodies, TSH levels and serum calcium and phosphorus are obtained. Cortisol status may also be included for testing. Occasionally, oocytes may still be present in the ovaries of these women even though follicular development is not occurring (resistant ovary syndrome).

If the second amenorrhea occurs early (<30 years), an incomplete form of gonadal dysgenesis should be sought by obtaining a karyotype. The importance of this test is to detect if there is Y material present, indicating a risk of dysgerminoma.

TREATMENT OF AMENORRHEA

The general principle of treatment is to replace estrogen and progesterone to prevent the consequences of long-term estrogen deficiency. Even short-term estrogen deficiency leads to bone loss, increasing the risk of osteoporosis.[27] More prolonged deficiency leads to cardiovascular risk. The mechanisms of these changes have been described in other chapters. Apart from these general principles, specific types of regimens and other options should be considered, depending on the specific diagnoses within the categories of primary and secondary amenorrhea. These treatments will be outlined below.

Primary amenorrhea

Delayed puberty might require no more treatment than reassurance. If thelarche has not occurred by age 14, for psychological reasons very low dose estrogen may be considered to begin the process of breast development, while being cautious to prevent premature closure of the long bone epiphyses. It is important to allow maximum growth as some of these girls may be short. Intermittent courses of three months can be considered; often only two courses are required. Doses of conjugated equine estrogens (CEE) 0.3 mg or micronized estradiol 0.5 mg may be considered. Very low dose initial exposure may give better breast development in the long term.

If FSH is elevated, gonadal dysgenesis is the diagnosis. Gonadectomy is necessary if Y chromosome material is present. Other than with this finding, routine hormonal replacement should be used, although many clinicians favor using combined oral contraceptives (COCS) for convenience and to enhance compliance. While oral contraceptives provide five-fold more estrogen than is necessary for substituting for estrogen deficiency in older women, in young healthy women it is a reasonable alternative and is the same as the way estrogen is used by women of the same age for contraception.

Women with Turner's syndrome are known to have increased risks of thyroid disease, diabetes,[28,29] osteoporosis, endometrial cancer (with unopposed estrogen) and cardiovascular disease. Recent evidence suggests that their cardiovascular system might not respond as well to conventional estrogen replacement.[30] Accordingly, oral contraceptives are a reasonable choice here as well. In women with Turner's syndrome, short stature is of concern. Recent studies have suggested a benefit in final height with the use of growth hormone supplements. In the past, limited success has also been achieved with the weak androgen, oxandrolone (0.1 mg/kg/day).[31]

In patients with normal or low FSH (hypothalamic failure), estrogen and progestogen replacement is prescribed once a CNS lesion has been ruled out. COCs may be used but, on theoretical grounds only, might not be as beneficial since the hypothalamic-pituitary axis is already suppressed.

In all these categories of patients, an important end point of therapy is normal breast development. If height is normal, doses equivalent to CEE 0.625–1.25 mg may be administered and there is no good evidence that higher doses are necessary. Time is what is required to progress through the Tanner stages of breast development. If full height has not been achieved, therapy should begin with only CEE 0.3 mg (to avoid premature epiphyseal closure) and the course of development is expected to take longer.

In hypogonadal individuals with dysgenetic ovaries, progeny may only be achieved through oocyte donation. The success and effectiveness of this treatment is excellent and is described in detail in chapter 42. In the other women with hypothalamic hypogonadism, i.v. or s.c. pulsatile GnRH therapy or i.m. gonadotropins can be used effectively. Use of gonadotropins (FSH and LH or purified FSH alone or, most recently, recombinant FSH) offers a practical advantage because of the ease of once daily administration and is a successful treatment in either hypothalamic or pituitary causes of anovulation and reproductive failure. However, much more intensive monitoring is required with injected gonadotropins to prevent hyperstimulation and multiple gestations.

In the rare case of 17α-hydroxylase deficiency, corticosteroid replacement normalizes the ACTH axis and then substitution estrogen/progestogen therapy can be prescribed. Pregnancies have been reported with in vitro fertilization (IVF) despite very low levels of sex steroids after gonadotropin stimulation.[32] In 46,XY individuals gonadectomy will be required to prevent dysgerminoma.

Androgen insensitivity (complete) is treated with gonadectomy and estrogen replacement. Mullerian agenesis does not require sex steroid therapy. An artificial vagina needs to be developed by dilatation therapy or by a neovaginoplasty procedure.[11,12] Pregnancy can be achieved by IVF and embryo transfer to another woman (gestational surrogacy).

The rare disorder of agonadism presents with no uterus or gonads. Estrogen treatment is necessary.

In 46,XY individuals with 17,20-desmolase deficiency, there is a defect in steroidogenesis that prevents the formation of dehydroepiandrosterone and androstenedione, but cortisol production is normal. Gonadectomy and estrogen-progestogen replacement is required.

In patients with primary amenorrhea with both breast and uterus present, the diagnostic categories and management principles are similar to those utilized in women with secondary amenorrhea.

Secondary amenorrhea (normal estrogen) PCOS

In women with PCOS, treatment usually consists of progestogens, used cyclically, to prevent endometrial hyperplasia and anovulatory dysfunctional uterine bleeding (DUB). Oral contraceptives and antiandrogens may be used to treat symptoms of hyperandrogenism, and induction of ovulation can be used (usually clomiphene citrate) when pregnancy is desired (see ch. 34).

Hypothalamic amenorrhea

Cyclical or intermittent progestogens can be used to induce withdrawal bleeding when serum E_2 levels are normal. Oral contraceptives may also be used.

Pregnancy may be achieved with induction of ovulation using clomiphene when estrogen status is normal. If clomiphene does not induce ovulation in doses up to 150 mg per day for five days, pulsatile GnRH or gonadotropins may be used effectively.

Hypothalamic failure

This is a more extreme degree of hypothalamic amenorrhea. Substitute estrogen and progestogen therapy is used once a CNS lesion is ruled out. Induction of ovulation usually requires pulsatile GnRH therapy or gonadotropins.

Premature ovarian failure

Substitute estrogen and progestogen therapy is used. If pregnancy is desired, oocyte donation is required (ch. 41). If the woman remains healthy, in our experience this procedure can be carried out at any age, and has been safely accomplished in women aged into the early 60s.

REFERENCES

1. Frisch RE, Revelle R 1971 Height and weight at menarche and a hypothesis of menarche. Archives of Diseases of the Child 46: 695–701
2. Mashchak CA, Kletzky OA, Davajan V et al 1981 Clinical and laboratory evaluation of patients with primary amenorrhea. Obstetrics and Gynecology 57: 715–721
3. Rosen DL, Kaplan B, Lobo RA 1988 Menstrual function and hirsutism in patients with gonadal dysgenesis. Obstetrics and Gynecology 17: 677–680
4. Biglieri EG, Herron MA, Brust N 1966 17-hydroxylation deficiency in man. Journal of Clinical Investigation 45: 1946–1954
5. Goldsmith O, Soloman DH, Horton R 1967 Hypogonadism and mineralocorticoid excess; the 17-hydroxylase deficiency syndrome. New England Journal of Medicine 277: 673–677

6. New MI 1970 Male pseudohermaphroditism due to 17-alpha-hydroxylase deficiency. Journal of Clinical Investigation 49: 1930–1941
7. Kletzky OA, Nicoloff JT, Davajan V et al 1978 Idiopathic hypogonadotropic hypogonadal primary amenorrhea. Journal of Clinical Endocrinology and Metabolism 46: 808–815
8. Reindollar RH, Byrd JR, McDonough PG 1981 Delayed sexual development: a study of 252 patients. American Journal of Obstetrics and Gynecology 140: 371–380
9. Kletzky OA, Costin G, Marrs RP et al 1979 Gonadotropin insufficiency in patients with thalassemia major. Journal of Clinical Endocrinology and Metabolism 48: 901–905
10. Morris JM, Mahesh VB 1963 Further observations on the syndrome 'testicular feminization.' American Journal of Obstetrics and Gynecology 87: 731–748
11. Frank RI 1938 The formation of an artifical vagina without operation. American Journal of Obstetrics and Gynecology 35: 1053–1055
12. Jones HW, Rock JA 1983 Reparative and constructive surgery of the female generative tract. Williams & Wilkins, Baltimore, p 146
13. Federman DD 1967 (ed): Abnormal sexual development: a genetic and endocrine approach in differential diagnosis. Philadelphia, WB Saunders
14. Goebelsmann U, Zachmann M, Davajan V et al 1976 Male pseudo-hermaphroditism consistent with 17,20 desmolase deficiency. Gynecological Investigation 7: 138–156
15. Kletzky OA, Davajan V, Nakamura RM et al 1975 Clinical categorization of patients with secondary amenorrhea using progesterone induced bleeding and measurement of serum gonadotropin levels. American Journal of Obstetrics and Gynecology 121: 695–703
16. Reindollar RH, Novak M, Tho SPT, McDonough PG 1981 Adult-onset amenorrhea: a study of 262 patients. American Journal of Obstetrics and Gynecology 140: 371–380
17. Schenker JG, Margalioth EJ 1982 Intrauterine adhesions: an updated appraisal. Fertility and Sterility 37: 593–610
18. Fries H, Nillus SJ, Pettersson F 1974 Epidemiology of secondary amenorrhea: a retrospective evaluation of etiology with special regard to psychogenic factors and weight loss. American Journal of Obstetrics and Gynecology 118: 473–479
19. Feicht CB, Johnson TS, Martin BJ et al 1978 Secondary amenorrhea in athletes. Lancet 2: 1145–1146
20. McArthur JW, Bullen BA, Beitins IZ et al 1980 Hypothalamic amenorrhea in runners of normal body composition. Endocrine Research Communications 7–13
21. Vigersky RA, Andersen AE, Thompson RG et al 1977 Hypothalamic dysfunction in secondary amenorrhea associated with simple weight loss. New England Journal of Medicine 297: 1141–1145
22. Mason HD, Sagle M 1988 Reduced frequency of luteinizing hormone pulses in women with weight loss-related amenorrhea and multifollicular ovaries. Clinical Endocrinology 28: 611–618
23. Warren MP, Jewelewicz R, Dyrenfurth I et al 1975 The significance of weight loss in the evaluation of pituitary response to LH-RH in women with secondary amenorrhea. Journal of Clinical Endocrinology and Metabolism 40: 601–611
24. Rebar RW, Connolly HV 1990 Clinical features of young women with hypergonadotropic amenorrhea. Fertility and Sterility 53: 804–810
25. Alper MM, Garner PR 1985 Premature ovarian failure: its relationship to autoimmune disease. Obstetrics and Gynecology 66: 27–30
26. Mignot MH, Schoemaker J, Kleingeld M et al 1989 Premature ovarian failure I. The association with autoimmunity. European Journal of Obstetrics, Gynecology and Reproductive Biology 30: 59–66
27. Schlechte JA, Sherman B, Martin R 1983 Bone density in amenorrheic women with and without hyperprolactinemia. Journal of Clinical Endocrinology and Metabolism 56: 1120–1123
28. Hamilton CR, Moldawer M, Rosenberg HS 1968 Hashimotos' thyroiditis and Turner's syndrome. Archive of Internal Medicine 122: 69–72
29. Forbes AO, Engel E 1963 The high incidence of diabetes mellitus in 41 patients with gonadal dysgenesis and their close relatives. Metabolism of Clinical and Experimental 12: 428–439
30. Biljan MM, Garden AS, Taylor CT, Fraser WD, Matijevic R, Diver MJ, Jones SV, Kingsland CR 1995 Exaggerated effects of progestogen on uterine artery pulsatility index in Turner's Syndrome patients receiving hormone replacement therapy. (Univ of Liverpool, England) Fertil Steril 64: 1104–1108
31. Rudman D, Goldsmith M, Kutner M, Blackston D 1980 Effect of growth hormone and oxandrolone singly and together on growth rate in girls with X chromosome abnormalities. J Pediatr Jan; 96(1): 132–135
32. Rabinovici J, Blankstein J, Goldman B et al 1989 In vitro fertilization and primary embryonic cleavage are possible in 17-alpha-hydroxylase deficiency despite extremely low intrafollicular 17-beta-estradiol. Journal of Clinical Endocrinology and Metabolism 68: 693–697

31. Primary dysmenorrhea

M. Åkerlund

Introduction

In women with primary dysmenorrhea no underlying anatomical cause of the symptoms can be established, and the condition can be regarded as 'functional'. The problem is common before the first birth, different Scandinavian studies having shown that about 50% of nulliparous women suffer from menstrual pain of some degree.[1–3] In 10–20%, the symptoms are so pronounced that women may be absent from work for 1–2 days each or every second menstruation.

The etiological mechanisms of the disease appear to include a subtle imbalance of estrogens and progestogens, and synthetic ovarian hormones have been used extensively in the therapy. In this overview, factors causing primary dysmenorrhea will be described in detail including the involvement of ovarian hormones. A broad discussion about present and possible future therapies, including the place of estrogens, progestogens and estrogen-progestogen combinations in the treatment will also be provided.

ETIOLOGICAL MECHANISMS IN PRIMARY DYSMENORRHEA

Uterine contractions and blood flow

In most women suffering from primary dysmenorrhea, myometrial hyperactivity can be demonstrated by intrauterine pressure recording.[4–6] A representative recording of intra-uterine pressure and local endometrial blood flow in a woman with painful menstruation[4] is shown in Figure 31.1. The pattern varies between individuals so that contractions of increased amplitude, very frequent contractions with no period of complete uterine relaxation in between and/or a high basal tone can be found, and as a whole the contractile pattern is chaotic in comparison to that in healthy women at the onset of menstruation.[4] In parallel with this increased contractile activity the uterine blood flow is decreased (Fig. 31.1), forceful contractions causing particularly well-demarked reductions in flow in the endometrium.[4]

The perception of pain in primary dysmenorrhea in relation to uterine activity was studied by recordings on a visual analogue scale performed by the women themselves in parallel to intra-uterine pressure recordings.[7] An example from those experiments is shown in Figure 31.2. There was frequently a time lag between individual peaks in pressure and maximal pain.[7] This suggests that the important mechanism by which intensive uterine activity causes pain is not the contractile force *per se*, but a factor in between, namely the reducing effect that these contractions may have on the blood flow.[4] The uterine ischemia resulting from intensive contractions would be expected to lead to accumulation of acid metabolites, which then cause pain.

Prostaglandins

Prostaglandins which stimulate contractions, particularly prostaglandin $F_{2\alpha}$, are also involved in mechanisms of dysmenorrhea. The effect of prostaglandin $F_{2\alpha}$ infusion on myometrial activity at the onset of menstruation is illustrated in Figure 31.3. Uterine prostaglandins may cause pain not only by stimulating contractions, but also by affecting afferent nerve fibers in the uterus. In animal trials it has been shown that the sensitivity of pain mediating nerves increases in the presence of prostaglandins.[8]

An increased endometrial synthesis of prostaglandin $F_{2\alpha}$ has been demonstrated in dysmenorrheic women.[9] Lumsden et al[10] found that the concentrations of both prostaglandin $F_{2\alpha}$ and prostaglandin E_2 in menstrual blood of women with dysmenorrhea were significantly increased compared to those of healthy controls on days 1 and 2 of the menstrual cycle. Furthermore, myometrial hyperactivity with accompanying circulatory changes in the uterus,

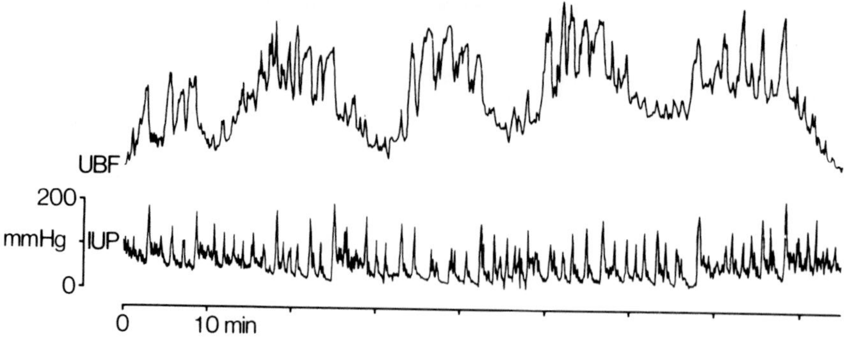

Fig. 31.1 Local endometrial blood flow (UBF) and intra-uterine pressure (IUP) on the first day of menstruation in a woman with severe dysmenorrhea.

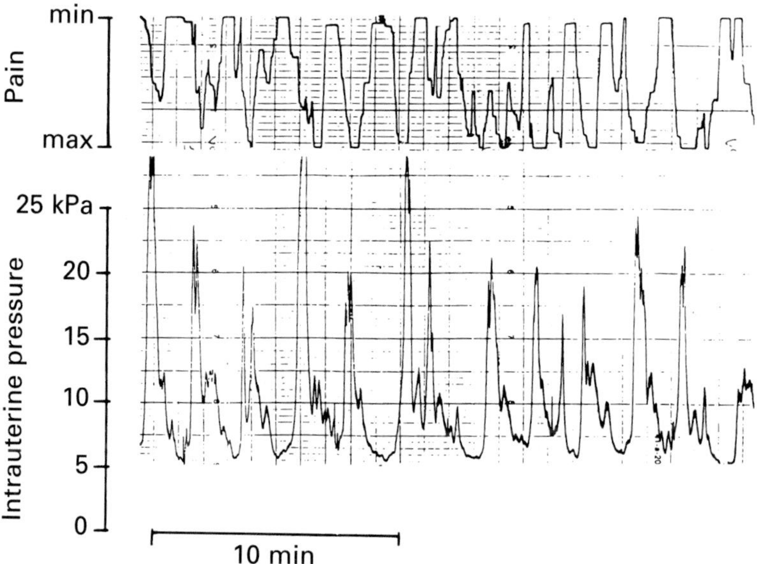

Fig. 31.2 Record of pain experienced (reversed visual analogue scale) and intra-uterine pressure in a woman with severe primary dysmenorrhea.

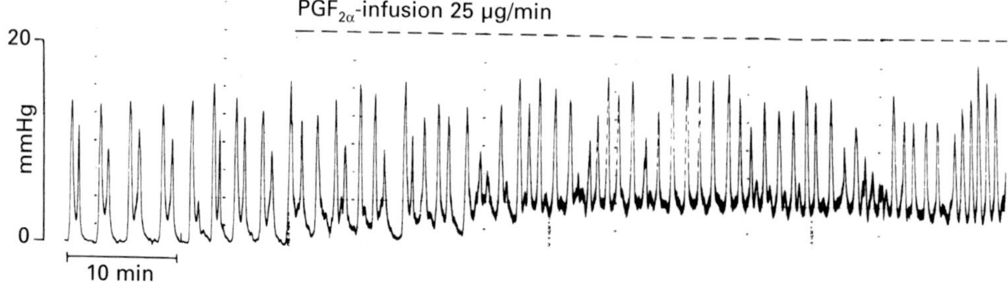

Fig. 31.3 Effect of prostaglandin $F_{2\alpha}$ infusion on uterine activity in a woman on the first day of menstruation.

which is caused by other factors, may lead to a secondary endometrial synthesis and release of prostaglandins.[11]

Vasopressin and other peptides

Women with primary dysmenorrhea have increased plasma concentrations of vasopressin,[12–15] and administration of this hormone causes the same pattern of myometrial hyperactivity and uterine ischemia as is seen in the condition.[16] Even a slight increase in the circulating level of vasopressin, which can be induced by infusion of hypertonic saline, increases uterine activity (Fig. 31.4).[15] The hormone has a pronounced effect not only on the myometrium, but also on the smooth muscle of arterial walls, particularly the resistance arteries near the endometrium.[17] Other peptides, such as oxytocin, endothelin and noradrenaline are also potent vasoconstrictors in the uterus, and may play some role.[17]

In experiments with infusion of hypertonic saline to dysmenorrheic women,[15] not only vasopressin but also oxytocin levels increased, and furthermore, both type V1a vasopressin and oxytocin receptors have been demonstrated in myometrium from nonpregnant women.[18] On the basis of these results, we have recently compared the effect of vasopressin and oxytocin on uterine activity *in vivo* in women in different ovarian hormonal states, who were due to undergo hysterectomy for benign gynecological disorders.[19] We also studied the *in vitro* myometrial

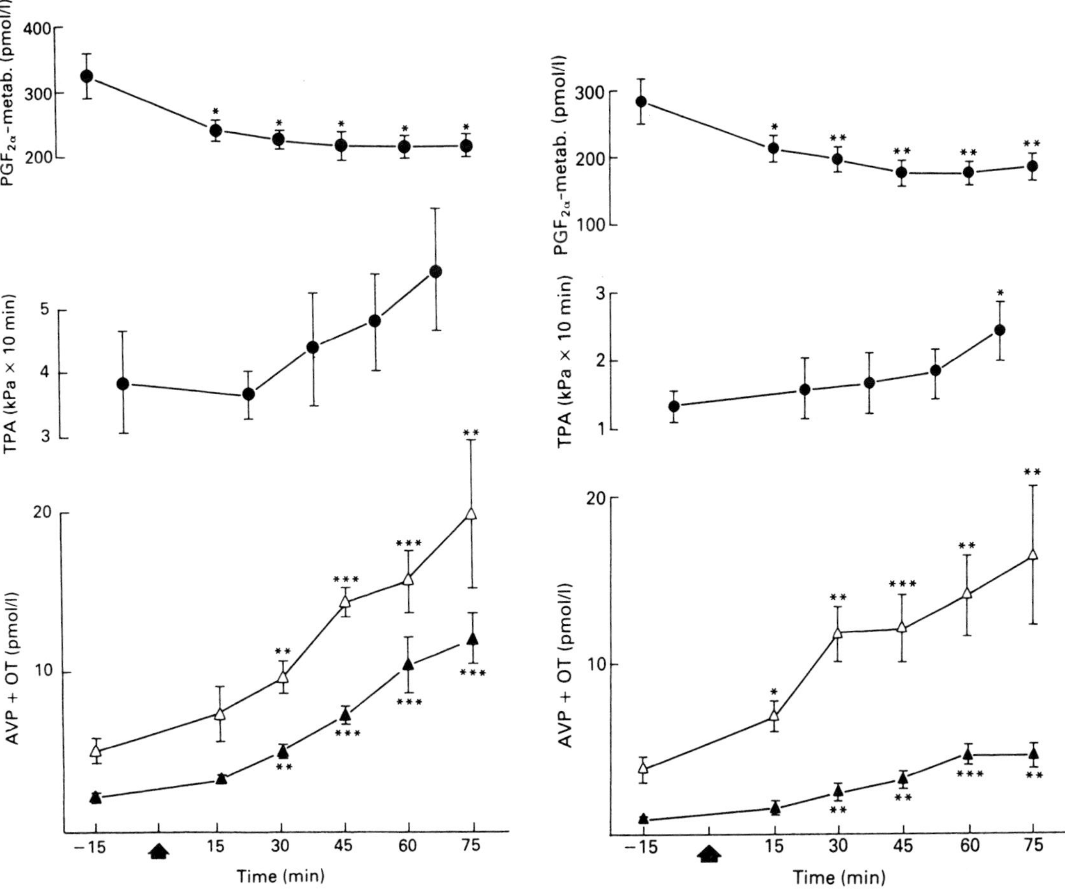

Fig. 31.4 Effect of hypertonic saline infusion on plasma levels of arginine vasopressin (AVP) (OT, the metabolite 15-keto-13,14-dihydro-PGF$_{2\alpha}$) and uterine activity measured as total pressure area (TPA) in nine women on the first day of bleeding and with primary dysmenorrhea (left), and without pain after one period of oral contraceptive treatment (right). Means and standard errors are shown and statistically significant differences in comparison to the observations before start of the infusion are indicated by asterisks (*$P<0.05$, ** = $P<0.01$). After the oral contraceptive treatment both vasopressin levels before and after infusion, as well as total pressure areas, were significantly reduced.

effects of the peptides after the operation as well as myometrial concentrations of vasopressin V1a and oxytocin receptors. The myometrial effects of oxytocin *in vivo* and the concentration of oxytocin receptors correlated, but such correlation was not seen for vasopressin. This may indicate that, in parallel to the situation in pregnancy,[20] vasopressin acts on both vasopressin V1a and oxytocin receptors, whereas oxytocin only influences its own receptor. The vasopressin receptor concentration was four times higher than that of oxytocin, with a mean of 216 versus 54 fmol/mg protein. The average potency of vasopressin on the uterus in women before the operation was also about four times higher than that of oxytocin and on isolated myometrium, 20 times greater. Furthermore, the effect of vasopressin was increased premenstrually. These observations emphasize the particular involvement of vasopressin in uterine activation and they are in agreement with an important but incompletely defined role for vasopressin in primary dysmenorrhea.

Uterine innervation

Nerves of adrenergic, cholinergic and peptidergic type have been demonstrated in the uterus, and there is an abundant innervation both of the myometrium and the smooth muscle of uterine arteries.[21–22] The resistance arteries are particularly well innervated, indicating that nerves are involved in the regulation of uterine blood flow. In connection with the hormonal changes during pregnancy a process of denervation takes place in the uterus, and the nerves regenerate only to a limited extent after delivery.[22] It has been hypothesized that this may be one of the reasons for the decreased incidence of dysmenorrhea after birth of a first child.[22]

Balance of ovarian hormones

Several clinical observations indicate an involvement of ovarian hormones and their balance in mechanisms of dysmenorrhea. Thus, women with amenorrhea, spontaneous or induced by oral contraceptive pills, rarely suffer from the condition and synthetic steroids in different combinations have a well established therapeutic effect. Ovarian hormones may not only influence the release of prostaglandins and vasopressin, but may also modulate the sensitivity of the uterus to these and other factors.

The content of prostaglandins in the endometrium normally varies during the menstrual cycle and rises considerably in the late luteal phase.[23] However, in a study of the influence of a combined oral contraceptive on the plasma level of the metabolite 15-ketodehydro-prostaglandin $F_{2\alpha}$, no significant change due to this treatment was observed.[24]

Ovarian hormones have a marked influence on the release of vasopressin. In healthy women a cyclical variation was observed with peak levels at the time of ovulation and usually the lowest circulating concentrations at the onset of menstruation.[25] Furthermore, experiments in postclimacteric women (Fig. 31.5) showed that the release of vasopressin is stimulated by estrogen, an effect which is counteracted by progestogen.[26,27] Progestogen by itself has no effect on vasopressin release. Estrogen also stimulated oxytocin release, but adding progestagen did not seem to inhibit this effect.[27] Instead, a further increase in the circulating level of this hormone is observed.[27]

The uterine sensitivity to vasopressin is also under ovarian hormonal influence, as a markedly reduced response is observed after oral contraceptive treatment.[28] This is in agreement with the lower receptor concentration found in women on oral contraceptive pills.[19]

In women with primary dysmenorrhea, an imbalance of ovarian hormones in comparison to healthy controls has been demonstrated. Different Scandinavian studies have demonstrated a significantly increased level of estradiol in plasma during the luteal phase of women with dysmenorrhea.[13,29]

Summary of etiological mechanisms

An illustration of the possible interaction of different factors in dysmenorrhea, including the involvement of ovarian hormones, is shown in Figure 31.6. Arginine vasopressin and prostaglandin $F_{2\alpha}$ are central causative factors in the condition. Estradiol stimulates and progesterone inhibits the release of vasopressin from the posterior pituitary. This peptide in turn has marked effects on the myometrium and on the smooth muscle of arterial walls, particularly the resistance arteries. Thereby, uterine hyperactivity and ischemia is caused. Ovarian hormones can also influence effects of vasopressin on the myometrium by changing the expression of receptors. Other peptides such as oxytocin, endothelin and noradrenalin and possibly substances like leukotrienes, could contribute to uterine ischemia. Cholinergic, adrenergic and peptidergic nerves may also influence blood flow. An excess of estradiol compared to progesterone secretion from the corpus luteum could exacerbate a number of these processes.

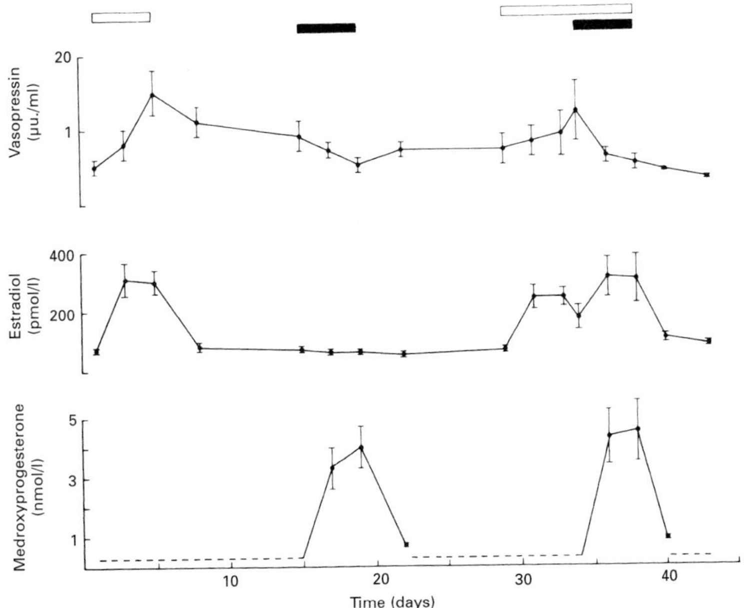

Fig. 31.5 Mean plasma concentrations (± SE) of vasopressin, estradiol and medroxyprogesterone in women during treatment with 2 mg estradiol valeriate per day (open bar) and 10 mg medoxyprogesterone acetate per day (solid bar).

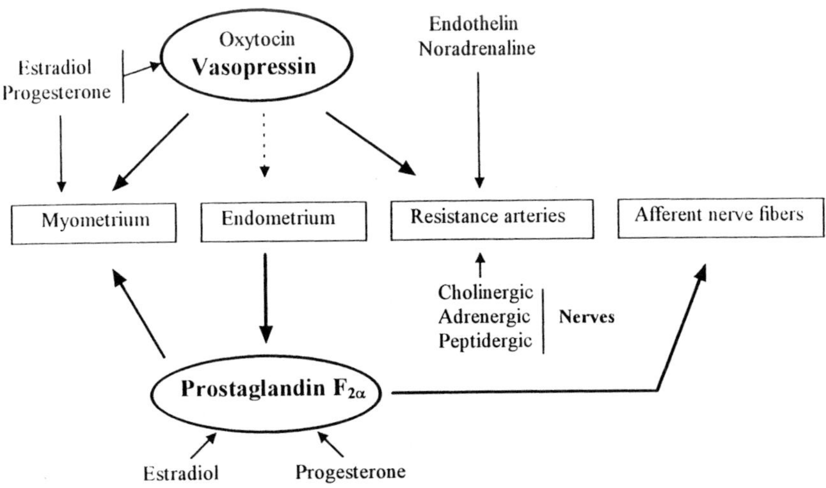

Fig. 31.6 Schematic representation of possible etiologic factors and effect or mechanisms in primary dysmenorrhea.

Prostaglandin $F_{2\alpha}$ is synthesized primarily in the endometrium. This synthesis is also under the influence of estradiol and progesterone. Prostaglandin $F_{2\alpha}$ causes pain by stimulating uterine contractility and afferent nerve fibers of the uterus. The responsiveness of the uterus to prostaglandins may be influenced by hormonal treatment.

THERAPEUTIC ASPECTS

Prostaglandin synthesis inhibitors

In the clinical management of both primary and secondary dysmenorrhea nonsteroid, antiinflammatory drugs, which inhibit prostaglandin synthesis and release, are well established.[6,30] Some may also have a partial end-organ blocking action. Ketoprofen is probably superior to naproxen in the condition, because of a more rapid uptake and action after oral administration.[31] Numerous prostaglandin-inhibiting agents have excellent demonstrated activity for primary dysmenorrhea.

Synthetic estrogens-progestogens

A combined and preferably monophasic oral contraceptive is the treatment of choice when dysmenorrheic women also require family planning. As illustrated in Figure 31.4, the plasma vasopressin level, the spontaneous uterine activity and the responsiveness of the uterus to vasopressin is reduced.[15,28] Decreased uterine sensitivity is probably due to a lowered myometrial concentration of vasopressin V1a and oxytocin receptors, vasopressin being active on both these types.[19] The myometrial response to prostaglandin $F_{2\alpha}$ in dysmenorrheic women is also decreased by oral contraceptive treatment.[28] In poorly responsive cases continuous use of a monophasic combination pill may effectively prevent menstruation and hence dysmenorrhea, but breakthrough bleeding may sometimes occur and can be accompanied by cramps.

In primary and secondary dysmenorrhea, the levonorgestrel-releasing IUD may also be of benefit, probably through a reduction of endometrial development with accompanying decreased prostaglandin synthesis.[32] Continuous intra-uterine progesterone is a well established treatment for primary dysmenorrhea.[33]

Other presently used therapies

Other pharmacological methods that may be tried in difficult-to-treat cases besides nonsteroidal, anti-inflammatory drugs and oral contraceptives, and which act by reducing the myometrial contractile activity in dysmenorrhea, are calcium channel blocking agents[35] and β_2-adrenoceptor stimulating drugs.[4] Both have been demonstrated as highly effective therapies, but side effects may be slightly commoner than with other therapies. Supportive alternative therapies such as acupuncture, behavioral modification therapies, naturopathy, traditional Chinese medicines, etc., may be of value in some individuals. Surgery to the uterosacral and presacral nerves has been advocated in resistant cases with severe symptoms, and probably has a small role.

New leads in treatment

Vasopressin V1a and oxytocin antagonists may have a therapeutic potential in primary dysmenorrhea. Our group, in collaboration with the Ferring Research Institute in Malmö, Sweden, have developed a series of oxytocin analogs, which inhibit the effect of vasopressin on the uterus.[34–36] An illustration of the inhibitory effect of the analog 1-deamino-2-D-Tyr(OEt)-4-Thr-8-Orn-oxytocin on vasopressin-

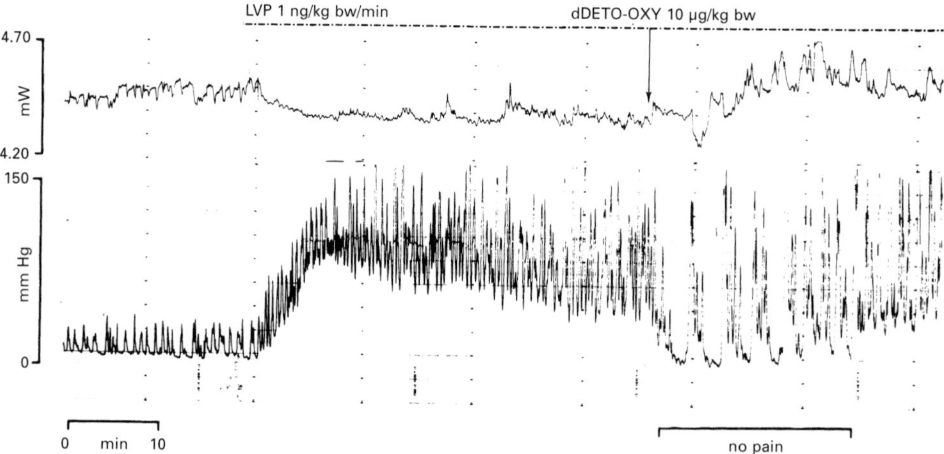

Fig. 31.7 Recording of uterine blood flow measured as added power and intra-uterine pressure in a nonpregnant woman on day 1 of menstruation. Infusion of lysine vasopressin (LVP) and bolus injection over 1 minute of the vasopressin and oxytocin antagonist, 1-deamino-2-D-Tyr(OEt)4-Thr-8-Orn-oxytocin (eDET-Oxy), are indicated. The LVP infusion induced dysmenorrhea-like pain in all subjects, which was completely relieved for about 15 minutes after antagonist injection.

induced contractile activity and uterine ischemia is shown in Figure 31.7. The compound blocks both the oxytocin and the vasopressin V1a receptor, and it inhibits both dysmenorrhea[37] and preterm labor.[38] However, this analog is not active by oral administration and absorption by the intranasal route is poor and variable. Other analogs, both peptide and nonpeptide compounds for inhibition of oxytocin and vasopressin V1a receptor effects, are under development.[39–42]

Acknowledgment Supported by the Swedish Medical Research Council (B 95-17-X6571-13) and the University and Hospital of Lund, Sweden.

REFERENCES

1. Bergsjö P, Jenssen H, Vellar OD 1975 Dysmenorrhoea in industrial workers. Acta Obstetrica Gynaecologica Scandinavica 54: 255–259
2. Andersch B, Milsom I 1982 An epidemiologic study of young women with dysmenorrhea. American Journal of Obstetrics and Gynecology 144: 655–660
3. Sundell G, Milsom E, Andersch B 1990 Factors influencing the prevalence and severity of dysmenorrhoea in young women. British Journal of Obstetrics and Gynaecology 97: 588–597
4. Åkerlund M, Andersson KE, Ingemarsson I 1976 Effect of terbutaline on myometrial activity, endometrial blood flow, and lower abdominal pain in women with primary dysmenorrhoea. British Journal of Obstetrics and Gynaecology 83: 673–678
5. Andersson KE, Ulmsten U 1978 Effects of nifedipine on myometrial activity and lower abdominal pain in women with primary dysmenorrhoea. British Journal of Obstetrics and Gynaecology 85: 142–148
6. Lundström V, Grèen K, Wiqvist N 1976 Prostaglandins, indomethacin and dysmenorrhoea. Prostaglandins 11: 893–904
7. Ekström P, Forsling M, Kindahl H, Åkerlund M 1990 Perception of pain in primary dysmenorrhoea in relation to uterine activity and plasma concentrations of vasopressin and $F_{2\alpha}$ metabolite. Journal of Neuroendocrinology, Fourth International Conference on the Neurohypophysis, pp 168–171
8. Ferreira SH, Nakamura M, de Abeu Castro MS 1978 The hyperalgesic effects of prostacyclin and prostaglandin E_2. Prostaglandins 16: 31–37
9. Lundström V, Grèen K 1978 Endogenous levels of prostaglandins $F_{2\alpha}$ and its main metabolites in plasma and the endometrium of normal and dysmenorreic women. American Journal of Obstetrics and Gynecology 130: 640–646
10. Lumsden MA, Kelly RW, Baird DT 1983 Primary dysmenorrhoea: the importance of both prostaglandins E_2 and $F_{2\alpha}$. British Journal of Obstetrics and Gynaecology 90: 1135–1140
11. Strömberg P, Åkerlund M, Forsling ML, Kindahl H 1983 Involvement of prostaglandins in vasopressin stimulation of the human uterus. British Journal of Obstetrics and Gynaecology 93: 332–337
12. Åkerlund M, Strömberg P, Forsling ML 1979 Primary dysmenorrhoea and vasopressin. British Journal of Obstetrics and Gynaecology 86: 484–487
13. Strömberg P, Åkerlund M, Forsling ML, Granström E, Kindahl H 1984 Vasopressin and prostaglandins in premenstrual pain and primary dysmenorrhoea. Acta Obstetrica Gynecologica Scandinavica 63: 533–538
14. Hauksson A, Strömberg P, Juchnicka E, Laudanski T, Åkerlund M 1989 The influence of a combined oral contraceptive on uterine activity and reactivity to agonists in primary dysmenorrhoea. Acta Obstetrica Gynecologica Scandinavica 68: 31–34
15. Ekström P, Åkerlund M, Forsling M, Kindahl H, Laudanski T, Mrugacz G 1992 Stimulation of vasopressin release in women with primary dysmenorrhoea and after oral contraceptive treatment — effect on uterine contractility. British Journal of Obstetrics and Gynaecology 99: 680–684
16. Åkerlund M, Andersson K-E 1976 Vasopressin response and terbutaline inhibition of the uterus. Obstetrics and Gynecology 47: 484–487
17. Ekström P, Alm P, Åkerlund M 1991 Differences in vasomotor responses between main stem and smaller branches of the human artery. Acta Obstetrica Gynecologica Scandinavica 70: 429–433
18. Maggi M, Magini A, Fiscella A, Giannini S, Fantoni G, Toffoletti F, Massi G, Serio M 1992 Sex steroid modulation of neurohypophyseal hormone receptors in human nonpregnant myometrium. Journal of Clinical Endocrinology and Metabolism 74: 385–392
19. Bossmar T, Åkerlund M, Szamatowicz J, Laudanski T, Fantoni G, Maggi M 1995 Receptor-mediated uterine effects of vasopressin and oxytocin in nonpregnant women. British Journal of Obstetrics and Gynaecology 102: 907–912
20. Bossmar T, Åkerlund M, Fantoni G, Szamatowicz J, Melin P, Maggi M 1994 Receptors for and myometrial responses to oxytocin and vasopressin in preterm and term human pregnancy: effects of the oxytocin antagonist atosiban. American Journal of Obstetrics and Gynecology 171: 1634–1642
21. Ekesbo R, Alm P, Ekström P, Lundberg L-M, Åkerlund M 1991 Innervation of the human uterine artery and contractile responses to neuropeptides. Gynecological and Obstetrical Investigation 31: 30–36
22. Thorbert G 1979 Regional changes in structure and functions of adrenergic nerves in guinea pig uterus during pregnancy. Acta Obstetrica Gyncecologica Scandinavica 79: 1–32
23. Maathius JB, Kelly RW 1978 Concentration of prostaglandins $F_{2\alpha}$ and E_2 in the endometrium throughout the human menstrual cycle, after the administration of clomiphene or an oestrogen-proestogen pill and in early pregnancy. Journal of Endocrinology 77: 361–371
24. Hauksson A, Åkerlund M, Forsling ML, Kindahl H 1987 Plasma concentrations of vasopressin and a prostaglandin $F_{2\alpha}$ metabolite in women with primary dysmenorrhoea before and during treatment with a combined oral contraceptive. Journal of Endocrinology 115: 355–361

25. Forsling ML, Åkerlund M, Strömberg P 1981 Variations in plasma concentrations of vasopressin during the menstrual cycle. Journal of Endocrinology 89: 263–266
26. Forsling ML, Strömberg P, Åkerlund M 1982 Effect of ovarian steroids on vasopressin secretion. Journal of Endocrinology 95: 147–151
27. Bossmar T, Forsling M, Åkerlund M 1995 Circulating oxytocin and vasopressin is influenced by ovarian steroid replacement in women. Acta Obstetrica Gynaecologica Scandinavica 74: 544–548
28. Ekström P, Juchnicka E, Laudanski T, Åkerlund M 1989 Effect of an oral contraceptive in primary dysmenorrhoea — changes in uterine activity and reactivity to agonists. Contraception 49: 39–47
29. Ylikorkala O, Puolakka J, Kauppila A 1979 Serum gonadotrophins, prolactin and ovarian steroids in primary dysmenorrhoea. British Journal of Obstetrics and Gynaecology 86: 648–653
30. Schwartz A, Zor U, Lindner HR, Naor S 1974 Primary dysmenorrhoea. Alleviation by an inhibitor of prostaglandin synthesis and action. Obstetrics and Gynecology 44: 709–712
31. Åkerlund M, Strömberg P 1989 Comparison of ketoprofen and naproxen in the treatment of dysmenorrhoea, with special regard to the time of onset of pain relief. Current Medical Research Opinion 11: 485–490
32. Sivin I, Stern J 1994 Health during prolonged use of levonorgestrel 20 micrograms/d and the copper Tcu 380Ag intra-uterine contraceptive devices: a multicenter study. International Committee for Contraception Research (ICOR). Fertility and Sterility 61: 70–77
33. Trobough G, Guderian AM, Erickson RR, Tillson SA, Leong P, Swisher DA, Phariss BB 1978 The effect of exogenous intrauterine progesterone on the amount and prostaglandin $F_{2\alpha}$ content of menstrual blood in dysmenorrheic women. Journal of Reproductive Medicine 21: 153–158
34. Åkerlund M, Hauksson A, Lundin S, Melin P, Trojnar J 1986 Vasotocin analogues which competitively inhibit vasopressin stimulated uterine activity in healthy women. British Journal of Obstetrics and Gynaecology 93: 22–27
35. Melin P, Trojnar J, Johansson B, Wilhardt H, Åkerlund M 1986 Synthetic antagonists of the myometrial response to oxytocin and vasopressin. Journal of Endocrinology 111: 125–131
36. Hauksson A, Åkerlund M, Melin P 1988 Uterine blood flow and myometrial activity at menstruation, and the influence of vasopressin and a synthetic antagonist. British Journal of Obstetrics and Gynaecology 95: 898–904
37. Åkerlund M 1987 Can primary dysmenorrhoea be alleviated by a vasopressin antagonist Acta Obstetrica Gynecologica Scandinavica 66: 459–461
38. Åkerlund M, Strömberg P, Hauksson A, Andersen LF, Lyndrup J, Trojnar J, Melin P 1987 Inhibition of uterine contractions of premature labour with an oxtocin analogue. British Journal of Obstetrics and Gynaecology 94: 1040–1044
39. Serradeil-Le-Gal C, Bagnon J, Garcia C, Lacour C, Guiraodou P, Christophe B et al 1993. Biochemical and pharmacological properties of SR 49059, a new, potent, nonpeptide antagonist of rat and human vasopressin V1a receptors. Journal of Clinical Investigation 92: 224–231
40. Yamamura Y, Ogawa WA, Chihara T 1991 OPC-21268, an orally effective, nonpeptide vasopressin V1a receptor antagonist. Science 252: 572–574
41. Bossmar T, Rasmusson T, Åkerlund M 1996 Effect of the nonpeptide vasopressin V1a receptor antagonist, SR 49059, and its enantiomer, SR 49770, on isolated human myometrium. Acta Obstetrica Gynecologica Scandinavica 75: 516–519
42. Bossmar T, Brouard R, Döberl A, Åkerlund M 1997 Effects of SR 49059, an orally active vasopressin V_{1a} receptor antagonist on vasopressin-induced uterine contractions in women. British Journal of Obstetrics and Gynaecology 104: 471–477

32. Secondary dysmenorrhea and chronic pelvic pain

O. A. Odukoya R. Atkinson I. D. Cooke

Introduction

Dysmenorrhea is a term which is derived from the Greek word meaning 'difficult monthly flow'. For many years it was a neglected condition although its presence has been recognized since early history, with cultural variations in social attitudes and beliefs. These attitudes and beliefs have resulted in differing responses to the condition, ranging from separation from families and friends to confinement at home and avoidance of all social engagement. Many taboos existed in various cultures for coping with women having dysmenorrhea.

Today, dysmenorrhea is regarded as a symptom complex which may arise from an alteration in prostaglandin production or from pelvic pathology and consists of severe cramping associated with menstruation. Approximately 45% of postpubertal females are affected, with about 10% being incapacitated for more than three days. It is not a life threatening condition but can be a source of significant morbidity. It affects one in seven women in the United States and is a major cause of economic loss from decreased productivity and loss of effective working hours: it is estimated that the equivalent of 140 million hours per week are lost.[1,2] However, the differentiation between a 'normal' and a 'painful' menstrual period is difficult because of subjectivity and individual and cultural variation in pain perception. Clinically, a woman is considered to suffer from painful menstrual periods if she seeks relief either in the form of consultation or self-medication.

Based on the cause, dysmenorrhea is commonly classified as primary or secondary. Primary dysmenorrhea refers to painful menstruation in which no abnormality is found in the history, physical examination or at investigative procedures. It is commonly associated with ovulatory cycles. Secondary dysmenorrhea refers to the condition in which a pathological cause is readily identifiable. Primary dysmenorrhea is discussed in chapter 31.

SECONDARY DYSMENORRHEA

Etiology

Uterine pathology or iatrogenic conditions, as well as parametrial pathology, may cause secondary dysmenorrhea (Table 32.1). The pathophysiologic mechanisms probably include excessive prostaglandin (PG) production, changes in intra-uterine pressure and blood flow in the pelvis or irritation of the pelvic peritoneum by pain inducing substances released during menstrual bleeding.[3] Increased release of certain prostaglandins induces incoordinate hyperactivity of the uterine muscle, resulting in reduced uterine blood flow, ischemia and pain. There is an increased concentration of endometrial prostaglandins in uterine myomas, in endometrium exposed to an intra-uterine contraceptive device

Table 32.1 Etiology of secondary dysmenorrhea.

1. Uterine
   - Congenital
     - Imperforate hymen
     - Noncommunicating uterine horn
     - Transverse vaginal septum
   - Acquired
     - Adenomyosis
     - Uterine myoma (typically pedunculated and submucous)
     - Intra-uterine contraceptive device
     - Large endometrial polyp
     - Intra-uterine synechiae resulting in haematometra
     - Cervical stenosis
2. Extra-uterine
   - Endometriosis
   - Pelvic inflammatory disease
   - Pelvic congestion syndrome
   - Ovarian cysts (especially endometriotic)
3. Psychological

(IUCD)[4–6,9] and in ectopic and eutopic endometrium of endometriosis sufferers.[7,8]

A variety of chemical substances such as bradykinins, 5-hydroxytryptophan, histamine and cytokines, which are present in inflammatory exudates and damaged tissues, act on sensory neurons or mobilize cellular arachidonic acid with the production of prostaglandins and secondary dysmenorrhea.[10,11] Intra-uterine contraceptive devices (IUCD) are known to provoke leucocytic infiltration which can activate the production of PG.[12] Furthermore, capsular distension or accident to an ovarian cyst, mechanical stimuli or tissue trauma may alter cell membrane stability causing PG production and pain. PG may also sensitize the nerve endings to other pain producing substances, e.g. substance P.[13]

Symptoms and signs

In secondary dysmenorrhea, the painful menstrual cramps begin usually many years after menarche, while in the primary type the pain begins soon after menarche. Dysmenorrhea associated with anovulatory cycles is almost always secondary in type. A detailed history with attention to the onset of pain, its severity, duration, character, site, radiation and any aggravating or relieving events is necessary. The characteristics of the pain often differ from those reported by women with primary dysmenorrhea, usually being more 'dragging' or 'congestive' in character and typically beginning well before the onset of menstruation and reaching a peak at the onset of bleeding. The relationship to menarche, menstrual cycle, previous pregnancy, coitus and sexual difficulties, physical and bowel movements, urinary voiding and associated systemic symptoms should be explored. Details of previous known or documented pelvic infections, endometriosis, pelvic masses and methods of contraception should be sought. The perception and role of the partner, the family and the patient's expectations are explored, taking cognizance of the cultural, educational and social background. Information regarding previous modalities of treatment, their effectiveness and her treatment expectations are important for adequate management.

In addition to a general examination to evaluate individual wellbeing, a pelvic examination is essential. In the adolescent with *virgo intacta*, a rectal examination coupled with pelvic ultrasound may be helpful. The aim of the examination is to detect any pelvic abnormalities which may be responsible for the pain. Evidence of an enlarged tender uterus of reduced mobility and nodules in the uterosacral ligaments may suggest adenomyosis, endometriosis or pelvic adhesions.

Investigations

The history and physical examination may influence the direction of investigation. A full blood count may show evidence of leucocytosis while the erythrocyte sedimentation rate and serum C-reactive protein may be elevated in patients with active infection. The latter, however, may be elevated in cases of nonspecific chronic inflammation. Swabs of the urethra, the posterior fornix and the endocervix for sexually transmitted organisms is mandatory in patients suspected of having pelvic inflammatory disease. It is important to investigate the sexual partner(s) of such patients. Further investigations in the form of pelvic (transvaginal) ultrasound may permit the diagnosis of uterine polyps, ovarian cysts and/or uterine myomata. It may identify a foreign body (IUCD) or diagnose rare congenital uterine anomalies such as a noncommunicating uterine horn. These investigations may be complemented by hysterosalpingogram, MRI or CT scan.[16] An intravenous urogram (IVU) is advised in patients with congenital uterine anomalies to exclude concomitant renal disorders.

Management

The treatment of patients with secondary dysmenorrhea depends on the cause: this can be medical, surgical, psychological or a combination of the above (Table 32.2).

Endometriosis

This condition is discussed in detail in chapter 37. The greater the number of implants in endometriosis the greater the severity of dysmenorrhea and chronic pelvic pain.[14] The pain is usually cyclical and worsened by intercourse. Severe cases may be associated with backache, rectal pain, tenesmus and urgency of micturition. Uterine tenderness, reduced mobility due to pelvic adhesions and a pelvic mass may be demonstrated. The presence of nodules in the uterosacral ligaments or a solitary, discrete mass in the rectovaginal septum is pathognomonic of endometriosis. Visualization and grading of the disease by careful and meticulous laparoscopy is the mainstay of diagnosis.[15]

The goal of treatment is to relieve symptoms, limit progression of disease and restore fertility. Treatments can be medical (combined oral contraceptive pill,

Table 32.2 Primary treatments of secondary dysmenorrhea.

Secondary dysmenorrhea	Treatment
Endometriosis Adenomyosis	Combined oral contraceptive, progestogens, Danazol, GnRH-a; surgery
Fibromas	Surgery
Ovarian cyst	Laparoscopic surgery; laparotomy
Endometrial polyp	Polypectomy
Pelvic infection (PID) and adhesions	Antibiotics; surgery
Intra-uterine devices (IUD)	NSAID; removal of device
Cervical strictures	Dilatation
Congenital obstructive Mullerian lesions	Surgery
Premenstrual syndrome	Medical; surgery

GnRH-a: gonadotropin-releasing hormone analog; NSAID: nonsteroidal anti-inflammatory drug

progestogen, danazol, gestrinone, gonadotropin-releasing hormone analogs with or without add-back therapy), surgical (laparoscopic or laparotomy) or a combination of medical and surgical.

Uterine myomata (fibroids)

This condition is discussed in detail in chapter 38. Although there are racial differences in the prevalence of uterine myomata, it is estimated that, overall, about 20% of women are affected, with increasing incidence up to menopause. About 50% of affected women are asymptomatic and many have myomata discovered during routine pelvic or antenatal examinations.[17]

The clinical presentation depends on the location and size of the fibroid. It may cause chronic, dragging pain, colicky labor-like abdominal pains and menorrhagia. Dysmenorrhea occurs when the myoma is submucous or protrudes into the uterine cavity. Pelvic (transvaginal) ultrasound scan and, where available, MRI are helpful in diagnosis and assessment. Outpatient hysteroscopy may be valuable to define location and resectability. Medical treatment using a GnRH agonist can reduce the fibroid volume by up to 50% as well as induce amenorrhea, although regrowth is common once the medication is stopped. Abdominal myomectomy is considered if the patient desires a future pregnancy or if psychological morbidity is envisaged following loss of the uterus. Hysterectomy is an option in women who have completed their family.

Intra-uterine contraceptive devices (IUCD)

The precise mechanism for the secondary dysmenorrhea occurring in some IUCD users is not known. It has been suggested that this could be due to distension of the endometrial cavity, myometrial irritability caused by low grade inflammatory responses in the endometrium or to the increased release of prostaglandins or other pain-inducing substances. Progesterone or progestogen-releasing intra-uterine systems are known to stabilize lysosomal membranes with a reduction in phospholipase A_2 and prostaglandin concentrations and these systems actually reduce dysmenorrhea. Furthermore, nonsteroidal anti-inflammatory agents (NSAIDs) inhibit prostaglandin, prostacyclin and thromboxane production with relief of menorrhagia and dysmenorrhea. Dysmenorrhea following IUCD insertion responds to NSAIDs although removal may be necessary if symptoms persist.[18]

Congenital abnormalities of the genital tract

Congenital anomalies of the genital tract, such as imperforate hymen or transverse vaginal septum, may cause outflow obstruction. These may present with cyclical menstrual pain without menstrual flow, while a noncommunicating uterine horn may cause pain coincident with menstrual flow by volume distension and PG production. Stenosis or occlusion of the cervix from conization or pelvic radiation may also present with dysmenorrhea or cyclical pain without menstruation. Such lesions may cause hematocolpos, hematometra and hematosalpinx. Clinical evaluation may be supplemented by vaginal ultrasound, hysteroscopy (with or without ultrasound guidance) and hysterosalpingography. The treatment is to relieve the obstruction by removal of the occluding membrane, vaginal septum or adhesions by conventional surgery or endoscopy.[19,20]

Fedele et al[21] evaluated dysmenorrhea in 90 patients with a septate or subseptate uterus before and after surgery. Sixty-two of the patients (69%) had hysteroscopic metroplasty and the frequency of dysmenorrhea fell from 55% to 18% at one year follow up.

Pelvic inflammatory disease (PID)

PID often follows a delayed or inadequately treated acute pelvic infection although in some cases the latter presents with low grade pyrexia and minor abdominal pain mimicking a transient flu-like infection. The infection may be pyogenic or gonococcal but is often chlamydial with an 'opportunist' secondary mixed infection. PID may also follow spontaneous or induced abortion, or normal delivery with retained products of conception. Dysmenorrhea secondary to pelvic inflammatory disease is exacerbated by coitus, is often maximal premenstrually and is sometimes relieved with the onset of menstrual bleeding. Mittelschmerz is also quite common while some patients complain of pelvic pain at defecation. There may be offensive vaginal discharge as well as abdominal tenderness. Examination of the pelvis may reveal a retroverted uterus of reduced mobility and pain if the uterus is moved during the examination. Adnexal tenderness with thickening may be present, as may a pelvic mass. Rectal examination may confirm adnexal thickening or swelling.

A full blood count is performed to assess the level of anemia and leucocytosis. In acute and subacute cases, there may be an increase in C-reactive protein and erythrocyte sedimentation rate. Microbiological swabs should be taken from the cervix, urethra and anal canal to try to identity sexually transmitted organisms such as gonorrhea and chlamydia. Diagnostic laparoscopy may be necessary to confirm and assess the condition.

Treatment is usually conservative and includes attention to general nutrition, analgesia, contact tracing and treatment of partners. Broad spectrum antibiotics such as third generation cephalosporins (ceftriaxone 250 mg i.m. or cefotaxime 1 g i.m. stat) with doxycycline 100 mg twice a day for 14 days are the treatment of choice.[22] In chronic cases, repeated doses of antibiotic treatment with oral analgesia (including NSAIDs) may be required. In a minority, major surgery, including hysterectomy and bilateral salpingo-oophorectomy, may ultimately be required.

Adenomyosis

Adenomyosis is a disease characterized by the presence of endometrial glands and stroma deep within the myometrium (see ch. 37). It is associated with inner myometrial distortion, hypertrophy and hyperplasia. It often affects the posterior uterine wall and may cause menorrhagia and dysmenorrhea. The severity of the dysmenorrhea is associated with the depth and extent of myometrial invasion of the glandular cells and the rate of invasion.[23] Although T2-weighted magnetic resonance imaging (MRI) is costly and not easily available, it is a more accurate and reliable noninvasive method of diagnosis than transvaginal ultrasound scan.[24]

The definitive treatment is hysterectomy, although myometrial reduction by electrocautery, laser, local excision of localized pathology or wedge resection of extensive areas of myometrium are alternative conservative methods that may ameliorate symptoms. GnRH analogs may sometimes be useful for temporary relief of symptoms as well as reducing the volume of the uterus while awaiting definitive surgery.

Psychogenic dysmenorrhea

In some patients, no specific diagnosis is established to account for the dysmenorrhea. In such a scenario psychological or psychiatric assessment may help to modulate the reactive component of the menstrual pain. However, the suggestion that such women are prone to develop significant neurotic tendencies with a higher level of anxiety and a greater tendency to express affective experiences by somatic reactions has not been substantiated by clinical trials.[25] The patient should be told that her pelvic organs are normal. Often a multidisciplinary approach involving a psychotherapist, nutritionist or hypnotherapist may be beneficial. The treatment of these patients is often prolonged and protracted. In the absence of any psychopathology, mild analgesics may be prescribed. As in primary dysmenorrhea, transcutaneous electrical nerve stimulation (TENS) and acupuncture have been successful in some cases.[26,27] Management of refractory dysmenorrhea often overlaps with the approach to management of chronic pelvic pain.

CHRONIC PELVIC PAIN

The literature does not provide a consistent definition of chronic pelvic pain (CPP). Some authors use the duration of symptoms, which varies from three to six months, others apply it to pelvic pain in the presence of normal pelvic anatomy while some apply it to pain that is accompanied by psychopathological disorders. Clinically, CPP can be defined as intermittent or constant pain which is present for at least six months and which is severe enough to interfere with the quality of life of the woman. Pain perception varies from one individual to another and is not related to the magnitude or duration of the pain-producing stimulus. A number of possible organic factors have been suggested but in many women no identifiable organic factor can be found, suggesting that the CPP population is a heterogeneous group. Factors such as social background, cultural differences, anxiety and stress levels which are known to affect personality also affect individual perception of pain.[28]

CPP represents one of the most difficult challenges confronting the gynecologist. The patients so afflicted are often angry, demanding and distraught. In a survey conducted by the Royal College of Obstetricians and Gynaecologists which involved 21 000 laparoscopies,[29] the primary indication was CPP in 11 000 (52%). In a similar study in the USA, 259 of 756 (34%) diagnostic laparoscopies were performed for CPP.[30] In an Australian study of 717 patients who had diagnostic laparoscopy for dysmenorrhea, 114 (16%) had CPP.[31] CPP was responsible for about 12% of hysterectomies performed in the USA between 1978–1981.[32] To understand the principles of the management of CPP the nerve supply of the pelvis will be briefly described and the theories of pain perception, the clinical presentation and the multidisciplinary approach to the management of such patients will be outlined.

Pelvic and lower abdominal nerve supply

Sympathetic and parasympathetic nerves supply the abdominopelvic organs carrying sensory as well as motor fibres. The sympathetic fibres arise mainly from the thoracolumbar (T5–L1) ganglia and pass down the celiac plexus into the intermesenteric (aortic) plexus and form the superior hypogastric plexus just below the bifurcation of the aorta. The latter gives rise to two main chains. The hypogastric nerves run inferolaterally on the pelvic side wall to merge with the pair of inferior hypogastric plexuses to form the pelvic plexuses. The plexuses are located on either side of the rectal ampulla with a forward extension to the base of the broad and transverse cervical ligaments. This extension is often referred to as the Lee-Frankenhauser plexus and supplies autonomic innervation to most of the pelvic organs. Parasympathetic fibers via S2–S5 are transmitted via the inferior hypogastric nerves and carry impulses from the cervix and lower uterus. They may be responsible for the lower backache experienced in certain diseases of these organs.

The lower anterior abdominal wall, anterior vulva, clitoris and urethra are innervated by mixed sensory and motor nerves from L1 and L2. The dorsal rami derived from these segments innervate the lower back, which is often a region of referred gynecological pain. The anus, perineum, and lower vagina are innervated by the nervi erigentes (S2–S4).

Damage to any of these nerve structures can cause pelvic pain. Pain impulses from the uterus, medial part of the Fallopian tube, broad ligament and upper vagina are conducted via afferents to Frankenhauser's paracervical plexus. The afferent pathway from the ovary, lateral part of the Fallopian tube and peritoneum enters the main sympathetic nerve chain at the fourth lumbar sympathetic ganglion and ascends with the sympathetic to enter the spinal cord at the ninth and tenth thoracic segments. Pain originating from the pelvic organs may be experienced as referred pain in the skin areas supplied by the somatic afferent fibers of the same spinal segment.

Pain perception (nociception)

The pelvis is supplied by somatic and visceral nerves. Pain initiation is dependent on the stimulation of nerve endings (nociceptors) with the transmission of impulses via the spinal cord to the cerebral cortex. The cortical perception of somatic structures is well established as representation of specific body areas to specific areas of the cortex. On the other hand, visceral structures have no discrete cortical representation and pain localization is poor. There are two types of afferents associated with nociceptors: the Aδ and the C types. The afferent axons of the Aδ receptors are associated with somatic fibers and are small rapid impulse conducting myelinated fibers.

The pain generated by this group of fibers is acute in onset, well localized and circumscribed. The impulses from the nociceptive fibers synapse in the grey matter of the dorsal horn of the spinal cord at the same or adjacent segment of the spinal cord and are relayed via ascending fibers in the contralateral spinothalamic tract to the reticular formation of the thalamus. The information processing is transferred to the postcentral gyrus of the cerebral cortex. The afferent visceral axons of the C fibers synthesize neuropeptide transmitters, such as vasoactive intestinal peptides (VIP), leucine enkephalin, substance P, serotonin, endorphins, cholecystokinin and methionine enkephalin at peripheral nerve endings.[33,34] Some of these transmitters are inhibitory (enkephalins) while others (substance P) are excitatory. The variation in the perception of pain is probably due to the degree of inhibitory modification rather than nociceptor activity.

Causes of CPP

An understanding of the etiology of CPP is important because of the damaging effect it may have on women. Women with CPP belong to a heterogeneous group (Table 32.3, Fig. 32.1). In 30–75% of the patients, no etiology can be found.[35,36] The demand of women to improve their quality of life coupled with the

Table 32.3 Etiology of chronic pelvic pain.

Gynecological	**Nongynecological**
Pelvis	Gastrointestinal
Pelvic adhesions (with bowel or ovarian involvement)	Irritable bowel syndrome
Endometriosis	Inflammatory bowel disease (Crohn's disease, ulcerative colitis, diverticulitis)
Pelvic congestion syndrome	Urinary
Neoplasms (myomata; or malignant)	Urinary tract infection (recurrent cystourethritis; interstitial cystitis)
Ovary	Ureteral obstruction: calculus; urinary tract malignancy
Benign cysts	Neurological
Polycystic ovarian disease (with enlarged ovaries)	Nerve entrapment syndrome
Ovarian remnant syndrome (with periovarian adhesions)	Neuroma
Uterus	Musculoskeletal
Dysmenorrhea (congestive and spasmodic)	Prolapsed intervertebral disc
Intra-uterine contraceptive devices	Spondylolisthesis
Uterovaginal prolapse	Degenerative spinal disease
Others	Pelvic injury
Vulvodynia	Systemic
	Lymphoma
	Systemic lupus erythematosus
	Acute intermittent porphyria
	Psychogenic
	Idiopathic

availability of better investigative technology, better understanding of the control of the reproductive system and the advent of multidisciplinary rather than 'single' treatment modalities have contributed to recent advances. Pain is a subjective phenomenon and the location may not correspond to anatomical pathology. Pains located in the lower pelvis in the reproductive age group are thought to be related to the reproductive organs and such patients are referred to the gynecologist. As such pain may have no demonstrable gynecological cause, the importance of meticulous history and examination cannot be overemphasized.

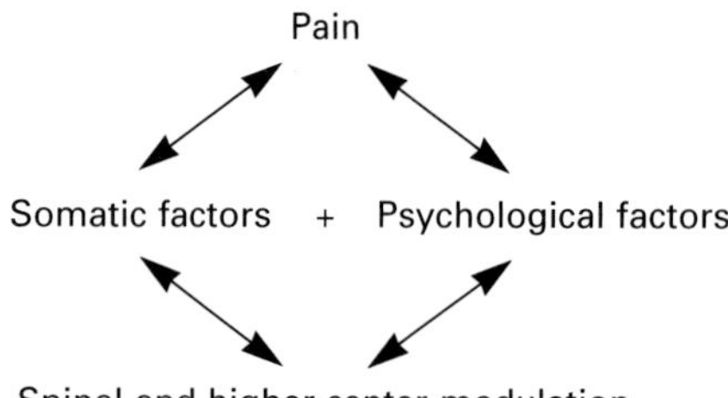

Fig. 32.1 Conceptual description of gate-control theory.

Mechanisms and endocrinology of CPP

The mechanism of causation of CPP follows the distribution of the pain pathways, visceral or somatic. Somatic fibers innervate the skin, abdominal muscles and parietal peritoneum while the sympathetic and the parasympathetic systems innervate the pelvic organs as well as the visceral peritoneum. Tissue damage mechanisms have defined local and distance changes. Local tissue ischemia with scarring, retraction, fibrosis and adhesion formation may produce pain on motion, exercise or at ovulation due to tension on tissues. Furthermore, the damage may involve nerve endings, causing irritation and nerve activation. This may explain the pain associated with pelvic adhesions following pelvic inflammatory disease and severe endometriosis.[37] In addition, fixity of the bowel with distension may cause colicky abdominal pain and simulate irritable bowel syndrome. Noxious irritation of the peritoneum and nerve endings by neoplastic or inflammatory mediators such as eicosanoids, serotonin and bradykinins can affect the morphology and physiology of central neurones, causing nociceptive pain.[13] It is believed that the spinal cord becomes reorganized as a consequence of the local damage and thereafter receives and handles impulses from normal tissue in an abnormal way.[38] Such central organization is triggered by impulses from unmyelinated afferents from the area of damage. It is postulated that these fibers release peptides from their spinal cord terminals which may produce long-term changes in spinal and reflex circuitry, causing intractable pain. This theory requires further elucidation. Other mechanisms include the distension and contraction of a hollow organ as well as capsular stretch of a 'solid' organ.

Pelvic congestion has been implicated as a cause of unexplained CPP. It is believed to be caused by distension and engorgement of the pelvic veins which are associated with relative stasis within the venous system. These changes are related in some way to the secretion of ovarian hormones. An 'imbalance' in serum estrogen and progesterone or their tissue effects may be responsible since the condition does not occur before puberty or after menopause. McCausland et al demonstrated a 30% increase in the distensibility of pelvic veins one week before menstruation and implicated progesterone as the cause of the condition although the importance of estrogen priming was not considered.[39] Furthermore, elimination of ovulatory cycles by continuous medoxyprogesterone acetate diminished the symptoms.[40] Vascular stasis may cause relative hypoxia and a build up of pain, producing substances such as ATP and substance P.[41]

Theories of pain perception

One of the major reasons for the divergent management of CPP is the different understanding of its pathogenesis and maintenance.

Cartesian theory

This is otherwise called the medical or classic theory. It sought to associate pain perception to direct tissue trauma and adduced the intensity of pain to the severity of tissue damage. The Cartesian theory proposed that identification and eradication of the source of pain may reduce if not completely ameliorate the symptom. With the widespread use of technologically intensive and invasive procedures such as ultrasound scan and laparoscopy, many clinicians have come to attribute the presence of an 'abnormal' pelvic condition, albeit unproved, as causative of pelvic pain. When no pathology is identified in the pelvis, the pain is often described as spurious or psychogenic. This model is, however, simplistic as removal of the supposed etiology has not been shown significantly to result in pain relief.[36,37] There is clinical evidence that multiple psychological factors including mood changes are commoner in patients with CPP.[42] The demonstration of the common neurotransmitters, serotonin and endorphins in the mediation of mood and pain perception led to the development of the gate control theory of pain perception.

Gate-control theory

This theory integrates peripheral signal nociceptive perception with cerebral cortical regulation of variables such as mood and anxiety in the perception of pain. This model proposed the simultaneous evolution of somatic and psychological factors as moderating or potentiating pain perception (Fig. 33.1). The concentrations of substance P and β-endorphin neurotransmitters are increased during anxiety and mood changes and are considered to play a major role in the processing and modulation of pain responses.[13] The model predicts short and long term outcomes of CPP populations better than the Cartesian theory. That theory fails to recognize the myriad social, cultural and environmental factors in the perception and maintenance of pain.

Biopsychosocial model

This model takes a more pragmatic view of the interaction between chronic nociceptive stimuli and multiple psychological and social determinants in pain perception (Fig. 32.2). The model was first proposed by Fordyce and suggested that since pain is not directly observable, what is known about it is from either verbal or nonverbal communication from the sufferer.[43] These communications are subject to reinforcement and modifications from social and environmental factors such as attention, avoidance of undesirable activities or perhaps financial compensation. The model presupposes that nociceptive stimuli do not lead to harmful outcomes in the absence of specific psychosocial conditions. As shown in Figure 32.2 eradication of one of these factors would lead to a temporary improvement in the symptoms with a disabling recurrence sometimes at a different site culminating in a complex referred to as 'symptom shifting'. In a cohort of 152 patients, 64 with chronic pelvic pain, 42 with headaches and 46 as controls, significant somatization and psychological morbidity were prevalent in the CPP group compared to the other groups.[44] In another study of 106 patients with CPP and 92 controls, the cumulative medication for the CPP sufferers was significantly more than in the

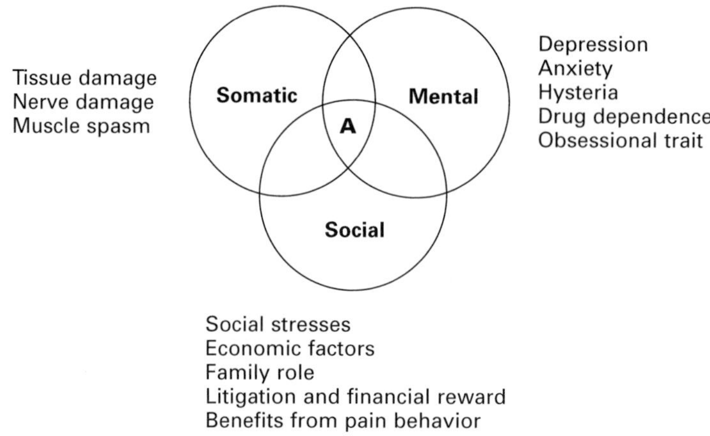

Fig. 32.2 Diagramatic representation of the theories and factors of chronic pelvic pain. The main factors are physical (somatic), mental and social. Zone A, chronic pelvic pain, marks the biopsychosocial theory and illustrates the need for a multidisciplinary approach to the management of chronic pelvic pain.

control group (160 versus 48), while 15 women (14%) had hysterectomy for CPP compared to three in the control group.[45] The development of the multidisciplinary approach to the management of CPP is based on this model. Failure to recognize and treat these factors often leads to recurrence and chronic ill-health.

Cognitive behavioral theory

This theory attempts to explain how individuals perceive pain and the impact of these cognitions on behavior and pain intensity. It highlights the importance of individual conceptualization of the cause of pain, its prognosis and the likelihood of effective treatment modalities. This theory recognizes the value of pain treatment through the alteration of cognitions held by the patient.

Overall, these theories provide a broad integrative team approach which simultaneously identifies and manages the somatic, psychological and social components of CPP. Secondly, it highlights the fact that the intensity of pain is not likely to be proportional to the severity of tissue damage. Thirdly, the treatment of only one factor out of many may result in a temporary relief of pain but with later recurrence and chronic ill health which may lead to frustration and loss of confidence by the patient and the clinician. In one six month randomized clinical trial of 106 patients, 49 were assigned to 'standard' treatment starting with an initial laparoscopy to exclude organic disease, 57 were assigned to integrative treatment with no initial laparoscopy and were clinically followed up for one year after treatment.[46] The group with the integrated approach had a significant reduction in pelvic pain, less disturbance in daily activities and fewer systemic abnormalities, which makes it a better and more effective approach than the 'standard' treatment, which predominantly seeks to diagnose or exclude somatic causes of chronic pelvic pain.

Evaluation of the patient with CPP

The initial assessment of the patient with CPP is an important one and a reasonable time should be allocated; in our experience this is about one hour. The clinic should be user-friendly with adequate space when necessary to accommodate the family. Ideally, information should be obtained from the patient and her partner or family. The aim of the visit is to identify any problem areas which are targets for intervention, develop a treatment plan for each patient and establish baseline information to allow progress in evaluation and treatment effectiveness. This initial visit should not be hurried but the physician should be a good listener, sympathetic and understanding, as many of these patients have passed through more than one practitioner. Particular attention is paid to composure, fluency of narration, derailment of thought and emotions, including 'body language', which may give valuable clues to the psychological state. For example pain may be a manifestation of the depressive illness first noticed by a flattened affect. Attitudes towards discussion of past history, including parental and sexual relationships, may give vital clues to hidden causes of pelvic pain.

A multidisciplinary clinic approach showed a greater reduction in pelvic pain when compared with a single therapy approach.[46] In our practice, we send the Hospital Anxiety and Depression (HAD) scale questionnaire[47] to the patient with the outpatient appointment letter (Table 32.4). This is received back and analyzed before the clinic appointment. When the patient is interviewed the characteristics of the pain, including the location, duration, and mode of onset, as well as the relationship to coitus, menstruation and preceding pregnancy may give an indication of probably cause. The previous treatment profile in chronological order with the results of investigations are documented. A history of unusual vaginal discharge and pelvic inflammatory disease are noted. Memories of childhood experiences and bereavement, including past psychiatric disturbances, are explored with caution and diplomacy. The relationship of the pain to aspects of the gastrointestinal tract such as diet,

Tabel 32.4 Hospital anxiety [A] and depression [D] scale.[47]

Item	Score
I feel tense or 'wound up' (A)	
Most of the time	3
A lot of the time	2
From time to time, occasionally	1
Not at all	0
I still enjoy the things I used to enjoy (D)	
Definitely as much	0
Not quite so much	1
Only a little	2
Hardly at all	3
I get a sort of frightened feeling as if something awful is about to happen (A)	
Very definitely and quite badly	3
Yes, but not too badly	2
A little, but it doesn't worry me	1
Not at all	0
I can laugh and see the funny side of things (D)	
As much as I always could	1
Not quite so much now	2
Definitely not so much now	3
Not at all	4
Worrying thoughts go through my mind (A)	
A great deal of the time	3
A lot of the time	2
From time to time, but not too often	1
Only occasionally	0
I look forward with enjoyment to things (D)	
As much as I ever did	0
Rather less than I used to	1
Definitely less than I used to	2
Hardly at all	3
I can sit at ease and feel relaxed (A)	
Definitely	0
Usually	1
Not often	2
Not at all	3
I feel as if I am slowed down (D)	
Nearly all the time	3
Very often	2
Sometimes	1
Not at all	0
I get a sort of frightened feeling like 'butterflies in the stomach, (A)	
Not at all	0
Occasionally	1
Quite often	2
Very often	3
I have lost interest in my appearance (D)	
Definitely	3
I don't take so much care as I should	2
I may not take quite as much care	1
I take just as much care as ever	0
I feel restless as if I have to be on the move (A)	
Very much indeed	3
Quite a lot	2
Not very much	1
Not at all	0
I feel cheerful (D)	
Not at all	3
Not often	2
Sometimes	1
Most of the time	0
I get sudden feelings of panic (A)	
Very often indeed	3
Quite offten	2
Not very often	1
Not at all	0
I can enjoy a good book or radio or TV programme (D)	
Often	0
Sometimes	1
Not often	2
Very seldom	3
A (Anxiety)	(8–10)
D (Depression)	(8–10)

Adapted from Zigmoid and Snaith 1983[47] with permission.

constipation, diarrhea, and to the genitourinary system as well as the impact of the pain on the daily function of the patient are explored. The intensity of the pain is assessed using a visual analog scale.

The general examination aims to exclude evidence of malignancy, such as dependent edema, lymphadenopathy and anemia. Abdominal examination is often normal although a 'trigger point' may be elicited. Tenderness over the ovarian point — the junction between the middle and the inner third of a line between the anterior superior iliac spine and the umbilicus — has been suggested to be characteristic of women with pelvic venous congestion,[41] although this is not a common finding in our experience. The sigmoid colon may be palpably enlarged and tender suggesting irritable bowel syndrome (IBS).

Speculum examination may show vaginal discharge with or without cervical pathology. Cervical tenderness may be present on bimanual examination. The uterus is assessed to determine the size, tenderness and the degree of mobility. The anatomy of the adnexa and the Pouch of Douglas is explored with emphasis on nodularity or thickening of the uterosacral ligaments. The uterosacral ligaments and rectovaginal septum may contain endometriotic nodules, which are better assessed by simultaneous vaginal and rectal examination.

The hip and lumbosacral spines are examined. In the absence of abnormal clinical signs, intravenous urography, barium enema, proctoscopy, cystoscopy and the like are seldom necessary. Although vaginal ultrasound scan, CT scan and MRI may play a role, albeit small, in the follow up of some causes of CPP, their role in primary evaluation in the absence of clinical signs is doubtful. Transuterine pelvic venography may be simple with few complications in unexplained CPP,[41] but it is moderately uncomfortable and involves exposure to x-rays, limiting its use in repeat studies. The inaccuracy of the history and physical examination has led to the acceptance of laparoscopy as the standard procedure in evaluation of acute and CPP.

Psychological assessment is essential in the evaluation of CPP. The aim is to identify factors other than somatic which may exacerbate or maintain the symptom of pain. There are various instruments available to assess psychological imbalance in the patient with pain but only a few have been tested in CPP.[48] These include the multidimensional character investigation of the McGill pain questionnaire, which takes into consideration sensory, emotional, practical and temporal aspects of pain, the Minnesota Multiphase Personality Inventory (MMPI) scale, Eysenck Personality Inventory, Middlesex Hospital questionnaire, National Institute of Mental Health Diagnostic Interview Schedule, the SCL-90, the structured sexual abuse interview and the Hospital Anxiety and Depression scale.[46–48] The psychosocial tests administered should be those that the clinic personnel are familiar with. In our practice we utilize the HAD questionnaire because it is simple, easy, sensitive and effective. It may be combined with either the McGill Pain Questionnaire or the SCL-90. A score of eight or greater on the HAD scale indicates a clinically significant score for depression or anxiety and justifies the use of antidepressants, which may be commenced on the first visit.

Treatment

The treatment approach should be multidisciplinary. In our practice we have a nurse clinician, a gynecologist, a health psychologist and a pain clinician. The patient should be made aware that treatment may be protracted and that the aim is to achieve a reduction in the pain and improve her quality of life. Although the physical and emotional treatments are concurrent, for the purposes of this discussion, they will be dealt with separately. Physical treatments are in the form of pharmacological agents, injections, surgery, stimulation techniques and general supportive measures (Table 32.5).

Table 32.5 Treatment modalities for chronic pelvic pain.

Pharmacological
Non-narcotic analgesics
Antidepressants
Anticonvulsants
Narcotic analgesics
Injections
Central (axonal) blockade
Local anesthetics
Neuronal blockade
(Opiates)
Surgery
Specific to etiology
Symptomatic
Psychological
Behavioral
Others
Transcutaneous electrical nerve stimulation (TENS); dorsal column stimulation
Acupuncture; cryotherapy; neurolysis

Pharmacologic agents

As noted, the pain may have no obvious cause, and some patients respond to conventional analgesics. These usually include paracetamol or NSAIDs, particularly when used in conjunction with nondrug therapies. There are no data on the use of narcotic analgesics in the treatment of CPP of nonmalignant origin. Protracted treatment may predispose to the fear of abuse, habituation and tolerance. Certain classes of drugs used in the adjunctive treatment of pelvic pain also have some analgesic properties. These are referred to as 'secondary analgesics' and include antidepressants, anticonvulsants, tranquilizers and hypnotics. Patients with CPP may be depressed either as a cause or consequence of their pain. Commonly used antidepressants include the tricyclic compounds, imipramine, prothiaden and the serotonin reuptake inhibitors.

These antidepressants improve pain tolerance, reduce depressive symptoms and restore normal sleep patterns.[49,50] If there is a disturbance of sleep pattern amitriptyline can be started at a dose of 25 mg at night and adjusted to suit individual patients. In cases with mild sleep disturbance nortriptyline 75–100 mg in divided doses or given at bedtime may be beneficial. If there is no sleep disturbance, fluoxetine 20–60 mg every morning or doxepin 50–75 mg daily may be appropriate.[51,52] The attending physician should be familiar with the side effects of these drugs. Anticonvulsants may have a small adjunctive role.

Sedatives and tranquilizers are rarely used because of habituation; their effects also wear off rapidly. Sex hormones, such as medoxyprogesterone acetate, either alone or in addition to psychotherapy, suppress ovarian function and may greatly alleviate the discomfort of pelvic congestion.[40] Bowel conditions such as chronic constipation and IBS may present with CPP. The management is dietary advice with supplementary psychotherapy. The latter is directed towards stress management. Dietary advice in the form of high fiber containing foods such as bran and cellulose is sensible. This may be supplemented during the hypermotile phase by drugs which directly alter bowel mobility such as diphenoxylate/atropine, loperamide or merbeverine.

Injections

The role of local 'anesthetic injection' in patients with chronic pain is two fold: diagnostic, when used for the identification of the source of pain, and prognostic in assessment of a more permanent therapeutic blockade. The anesthetic agent may be combined with other pharmacologic agents (e.g. steroids) to provide longer-term pain relief. The local anesthetic agent produces an axonal blockade which makes the painful area numb. If there is effective blockade without any relief of pain then a referred pain is likely. This approach is used in the treatment of a lower abdominal wall trigger spot by injecting 3–5 ml of a dilute solution of bupivacaine using a 25-gauge needle. Local cryotherapy to freeze the involved nerves may result in cell disruption and potential loss of function, but is less destructive than neurolysis. This has not been used in pelvic pain but has been used effectively in neuralgia following thoracotomy.[53] Furthermore, sympathetic blockade of the superior hypogastric nerves just below the sacral promontory using CT guidance[54] or neurolytic block with chemical irritants such as alcohol or phenolic agents to destroy nerve fibers have been described as having limited success.[55] However, this mode of therapy should be supported by coping strategies.[55]

Surgery

The aim of surgery in the treatment of CPP is to remove the source of pain and prevent nociceptive transmission to the brain, with conservation of the gynecological structures, or to remove certain pelvic organs on the premise that the pain will then subside. None of these aims has been achieved. Adhesiolysis for abdominopelvic adhesions has been undertaken by laparotomy or laparoscopy with various results. Chan and Wood performed adhesiolysis by laparotomy in 100 patients with CPP and described relief in 65% of the patients[56] while Daniell described relief in 28 of 42 (67%) patients after laparoscopic adhesiolysis.[57] The amount of pelvic adhesive disease has no consistent relationship to the self-report of pelvic pain.[58] Adhesions which cause significant restriction of movement or bowel distension are associated with CPP. In a randomized controlled trial of 48 patients with CPP and pelvic adhesions, benefit from adhesiolysis was demonstrated only in those with severe adhesions involving the serosa of the small bowel or colon.[59]

When adhesive pelvic disease is considered a probable cause of CPP, adhesiolysis by laparoscopy in competent hands rather than laparotomy has a lower incidence of adhesion reformation and pain recurrence. Using proportional regression analysis in 123 patients who had microsurgical or laparoscopic surgery for the treatment of chronic pelvic pain, the cumulative probability of recurrence or persistence of pain was three times more common following surgery by laparotomy compared to laparoscopy.[60] Adhesion reformation can sometimes be reduced by intraperitoneal barrier devices either in the form of fluids (dextran, crystalloids), solids (Interceed®, Preclude®) or natural tissues such as omentum applied on the raw surfaces at the time of operation.[61] Premature resort to hysterectomy as 'quick fix' surgery is a common clinical error in the management of CPP. Among 99 patients who had hysterectomy for unexplained CPP, 22 had persistent pain after a mean follow up of 22 months.[62] Cautious counseling should emphasize the high failure rate as surgery should only be performed in special clinical circumstances. The value of other procedures, such as presacral neurectomy or uterosacral ligament resection, which are often used in the treatment of endometriosis-related pelvic pain are discussed in chapter 37.

Psychological

Various psychological treatment modalities may offer benefit depending on the initial and ongoing assessments. These techniques involve a reconceptualization of the pelvic pain and its associated problems. The process aims to explore and understand the affective state, the coping resources and the psychosocial state of the patient so that an appropriate plan can be made in conjunction with medical options. Psychological treatment can be employed in one of two ways: either as a single approach, in which it serves as the sole treatment after all other options have failed, or as a mixed approach, in which it is used as one among many other treatments. The latter is the preferred option as this has been shown to be an effective multidisciplinary strategy in the management of CPP with or without obvious pathology.[46] In this approach diminution of the nociceptive stimulation is enhanced by traditional medical methods such as TENS, or myofascial anesthetic local injections of 'trigger spots' as well as the treatment of specific psychological issues identified during the initial assessment. We prescribe antidepressant or anxiolytic drugs if the HAD score is abnormal at the initial visit. The behavioral treatment approach includes relaxation, biofeedback, stress management, sex therapy, marital and family counseling and hypnosis, as well as cognitive therapy aimed at reducing the thoughts that maintain negative feelings and exacerbate the pain. These are provided by the nurse counselor. The identification of an abnormal psychological morbidity may be treated by a specific psychotherapeutic modality. Assessment is carried out at regular intervals to determine the progress of the patient using the same questionnaire as at the beginning.

Conclusion

The narrow view of the biomedical theory as a cause of chronic pelvic pain is no longer appropriate. There is a plethora of organic, functional and psychologically-related causes with great interdigitation. Patients must be counseled about realistic expectations when undergoing treatment for CPP. Most patients are unwilling to undertake a nonsurgical, often prolonged approach, as they feel surgery will serve as a 'quick fix' to relieve the symptoms. There is a need to formulate and evaluate an acceptable, patient friendly psychological assessment questionnaire for patients with chronic pelvic pain. Such an assessment should be interdisciplinary with the aim of dissecting the role and various interactions between the multiple etiologies of chronic pelvic pain, and should be aimed at formulating an individualized treatment plan. Conventional medical approaches are inadequate to treat many of these conditions and this may lead to frustration and distrust between the patient and physician. The multidisciplinary approach which incorporates behavioral, medical and psychosocial treatment modalities is more effective than the single therapy Cartesian approach.

REFERENCES

1. Ylikorkala O, Dawood Y 1978 New concepts in dysmenorrhea. American Journal of Obstetrics and Gynecology 130: 833–847
2. Mathias S, Kuppermann M, Liberman R, Lipschutz R, Steege J 1996 Chronic pelvic pain: prevalence, health-related quality of life, and economic correlates. Obstetrics and Gynecology 87: 321–327
3. Smith R 1993 Cyclic pelvic pain and dysmenorrhea. Obstetric and Gynecology Clinics of North America 20: 753–764
4. Williams EA, Collins WP, Clayton SG 1976 Studies in the involvement of prostaglandins in uterine symptomatology and pathology. British Journal of Obstetrics and Gynaecology 83: 337–341
5. Rees MC, Turnbull A 1985 Leiomyoma release prostaglandins. Prost Leuk 18: 65–68
6. Chaudhuri G 1973 Release of prostaglandin by the IUCD. Prostaglandins 3: 773–777
7. Moon YS, Leung PC, Ho Yuen B, Gomel V 1981 Prostaglandin F in human endometriotic tissue. American Journal of Obstetrics and Gynecology 141: 344–345
8. Vernon MW, Beard JS, Graves K, Wilson EA 1986 Classification of endometriotic implants by morphologic appearance and capacity to synthesize prostaglandin F. Fertility and Sterility 46: 801–806

9. Åkerlund M 1979 Pathophysiology of dysmenorrhea. Acta Obstetrica Gynecologica 87: 27–35
10. Bevan S, Yeats J 1991 Protons activate a cation conductance in a subpopulation of rat dorsal root ganglion neurons. Journal of Physiology 433: 145–161
11. Weinreich D 1986 Bradykinin inhibits a slow spike after hyperpolarization in visceral sensory neurones. Journal of Pharmacology 132: 61–63
12. van Os 1983 Intra-uterine devices. In: Studd J (ed) Progress in obstetrics and gynaecology. Churchill Livingstone, Edinburgh, pp 292–304
13. Rang HP, Bevan S, Dray A 1991 Chemical activation of nociceptive peripheral neurones. British Medical Bulletin 47: 534–548
14. Perper MM, Nezhat F, Goldstein H, Nezhat C 1995 Dysmenorrhea is related to the number of implants in endometriosis. Fertility and Sterility 63: 500–503
15. Odukoya OA, Cooke ID 1996 Endometriosis: a review. In: Studd J (ed) Progress in obstetrics and gynaecology. vol 12 1996 Churchill Livingstone, Edinburgh 327–344
16. Takahashi K, Okada S, Ozaki T, Kitao M, Sugimura K 1994 Diagnosis of pelvic endometriosis by magnetic resonance imaging using 'fat saturation' technique. Fertility and Sterility 62: 973–977
17. Buttram VC, Reiters RC 1981 Uterine leiomyomata: etiology, symptomatology, and management. Fertility and Sterility 36: 443–445
18. Roy S, Shaw ST 1981 Role of prostaglandin in IUD-associated uterine bleeding — effect of a prostaglandin synthethase inhibitor (ibuprofen). Obstetrics and Gynecology 58: 101–105
19. Canis M, Wattiez A, Pouly JL, Mage G, Manhes H, Bruhat MA 1990 Laparoscopic management of unicornuate uterus with rudimentary horn and unilateral extensive endometriosis: case report. Human Reproduction 5: 819–820
20. Perino A, Chianchiano N, Simonaro C, Cittadini E 1995 Endoscopic management of a case of 'complete septate uterus wirh unilateral haematometra'. Human Reproduction 10: 2171–2173
21. Fedele L, Bianchi S, Bocciolone L, Di Nola G, Arcaini L, Franchi D 1994 Relief of dysmenorrhoea associated with septate uteri after abdominal or hysteroscopic metroplasty. Acta Obstetrica Gynecologica Scandinavica 73: 56–59
22. McCormack WM 1994 Pelvic inflammatory disease: current concepts. New England Journal of Medicine 330: 115–119
23. Nishida M 1991 Relationship between the onset of dysmenorrhea and histologic finding in adenomyosis. American Journal of Obstetrics and Gynecology 165: 229–234
24. Brosens JJ, De Souza NM, Baker F, Paraschos T, Winston R 1995 Endovaginal ultrasonography in the diagnosis of adenomyosis uteri: identifying the predictive characteristics. British Journal of Obstetrics and Gynaecology 102: 471–474
25. Coppen A, Kessel N 1963 Menstruation and personality. British Journal of Psychiatry 711–721
26. Helme JM 1987 Acupuncture for the management of primary dysmenorrhea. Obstetrics and Gynecology 69: 51–56
27. Dawood MY, Ramos J 1990 Transcutaneous electrical nerve stimulation (TENS) for the treatment of primary dysmenorrhea — a randomized crossover comparison with placebo, TENS, and ibuprofen. Obstetrics and Gynecology 75: 656–660
28. Editorial 1994 Chronic pelvic pain. British Journal of Anaesthesia 73(5): 571–573
29. Chamberlain G, Brown JC 1978 Gynaecological laparoscopy: report of the working party of the confidential enquiry into gynaecological laparoscopy. Royal College of Obstetrics and Gynaecology 1–27, London
30. Reiter CR 1990 A profile of women with chronic pelvic pain. Clinical Obstetrics and Gynecology 33: 130–136
31. O'Connor DT 1987 Clinical features in diagnosis. In: Jordan A, Singer A (eds) Endometriosis 21–33. Churchill Livingstone, Edinburgh
32. Lee NC, Dicker RC, Rubin GL, Ory HW 1984 Confirmation of the preoperative diagnosis for hysterectomy. American Journal of Obstetrics and Gynecology 150: 283–287
33. Rapkin A 1990 Neuroanatomy, neurophysiology and neuropharmacology of pelvic pain. Clinical Obstetrics and Gynecology 33: 119–129
34. De Groat WC 1989 Neuropeptides in pelvic afferent pathways. Experientia 56: 334–361
35. Peters A, van Dorst E, Jellis B, van Zuuren, Hermans J, Trimbos A 1991 A randomized clinical trial to compare two different approaches in women with chronic pelvic pain. Obstetrics and Gynecology 77: 740–744
36. Reiter RC, Gambone JC 1991 Nongynecologic somatic pathology in women with idiopathic chronic pelvic pain. Journal of Reproductive Medicine 36: 253–258
37. Steege JF, Stout A 1991 Resolution of chronic pelvic pain after laparoscopic lysis of adhesion. American Journal of Obstetrics and Gynecology 165: 278–285
38. Wall PD 1986 Causes of intractable pain. Hospital Update, Dec., pp 969–974
39. McCausland A, Holmes F, Trotter A 1966 Venous distensibility during menstrual cycle. American Journal of Obstetrics and Gynecology 68: 640–643
40. Reginald PW, Adams J, Franks S, Wadsworth J, Beard R 1989 Medoxyprogesterone acetate in the treatment of pelvic pain due to venous congestion. British Journal of Obstetrics and Gynaecology 96: 1148–1152
41. Beard RW, Highman JW, Pearse S, Reginald PW 1984 Diagnosis of pelvic varicosities in women. Lancet 2: 946–949
42. Walker E, Katon W, Harrop-Griffith J, Holm L, Russo J, Hickok R 1988 Relationship of chronic pelvic pain to psychiatric diagnoses and childhood sexual abuse. American Journal of Psychiatry 145: 75–80
43. Fordyce WE 1976 Behavioural methods of control of chronic pelvic pain and illness 63–72. CV Mosby, St Louis
44. Walling MK, O'Hara MW, Reiter RC, Milbulin AK, Lilly G, Vincent SD 1994 Abuse history and chronic pelvic pain in women II. A multivariate analysis of abuse and psychological morbidity. Obstetrics and Gynecology 84: 200–206
45. Reiter RC, Gambode JC 1990 Demographic and historic variables in women with idiopathic chronic pelvic pain. Obstetrics and Gynecology 75: 428–432
46. Kames LD, Rapkin AJ, Naliboff BD, Afifi S, Ferrer-Brechner T 1990 Effectiveness of an interdisciplinary pain management program for the treatment of chronic pelvic pain. Pain 41: 41–46

47. Zigmoid AS, Snaith RP 1983 The Hospital Anxiety and Depression Scale. Acta Psychiatrica Scandinavica 67: 361–370
48. Magni G, Andreoli C, de Leo D, Martinotti G, Rossi C 1986 Psychological profile of women with chronic pelvic pain. Archives of Gynecology 237: 165–169
49. Hameroff SR, Cook RC, Scherer K 1982 Doxepin effects on chronic pain, depression and plasma opioids. Journal of Clinical Psychiatry 43: 22–25
50. Beresin EV 1986 Imipramine in the treatment of chronic pelvic pain. Psychosomatics 27: 294–297
51. McQuay HJ, Carroll D, Glynn CJ 1993 Low dose amitriptyline in the treatment of chronic pain. Anaesthesia 47: 646–652
52. Milburn A, Reiter RC, Rhomeberg AT 1993 Multidisciplinary approach to chronic pelvic pain. Obstetric and Gynecology Clinics of North America 20: 643–659
53. Conacher ID 1986 Percutaneous cryotherapy for post-thoracotomy neuralgia. Pain 25: 227–228
54. Wechsler RJ, Maurer PM, Halpern EJ, Frank ED 1995 Superior hypogastric plexus block for chronic pelvic pain in the presence of endometriosis: CT techniques and results. Radiology 196: 103–106
55. Hanks GW 1991 Opioid-responsive and opioid-nonresponsive pain in cancer. British Medical Bulletin 47: 718–731
56. Chan CLK, Wood C 1985 Pelvic adhesiolysis — the assessment of symptom relief by 100 patients. Australian and New Zealand Journal of Obstetrics and Gynaecology 25: 295–298
57. Daniell JF 1989 Laparoscopic enterolysis for chronic pelvic pain. Journal of Gynecological Surgery 5: 61–65
58. Stout AL, Steege FJ 1991 Relationship of laparoscopy finding to self report of pelvic pain. American Journal of Obstetrics and Gynecology 164: 73–79
59. Peters AW, Trimbos-Kemper CG, Admiraal C, Trimbos JB 1992 A randomized clinical trial on the benefit of adhesiolysis in patients with intraperitoneal adhesions and chronic pelvic pain. British Journal of Obstetrics and Gynecology 99: 59–62
60. Saravelos H, Li TC, Cooke ID 1995 An analysis of the outcome of microsurgical and laparoscopic adhesiolysis for chronic pelvic pain. Human Reproduction 10: 2895–2901
61. Li TC, Cooke ID 1994 The value of absorbable adhesion barrier, Interceed, in the prevention of adhesion formation in infertility and endometriosis surgery. British Journal of Obstetrics and Gynaecology 101: 281–366
62. Stoval TG, Ling FR, Crawford DA 1990 Hysterectomy for chronic pelvic pain of presumed uterine origin. Obstetrics and Gynecology 75: 676–679

33. Premenstrual syndrome

William R. Keye Jr

Introduction

The concept that premenstrual syndrome (PMS) is the result of alterations in the secretion of sex steroids by the ovary was first suggested in the scientific literature by Frank in 1931.[1] On the basis of his study of 15 women, he concluded that 'premenstrual tension' is caused by the accumulation of hormones produced by the ovary. Efforts to isolate and identify the gonadal steroids responsible for premenstrual syndrome have been based largely on this early hypothesis. Unfortunately, now almost 70 years after this landmark article by Frank, researchers and clinicians alike are still searching for the etiologic agent(s) and pathophysiologic mechanism(s) that underlie PMS. The uncertainties and confusions surrounding this variable condition will be placed in context with our present knowledge in this chapter.

PREMENSTRUAL SYNDROME

Definition

Despite many proposed definitions of PMS over the years, the definition by Reid and Yen in 1981 is one of the most practical for the clinician.[2] They defined PMS as 'the cyclic recurrence in the luteal phase of the menstrual cycle of a combination of distress and physical, psychological and/or behavioral changes of sufficient severity to produce the deterioration of interpersonal relationships and/or interference with normal activities'. A variant of PMS known as premenstrual dysphoric disorder (PDD) was proposed by The American Psychiatric Association in its fourth edition of the Diagnostic and Statistical Manual of Mental Disorders (DSM-IV).[4] This disorder as defined by The American Psychiatric Association applies to some but not all women who meet the criteria proposed by Reid and Yen. However, it contains several key elements which are important for the clinician. At least one of the following four symptoms or symptom clusters should be present:

1. Marked affective lability
2. Persistent and marked anger or irritability
3. Marked anxiety, tension, feelings of being keyed up or on edge
4. Marked depressed mood, feelings of hopelessness, or self-deprecating thoughts.

In addition, one or more of the following should be present:

1. Decreased interest in usual activities
2. Lethargy, easy fatigability or marked lack of energy
3. Subjective change of difficulty in concentrating
4. Marked change in appetite
5. Hypersomnia or insomnia
6. Other physical symptoms such as bloating, breast tenderness, headache or joint or muscle pain
7. Avoidance of social activity
8. Decreased productivity and efficiency at work and at home
9. Increased sensitivity to rejection
10. Subjective sense of being overwhelmed
11. Subjective sense of feeling out of control
12. Increased interpersonal conflicts.

In addition to listing specific symptoms, the definition proposed by The American Psychiatric Association also notes that these symptoms must be clustered in the luteal phase and disappear within the first few days of the onset of menstruation. These symptoms must be serious enough that they interfere with the sufferer's quality of life. Finally, it requires that the symptoms are not the exacerbation of another underlying psychiatric disorder.

The essence of this definition is that it emphasizes the timing and the severity of symptoms as much as it does the individual symptoms themselves. However, it focuses on emotional symptoms and does not include women with only premenstrual physical symptoms, such as those who may experience premenstrual migraine headaches or seizures, or recurring premenstrual gastrointestinal, cardiac or pulmonary symptoms.

Epidemiology

Since the presence or absence of PMS is determined solely by the patient's subjective experience of symptoms, it is difficult to establish its true prevalence. This is also complicated by the fact that until recently there has been an absence of a standardized and well-accepted definition for PMS and the absence of validated methods for establishing the diagnosis. On these bases, recent studies have suggested that only about 3–5% of women of reproductive age suffer from this condition.[4]

An association between PMS and a history of postpartum depression, intolerance to birth control pills, spontaneous miscarriages, pregnancy-induced hypertension and hyperemesis gravidarum has been suggested[5] but prospectively controlled studies have not confirmed these clinical impressions.[6] In a recent, well designed study, Rojansky and Halbreich failed to confirm the suggested clinical association between tubal ligation and PMS.[7] There were no significant differences in estradiol, progesterone, testosterone, prolactin, TSH and thyroxin values between those who had a tubal ligation and those who had not.

Adolescent daughters of mothers with PMS have reported more menstrual and premenstrual symptoms than the mothers without PMS,[8] but it is unclear whether this is a biological, psychosocial or learned experience.

Clinical features

The symptoms of PMS are well known to most clinicians. They consist of physical and emotional symptoms as well as behavioral changes (Table 33.1). Common physical symptoms experienced by women with PMS are breast tenderness, fatigue, joint pain, headache and bloating. The emotional symptoms most commonly reported include depression, irritability and anxiety. Finally, the behavioral changes often reported by women with PMS are binge eating (especially carbohydrate craving), the avoidance of social activities, crying episodes and physical or emotional abuse of those around them. Well over 150 symptoms have been reported to comprise the syndrome of PMS.

Some researchers have attempted to subtype PMS by carrying out factor analyses of symptoms recorded by women on standardized questionnaires. For example, Moos described eight factors or symptom groups derived from 47 symptoms on the Menstrual Distress Questionnaire.[9] These symptom groups were labeled: negative affect, water retention, arousal, control, behavioral change, autonomic reactions, concentration and pain. While the concept of defining subgroups of the premenstrual syndrome based on symptom patterns is appealing, at the present time there is no evidence to suggest that these subgroups represent different etiologies or different pathophysiologic mechanisms.

As noted above, it is also of value to collect more than a single month of prospective charting. A study by Ekholm demonstrated that one out of every three patients will have a significant change in their pattern from one month to another.[10] The degree of confidence in the diagnosis is usually substantially improved by the collection of more than one month of prospective data.

There have been numerous attempts to validate the subjective symptoms of women with PMS. Kuczmierczyk et al evaluated pain threshold and ability

Table 33.1 Clinical features of premenstrual syndrome.

Physical symptoms	
Fatigue	Backache
Bloating	Sensitivity to light, noise or touch
Breast tenderness	Food cravings
Headache	Clumsiness
Emotional symptoms	
Emotional lability	Anxiety or tension
Hopelessness or depressed mood	Feeling overwhelmed
Hostility or irritability	Feeling out of control
Desire to withdraw	Feelings of inadequacy and rejection
Loss of patience	
Cognitive changes	
Forgetfulness	Confusion
Inability to concentrate	Inability to problem solve

to tolerate pain in the follicular and the luteal phases of the menstrual cycle of PMS subjects & controls.[11] They found no difference between the groups with respect to pain sensitivity. However, ratings for pain intensity were higher in both the phases of the menstrual cycle for women with premenstrual syndrome, suggesting that the subjective experience of pain and discomfort by women with premenstrual syndrome may be indicative of a heightened perceptual sensitivity.

A prospective study of manual dexterity and perception found that women without premenstrual syndrome noted an improvement in fine motor function in the luteal phase of the menstrual cycle, while women with premenstrual syndrome experienced a deterioration.[12] However, there were no significant differences between the groups using other tests of function ability. It appears that the physical and behavioral changes reported in the luteal phase in women with premenstrual syndrome are sometimes difficult to verify.

Features of the premenstrual syndrome that are often overlooked include the interpersonal and social problems that may occur as a result of the recurring premenstrual behavior changes and emotional and physical symptoms. Women with PMS, as well as their husbands, will often describe an increased frequency of disagreements and arguments during the luteal phase of the menstrual cycle.[13] Women with PMS may also report more verbal abuse of their children and an increase in conflicts with friends and coworkers during the luteal phase of the menstrual cycle. As a result, women with PMS may become socially withdrawn and experience a decrease in self-esteem and self-confidence as well as separation, divorce and job loss.

Diagnosis

At the present time the diagnosis of PMS is made on the basis of self-report of symptoms and behavioral changes. In a clinical setting the diagnosis is usually made by history alone. However, studies show that less than 50% of women presenting with the 'self-made' diagnosis of PMS will actually meet the criteria for the diagnosis.[14,15] Therefore, it is important that some form of prospective daily calendar, diary, chart or scale be obtained.

There is general agreement that there should be a relative absence of symptoms during the follicular phase of the menstrual cycle with at least a 30% increase in the severity of symptoms in the luteal phase. Detailed devices are useful in a research setting, but are often cumbersome in a clinical setting where patient compliance is often poor. None of these measurement tools has yet been externally well validated nor shown to be associated with biological or behavioral markers of PMS.

As yet, there is no biological marker for PMS. Therefore there is no single laboratory test that can be ordered to confirm the diagnosis. The role of the physical examination and laboratory and radiologic studies is to rule out other underlying psychological and physical disorders which may mimic PMS. Table 33.2 is a list of physical and psychiatric conditions that may mimic premenstrual syndrome.

From a practical standpoint, it is sometimes necessary to initiate therapy without prospective data. Many women seeking care within a physician's office for PMS are convinced of the validity of their own self-made diagnosis of premenstrual syndrome and are often unwilling to delay therapy for two or three months to accumulate prospective data. In addition, the clinical history may be clear cut enough that the physician has little doubt about the validity of the patient's diagnosis. In this setting the clinician has to make a clinical judgement as to the need to collect prospective data.

Table 33.2 Conditions that may mimic premenstrual syndrome.

Psychiatric disorders	
Dysthymia	Unipolar or bipolar affective disorder
Phobias	Personality disorder
Obsessive compulsive disorder	Anxiety neurosis
Alcohol abuse or dependence	Multiple personality disorder
Physical disorders	
Hypo- or hyperthyroidism	Lyme disease
Systemic lupus erythematosus	Migraine syndrome
CNS neoplasm	Endometriosis
Mitral valve prolapse	Irritable bowel syndrome
Chronic fatigue syndrome	Idiopathic edema
Seizure disorder	Anemia

Natural history of premenstrual syndrome

Little is known about the natural history of PMS and there have been few follow-up studies. Freeman and her colleagues reported a one year follow-up of 129 subjects who had participated in a prospective blinded study of progesterone suppository therapy.[16] They reported that the severity of symptoms one year following participation in the study was less than at the time of enrollment but greater than at the end of the study.

In a six year follow-up study of women who had participated in a survey of 730 female nursing school graduates Johnson & Milburn[17] categorized the women into five groups according to severity of their premenstrual symptoms at the time of the initial survey and then resurveyed them six years later. They concluded that few women had a progression and most women had a regression of their symptoms. In addition, they found that women with coexisting depression had a greater tendency to progress while those without had a greater tendency to regress. However, they did not analyze such complicating factors as the onset of menopause, birth control pill use, hysterectomy or method of treatment, and it is uncertain from these preliminary results whether such regression was the result of a natural course of the disease or the result of interval factors.

Finally, a nine year follow-up study of 43 women by Keye and colleagues found that while all 37 premenopausal women who still had their ovaries in place still reported PMS, 71% reported that their symptoms were less severe and only 13% reported that they were more severe.[18] While the original diagnosis had been made using a prospective calendar as well as psychometric tests administered in both the luteal and follicular phases of the menstrual cycle, the follow-up data were collected from surveys and therefore not validated with prospective measurements. In addition, not all of the individuals who were surveyed responded and therefore there may have been selection bias in the follow-up.

It has been suggested by a number of authors and women with PMS that the regression and improvement of symptoms is often the result of validation of the premenstrual syndrome, education, support and caring as well as medication. Prospective studies are needed to confirm this hypothesis.

Etiology

Psychosocial etiologies

The bulk of research into the etiology of PMS has focused on hormonal fluctuations throughout the menstrual cycle. Despite decades of research into possible endocrinopathies or hormonal triggers for premenstrual symptoms, none has been supported by conclusive evidence.

Koeske and Koeske evaluated the possible role of women's beliefs about menstruation as a factor in the etiology of PMS.[19] They studied the possibility that women in the United States have certain beliefs about menstruation and behavior and that these beliefs influence how they interpret the relationship between mood swings and the approach of menstruation. They found that women attributed their negative but not their positive moods to their biology. This was in contrast to men who were not as likely to attribute negative moods to their biology. They hypothesized that women who were in upsetting situations in the luteal phase of the menstrual cycle were more likely to accept responsibility for the situation and their emotional reaction to it than to try and alter the situation through positive action.

AuBuchon and Calhoun evaluated the effects of social expectations on psychological and psychosomatic symptoms.[20] When women were told that a study involved premenstrual mood changes, they reported significantly more negative psychological and psychosomatic symptoms during their premenstrual and menstrual phases than a group of women who were not told the nature of the study. The authors concluded that the reporting of premenstrual symptoms by some women is influenced by the fact that they have been taught that the premenstrual part of the menstrual cycle is associated with negative physical and emotional symptoms.

Finally, a minority of investigators argue that premenstrual syndrome is simply a variant of more classic psychiatric diseases that have become entrained to the luteal phase of the menstrual cycle.

Biological etiologies

While most serious students of PMS acknowledge the role of cultural and psychological factors, there is a widespread belief that cyclic biological changes during the menstrual cycle somehow act to trigger negative moods and the other symptoms and behavioral changes of PMS. Numerous studies have been performed looking for the specific hormonal profile or biological trigger responsible for premenstrual symptoms. While, thus far, there have been no data supporting the central role of any one specific biological factor, there are a number of promising leads.

Gonadal steroids and gonadotropins. There is indirect evidence that gonadotropins and/or gonadal steroids are related to the etiology of premenstrual syndrome. First, premenstrual syndrome occurs during the luteal phase of the menstrual cycle when blood levels of estradiol and progesterone are elevated. Second, premenstrual syndrome is absent prior to menarche and after the menopause when estradiol and progesterone levels are very low. Third, premenstrual syndrome persists in women who have had their ovaries left *in situ* at the time of a hysterectomy but is absent when the ovaries are removed at hysterectomy.[21]

The relationship between mood states and progesterone levels was first studied and reported in 1972 by Kyger and Webb.[22] They administered psychological tests to 30 normal women during menstruation and again during periods of elevated progesterone (in the luteal phase, during oral contraceptive therapy and during the third trimester of pregnancy). They studied 57 variables but found only two that were indicative of increasing emotional vulnerability during periods of elevated progesterone. They decided that these findings could be explained by chance and that it was unlikely that increased progesterone levels are responsible for serious physiological disturbances.

O'Brien et al found that progesterone concentrations in women with PMS were significantly higher than those in a control group during the luteal phase,[23] and concluded that there is no evidence that progesterone deficiency causes PMS. Additional studies have been contradictory and inconsistent. In perhaps the most elegant and elaborate study done to date, Rubinow et al[24] were unable to demonstrate any difference in circulating concentrations of several hormones between women with and without PMS.

To eliminate the influence of the episodic secretion of these hormones, Dennerstein and colleagues compared urinary profiles of estrogen and pregnanediol in 65 women with documented PMS and 18 asymptomatic volunteers.[25] They, too, were unable to find any significant differences between the two groups with respect to levels of urinary estrogen or pregnanediol, although the day of pregnanediol peak occurred significantly later in the luteal phase for women with PMS than asymptomatic volunteers.

In a novel study, using the antiprogesterone agent mifepristone, Schmidt and colleagues truncated the luteal phase of the menstrual cycle without altering premenstrual symptoms.[26] From these observations they concluded that the endocrine events of the late luteal phase of the menstrual cycle, primarily those of falling progesterone levels, were not directly responsible for creating the symptoms of PMS. They suggested that the symptoms of PMS may be triggered by hormonal events that occurred before the late luteal phase or that PMS is an autonomous cyclic disorder that is linked to, but can be disassociated from, the menstrual cycle itself.

Finally, a study by Lewis and co-workers sampled the pulsatile release of LH and progesterone in six women with PMS and compared it to that of six age-matched control volunteers.[27] They found there were no differences between the two groups with respect to the mean concentration or to the frequency or amplitude of LH or progesterone pulses. By contrast, Facchinetti et al found some differences in the episodic secretion of LH and progesterone, with an increased frequency but decreased amplitude of both LH and progesterone in women with PMS.[28] These findings suggested that there may be greater sensitivity of the corpus luteum to LH stimulation at the time of the onset of symptoms in women with PMS.

Prolactin. Prolactin has been implicated as a possible etiologic agent or trigger for PMS because of its small rise at midcycle. While several studies have reported a greater elevation in prolactin levels in the luteal phase in women with PMS as compared to controls, others have found that there is no difference.[24,29]

Thyroid hormone. In 1987 Brayshaw and Brayshaw reported that women with PMS demonstrated increased thyroid stimulatory hormone (TSH) responses to thyrotropin releasing hormone (TRH) and that therapy with levothyroxine was effective in many of their patients.[30] In contrast, Roy-Byrne and colleagues in 1987 were unable to find any significant differences in TSH after TRH in women with PMS when compared to normal volunteers.[31] Likewise, Casper and colleagues[32] and Nikolai and colleagues[33] were unable to find any differences in levels of thyroxine, T3 or TSH both before and after stimulation with TRH. Finally, Schmitt and colleagues at the National Institute of Mental Health have looked at basal thyroid function tests, thyroid autoantibody levels, TRH stimulation tests and the efficacy of thyroxine in the treatment of premenstrual syndrome.[34] They found that approximately 10% of women had evidence of either hypothyroidism or hyperthyroidism. Thirteen percent of women had elevated thyroid autoantibody titers and 30% of women who had normal basal TSH levels had abnormal TSH responses to TRH. They also found that treatment with thyroxine was not superior to placebo in a double blind, controlled cross-over trial. They concluded that basal thyroid function testing was abnormal in only a small percentage of women with prospectively confirmed PMS. Their finding that 10% of subjects with PMS had subclinical hypothyroidism was comparable to the prevalence of subclinical hypothyroidism in the general population (4.6–7.5%). They concluded that PMS was not the result of 'masked' or subclinical hypothyroidism.

Most investigators have been unable to demonstrate any differences between PMS sufferers and controls in serum levels of TSH or thyroid hormones, in response to TRH or in response to thyroxine treatment.[32,34] although one study suggested some differences and responses to treatment.[30]

Cortisol. Several mood disorders including depression and anorexia nervosa have been associated with elevations of basal evening cortisol and a blunted adrenocorticotropic hormone (ACTH) response to corticotropin-releasing hormone (CRH) stimulation. Several reports have suggested that morning plasma cortisol concentrations, but not urinary free cortisol secretion, may be elevated in patients with PMS when compared to normal volunteers without PMS. Rubinow et al were unable to find any abnormalities in cortisol secretion in women with PMS,[24] but a more detailed study by the same group found subtle increase in response of the pituitary-adrenal axis to CRH.[35]

Glucose. Many women with premenstrual syndrome are concerned that they also suffer from hypoglycemia. Reid et al performed oral glucose tolerance tests in six women with PMS and five control subjects,[36] and found no difference in glucose tolerance nor glucose, insulin or glucagon responses to naloxone between the two groups. Other groups have also found no statistically significant difference in plasma glucose or insulin levels between PMS sufferers and controls.[37]

Melatonin. Parry et al examined melatonin secretion in eight women with PMS and eight matched controls.[38] Women with PMS demonstrated significantly lower levels of melatonin than control subjects and a significantly earlier nocturnal onset of melatonin secretion throughout the menstrual cycle. These findings suggest the possibility of disturbances in biorhythms involving melatonin in women with PMS.

Androgens. Rubinow et al were unable to demonstrate any differences in the concentrations of several circulating androgens in PMS sufferers.[24]

Calcium-regulating hormones. In a small study of seven women with documented PMS and five women who were asymptomatic controls total and ionized calcium declined significantly in both groups at midcycle with the increase in estradiol.[39] In the PMS group peak midcycle parathyroid hormone (PTH) was elevated by approximately 30% above early follicular phase levels, while in the asymptomatic controls, PTH did not vary throughout the menstrual cycle. They also found significant differences between the groups with respect to total calcium, 25 OHD and 1,25-$(OH)_2$ D. This suggests that women with PMS may have a midcycle elevation of PTH with a transient secondary hyperparathyroidism. These results support the possible value of daily vitamin D and calcium replacement in women with PMS.

Atrial natriuretic peptide (ANP). One of the classic theories of PMS has been that of premenstrual fluid retention. To study this phenomenon, Hussain et al measured circulating concentrations of ANP in 11 women with PMS and 12 asymptomatic controls.[40] The asymptomatic women demonstrated no change in ANP concentrations throughout the menstrual cycle. However, in the women with premenstrual syndrome, ANP levels showed a significant fall in the midluteal phase compared to levels in the follicular phase. Throughout the cycle ANP levels were consistently lower in the premenstrual syndrome group than in the control group. These decreased ANP concentrations in the group with premenstrual syndrome in the luteal phase may indicate either a lower plasma volume or a decrease in the total body sodium content, or both.

Serotonin and other neurotransmitter systems. Serotonin is known to play a mediating role in the origin of mood and behavioral disorders in which depression, irritability and aggression are prominent. As a result, it has been speculated that serotonin may play a central role in premenstrual syndrome. Rapkin et al[41] found that whole blood serotonin levels were significantly lower during the last 10 days of the menstrual cycle in women with PMS, when compared to controls. This occurred despite the fact that there was no significant decrease in circulating concentrations of serum estradiol or progesterone. In subjects with PMS, there was also a decrease in whole body serotonin after tryptophan loading in the late luteal phase.

Additional evidence that there may be abnormalities of the serotoninergic system in women with PMS comes from two studies of imipramine-binding sites which have demonstrated that imipramine receptor binding was lower in women with PMS characterized by severe mood changes than in a group of controls.[42,43] They noted this difference in the early luteal phase and suggested that the development of premenstrual mood changes might be related to gonadal hormone modulation of the serotoninergic system.

In contrast to these studies, Malmgren and colleagues failed to demonstrate any difference in serotonin metabolism.[44] However, this study was criticized for not using daily symptom ratings. The role of the serotoninergic system clearly deserves additional study.

Beta-endorphin. Several studies have consistently shown low β-endorphin levels in PMS subjects. Chuong et al reported that β-endorphin levels throughout the periovulatory phase were lower in women with PMS than in controls.[45] Facchinetti et al reported that women with premenstrual symptoms had a marked decrease in β-endorphin levels before and during menstruation, whereas no changes were observed in the control subjects.[46]

Other potential biological factors. Jakubowicz et al were unable to demonstrate changes in prostaglandin levels during the menstrual cycle but they found that circulating prostaglandin levels were lower in women with PMS than control subjects.[47] Piccoli found that there was a significant reduction in the urinary secretion of prostaglandin E_2 and prostaglandin $F_{2\alpha}$ in women with PMS when compared to the control group.[48] These authors suggested that there is reduced renal synthesis of PGE_2 and $F_{2\alpha}$ in women with PMS. They concluded that there may be differences in the manner in which the kidneys handle water and electrolytes in women with premenstrual syndrome when compared to healthy controls.

Mira et al[49] found no differences between PMS and control groups for serum levels of magnesium, zinc and vitamins A, E and B_6, and Chuong was similarly unable to find any differences in vitamin A levels.[50]

On the other hand, Abraham reported lower serum and intracellular magnesium levels[51] and Chuong & Dawson[52] noted lower levels of zinc and higher levels of copper during the luteal phase in women with PMS compared to controls. They pointed out that essential minerals may play physiologic roles in regulating the release and/or biological activity of hormones and neuropeptides involved in the menstrual cycle, and thus these observations may be clinically significant.

Harrison and colleagues found that women with PMS were more sensitive to the anxiety-stimulating properties of CO_2 inhalation and lactate infusion than asymptomatic controls.[53] These observations have been summarized in a hypothesis by Donald Klein called 'The Suffocation False Alarm Theory'.[54] He suggested that in PMS characterized by panic there is a hypersensitivity to CO_2 so that the body believes it is suffocating and triggers the 'suffocation alarm system'. This produces the sudden sensation of respiratory distress followed by a brief hyperventilation, panic and the urge to flee. Finally, Schmidt et al evaluated circulating levels of 'anxiolytic steroids'.[55] They postulated that premenstrual anxiety may be the result of a deficiency in metabolites of progesterone (which have sedative and hypnotic effects) that bind with high affinity to the gamma amino-butyric acid (GABA) receptor complex in the central nervous system but were unable to find any significant correlations between the severity of mood and plasma levels of progesterone, allopregnanolone or pregnenolone in humans.

Conclusions

When these studies are viewed together, it appears as though they do not support the hypothesis that there are consistent alterations of hormones, prostaglandins, vitamins or trace elements or electrolytes in women with premenstrual syndrome. The work regarding CO_2 inhalation suggests that there may be similarities between women with premenstrual syndrome and those with anxiety or panic disorders. If there is a biological difference between women with PMS and those without, it is likely to reside within the central nervous system rather than within the ovaries.

Biopsychosocial hypothesis

If an attempt is made to tie these varied observations together, then it is tempting to consider the biopsychosocial model of Engel.[56] Rather than propose that there is a single biological, psychological or cultural abnormality that accounts for premenstrual symptoms, the biopsychosocial model would suggest that PMS is the result of the interaction of all of these factors (Fig. 33.1). It is possible that women with premenstrual syndrome are in some way biologically vulnerable and that this biological vulnerability may be induced by past or influenced by contemporary psychosocial factors. During the menstrual cycle, normal biological changes may act as triggers to induce premenstrual symptoms in these biologically vulnerable individuals. It is unlikely that there is a single etiologic factor to explain PMS. It is more likely that the interaction of gonadal steroids with neurotransmitter, neuroendocrine and biorhythms influence mood, behavior and cognition. In addition, cultural and social factors are also important and may sensitize the individual to these biological changes. Future research should concentrate on the interaction of these biopsychosocial factors.

THERAPY

Since the original description of premenstrual syndrome by Frank in 1931,[1] dozens of therapies have

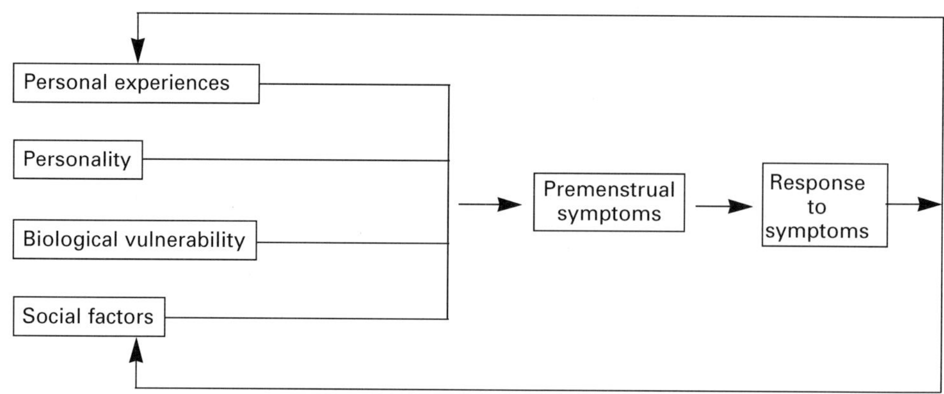

Fig. 33.1 Biopsychosocial model of PMS.

been proposed for PMS. The reasons for this include the possibility that PMS is not a single disorder but a group of disorders that do not all respond to a single treatment. Fortunately, several therapies appear to be effective for women with PMS. While this review will summarize the findings of many of the therapies currently used today, it will emphasize those therapies which have been shown to be effective from well-designed, placebo-controlled prospective studies.

The therapies of premenstrual syndrome could be categorized in many ways. I have chosen to categorize them separately into medical and psychosocial therapies (Table 33.3).

Medical therapies

Estrogen

Estrogen alone has been used to suppress cyclic ovarian activity in the belief that the hormonal changes that occur at ovulation act to trigger premenstrual symptoms. Using subcutaneous implants of estradiol, Magos et al treated 92 women with premenstrual syndrome, including 16 who suffered from menstrual migraine headaches.[57] They followed these patients for an average of two years and noted complete or almost complete relief of symptoms of PMS in 84% of the women. To avoid endometrial hyperplasia a progestogen was given for 7–10 days to induce

Table 33.3 Therapies for premenstrual syndrome.

Lifestyle changes	**Miscellaneous medical therapies**
Diet	Melatonin inhibitors
Exercise	Clonidine
Avoiding stressful situations	Doxycycline
Nutritional (vitamin B_6, magnesium, calcium, gammalinolenic acid)	Naltrexone
Sex hormonal therapies	**Psychotropic therapies**
Estrogen	Anxiolytics
Progesterone	Alprazolam
Ovulation suppression or elimination	Buspirone
Danazol	Antidepressants
GnRH agonist	Serotonin selective reuptake inhibitors (SSRIs)
Progestogen	Monoamine oxidase inhibitors (MAOIs)
Combined estrogen-progestogen	Tricyclics (TCAs)
Oophorectomy	Others (Valproate)
Antiprogesterone	
Other hormone therapy	
Antiprostaglandins	
Thyroid hormone	
Dopamine agonist	

regular withdrawal bleeding. Interestingly, the authors noted that there was a return of premenstrual symptoms in 45% of women at the time the progestogen was given.

Prospective and placebo-controlled studies of continuous estradiol implants or skin patches with cyclical progestogen demonstrated substantial or complete relief of symptoms throughout treatment.[58,59]

Progesterone

Green and Dalton first suggested progesterone therapy for premenstrual syndrome in 1953.[60] They administered progesterone intramuscularly on alternate days for 12 days before the onset of bleeding. They found that progesterone was effective in relieving the symptoms of premenstrual tension. On the basis of these observations and earlier reports from South Africa and France on trials of progesterone, Dalton advocated the use of progesterone for the treatment of premenstrual syndrome. More than a dozen studies have now been performed using progesterone or its optical isomer dydrogesterone. (For a review see reference 61.) Ten studies utilized a vaginal suppository in doses ranging from 200–800 mg a day. Two studies evaluated oral progesterone. Only two studies demonstrated a benefit of progesterone over that of placebo.

The study conducted by Freeman et al had perhaps the strongest design.[62] Subjects were selected on the basis of two months of prospective ratings of symptoms followed by two months of placebo treatment. Subjects were then randomly assigned to groups receiving either placebo or active treatment with progesterone suppositories, 400 or 800 mg daily. Each group continued treatment for two months for a total of six months of double blind, cross-over treatment. Daily symptom reports as well as subject's global symptom ratings demonstrated that neither dose of progesterone was more effective than the placebo.

Similarly, Corney et al found no significant difference between progesterone, placebo and behavioral psychotherapy for the treatment of premenstrual syndrome.[63] Many of the women taking progesterone or placebo mentioned minor side effects and compliance rates for treatment were low. Many found that insertion of the suppositories was messy and inconvenient.

In contrast of these studies there are two that have demonstrated a therapeutic effect of progesterone. In the first by Dennerstein et al 23 women were treated with 300 mg oral micronized progesterone or placebo each day for two months followed by cross-over therapy for 2 months.[64] Statistical analysis found significant differences in the means for nearly all the variables. They found that after only one month of treatment, patients receiving progesterone could be distinguished clearly from those receiving placebo on measures of stress, anxiety and concentration. Daily symptom scores were also calculated for both the progesterone and the placebo groups and 12 women clearly responded to the progesterone whereas only four responded to the placebo. The only serious side effect was reported by a 36-year-old women who developed a migraine headache premenstrually while taking the progesterone during the last month of the clinical trial.

Recently, Baker et al studied 17 women through a double-blind, placebo-controlled trial using vaginal suppositories containing 200 mg of 65 progesterone.[65] While overall scores of menstrual distress were not significantly different between the two groups, progesterone reduced the symptoms of tension, mood swings, irritability, anxiety and lack of control.

Dydrogesterone, the optical isomer of progesterone, has also been investigated in three studies and has not been found to be superior to placebo.[61]

Ovulation suppression

Ovulation can be effectively suppressed with a variety of medications including oral contraceptives, danazol, MPA, GnRH agonists, and oophorectomy. Danazol, 200–400 mg per day, appears to be effective for the treatment of most symptoms of PMS,[66,68] and this appears to be associated with its ability to suppress ovulation. Twenty of 23 anovulatory cycles were symptom-free, while only six of 32 ovulatory cycles were symptom-free.[68] Unfortunately, some patients will experience the typical side effects of danazol on these regimens. Luteal phase danazol, 200 mg daily, was effective in the treatment of premenstrual mastalgia.[67]

GnRH agonists may also be substantially superior to placebo in suppressing most symptoms of PMS, especially when ovulation is inhibited.[69–71] Unfortunately the prolonged use of GnRH-agonists alone to reduce the symptoms of PMS may be accompanied by significant vasomotor symptoms as well as decreased bone density (see ch. 37). To prevent these side effects several studies have been performed utilizing GnRH agonists coupled to hormone replacement using estrogen and a progestogen (so-called 'add-back' therapy). For example, Muse added estradiol valerate, 2 mg intramuscularly at four week intervals, and a progestogen, medroxyprogesterone acetate, to the leuprolide acetate.[72] He noted that the estrogen tended to induce a recurrence of the emotional component of the premenstrual symptom profile whereas the progestogen recreated physical complaints such as bloating and headache. These disappointing results suggested that the combination of hormone replacement therapy and GnRH agonists was not useful in treating premenstrual syndrome. However, Mortola et al treated PMS sufferers with placebo or with leuprolide acetate and either estrogen plus progestogen or estrogen alone or a progestogen alone.[73] Subjects in all of the active treatment groups reported a reduction of their symptoms.

Experience regarding the use of oral contraceptives to treat premenstrual symptoms is largely anecdotal. Backstrom et al studied women with either pure PMS or the premenstrual exacerbation of preexisting symptoms who were randomly placed on either a monophasic or triphasic oral contraceptive.[74] They demonstrated a lower incidence of tension, irritability and swelling if the monophasic oral contraceptive contained desogestrel but not when it contained levonorgestrel. In addition, the group of women taking the monophasic oral contraceptive containing desogestrel also experienced less tension, irritability and depression than those on a triphasic oral contraceptive containing levonorgestrel.

Other studies have been methodologically flawed and therefore provide little insight into the value of oral contraceptives to treat premenstrual mood changes. Clinical experience would suggest that while some women may note significant improvement in their premenstrual symptoms while on oral contraceptives, others will note no effect and a significant number will note an exacerbation of their depression, anxiety and physical symptoms. Continuous use of a monophasic pill should be effective, but has not been objectively evaluated.

The abolition of ovulation and menstruation with the long-acting progestogen, depomedroxyprogesterone acetate (DMPA), has been anectotally reported by clinicians to be helpful in treating premenstrual symptoms of both a physical and physiological nature. In an open clinical trial, DeLia et al found that 85% of their patients reported greater than 75% relief of their symptoms.[75] Minor side effects included unpredictable bleeding, headache, weight gain, decreased libido and others have reported reduced bone density. My own experience would suggest that this therapeutic option is potentially worthwhile and should be studied in a prospective fashion.

The ultimate method of eliminating ovulation is to perform bilateral ovariectomy. Bilateral ovariectomy has been performed in two studies in women with severe premenstrual symptoms that were unresponsive to conservative medical therapy and followed with low dose estrogen replacement therapy.[76,77] Each of the women noted lasting relief from their cyclic premenstrual symptoms. These investigators have suggested that this option is an effective final alternative for women with debilitating premenstrual syndrome who do not respond to conventional interventions.

By contrast, simple hysterectomy without removal of the ovaries was followed by significant improvement in ratings of premenstrual tension, irritability and depression, but late luteal phase symptoms remained significantly more severe than follicular phase symptoms.[78] It is clear that removal of the ovaries at the time of hysterectomy is necessary to eliminate premenstrual symptoms.

Antiprogesterone: RU-486

Since progestational agents will often trigger premenstrual symptoms in women undergoing hormone replacement therapy, progesterone receptor blockade might be expected to reduce the severity of symptoms. Chan et al performed a six month randomized, double-blind, placebo-controlled, cross-over study utilizing three months of low dose mifepristone (RU-486), a progesterone antagonist, or placebo, but found that luteal phase administration did not significantly reduce the physical or emotional symptoms of PMS.[79] Although the suppression of ovarian hormone secretion often eliminates premenstrual symptoms, a specific role for progesterone is still uncertain.

Psychotropic agents: antidepressants and anxiolytics

Anxiety is a common symptom of PMS and several recent double-blind randomized trials of the anxiolytic drug alprazolam have found it to be superior to placebo in the relief of a wide range of emotional and physical premenstual symptoms.[80,81] The therapeutic benefit of alprazolam for the physical symptoms such as headache and abdominal bloating and cramping is unexplained. It may, however, represent a 'domino effect' associated with the decreased emotional symptoms with a resulting decrease in sensitivity to physical symptoms. Minor side-effects have included wild daytime sedation. In a recent three group study, Freeman et al concluded that luteal phase alprazolam

(0.25 mg four times daily) was more effective than placebo or oral micronized progesterone (300 mg daily) for relief of premenstrual symptoms.[82]

Depression is a frequent and, for some women, the most significant symptom of PMS, but antidepressant therapy has never been popular among patients with PMS because of side-effects. Nevertheless, prospective, double-blinded studies of clomipramine and nortriptyline have shown that these agents were superior to placebo,[61] whereas lithium was of no benefit.[67] Limited evidence from small numbers of patients suggests that a luteal phase increase in dose of nortriptyline may be beneficial in women with only partial relief of premenstrual depression on standard doses.[83] Similar benefits may be seen with varying of lithium dosage.[84]

Increasing evidence points to a disturbance of serotonin metabolism underlying the mood changes of PMS and several recent randomized double-blind, placebo-controlled trials of selective serotonin reuptake inhibitors (SSRIs) have demonstrated a dramatic and maintained benefit in severe PMS sufferers.[85–89] The agent studied most widely has been fluoxetine in a dose of 20–60 mg daily. The women treated with fluoxetine have demonstrated complete or partial relief of a wide variety of symptoms, including affective lability, irritability, anxiety, depression, fatigue, difficulty concentrating, increased appetite, hypersomnia and physical symptoms, generally without significant side effects. At higher doses, a minority of women may experience loss of libido. Most of the subjects taking fluoxetine have elected to continue with this treatment after completion of the studies. Anecdotally, luteal phase fluoxetine may also be of benefit in some women.

Other SSRIs such as D-fenfluramine, sertraline and paroxetine may also provide substantial symptomatic benefit in the majority of PMS sufferers.[90–93] D-fenfluramine may offer particular benefits for premenstrual depression and for the premenstrual rise in intake of carbohydrates, fat and total calories.[90]

The anti-convulsant valproate has been demonstrated to improve the behavior and mood of individuals suffering from bipolar and schizo-affective disorders. Jacobsen investigated whether low doses of valproate may be useful in stabilizing mood in women with mild rapid cycling disorders and premenstrual syndrome.[94] Five of the 19 women reported complete elimination of the symptoms and eight women reported partial improvement while on valproate. In contrast, three of eight women with the chief complaint of premenstrual syndrome alone reported a good response, while five reported no response.

Nutritional supplements and dietary changes

Several double-blind controlled studies of vitamin B_6 (pyridoxine) have demonstrated that treatment with this vitamin is significantly more effective than placebo in the management of most PMS symptoms, especially depression,[95,96] whereas one has not.[97]

There was a slight but not statistically significant benefit from vitamin E treatment in a randomized double-blind placebo-controlled study by London et al.[98] A double-blind, placebo-controlled cross-over study by Thys-Jacobs et al also demonstrated some efficacy of 1000 mg of calcium a day for premenstrual symptoms,[99] however, nausea, constipation, flatulence and gastrointestinal discomfort were common in those receiving the calcium.

Several studies have been performed to evaluate the efficacy of evening primrose oil, a preparation which has been widely promoted to the general public. This substance contains gamma linoleic acid which is a critical precursor of prostaglandin E_1. The evidence from three double-blind studies suggest that evening primrose oil is no more effective than placebo for the treatment of premenstrual symptoms.[61]

Diuretics

The use of diuretics in the treatment of premenstrual syndrome has been studied extensively. These include ammonium chloride plus caffeine, chlorthalidone, metolazone and spironolactone. The results of these studies suggest that diuretics may be effective for the treatment of premenstrual 'bloating' or weight gain but not the emotional symptoms of the premenstrual syndrome.[61]

Other agents which may have some beneficial effects on PMS

Bromocriptine is a dopamine agonist that inhibits the secretion and release of prolactin, and may also stimulate the excretion of electrolytes and thereby cause diuresis. Six of the eight studies of bromocriptine were performed in a double-blind, cross-over fashion,[61] but the majority failed to show any benefit of bromocriptine over placebo except for the relief of breast tenderness.

Sayegh et al studied the benefits of a carbohydrate-rich beverage on premenstrual symptoms.[100] They hypothesized that the dietary intake of carbohydrates may increase tryptophan uptake and serotonin synthesis in the brain, which in turn may improve mood. Using a double-blind, cross-over design, they found that the carbohydrate intervention decreased self-reported depression, anger, confusion and carbohydrate cravings within 90–180 minutes.

There have been four studies which have evaluated the role of the melatonin inhibitors, propranolol and atenolol, or the controlled use of bright light because it tends to suppress melatonin secretion in the early evening. All three of these therapies may sometimes exhibit benefit for the treatment of depressive symptoms of PMS,[101] although there was no difference between the beneficial effects of the administration of light during the morning or the evening. Other studies have not been able to confirm these benefits.[102,103] While these studies demonstrate some promise for this approach to the treatment of premenstrual syndrome, additional studies which are free of methodologic deficiencies need to be performed.

Clonidine, which decreases norepinephrine release, was found to be effective in decreasing emotional symptoms in doses of 17 mg per kg per day, but methodologic deficiencies limit the strength of the conclusions.[104]

Toth et al postulated an infectious etiology for PMS and proposed that doxycycline would eliminate the infectious agent and decrease premenstrual symptoms.[105] Each of the women received either doxycycline 200 mg or a placebo for two months on a double-blind basis, and doxycycline was found to be significantly more effective than placebo in relieving premenstrual symptoms even up to six months after the treatment had ceased.

All four studies of the luteal phase administration of the prostaglandin inhibitor, mefenamic acid (750–2000 mg/day) have demonstrated that it is superior to placebo in the treatment of most premenstrual symptoms.

Chuong et al reported the results of a double-blind, placebo cross-over study of the narcotic antagonist, naltrexone.[106] While it was superior to placebo, significant side effects such as nausea, decreased appetite and dizziness occurred. No benefit was demonstrated with either L-thyroxine or placebo after two months of treatment in a double-blind placebo-controlled study by Nikolia et al.[107]

Psychosocial therapies

Many of the symptoms of premenstrual syndrome are emotional. Therefore, it is logical to believe that behavioral therapies may be effective in treating these symptoms, and various psychosocial treatments have been suggested (Table 33.4).

Table 33.4 Psychosocial treatments for premenstrual syndrome.

Insight therapy
Relaxation therapy
Anxiety/anger management
Biofeedback
Relaxation/motive therapy
Cognitive/behavior therapy
Stress management
Physical exercise
Self-hypnosis
Support groups
Marital and family therapy

Although studies of cognitive and behavior therapy, relaxation groups and support groups have demonstrated variable results, additional studies are needed.[61] The use of psychological therapies either alone or in combination with medication may be a valuable part of our armamentarium in the future.

A practical approach

Because of the conflicting results of many studies regarding the efficacy of various treatments for PMS, it is frustrating and often confusing for the clinician who must respond to his or her patient's requests for evaluation and treatment. As a result of the complex nature of this condition and the methodologic difficulties that still plague studies of premenstrual syndrome, there is no universal agreement with respect to the diagnosis, investigation or treatment of women with this disorder.

Therefore, reliance has to be placed on the extensive clinical experience of physicians and allied health workers who care for women with premenstrual syndrome, as well as the evidence from the best studies of treatments for the premenstrual syndrome. What follows is one approach to the evaluation of women with premenstrual syndrome and suggestions with respect to therapy.

Whether an individual presenting for the treatment of PMS voices it or not, she is often there for confirmation and validation of her self-made diagnosis of premenstrual syndrome. The more severe the symptoms the greater the need, for many of these women fear that they are 'going crazy'. As a result, the first step is to attempt to validate the woman's claim that she has premenstrual syndrome. This is best accomplished by the taking of a detailed history of her symptoms and their temporal relationship to the menstrual cycle. It should also include a discussion of the events that may have precipitated or exacerbated the premenstrual syndrome. To validate or confirm her diagnosis, the use of a prospective calendar or chart is necessary. In cases in which significant emotional symptoms exist and the pattern is not so obvious, the administration of psychometric tests in both the follicular and luteal phases of the cycle may be of additional help. The results of these tests are not only of help to the clinician but may also provide an insight for the patient.

While these data are being gathered, it is often necessary to begin therapy. The initial approach may be as simple as discussing lifestyle changes such as aerobic exercise for 20–30 minutes a day and modification of diet. While there have been many articles and books which have suggested specific dietary recommendations, objective evidence indicates that the effect of diet on premenstrual symptoms is not uniform and therefore each woman should decide for herself whether such nutritional substances such as salt, caffeine or sugar aggravate or improve her symptoms. It is through the process of self-discovery and the evaluation of the impact of these lifestyle changes that many women will actually begin to feel better, for this process gives many women a sense of control over their symptoms.

To determine the nature of the woman's symptoms further, a physical examination and appropriate laboratory and radiologic studies may sometimes be necessary to rule out other causes for her symptoms. There is no investigation or combination of investigations that must be ordered for each woman. Each individual symptom should be evaluated and laboratory and radiologic studies performed as necessary to rule in or rule out possible medical or psychiatric conditions which may occasionally mimic premenstrual syndrome. For example, thyroid studies to evaluate the possibility of hypothyroidism or hyperthyroidism may be of value. In patients with significant fatigue and joint pains or skin rashes, studies to evaluate the possibility of systemic lupus erythematosus may be useful. Finally, in women with premenstrual headaches a neurological evaluation and possible radiologic studies of the central nervous system may be of value to rule out the possibility of a central nervous system neoplasm.

The last and perhaps most important aspect of the evaluation of women with premenstrual syndrome is to begin to explore psychological and social factors. Many women find that their premenstrual symptoms are more severe during periods of significant stress or following some major emotional or physical event. A detailed history of the woman's lifestyle and social stresses may often shed light on factors that are influencing her symptoms. Such experiences as living with an abusive spouse, undergoing severe financial distress or past experiences of abuse may play a role in perpetuating or triggering PMS. A review of the impact of the premenstrual symptoms on the individual's self-esteem as well as her relationship with others is important.

Treatment has become easier in recent years because of the demonstration in well-designed prospective studies of the value of certain psychopharmacologic agents. For example, many women who complain primarily of emotional symptoms may benefit greatly from the administration of low doses of SSRIs. The administration of 20 mg of fluoxetine, 50 mg of sertraline or 20 mg of paroxetine continuously through the menstrual cycle is an effective therapy for most women. Fortunately, the stigma attached to the use of these medications is not as great in today's society and more women are willing to use psychotropic medications than ever before. For those women who may experience a greater degree of anxiety and tension, alprazolam 0.25 mg three times a day during the luteal phase is often effective. However, some women find that they don't like the side effects of these medications or they do not feel comfortable using them. In this situation the use of hormonal therapy may be of benefit. While the vast majority of studies of progesterone supplementation have failed to demonstrate benefit over placebo, a short trial of oral micronized progesterone, 200–400 mg a day in divided doses in the luteal phase may benefit some women with premenstrual symptoms. For those women who have premenstrual and perimenstrual symptoms such as severe dysmenorrhea or headaches, abolition of the menstrual cycle with the use of medroxyprogesterone acetate, 20–30 mg a day or depomedroxyprogesterone acetate 150 mg every three months, may be effective. Finally, for those women with severe premenstrual symptoms who do not tolerate the other medications, the use of a GnRH agonist followed by 'add-back' hormone replacement therapy may be indicated if cost is not a major issue. Other agents such as prostaglandin inhibitors as the oral contraceptive pill may sometimes have a role.

Conclusion

The process of treating premenstrual syndrome is often one of trial and error and during the course of therapy it may sometimes become obvious that the diagnosis is erroneous and that other conditions requiring different therapy are contributing. The exciting news is that the vast majority of women will find substantial benefit from some form of active therapy and for many women there will be no need to continue therapy for the long term. Medical therapy should usually be thought of as an adjunct to psychosocial therapies, which may have a significant long-term impact.

REFERENCES

1. Frank RT 1931 The hormonal causes of premenstrual syndrome. Archives of Neurology and Psychiatry 36: 1053–1057
2. Reid RL, Yen SSC 1981 Premenstrual syndrome. American Journal of Obstetrics and Gynecology 139: 85–91
3. American Psychiatric Association 1995 Diagnostic and statistical manual of mental disorders, 4th edn. American Psychiatric Association, Washington DC
4. Rivera-Tovor AD, Frank E 1990 Late luteal phase dysphoric disorder in young women. American Journal of Psychiatry 147: 1634–1636
5. Dalton K 1984 The premenstrual syndrome and progesterone therapy, 2nd edn. Chicago Year Book Medical Publishers,
6. Dennerstein L, Morse CA, Varnavides K 1987 Mood changes in the premenstrum and postpartum. In: Burrows GD, Petrucco OM, Llewelyn-Jones D (eds) Psychosomatic aspects of reproductive medicine and family planning, York Press, Abbotsford, Victoria, pp 73–77
7. Rojansky N, Halbreich U 1991 Prevalence and severity of premenstrual syndrome after tubal ligation. Journal of Reproductive Medicine 36: 551–555
8. Wilson CA, Turner CW, Keye Jr WR 1991 Firstborn adolescent daughters and mothers with and without premenstrual syndrome: a comparison. Journal of Adolescent Health 12: 130–137
9. Moos RH 1968 The development of a menstrual distress questionnaire. Psychosomatic Medicine 30: 853–865
10. Ekholm UB, Hammarback S, Backstrom T 1992 Premenstrual syndrome: changes in symptom pattern between two menstrual cycles. Journal of Psychosomatic Obstetrics and Gynecology 13: 107–119
11. Kuczmierczyk AR, Adams HE, Calhoun KS, Naor S, Giombetti R, Cattalani M, McCann P 1986 Pain responsivity in women with premenstrual syndrome across the menstrual cycle. Perceptual Motor Skills 63: 387–393
12. Posthuma BW, Bass MJ, Bull SB, Nisker JA 1987 Detecting changes in functional ability in women with premenstrual syndrome. American Journal of Obstetrics and Gynecology 156: 275–278
13. Unpublished data
14. Hurt SW, Schnurr PP, Severino SK 1992 Late luteal phase dysphoric disorder in 670 women evaluated for premenstrual complaints. American Journal of Psychiatry 149: 525–530
15. Gise LH, Lebovits AH, Paddison DL, Strain JJ 1990 Issues in the identification of premenstrual syndrome. Journal of Nervous and Mental Disorders 178: 228–234
16. Freeman EW, Rickels K, Sondheimer SJ 1992 Course of premenstrual syndrome symptom severity after treatment. American Journal of Psychiatry 149: 531–533
17. Johnson SR, Milburn A 1992 A longitudinal study of premenstrual symptoms in a nonclinical sample. Proceedings of the 20th Annual Meeting of the American Society of Psychosomatic Obstetrics and Gynecology, February 26, Seattle, WA. Abstract p 27
18. Keye WR, Keye DS, Shanteau RE, Trunnell EP 1993 A longitudinal study of women treated for premenstrual syndrome (PMS) by a multidisciplinary team. Proceedings of the 49th Annual Meeting of the American Fertility Society, October 11, Montreal, Abstract
19. Koeske RK, Koeske GK 1975 An attributional approach to moods and the menstrual cycle. Journal of Personal and Social Psychology 31: 473–478
20. AuBuchon PG, Calhoun KS 1985 Menstrual cycle symptomatology: the role of social expectancy and experimental demand characteristics. Psychosomatic Medicine 47: 35–45
21. Backstrom CT, Boyle H 1981 Persistence of symptoms of premenstrual tension in hysterectomized women. British Journal of Obstetrics and Gynecology 88: 530–536
22. Kyger K, Webb WW 1972 Progesterone levels and psychological state in normal women. American Journal of Obstetrics and Gynecology 113: 759–762
23. O'Brien PMS, Selby C, Symonds EM 1980 Progesterone, fluid and electrolytes in premenstrual syndrome. British Medical Journal 1: 1161–1163
24. Rubinow DR, Hoban C, Grover GN, Galloway DS, Roy-Byrne P, Anderson R, Merriam GR 1988 Changes in plasma hormones across the menstrual cycle in patients with menstrually related mood disorder and in control subjects. American Journal of Obstetrics and Gynecology 158: 5–11
25. Dennerstein L, Brown JB, Gotts G, Morse CA, Farley TMM, Pinol A 1993 Menstrual cycle hormone profiles of women with and without premenstrual syndrome. Journal of Psychosomatic Obstetrics and Gynecology 14: 259–268
26. Schmidt PJ, Nieman LK, Grover GN, Mulla KL, Merriam GR, Rubinow DR 1991 Lack of effect of induced menses on symptoms in women with premenstrual syndrome. New England Journal of Medicine 324: 1174–1179
27. Lewis LL, Greenblatt EM, Rittenhouse CA, Veldhuis JD, Jaffe RB 1995 Pulsatile release patterns of luteinizing hormone and progesterone in relation to symptom onset in women with premenstrual syndrome. Fertility and Sterility 64: 288–292
28. Facchinetti F, Genazzani AD, Martignoni E, Floroni L, Nappi G, Genazzani AR 1993 Neuroendocrine changes in luteal function in patients with premenstrual syndrome. Journal of Clinical Endocrinology and Metabolism 76: 1123–1127
29. Parry BL, Gerner RH, Wilkins JN 1991 CSF and neuroendocrine studies of premenstrual syndrome. Neuropsychopharmacology 5: 127–137
30. Brayshaw ND, Brayshaw DD 1987 Premenstrual syndrome and thyroid dysfunction. Integrative Psychiatry 5: 179–193

31. Roy-Bryne PP, Rubinow DR, Hoban MC, Grover GN, Blank D. TSH and prolactin responses to TRH in patients with premenstrual syndrome. American Journal of Psychiatry 144: 480–484
32. Casper RF, Patel-Christopher A, Powell AM 1989 Thyrotropin and prolactin responses to thyrotropin-releasing hormone in premenstrual syndrome. Journal of Clinical Endocrinology and Metabolism 68: 608–612
33. Nikolai TF, Mulligan GM, Gribble RK, Harkins PG, Meier PR, Roberts RC 1990 Thyroid function and treatment in premenstrual syndrome. Journal of Clinical Endocrinology and Metabolism 70: 1108–1113
34. Schmidt PJ, Grover GA, Roy-Byrne PP, Rubinow DR 1993 Thyroid function in women with premenstrual syndrome. Journal of Clinical Endocrinology and Metabolism 76: 671–674
35. Rabin DS, Schmidt PJ, Campbell G, Gold PW, Jensvold M, Rubinow DR, Chrouos GP 1990 Hypothalamic-pituitary adrenal function in patients with the premenstrual syndrome. Journal of Clinical Endocrinology and Metabolism 71: 1158–1162
36. Reid RL, Greenaway-Coates A, Hahn PM 1986 Oral glucose tolerance during the menstrual cycle in normal women and women with alleged premenstrual 'hypoglycemic' attacks: effects of naloxone. Journal of Clinical Endocrinology and Metabolism 62: 1167–1172
37. Spellacy WN, Ellingson AB, Keith G, Khan-Dawood FS, Tsibris JCM 1990 Plasma glucose and insulin levels during the menstrual cycles of normal women and premenstrual syndrome patients. Journal of Reproductive Medicine 35: 508–511
38. Parry BL, Berga SL, Kripke DF 1990 Altered waveform of plasma nocturnal melatonin secretion in premenstrual depression. Archives of General Psychiatry 47: 1139–1146
39. Thys-Jacobs S, Alvir MAJ 1995 Calcium regulating hormones across the menstrual cycle: evidence of a secondary hyperparathyroidism in women with PMS. Journal of Clinical Endocrinology and Metabolism 80: 2227–2232
40. Hussain SY, O'Brien PMS, DeSouza V, Okonofua F, Dandona P 1990 Reduced atrial natriuretic peptide concentrations in premenstrual syndrome. British Journal of Obstetrics and Gynecology 97: 397–401
41. Rapkin AJ, Edelmuth E, Chang LC, Reading AE, McGuire MT, Su T-P 1987 Whole-blood serotonin in premenstrual syndrome. Obstetrics and Gynecology 70: 533–537
42. Rojansky N, Halbreich U, Zander K 1991 Imipramine receptor binding and serotonin uptake in platelets of women with premenstrual changes. Gynecological and Obstetrical Investigation 31: 146–152
43. Steege JF, Stout AL, Night DL, Nemeroff CB 1992 Reduced platelet tritium-labeled imipramine binding sites in women with premenstrual syndrome. American Journal of Obstetrics and Gynecology 167: 168–172
44. Malmgren R, Collins A, Milsson CG 1987 Platelet serotonin uptake and effects of Vitamin B_6 treatment in premenstrual tension. Neuropsychobiology 18: 83–88
45. Chuong CJ, Hsi BP, Gibbons WE 1994 Periovulatory β-endorphin levels in premenstrual syndrome. Obstetrics and Gynecology 83: 755–760
46. Facchinetti F, Martignoni E, Petraglia F 1987 Premenstrual fall of plasma β-endorphin in patients with premenstrual syndrome. Fertility and Sterility 47: 570–573
47. Jakubowicz DL, Godard E, Dewhurst J 1984 The treatment of premenstrual tension with mefenamic acid: analysis of prostaglandin concentrations. British Journal of Obstetrics and Gynecology 91: 78–84
48. Piccoli A, Modena F, Calo L, Cantaro S, Avogadro A, Nardo G, Cerutti R 1993 Reduction in urinary prostaglandin excretion in the premenstrual syndrome. Journal of Reproductive Medicine 38: 941–944
49. Mira M, Steward PM, Abraham SF 1988 Vitamin and trace element status in premenstrual syndrome. American Journal of Clinical Nutrition 47: 636–641
50. Chuong CJ, Dawson EB, Smith ER 1990 Vitamin A levels in premenstrual syndrome. Fertility and Sterility 54: 643–647
51. Abraham GE 1983 Nutritional factors in the etiology of the premenstrual tension syndrome. Journal of Reproductive Medicine 28: 446–464
52. Chuong CJ, Dawson EB 1994 Zinc and copper levels in premenstrual syndrome. Fertility and Sterility 62: 313–320
53. Harrison WM, Sandberg D, Gorman JM 1989 Provocation of panic with carbon dioxide inhalation in patients with premenstrual dysphoria. Psychiatry Research 27: 183–192
54. Klein D 1993 False suffocation alarms, spontaneous panics and related conditions. Archives of General Psychiatry 50: 306–317
55. Schmidt PJ, Purdy RH, Moore PH, Paul SM, Rubinow DR 1994 Circulating levels of anxiolytic steroids in the luteal phase in women with premenstrual syndrome and in control subjects. Journal of Clinical Endocrinology and Metabolism 79: 1256–1260
56. Engel GI 1977 The need for a new medical model: a challenge for biomedicine. Science 19: 129–136
57. Magos AL, Collins WP, Studd JWW 1984 Management of premenstrual syndrome by subcutaneous implants of oestradiol. Journal of Psychosomatic Obstetrics and Gynecology 3: 93–99
58. Magos AL, Brincat M, Studd JWW 1986 Treatment of the premenstrual syndrome by subcutaneous oestradiol implants and cyclical oral norethisterone: placebo controlled study. British Medical Journal 292: 1629–1633
59. Watson NR, Savvas M, Studd JWW 1989 Treatment of severe premenstrual syndrome with oestradiol patches and cyclical oral norethisterone. Lancet 2: 730–732
60. Greene R, Dalton K 1953 The premenstrual syndrome. British Medical Journal 187: 1007–1014
61. Rivera-Tovar A, Rhodes R, Pearlstein TB, Frank E 1994 Treatment efficacy. In: Gold JH, Severino SK (eds) Premenstrual dysphorias: myths and realities. American Psychiatric Press, Washington DC, 99–148
62. Freeman E, Rickels K, Sonaheimer SJ, Polansky M 1990 Ineffectiveness of progesterone suppository treatment for premenstrual syndrome. Journal of the American Medical Association 264: 349–353
63. Corney RH, Stanton R, Newell R, Clare AW 1990 Comparison of progesterone, placebo and behavioral psychotherapy in the treatment of premenstrual syndrome. Journal of Psychosomatic Obstetrics and Gynecology 11: 211–220

64. Dennerstein L, Spencer-Gardner C, Gotts G, Brown JB, Smith MA, Burrows GD 1985 Progesterone and the premenstrual syndrome: a double-blind cross-over trial. British Medical Journal 290: 1617–1620
65. Baker ER, Best RG, Manfredi RL, Demers LM, Wolf GC 1995 Efficacy of progesterone vaginal suppositories in alleviations of nervous symptoms in patients with premenstrual syndrome. Journal of Assisted Reproduction and Genetics 12: 205–209
66. Gilmore DH, Hawthorne RJS, Hart OM 1985 Danazol for premenstrual syndrome: a preliminary report of a placebo-controlled double-blind study. Journal of Internal Medicine Research 13: 129–133
67. Sarno AP, Miller EJ, Lundblad EG 1987 Premenstrual syndrome: beneficial effects of periodic, low dose danazol. Obstetrics and Gynecology 70: 33–36
68. Halbreich U, Rojansky N, Patter S 1991 Elimination of ovulation and menstrual cyclicity (with danazol) improves dysphoric premenstrual syndromes. Fertility and Sterility 56: 1066–1069
69. Hammarback S, Backstrom T 1988 Induced anovulation as a treatment of premenstrual tension syndrome: a double-blind crossover study with GnRH-agonist versus placebo. Acta Obstetrica Gynecologica Scandinavica 67: 159–166
70. Bancroft J, Boyle H, Warner P, Fraser HM 1987 The use of a LHRH agonist, Buserelin, in the long term management of premenstrual syndromes. Clinical Endocrinology 27: 171–182
71. Brown CS, Ling FW, Andersen RN, Farmer RG, Arheardt KL 1994 Efficacy of depoleuprolide in premenstrual syndrome: effect of symptom severity and type in a controlled study. Obstetrics and Gynecology 84: 779–786
72. Muse KA 1989 Gonadotropin releasing hormone agonist suppressed premenstrual syndrome (PMS): PMS symptoms induction by estrogen, progestin or both. Proceedings of the 36th Annual Meeting of the Society for Gynecological Investigation, Abstract 75
73. Mortola JF, Girton L, Fischer U 1991 Successful treatment of severe premenstrual syndrome by combined use of gonadotropin-releasing hormone agonist and estrogen/progestin. Journal of Clinical Endocrinology and Metabolism 71: 252A–252F
74. Backstrom T, Hanson-Malmstrom Y, Lindke BA 1992 Oral contraceptives in premenstrual syndrome: a randomized comparison of triphasic and monophasic preparations. Contraception 46: 253–258
75. DeLia J, Keye WR, Worley RJ, Deneris A 1983 Preliminary report of the effects of depo-medroxyprogesterone acetate on premenstrual tension syndrome. Proceedings of the First International Symposium on Premenstrual Syndrome and Dysmenorrhea. Charleston, South Carolina, Abstract 14
76. Casson P, Hahn PM, VanVugt DA, Reid RL 1990 Lasting response to ovariectomy in severe intractable premenstrual syndrome. American Journal of Obstetrics and Gynecology 162: 99–105
77. Casper RF, Hearn HT 1990 The effect of hysterectomy and bilateral oophorectomy in women with severe premenstrual syndrome. American Journal of Obstetrics and Gynecology 162: 105–109
78. Backstrom CT, Boyle H, Baird HT 1981 Persistence of symptoms of premenstrual tension in hysterectomized women. British Journal of Obstetrics and Gynaecology 88: 530–536
79. Chan AF, Mortola JF, Wood SH, Yen SSC 1994 Persistence of premenstrual syndrome during low dose administration of the progesterone antagonist RU 486. Obstetrics and Gynecology 84: 1001–1005
80. Harrison WM, Endicott J, Rabkin JG 1987 Treatment of premenstrual dysphoria with alprazolam and placebo. Psychopharmacology Bulletin 23: 150–153
81. Smith J, Rinehart JS, Ruddock VE, Schiff I 1987 Treatment of premenstrual syndrome with alprazolam: results of a double-blind, placebo-controlled, randomized cross-over clinical trial. Obstetrics and Gynecology 70: 37–43
82. Freeman EW, Rickels K, Sondheimer SJ, Polansky M 1995 A double-blind trial of oral progesterone, alprazolam and placebo in treatment of severe premenstrual syndrome. Journal of the American Medical Association 274: 51–57
83. Jensvold MF, Reed K, Jarrett DB, Hamilton JA 1992 Menstrual cycle-related depressive symptoms treated with variable antidepressant dosage. Journal of Womens Health 1: 109–115
84. Conrad CD, Hamilton JA 1986 Recurrent premenstrual decline in serum lithium concentration: clinical correlated and treatment implications. Journal of the American Academy of Child Psychiatry 26: 852–857
85. Stone AB, Pearlstein TB, Brown WA 1991 Fluoxetine in the treatment of late luteal phase dysphoric disorder. Journal of Clinical Psychiatry 52: 290–293
86. Wood SH, Mortola JF, Chan Y-F, Moossazadeh F, Yen SSC 1992 Treatment of premenstrual syndrome with fluoxetine: a double-blind, placebo-controlled cross-over study. Obstetrics and Gynecology 80: 339–344
87. Menkes DB, Taghavi E, Mason PA, Spears GFS, Howard RC 1992 Fluoxetine treatment of severe premenstrual syndrome. British Medical Journal 305: 346–347
88. Pearlstein TB, Stone AB 1994 Long-term fluoxetine treatment of late luteal phase dysphoric disorder. Journal of Clinical Psychiatry 55: 332–335
89. Steiner M, Steinberg S, Stewart D, Carter D, Berger C, Reid R, Grover O, Streiner D 1995 Fluoxetine in the treatment of premenstrual dysphoria. New England Journal of Medicine 332: 1529–1534
90. Brzezinski AA, Wurtman JJ, Wurtman RJ, Gleason R, Greenfield J, Nader T 1990 D-flenfluamine suppresses the increased calorie and carbohydrate intakes and improves the mood of women with premenstrual depression. Obstetrics and Gynecology 76: 296–301
91. Frank E, Haskett RF, Yonkers KA, Halbreich U, Freeman EW, Grudy TA 1995 Efficacy of sertraline in premenstrual dysphoria. Presented at the 34th Annual Meeting of the American College of Neuropsychopharmacology, Puerto Rico
92. Yonkers KA, Gullian C, Williams A, Novak K, Rush AR 1996 Paroxetine as a treatment for premenstrual dysphoric disorder. Journal of Clinical Psychopharmacology 16: 3–8
93. Eriksson E, Hedber MA, Andersch B, Sundblad C 1996 The serotonin reuptake inhibitor paroxetine is superior to the noradrenaline reuptake inhibitor maprotiline in the treatment of premenstrual syndrome: a placebo-controlled trial. Neuropsychopharmacology 12: 169–176

94. Jacobsen FM 1993 Low dose valproate: a new treatment for cyclothymia, mild rapid cycling disorders and premenstrual syndrome. Journal of Clinical Psychiatry 54: 229–234
95. Abraham GE, Hargrove JT 1980 Effect of vitamin B_6 on premenstrual symptomatology in women with premenstrual tension syndromes: a double-blind crossover study. Infertility 3: 155–165
96. Doll H, Brown S, Thurston A, Vessey M 1989 Pyridoxine and the premenstrual syndrome: a randomized crossover trial. Journal of the Royal College of General Practitioners 39: 364–368
97. Berman MK, Taylor ML, Freeman E 1990 Vitamin B_6 in premenstrual syndrome. Journal of the American Dietetic Association 90: 859–861
98. London RS, Murphy C, Kitlowski KE 1987 Efficacy of alpha-tocopherol in the treatment of the premenstrual syndrome. Journal of Reproductive Medicine 32: 400–404
99. Thys-Jacobs S, Ceccarelli S, Bierman A 1989 Calcium supplementation in premenstrual syndrome: a randomized crossover trial. Journal of General Internal Medicine 4: 183–189
100. Sayegh R, Schiff I, Wurtman J, Spiers P, MacDermott J, Wurtman R 1995 The effect of a carbohydrate-rich beverage on mood, appetite and cognitive function in women with premenstrual syndrome. Obstetrics and Gynecology 86: 520–528
101. Parry BL, Berger SL, Mostofi N 1989 Morning versus evening bright light treatment of late luteal phase dysphoric disorder. American Journal of Psychiatry 146: 1215–1217
102. Rausch JL, Jarowsky DS, Golshan S 1988 Atenolol treatment of late luteal phase dysphoric disorder. Journal of Affective Disorders 15: 141–147
103. Parry BL, Rosenthal NE, James SP 1991 Atenolol in premenstrual syndrome: a test of the melatonin hypothesis. Psychiatry Research 37: 131–138
104. Giannini AJ, Sullivan B, Sarachene J 1988 Clonidine in the treatment of premenstrual syndrome: a subgroup study. Journal of Clinical Psychiatry 49: 62–63
105. Toth A, Lesser M, Naus G 1988 Effect of doxycycline on premenstrual syndrome: a double-blind randomized clinical trial. Journal of Internal Medicine Research 16: 270–279
106. Chuong C, Coulam C, Bergstrath E 1988 Clinical trial of natrexone in premenstrual syndrome. Obstetrics and Gynecology 72: 332–336
107. Nikolai TF, Mulligan GM, Gribble RK, Harkins PG, Meier DR, Roberts R 1990 Thyroid function and treatment in premenstrual syndrome. Journal of Clinical Endocrinology and Metabolism 70: 1108–1113

34. Polycystic ovary syndrome (PCOS)

Rogerio A. Lobo

Introduction

Polycystic ovary 'syndrome' (PCOS) or polycystic ovarian 'disease' is an endocrinopathy and is characterized by anovulation (menstrual irregularity) and hyperandrogenism. The finding of polycystic ovaries, typically by ultrasound, is extremely common, but may occur without the symptoms of the syndrome, and does occasionally occur in other disorders. In this setting the diagnosis of the syndrome (PCOS) should not be made, although the presence of this ovarian morphology is noteworthy and may be a risk factor for the development of symptoms and signs at a later time.[1]

The syndrome is characterized by anovulation; thus progesterone secretion is lacking and needs to be replaced by stimulating its production endogenously (ovulation induction) or by exogenous replacement. Estrogen secretion is normal and total estrogen status is often increased, as will be discussed below. This chapter will begin with a description of the syndrome (PCOS) and will be followed by various treatment options.

CLINICAL FEATURES OF PCOS

The classic clinical signs of PCOS are hyperandrogenism, frequently presenting with hirsutism and/or acne, and menstrual disturbances (oligomenorrhea or amenorrhea). Obesity is also an extremely common finding. However, the syndrome is extremely heterogenous, and in most women considered to have PCOS only one or two clinical signs may be present.

The most common clinical feature is that of menstrual irregularities, which generally appear at menarche or immediately thereafter. Although oligomenorrhea (with or without menorrhagia) and amenorrhea are the most common findings, polymenorrhea or even 'normal' menses may be present.[2,3] We recently reviewed data on 240 patients with PCOS (defined by the clinical findings of hyperandrogenism and anovulation) and found that 15% of these patients had regular menses but evidence of chronic anovulation.[4] Hirsutism is not synonymous with hyperandrogenism and a minority of PCOS patients (in the US about 30%) do not have hirsutism in spite of elevated androgen levels. Skin 5α-reductase activity largely determines the presence or absence of hirsutism[5] and 5α-reductase activity is also influenced by racial characteristics of patients; therefore, the prevalence of hirsutism (70%) reported in the US and Europe decreases to 10% or less when Oriental populations are studied.[6] Obesity *per se* may be present only in 40% of women with PCOS; however, when obesity is present, it accentuates the endocrine disturbance and increases the long-term consequences and cardiovascular risk of the syndrome. Although it has been suggested that obesity may play a major role in the pathogenesis of PCOS, the relatively low prevalence of obesity in PCOS (particularly outside of the US) argues against this hypothesis.

Other clinical signs of PCOS are less frequently encountered. Acne represents a manifestation of hyperandrogenism, and in the more unusual patient, acne may represent the only clinical sign of PCOS. Acanthosis nigricans, a skin alteration associated with hyperinsulinemia, is often observed but is not a marker of PCOS or of the severity of insulin abnormalities in the syndrome.

Morphologic alterations and the role of the ultrasound appearance of the ovaries in PCOS

Classically, polycystic ovaries are enlarged and have an increased number of follicles (2–10 mm diameter) arranged peripherally around an increased mass of stroma.[7] In the past, laparoscopy has been used to visualize this ovarian morphology, but ultrasound has been used increasingly and is now considered routine for evaluating ovarian morphology. The ultrasound appearance also has been shown to correlate well with ovarian histology. Transvaginal ultrasound is currently the preferred method;[8] however, the criteria of Adams et al[9] cited above for the ultrasonographic diagnosis of polycystic ovaries was based on transabdominal ultrasound scans. The ultrasound appearance is heterogenous,[10,11] and many patients with PCOS (defined on the basis of hyperandrogenism and anovulation) do not have the 'classic' PCO pattern. The most specific criterion is probably the increase in ovarian stroma, which is absent in the multifollicular ovaries that are often seen in other diseases and during adolescence.[8,12] However, consistent with the known heterogeneity of the ultrasonographic appearance, it is not always possible to demonstrate stromal hypertrophy in patients with PCOS, and in a recent study 26% of patients did not have an increase of ovarian stroma.[13] These data suggest that ultrasound, while being useful for evaluation of the ovaries when PCOS is suspected, should not be considered the gold standard for making the diagnosis of PCOS.

Polycystic ovaries may be found in many other endocrine disorders generally associated with some degree of hyperandrogenism (Cushing's syndrome, congenital forms of adrenal enzymatic deficiencies, some ovarian or adrenal tumors).[14] However, polycystic appearing ovaries also can be found occasionally in other disorders not associated with hyperandrogenism, including hypogonadotropic hypogonadism,[14] thyroid disorders and bulimia nervosa.[15] In all these subjects, the presence of this ovarian morphology is associated with exaggerated responses to gonadotropin stimulation.[16] This response is similar to that of women with PCOS. Thus, as stated earlier the finding on ultrasound of polycystic ovaries in women without relevant symptoms should not lead to an automatic diagnosis of PCOS.

We have been particularly interested in the finding of polycystic ovaries in normal women (Fig. 34.1), reported initially by Polson et al[7] and then confirmed by several other groups.[14,16–18] Although this has not been exhaustively studied, it may represent a very common finding occurring in 20–25% of the general population and first noted during childhood and early adolescence.[19] The significance and the possible clinical relevance of such a common finding is unclear. To date, some minor endocrine abnormalities have been reported in these apparently normal women. We recently evaluated 15 apparently normal women who had polycystic appearing ovaries (PAO), and although we did not find evidence of LH alterations, there were some minor androgenic abnormalities consistent with a recent published report.[20] We found low circulating levels of IGF-BP1 and a mild degree of insulin resistance in these nonobese women. Others have also observed a derangement in insulin secretion and metabolism in women with multifollicular ovaries.[21] Therefore, some degree of insulin resistance may actually contribute to the genesis of polycystic ovaries.

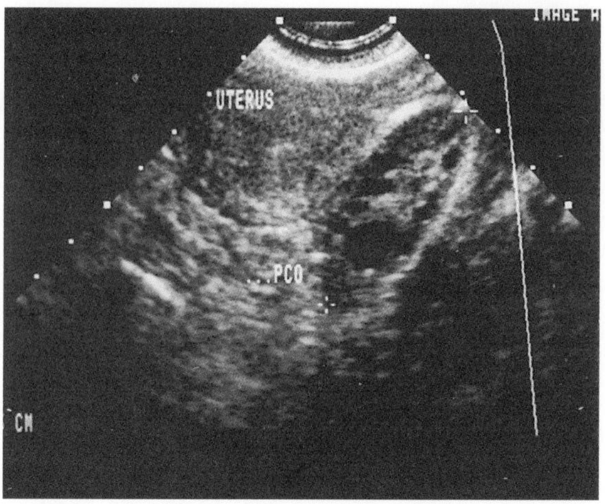

Fig. 34.1 Vaginal ultrasound on a woman without evidence of hyperandrogenism or anovulation.

Endocrine features of PCOS

For many years, the frequently observed increase of serum LH was considered to be a reliable biochemical marker of PCOS.[22] However, it is evident that gonadotropin secretion in PCOS is extremely heterogenous and lacks uniformity in individual patients studied at different times, as well as not being consistently elevated in many women.[22,23] Nevertheless, what may be more frequently encountered is the finding of increased pituitary sensitivity.[24]

An exaggerated response of serum LH, but not FSH, to gonadotropin-releasing hormone (GnRH) as compared with that occurring in various phases of the normal menstrual cycle (Fig. 34.2) has been well documented. Because serum FSH may be low and LH may not always be elevated, it has been suggested that the use of the LH:FSH ratio would be most discriminatory for a hormonal diagnosis.

In the past, we have used an LH:FSH ratio of over 3 to diagnose PCOS, provided the serum LH level is not below 8 mIU/mL. Others have used different ratios (1.5 or 2), but there is actually a general consensus that, although an altered ratio is common in PCOS, it

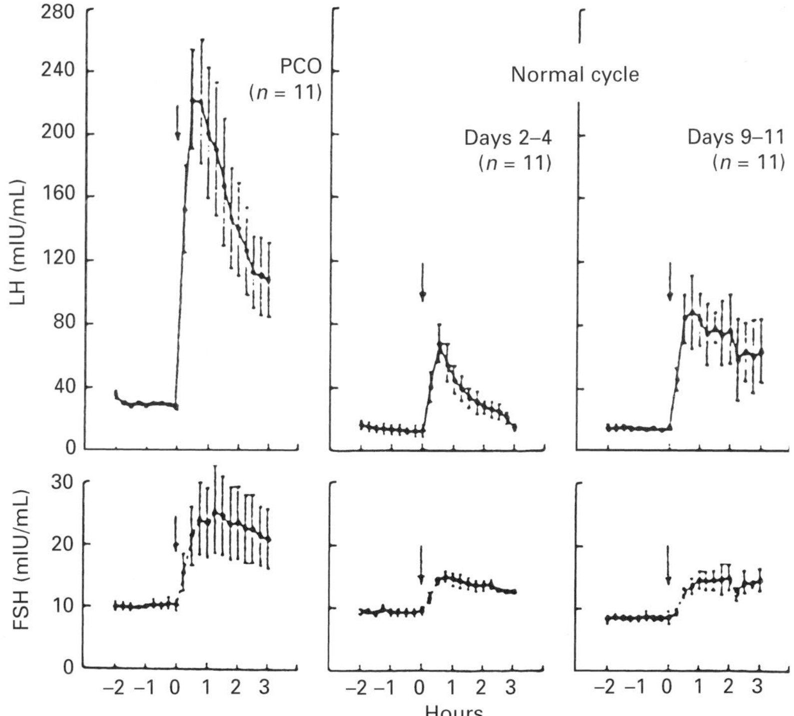

Fig. 34.2 Comparison of quantitative LH and FSH release in response to a single bolus of 150 μg of GnRH in PCOS patients and in normal women during low estrogen (early follicular) and high estrogen (late follicular) phases of their cycles. (Reproduced from Rebar R, Judd HL, Yen SSC et al 1976. Characterization of the inappropriate gonadotropin secretion in polycystic ovary syndrome. Journal of Clinical Investigation 57: 1320, by copyright permission of the American Society of Clinical Investigation.)

is not a criterion needed to make the diagnosis of PCOS. We have also assessed the measurement of bioactive LH in serum, using a sensitive *in vitro* assay and have compared this measurement with serum LH and the LH:FSH ratio[23] (Fig. 34.3). In this study, an elevation of serum immunoreactive LH and LH:FSH ratio was present in about 70% of PCOS patients. However, serum bioactive LH was elevated in all but one patient. Our observation would suggest that an abnormality of gonadotropin secretion, as assessed by circulating bioactive LH, is present in almost all PCOS patients and could be used to characterize PCOS. However, serum LH bioactivity cannot be evaluated routinely because of high costs and difficult methodology. The increased LH in PCOS results, at least in part, from a heightened pituitary sensitivity to GnRH stimulation probably secondary to hyperestrogenism.[25–27] In fact, PCOS should be viewed as a hyperestrogenic syndrome as well as a hyperandrogenic syndrome. Whereas serum total estradiol (E_2) is normal, levels of serum estrone and E_2 not bound to sex hormone-binding globulin (unbound E_2) are elevated.[25] We have observed statistical correlations between estrogens and both LH and the LH:FSH ratio in PCOS. Elevations of estrone also may be responsible for the disparity between LH and FSH levels in PCOS.[28]

The careful evaluation of LH levels has shown that the pulsatility of LH secretion is characterized not only by increased amplitude of LH pulse but also by an increased frequency of LH pulses.[29,30] This is different from what happens in late onset 21-hydroxylase deficiency, a syndrome that mimics PCOS and has similar increases in estrogens, serum LH and increased amplitude of LH pulses but without an increased frequency of LH pulses.[31] It is clear that factors other than estrogen alone explain the LH abnormalities in PCOS; the data in women with an adrenal enzymatic deficiency suggest further that other factors may be involved in PCOS.

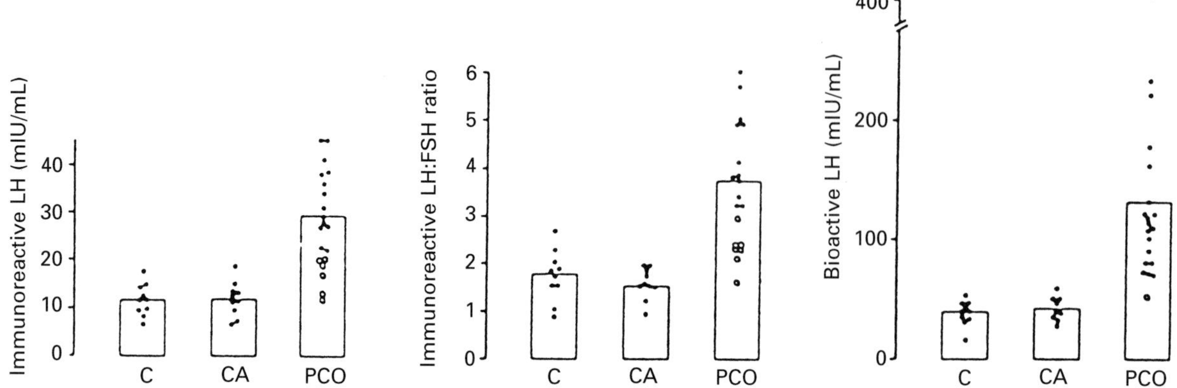

Fig. 34.3 Serum measurements of immunoreactive LH, immunoreactive LH:FSH ratios, and bioactive LH in control subjects (C), women with chronic anovulation (CA) and women with PCO. Solid circles for women with PCO indicate values exceeding 3 SD of mean control levels.[23] (Reproduced by permission from the American Society for Reproductive Medicine (formerly the American Fertility Society.)

An elevation of LH in patients is not needed to make the diagnosis of PCOS, but it may be an important factor in impairing fertility or causing pregnancy wastage. After ovulation induction in women with PCOS, the miscarriage rate is increased overall. A hypothesis has emerged regarding the adverse effects of LH[32] that suggests that LH levels as high as 10 mIU/mL in the early follicular phase can have a deleterious effect on the oocyte, the embryo and/or the endometrium and may result in an increased rate of miscarriage.

Finally, it must be noted that normalization of serum LH may occur spontaneously after induced ovulation and progesterone elevation.[33] Indeed, although chronic anovulation is a characteristic feature of PCOS, occasional ovulatory cycles may occur. These sporadic occurrences are unexpected and may lead to changes in the hormonal profile and confound the interpretation of the endocrine pattern in certain patients.

Ovarian hyperandrogenism

Ovarian hyperandrogenism is a cardinal feature of PCOS. Many investigators who do not use elevations in serum androgens as a criterion for the diagnosis of PCOS agree that hyperandrogenism is an important facet of the syndrome. In this disorder, the ovaries produce increased amounts of testosterone (T), androstenedione (A) and dehydroepiandrosterone (DHEA), but the elevation of serum T is the most frequently encountered finding. Because of the effect of androgens and insulin on SHBG, unbound or free testosterone is almost always elevated and is used by some as a diagnostic criterion. Also, obesity may contribute to the rise of serum T and unbound T because of increased peripheral conversion of A to T and lower levels of SHBG.

An important contribution to our understanding of the ovarian hyperandrogenism in PCOS has been the data obtained from the use of a GnRH agonist (Fig. 34.4). The agonist causes an exaggerated response of the Δ_4 steroidogenic pathway at the level of 17α-hydroxylase and involving 17,20 lyase. There are small changes of serum pregnenolone, progesterone and DHEA with stimulation, but significantly elevated responses of 17-hydroxyprogesterone (17OHP) and also of A, T, and estrone.[34,35]

Adrenal hyperandrogenism

In most patients with PCOS adrenal androgenism (AA excess) coexists with ovarian hyperandrogenism. This has been shown by a variety of means, including the findings of elevations in basal levels of specific AA markers dehydroxyepiandrosterone sulfate (DHEAS) and 11β-hydroxyandrostenedione (11A),[6,36] increased response to tests of adrenal secretion (ovine CRH, ACTH, metyrapone),[37] and augmented adrenal uptake of iodomethynor-cholesterol.[38] With all these methods, the prevalence of AA excess in PCOS is about 50–60% and appears to be similar in ethnically divergent populations.[6] Most patients who are deemed to have AA excess have increased levels of both DHEAS and

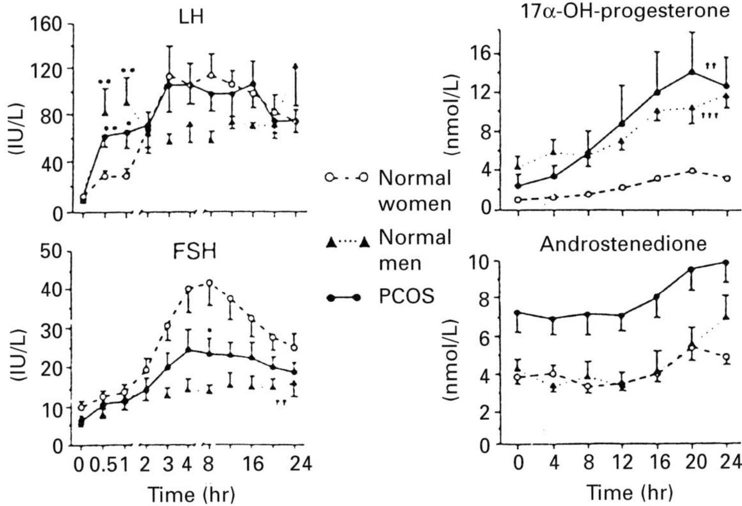

Fig. 34.4 Responses of LH, FSH, 17α-hydroxyprogesterone (17α-OH-progesterone) and androstenedione to the gonadotropin-releasing hormone agonist nafarelin in five women with PCO, nine normal women and five normal men (**P* <0.05; ***P* <0.01, ††*P* <0.01, †††*P* <0.001.)[34] (Reprinted with permission from The New England Journal of Medicine)

11A, but about one-third have increased serum levels of only one of these adrenal steroids.[6,36,39] This finding, which is probably due to the heterogeneity of the mechanisms influencing AA secretion in PCOS, suggests that the prevalence of AA excess is similar to that of other characteristic features of the syndrome, such as the increase in serum LH.

It has been suggested that, in a fashion similar to that in the ovary, AA excess could be due to selective activation of the Δ_4 androgenic pathway involving 17α-hydroxylase and 17,20 lyase.[35] A single gene encodes the production of cytochrome P_{450} 17α/17-20 desmolase in both ovary and adrenal. Alternatively, the enhanced activity may not be due to gene overexpression; other factors, including estrogen, opioids and insulin may be involved and determine a generalized increase of adrenal androgen secretion.[37,40,41,42]

Hyperandrogenism and insulin resistance

The association of hyperandrogenism and insulin resistance has been known for a long time,[43] but it was considered an uncommon occurrence and attention was concentrated on rare genetic syndromes of extreme insulin resistance and hyperandrogenism.[44,45] Only recently was it realized that mild hyperinsulinemia and insulin resistance are a common finding in PCOS[46,47] and that a derangement of insulin secretion may represent a main component of the pathogenesis and the clinical expression of the syndrome. Insulin resistance occurs not only in obese women with PCOS, where it might be expected because obesity is often associated with insulin resistance, but also in 50% of normal-weight women with PCOS.[6,47,48] In those patients, fasting serum insulin levels are higher when compared to controls of the same body weight. The overall prevalence of documented insulin resistance is approximately 70–75% in PCOS women patients[6] and appears to be independent of ethnic background (Fig. 34.5).

The molecular mechanism of insulin resistance in PCOS is not known, but appears to be different from that found in other syndromes of insulin resistance. Dunaif et al[49] have recently reported a novel abnormality of excessive insulin receptor phosphorylation in 50% of women with PCOS. It is suggested that perhaps another 30% may have a defect in postreceptor signal transduction between the receptor kinase and the glucose transporter system. Therefore, several alterations in different steps of insulin action may be the causes of hyperinsulinemia in patients with PCOS; the defects are probably heterogeneous.

In turn, excess circulating insulin influences the clinical presentation of PCOS in several major ways:

1. Directly increasing ovarian androgen secretion.
2. Reducing IGF-BP1 production and, as a

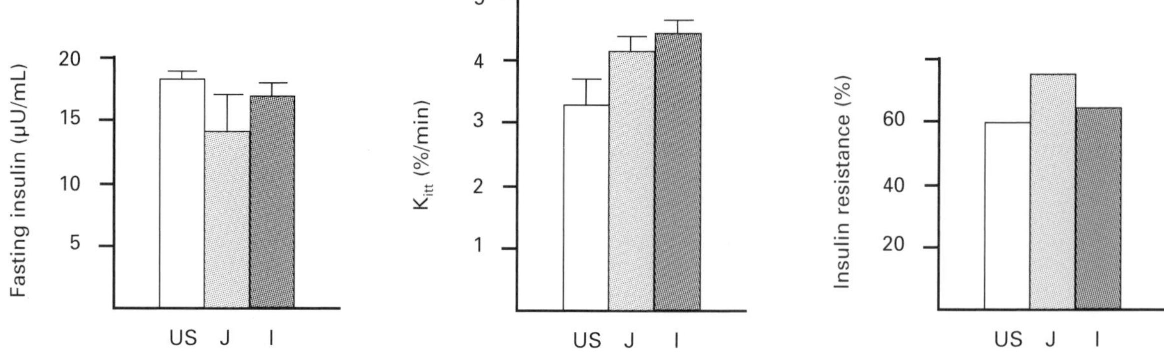

Fig. 34.5 Prevalence of insulin resistance of PCOS patients in different ethnic groups. (US = United States; J = Japan; I = Italy)[6] (Reproduced by permission from the American Journal of Obstetrics and Gynecology.)

consequence, increasing bioavailable IGF-1 activity

3. Elevation in insulin and bioavailable IGF-1 influencing gonadotropin-secretion, adrenal androgen secretion and also contributing to abnormalities in lipids and lipoproteins (Fig. 34.6).

It has been shown that insulin stimulates ovarian androgen secretion; and this effect perpetuates the chronicity of ovarian hyperandrogenism in PCOS. This effect is partially dependent on an increase of LH receptors but may also be linked to a direct effect of insulin on steroidogenesis. Because of peripheral insulin resistance, the effects of insulin on ovarian steroidogenesis have been ascribed to insulin binding to ovarian IGF-1 receptors. Although this is possible, it is improbable given the low affinity of insulin for IGF-1 receptors (100–1000-fold less than IGF-1). Insulin most likely binds to its own receptor,[50] which in the ovary is functioning normally. Insulin also decreases levels of IGF-BP1, thus acting on hepatic cells that function normally.[51,52] These and other data suggest that insulin resistance in PCOS is only partial and does not affect the action of insulin on the ovary and other tissues.

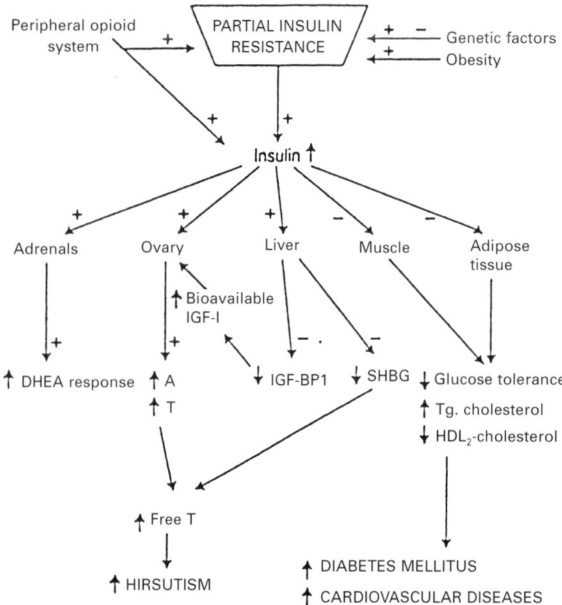

Fig. 34.6 Model of how insulin influences PCOS presentation.

Nevertheless, the importance of insulin resistance in PCOS is exemplified by trials using diazoxide, metformin and troglitazone.[53,54,55] With prolonged treatment, metformin reduces LH levels and it may mediate a decrease of T (–40%) and A (–30%).[53] Approaches such as the several trials now completed using metformin or troglitazone offer promise in terms of primary or adjunctive treatment for PCOS.

Other endocrine features of PCOS

A major endocrine feature of PCOS is hyperestrogenism which, as previously observed, may contribute to the characteristic gonadotropin abnormalities of the syndrome[25–28] (Fig. 34.7). The increase of serum unbound E_2[25] is the consequence of low SHBG levels, but the increase of serum estrone (E_1) has been viewed as secondary to peripheral conversion of increased adrenal and ovarian A. Recent studies with GnRH agonists have also suggested some direct secretion of E_1 from the ovary.[34,35]

A mild increase of serum PRL (mean PRL levels <50 ng/mL, where normal range is 5–20 ng/mL) may

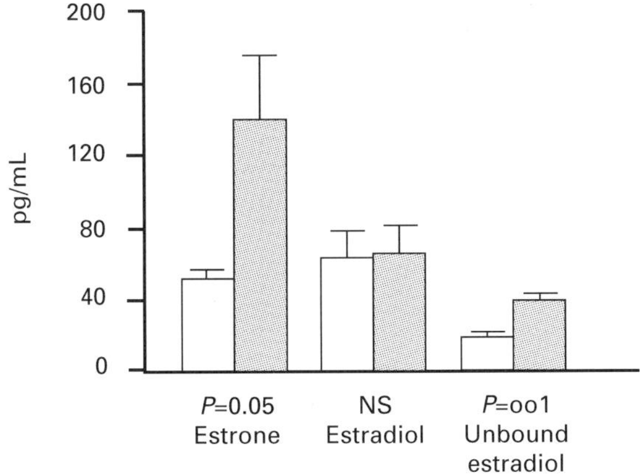

Fig. 34.7 Serum estrogen concentrations in 13 normal women and 22 PCO patients (shaded areas). (NS = not significant).[25] (Reproduced by permission from The Endocrine Society)

be found in some women with PCOS. Although it was suggested that the hyperprolactinemia of PCOS could be a sign of reduced inhibitory dopaminergic tone, most evidence indicates that it is a consequence of chronic hyperestrogenism. Because PRL may increase adrenal androgen (AA) secretion[56] and treatment with bromocriptine reduces serum DHEAS, we have previously suggested that hyperprolactinemia may contribute to the adrenal hyperandrogenism of PCOS. Our own data suggest that hyperprolactinemia in PCOS is relatively uncommon, and was found in only 12% of 94 of our patients with PCOS.

Another endocrine feature of PCOS which has been related to the AA excess is the presence in blood of elevated levels of β-endorphin (β-EP).[41] This increase in plasma β-EP does not appear to be pituitary in origin, in that corticotropin-releasing hormone (CRH) levels are not increased. The increase of β-endorphin secretion in PCOS has been also correlated with insulin resistance.[57] Increased endogenous opiates may have a role in inducing or in worsening the insulin resistance of PCOS. The data, however, remain unclear.

Some abnormalities of GH secretion in PCOS have been reported. It is improbable that such alterations are clinically relevant because IGF-1 and IGF-BP3 serum levels are normal. Indeed, many features of PCOS, such as obesity or hyperestrogenism, which are well known to result in mild abnormalities of GH secretion, may explain these reported findings.

Metabolic alterations and late complications

Recent evidence has suggested that women with PCOS have a significant risk for cardiovascular (CV) disease and myocardial infarction and that frank diabetes mellitus occurs with increased frequency by the fourth and fifth decade.[58,59] Several markers represent overlapping risk factors: obesity, hyperandrogenism, and lipid and lipoprotein abnormalities.[60] The hyperinsulinemia consequent to insulin resistance may also have direct effects on the CV system, inducing cardiac hypertrophy, hypertension and atherosclerosis.[61–63] It is possible that some of the serious effects are mediated by other mechanisms, occasioned by insulin resistance. A complete discussion of the metabolic and cardiovascular effects of insulin resistance is beyond the scope of this chapter (some aspects are addressed in ch. 61) but it is important to recognize and treat the metabolic features of PCOS. Thus, identifying women with PCOS and acknowledging their increase in CV risk will be important for developing a preventative health care strategy.

The most common lipid abnormalities are an increase of triglycerides and cholesterol and a decrease in HDL-cholesterol.[64,65] Although a decrease of total HDL-cholesterol has not been found in most studies, a reduction of the HDL2 cholesterol and apo-protein A1 notably is important in determining cardiovascular alterations, and is present in most patients (Fig. 34.8). The lipid and lipoprotein findings, nevertheless, are diverse and are influenced by diet, life style and ethnicity. Androgen *per se* plays less of a role here than insulin and diet.

As a result of all these risk factors, the relative risk for myocardial infarction is much increased in PCOS compared to normal women of the same age, and it has been calculated to be 4.2 between 40–49 years, and 11.0 between 50–61 years of age.[66]

Another possible late complication of PCOS is endometrial carcinoma, the prevalence of which is higher in women with PCOS.[58] We have been impressed by the common finding of hyperplastic endometrium in routine ultrasound scans in the absence of clinical symptomatology. Chronic, unopposed hyperestrogenism favors endometrial hyperplasia, together with other risk factors such as obesity and hyperinsulinemia, and it places all patients with PCOS at risk for endometrial carcinoma.

Pathophysiology

A detailed description of pathophysiology is beyond the scope of this review. No defining cause has been uncovered to explain the disorder, although a genetic component is important. In that PCOS exhibits such

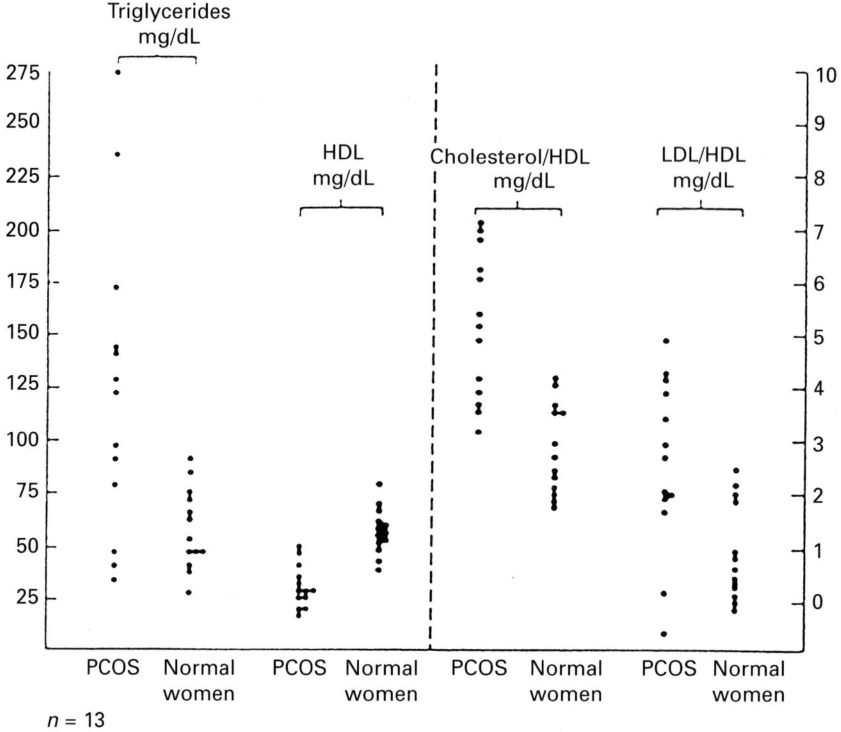

Fig. 34.8 Lipid and lipoprotein profiles in 13 women with polycystic ovary syndrome (PCOS) versus control group when matched for percent ideal body weight. Differences are evident in all measures ($P < 0.01$). (Reproduced by permission from Wild RA, Bartholomew MJ 1988 The influence of body weight on lipoprotein lipids in patients with polycystic ovary syndrome. American Journal of Obstetrics and Gynecology 58: 423)

marked heterogeneity, it is unlikely that any one cause explains the abnormality. Our view on this may be found in one of our more comprehensive reviews.[4,67] Among the various pathophysiological processes, an important variable is the high prevalence of insulin resistance. This is important in discussing options for treatment, which is otherwise only directed at ameliorating specific complaints.

TREATMENT

Patients with PCOS present with three major categories of symptoms: abnormal bleeding (DUB), signs of hyperandrogenism (skin manifestations, e.g. hirsutism) and infertility. Each of these requires a different treatment perspective. However, the first two abnormalities require suppression of the hypothalamic-pituitary axis and the third (anovulation), which is caused by abnormal endocrine feedback (and/or inherent ovarian dysfunction), is treated by induction of ovulation.

Apart from these specific entities, PCOS is a lifelong disorder which carries with it a significant metabolic and CV risk in terms of morbidity and mortality. Therefore strategies should be developed to normalize these abnormalities as much as possible.

The reduction of body weight should be considered in all protocols of PCOS treatment. In fact, it has been shown that a normalization of body weight reduces insulin resistance and permits an improvement of many clinical and endocrine parameters of the syndrome[68] (Fig. 34.9). Although it is often difficult to get a prolonged normalization of body weight, and many women with PCOS rapidly regain the lost weight, a dietetic treatment with coordinated exercise program has to be suggested to the patients to improve the lipid profile and to reduce insulin resistance and the possible glucose intolerance.

Recently some attempts have been made to intervene on what has been considered the main pathogenetic mechanism, insulin resistance. An analog of somatostatin, octreotide, which produces a

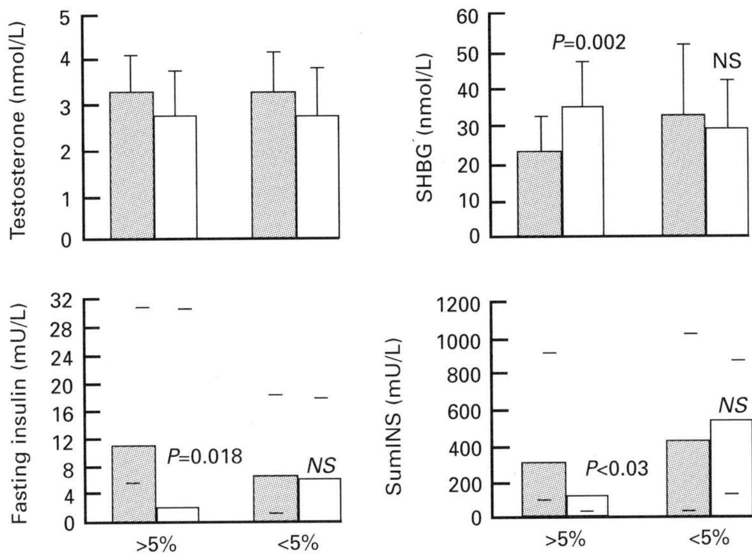

Fig. 34.9 Effect of weight loss on endocrine pattern of PCOS.[68] (Hatched bars: before treatment; Open bars: after weight loss. Comparing greater than 50% with less than 5% weight reduction. (Reproduced by permission from Clinical Endocrinology)

prolonged decrease of insulin secretion, has been used in PCOS; it has been shown to decrease LH and androgen secretion[69] and to improve the ovarian response to HMG.[70] An improvement of clinical and endocrine features of the syndrome also has been obtained by using metformin, an agent that increases the peripheral sensitivity to insulin as discussed earlier. Troglitazone is the latest product of this type to undergo successful clinical trials. However, all these therapies are still considered experimental and will require further evaluation.

DUB and anovulation should be aggressively evaluated (biopsy) and treated with progestogens. In anovulatory patients, hyperplasia may be present even without the history of abnormal bleeding.

Medroxyprogesterone acetate (MPA) or norethindrone (NET) 5–10 mg may be administered for 10–14 days each month to induce menses. This is the preferred approach if DUB has been a problem due to anovulation. However, if there has been no complaint of excessive bleeding, the regimen can be administered every other month. An alternative is to use oral contraceptives (COCs).

Oral contraceptives have some long-term therapeutic benefits. Apart from suppression of androgen secretion, the newer COCs tend to raise HDL-C, which is often low in PCOS. Insulin resistance on the other hand is not improved with COCs, but probably is not affected adversely either. In this setting the preference has been to administer the least androgenic COC, such as those containing desogestrel, norgestimate cyproterone acetate or gestodene. Because of recent concerns with a small risk of thrombosis, a second generation COC containing norethindrone or ethynodiol diacetate may be equally acceptable.

Skin manifestations of androgen excess (both ovarian and/or adrenal excess) in PCOS occur in conjunction with skin sensitivity to androgens. This is explained by enhanced 5α-reductase activity. Accordingly, successful regimens for hirsutism in particular may require the addition of an antiandrogen. While COCs (as above) may be used initially, an antiandrogen should be considered as well. COCs are able to decrease mild to moderate degrees of adrenal hyperandrogenism, as reflected by elevated levels of DHEA-S. Levels are decreased by about 30%.

For significant complaints of hirsutism and acne, antiandrogen therapy is often necessary. A COC containing an antiandrogenic progestogen (cyproterone acetate 2 mg) may be an effective regimen for acne. Alternatively, spironolactone 100–200 mg/day or flutamide 250 mg twice to three times/day have been found to be effective. Inhibition of 5α-reductase has also been found to be beneficial. Specific treatment would require an inhibition of both isoenzymes of 5α-reductase. However, only finasteride has been used in clinical trials and is a specific 5α-2 inhibitor. The magnitude of benefit with this agent is similar to that of spironolactone 100 mg/day.

Progestogen therapy, used alone, has been an option for patients with PCOS to suppress LH and the ovary. Here, doses as high as MPA 30 mg daily have been used for the treatment of hirsutism. Regimens such as this have been used with some success. However, this regimen is less desirable from the standpoint of efficacy as well as metabolic benefit. High doses of progestogens, used alone, lower HDL-C and enhance hyperinsulinemia.

Other agents for more severe cases of acne and hirsutism include high dose cyproterone acetate (50–100 mg) in a reverse sequential regimen (with ethinyl estradiol) or the use of a GnRH agonist for more complete ovarian suppression coupled with estrogen replacement or a COC to counteract the induced hypoestrogenism. A more detailed description of treatment options may be found elsewhere.[71]

Induction of ovulation is quite effectively carried out with clomiphene citrate, which is a mixture of the en- and z-isomers of clomiphene with an effect which is predominantly antiestrogenic. It is important that women with PCOS begin treatment after preconceptual counseling in order to enter pregnancy in as healthy a state as possible. A success rate with clomiphene in terms of pregnancy has been reported in up to 75% after six cycles. Up to 10% of women will not ovulate with doses as high as 150 mg/day, although a few more will ovulate with doses up to 250 mg/day. Defective luteal function is sometimes seen. Dexamethasone has sometimes been added to clomiphene to enhance efficacy if adrenal androgen levels are markedly elevated. In PCOS, resistance to clomiphene is thought to be at the level of the ovary.

Despite increased endogenous GnRH pulse frequency in many patients with PCOS, clomiphene further augments pulse amplitude. In addition, clomiphene may have other pituitary and perhaps ovarian effects as well.[72]

If clomiphene is ineffective, then low dose gonadotropin therapy is appropriate. Some enthusiasm has been mounted for use of pulsatile GnRH therapy here as well, particularly with prior pituitary down-regulation with a GnRH agonist. In our experience, however, low dose gonadotropin therapy is more effective than pulsatile GnRH therapy. It is important to emphasize that patients with PCOS as well as other women with polycystic ovaries may be extremely, but variably, sensitive to gonadotropins and although lower doses are used they require much closer monitoring (ultrasound and serum E_2). Whether urinary gonadotropins (LH and FSH), purified urinary FSH or recombinant FSH is used, a starting dose of 1 ampoule (75 U) per day is recommended with half ampoule increments after 5–7 days depending on response.

Wedge resection has been advocated by some authors for polycystic ovaries. Although the results are extremely poor for the symptom of hirsutism (16% overall), induction of ovulation, at least in the short term, may be achieved 60–70% of the time. These techniques have recently been popularized with laparoscopic and laser techniques[73–75] (Fig. 34.10). In clomiphene-resistant patients, ovulatory cycles have been reported in up to 90% so treated. The endocrine changes reported are similar to older data of wedge resections with decreased ovarian androgen secretion although LH pulse frequency may not be normalized. It is not clear whether the newer laparoscopic techniques may help to avoid or reduce ovarian-pelvic adhesion formation, one of the major problems encountered with the laparotomy wedge resections.[76,77] We now reserve laparoscopic resections only for the few patients who have large ovaries and who have failed most attempts to achieve ovulation with conventional medical therapy. This we feel to be a prudent view, particularly for those patients with hyperandrogenic chronic anovulation who may not have abnormal ovaries.

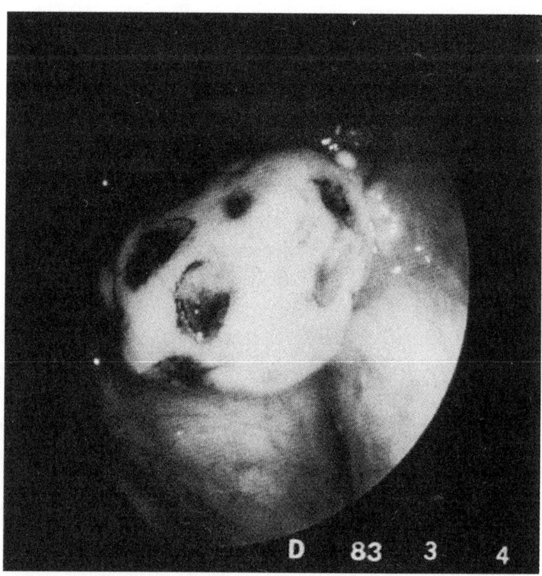

Fig. 34.10 The ovary after electrocautery for the treatment of PCO.[73] (Reproduced by permission from the American Society for Reproductive Medicine (formerly the American Fertility Society))

REFERENCES

1. Lobo RA 1995 A disorder without identity. 'HCA,' 'PCO,' 'PCOD,' 'PCOS,' 'SLS.' What are we to call it? Fertility and Sterility 63: 1158
2. Goldzieher JW, Axelrod LR 1963 Clinical and biochemical features of polycystic ovarian disease. Fertility and Sterility 14: 631–653
3. Balen AH, Conway GS, Kaltsas G et al 1995 Polycystic ovary syndrome: the spectrum of the disorder in 1741 patients. Human Reproduction 10: 2107–2111
4. Lobo RA, Carmina E 1997 Polycystic ovary syndrome. In: Lobo RA, Mishell DR, Paulson RJ, Shoupe D (eds) Mishell's textbook of infertility, contraception and reproductive endocrinology, 4th edn. Blackwell Scientific Publications, Malden, Massachusetts, pp 363–383
5. Lobo RA, Gobelsmann U, Horton R 1983 Evidence for the importance of peripheral tissue events in the development of hirsutism in polycystic ovary syndrome. Journal of Clinical Endocrinology and Metabolism 57: 393–397
6. Carmina E, Koyama T, Chang L et al 1992 Does ethnicity influence the prevalence of adrenal hyperandrogenism and insulin resistance in polycystic ovary syndrome? American Journal of Obstetrics and Gynecology 167: 1807–1812
7. Polson DW, Wadsworth J, Adams J, Franks S 1988 Polycystic ovaries: a common finding in normal women. Lancet 1: 870–872
8. Ardaens Y, Robert Y, Lemaire L, Fossati P, Dewailly D 1991 Polycystic ovarian disease: contribution of vaginal endosonography and reassessment of ultrasonic diagnosis. Fertility and Sterility 55: 1062–1068
9. Adams J, Polson DW, Franks S 1986 Prevalence of polycystic ovaries in women with anovulation and idiopathic hirsutism. British Medical Journal 293: 355–359
10. Hann LE, Hall DA, McArdle CR, Seibel M 1984 Polycystic ovarian disease: sonographic spectrum. Radiology 150: 531–534
11. Yeh HC, Futterweit W, Thornton JC 1987 Polycystic ovarian disease: US features in 104 patients. Radiology 163: 111–116
12. Adams J, Polson DW, Abulwadi N et al 1985 Multifollicular ovaries: clinical and endocrine features and response to gonadotropin releasing hormone. Lancet 2: 1375–1378
13. Roberts Y, Dubrulle F, Gaillandre L et al 1995 Ultrasound assessment of ovarian stroma hypertrophy in hyperandrogenism and ovulation disorders: visual analysis versus computerized quantification. Fertility and Sterility 64: 307–312
14. Abdel-Gadir A, Khatim MS, Mowafi RA et al 1992 Implications of ultrasonically diagnosed polycystic ovaries I. Correlation with basal hormone profiles. Human Reproduction 7: 453–457
15. Raphael FJ, Rodin DA, Peattie A et al 1995 Ovarian morphology and insulin sensitivity in women with bulimia nervosa. Clinical Endocrinology 43: 451–454
16. Clayton RN, Ogden V, Hodgkinson J et al 1992 How common are polycystic ovaries in normal women and what is their significance for the fertility of the population? Clinical Endocrinology 37: 127–134
17. Farquhar CM, Birdsall M, Manning P et al 1994 The prevalence of polycystic ovaries on ultrasound scanning in a population of randomly selected women. Australian and New Zealand Journal of Obstetrics and Gynaecology 34: 67–72
18. Wong LI, Morris RS, Legro R et al 1995 Isolated polycystic morphology in ovum donors predicts response to controlled hyperstimulation. Human Reproduction 10: 524–528
19. Bridges NA, Cooke A, Healy MJR et al 1993 Standards for ovarian volume in childhood and puberty. Fertility and Sterility 60: 456–460
20. Carmina E, Wong LI, Chang L et al 1997 Endocrine abnormalities in ovulatory women with polycystic ovaries on ultrasound. Human Reproduction 12: 905–909
21. Filicori M, Flamigni C, Cognini G et al 1994 Increased insulin secretion in patients with multifollicular and polycystic ovaries and its impact on ovulation induction. Fertility and Sterility 62: 279–285
22. Rebar R 1984 Gonadotropin secretion in polycystic ovary syndrome. Reproductive Endocrinology 2: 23
23. Lobo RA, Kletzky OA, Campeau JD, Di Zerega G 1983 Elevated bioactive luteinizing hormone in women with polycystic ovary syndrome. Fertility and Sterility 39: 674–678
24. Waldstreicher J, Santoro NF, Hall JE 1988 Hyperfunction of the hypothalamic pituitary axis in women with polycystic ovarian disease: indirect evidence for partial gonadotroph desensitization. Journal of Clinical Endocrinology and Metabolism 66: 165–172
25. Lobo RA, Granger L, Goebelsmann U 1981 Elevation in unbound serum estradiol as a possible mechanism for inappropriate gonadotropin secretion in women with PCO. Journal of Clinical Endocrinology and Metabolism 52: 156–158
26. Lobo RA, Shoupe D, Chang SP 1984 The control of bioactive luteinizing hormone secretion in women with polycystic ovary syndrome. American Journal of Obstetrics and Gynecology 148: 423
27. Lobo RA, Granger L, Goebelsmann U 1982 Effect of androgen excess on inappropriate gonadotropin secretion as found in the polycystic ovary syndrome. American Journal of Obstetrics and Gynecology 142: 394–401
28. Chang RJ, Mandel FP, Lu JK, Judd HL 1982 Enhanced disparity of gonadotropin secretion by estrone in women with polycystic ovarian disease. Journal of Clinical Endocrinology 50: 490–494
29. Rosen GF, Lobo RA 1987 Further evidence against dopamine efficiency as the cause of inappropriate gonadotropin secretion in patients with polycystic ovary syndrome. Journal of Clinical Endocrinology and Metabolism 65: 891–895
30. Hall JK, Taylor AE, Martin KA, Crowley WI 1992 Neuroendocrine investigation of polycystic ovary syndrome: new approaches in polycystic ovary syndrome. In: Dunaif A, Given JR, Haseltine FP, Merriam GR (eds) Blackwell Scientific, Oxford, pp 39–50
31. Levin JH, Carmina E, Lobo RA 1991 Is the inappropriate gonadotropin secretion of patients with polycystic ovary syndrome similar to that of patients with adult onset congenital adrenal hyperplasia? Fertility and Sterility 56: 635–640

32. Balen AH, Tan SL, Jacobs HS 1993 Hypersecretion of luteinizing hormone: a significant cause of infertility and miscarriage. British Journal of Obstetrics and Gynaecology 100: 1082–1089
33. Buckler HM, Phillips SE, Cameron IT et al 1988 Vaginal progesterone administration before progesterone induction with exogenous gonadotropin polycystic ovarian syndrome. Journal of Clinical Endocrinology and Metabolism 67: 300–306
34. Barnes RB, Rosenfield RL, Burnstein S, Ehrmann DA 1989 Pituitary-ovarian responses to nafarelin testing in the polycystic ovary syndrome. New England Journal of Medicine 320: 559–565
35. Ehrmann DA, Barnes RB, Rosenfield RL 1995 Polycystic ovary syndrome as a form of functional ovarian hyperandrogenism due to dysregulation of androgen secretion. Endocrine Reviews 16: 322–353
36. Carmina E, Stanczyk FZ, Chang L et al 1992 The ratio of androstenedione: 11β-hydroxyandrostenedione is an important marker of adrenal androgen excess in women. Fertility and Sterility 58: 148–152
37. Carmina E, Lobo RA 1990 Pituitary adrenal responses to ovine corticotropin releasing factor in polycystic ovary syndrome and in other hyperandrogenic patients. Gynecological Endocrinology 4: 225–232
38. Gross MD, Wortsman J, Shapiro B 1986 Scintigraphic evidence of adrenal cortical dysfunction in the polycystic ovary syndrome. Journal of Clinical Endocrinology and Metabolism 62: 197–201
39. Carmina E, Gonzalez F, Chang L, Lobo RA 1995 Reassessment of adrenal androgen secretion in women with polycystic ovary syndrome. Obstetrics and Gynecology 85: 971–976
40. Ditkoff EC, Fruzzetti F, Chang L et al 1995 The impact of estrogen on adrenal androgen sensitivity and secretion in polycystic ovary syndrome. Journal of Clinical Endocrinology and Metabolism 80: 603–607
41. Chang RJ, Nakamura RM, Judd HL, Kaplan SA 1983 Insulin resistance in nonobese patients with polycystic ovarian disease. Journal of Clinical Endocrinology and Metabolism 57: 356–359
42. Moghetti P, Castello R, Negri C et al 1996 Insulin infusion amplifies 17α-hydroxycorticosteroid intermediates response to adrenocorticotropin in hyperandrogenic women: apparent relative impairment of 17,20-lyase activity. Journal of Clinical Endocrinology and Metabolism 81: 881–886
43. Achard C, Thiers J 1921 Le virilisme pilaire et son association a l'insuffisance glycolytique (diabetes a femme de barbe) Bulletin of the National Medical Academy (Paris) 86: 51–53
44. Kahn CR, Flier JS, Bar RS et al 1976 The syndromes of insulin resistance and acanthosis nigricans. New England Journal of Medicine 204: 739–742
45. Barbieri RL, Ryan KJ 1983 Hyperandrogenism, insulin resistance and acanthosis nigricans: a common endocrinopathy with distinct pathophysiological features. American Journal of Obstetrics and Gynecology 147: 90–101
46. Shoupe D, Kumar DD, Lobo RA 1983 Insulin resistance in polycystic ovary syndrome. American Journal of Obstetrics and Gynecology 147: 588–592
47. Chang RJ, Nakamura RM, Judd HL, Kaplan SA 1983 Insulin resistance in nonobese patients with polycystic ovarian disease. Journal of Clinical Endocrinology and Metabolism 57: 356–359
48. Grulet H, Hecart AC, Delemer B et al 1993 Roles of luteinizing hormone and insulin resistance in lean and obese polycystic ovary syndrome. Clinical Endocrinology 38: 621–626
49. Dunaif A, Xia J, Book CB 1995 Excessive insulin receptor serine phosphorylation in cultured fibroblasts and in skeletal muscle: a potential mechanism for insulin resistance in the polycystic ovary syndrome. Journal of Clinical Investigation 96: 801–810
50. Willis D, Franks S 1995 Insulin action in human granulosa cells from normal and polycystic ovaries is mediated by the insulin receptor and not the type-insulin-like growth factor receptor. Journal of Clinical Endocrinology and Metabolism 80: 3788–3790
51. Carmina E, Stanczyk FZ, Morris RA et al 1995 Altered regulation of insulin-like-growth factor binding protein-1 in patients with polycystic ovary syndrome. Journal of the Society for Gynecological Investigation 2: 743–747
52. Geffner ME, Golde DW 1988 Selective insulin action on skin, ovary and heart in insulin-resistant states. Diabetes Care 11: 500–505
53. Wilcox JG, Najmabadi S, Gentzschein EK et al 1996 Metformin improves the hormonal profiles of patients with polycystic ovary syndrome. Journal of the Society for Gynecological Investigation 3(Suppl): 165A, Abs 21
54. Dunaif A, Scott D, Finegood D et al 1996 The insulin-sensitizing agent troglitazone improves metabolic and reproductive abnormalities in the polycystic ovary syndrome. Journal of Clinical Endocrinology and Metabolism 81: 3299–3306
55. Ehrmann DA, Schneider DJ, Sobel BE, Cavaghan MK et al 1997 Troglitazone improves defects in insulin action, insulin secretion, ovarian steroidogenesis and fibrinolysis in women with polycystic ovary syndrome. Journal of Clinical Endocrinology and Metabolism 82: 2108–2116
56. Lobo RA, Kletzky DA, Kaptein EM, Goebelsmann U 1980 Prolactin modulation of dehydroepiandrosterone sulfate secretion. American Journal of Obstetrics and Gynecology 138: 632–636
57. Hatch LE, Spahn MA, Wilcox JG et al 1995 Opiate regulation of insulin sensitivity and the IGF-1 axis in polycystic ovary syndrome (PCO). Journal of the Society for Gynecological Investigation 2(Suppl): 203, Abs 0133
58. Dahlgren E, Johansson S, Lindstedt G et al 1992 Women with polycystic ovary syndrome wedge resected in 1956–65. A long term follow-up focusing on natural history and circulating hormone. Fertility and Sterility 57: 505–513
59. Conway GS, Jacobs HS 1993 Clinical implications of hyperinsulinemia in women. Clinical Endocrinology 29: 623–632
60. Wild RA, Grubb B, Hartz A et al 1990 Clinical signs of androgen excess as risk factors for coronary artery disease. Fertility and Sterility 54: 255–259
61. Fontbonne A, Charles MA, Thibault N et al 1991 Hyperinsulinemia as a predictor of coronary heart disease in a healthy population. The Paris prospective study 15 years follow-up. Diabetologia 34: 356–361
62. Edelson GW, Sowers JR 1993 Insulin resistance in hypertension: a focused review. American Journal of Medical Science 306: 345–347

63. Stout RW 1994 The impact of insulin upon atherosclerosis. Hormone Metabolism Research 26: 125–128
64. Conway GS, Agawal R, Betteridge DJ, Jacobs HS 1992 Risk factors for coronary artery disease in lean and obese women with polycystic ovary syndrome. Clinical Endocrinology 32: 119–125
65. Legro RS, Blanche P, Krauss RM, Lobo RA 1993 Alterations in atherogenic lipoproteins among hyperandrogenic women: influence of insulin and genetic factors. 40th Annual Meeting of the Society for Gynecological Investigation, Toronto, Abstract P 355
66. Dahlgren E, Janson PO, Johansson S et al 1992 Polycystic ovary syndrome and risk for myocardial infarction. Acta Obstetrica Gynaecologica Scandinavica 71: 599–604
67. Lobo RA 1996 A unifying concept for polycystic ovary syndrome. In: Chang JR (ed) Serono symposia USA. Polycystic ovary syndrome. Springer-Verlag, New York, pp 334–352
68. Kiddy DS, Hamilton-Fairley D, Bush A et al 1992 Improvement in endocrine and ovarian function during dietary treatment of obese women with polycystic ovary syndrome. Clinical Endocrinology 36: 105–111
69. Morris R, Carmina E, Vijod MA et al 1995 Alterations in the sensitivity of serum IGF-1 and IGF-BP3 to octreotide in polycystic ovary syndrome. Fertility and Sterility 63: 742–746
70. Prelevic GM, Ginsburg J, Maletic D et al 1995 The effect of somatostatin analogue octreotide on ovulatory performance in women with polycystic ovaries. Human Reproduction 10: 28–32
71. Lobo RA, Carmina E 1997 Androgen excess. In: Lobo RA, Mishell DR, Paulson RJ, Shoupe D (eds) Mishell's textbook of infertility, contraception and reproductive endocrinology, 4th edn. Blackwell Scientific Publications, Malden, Massachusetts, pp 342–362
72. Adashi EY 1993 Clomiphene citrate: the case for a monoisomeric preparation. Baillières Clinical Obstetrics and Gynecology 7: 331–347
73. Gjonnaes H 1984 Polycystic ovarian syndrome treated by ovarian electrocautery through the laparoscope. Fertility and Sterility 41: 20–25
74. Kovacs G, Buckler H, Bangah M et al 1991 Treatment of anovulation due to polycystic ovarian syndrome by laparoscopic ovarian electrocautery. British Journal of Obstetrics and Gynaecology 98: 30–35
75. Naether OG, Fischer RM, Weise HC et al 1993 Laparoscopic electrocoagulation of the ovarian surface in infertile patients with polycystic ovarian syndrome. Fertility and Sterility 60: 88–94
76. Dabirashrafi H, Mohamad K, Behjatnja T, Moghadami-Tabrizi N 1991 Adhesion formation after ovarian electrocauterization on patients with polycystic ovary syndrome. Fertility and Sterility 55: 1200–1201
77. Greenblatt EM, Casper RF 1993 Adhesion formation after laparoscopic ovarian cautery for polycystic ovarian syndrome: lack of correlation ovarian cautery for polycystic ovarian syndrome: lack of correlation with pregnancy rate. Fertility and Sterility 60: 766–770

35. Dysfunctional uterine bleeding

Ian S. Fraser   Martha Hickey

Introduction

Disturbances of menstrual bleeding are a major social and medical problem for women, their families and the health services. Menstrual disorders are the second most common gynecological condition resulting in hospital referral,[1] and affect up to one third of women of childbearing age.[2,3] In the UK, for example, it has been estimated that menstrual disorders cost the Health Service £800 million per annum.[4] Women now represent a major sector of the paid workforce in the developed world, and any source of regular debility has important economic and personal consequences. These women are now exposed to a ten fold increase in the number of menstrual cycles in an average lifetime,[5] as the age of menarche is falling, birth spacing is commonly practiced and lactational amenorrhea is less customary. A large Swedish study[6] found that 88% of women worked full-time or part-time and that 10% had been absent from work at some time due to excessive menstrual bleeding. Heavy menstrual bleeding is also the commonest cause of iron deficiency anemia in the Western world[7] and a source of chronic ill health for women in developing countries.

The term 'dysfunctional uterine bleeding' (DUB) will be taken to mean 'excessively heavy, prolonged or frequent bleeding of uterine origin that is not due to pregnancy or to recognizable pelvic or systemic disease'.[8] This diagnosis is, therefore, one of exclusion and applies to 40–60% of cases of excessive menstrual bleeding.[9,10] Ovarian cycles associated with bleeding may be ovulatory or anovulatory, and the condition may be acute or chronic. In modern western society, dysfunctional bleeding is regular and ovulatory in approximately 80% of cases.[10]

Definitions of DUB vary. In the USA the term is associated with irregular bleeding, which is secondary to anovulation in the majority of cases.[11] Women from adolescent years to the perimenopause can be affected,[12,13] and anovulatory DUB occurs most commonly at the extremes of reproductive life.

MECHANISMS OF OVULATORY DYSFUNCTIONAL UTERINE BLEEDING

Excessive menstrual bleeding can occur as a secondary event to pelvic pathology, such as myomata, adenomyosis or polyps, or systemic disease, such as hypothyroidism or a coagulopathy.[14] Uncommonly, premenopausal endometrial carcinoma presents with regular excessive bleeding.[15] In 45–60% of cases, no pelvic or systemic abnormality is detected on clinical history or examination, and the descriptive term 'dysfunctional' bleeding is applied. On subsequent detailed pelvic inspection and pathological examination of the uterus, pathology not capable of explaining the bleeding pattern can be found in up to 40% of cases.[16] With modern techniques of high resolution transvaginal ultrasonography, hysteroscopy and laparoscopy these figures may be much less.[17,18]

Normal values for menstrual blood loss (MBL) have been determined[2,19] on white European populations. The distribution curve of normal blood loss is positively skewed, with a mean monthly MBL of 35 mL. An 80 mL blood loss represents the 90th centile. One fifth of women have a mean MBL of over 60 mL, but blood loss varies by up to 40% between cycles, especially in menorrhagia.[2] With a monthly blood loss of greater than 50–60 mL per cycle, most women consuming an average Western diet will be in negative iron balance.[20]

Estrogens and progesterone in ovulatory DUB

The mechanisms of excessive menstrual bleeding in ovulatory DUB are still largely unexplained, and no consistent abnormality of circulating pituitary ovarian steroid hormones has been observed.[21] Human ovarian steroid hormones are known to be vasoactive. The endometrial basal arterioles appear to be relatively unaffected by steroid hormones, but vessels in the functional layer show marked changes under the influence of steroid hormones.[22] Estrogen causes a fall in uterine vascular resistance, and an increase in uterine blood flow,[23] and this effect is lost with the addition of progesterone. In postmenopausal women receiving transdermal estradiol and sequential progestogens, estradiol reduces uterine arterial tone, and the addition of progestogens partially antagonizes this effect.[24]

The influence of ovarian steroid hormones on the endothelial cells is unlikely to be direct, because receptors to estrogen and progesterone have not been demonstrated on endothelial cells of vessels in the functional layer.[25] However, ovarian steroid hormones might act directly and indirectly to modulate vascular tone. Progesterone directly modulates calcium-controlled smooth muscle contraction in the uterine artery[26] and stimulates the degradation of endothelin, a potent vasoconstrictor.[27] Vasopressin, which acts to decrease endometrial blood flow, is stimulated by estradiol and inhibited by progesterone.[28]

Despite normal levels of circulating ovarian steroids, the action of estrogen and progesterone at an endometrial level could be altered in women with DUB. Levels of endometrial estrogen receptors (ER) and progesterone receptors (PR) are higher in the late secretory phase in women with DUB compared with women with normal menstrual loss.[29] This is particularly marked for ER, implying that an increased local estrogen effect could be present in premenstrual endometrium. In women with DUB there is an increase in endometrial flow corresponding with a raised estradiol secretion in the follicular phase, and a decrease in flow in the secretory phase. In women with anovulatory DUB, flow rates are variable, but tend to be high.[23]

The endometrial vasculature

The site of bleeding in excessive menstrual loss is not known. It might be imagined that regular menorrhagic bleeding represents increased loss from a normal bleeding location and that irregular and intermenstrual bleeding represents bleeding from 'abnormal' sites, but this has not been explored. Morphometric analysis of uterine spiral arteriole density has shown no correlation with MBL,[30] but myometrial venous density can be increased in DUB.[31] However, it can be functional rather than anatomical changes in the endometrial vasculature that are mainly responsible for excessive menstrual bleeding.

Endometrial vasoactive substances

Prostaglandins

Prostaglandins (PGs) are powerful local vasoactive substances in the control of menstrual blood loss. Prostaglandin production is regulated by circulating estrogen and progesterone concentrations; progesterone acts as an inhibitor of endometrial PG synthesis, and progesterone withdrawal will enhance PG production.[32]

Ovulatory DUB is associated with a shift in the ratio of endometrial vasoconstricting $PGF_{2\alpha}$ to vasodilatory PGE_2,[33] and an increase in total endometrial concentration of PG.[34] Increased PGI_2 comes from myometrial prostacyclin synthetase acting on endometrial endoperoxidases (PGG_2 and PGH_2), which are increased in ovulatory DUB.[33] In persistently proliferative endometrium seen in anovulatory DUB, the availability of arachidonic acid is reduced and prostaglandin production is impaired.[34] Endometrial tissues could be more responsive to the action of vasodilatory prostaglandins (PGE_2 and prostacyclin) via increased receptor concentrations in women with menorrhagia.[35] Successful treatment of ovulatory DUB with prostaglandin synthetase inhibitors (PGSIs) leads to a reduction in endometrial concentrations of $PGF_{2\alpha}$ and PGE_2,[36] and inhibits binding of PGE to its receptors.[37]

Endothelins

Adequate and timely vasoconstriction of the spiral arterioles is an essential component of menstrual hemostasis.[38] Endometrial endothelins are powerful vasoconstrictors, but they also stimulate the release of endothelial relaxing factors such as nitric oxide, atrial naturetic peptide and prostacyclin.[39] Depending on endothelin concentrations, other vasoconstrictor release can also be stimulated (e.g. $PGF_{2\alpha}$[40]). Receptors for endothelins are predominantly located at the endometrial–myometrial junction[41] and are present at increased concentrations just before menstruation. Deficient endothelin production can prolong or increase MBL and facilitate menorrhagia. Endothelin activity is influenced by ovarian steroids: estradiol increases endothelin receptors and sequential estradiol and progesterone will reduce receptor concentrations.[42] Endometrial endothelin can initiate the vasospasm which characteristically precedes normal menstruation.[43] However, vasospasm is still observed in endometrial explants where there is no endomyometrial junction.[43,44]

Nitric oxide (endothelium derived relaxing factor)

Nitric oxide is a highly potent vasodilator derived from the endothelium and other cell types and plays a major role in modulating vascular resistance.[45] Nitric oxide inhibits the action of platelets and is an important component of antithrombogenic actions of the endothelium.[46] The actions of nitric oxide are localized and short-lived. In the endometrium, nitric oxide can be produced from endothelial cells or from infiltrating cells such as macrophages, neutrophils and platelets.[47] Factors which modulate the synthesis and action of nitric oxide might also influence vascular hemostasis, so that an increase in endometrial nitric oxide could lead to an increase in menstrual bleeding. This might be an important mechanism in anovulatory DUB.

Abnormalities of tissue breakdown and remodeling

Abnormalities in the process of endometrial destruction and remodeling may contribute to changes in the quantity and quality of menstrual loss. Endometrial breakdown and repair are largely controlled by local factors.

Lysosomes

Lysosomes are intracellular membrane-bound vacuoles containing destructive hydrolytic enzymes, and are vital to tissue remodeling and regeneration.[48] Endometrial lysosomes show cyclical variation, with a marked rise in lysosomal enzyme activity in the late secretory phase and during early menstruation.[49] Progressive accumulation and release of hydrolytic enzymes in secretory endometrium may be a principle mechanism in cell separation, endometrial bleeding, remodeling and subsequent regeneration in normal menstruation.[49,50] Tissue hypoxia following spiral artery coiling and endometrial regression and vascular stasis stimulates lysosomal activation.[49] Lysosomal enzyme activity in the endometrium is increased in women with ovulatory dysfunctional uterine bleeding and with heavy menstrual bleeding secondary to the use of intra-uterine contraceptive devices (IUCDs).[51]

Matrix metalloproteinases

Matrix metalloproteinases (MMPs) are a highly regulated family of enzymes that together can degrade most components of the extracellular matrix. They are active in the normal and pathological processes involved in tissue remodeling. Endometrial MMPs are expressed cyclically,[52] consistent with regulation by ovarian steroid hormones and with specific roles in tissue remodeling. Menstruation is associated with a change in the balance between the expression of MMPs and their tissue inhibitors, leading to tissue degradation.[53] Little is known about the role of MMPs in excessive and irregular menstrual bleeding, but it is possible that excessive or prolonged tissue degradation due to MMP activity may result in increased MBL.

Macrophages and other migratory leukocytes

Macrophages are common in the endometrium, particularly in the endometrial stroma.[54] These leukocytes are known to be involved in phagocytosis, antigen processing and the release of cytokine mediators. During the normal menstrual cycle there is a premenstrual increase in endometrial stromal macrophages and other leukocytes.[54,55] Polymorphonuclear leukocytes only appear in normal uterine tissues at the onset of menstruation[54,55] and are located near blood vessels in the endometrium, where they can influence vascular permeability and integrity. Polymorphs also appear in focal endometrial necrosis associated with prolonged use of high-dose progestogens.[56] Polymorphs may contain a large number of lysosomes from which proteolytic enzymes can be released into endometrial tissue and cause cellular breakdown. Leukocytes can release a variety of other potentially vasoactive and tissue regulatory substances in various circumstances.

Macrophages and other migratory leukocytes may be implicated in the control of MBL and contribute to mechanisms of excessive loss. An excessive leukocyte infiltrate has been associated with use of the copper IUCD.[57] Macrophages can release platelet-activating factor and PGE, potent vasodilators that could augment MBL. They may also stimulate release of free oxygen radicals which can contribute to the local destruction of tissue. Endometrial granulated lymphocytes secrete perforins, which can degrade endometrial cellular and vascular structures and promote bleeding.

Mast cells degranulate premenstrually to secrete heparin, histamine and a number of other potentially vasoactive substances. Heparin stimulates endometrial fibrinolysis via the secretion of tissue plasminogen activator, and histamine causes endothelial cell contraction creating gaps between vascular endothelial cells. In DUB, endometrial secretion of heparin-like substances is increased.[58]

Intercellular adhesion molecules

The expression of adhesion molecules is crucial for the maintenance of tissue integrity. Cell to cell contacts are important in the normal physiology of growing and developing tissues. Adhesion molecules in the endometrium modulate the influx and aggregation of leukocytes into the endometrium from the circulation.[59] Intercellular adhesion molecule-1

(ICAM-1) and platelet-endothelial cell adhesion molecule (PECAM) are thought to control binding of leukocytes to endothelial cells and the maintenance of cell to cell contacts. Breakdown of intercellular bonds may contribute to dysfunctional bleeding. ICAM-1 expression is maximal in the endothelial cells of endometrial blood vessels at the menstrual stage, and can play an important role in the migration of leukocytes across the endothelial cell layer of blood vessels, thus facilitating menstruation.[60] PECAM is expressed throughout the cycle at cell to cell contacts between endothelial cells, and may contribute to the maintenance of the endothelial cell layer of endometrial blood vessels. Altered expression or action of adhesion molecules in the endometrium may therefore contribute to changes in menstrual bleeding patterns.

Endometrial repair and regeneration

For menstrual bleeding to stop, there must be repair of the epithelium and vascular endothelium, initiated from the remaining basal endometrial tissue. Local factors are likely to play a central role in this reparative process.

Cytokines

A cytokine is a specific type of cell product that affects the behaviour of other cells, usually in an autocrine or paracrine fashion. Cytokines such as interleukins, tumor necrosis factor and interferons can all be important in endometrial remodelling and repair. Cytokines are chemotaxic for leukocytes. The chemokine interleukin-8 can selectively induce neutrophil chemotaxis and can activate leukocytes in the endometrium.[61] Interleukin-8 is strategically located in the perivascular endometrium.[62] Production of interleukin-8 is inhibited by progesterone,[63] thus sex steroids may act indirectly to control leukocyte changes in the endometrium. In the regulation of MBL, cytokines may influence vasoconstriction, hemostatic plug formation and angiogenesis.

Epithelial regeneration

During menstruation the superficial endometrial layers are lost. Regeneration begins within 24 hours and is complete within 4–5 days of the onset of menstruation.[64,65] Growth factors in the endometrium may be crucial to the speed and efficacy of the reparative process. The secretion of potent growth factors such as vascular endothelial growth factor (VEGF), basic fibroblast growth factor (b-FGF) and epidermal growth factor is influenced by circulating ovarian steroid hormones.[66] In DUB, delayed or incomplete endometrial repair may prolong menstrual bleeding episodes. These growth factors are also potent stimulators of angiogenesis in the endometrium. Estrogen and progesterone act to stimulate the release of b-FGF and VEGF, and thus can control the rate of endometrial repair and regeneration.[67]

Endometrial hemostasis

Active fibrinolysis within the uterine cavity prevents organized clot formation and the development of intra-uterine adhesions. The defective hemostasis seen in normal menstruation may be exaggerated in ovulatory DUB. Vascular plugs are loose and solely located inside vessels, and reduced fibrin concentrations make them unstable.[68] Fibrinolysis will occur according to the balance of plasminogen activators, plasminogen inhibitors and plasmin. Excessive menstrual blood loss is associated with an increase in endometrial fibrinolysis in ovulatory DUB.[29] Estrogens stimulate and progesterone inhibits the release of tissue plasminogen activators, and progesterone also stimulates the release of fibrinolytic inhibitors.[69] An increased concentration of tissue plasminogen activator has been observed in women with ovulatory DUB and menorrhagia due to an IUCD.[70] Over-activation of the fibrinolytic system may unbalance the hemostatic system, causing early breakdown of thrombi in the endometrial vessels and excessive blood loss. Estrogen stimulates fibrinolysis and progesterone inhibits this process by creating a decidual reaction with an increased concentration of fibrinolytic inhibitors.[71]

It seems likely that there is a common mechanism underlying these numerous changes in endometrial vasoactive factors, leukocytes and blood flow in ovulatory DUB, such that these changes represent a cascade of events from a trigger. If a unifying mechanism exists, it is likely to be located prior to the chain of reactions following the late luteal decline in estradiol and progesterone. It is almost certainly a local endometrial mechanism, and may be expressed via estrogen and progesterone receptors. This abnormality appears not to affect endometrial histology nor glandular and stromal growth or morphology.

MECHANISMS OF ANOVULATORY DYSFUNCTIONAL UTERINE BLEEDING

Estrogens and progesterone in anovulatory DUB

In the normal menstrual cycle, progesterone withdrawal from an estrogen-primed endometrium leads to menstrual bleeding. Bleeding only happens if the endometrium is primed with estrogen[72] and it can be prevented by the continued administration of progesterone. Sudden withdrawal of estrogen may lead to bleeding, but bleeding will not usually occur if the withdrawal is gradual.[73] Excessive and irregular menstrual bleeding usually occurs from a proliferative or hyperplastic endometrium exposed to unopposed and excessive estradiol levels following an anovulatory cycle.

Changes in the length of the menstrual cycle generally imply disturbances of the hypothalamo-pituitary-ovarian axis. In anovulatory DUB with acyclic estrogen production there will be no progesterone withdrawal from estrogen-primed endometrium and hence cycles are irregular. Endometrial histology can demonstrate cystic glandular hyperplasia if estrogen stimulation is prolonged and excessive.[74] Endometrial blood flow can be increased in anovulatory DUB.[23] Bleeding may be light and intermittent or infrequent and heavy. Metropathia hemorrhagica is one end of the anovulatory DUB spectrum.

The mechanism of irregular bleeding in anovulatory cycles is unclear: prolonged estrogen stimulation may cause endometrial proliferation and eventual erratic breakdown. Estrogen might act via the stimulation of excessive endothelial production of nitric oxide in the endometrium. This is a pattern seen in polycystic ovary syndrome (PCOS) and in DUB at the extremes of reproductive life.

CLINICAL ASSESSMENT

Tolerance and perception of irregular and heavy menstrual bleeding

Menstrual bleeding that fails to occur at regular and predictable times or bleeding that is of markedly reduced or excessive quantity is poorly tolerated by most women.[75] Similarly, vaginal bleeding patterns are a major factor in dictating patient tolerance of exogenous hormone preparations. Irregular menstrual bleeding in the absence of exogenous hormones may occur with genital tract lesions, including trauma, tumors or infection, or as a complication of pregnancy. Rarely, systemic disease or concomitant medications may be the cause. The diagnosis of DUB can only be made after excluding these causes.

Many women will interpret prolonged or frequent bleeding as heavy, even when their total blood loss is not increased.[76] This can augment feelings of ill health associated with disrupted menstrual bleeding patterns. Of those with regular menstrual bleeding, approximately 50% presenting to the gynecology outpatient clinic with a convincing complaint of excessive bleeding will be shown to have a normal quantity of MBL.[77,78,79]

The clinical history

Abnormal vaginal bleeding is a common gynecological symptom, with an extensive list of potential causes.[14] The aims of the clinical history and examination are to exclude organic disease, and also to assess both the extent of disruption and the distress to the patient attributable to her bleeding complaint, as well as her expectations from treatment.

Objective assessment of MBL is really only warranted in research studies, but clinical diagnostic accuracy can be improved by careful questioning[9] (Table 35.1). With a history of regular bleeding, it is likely that cycles are ovulatory. Premenstrual symptoms and dysmenorrhea also suggest ovulation. Heavy, irregular and painless menstrual bleeding, particularly at the extremes of reproductive life, suggests dysfunctional ovulation (such as PCOS) or a perimenopausal state.

Evidence of systemic or pelvic pathology to explain the bleeding should be sought. Since many women complaining of heavy or irregular bleeding will eventually come to hysterectomy,[80] it is also pertinent to enquire about associated gynecological pathology (such as urinary incontinence or premenstrual symptoms), which could indicate the need for additional surgical procedures. The clinician should enquire about previous medical history, including conditions that may preclude treatment with nonsteroidal anti-inflammatory drugs, hormonal treatments or antifibrinolytics.

Finally, the clinician should establish the aspect(s) of the heavy or irregular bleeding that are most

Table 35.1 Direct questioning which may improve the precision of an assessment of menorrhagia.

Does the patient use 'super' pads or tampons?
Does she regularly need to use two pads, or a pad and tampon simultaneously?
How often does she need to change her sanitary protection during the heaviest days of bleeding? (Changing protection every half to two hourly implies menorrhagia).
Does she ever soak the bedclothes with blood, or deeply stain or soak her underclothes and overclothes.

troublesome for the patient and her expectations of treatment. Tolerance of bleeding patterns varies substantially between women. For some, the reassurance that there is no serious medical abnormality, specifically cancer, is adequate treatment. Others desire permanent amenorrhea and expect that hysterectomy is the only solution to their problems. It is important that these beliefs and preconceptions are discussed before therapy is commenced, as they will certainly influence compliance and satisfaction with treatment.

Patient examination

General physical examination should search for evidence of pelvic and systemic pathology that may account for the bleeding pattern. Bimanual pelvic examination should not be performed if the patient is an adolescent and has never been sexually active; information on possible pelvic causes can then usually be gained by other means.

A Pap smear should be taken if there has been irregular bleeding or according to local guidelines for routine repeats.

Investigations

An estimation of circulatory hemoglobin levels and red blood cell indices should be performed on all women complaining of menorrhagia. Ferritin estimation is indicated if there is hypochromic anemia. In irregular DUB, serum LH and FSH changes might indicate PCOS or a perimenopausal state. If there is irregular or acute bleeding, pregnancy should be excluded.

Special blood tests that are occasionally indicated include:

- Serum TSH and thyroid function tests if thyroid disease is suspected
- Serum biochemical analysis if renal or liver disease is suspected
- Antinuclear antibody, DNA binding and lupus inhibitor if SLE is suspected
- A coagulation screen, or special tests of platelet function if there is a history of easy bruising or excessive bleeding at minor surgery. This is particularly important for the adolescent with DUB where platelet abnormalities, von Willebrand's disease (factor VIII dysfunction), Christmas disease (factor IX deficiency) and, rarely, factor XIII deficiency may need to be excluded.

Transvaginal ultrasound scanning in the follicular phase, with or without the use of color Doppler, often gives valuable information about the endometrium, as well as imaging the myometrium (see ch. 30). Submucous fibroids can usually be detected using ultrasound, but polyps are less easily identified, unless saline is instilled in cases of endometrial echogenicity. There could be a role for transvaginal ultrasound in the diagnosis of moderate or severe adenomyosis,[84] although magnetic resonance imaging might be more accurate.

Using diagnostic hysteroscopy and endometrial biopsy, it is possible to estimate the size and characteristics of the uterine cavity, and to exclude intra-uterine pathology that may influence further management.[81] Endometrial carcinoma presents in only 1 in 1000 to 1 in 10 000 women below 40 years of age,[82] but endometrial histology may indicate other pathology such as endometritis which may influence treatment. Approximately 1% of perimenopausal women with apparent 'DUB' will have an endometrial adenocarcinoma, and 40% of endometrial malignancies in premenopausal women present with regular excessive menstrual bleeding.[15] Endometrial tissue can be obtained by blind sampling or, preferably, by endometrial biopsy following diagnostic hysteroscopy. Dilatation and blind curettage is not a sensitive or specific diagnostic tool and should not normally be performed without hysteroscopy.[83] Myometrial biopsy at hysteroscopy could also have a role in the diagnosis of adenomyosis,[84] but there is a high incidence of false negatives. The presence of adenomyosis has important management implications, and an attempt should be made to provisionally exclude this diagnosis if the history is suggestive (see ch. 38).

Since history alone will not discriminate well between those with excessive and those with normal MBL, the clinician can consider using the pictorial blood loss assessment chart (PBAC)[85] to clinically assess menstrual blood loss. This correlates well with the results of the 'gold standard' alkaline hematin[86] method of MBL measurement, without the tedious collection or analysis of pads and tampons. A problem with both of these methods is that they only assess the blood component of menstrual loss, which constitutes about 40–50% of total menstrual loss.[9] This could help to explain part of the poor correlation between perceived menstrual loss and MBL as objectively measured.

Following investigation, the patient should be reviewed and offered reassurance that there is no evidence of malignancy, and be given an opportunity to discuss the options for treatment. Even if measured or objectively assessed MBL is normal, the patient might still perceive that she has a problem that requires management. For those who still request treatment after reassurance, it is usually appropriate to begin with medical therapy.

TREATMENT OPTIONS

The wide range of treatment options for DUB reflects a lack of understanding of the underlying pathophysiology.

Acute DUB

Rarely, a woman might present with torrential vaginal bleeding requiring emergency hospital admission and parenteral hormonal or surgical management. In such a circumstance the possibility of complications of an undiagnosed pregnancy, myoma, adenomyosis or malignancy must be considered. A history of severe pain accompanying the bleeding may suggest necrosis or cervical extrusion of a submucous fibroid or polyp.

Bimanual pelvic examination may reveal a fibroid uterus or other pelvic mass, but is unlikely to provide precise information on the cause of the bleeding. With heavy bleeding it can be difficult to exclude a cervical lesion, and a Pap smear is unlikely to be accurately interpreted. If the cervix is not inspected for local lesions during an acute bleeding episode then this examination should be performed before discharge from the hospital.

Ultrasound may indicate myometrial pathology. Hysteroscopy and curettage are required to exclude intra-uterine pathology. Hysteroscopy may reveal a thickened, irregular proliferative or hyperplastic endometrium characteristic of prolonged unopposed estrogen stimulation. This tissue may sometimes show cellular and architectural atypia. Heavy bleeding can obscure the hysteroscopic view of the uterine cavity, even if dextran, saline or glycine distension media are used. Directed biopsy of any tissue with an abnormal appearance should be performed. Curettage often provides a temporary reduction in bleeding, but it is rarely a long-term treatment for DUB.[87,88]

In extreme circumstances, parenteral therapy with intravenous conjugated estrogens (25 mg) will usually arrest an acute bleeding episode.[89] GnRH agonists have also been used in these circumstances;[90] their efficacy may be due to an initial stimulation of endogenous estrogen. Estrogens probably act initially on local coagulation factors and then by promoting re-epithelialization of the endometrium. Parenteral therapy should be followed by 2–3 weeks of oral progestogens.

In less extreme cases, oral progestogens will usually slow or halt bleeding within 6–8 hours. A 2–3 week course of oral progestogen, such as norethindrone acetate (5 mg) or medroxyprogesterone acetate (10 mg), three to four times daily, will usually be effective.

Chronic DUB

Any known cause underlying or exacerbating the bleeding should be addressed. Further treatment may be considered in terms of medical and surgical methods. It is usual for patients to be initially managed with medical treatment, and for surgery to be reserved for those with failed medical management. Patterns of medical treatment for DUB have followed national and regional trends, and the absence of a definitive medical treatment reflects a lack of understanding of the underlying mechanisms of bleeding.

Of those women who present at a gynecology outpatient clinic complaining of menorrhagia in the UK, up to 60% will come to hysterectomy.[80] With the introduction of more effective medical treatment, and with the availability of conservative surgical treatment, there is now a move away from hysterectomy as the most common long-term management for chronic excess bleeding. Those women who complain of menorrhagia, but who are shown to have MBL within the normal range, may be reassured that their loss is normal, and that medical or surgical therapy is not essential.[91]

Medical treatments

Hormonal treatments

Hormonal therapy with progestogens or estrogen–progestogen combinations has been the mainstay of therapy of DUB for several decades, but little objective testing of their efficacy has been carried out until recently. They still have a major role, but a variety of alternative approaches with variable effects are also now available.

The combined oral contraceptive pill (COCP)

Modern low-dose pills can be safely prescribed to most premenopausal women,[92] provided that contraindications to these preparations (see chs 59–68) are excluded.

An objective reduction of about 50% in menstrual blood loss has been shown with medium and high dose monophasic COCP in both ovulatory and anovulatory DUB.[87] No large scale randomized and comparative trials have been carried out, but one small scale randomized study has shown some benefits in objective menstrual blood loss reduction with a modern low-dose monophasic pill compared with mefenamic acid.[93] However, 3 out of 12 subjects did not experience worthwhile objective improvement. Unfortunately, some women were unsuitable for this treatment and a further 20% do not respond well. It is not clear why some women continue to have heavy bleeding whilst taking the COCP. It is possible that women in published studies may have had undiagnosed intra-uterine pathology.

Some women may also reject the option of treatment with a drug that they know as a contraceptive, when they have already made a permanent decision about further pregnancies (such as tubal ligation), or when they see the COCP as inappropriate or unsafe for women of their age, despite reassurance.

Progestogens

Progestogens are molecules that bind to progestogen receptors and simulate some or all of the hormonal actions of progesterone.[94] Their actions on the estrogen-primed endometrium include the inhibition of proliferation, secretory transformation, decidualization of the stroma and, eventually, the suppression of endometrial growth to a state indistinguishable from atrophy.[95] On high-dose, long-term progestogens, follicular growth and ovulation are inhibited. In the treatment of DUB, progestogens can be given by a variety of routes,[19] and might be suitable for many women who are unable to take estrogen-containing compounds.

Oral progestogens

Although their efficacy is poorly established in the treatment of ovulatory and anovulatory DUB, oral progestogens are the most widely used medical treatment for DUB in the UK.[96] Many regimens of oral progestogens have been used. The drug dosage, as well as the duration of use, will influence the effect on the endometrium and the consequent pattern of bleeding[19] (Table 35.2).

In the adolescent with anovulatory DUB, cyclical oral progestogens may be required until spontaneous regular ovulation occurs. Some of the poor confidence in medical treatment for DUB may stem from the inappropriate use of oral progestogens. Luteal supplementation (days 16–25) by oral progestogens is of no objective benefit in ovulatory DUB[19] and can increase MBL,[96] but such luteal phase replacement works well in women with anovulatory bleeding.[97] Longer term regimens such as three weeks out of four (days 5–25) work reasonably well with ovulatory DUB.[97]

The disadvantages of oral progestogen regimens for DUB include the need for long-term oral medication and the possibility of unwanted premenstrual symptoms, including bloating, edema, headache, depression and reduced libido; androgenic effects (depending on the progestogen used), such as acne and hirsutism; irregular breakthrough bleeding, and a change in carbohydrate tolerance and lipid balance[9] (see chs 61 and 62).

Intramuscular progestogens

A contraceptive depot preparation of medroxyprogesterone actetate will induce amenorrhea in 50% of users by one year of use.[98] For those who can accept the 15–20% rate of irregular or prolonged BTB, this may provide a safe and effective treatment regimen.

Intra-uterine progestogens

Since the systemic effects of progestogens often reduce long-term acceptability, while it is the endometrial effects that actually reduce bleeding, it is logical to consider the direct intra-uterine administration of progestogen therapy. This results in high endometrial

Table 35.2 The endometrial effects and clinical applications of different oral progestogen regimens.

Days of menstrual cycle	Endometrial effect	Clinical application
16–25	Secretory transformation	Anovulatory DUB
5–25	Inhibits growth	Ovulatory DUB
Continuous	Endometrial suppression	Ovulatory and anovulatory DUB*
Combined with estrogen	Endometrial suppression	Ovulatory and anovulatory DUB*

*Breakthrough bleeding may occur

concentrations of progestogen, but limited systemic absorption. An intra-uterine implant system (IUS) releasing 20 μg of levonorgestrel/day (LNG-IUS 20) has demonstrated an 86% reduction in MBL at three months and a 97% reduction at 12 months in women with ovulatory DUB,[99] an improvement that continues over a five year period. MBL will be dramatically reduced in both anovulatory and ovulatory DUB. The system also acts as a highly effective and reversible contraceptive.

The endometrial effect of this intra-uterine levonorgestrel seems to be one of profound suppression.[100] Irregular bleeding and spotting, particularly in the early months, are the main source of patient disatisfaction with the IUS.[101] The mechanism of this bleeding is not clearly understood. There is some evidence that supplemental estrogen may regulate bleeding patterns with progestogen-only contraceptives, at least for the duration of estrogen use.[76,102] However, the addition of estrogens may limit the application of these progestogen-only therapies. Estrogens may regulate bleeding by stimulating angiogenesis in endothelial cells[103] and may promote the repair of progestogen-induced defects in the overlying epithelium.

Long-term progestogen use

Women treated with long-term progestogen therapy should be reviewed at regular intervals (at three months initially and then at 6–12 monthly intervals) for consideration of efficacy and side-effects, with the usual examination of blood pressure, breasts, abdomen and pelvis. Some alteration and adjustment of dosage is often required. Cervical smears should be taken at the recommended screening intervals. Progestogens may be used safely for the long-term treatment of DUB, but attention should be paid to regimens and possible long-term metabolic effects.

Danazol and gestrinone

Danazol in an isoxazol derivative of 17α-ethinyl testosterone. Its effects on the reproductive system are numerous: it alters the pulsatile secretion of GnRH, it inhibits the LH and FSH surge and it causes abnormal follicular maturation and thus reduces estrogen production. Direct endometrial effects include atrophy through suppression of estrogen and progesterone receptors, rendering the endometrium functionally hypoestrogenic and hypoprogestogenic.[104]

The effects of danazol in DUB are dose-dependent. On 800 mg/day the majority of women will be amenorrheic, regardless of their previous ovulatory status.[105,106] This dosage can be associated with a significant level of unwanted effects in some women, sufficient to reduce compliance in many. On 200 mg/day there is a highly significant decrease in MBL over a three month period, and side-effects are considerably less.[105,107] Direct comparison with oral norethindrone, the combined OCP and two prostaglandin inhibitors in ovulatory DUB[36,93,107] has shown danazol to be the most effective in reducing objective MBL in the medium-term, and it will also reduce or eliminate dysmenorrhea.

Danazol is unusual amongst medical therapies for menorrhagia in that there is a persistent suppression of MBL for 2–3 cycles after treatment is discontinued. Blood loss then returns to pretreatment levels.[105,106] Danazol is rarely used for more than six months continuously because of its androgenic effect on serum lipids, with a relative depression of high density lipoprotein levels and an elevation of low density lipoproteins.[108] An increase in platelet numbers, but no change in platelet function, has been observed with prolonged use.[109] In practice, danazol can be considered as limited duration therapy for severe menorrhagia for women who require 'thinking time' before scheduling more definitive long-term therapy.

Gestrinone has been used with similar effect to danazol in the management of menorrhagia.[110] It has some of the unwanted effects of danazol, but has the advantage of a twice weekly treatment regimen.

GnRH agonists

Continuous use of GnRH agonists down-regulates pituitary receptors after an initial stimulatory effect, and produces hypogonadotropic hypogonadism.[111] Depot preparations are the most effective in suppressing ovarian function and menstruation, and most women with DUB will become amenorrheic within two to three months of treatment.[90] Menses will return to their pretreatment volume 7–10 weeks after the last depot injection.

Treatment duration must be limited because of bone demineralization associated with prolonged ovarian suppression. This effect is not completely reversible on cessation of use in all women.[112] An add-back regimen of low-dose estrogen and progestogen produces a substantial reduction in MBL.[113] When used alone, the main application of GnRH agonists is likely to be as a short-term measure before a definitive surgical procedure, such as endometrial ablation. The high cost is likely to limit long-term use with add-back therapy.

Nonhormonal drug therapies

Prostaglandin synthetase inhibitors

In women with DUB, mefenamic acid,[97,105,114–117,119,120] meclofenamic acid,[121] ibuprofen,[118] and naproxen[97,119] have been shown to be effective in reducing MBL. Mean reductions in MBL have varied between 20–40%. A reduction in MBL with mefenamic acid has been observed with ovulatory and anovulatory DUB.[116]

The mode of action of PGSIs in reducing MBL is not fully understood. Mefenamic and meclofenamic acids have been shown to inhibit the binding of vasodilatory PGE to its receptor in the myometrium,[37] as well as inhibiting prostaglandin synthesis. Increased platelet aggregation and degranulation and additional vasoconstriction in the endometrium follows treatment with mefenamic acid.[120] The degree of MBL reduction may be greater in women with the highest original blood loss.[115,116] Mefenamic acid given at doses of 500 mg tds during menstruation can reduce the number of bleeding days.[116]

PGSIs reduce the dysmenorrhea that may accompany ovulatory DUB,[107,116] and may relieve menstrually-related headaches and diarrhea.[116] This can help to increase treatment acceptability, but it is vital that the need for regular and routine use every cycle is explained to the patient, otherwise many women will take the medication on a haphazard rather than regular basis. A further advantage in terms of compliance and cost is that PGSIs need only be taken during days 1–5 of menstruation, rather than through the whole month. There might be an occasional problem with long-term patient acceptance of this treatment, especially in women who experience side-effects such as nausea, vomiting, abdominal discomfort, diarrhea, headaches, dizziness or edema.[107]

Antifibrinolytic agents

Tranexamic acid is an omega-aminocarboxylic, antifibrinolytic drug that inhibits the transformation of plasminogen to plasmin. Menstrual fibrinolytic activity is reduced in women taking tranexamic acid[122,123] and MBL is significantly reduced in DUB,[87,96,124,125] with an average reduction in MBL of 45–60%. In a comparison with mefenamic acid, tranexamic acid and ethamsylate for objectively measured menorrhagia,[122] the greatest reduction in MBL occurred with tranexamic acid (58%), compared to mefenamic acid (25%) and ethamsylate (no change).

Rare case reports of thrombosis associated with the use of tranexamic acid may account for the reluctance of some gynecologists to use this drug. These have included one case of cerebral thrombosis and death.[126] Vast clinical experience in Scandinavian women and large trials in men, however, have disputed a causal association with tranexamic acid.[127] Tranexamic acid does not constitute a significant risk factor for thrombosis for women with DUB who do not have other risk factors.

Patient acceptability of tranexamic acid is high, despite the awkward 4–6 g/day dosage and the (infrequent) unwanted effects of nausea, dizziness, tinnitus, rashes and abdominal cramps.[128] The possibility of vaginal administration of tranexamic acid has been explored.[129] With appropriate modifications of prodrugs this could allow improved systemic and local absorption with a reduction in unwanted effects.

Summary of medical treatments

A medical approach should be considered first line treatment in the management of most cases of DUB. In irregular bleeding secondary to anovulatory cycles, cyclical two-weekly courses of progestogens can regulate bleeding patterns. Oral progestogens have not proven useful therapy in ovulatory DUB when given as a luteal phase supplement, and progestogens must be given for at least 21 days per month or via the intra-uterine route to reduce MBL. Intra-uterine progestogen delivery has great promise because of its ability to induce a dramatic reduction in MBL.

When bleeding is heavy and regular, PGSIs taken during menstruation can decrease bleeding and relieve dysmenorrhea. Tranexamic acid is an alternative therapy, but should be avoided in women with significant risk factors for thrombosis. Hormonal treatment should include a trial of a monophasic COCP, if there are no contraindications. Because of their side-effects, danazol, gestrinone and GnRH agonists are only suitable for short-term therapy.

Medical treatment can reduce excessive MBL by over 50%, but as only 40–50% of women referred to specialist care with a convincing history of menorrhagia actually lose more than 80 mL,[78] it is not surprising that medical treatment can appear to fail. Apparent failure should prompt the clinician to reconsider the diagnosis in the first instance rather than to immediately consider surgery.

Surgical treatments

A large proportion of those women referred for gynecological specialist advice for heavy or irregular menstrual bleeding will eventually undergo an operation for their complaint,[80] mostly without prior objective confirmation of their MBL. One in five women in the UK[130] and up to 50% in some parts of the USA[131] have had a hysterectomy by the age of 65 years. Menstrual disorders are the most common indication for hysterectomy in these countries.[130,132] The prevalence of hysterectomy varies substantially between countries, despite the relatively stable rate of the common indications for this operation.[130]

Endometrial resection and ablation techniques have now increased the range of surgical options for bleeding disturbances. Similarly, widespread availability of the levonorgestrel IUS will expand the possibility of long-term medical treatment. It is likely that hysterectomy rates will fall with the introduction of these new therapies, even though the role of new surgical options for DUB is not fully established. In the UK, it is disappointing to note that dilatation and curettage is still commonly offered as surgical 'treatment' for menorrhagia,[133] despite its objectively poor therapeutic and diagnostic value.[83,87,133]

Hysterectomy

Hysterectomy is the only definitive treatment for DUB that guarantees amenorrhea. It is associated with a high level of patient satisfaction,[134,135] superior to that seen following endometrial resection in one recent study.[136] There is no evidence that hysterectomy is associated with a long-term increase in psychological morbidity, and some indication that it may improve psychological state.[137] Hysterectomy allows the simultaneous removal of the ovaries if this is medically indicated and desired by the patient. Bilateral oophorectomy usually provides relief for severe cyclical premenstrual symptoms, the pelvic pain syndrome and menstrual migraine, all of which can accompany DUB.[138] When medical treatments for DUB fail, hysterectomy has thus been the traditional surgical approach, and it remains the most common definitive treatment for menstrual problems despite efforts to identify an effective medical alternative.

The safety of hysterectomy depends on the route of surgery, the patient's age and general condition, and the skill of the surgeon and anesthetist. A mortality rate of up to 1–2 per 1000 is quoted,[139] and a morbidity of over 40% if all complications are considered.[132] The current mortality and morbidity figures for hysterectomy in a fit premenopausal woman with a benign condition, performed by an experienced operator with anticoagulant and antibiotic prophylaxis is unknown, but is considerably less than these figures.

Disruption of the ovarian blood supply at hysterectomy can induce premature ovarian failure.[140] Without estrogen replacement, ovarian removal will often have important long-term harmful consequences for health. The incidence of cardiovascular disease posthysterectomy was trebled in one study in women under the age of 50 years,[141] and in the past many women have chosen not to take cardioprotective hormone therapy after oophorectomy. Studies are lacking on other possible long-term consequences of hysterectomy, such as micturition difficulties, prolapse and pelvic pain.

The great majority of hysterectomies are performed via the abdominal route,[142] despite good evidence that morbidity (as well as cost) of the procedure is less with vaginal hysterectomy.[132] For women with DUB the uterus is (by definition) not enlarged by fibroids and there is no other known pelvic pathology. There does not always need to be demonstrable preoperative uterine descent before vaginal hysterectomy, and the ovaries can often be removed at vaginal hysterectomy if required, dependent on the skill and experience of the surgeon.

There is much current interest in applying the techniques of minimal access surgery to hysterectomy. Although laparoscopic methods might have an advantage over abdominal hysterectomy in terms of the duration of hospital stay and speed of recovery,[143,144] there is little to support the advantage of adding laparoscopy to vaginal hysterectomy in the majority of cases.[145] The main aim of laparoscopic hysterectomy techniques is to convert an abdominal hysterectomy into a vaginal procedure or avoid the vaginal procedure completely, but the problems of prolonged duration of surgery and small risks of serious complications (such as ureteric damage) are unresolved.[145]

A small proportion of women with failed conservative surgical management, such as endometrial ablation or resection (see below), will eventually come to hysterectomy. With time the size of this group will be established, as well as the prognostic factors in menstrual complaints that should lead the clinician to best advise initial management.

Endometrial ablation

Applying the principle that pathological endometrial destruction and intra-uterine adhesions as seen with Asherman's Syndrome[146] are associated with amenorrhea, techniques of deliberate endometrial resection and ablation have been refined over the last decade. Many women wish to have a definitive solution to their menstrual problems without a major operation. This has become possible with the development of improved endoscopic optics, controlled irrigation fluid systems and instruments for hysteroscopic destruction of the endometrium under direct vision.

The three main methods of removing the endometrium have been Nd-YAG laser ablation, diathermy loop resection and diathermy rollerball ablation. Various other potential methods using radiofrequency current or application of heat or cold are currently being explored. It is unclear which of these techniques is most effective in short and long-term outcome, but it appears that rollerball ablation is associated with fewer intraoperative complications, while there is a comparable outcome in reduction in MBL.[147,148] If a destructive technique is used, some tissue should be resected for histology, preferably at preliminary hysteroscopy, as there have been reports of endometrial adenocarcinoma found unexpectedly at resection.[149]

The major advantages of these techniques are that they can usually be managed as day case procedures, and that most patients are able to return to work only a few days later.[148] The short-term costs of endometrial ablation are less than hysterectomy, but since some women will require hysterectomy or repeat ablation, the true cost differential requires long-term comparison. In a large audit of 987 endometrial ablations, almost 20% of those treated by laser ablation and 11% treated using diathermy required repeat surgery within twelve months.[150] It is unclear how much repeat surgery is caused by insufficiently skilled surgery, by inappropriate selection of patients or by inherent limitations of the techniques themselves. There may be a small number of women with undiagnosed adenomyosis who experience increased pain after resection or ablation treatments, or adenomyosis may rarely be caused by the procedure.

The major complications of transcervical endometrial resection techniques are perforation of the uterus and intravasation of large volumes of hypotonic glycine solution causing pulmonary or cerebral edema.[150] There have been deaths after endometrial resection following trauma, often unrecognized, to intra-abdominal organs, hemorrhage and infection, as well as fluid overload, but these are rare. Preoperative thinning of the endometrium with a priming agent such as danazol (400–600 mg daily for 4–6 weeks) or injection of subcutaneous GnRH agonist appear to improve success and reduce the complications of endometrial ablation to a greater extent than danazol, but prospective randomized trials are limited.[151,152] Progestogens can be used but take longer to produce thinning of the endometrium and the long-term outcome is inferior to pretreatment with danazol.[153]

Hysteroscopic endometrial ablation does not guarantee amenorrhea and patients should be aware of this. Up to 50% may continue to have some bleeding.[154] Irregular bleeding can develop, particularly in the perimenopause. This has important implications in terms of management, because cervical cancer and (rarely) endometrial cancer can still occur after ablation. In theory, residual endometrium or adenomyosis could become neoplastic and might fail to present early with postmenopausal bleeding following endometrial ablation because of intra-uterine adhesions. Progestogens should be offered in conjunction with estrogens for any hormone replacement therapy given following endometrial ablation.

Patient selection plays a crucial role in optimizing the success of endoscopic techniques. Ablation may be less successful in women under 35 years because of the greater tendency for the endometrium to regenerate in these women.[150] Poor outcome is also associated with a uterine cavity of more than 10 cm in length, with a submucous myomata or with adenomyosis. Like hysterectomy, the procedure is unsuitable for women who have not completed their families, yet it is not a completely reliable contraceptive. Pregnancies occurring after ablation are rare but are associated with a poor obstetric prognosis; the issue of contraception should be resolved in preoperative counseling. Better results may be achieved in women with ovulatory DUB than those with irregular and anovulatory bleeding.[150]

Audit plays an important role in the assessment of any new surgical technique, by directing attention away from the successful figures of individual enthusiasts to a realistic appraisal of the likely outcome for the majority of women managed by a number of surgeons using different techniques. Since there is an indication that the success of endometrial ablation may diminish with time,[154] conclusions cannot be drawn without large studies of long-term outcome. Information is also needed on the long-term effects of ablation, hysterectomy and medical therapy for DUB on quality of life.

Summary of surgical treatments

Abdominal hysterectomy has been the traditional surgical management option for DUB when medical treatments fail. Despite the many patient benefits of performing hysterectomy via the vaginal route, abdominal hysterectomy remains one of the commonest major surgical procedures in the developed world.

Endoscopic endometrial ablation and resection techniques have increased the range of permanent surgical treatments for DUB. They have a number of short-term advantages over hysterectomy in terms of morbidity and cost, but their long-term role in the management of DUB is not yet fully established. Progestogens have little role in preoperative thinning of the endometrium compared with GnRH analogs.

The development of laparoscopic techniques for hysterectomy may increase the number of procedures that can safely be performed via the vaginal route. Dilatation and curettage does not have a place in the treatment of chronic DUB, and should not normally be performed for diagnosis without simultaneous hysteroscopy.

Conclusions

Dysfunctional uterine bleeding is a common problem in most developed countries, particularly for women between 35–50 years of age. Of this group, 80% are ovulating regularly and have no apparent abnormality of the hypothalamo-pituitary-ovarian axis. The diagnosis of DUB is one of exclusion, and uterine pathology should be excluded by transvaginal ultrasound scanning and by hysteroscopy and endometrial biopsy.

The mechanism of DUB in ovulatory and anovulatory states is not fully understood. It is likely that local endometrial mechanisms are important in the pathophysiology of DUB. These local mechanisms probably to involve the uterine vasculature, possibly influenced by prostaglandins and other vasoactive substances, altered mechanisms of hemostasis, and changes in the process of tissue breakdown and remodeling. The influence of ovarian or exogenous steroids upon these processes is likely to be indirect.

Medical treatments for DUB include many hormonal regimens based on progestogens, estrogens, combinations of estrogens and progestogens, danazol and GnRH analogs. Prostaglandin synthetase inhibitors and antifibrinolytic agents have also proved to be successful at reducing MBL. Approaches to medical management have been hindered by a lack of understanding of the mechanisms causing DUB and by highly variable and non-evidence-based prescribing habits. Wider availability of the levonorgestrel-releasing intra-uterine system could greatly improve the options for long-term medical management of DUB.

The surgical management of DUB is moving away from abdominal hysterectomy towards more conservative techniques involving endoscopy. The place of these methods with regard to other medical and surgical therapies is yet to be established.

REFERENCES

1. Coulter A, Noone A, Goldacre M 1989 General practitioner's referrals to specialist outpatient clinics. British Medical Journal 299: 304–308
2. Hallberg L, Hogdahl AM, Nilsson L, Rybo G 1966 Menstrual blood loss — a population study. Acta Obstetrica Gynecologica Scandinavica 45: 320–351
3. Gath D, Osborn M, Bungay G 1987 Psychiatric disorder and gynaecological symptoms in middle-aged women: a community survey. British Medical Journal 294: 213–218
4. Cameron IT 1994 Endocrinology in dysfunctional uterine bleeding. In: Dysfunctional uterine bleeding. Key Paper Conferences. Royal Society of Medicine Press, London, pp 38–39
5. Short RV 1984 Oestrus and menstrual cycles. In: Austin CR, Short RV (eds) Hormonal control of reproduction. Cambridge University Press, Cambridge, pp 115–152
6. Edlund M, Magnusson C, Von Schoultz B 1994 Quality of life — a Swedish survey of 2200 women. In: Dysfunctional uterine bleeding. Key Paper Conferences. Royal Society of Medicine Press, London, pp 36–37
7. Cohen BJB, Gibor Y 1983 Metabolic and endocrine effects of medicated intra-uterine devices. In: Benagiano G, Diczfalusy E (eds) Endocrine mechanism in fertility regulation. Raven Press, New York, pp 71–124
8. Fraser IS 1985 The dysfunctional uterus: dysmenorrhoea and dysfunctional uterine bleeding. In: Shearman RP (ed) Clinical reproductive endocrinology. Churchill Livingstone, Edinburgh, pp 579–598
9. Fraser IS 1989 Treatment of menorrhagia. In: Drife JO (ed) Dysfunctional uterine bleeding. Baillière's Clinical Obstetrics and Gynaecology: Baillière Tyndall, London. 3: 391–402
10. Cameron IT 1989 Dysfunctional uterine bleeding. In: Drife JO (ed) Dysfunctional uterine bleeding and menorrhagia. Baillière's Clinical Obstetrics and Gynaecology. Baillière Tyndall, London. 3: 315–328
11. Bayer SR, DeCherney AH 1993 Clinical manifestations and treatment of dysfunctional uterine bleeding. Journal of the American Medical Association 269: 1823–1828
12. Cowan BD, Morrison JC 1991 Management of abnormal genital bleeding in girls and women. New England Journal of Medicine 324: 1710–1715
13. Murram D 1990 Vaginal bleeding in childhood and adolescence. Obstetric and Gynecology Clinics of North America 17: 380–408
14. Fraser IS 1994 Menorrhagia — a pragmatic approach to the understanding of causes and the need for investigations. British Journal of Obstetrics and Gynaecology 10 (Suppl 11): 3–7

15. Quinn M, Neale BJ, Fortune DW 1985 Endometrial carcinoma in premenopausal women: a clinicopathological study. Gynecological Oncology 20: 298–306
16. Beazley JM 1972 Dysfunctional uterine haemorrhage. British Journal of Hospital Medicine 7: 573–578
17. Fraser IS 1990 Hysteroscopy and laparoscopy in women with menorrhagia. American Journal of Obstetrics and Gynecology 162: 1264–1269
18. Rudigoz RC, Frobert C, Chassagnard F, Gaucherand P 1992 The role of vaginal echography in the investigation of menorrhagia and metrorrhagia in the reproductive years. J Gynecol Obstet Biol Reprod Paris 34: 644–650
19. Cole SK, Billewicz WZ, Thomson AM 1971 Sources of variation in menstrual blood loss. Journal of Obstetrics and Gynaecology of the British Commonwealth 78: 933–939
20. Rybo G 1966 Clinical and experimental studies on menstrual blood loss. Acta Obstetrica Gynecologica Scandinavica Suppl. pp 1–23
21. Eldred JM, Thomas EJ 1994 Pituitary and ovarian hormone levels in unexplained menorrhagia. Obstetrics and Gynecology 84: 775–778
22. Fraser IS, Peek MJ 1992 Effects of exogenous hormones on endometrial capillaries. In: Alexander NJ, d'Arcangues C (eds) Steroid hormones and uterine bleeding. American Association for the Advancement of Science, Washington, pp 67–79
23. Fraser IS, McCarron G, Hutton B, Macey D 1983 Endometrial blood flow measured by xenon-133 clearance in women with normal menstrual cycles and dysfunctional uterine bleeding. American Journal of Obstetrics and Gynecology 156: 158–166
24. Hilliard TC, Crayford TB, Bourne TH, Collins WP, Whitehead MI, Campbell S 1995 Differential effects of transdermal oestradiol and sequential progestagens on impedance to flow within the uterine arteries of postmenopausal women. Fertility and Sterility 58: 959–963
25. Perrot-Applanat M, Groyer-Pickard MT, Garcia E, Lorenzo F, Milgrom E 1988 Immunocytochemical demonstration of estrogen and progesterone receptors in muscle cells of uterine arteries in rabbits and humans. Endocrinology 123: 1511–1519
26. Ford SP, Reynolds LP, Farley DB, Bhatnager RK, Van Orden DE 1984 Interaction of ovarian steroids and periarterial α-1 adrenergic receptors in altering uterine blood flow during the oestrus cycle of gilts. American Journal of Obstetrics and Gynecology 150: 480–484
27. Economos K, MacDonald PC, Casey ML 1992 Endothelin-1 gene expression and protein biosynthesis in human endometrium: potential modulator of endometrial blood flow. Journal of Clinical Endocrinology and Metabolism 74: 14–19
28. Akerlund M, Bengtsson LP, Carter AM 1975 A technique for monitoring endometrial or decidual blood flow with an intra-uterine thermistor probe. Acta Obstetrica Gynecologica Scandinavica 54: 469–477
29. Gleeson N, Devitt M, Sheppard BL, Bonnar J 1993 Endometrial fibrinolytic enzymes in women with normal menstruation and dysfunctional uterine bleeding. British Journal of Obstetrics and Gynaecology 100: 768–771
30. Rees MCP, Dunhill MS, Anderson ABM, Turnbull AC 1984 Quantitative uterine histology during the menstrual cycle in relation to measured menstrual blood loss. British Journal of Obstetrics and Gynaecology 91: 662–666
31. Farrer-Brown G, Beilby JOW, Tarbit MH 1970 The blood supply of the uterus. 1: Arterial vasculature. Journal of Obstetrics and Gynaecology of the British Commonwealth 77: 672–681
32. Smith SK, Kelly RW 1987 The effect of the antiprogestins RU486 and ZK on the synthesis and metabolism of $PGF2_{\alpha}$ and PGE_2 in separated cells from early human decidua. Journal of Clinical Endocrinology and Metabolism 63: 527–537
33. Smith SK, Abel MH, Kelly RW, Baird DT 1981 Endometrial prostaglandins in women with ovular dysfunctional uterine bleeding. British Journal of Obstetrics and Gynaecology 88: 434–442
34. Smith SK, Abel MH, Kelly RW, Baird DT 1982 The synthesis of prostaglandins from persistent proliferative endometrium. Journal of Clinical Endocrinology and Metabolism 55: 284–289
35. Adelentado JM, Rees MCP, Lopez Bernal A, Turnbull AC 1988 Increased uterine prostaglandin E receptors in menorrhagic women. British Journal of Obstetrics and Gynaecology 95: 162–165
36. Cameron IT, Leask R, Kelly RW, Baird DT 1987 The effects of danazol and mefenamic acid, norethisterone and a progestogen-impregnated coil on endometrial prostaglandin concentration in women with menorrhagia. Prostaglandins 34: 99–100
37. Rees MCP, Canete-Soler R, Lopez-Bernal A, Turnbull AC 1988 Effect of fenamates on prostaglandin E receptor binding. Lancet ii: 541–542
38. Christiaens GCML, Sixma JJ, Haspels AA 1980 Morphology of haemostasis in the normal endometrium. British Journal of Obstetrics and Gynaecology 87: 425–439
39. Goetz KL, Wang BC, Madwell JB 1988 Cardiovascular, renal and endocrine responses to intravenous endothelin in conscious dogs. American Journal of Physiology 255: 1064–1068
40. Cameron IT, Davenport AP, Brown MJ, Smith SK 1991 Endothelin-1 stimulates $PGF2_{\alpha}$ release from human endometrium. Prostaglandins, Leukotrienes and Essential Fatty Acids 42: 155–158
41. Cameron IT, Davenport AP, van Papendorp C et al 1992 Endothelin-like immunoreactivity in human endometrium. Journal of Reproduction and Fertility 95: 623–628
42. Maggi M, Vannelli GB, Peri A et al 1991 Immunolocalization, binding and biological activity of endothelin in rabbit uterus: effect of ovarian steroids. American Journal of Physiology 260: E292–E305
43. Markee JE 1940 Menstruation in intraocular endometrial transplants in the rhesus monkey. Contributions in embryology. Carnegie Institute of Washington, Publication No. 518, 28: 219–308
44. Abel MH, Zhu C, Baird DT 1982 An animal model to study menstrual bleeding. Research and Clinical Forums 4: 25–34
45. Cooke JP, Santosa AC 1992 Endothelium-derived relaxing factor (nitric oxide) and vascular tone. In: Alexander N J, Arcangues CD (eds) Steroid hormones and uterine bleeding. American Association for the Advancement of Science, Washington, pp 225–240

46. Stamler JS, Mendelsohn ME, Amaranate P 1989 N-acetylcysteine potentiates platelet inhibition by endothelium-derived relaxing factor. Circulation Research 65: 789–795
47. Vane JR, Botting RM 1991 Endothelium-derived vasoactive substance and the control of the circulation. Seminars in Perinatology 15: 4–10
48. De Duve C, Wattiaux R 1966 Functions of lysosomes. American Review of Physiology 28: 435–492
49. Henzl MR, Smith RE, Boost G, Tyler ET 1972 Lysosomal concept of menstrual bleeding in humans. Journal of Clinical Endocrinology and Metabolism 34: 860–875
50. Christiaens GCML, Sixma JJ, Haspel AA 1982 Haemostasis in menstrual endometrium: a review. American Journal of Reproductive Immunology 5: 78–83
51. Wang IYS, Fraser IS, Manconi F, Barsamian S, Street D 199• Endometrial lysosomal enzyme activity in women with menorrhagia due to ovulatory dysfunctional uterine bleeding or intra-uterine contraceptive devices. Submitted for publication
52. Rogers WH, Matrisian LM, Giudice LC, Dsupin B, Cannon P, Svitek C, Gorstein F, Osteen KG 1994 Patterns of matrix metalloproteinases expression in cycling endometrium imply differential functions and regulation by steroid hormones. Journal of Clinical Investigation 94: 946–953
53. Hampton AL, Salmonsen LA 1994 Expression of messenger ribonucleic acid encoding matrix metalloproteinases and their tissue inhibitors is related to menstruation. Journal of Endocrinology 141(1): R1–3
54. Bulmer JN, Johnson PM, Bulmer D 1987 Leucocyte populations in human decidua and endometrium. In: Gill TJ III, Wegmann TJ (eds) Immunoregulation and fetal survival. Oxford University Press, New York, pp 111–134
55. Kamat BR, Isaacson PG 1987 The immunocytochemical distribution of leucocyte subpopulations in human endometrium. American Journal of Pathology 127: 66–73
56. Song JY, Markham R, Russell P, Wong T, Young L, Fraser IS 1995 The effect of high dose medium and long-term progestogen exposure on endometrial vessels. Human Reproduction 10: 797–800
57. Sheppard BL 1987 Endometrial morphology changes in IUD users: a review. Contraception 36: 1–10
58. Foley ME, Griffin BD, Zugel M 1978 Heparin-like activity in uterine fluid. British Medical Journal ii: 322–324
59. Tabibzadeh SS, Poubouridis D 1990 Expression of leukocyte adhesion molecules in human endometrium. American Journal of Clinical Pathology 93: 183–188
60. Tawia SA, Beaton LA, Rogers PAW 1983 Immunolocalisation of the cellular adhesion molecules, ICAM-1 and PECAM in human endometrium through the normal menstrual cycle. Human Reproduction 8: 175–181
61. Clark DA 1993 Cytokines, decidua and pregnancy. Oxford Review of Reproductive Biology 15: 83–111
62. Critchley HOD, Kelly RW, Kooy J 1994 Perivascular expression of chemokine interleukin-8 in human endometrium: a preliminary report. Human Reproduction 9: 1406–1409
63. Kelly RW, Illingworth P, Baldie G, Leask R, Brouwer S, Calder AA 1994 Progestogen control of interleukin-8 production in the endometrium and choriodecidual cells underlines the role of the neutrophil in menstruation and parturition. Human Reproduction 9: 253–258
64. Ferenczy A 1976 Studies on the cytodynamics of human endometrial regeneration 1. Scanning electron microscopy. American Journal of Obstetrics and Gynecology 124: 64–74
65. Ferenczy A 1976 Studies on the cytodynamics of human endometrial regeneration 11. Transmission electron microscopy and histochemistry. American Journal of Obstetrics and Gynecology 124: 582–595
66. Smith SK 1989 Prostaglandins and growth factors in the endometrium. In: Drife JO (ed) Baillière's Clinical Obstetrics and Gynaecology. Dysfunctional uterine bleeding. 3(2): 249–270. Baillière Tyndall, London
67. Findlay JK 1986 Angiogenesis in reproductive tissues. Journal of Endocrinology 111: 357–366
68. Sheppard BL 1990 Coagulation and electron microscopy studies in menorrhagia. In: Shaw RW (ed) Advances in reproductive endocrinology, vol 2. Dysfunctional uterine bleeding. Parthenon, Lancs, England, pp 25–42
69. Cässlen B, Andersson A, Nilsson IM 1986 Hormonal regulation of the release of plasminogen activators and of a specific activator inhibitor from endometrial tissues in culture. Proceedings of the Society of Experimental Biology and Medicine 182: 419–424
70. Kasonde JM, Bonnar J 1976 Plasminogen activators in the endometrium of women using intra-uterine contraceptive devices. British Journal of Obstetrics and Gynaecology 83: 315–319
71. Casslén B, Åstedt B 1983 Reduced plasminogen activator content of endometrium in oral contraceptive users. Contraception 28: 181–188
72. Padwick ML, Pryse-Davies MI, Whitehead M 1986 A simple method for determining the optimal dose of progestin in women receiving estrogens. New England Journal of Medicine 315: 930–933
73. Corner GW 1942 The hormones in human reproduction. Princeton University Press, Princeton
74. Brown JB, Kellar RJ, Mathew GD 1959 Urinary oestrogen excretion in certain gynaecological disorders. Journal of Obstetrics and Gynaecology of the British Empire 66: 177–211
75. Snowden R, Christaens B 1983 Patterns and perception of menstruation. Croom Helm, London
76. Fraser IS 1983 A survey of approaches to management of menstrual disturbances in women using injectable contraceptives. Contraception 28: 385–397
77. Chimbira TH, Anderson BM, Turnbull AC 1980 Relationship between measured menstrual blood l oss and patient's subjective assessment of loss, duration of bleeding, number of sanitary towels used, uterine weight and endometrial surface area. British Journal of Obstetrics and Gynaecology 87: 603–609

78. Fraser IS, McCarron G, Markham R 1984 A preliminary study of factors influencing perception of menstrual blood loss volume. American Journal of Obstetrics and Gynecology 149: 788–793
79. Lee NC, Dicker RC, Rubin GL, Ory HW 1984 Confirmation of preoperative diagnosis for hysterectomy. American Journal of Obstetrics and Gynecology 150: 283–287
80. Coulter A, Bradlow J, Agass M, Martin-Bates C, Tulloch A 1991 Outcomes of referrals to gynaecology outpatient clinics for menstrual problems: an audit of general practice. British Journal of Obstetrics and Gynaecology 98: 789–796
81. Fraser IS 1993 My personal techniques and results for outpatient diagnostic hysteroscopy. Gynaecological Endoscopy 2: 29–34
82. Mackenzie JZ, Bibby JG 1978 Critical assessment of dilatation and curettage in 1029 women. Lancet ii: 566–569
83. Gimpelson RJ 1984 Panoramic hysteroscopy with directed biopsy versus dilatation and curettage for accurate diagnosis. Journal of Reproductive Medicine 29: 575–578
84. McCausland AM 1992 Hysteroscopic myometrial biopsy: its use in diagnosing adenomyosis and its clinical application. American Journal of Obstetrics and Gynecology 166(6 pt 1): 1619–1626
85. Higham JM, O'Brien PMS, Shaw RW 1990 Assessment of menstrual blood loss using a pictorial chart. British Journal of Obstetrics and Gynaecology 97: 734–739
86. Hallberg L, Nilsson L 1964 Determination of menstrual blood loss. Scandinavian Journal of Clinical Laboratory Investigation 16: 244–248
87. Nilsson L, Rybo G 1971 Treatment of menorrhagia. American Journal of Obstetrics and Gynecology 110: 713–720
88. Haynes PJ, Hodgson H, Andersson ABM, Turnbull AC 1977 Measurement of menstrual blood loss in patients complaining of menorrhagia. British Journal of Obstetrics and Gynaecology 84: 763–768
89. De Vore GR, Owens O, Kase N 1982 Use of intravenous Premarin in the treatment of dysfunctional uterine bleeding — a double blind randomized controlled study. Obstetrics and Gynecology 59: 285–291
90. Shaw RW 1990 Menorrhagia treatment with LHRH analogues. In: Shaw RW (ed) Advances in reproductive endocrinology, vol 2. Dysfunctional uterine bleeding. Parthenon, Lancs, England, pp 149–160
91. Rees MCP 1991 Role of menstrual blood loss measurement in the management of menorrhagia. British Journal of Obstetrics and Gynaecology 90: 327–328
92. Robinson GE 1994 Low-dose combined oral contraceptives. British Journal of Obstetrics and Gynaecology 101: 1036–1041
93. Fraser IS, McCarron G 1991 Randomised trial of two hormonal and two prostaglandin-inhibiting agents in women with a complaint of menorrhagia. Australian and New Zealand Journal of Obstetrics and Gynaecology 31: 66–70
94. Rozenbaum H 1982 Relationships between chemical structure and biological properties of progestogens. American Journal of Obstetrics and Gynecology 142: 719–724
95. Roberts DK, Morbelt DV, Powell LC 1975 The ultrastructural response of human endometrium to medroxyprogesterone acetate. American Journal of Obstetrics and Gynecology 123: 811–818
96. Preston JT, Cameron IT, Adams EJ, Smith SK 1995 Comparative study of tranexamic acid and norethisterone in the treatment of ovulatory menorrhagia. British Journal of Obstetrics and Gynaecology 102: 410–416
97. Fraser IS 1990 Treatment of ovulatory and anovulatory menorrhagia with oral progestogens. Australian and New Zealand Journal of Obstetrics and Gynaecology 30: 353–356
98. Odlind V, Fraser IS 1990 Hormonal contraception and bleeding disturbances: a clinical overview. In: d'Arcangues C, Fraser IS, Newton JR, Odlind V (eds) Contraception and mechanisms of endometrial bleeding. Cambridge University Press, Cambridge, England, pp 5–29
99. Anderson JK, Rybo G 1990 The levonorgestrel releasing intra-uterine contraceptive device in the treatment of menorrhagia. British Journal of Obstetrics and Gynaecology 97: 690–694
100. Nilsson CG, Luukkainen T, Arko H 1978 Endometrial morphology of women using the D-norgestrel releasing intra-uterine device. Fertility and Sterility 29: 397–401
101. I-Cheng Chi PH 1991 An evaluation of the levonorgestrel IUD: its advantages and disadvantages when compared with copper releasing IUDs. Contraception 44: 573–588
102. Diaz S, Croxatto HB, Pavez M, Belhadj H, Stern J, Sivin I 1990 Clinical assessment of treatments for prolonged bleeding in users of Norplant implants. Contraception 42: 97–109
103. Smith SK 1990 The physiology of menstruation. In: d'Arcangues C, Fraser IS, Newton JR, Odlind V (eds) Contraception and mechanisms of endometrial bleeding. Cambridge University Press, Cambridge, England, pp 33–41
104. Jeppson S, Mellquist P, Rannevik G 1984 Short-term effects of danazol on endometrial histology. Acta Obstetrica Gynecologica Scandinavica 123: 41–44
105. Chimbira TH, Cope E, Anderson ABM, Bolton FG 1979 The effects of danazol on menorrhagia, coagulation mechanisms, haematological indices and body weight. British Journal of Obstetrics and Gynaecology 86: 46–50
106. Fraser IS 1985 Treatment of dysfunctional uterine bleeding with danazol. Australian and New Zealand Journal of Obstetrics and Gynaecology 25: 224–226
107. Dockeray CJ, Shepperd BL, Bonnar J 1989 Comparison between mefenamic acid and danazol in the treatment of established menorrhagia. British Journal of Obstetrics and Gynaecology 96: 840–844
108. Allen JK, Fraser IS 1981 Cholesterol, high-density lipoproteins and danazol. Journal of Clinical Endocrinology and Metabolism 53: 149–152
109. Burridge J, Fraser IS 1980 Danazol treatment and platelet function. Medical Journal of Australia 1: 313–314

110. Turnbull AC, Rees MCP 1990 Gestrinone in the treatment of menorrhagia. British Journal of Obstetrics and Gynaecology 97: 713–715
111. Meldrum D, Chang R, Lu J, Vale W, Rivier J, Judd H 1982 Medical oophorectomy using a long-acting GnRH agonist — a possible new approach to the treatment of endometriosis. Journal of Clinical Endocrinology and Metabolism 54: 1081–1083
112. Fraser IS 1991 Relationship between gonadotrophin-releasing hormone analogue therapy and bone loss; a review. Reproduction, Fertility and Development 3: 61–69
113. Thomas EJ, Okuda KJ, Thomas NM 1991 The combination of a depot gonadotrophin releasing hormone agonist and cyclical hormone replacement therapy for dysfunctional uterine bleeding. British Journal of Obstetrics and Gynaecology 98: 1155–1159
114. Anderson ABM, Haynes PJ, Guillebaud J, Turnbull AC 1976 Reduction of menstrual blood loss by prostaglandin synthetase inhibitors. Lancet i: 774–776
115. Haynes PJ, Flint AP, Guillebaud J, Turnbull AC 1990 Studies in menorrhagia, (a) Mefenamic acid, (b) Endometrial prostaglandin concentrations. International Journal of Gynecology and Obstetrics 17: 567–572
116. Fraser IS, Pearce C, Shearman RP, Elliot PM, McIlveen J, Markham R 1981 Efficacy of mefenamic acid in patients with a complaint of menorrhagia. Obstetrics and Gynecology 58: 543–551
117. Muggeridge J, Elder MG 1983 Mefenamic acid in the treatment of menorrhagia. Research and Clinical Forums 5(3): 83–88
118. Mäkäräinen L, Ylikorkala O 1986 Ibuprofen prevents IUCD-induced increases in menstrual blood loss. British Journal of Obstetrics and Gynaecology 93: 285–288
119. Hall P, McLachan N, Thorn N 1987 Control of menorrhagia by the cyclo-oxygenase inhibitors naproxen sodium and mefenamic acid. British Journal of Obstetrics and Gynaecology 94: 554–558
120. van Eijkeren MA, Christaens GC, Geuze HJ, Haspels AA, Sixma JJ 1992 Effects of mefenamic acid on menstrual haemostasis in essential menorrhagia. American Journal of Obstetrics and Gynecology 160: 1419–1428
121. Vargyas JM, Campeau JD, Mishell DR Jr 1987 Treatment of menorrhagia with meclofenamate sodium. American Journal of Obstetrics and Gynecology 157: 944–950
122. Gleeson NC, Buggy F, Sheppard BL, Bonnar J 1994 The effect of tranexamic acid on measured menstrual blood loss and endometrial fibrinolytic enzymes in dysfunctional uterine bleeding. Acta Obstetrica Gynecologica Scandinavica 73(3): 274–277
123. Dockeray CJ, Sheppard BL, Daly L, Bonnar J 1987 The fibrinolytic enzyme system in normal menstruation and excessive uterine bleeding and the effects of tranexamic acid. European Journal of Obstetrics, Gynecology and Reproductive Biology 24: 309–318
124. Vermylen J, Verhaegen-Declercq ML, Verstraete M, Fierens F 1978 A double blind study on the effect of tranexamic acid in essential menorrhagia. Thromb Diath Haemorrh 20: 583–587
125. Callender ST, Warner GT, Cope E 1970 Treatment of menorrhagia with tranexamic acid. A double blind trial. British Medical Journal 4: 214–216
126. Rydin E, Lundberg PO 1976 Tranexamic acid and intracranial thrombosis. Lancet ii: 49
127. Hedlund PO 1975 Postoperative venous thrombosis in benign prostatic disease. A study of 316 patients using ^{125}I-fibrinogen uptake test. Scandinavian Journal of Urology and Nephrology 27: 1–100
128. Smith SK, Haining REB 1994 Investigation and management of excessive menstrual bleeding. In: Dysfunctional uterine bleeding. Key Paper Conferences. Royal Society of Medicine Press, London, pp 109–135
129. Moodley J, Cohen M, Devray K, Dutton M 1992 Vaginal absorption of tranexamic acid from impregnated tampons. South African Medical Journal 81: 150–152
130. Coulter A, McPherson K, Vessey M 1988 Do British women undergo too many or too few hysterectomies? Social Science and Medicine 27(9): 987–994
131. Bunker JP, Brown B 1974 The physician-patient as an informed consumer of surgical services. New England Journal of Medicine 290: 1051–1055
132. Dicker RC, Greenspan JR, Strauss LT 1982 Complications of abdominal and vaginal hysterectomy amongst women of reproductive age in the United States. American Journal of Obstetrics and Gynecology 144: 841–848
133. Coulter A, Klasses A, Mackenzie I, McPherson K 1993 Diagnostic dilatation and curettage: is it used appropriately? British Medical Journal 306: 236–239
134. vanKeep PA, Wildemeersch D, Lehert P 1983 Hysterectomy in six European countries. Maturitas 5(2): 69–75
135. Webb C 1983 A study of recovery from hysterectomy. In: Wilson-Barnett J (ed) Nursing research — studies in patient care. Baillière Tindall, London, pp 7–22
136. Dwyer NA, Hutton J, Stirrat GM 1993 Randomised controlled trial comparing endometrial resection with abdominal hysterectomy for the surgical treatment of menorrhagia. British Journal of Obstetrics and Gynaecology 100: 237–243
137. Gath D, Cooper P, Day A 1982 Hysterectomy and psychiatric disorder: levels of psychiatric morbidity before and after hysterectomy. British Journal of Psychiatry 140: 335–342
138. Studd JWW 1989 Hysterectomy and menorrhagia. In: Drife JO (ed) Baillière's Clinical Obstetrics and Gynaecology. Dysfunctional uterine bleeding. Baillière Tyndall, London 3(2): ch 13, pp 415–424
139. Bunker JP, McPherson K, Hennerman PL 1977 Elective hysterectomy. In: Bunker JP, Barnes BA, Mosteller F (eds) Costs, risks and benefits of surgery. Oxford University Press, Oxford, pp 262–276
140. Siddle N, Sarrel P, Whitehead MI 1987 The effect of hysterectomy on the age of ovarian failure: identification of a subgroup of women with premature loss of ovarian function, and literature review. Fertility and Sterility 47: 94–100
141. Centerwall BS 1981 Premature hysterectomy and cardiovascular disease. American Journal of Obstetrics and Gynecology 139: 58–61

142. Lalonde A 1994 Evaluation of surgical options in menorrhagia. British Journal of Obstetrics and Gynaecology 101: 8–14
143. Hunter RW, McCartney A 1993 Can laparoscopic assisted hysterectomy safely replace abdominal hysterectomy? British Journal of Obstetrics and Gynaecology 100: 932–934
144. Phipps J, Nayak K 1993 Comparison of laparoscopically assisted vaginal hysterectomy and bilateral salpingo-oophorectomy with conventional abdominal hysterectomy and bilateral salpingo-oophorectomy. British Journal of Obstetrics and Gynaecology 100: 698–700
145. Summit RL Jr, Stovall TJ, Lipscomb GH, Ling FW 1992 Randomised comparison of laparoscopy assisted hysterectomy with standard vaginal hysterectomy in an outpatient setting. Obstetrics and Gynecology 80: 895–901
146. Asherman JG 1948 Amenorrhoea traumatica (atretica). Journal of Obstetrics and Gynaecology of the British Empire 55: 23–30
147. Fraser IS, Angsuwathana S, Mahmoud F, Yezerski S 1993 Short and medium term outcomes after rollerball endometrial ablation for menorrhagia. Medical Journal of Australia 158(7): 454–457
148. Magos AL, Baumann R, Lockwood GM, Turnbull AC 1991 Experience with the first 250 endometrial resections for menorrhagia. Lancet 337: 1074–1078
149. Dwyer NA, Stirrat GM 1991 Early endometrial cancer: an incidental finding after endometrial ablation. British Journal of Obstetrics and Gynaecology 98: 733–734
150. Lumsden MA 1995 Audit of transcervical endometrial ablation. British Journal of Obstetrics and Gynaecology 102: 87–89
151. Sutton CJG, Ewen SP 1994 Thinning the endometrium prior to ablation: is it worthwhile? British Journal of Obstetrics and Gynaecology 101(Suppl 10): 10–12
152. Fraser IS, Healy D, Torode H, Wilde F, Mamers P, Song JY 1996 Depot goserelin and danazol pretreatment before rollerball endometrial ablation for menorrhagia. Obstetrics and Gynecology 87: 544–550
153. Brooks PG, Serden MD, Scott P, Daros I 1991 Hormonal inhibition of the endometrium for resectoscopic endometrial ablation. American Journal of Obstetrics and Gynecology 164: 1601–1608
154. Chullapram T, Song JY, Fraser IS 1996 Medium term follow-up of women with menorrhagia treated by rollerball endometrial ablation. Obstetrics and Gynecology 88: 71–76

36. Defective luteal function

Bruce A. Lessey Marc A. Fritz

Introduction

Luteal phase deficiency (LPD) is a disorder characterized by a delayed or otherwise abnormal pattern of secretory endometrial development caused by inadequate corpus luteum (CL) progesterone production.[1] Subfertility and early pregnancy wastage have long been regarded as clinical consequences of LPD,[2,3] presumably due to failed or defective implantation or a premature luteal-placental shift.[4,5] The concept is relatively simple and certainly a plausible one. Unfortunately, the pathophysiology which underlies this disorder has proven elusive. Exactly why or how the functional capacity of the CL is reduced in LPD remains unclear. Although frustrating, our ignorance is understandable because the mechanisms of luteolysis that operate in the normal menstrual cycle are also still undefined. Recent evidence that embryo implantation occurs within a distinctly finite and relatively narrow 'window' of time has again focused attention on the CL and its influence on endometrial development and function. The mechanisms that render the endometrium receptive to embryo implantation are key to understanding the cascade of events involved in the implantation process. Understandably, LPD is once again a topic of interest and active debate.

Historical perspective

The idea that progesterone deficiency might predispose to pregnancy wastage emerged from the work of Allen and Corner on the physiology of the CL.[6] The significance of morphological changes in the secretory endometrium was first suggested by Rock and Bartlett in 1937,[1] but it was not until 1949 that Georgeanna Seegar Jones hypothesized that a disruption in this sequence of changes, a delay in endometrial maturation, might be a cause of infertility.[7] The seminal work of Noyes, Hertig and Rock was published in 1950 and established criteria to 'date' the endometrium.[8] Those criteria have endured, despite their many shortcomings, and histological dating remains the 'gold standard' against which all other methods for assessing the quality of luteal function must be compared (Fig. 36.1).[9] Other methods of diagnosis have been proposed and each has its own proponents. Unfortunately, progress in resolving the many controversies surrounding this disorder has been hampered by this lack of uniformity in approach to its diagnosis, and by our inability to define the regulatory mechanisms that govern the normal CL. Recent efforts aimed at defining the implantation process have provided new insights and offered new perspectives on the pathophysiology of LPD and now promise to further our understanding of this enigmatic reproductive endocrinopathy.

Although LPD has been the focus of a great many clinical investigations, there remains no consensus on the prevalence of this disorder nor its impact on fertility. Reports on the prevalence of LPD in infertile women have varied widely. Jones, drawing from her own large body of experience, found evidence of LPD in less than 4% of the infertile women in her practice.[4] Summarizing the results of 12 early studies involving more than 4000 patients, Noyes concluded that endometrial development was abnormal in nearly 32% of infertile women.[10] In some studies, the prevalence of LPD has been as high as 60%.[4,5,7,11-16] These differences largely can be attributed to differences in diagnostic criteria; the true prevalence of LPD is probably in the range of 5–10%.

PATHOPHYSIOLOGY

LPD is best viewed not as a single distinct entity, but rather as a final common pathway with a variety of predisposing factors or causes. Although inadequate luteal function can ultimately be traced to the ovary, its endometrial consequences are largely responsible for

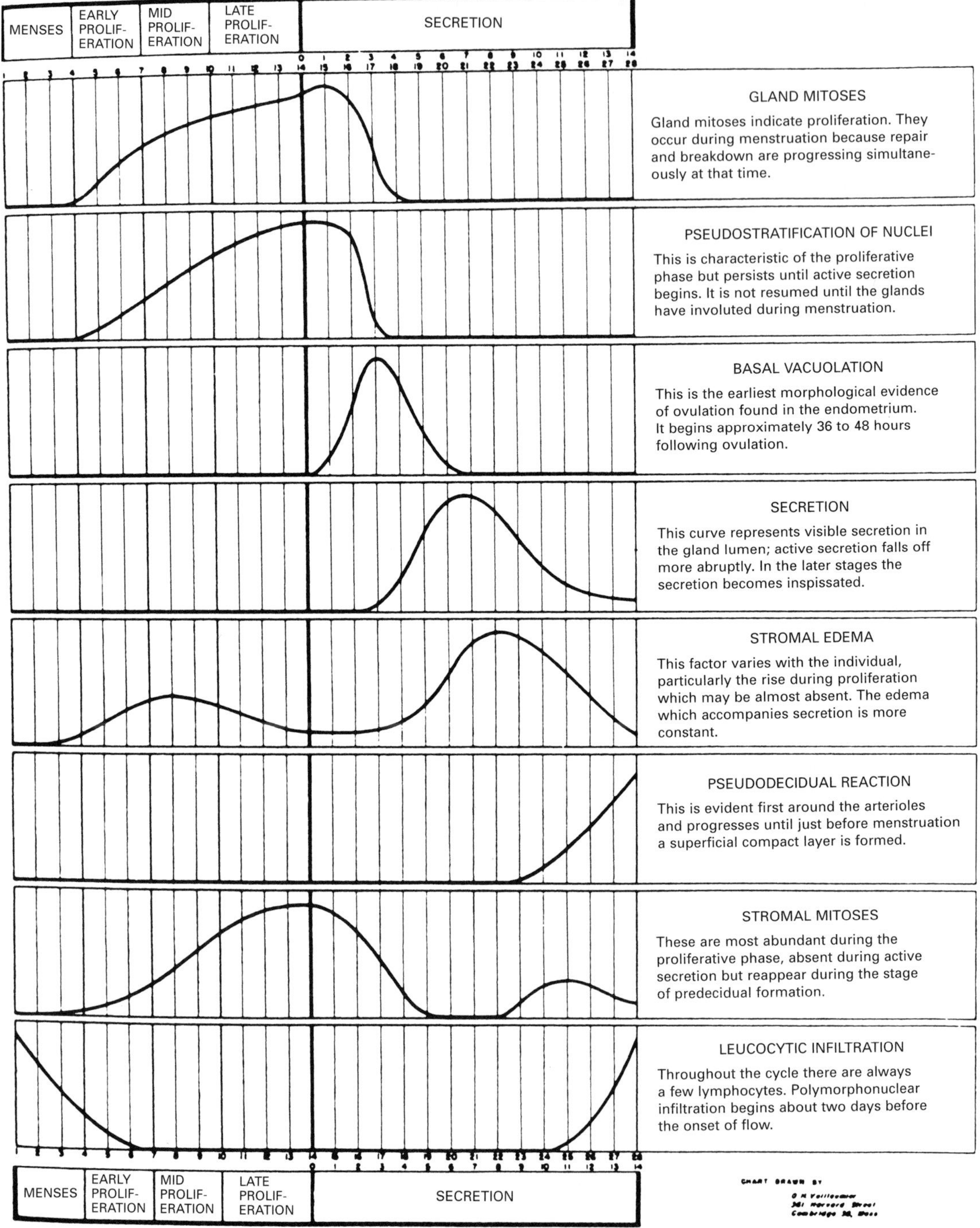

Fig. 36.1 The dating criteria of Noyes et al used to assess the maturation of the endometrium.[8] (Reproduced with permission of the American Society for Reproductive Medicine)

any adverse effects the disorder has on reproductive function. The infertility and early pregnancy wastage associated with LPD, at least in theory, might involve two different but closely related mechanisms. Timely and optimal development of the secretory endometrium clearly depends on steroid hormones produced by the CL. Inadequate levels of steroid production may thus delay or otherwise disturb endometrial maturation. Given recent evidence that implantation occurs only within a narrow 'window' of endometrial receptivity,[17,18] an arriving embryo may encounter an endometrium not yet prepared to receive it. If that delay is sufficiently prolonged, implantation may fail altogether. Lesser degrees of immaturity may allow the embryo to implant, albeit late, with other consequences such as recurrent pregnancy loss. Inevitably, the resulting delay in the embryo's 'rescue' signal will be delivered only after the CL has passed its functional prime and entered the early stages of regression.

A number of factors that can affect CL function and influence the pattern of secretory endometrial development, directly or indirectly, have been identified. These 'causes' of LPD have been reviewed by Jones,[5] more recently by Nakajima and Gibson,[19] and are summarized in Table 36.1. It is important to realize that, to a large degree, the functional capacity of the CL depends on the relative health and maturity of the preovulatory ovarian follicle from which it derives. If nothing else, the extent of granulosa proliferation in the preovulatory follicle and the quality of its luteinization largely determine the size of the luteal cell mass. Ovarian follicular development and steroid production are driven by pituitary gonadotropins which, in turn, are secreted in a pattern influenced by the frequency and amplitude of hypothalamic gonadotropin-releasing hormone (GnRH) secretion.[20] Any disturbance in this highly coordinated and delicately balanced hypothalamic-pituitary-gonadal axis may adversely affect the course or quality of ovarian follicular development. If it does not cause overt ovulatory failure, that disturbance may still compromise the quality or duration of CL function. In this context, luteal phase deficiency can be viewed as a subtle but distinct form of ovulatory dysfunction.

Factors affecting the follicular phase

Several lines of evidence support this concept of LPD. It seems clear that even subtle alterations in gonadotropin secretion during the follicular phase can compromise the quality and duration of luteal function.[21] Early studies by Strott et al in women with a naturally occurring short luteal phase demonstrated significantly lower follicular phase FSH/LH ratios and reduced magnitude of the LH surge in such cycles, compared to those with a normal luteal phase duration.[22] Similarly, Sherman and Korenman found

Table 36.1 Causes of luteal phase defect.

Cause	*Suspected mechanism*
Medications	
Opioids	Suppression of GnRH
NSAIDs	Disruption of ovulation
Clomiphene citrate	Altered endometrial receptivity
Phenothiazines	Elevated prolactin (inhibition of PIF)
Endocrinopathy	
Hyperprolactinemia	Altered GnRH, pituitary or ovarian function
Hyperandrogenism	Alteration in ovarian or endometrial function
Thyroid disease	Elevation of prolactin
Systemic disease	
Stress, eating disorders, chronic disease, excessive exercise	Opioids, weight loss alterations in GnRH pulsatility or opioid tone
Idiopathic/miscellaneous	
Endometrial abnormalities	Altered receptivity
Inhibin abnormalities	Altered FSH/folliculogenesis
Early luteolysis	Direct or indirect CL effect
Poor CL rescue	Delayed or inadequate implantation

that abnormally low luteal phase estradiol and progesterone concentrations were often associated with lower than expected midfollicular phase FSH levels.[23] The inferences drawn from these early observations have since been tested by direct experiments, conducted in both nonhuman primates and women. In monkeys, selective suppression of FSH, achieved by infusion of porcine follicular fluid (a rich source of inhibin), results in lower preovulatory estradiol levels, reduced midluteal progesterone concentrations and a significant decrease in luteal cell mass.[24] In women, administration of a long-acting GnRH agonist for a brief interval in the early follicular phase induces a similar decline in midfollicular phase FSH levels, followed by an abbreviated luteal phase in which both estradiol and progesterone concentrations are significantly reduced.[25] The clinical significance of these observations is suggested by the fact that abnormally low follicular phase FSH and estradiol levels, and reduced luteal phase serum progesterone concentrations, have been observed in women with otherwise unexplained infertility. Contradictory evidence does exist, however.

The aberrant patterns of follicular phase gonadotropin secretion associated with poor luteal function are not limited to inadequate FSH levels. Soules et al have demonstrated that midcycle bioactive and immunoactive LH levels are frequently reduced in women with documented LPD,[26] an observation also made by Ayabe et al.[27] The work of Schweiger et al indicates that abnormally slow pulsatile LH rhythms can also be seen in cycles that exhibit low luteal phase steroid concentrations.[28] Taken together, since the pattern of pulsatile LH secretion presumably reflects that of hypothalamic GnRH, and since the frequency and amplitude of pulsatile GnRH secretion influence the relative quantities of pituitary FSH and LH release, these data suggest that inadequate luteal function can be caused by a variety of factors. Such factors can be both intrinsic and extrinsic, influencing the activity of the hypothalamic GnRH pulse generator or the pituitary response to GnRH secretion.

Endocrinopathies

Endocrinopathies, their metabolic consequences, or the homeostatic mechanisms they trigger, can disturb the delicate balance of the hypothalamic-pituitary-ovarian axis. Thyroid disease is one example. Both hyperthyroidism and hypothyroidism are relatively common in reproductive aged women. The metabolic clearance of steroid hormones, and thus the feedback signals they communicate, is altered in these disorders.[29] Elevated levels of total and free estradiol are common in thyroid disease and may exert a feedback inhibition on gonadotropin secretion. Primary hypothyroidism may also be associated with a secondary hyperprolactinemia, the result of increased levels of hypothalamic thyrotropin-releasing hormone (TRH) secretion (which also stimulates pituitary lactotropes), the effects of increased circulating estrogens (which stimulate prolactin production by activating gene transcription, interfering with the inhibitory action of hypothalamic dopamine, and upregulating the TRH receptor) and the lower metabolic clearance of prolactin in hypothyroid individuals. The reproductive implications of hyperprolactinemia are well known and include LPD.

Hyperprolactinemia, of course, has many other causes including expanding hypothalamic tumors (that compress the pituitary stalk and interfere with effective delivery of hypothalamic dopamine), prolactin-secreting pituitary adenomas, a wide variety of drugs (that alter the synthesis, metabolism, re-uptake, or receptor binding of dopamine) and chronic renal failure (due to a reduced metabolic clearance and increased production of prolactin). Whatever its cause, hyperprolactinemia is frequently associated with hypogonadism of varying degrees. The fact that even the profound hypoestrogenism that frequently accompanies hyperprolactinemia is not associated with hot flushes strongly suggests that neurotransmitter mechanisms are altered in this disorder. The available evidence indicates that high prolactin levels induce an increase in the levels of hypothalamic dopamine and opioid peptides,[30] both of which serve as inhibitory neuromodulators of pulsatile hypothalamic GnRH secretion.

When pronounced, hyperprolactinemia frequently results in anovulation or even amenorrhea, but the effects of lesser elevations are often more subtle.[31,30] Cycle characteristics after discontinuation of bromocriptine treatment in hyperprolactinemic women suggest that inadequate luteal function may be one of the earliest manifestations of an underlying prolactin disorder. A shortening of the luteal phase is the first observation followed, in sequence, by a return of galactorrhea, frank anovulation and, finally, amenorrhea.[32] Indeed, a causal link between elevated prolactin levels and LPD is now rather well established. Wenner was the first to suggest an association between hyperprolactinemia and infertility.[33] Numerous authors have since observed a relatively high incidence of short luteal phase or otherwise inadequate luteal function in hyperprolactinemic women.[32–40] Conversely, Daly et al found that 16% of women with documented LPD also had hyperprolactinemia.[41] Induction of hyperprolactinemia by metoclopramide in normal, healthy women was shown to result in smaller peak follicular diameter and serum LH at midcycle and reduced luteal progesterone levels.[42] Transient, but exaggerated, nocturnal elevations of prolactin levels may be one cause of galactorrhea in women who otherwise appear euprolactinemic. This same phenomenon, undetected in random daytime determinations, has been observed in some women with LPD or unexplained infertility.[43–45]

Elevated circulating androgen concentrations have also been implicated as a possible cause of LPD. Evidence suggests they may act centrally to alter patterns of gonadotropin secretion, on the ovary where they may compromise the quality of follicular development, or in the endometrium where they may interfere with estrogen-mediated progesterone receptor induction. Sherman and Korenman found that progesterone concentrations in ovulatory, obese, hirsute women were significantly lower than in normal individuals. This is one of the very few studies that have addressed the effects of hyperandrogenism on luteal function.[46] Clearly, women with polycystic ovarian syndrome (PCOS) associated with hyperandrogenism and oligo-ovulation have lower fecundity and a higher frequency of spontaneous abortion.[47,48] Given that LPD is merely one manifestation of ovulatory dysfunction, it is quite possible that inadequate luteal function may contribute to their poor reproductive performance.

Medications

Certain classes of medications have also been associated with poor luteal function. Their effects may often be attributed to altered levels of neurotransmitters or interference with their actions at the pituitary level.[49] Others, like the nonsteroidal anti-inflammatory agents which inhibit prostaglandin synthesis, may have more direct actions on the ovary or endometrium.[50] The potent inhibitory effects that opioid peptides have on hypothalamic GnRH neurosecretory cells may explain why female heroin addicts so often have abnormal menstrual cycle characteristics, ranging from a short luteal phase to complete amenorrhea.[51,52] Levels of endogenous opioids, specifically β-endorphins, increase with physical activity. Thus, the same mechanism may explain the apparent link between LPD and strenuous physical exercise and other forms of environmental stress, including the weight loss associated with crash dieting and other eating disorders.[53–55]

Normal mechanisms of corpus luteum function

The CL itself is a remarkable endocrine organ. In the nonfertile cycle it survives only briefly, 14–16 days on average, then regresses. The cause of its demise in humans is still a mystery. In the fertile cycle, stimulated by the exponential rise in chorionic gonadotropin, the CL persists, its continued function crucial until such time as the trophoblast matures and becomes self-sufficient. The CL is governed by a number of complex regulatory mechanisms and normal luteal function has several requirements.[56]

It is difficult to deny that the first and foremost requirement of normal luteal function is optimal development of the preovulatory follicle. Clearly, inadequate luteal function may often be simply the natural consequence of poor follicular development. The lifespan and steroidogenic capacity of the CL also depends on continuation of at least a tonic level of pituitary LH secretion. In nonhuman primates, administration of an LH antiserum in the early luteal phase is followed by a prompt decline in circulating progesterone levels and the early onset of menses.[57] A short luteal phase and low levels of progesterone production follow ovulation induction in hypophysectomized women, unless further exogenous gonadotropin support is provided.[58] Similar observations have been made in normal women when luteal phase LH secretion is inhibited by use of a GnRH antagonist.[59] Whereas a pulsatile infusion of exogenous GnRH can restore gonadotropin secretion and induce ovulation in monkeys with hypothalamic lesions that eliminate endogenous GnRH production, discontinuation of that infusion during the luteal phase brings about a prompt fall in progesterone levels and the onset of menses.[60] Studies involving frequent blood sampling have demonstrated that the CL secretes progesterone in distinct pulses that closely correlate with LH pulses.[61,62] These data indicate that LH plays not just a supportive role but is also an acute regulator of CL function. Soules et al have observed reduced levels of both bioactive and immunoactive LH at midcycle and during the mid- to late luteal phase in women with documented LPD.[63] A subtle deficiency in luteal phase LH secretion, although insufficient to cause a premature luteolysis, could well compromise the quality of luteal function. Indeed, any of the factors which disturb gonadotropin secretion and adversely affect development of the preovulatory follicle may also have consequences for the CL.

Given the similar structure and actions of LH and hCG, it is easy to envision how and why rapidly rising levels of hCG might 'rescue' the CL in the conception cycle. What may be less clear is why the CL regresses in the first place when there is no dramatic fall in the levels of endogenous LH. Current evidence suggests that luteolysis is the result of a progressive decrease in sensitivity to LH stimulation. Consequently, rescue can only be effected by the dramatic increases in stimulation provided by the exponential rise of hCG in conception cycles.

In the fertile cycle, the first appearance of hCG exactly coincides with the peak in CL development and function. Evidence indicates that this temporal association may be crucial to a successful rescue of the CL. Studies in the nonhuman primate demonstrate that the patterns and amounts of estrogen and progesterone secretion that accompany a course of incremental exogenous hCG vary significantly with the postovulatory age of the CL.[64,65] The steroidogenic response to hCG is modest in the early luteal phase, greatest at midluteal phase and decreases again in the late luteal phase. Very similar observations have been made in women.[66] If the onset of the exponential rise in hCG production in early pregnancy is postponed, even by a few days when luteolysis may already be underway, it may be too late to ensure that the CL can provide the requisite level and duration of steroidogenic support. This mechanism might explain the association between LPD and recurrent pregnancy loss, and focuses attention on the endometrium and the factors which determine the rate and quality of its preimplantation development.

Physiologic consequences of an inadequate luteal phase

Progesterone is critical to development of a receptive endometrium. Under its influence, proliferating endometrial epithelial cells undergo a characteristic secretory transformation and begin synthesis and secretion of proteins now thought to play a vital role in the implantation process.[67–69] Over the course of the luteal phase, progesterone also converts the endometrial stroma into the decidua, a highly specialized compartment that produces extracellular matrix, cytokines and growth factors which facilitate but also limit invasion of the trophoblast. One important feature of progesterone's action is that it down-regulates its own receptor (PR) in epithelial cells while concentrations in the decidua are maintained.[70–72] This is arguably a key event in endometrial development since it signals a shift from epithelial activity to stromal/decidual function. Inadequate luteal phase progesterone production, by causing a delay in epithelial PR down-regulation, may alter patterns of protein expression and render the endometrium nonreceptive to embryo implantation.

Abnormalities of endometrial maturation may be identified even when progesterone concentrations are not clearly low.[73,74] Balasch and Vanrell found that endometrial maturation was delayed by two or more days in 13.5% of infertile women and 32.5% of patients with a history of recurrent pregnancy loss, even though 86% overall had what they considered a normal hormone profile.[73] In a more recent study by Batista et al, abnormal pre-implantation endometrial development was nearly five times more common in women with unexplained infertility than in fertile controls, but in most cases progesterone concentrations were again normal.[75] Keller coined the term 'pseudo corpus luteum insufficiency' to describe this phenomenon and speculated that it reflects a poor endometrial response to otherwise normal luteal function.[76] Theoretically, inadequate preovulatory estrogen-induced endometrial proliferation and PR induction might preclude a normal and timely sequence of secretory maturation, but this would likely be accompanied by poor follicular development. It is also quite possible that entirely normal variations in histologic maturation among women or simple differences in the day of sampling might account for these observations. In a recent study of 36 normal fertile volunteers who underwent endometrial biopsy 8–10 days following detection of a urinary LH surge, 12 specimens (33%) exhibited glandular/stromal dyssynchrony; epithelial development was delayed by three or more days, but stromal maturation was normal. On closer inspection, however, dyssynchrony was observed only in specimens obtained on luteal day 8.[56] This pattern has often been interpreted as abnormal, but the frequency of this finding in a group of normally cycling parous women and its absence in specimens obtained only slightly later in the luteal phase suggest that the histologic features of normal midsecretory phase endometrium may vary more than has been previously recognized.

Numerous studies have attempted to define the endometrial steroid receptor profile in normal cycles and in LPD but results have been conflicting. Reduced, normal and even higher PR concentrations have been reported in women with delayed endometrial maturation.[76–80] These inconsistent results might reflect the fact that there is more than one cause for LPD, but the dynamic changes in PR levels during the luteal phase and the different patterns of PR expression in glands and stroma are a more likely explanation. Immunohistochemical analyses, which examine PR expression *in situ*, have revealed that delayed endometrial maturation is associated with a delay in epithelial PR down-regulation and that both abnormalities can be corrected with appropriate treatment.[81]

A delay in histologic endometrial development is the *sine qua non* of LPD. Presumably, this morphologic abnormality has a functional consequence — a decrease or loss of endometrial receptivity.[82] From the embryo's perspective, the absolute concentrations of circulating progesterone are of little importance; whatever level or pattern of secretion effectively prepares the endometrium for its arrival is sufficient. Data derived from highly sensitive assays for hCG suggest that embryo implantation occurs between cycle days 20 and 24 (luteal days 6–10).[83] This putative 'window of endometrial receptivity' is consistent with the early observations of Hertig et al. After careful examination of 34 hysterectomy specimens obtained in cycles of conception, embryos were uniformly unattached before cycle day 19 and all were implanted after cycle day 21.[84] Taken together, these data suggest that implantation occurs within a relatively narrow interval of time that is both specific and precise. Animal data from studies by Pope suggest that abortion may indeed be a consequence of dyssynchronous embryo and endometrial development.[85] Thus they may also offer an explanation for the association between LPD and recurrent pregnancy loss.

Recently, considerable efforts have been directed towards identification of biochemical markers which can define the receptive endometrium (see references 69, 86 and 87 for review). Candidate markers have included steroid receptors, lectins, mucins and other glycoproteins. One particular glycoprotein, placental protein 14 (PP14), has been studied extensively. First described by Joshi[68] and originally called progestogen-dependent endometrial protein (PEP), its early promise as a serum marker for LPD in the evaluation of infertility and recurrent pregnancy loss has not been realized.[88]

Increasing attention has focused on another class of cell adhesion proteins known as integrins. Whereas integrins are by no means unique to the endometrium, certain members of this family exhibit distinct cycle-specific patterns of endometrial expression that suggest they may serve effectively as markers of endometrial receptivity. The putative implantation window, as defined by the histological criteria of Noyes et al,[8] spans the interval from cycle days 20–24. Three specific integrins αvβ3, α1β1, α4β1 are conspicuously coexpressed in endometrial epithelium only during this same five-day period. One of these, the αvβ3 integrin, abruptly appears on cycle day 20, when the endometrium presumably may first become receptive (Fig. 36.2). It is also the only epithelial integrin that is

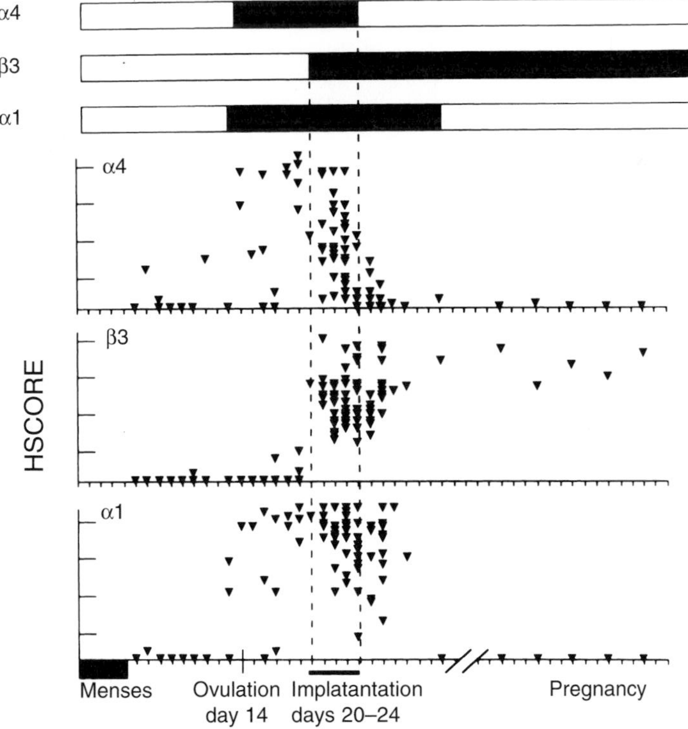

Fig. 36.2 Relative intensity of staining for the epithelial α4, β3 and α1 integrin subunits throughout the menstrual cycle and in early pregnancy. The negative staining (open bars) was shown for immunostaining of an average HSCORE ≤ 0.7, for each of the three integrin subunits. Positive staining for all three integrin subunits was seen only during a five day interval corresponding to the putative window of implantation.[18] (Reproduced with permission of the American Society for Reproductive Medicine)

expressed in pregnant endometrium. Patterns of integrin expression closely correlate with traditional histologic dating criteria in both normal and abnormal cycles. Subsequent investigations have revealed delayed or absent expression of αvβ3 in women with LPD (Fig. 36.3) and demonstrated that treatment which corrects a histologic delay in endometrial maturation also restores a normal pattern of integrin expression. Whereas these observations indicate that poor luteal function may indeed have functional endometrial consequences, they do not establish a causal link with infertility or recurrent spontaneous abortion.

Taken together, the available data suggest that each of the essential steps in the implantation process must take place within a unique and very precise 'window' of opportunity (Fig. 36.4). The embryo must attach and invade soon after it achieves that capacity or risk losing its developmental momentum. The endometrium must mature in a normal and timely fashion or its interval of receptivity will not coincide with that of the conceptus. The CL must receive a timely rescue signal, one delivered at the peak of its development, or its functional response to rising levels of hCG may be insufficient in amount or duration to ensure the success of early pregnancy. That delayed endometrial maturation may cause a temporal shift in endometrial receptivity and thereby predispose to failed or late implantation or unsuccessful CL rescue is a plausible concept that has much evidence to support it.

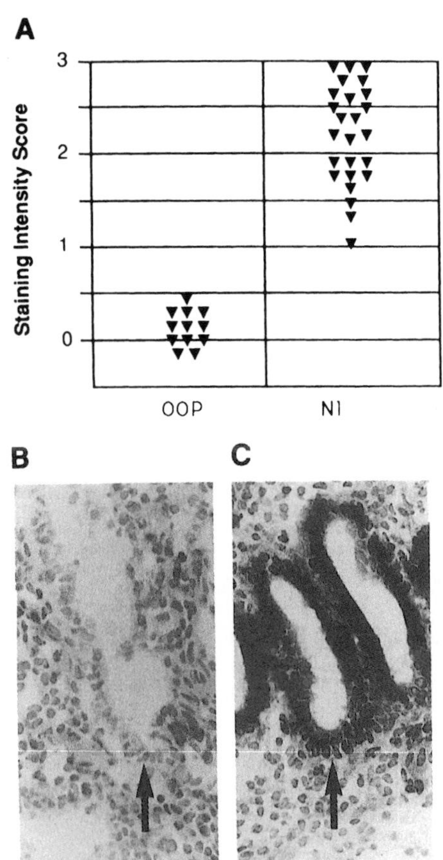

Fig. 36.3 Staining intensity of epithelial β3 in 12 infertility patients with delayed endometrial maturation. Patients with endometrial biopsies three or more days 'out of phase' (OOP group) were compared with 25 endometrial biopsies that were 'in phase' (Normal) and shown in (**A**) with negative (**B**) and positive (**C**) immunostaining for β_3 (magnification ×400).[82] Reproduced with permission of the Rockefeller Press, New York)

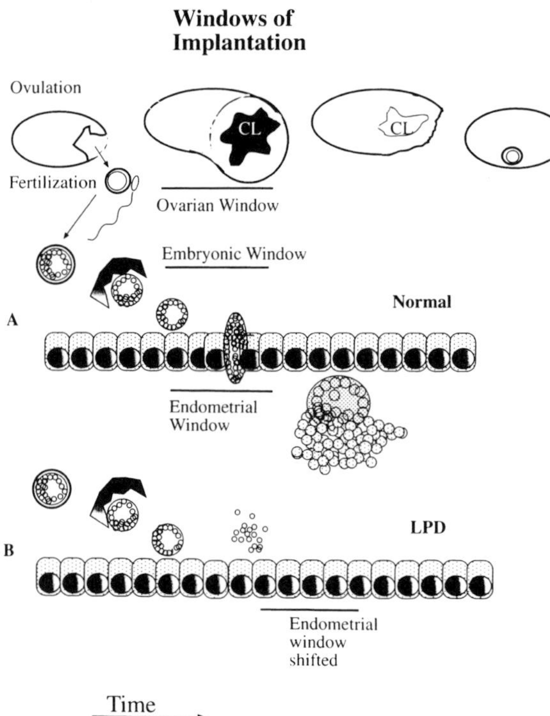

Fig. 36.4 Schematic representation of three different 'windows' of receptivity. The endometrium undergoes developmental changes that reflect the adequacy of hypothalamic/pituitary and ovarian influences. The timing of implantation based on endometrial receptivity is presumed to be synchronous with the embryonic and corpora luteum requirements. As described in the text, a delay in the timing of implantation (**B**) could compromise the ability of the embryo to survive directly, or indirectly, by failure to adequately rescue the waiting CL which begins to undergo luteolysis in the later stages of the luteal phase.

DIAGNOSIS OF LPD

The various methods that have been proposed to assess the quality of luteal function have previously been reviewed.[3,89] It is clear that a reliable test for LPD is not yet available. The poor correlation between methods and the widely varying estimates of the prevalence of this disorder reflect this fact. Nevertheless, it is helpful to review each of the methods currently used in clinical practice, if only to better understand their relative strengths and weaknesses.

Basal body temperature

Basal body temperature (BBT) charting is a time-honored method for assessing ovulatory function. Because the 'thermogenic shift' in BBT is a progesterone-induced phenomenon it has also been used as a measure of CL function. Cycles exhibiting a temperature elevation less than 11 days in duration are considered to have a short, and therefore inadequate, luteal phase. Some have suggested a gradual, staggered rise in BBT as another indication of poor luteal function.

As a method for assessing the quality of luteal function, BBT is both noninvasive and inexpensive. Unfortunately, it lacks both sensitivity and specificity. Soules has suggested that short intermenstrual intervals or abnormal BBT characteristics can be identified in up to 80% of women with histologic evidence of LPD,[90] but Downs and Gibson found that BBT recordings revealed a short luteal phase in only 6 of 20 (30%) infertile women with histologically documented LPD.[91] Others have found a similarly poor correlation between BBT recordings and endometrial histology or serum progesterone determinations.[91–93] A short luteal phase may suggest LPD but is also often observed in normal fertile women whose luteal function is normal by any other measure. In one prospective controlled study in which the midcycle LH surge was carefully identified, Smith et al found that a short luteal phase occurred with equal frequency in fertile and infertile women.[94]

Serum progesterone determinations

Quite obviously, the amount of progesterone produced by the CL is a valid measure of its functional capacity. Not surprisingly, serum progesterone determinations are often used to assess the quality of luteal function.[26,95–98] In studies involving daily measurements or even more frequent determinations, Li et al and Soules et al have demonstrated that integrated serum progesterone concentrations correlate with the quality of secretory endometrial development.[63,99] Others, however, have failed to confirm these findings. Even if it was proven as a valid and reliable approach to the diagnosis of LPD, few would argue that daily luteal phase progesterone determinations are practical or cost-effective in clinical practice. Abraham has suggested that a sum of three determinations obtained between cycle days 18 and 26 greater that 15 ng/ml is satisfactory for diagnosis.[100] A number of others have attempted to define LPD with a single midluteal serum progesterone determination.[101] Unfortunately, there is no consensus on the minimum progesterone concentration that may be confidently considered as adequate.

Levels as low as 3 ng/ml and as high as 10 ng/ml have been proposed, but all have found considerable overlap in the concentrations observed in normal and LPD cycles and in conception and nonconception cycles in proven fertile women. Given that even daily integrated progesterone levels cannot reliably predict endometrial histology, it is not surprising that single serum determinations also correlate poorly with the quality of endometrial maturation.[75]

One obvious explanation for our inability to define the minimum normal serum concentration of progesterone is the fact that CL progesterone secretion is pulsatile in nature.[102] Studies by Ellinwood et al in the nonhuman primate[61] and by Filicori et al in women[62] have clearly demonstrated that progesterone levels fluctuate widely during the luteal phase, closely correlating with distinct pulses in pituitary LH release. Levels as low as 5 and as high as 40 ng/ml can be observed within an interval of only hours. Syrop and Hammond have suggested that the impact of these variations can be minimized by sampling during the morning hours when concentrations are highest and less erratic than at other times of day, but for most, these observations all but invalidate the use of serum progesterone concentrations for diagnosis of LPD.[102]

Endometrial biopsy

Histologic 'dating' of the secretory phase endometrium has endured as the method of choice for diagnosis of LPD. Since the extent of endometrial development and maturation reflects both CL functional capacity and the end organ tissue response, this approach has been considered as a bioassay of luteal function. Clearly, it is the only method able to detect abnormalities that arise within the endometrium itself.

When the quality of luteal function is defined by the histologic characteristics of endometrial development,

LPD is more commonly found in women with unexplained infertility or advanced reproductive age (over 35 years) than in those with tubal factor infertility or in normal fertile individuals.[103,104] It is also more common in women with primary infertility than in those who have conceived before. In patients with history of recurrent pregnancy loss, the incidence of LPD is even higher, ranging from 23% to as high as 60%.[105,106] Few studies have examined the incidence of LPD in fertile women. In one study of parous women seeking elective sterilization, sterilization reversal, or donor insemination, none had evidence of LPD.[107] However, Aksel et al have demonstrated that LPD does occur, at least sporadically, in normal women.[108] Li et al detected LPD in 4% of a group of proven fertile women.[109] Batista et al made the diagnosis in 14 of 50 normally cycling women (28%), 33 (66%) of whom were parous. In another study by the same investigators, 9% of fertile controls had evidence of LPD.[75] Davis found that a random cycle may reveal evidence of LPD in more than 30% of fertile subjects, although a subsequent cycle is again abnormal in less than 7% of patients.[110] Taken together, these studies indicate that at least on occasion, endometrial maturation is delayed or otherwise abnormal even in proven fertile individuals. They also serve to demonstrate why the diagnosis of LPD should be made only when such abnormalities are repeatedly observed.

The traditional criteria of Noyes et al are the basis for histologic dating of the endometrium.[83] As mentioned earlier, the data on which those criteria are based were collected entirely within the context of evaluation and care of an infertile population. This approach to the diagnosis of LPD has also demonstrated a rather high degree of intra- and inter-observer variation. The clinical implications of such variations have been demonstrated by Scott et al.[111] With a calculated intra-observer variation of 0.69 ± 0.05 days in their institution, re-examination of the same tissue specimen could result in a change in interpretation, and in clinical management, in up to 30% of patients.

The optimal time to perform endometrial biopsy for diagnosis of LPD is controversial. Late luteal phase sampling within the three days preceding expected onset of menses has traditionally been recommended. However, many now believe that the results of midluteal or 'peri-implantation' phase endometrial sampling are more relevant.[16] When two biopsies from the same cycle were compared, the apparent incidence of LPD based on endometrial histology was greater in the midluteal biopsy compared to the traditional late biopsy,[112] consistent with previous reports showing greater variability in the early biopsy.[95,113–115] These observations suggest that the timing of endometrial sampling is an important consideration and deserves further study and clarification.

Interpretation of the biopsy is also directly influenced by the method used to determine or define the day of sampling. Traditionally, the expected histologic date was determined in retrospect by counting backwards from the onset of the subsequent menses.[13] This relatively imprecise method assumes an idealized 14 day luteal phase duration and ignores any effects that biopsy itself may have on the onset of menses. Shoupe et al have demonstrated a relatively poor correlation (+/– 2 days) between observed and expected histologic dates with this method (65%). Correlation is much improved when the day of ovulation, and therefore the day of sampling, is defined prospectively, based on detection of the midcycle LH surge (85%) or on ultrasound evidence of follicular collapse (96%).[116] The latter reference point is the most accurate, but serial ultrasound examinations can be expensive and difficult to schedule. Urinary LH determinations using widely available over-the-counter ovulation predictor kits offer a convenient and more cost-effective alternative only slightly less accurate.

Other methods

Still other methods have been proposed for the diagnosis of LPD. These include serial sonograms to evaluate the quality of follicular development or measure endometrial thickness,[117] and hysteroscopic inspection.[118] More recently, color flow Doppler ultrasound has been used to examine the characteristics of blood flow into and around the CL[119] or endometrium.[120] Quite clearly, an ideal method has yet to be found. Each of the techniques currently available has its own advantages, disadvantages and pitfalls. Newly identified biochemical markers of endometrial receptivity represent yet another possible approach to the diagnosis of LPD, but will require additional careful study before they can be recommended for use in clinical practice.

TREATMENT

Although early uncontrolled and nonrandomized studies noted an increase in cycle fecundity following treatment of luteal phase defect,[1,45,92] the benefit of treatment on this disorder has not been convincingly shown.[121] The many treatment strategies devised reflect the many potential causes of LPD. Choice of treatment is generally one of individual preference, although certain causes dictate the form of therapy.

Treatment options include exogenous progesterone supplementation, hCG, clomiphene citrate (CC), bromocriptine and human menopausal gonadotropins. It is both interesting and helpful to examine the principles that underlie the use of each. In a novel study by Daly,[41] sequential treatment was undertaken in 36 infertility patients with biopsy proven LPD. Patients with hyperprolactinemia or hypothyroidism received specific therapy but 29 others received progesterone vaginal suppositories (25 mg BID), clomiphene citrate or human menopausal gonadotropins, each for a defined interval. Pregnancies were achieved with all of these regimens, but only by those whose treatment normalized histologic dating.

Clomiphene citrate (CC)

Since its introduction in 1960,[122] CC has become the most frequently used drug for ovulation induction. It is also often chosen as treatment for LPD. CC may be particularly useful in patients with a grossly short luteal phase which is characteristically associated with low follicular phase FSH levels. As an anti-estrogen, CC interferes with estrogen feedback signals centrally and stimulates pituitary gonadotropin secretion by altering the pattern of hypothalamic GnRH release.[93] When given to ovulatory women with LPD, the intent of CC treatment is to enhance follicular development and, in turn, the functional capacity of the resultant corpus luteum,[123,124] although some suggest it acts by increasing the number of preovulatory follicles and corpora lutea.[125] Paradoxically, Cook and colleagues reported that ovulatory women frequently develop LPD after receiving CC, an observation that suggests CC treatment may be detrimental in cycling women.[126] Downs and Gibson have suggested that CC can be effective, but only in women with profound degrees of histologic delay (≥ 5 days out of phase).[127] Others have reported excellent results in women with a short luteal phase.[93,128,129] In women with unexplained infertility, CC treatment can reduce the incidence of ovarian cyst formation and endometrial maturation delay consistent with LPD.[130]

It is important to recognize that CC treatment is systemic and may therefore affect all estrogen-receptor positive tissues, including the pituitary, ovary, endometrium and cervix. Besides possibly inducing LPD,[126] adverse effects of CC on ovarian and cervical function have also been suggested. At the ovarian level, CC may attenuate the follicular response to FSH[131] or compromise developmental potential of the ovum.[132] Reduced quantity and quality of cervical mucus have long been associated with CC, presumably the result of interference with the local actions of estrogen. At least in the endometrium, CC does not appear to alter endometrial estrogen and progesterone receptor concentrations.[133] However, alterations in the action of these steroids in the presence of CC cannot be excluded.

Progesterone therapy

Since LPD is characterized by insufficient progesterone production or an inadequate response to this steroid, treatment with exogenous progesterone supplementation is both logical and common. Progesterone can be used in a variety of ways, including vaginal suppositories,[92,134] micronized oral administration,[135] intramuscular injection and now even nasal[136] or sublingual administration.[137] Transdermal therapy is not practical because of the relatively large surface areas required to achieve physiologic progesterone concentrations. Nillius and Johansson compared plasma progesterone levels after vaginal, rectal and i.m. administration.[138] Each route can promptly achieve plasma concentrations typical of those seen during the midluteal phase. Levels decline more slowly after i.m. injection than with other routes of administration. Recently, Bulletti and colleagues demonstrated that progesterone absorbed from vaginal suppositories rapidly reaches the endometrium in what the authors described as a 'first uterine pass effect'.[139] These observations suggest that effective endometrial levels might be well above measured serum concentrations after vaginal administration of progesterone.

Vaginal suppositories are the preferred form of treatment for LPD for a number of investigators.[5,14,92] Soules and coworkers reported a 50% pregnancy rate in 16 women with documented LPD; treatment began on the third day after the post ovulatory rise in BBT. In one of the few controlled randomized studies to examine treatment efficacy with progesterone,[140] Balash demonstrated improved fecundity in women who received adequate treatment compared to those who were not treated. Huang compared the efficacy of CC and progesterone supplementation in the treatment of LPD and found no difference in pregnancy rates between the two groups.[113] Murray et al obtained similar results.[141] In ART cycles, progesterone supplementation was associated with a thicker endometrium, which in turn correlated with a higher pregnancy rate.[142]

hCG

Exogenous human chorionic gonadotropin (hCG) stimulates the corpus luteum directly and represents an alternative to progesterone supplementation and CC for the treatment of LPD, although inadequate luteal function that results from an intrinsic insensitivity to tropic stimulation may not respond. Supplemental hCG is most appropriate when specific defects in pre- or postovulatory LH secretion can be identified or in the management of recurrent pregnancy loss when delayed implantation is suspected.[142,143]

Recommendations regarding the dosage of exogenous hCG range widely.[13,144] Some clinicians advocate administration of 5000–10 000 IU at the time of ovulation followed by an additional 5000 IU 5–7 days later. Alternatively, 10 000 IU can be given in divided doses every three days after ovulation. Few studies have compared the use of hCG with other forms of treatment for LPD. In general, treatment should not extend beyond postovulatory day 12 and patients should be advised that menstrual delay and a false positive pregnancy test are possibilities. In a conception cycle, successive hCG determinations will document a rising titer of hCG; if the patient fails to conceive, levels will naturally decline.

Bromocriptine

Several studies have documented an association between hyperprolactinemia and LPD.[32,37,40,145] Nearly 17% of an infertility population studied by Daly had elevated prolactin, most of whom conceived after treatment with bromocriptine.[41] Bromocriptine, a potent dopamine agonist, lowers prolactin production by direct action on pituitary lactotrophs and is the drug of choice for hyperprolactinemic patients with LPD.[146–150] Gastrointestinal upset and postural hypotension are common and often troublesome side effects that can be minimized by starting treatment with small doses (1.25 mg or less) at bedtime, with small increments at intervals if needed. In highly sensitive patients, vaginal administration is helpful and still effective. Oversuppression of prolactin should be avoided.[151] The effectiveness of any given dose can be determined after 7–14 days of therapy. Once euprolactinemia is restored, a return of ovulatory function can be expected. Treatment is continuous and generally discontinued only once pregnancy occurs. Although large scale follow-up studies of pregnancies achieved during bromocriptine treatment have revealed no evidence of increased risk of congenital malformation,[152] most clinicians discontinue treatment once pregnancy is documented and fetal heart activity is observed.

Choice of therapy

In the absence of identifiable endocrinopathies such as hypothyroidism or hyperprolactinemia, the treatment of LPD usually begins with either CC or progesterone supplementation, which appear to be equally effective. Many clinicians prefer to begin with CC given its ease of use. Some clinicians base their choice of therapy on endometrial histologic characteristics or the quality of follicular development as determined by ultrasound. Reasoning that endometrial gland/stromal dyssynchrony suggests a gonadotropin deficiency and poor folliculogenesis, Witten and Martin favor CC treatment in such patients, reserving progesterone supplementation for those with synchronous maturation delay. Check et al recommend progesterone when follicular growth and midcycle estradiol levels are normal and CC treatment when they are not. Regardless what form of treatment is used, its effectiveness should be documented and not simply assumed.

Conclusion

Although in many ways still controversial, inadequate corpus luteum function may be regarded as a subtle but relatively common reproductive endocrinopathy. When it is a consistent finding, LPD may hinder reproductive function by reducing fecundity and predisposing to recurrent spontaneous abortion. Available evidence indicates it may have several causes. Delayed endometrial maturation is the final common denominator and its demonstration remains the gold standard of diagnostic methods. Unfortunately, until diagnostic criteria became more universal and firmly established, the true prevalence of LPD will remain unclear and its treatment largely empiric. The mechanisms which govern the interaction of the corpus luteum, endometrium and the conceptus are clearly complex and represent one of the frontiers in reproductive medicine. Newly identified markers of endometrial receptivity provide a tool for probing this frontier with the promise of new insights and a greater understanding of the implantation process.

REFERENCES

1. Rock J, Bartlett MK 1937 Biopsy studies of human endometrium, criterion of dating and information about amenorrhea, menorrhea, and tissue ovulation. Journal of the American Medical Association 108: 2022
2. McNeely MJ, Soules MR 1988 The diagnosis of luteal phase deficiency: a critical review. Fertility and Sterility 50: 1–15
3. Gibson M 1990 Clinical evaluation of luteal function. Seminars in Reproductive Endocrinology 8: 130–141
4. Jones GS 1973 Luteal phase insufficiency. Clinical Obstetrics and Gynecology 16: 255–273
5. Jones GS 1976 The luteal phase defect. Fertility and Sterility 27: 351–356
6. Allen WM, Corner GW 1929 Physiology of the corpus luteum III. Normal growth and implantation of embryos after very early ablation of the ovaries, under the influence of extracts of the corpus luteum. American Journal of Physiology 88: 340–346
7. Jones GS 1949 Some newer aspects of management of infertility. Journal of the American Medical Association 141: 1123–1129
8. Noyes RW, Hertig AI, Rock J 1950 Dating the endometrial biopsy. Fertility and Sterility 1: 3–25
9. Key JD, Kempers RD 1987 Citation classics: most-cited articles from Fertility and Sterility. Fertility and Sterility 47: 910–915
10. Noyes RW 1959 The underdeveloped secretory endometrium. American Journal of Obstetrics and Gynecology 77(5): 929–945
11. Grant A, McBride WG, Moyes JM 1959 Luteal phase defects in sterility. International Journal of Fertility 4: 315
12. Murthy YS, Arronet GH, Parekh MC 1970 Luteal phase inadequacy: its significance in infertility. Obstetrics and Gynecology 36: 758–761
13. Wentz AC 1979 Physiologic and clinical considerations in luteal phase defects. Clinical Obstetrics and Gynecology 22: 169–185
14. Gillam JS 1955 Study of the inadequate secretory phase of endometrium. Fertility and Sterility 6: 18–36
15. Bottella-Llusia J 1959 Endometrial biopsy in 2000 infertile women. International Journal of Fertility 4: 300–305
16. Li TC, Cooke ID 1991 Evaluation of the luteal phase. Human Reproduction 6: 484–499
17. Navot D, Bergh PA, Williams M, Garrisi GJ, Guzman I, Sandler B, Fox J, Schreiner-Engel P, Hofmann GE, Grunfeld L 1991 An insight into early reproductive processes through the in vivo model of ovum donation. Journal of Clinical Endocrinology and Metabolism 72: 408–414
18. Lessey BA, Castelbaum AJ, Buck CA, Lei Y, Yowell CW, Sun J 1994 Further characterization of endometrial integrins during the menstrual cycle and in pregnancy. Fertility and Sterility 62: 497–506
19. Nakajima ST, Gibson M 1991 Pathophysiology of luteal-phase defiency in human reproduction. Clinical Obstetrics and Gynecology 34: 167–179
20. Belchetz PE, Plant TM, Nakait Y, Keogh EJ, Knobil E 1978 Hypophyseal responses to continuous and intermittent delivery of hypothalamic gonadotropin-releasing hormone. Science 202: 631–633
21. DiZerega GS, Hodgen GD 1981 Luteal phase dysfunction infertility: a sequel to aberrant folliculogenesis. Fertility and Sterility 35: 489–499
22. Strott CA, Cargille CM, Ross GT, Lipsett MB 1970 The short luteal phase. Journal of Clinical Endocrinology and Metabolism 30: 246–251
23. Sherman BM, Korenmann SG 1974 Measurement of plasma LH, FSH, estradiol and progesterone in disorders of the human menstrual cycle: the short luteal phase. Journal of Clinical Endocrinology and Metabolism 38: 89–93
24. Stouffer RL, Hodgen GD, Ottobre AC, Christian CD 1984 Follicular fluid treatment during the follicular versus luteal phase of the menstrual cycle: effects on corpus luteum function. Journal of Clinical Endocrinology and Metabolism 58(6): 1027–1033
25. Sheehan KL, Casper RF, Yen SSC 1982 Luteal phase defects induced by an agonist of luteinizing hormone releasing factor: a model for fertility control. Science 215: 170–172
26. Soules MR, McLachlan RI, Marit EK, Dahl KD, Cohen NL, Bremner WJ 1989 Luteal phase deficiency: characterization of reproductive hormones over the menstrual cycle. Journal of Clinical Endocrinology and Metabolism 69: 804–812
27. Ayabe T, Tsutsumi O, Momoeda M, Yano T, Mitsuhashi N, Taketani Y 1994 Impaired follicular growth and abnormal luteinizing hormone surge in luteal phase defect. Fertility and Sterility 61: 652–656
28. Schweiger U, Laessle RG, Tuschl RJ, Broocks A, Krusche T, Pirke CM 1989 Decreased follicular phase gonadotropin secretion is associated with impaired estradiol and progesterone secretion during the follicular and luteal phase in nornally menstruating women. Journal of Clinical Endocrinology and Metabolism 68(5): 888–892
29. Burrow GN 1991 The thyroid gland and reproduction. In: Yen SSC, Jaffe RB (eds) Reproductive endocrinology. WB Saunders Co., Philadelphia, pp 555–575
30. Yen SSC 1991 Prolactin in human reproduction. In: Yen SSC, Jaffe RB (eds) Reproductive endocrinology. WB Saunders Co., Philadelphia, p 379
31. Chang RJ 1983 Hyperprolactinemia and menstrual dysfunction. Clinical Obstetrics and Gynecology 26: 736–748
32. Seppala M, Hiroven E, Ranta T 1976 Hyperprolactinemia and luteal insufficiency. Lancet 1: 229–230
33. Wenner R 1975 Les antiprolactines. Actual Gynecology 6: 91
34. Franks S, Murray MAF, Jequier AM, Steele SJ, Nabarro JDN, Jacobs HS 1975 Incidence and significance of hyperprolactinaemia in women with amenorrhoea. Clinical Endocrinology 4: 597–607
35. Corenblum B, Pairandeau N, Shewchuk AB 1976 Prolactin hypersecretion and short luteal phase defects. Obstetrics and Gynecology 47: 486–488
36. Spark RF, Pallotta J, Naftoen F, Clemens R 1976 Galactorrhea-amenorrhea syndromes: etiology and treatment. Annals of Internal Medicine 84: 532–537

37. Muhlenstedt D, Bohnet HG, Hanker JP, Schneider HPG 1978 Short luteal phase and prolactin. International Journal of Fertility 23: 213–218
38. El-Mahgoub S, Yaseen S 1980 A positive proof for the theory of coelomic metaplasia. American Journal of Obstetrics and Gynecology 137: 137–140
39. Bahamondes L, Saboya W, Tambascia M, Trevisani M 1979 Galactorrhea, infertility, and short luteal phases in hyperprolactinemia women: early stage of amenorrhea-galactorrhea? Fertility and Sterility 32: 476–477
40. del Pozo E, Wyss H, Tolis G, Alcaiz J, Campana A, Naftolin F 1979 Prolactin and deficient luteal function. Obstetrics and Gynecology 53: 282–286
41. Daly DC 1983 The endometrium and the luteal phase defect. Seminars in Reproductive Endocrinology 1(3): 237–247
42. Kauppila A, Leinonen P, Vihko R, Ylöstalo P 1982 Metoclopramide-induced hyperprolactinemia impairs ovarian follicular maturation and corpus luteum function in women. Journal of Clinical Endocrinology and Metabolism 54: 955–960
43. Board JA, Storlazzi E, Schneider V 1981 Nocturnal prolactin levels in infertility. Fertility and Sterility 36: 720–724
44. Ben David M, Schenker JG 1983 Transient hyperprolactinemia: a correctable cause of idiopathic infertility. Journal of Clinical Endocrinology and Metabolism 57: 442–444
45. DeVane GW, Guzick DS 1986 Bromocriptine therapy in normoprolactinemic women with unexplained infertility. Fertility and Sterility 46: 1026–1031
46. Sherman BM, Korenman SG 1974 Measurement of serum LH, FSH, estradiol and progesterone in disorders of the human menstrual cycle: the inadequate luteal phase. Journal of Clinical Endocrinology and Metabolism 39: 145–149
47. Farhi J, Homburg R, Lerner A, Ben-Rafael Z 1993 The choice of treatment for anovulation associated with polycystic ovarian syndrome following failure to conceive with clomiphene citrate. Human Reproduction 8: 1367–1391
48. Homburg R 1996 Polycystic ovary syndrome — from gynaecological curiosity to multisystem endocrinopathy. Human Reproduction 11: 29–39
49. Dickey RP, Stone SC 1975 Drugs that affect the breast and lactation. Clinical Obstetrics and Gynecology 18: 95–111
50. Souka AR, Medhat M, Rahman HA, Osman M, Sokkary HE 1984 Effect of aspirin on the luteal phase of human menstrual cycle. Contraception 29(2): 181–188 (Abstract)
51. Carr DB, Bullen BA, Skrinar GS, Arnold MA 1981 Physical conditioning facilitates the exercise-induced secretion of beta-endorphin and beta-lepotropin in women. New England Journal of Medicine 305: 560–563
52. Pontiroli AE, Baco G, Stella L, Crescenti A 1982 Effects of naloxone on prolactin, luteinizing hormone, and cortisol response to surgical stress in humans. Journal of Clinical Endocrinology and Metabolism 55: 378–380
53. Shangold M, Freeman R, Thysen B, Gatz M 1979 The relationship between long-distant running, plasma progesterone and luteal phase length. Fertility and Sterility 31: 130–133
54. Prior JC, Vigna YM 1991 Ovulation disturbances and exercise training. Clinical Obstetrics and Gynecology 34: 180–190
55. Schweiger U 1991 Menstrual function and luteal-phase deficiency in relation to weight changes and dieting. Clinical Obstetrics and Gynecology 34: 191–197
56. Wolf LJ, Novotny DB, Meyer WR, Lessey BA, Fritz MA 1996 Dyssynchronous glandular/stromal endometrial maturation: prevalence in normally cycling proven or presumed fertile women. Soc Gynecol Invest 3: 269 (Abstract)
57. Wathen NC, Perry L, Lilford RJ, Chard T 1984 Interpretation of single progesterone measurement in diagnosis of anovulation and defective luteal phase: observations on analysis of the normal range. British Medical Journal 288: 7–9
58. Vande Wiele RL, Bogumil J, Dyrenfrith I, Ferin M, Jewelewicz R, Warren M, Rizkallah T, Mikhail G 1971 Mechanisms regulating the menstrual cycle in women. Recent Progress in Hormone Research 26: 63–103
59. Filicori M, Flamigni C 1988 GnRH agonists and antagonists. Current Clinical Status Drugs 35: 63–82
60. Belchetz PE, Plant TM, Nakait Y, Keogh EJ, Knobil E 1978 Hypophyseal responses to continuous and intermittent delivery of hypothalamic gonadotropin-releasing hormone. Science 202: 631–633
61. Ellinwood WE, Norman RL, Spies HG 1984 Changing frequency of pulsatile luteinizing hormone and progesterone secretion during the luteal phase of the menstrual cycle of rhesus monkeys. Biology of Reproduction 1984; 31: 714–722
62. Filicori M, Butler JP, Crowley WF Jr 1984 Neuroendocrine regulation of the corpus luteum in the human: evidence for pulsatile progesterone secretion. Journal of Clinical Investigation 73: 1638–1644
63. Soules MR, McLachlan RI, Ek M, Dahl KD, Cohen NL, Bremner WJ 1989 Luteal phase deficiency: characterization of reproductive hormones over the menstrual cycle. Journal of Clinical Endocrinology and Metabolism 69: 804–812
64. Wilks JW, Noble AS 1983 Steroidogenic responsiveness of the monkey corpus luteum to exogenous chorionic gonadotropin. Endocrinology 113: 1256–1266
65. Dhont M, Vandekerckhove D, Vermeulen A, Vandeweghe M 1974 Daily concentrations of plasma LH, FSH, estradiol, estrone and progesterone throughout the menstrual cycle. European Journal of Obstetrics, Gynecology and Reproductive Biology 4(Suppl): S153–159
66. Fritz MA, Hess DL, Patton PE 1992 Influence of corpus luteum age on the steroidogenic response to exogenous human chorionic gonadotropin in normal cycling women. American Journal of Obstetrics and Gynecology 167: 709–716
67. Fazleabas AT, Hild-Petito S, Verhage HG 1994 Secretory proteins and growth factors of the baboon (Papio anubis) uterus: potential roles in pregnancy Cell Biology International 18: 1145–1154

68. Joshi SG 1983 Progestin-regulated proteins of the human endometrium. Seminars in Reproductive Endocrinology 1: 221–236
69. Ilesanmi AO, Hawkins DA, Lessey BA 1993 Immunohistochemical markers of uterine receptivity in the human endometrium. Microscopy Research Techniques 25: 208–222
70. Lessey BA, Killam AP, Metzger DA, Haney AF, Greene GL, McCarty KS Jr 1988 Immunohistochemical analysis of human uterine estrogen and progesterone receptors throughout the menstrual cycle. Journal of Clinical Endocrinology and Metabolism 67: 334–340
71. Garcia E, Bouchard P, De Brux J, Berdah J, Frydman R, Schaison G, Milgrom E, Berrot-Applanat M 1988 Use of immunoctyochemistry of progesterone and estrogen receptors for endometrial dating. Journal of Clinical Endocrinology and Metabolism 67: 80–87
72. Press MF, Udove JA, Greene GL 1988 Progesterone receptor distribution in the human endometrium. Analysis using monoclonal antibodies to the human progesterone receptor. American Journal of Pathology 131: 112–124
73. Balasch J, Vanrell JA 1986 Luteal phase deficiency: an inadequate endometrial response to normal hormone stimulation. International Journal of Fertility 31: 368–371
74. Grunfeld L, Sandler B, Fox J, Boyd C, Kaplan P, Navot D 1989 Luteal phase deficiency after completely normal follicular and periovulatory phases. Fertility and Sterility 52: 919–923
75. Batista MC, Cartledge TP, Zellmer AW, Merino MJ, Nieman LK, Loriaux DL, Merriam GR 1996 A prospective controlled study of luteal and endometrial abnormalities in an infertile population. Fertility and Sterility 65: 495–502
76. Keller DW, Wiest WG, Askin FB, Johnson LW, Strickler RC 1979 Pseudo corpus luteum insufficiency: a local defect of progesterone action on endometrial stroma. Journal of Clinical Endocrinology and Metabolism 48: 127–132
77. Jacobs MH, Balasch J, Gonzalez Merlo JM, Vanrell JA, Wheeler C, Strauss JF, Blasco L, Wheeler JE, Lyttle CR 1987 Endometrial cytosolic and nuclear progesterone receptors in the luteal phase defect. Journal of Clinical Endocrinology and Metabolism 64: 472–475
78. McRae MA, Blasco L, Lyttle CR 1984 Serum hormones and their receptors in women with normal and inadequate corpus luteum function. Fertility and Sterility 42: 58–63
79. Gravanis A, Zorn JR, Tanguy G, Nessmann C, Cedard L, Robel P. The 'dysharmonic luteal phase' syndrome: endometrial progesterone receptor and estradiol dehydrogenase. Fertility and Sterility 42: 730–736
80. Hirama Y, Ochiai K 1995 Estrogen and progesterone receptors of the out-of-phase endometrium in female infertile patients. Fertility and Sterility 63: 984–988
81. Lessey BA, Yeh IT, Castelbaum AJ, Fritz MA, Ilesanmi AO, Korzeniowski P, Sun H, Chwalisz K 1996 Endometrial progesterone receptors and markers of uterine receptivity in the window of implantation. Fertility and Sterility 65: 477–483
82. Lessey BA, Damjanovich L, Coutifaris C, Castelbaum A, Albelda SM, Buck CA 1992 Integrin adhesion molecules in the human endometrium. Correlation with the normal and abnormal menstrual cycle. Journal of Clinical Investigation 90: 188–195
83. Bergh PA, Navot D 1992 The impact of embryonic development and endometrial maturity on the timing of implantation. Fertility and Sterility 58: 537–542
84. Hertig AT, Rock J, Adams EC 1956 A description of 34 human ova within the first 17 days of development. American Journal of Anatomy 98: 435–493
85. Horta JLH, Fernandex JG, de Leon BS, Cortes-Gallegos V 1977 Direct evidence of luteal phase insufficiency in women with habitual abortion. Obstetrics and Gynecology 49: 705–708
86. Yaron Y, Botchan A, Amit A, Kogosowski A, Yovel I, Lessing JB 1993 Endometrial receptivity: the age-related decline in pregnancy rates and the effect of ovarian function. Fertility and Sterility 60: 314–318
87. Anderson TL, Hodgen GD 1989 Uterine receptivity in the primate. Prog Clin Biol Res 294: 389–399
88. Batista MC, Bravo N, Cartledge TP, Loriaux DL, Merriam GR, Nieman LK 1993 Serum levels of placental protein 14 do not accurately reflect histologic maturation of the endometrium. Obstetrics and Gynecology 81: 439–443
89. Somkuti S, Appenzeller MF, Lessey BA 1995 Advances in the assessment of endometrial function. Infertility and Reproductive Medicine Clinics of North America 6: 303–328
90. Garcia J, Jones GS, Wentz AC 1977 The use of clomiphene citrate. Fertility and Sterility 28: 707–717
91. MacLaughlin DT, Santoro NF, Bauer HH, Lawrence D, Richardson GS 1986 Two-dimensional gel electrophoresis of endometrial protein in human uterine fluids: qualitative and quantitative analysis. Biology of Reproduction 34: 579–585
92. Soules MR, Wiebe RH, Aksel S, Hammond CB 1977 The diagnosis and therapy of luteal phase deficiency. Fertility and Sterility 28: 1033–1037
93. Annos T, Thompson IE, Taymor ML 1980 Luteal phase deficiency and infertility: difficulties encountered in diagnosis and treatment. Obstetrics and Gynecology 55: 705–710
94. Smith SK, Lenton EA, Landgren BM, Cooke ID 1984 The short luteal phase and infertility. British Journal of Obstetrics and Gynaecology 91: 1120–1122
95. Cummings DC, Honore LH, Scott JZ, Williams KP 1985 The late luteal phase in inferile women: comparison of simultaneous endometrial biopsy and progesterone levels. Fertility and Sterility 43: 715–719
96. Daya S, Ward S, Burrows E 1988 Progesterone profiles in luteal phase defect cycles and outcome of progesterone treatment in patients with recurrent spontaneous abortion. American Journal of Obstetrics and Gynecology 158: 225–232
97. Hecht BR, Bardawil WA, Khan-Dawood FS, Dawood MY 1990 Luteal insufficiency: correlation between endometrial dating and integrated progesterone output in clomiphene citrate-induced cycles. American Journal of Obstetrics and Gynecology 163: 1986–1991
98. Shepard MK, Senturia YD 1977 Comparison of serum progesterone and endometrial biopsy for confirmation of ovulation and evaluation of luteal function. Fertility and Sterility 28: 541–548

99. Li TC, Lenton EA, Dockery P, Cooke ID 1990 A comparison of some clinical and endocrinological features between cycles with normal and defective luteal phases in women with unexplained infertility. Human Reproduction 5: 805–810
100. Abraham GE, Margoulis GB, Marshall JR 1974 Evaluation of ovulation and corpus luteum function using measurements of plasma progesterone. Obstetrics and Gynecology 44: 522–525
101. Hull MGR, Savage PE, Bromham DR, Ismail AAA, Morris AF 1982 The value of a single serum progesterone measurement in the midluteal phase as a criterion of a potentially fertile cycle ('ovulation') derived from treated and untreated conception cycle. Fertility and Sterility 37: 355–360
102. Syrop CH, Hammond MG 1987 Diurnal variations in midluteal serum progesterone measurements. Fertility and Sterility 47: 67–70
103. Graf MJ, Reyniak JV, Battle Mutter P, Laufer N 1988 Histologic evaluation of the luteal phase in women following follicle aspiration for oocyte retrieval. Fertility and Sterility 49: 616–619
104. Lessey BA, Castelbaum AJ, Sawin SJ, Sun J 1995 Integrins as markers of uterine receptivity in women with primary unexplained infertility. Fertility and Sterility 63: 535–542
105. Jones GS 1974 Luteal phase insufficiency. Clinical Obstetrics and Gynecology 44: 255–273
106. Fritz MA 1988 Inadequate luteal function and recurrent abortion: diagnosis and treatment of luteal phase deficiency. Seminars in Reproductive Endocrinology 6: 129–143
107. Hague WE, Maier DB, Schmidt CL, Randolph JF 1987 An evaluation of late luteal phase endometrium in women requesting reversal of tubal ligation. Obstetrics and Gynecology 69: 926–928
108. Aksel S 1980 Sporadic and recurrent luteal phase defects in cycling women: comparison with normal cycles. Fertility and Sterility 33: 372–377
109. Li TC, Dockery P, Cooke ID 1991 Endometrial development in the luteal phase of women with various types of infertility: comparison with women of normal fertility. Human Reproduction 6: 325–330
110. Davis OK, Berkeley AS, Naus GJ, Cholst IN, Freedman KS 1989 The incidence of luteal phase defect in normal, fertile women, determined by serial endometrial biopsies. Fertility and Sterility 51: 582–586
111. Scott RT, Snyder RR, Bagnall JW, Reed KD, Adair CF, Hensley SD 1993 Evaluation of the impact of intraobserver variability on endometrial dating and the diagnosis of luteal phase defects. Fertility and Sterility 60: 652–657
112. Castelbaum AJ, Wheeler J, Coutifaris CB, Mastroianni L Jr, Lessey BA 1994 Timing of the endometrial biopsy may be critical for the accurate diagnosis of luteal phase deficiency. Fertility and Sterility 61: 443–447
113. Huang KE 1986 The primary treatment of luteal phase inadequacy: progesterone versus clomiphene citrate. American Journal of Obstetrics and Gynecology 155: 824–828
114. Rosenfeld DL, Chudow S, Bronson RA 1980 Diagnosis of luteal phase inadequacy. Obstetrics and Gynecology 56: 193–196
115. Wentz AC 1980 Endometrial biopsy in the evaluation of infertility. Fertility and Sterility 33: 121–124
116. Shoupe D, Mishell DR Jr, Lacarra M, Lobo RA, Horenstein J, d'Ablaing G, Moyer D 1989 Correlation of endometrial maturation with four methods of estimating day of ovulation. Obstetrics and Gynecology 73: 88–92
117. Grunfeld L, Walker B, Bergh PA, Sandler B, Hofmann G, Navot D 1991 High-resolution endovaginal ultrasonography of the endometrium: a noninvasive test for endometrial adequacy. Obstetrics and Gynecology 78: 200–204
118. Sakumoto T, Inafuku K, Miyara M, Takamiyagi N, Miyake A, Shinkawa T, Nakayama M 1992 Hysteroscopic assessment of midsecretory-phase endometrium, with special reference to the luteal-phase defect. Hormone Research 37 (Suppl 1): 48–52
119. Glock JL, Brumsted JR 1995 Color flow pulsed doppler ultrasound in diagnosing luteal phase defect. Fertility and Sterility 64(3): 500–504
120. Steer CV, Tan SL, Dillon D, Mason BA, Campbell S 1995 Vaginal color doppler assessment of uterine artery impedance correlates with immunohistochemical markers of endometrial receptivity required for the implantation of an embryo. Fertility and Sterility 63: 101–108
121. Karamardian LM, Grimes DA 1992 Luteal phase deficiency: effect of treatment on pregnancy rates. American Journal of Obstetrics and Gynecology 167: 1391–1398
122. Montes M, Roberts D, Berkowitz RS, Genest DR 1996 Prevalence and significance of implantation site trophoblastic atypia in hydatidiform moles and spontaneous abortions. American Journal of Clinical Pathology 105: 411–416
123. Dodson KS, McNaughton MC, Coutts JRT 1975 Infertility in women with apparently ovulatory cycles II. The effects of clomiphene treatment on the profiles of gonadotropins and sex steroid hormones in peripheral plasma. British Journal of Obstetrics and Gynaecology 82: 625–633
124. Soules MR, Hughes CL, Aksel S, Tyrey L, Hammond CB 1981 The function of the corpus luteum of pregnancy in ovulatory dysfunction and luteal phase deficiency. Fertility and Sterility 36(1): 31–36
125. Fleming R, Coutts JR 1982 Effects of clomiphene treatment on infertile women with normal menstrual rhythm. British Journal of Obstetrics and Gynaecology 89: 749–753
126. Cook CL, Schroeder JA, Yussman MA, Sanfilippo JS 1984 Induction of luteal phase defect with clomiphene citrate. American Journal of Obstetrics and Gynecology 149: 613–616
127. Downs KA, Gibson M 1983 Clomiphene citrate therapy for luteal phase defect. Fertility and Sterility 39: 34–38
128. Quagliarello J, Weiss G 1979 Clomiphene citrate in the management of infertility associated with shortened luteal phase. Fertility and Sterility 31: 373–377
129. Guzick DS, Zeleznik A 1990 Efficacy of clomiphene citrate in the treatment of luteal phase deficiency: quantity versus quality of preovulatory follicles. Fertility and Sterility 54: 206–210

130. Rodin DA, Fisher AM, Clayton RN 1994 Cycle abnormalities in infertile women with regular menstrual cycles: effects of clomiphene citrate treatment. Fertility and Sterility 62: 42–47
131. Marut EL, Hodgen GD 1982 Antiestrogenic action of high-dose clomiphene in primates; pituitary augmentation but with ovarian attenuation. Fertility and Sterility 38: 100–104
132. Yoshimura Y, Hosoi Y, Atlas SJ, Wallach EE 1986 Effect of clomiphene citrate on in vitro ovulated ova. Fertility and Sterility 45: 800–804
133. Fritz MA, Holmes RT, Keenan EJ 1991 Effect of clomiphene citrate treatment on endometrial estrogen and progesterone receptor induction in women [see comments]. American Journal of Obstetrics and Gynecology 165: 177–185
134. Rosenberg SM, Luciano AA, Riddick DH 1980 The luteal phase defect: the relative frequency of and encouraging response to, treatment with vaginal progesterone. Fertility and Sterility 34(1): 17–20
135. Maxson WS, Hargrove JT 1985 Bioavailability of oral micronized progesterone. Fertility and Sterility 44: 622–626
136. Steege JF, Rupp SL, Stout AL, Bernhisel M 1986 Bioavailability of nasally administered progesterone. Fertility and Sterility 46: 727–729
137. Stovall DW, Van Voorhis BJ, Mattingly KL, Sparks AET, Chapler FK, Syrop CH 1996 The effectiveness of sublingual progesterone administration during cryopreserved embryo transfer cycles: results of a matched follow-up study. Fertility and Sterility 65: 986–991
138. Nillius SJ, Johansson EDB 1971 Plasma levels of progesterone after vaginal, rectal and intramuscular administration of progesterone. American Journal of Obstetrics and Gynecology 110: 470–477
139. Bulletti C, de Ziegler D, Giacomucci E, Franceschetti F, Boletti GF, Flamigni C 1995 Direct transport to the uterus of vaginally administered P (first uterine pass effect). Journal of the Society for Gynecological Investigation 2: 357–P362
140. Balasch J, Vanrell JA, Marquez M, Burzaco I, Gonzalez-Merlo J 1982 Dehydrogesterone versus vaginal progesterone in the treatment of the endometrial luteal phase deficiency. Fertility and Sterility 37: 751–754
141. Murray DL, Reich L, Adashi EY 1989 Oral clomiphene citrate and vaginal progesterone suppositories in the treatment of luteal phase dysfunction: a comparative study. Fertility and Sterility 51: 35–41
142. Segal S, Casper RF 1992 Progesterone supplementation increases luteal phase endometrial thickness and oestradiol levels in in-vitro fertilization. Human Reproduction 7: 1210–1213
143. Jones GS, Aksel S, Wentz AC 1974 Serum progesterone values in the luteal phase defects. Obstetrics and Gynecology 44: 26–34
144. Jones GS 1986 Editorial comment. Obstetrics and Gynecology Survey 41: 706–709
145. Fredricsson B, Bjork G, Carlstrom K 1977 Short luteal phase and prolactin [letter]. Lancet 1: 1210
146. Andersen AN, Larsen JF, Eskildsen PC, Knoth M, Micic S, Svenstrup B, Nielsen J 1979 Treatment of hyperprolactinemic luteal insufficiency with bromocriptine. Acta Obstetrica and Gynecologica Scandinavica 58: 379–383
147. Lehtovirta P, Arjomaa P, Ranta T, Laatikainen T, Hirvonen E, Seppala M 1979 Prolactin levels and bromocriptine treatment of short luteal phase. International Journal of Fertility 24: 57–60
148. Saunders DM, Hunter JC, Haase HR, Wilson GR 1979 Treatment of luteal phase inadequacy with bromocriptine. Obstetrics and Gynecology 53: 287–289
149. Fredricsson B, Carlstrom K, Bjork G, Messinis I 1981 Effects of prolactin and bromocriptine on the luteal phase in infertile women. European Journal of Obstetrics and Gynecology and Reproductive Biology 11: 319–333
150. Borenstein R, Katz Z, Lancet M, Caspi B, Ben David M 1980 Bromocriptine treatment of hyperprolactinemic infertility with ovulatory disturbances. International Journal of Gynecology and Obstetrics 18: 195–199
151. Bohnet HG, Muhlenstedt D, Hanker JP, Schneider HP 1977 Prolactin over suppression. Archives of Gynecology 2223: 173–178
152. Griffith RW, Turkalj I, Braun P 1978 Outcome of pregnancy in mothers given bromocriptine. British Journal of Clinical Pharmacology 5: 227–231

37. Endometriosis and adenomyosis

Robert L. Barbieri

Introduction

Endometriosis and adenomyosis are two of the most common gynecologic disorders of women. Endometriosis is the presence of tissue that resembles endometrial glands and/or stroma outside of the uterus.[1] Endometriosis is found most often on the pelvic peritoneal surface in the region of the uterosacral ligaments, the posterior leaf of the broad ligament and on the ovary. Adenomyosis is the presence of tissue that resembles endometrial glands in the myometrium without any clear connection between these abnormally located glands and the endometrial cavity.[2] Both disease processes are steroid dependent, but each disease has its own unique etiologic and epidemiologic features.

Endometriosis has a peak incidence between 20–30 years of age. The prevalence of endometriosis is difficult to determine precisely because it requires surgery for diagnosis; it is estimated to be approximately 5% in women of reproductive age.[1] Adenomyosis has a peak incidence between 35–45 years of age. Based on data from hysterectomy specimens, the prevalence of adenomyosis is approximately 20% of women undergoing hysterectomy and 5% of women of reproductive age.[2] In this chapter the evidence that supports the steroid dependence of each disease will be reviewed and the most common steroid treatments will be discussed.

ENDOMETRIOSIS

Numerous clinical observations suggest that endometriosis is steroid dependent.[3] New cases of endometriosis are seldom diagnosed before menarche or after menopause, two reproductive states associated with low estradiol and progesterone levels. In women with proven endometriosis, surgical removal of both ovaries is usually associated with cure of the disease. In addition, treatment of endometriosis with medications that suppress ovarian steroid production, such as the gonadotropin releasing hormone agonist analogs (GnRH agonists) typically results in atrophy of the endometriosis lesions. Men who are administered high doses of the synthetic estrogen, diethylstilbestrol (DES) for the treatment of prostate cancer can develop endometriosis-like glands in their reproductive tracts. These clinical observations, which demonstrate the central role of estrogen in the development of endometriosis, are supported by many laboratory studies that suggest that endometriosis lesions are steroid dependent.

Many investigators have demonstrated that endometriosis lesions contain estradiol, progesterone and androgen receptors.[4] In normal endometrium, estradiol receptors (ER) and progesterone receptors (PR) increase throughout the proliferative phase. The highest concentration of ER and PR are observed during the late proliferative phase of the menstrual cycle. In endometriosis lesions a similar observation has been made.[5] In normal endometrium, ER and PR decline throughout the secretory phase. Similar observations have been made in endometriosis lesions.[5] Two independent investigators have reported that ER and PR concentrations are slightly lower in endometriosis lesions than in normal endometrium[5,6] but the clinical importance of this observation is unclear. Androgen receptors are also present in endometrium and endometriosis lesions.[7]

The precise mechanisms by which steroids regulate growth and differentiation in reproductive tissues remain to be completely defined. Growth factors such as epidermal growth factor (EGF) and insulin-like growth factors (IGFs) probably play important roles in mediating the effects of steroids on the endometrium. For example, both estradiol and EGF have been demonstrated to promote cell growth in the endometrium.[8,9] In human endometrium, estradiol over a broad range of concentrations appears to promote growth of the endometrium. In contrast, androgens tend to block the growth promoting effects of estradiol.[10] The effects of progesterone are complex, and dependent on the previous hormone exposure of the endometrium and the dose of progestogen utilized. In the normal menstrual cycle, progesterone will act on the estrogen primed endometrium to induce differentiation and reduce cell growth. An exception is the small increase in stromal mitoses induced by progesterone late in the luteal phase. At high doses, progestogens are associated with atrophic changes in the endometrial glands and pseudodecidualization in the endometrial stroma. These characteristic responses of the endometrium to estradiol, androgen and progesterone are the basis for all current hormone strategies to control endometriosis implants.

In addition to hormonal factors, the growth and activity of endometriosis lesions are regulated by the immune system. Women with endometriosis have been demonstrated to have an increased volume of peritoneal fluid, increased macrophage concentration and function, and increased peritoneal fluid concentration of prostaglandins, interleukin-1, tumor necrosis factor and proteases. These alterations may impair oocyte, sperm, embryo and fallopian tube function, contributing to the relationship between endometriosis and diminished fecundity.[11]

Clinical problems common in endometriosis

Women with endometriosis tend to present to clinicians for treatment of one of three problems: pelvic pain, a pelvic mass or infertility. For women with a pelvic mass, surgical intervention is simultaneously both diagnostic and therapeutic. For women with a pelvic mass due to an endometrioma, surgery is the preferred therapy because of the poor efficacy of hormonal therapy in the treatment of endometriomas. In most series, approximately 50% of endometriomas respond to hormonal therapy with a significant reduction in size. Of those endometriomas that do respond to hormonal therapy, the majority return to their original size once hormone treatment is discontinued.[12] Most authorities believe that hormonal treatment has no significant role in the treatment of endometriomas.

For couples with infertility, where the female partner is known to have endometriosis, there is no evidence that hormonal treatment of the endometriosis increases fecundity. Numerous investigators have studied the effects of hormonal treatment of the infertility associated with endometriosis, and no randomized study has demonstrated increased fecundity.[13,14,15] Most authorities do not recommend hormonal treatment of endometriosis as a method of increasing fecundity. Clinical trials suggest that *in vitro* fertilization and controlled ovarian hyperstimulation with or without intra-uterine insemination improves fecundity in infertile couples where the female partner has endometriosis.[11]

For women with endometriosis, a major clinical problem is pelvic pain. Pelvic pain caused by endometriosis is often characterized under three major headings: dysmenorrhea, dyspareunia and pelvic pain not associated with menses. Numerous studies demonstrate that hormonal treatment is efficacious in the treatment of pelvic pain due to endometriosis. All three types of pelvic pain, dysmenorrhea, dyspareunia and noncyclic pelvic pain respond to hormonal treatment.[1] Since endometriosis requires a surgical procedure such as laparoscopy to make a definitive diagnosis, it is most efficient to attempt to ablate or excise endometriosis lesions at the time of the initial laparoscopy procedure. For many women, excision or ablation of the endometriosis lesions will result in improvement in their pain. However, for those women who have persistent pain after the initial surgical diagnosis and treatment of endometriosis, hormone therapy is an effective alternative to a second surgical procedure. Additional well designed randomized studies of surgical versus hormone treatment of pelvic pain associated with endometriosis are required to fully understand the optimal role for each approach.

Numerous hormonal strategies are available for the treatment of pelvic pain associated with endometriosis. The most commonly used strategies include: androgens, such as danazol; the GnRH agonists, such as leuprolide, nafarelin and goserelin; combination estrogen–progestogen medications; and progestogen-only regimens. These hormonal strategies are discussed in detail below.

Hormone treatment of endometriosis: the historical perspective

As noted above, the yin and yang of the steroid control of endometriosis lesions is that estradiol promotes growth and androgens and high dose synthetic progestogens induce regression (Fig. 37.1). The first agents to be used to treat endometriosis were methyl testosterone and testosterone.[16] Preston and colleagues[16] demonstrated that the administration of methyl testosterone caused a decrease in pelvic pain and a regression in endometriosis lesions in women with advanced endometriosis. In a case series using parenteral testosterone, serial biopsy of cul-de-sac and

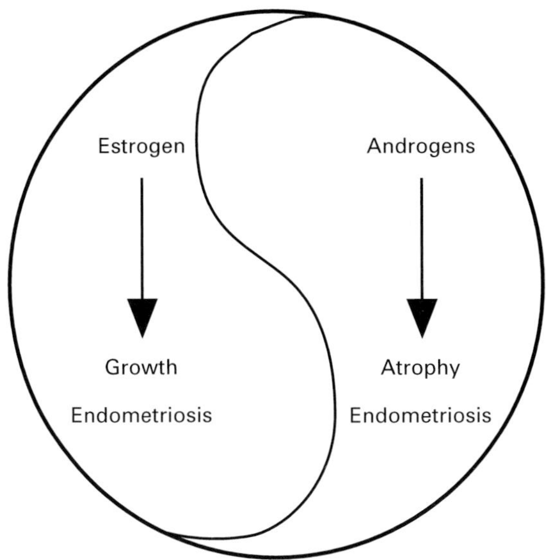

Fig. 37.1 Estrogen and androgens are the yin and yang controlling the growth of endometriosis lesions.

vaginal endometriosis lesions demonstrated atrophy of the lesions after treatment. Not unexpectedly, the women treated with parenteral testosterone became virilized and treatment was discontinued due to the severity of the side effects.

The next hormone treatment of endometriosis to be developed was the high dose diethylstilbestrol (DES) therapy of Karnaky.[17] DES is a nonsteroidal estrogen and at high doses it can cause a paradoxical regression of estrogen-dependent neoplasms such as breast tumors and endometriosis lesions. Karnaky[17] recommended the administration of up to 100 mg of DES daily. This treatment was never evaluated in a randomized controlled clinical trial, but approximately 50% of women treated with this regimen reported a decrease in pelvic pain. Unfortunately, high-dose DES therapy was associated with intolerable nausea and vomiting, and this treatment never become widely utilized.

As noted above, high dose progestogen therapy is effective in the treatment of endometriosis. High doses of progestogens produce pseudodecidualization in endometriosis implants by a direct action on the lesions and by suppression of ovarian estrogen production. High doses of synthetic progestogens saturate the progesterone receptor systems in the endometrial stroma and produce changes ordinarily seen only in pregnancy. These histopathologic changes, including enlargement of the stromal cells and atrophy of the endometrial glands, are referred to as pseudodecidualization. In addition to this direct effect, progestogens also suppress pituitary LH secretion, which can result in a decrease in ovarian follicular development and estradiol production. In 1958 Kistner[18] reported his experience with the use of medroxyprogesterone acetate and other synthetic progestogens to treat endometriosis. At high doses these agents produce amenorrhea and a decrease in pelvic pain in up to 75% of women with endometriosis.

In 1959 Kistner[19] reported that combination estrogen–progestogen oral contraceptives were effective in the treatment of pelvic pain caused by endometriosis when used in a continuous 'pseudopregnancy regimen'. Like progestogen only regimens, pseudopregnancy therapy can produce pseudodecidualization in the endometriosis lesions.

In 1976 danazol was approved for the treatment of endometriosis. Danazol is an attenuated androgen that can directly suppress cell metabolism in implants of endometriosis and can suppress gonadotropin secretion, thereby decreasing ovarian estrogen production.[20] This two pronged approach results in an intracellular milieu characterized by a high androgen and low estrogen effect, which results in the atrophy of the endometriosis lesion.

In the late 1980s gonadotropin releasing hormone (GnRH) agonists were approved for the treatment of endometriosis.[21] GnRH agonists produce an initial rise in gonadotropin secretion, followed by a prolonged block in pituitary gonadotropin secretion and a near complete suppression of ovarian estradiol production. The marked hypoestrogenic state produced by chronic GnRH agonist treatment causes regression in endometriosis implants. One disadvantage of GnRH agonists is that they increase estradiol during the first few days of treatment, prior to full pituitary desensitization. This initial rise in estradiol can cause an increase in pelvic pain for the first few weeks of treatment. In the next few years, GnRH antagonists will be introduced: they can immediately suppress ovarian estradiol production without the agonist phase.[22]

In the early 1990s, antiprogestogens were reported to be effective in the treatment of the pelvic pain associated with endometriosis.[23] Unlike GnRH agonists the antiprogestogens do not cause the severe symptoms of hypoestrogenism. In addition, they are not associated with the marked decrease in bone density that is caused by the GnRH agonists. Although not yet approved for the treatment of endometriosis, many pharmaceutical firms are developing antiprogestogens which may become the first line hormone treatment for the pain caused by endometriosis in the next millennium.

Danazol

Danazol is an isoxazole derivative of 17α-ethinyltestosterone (Fig. 37.2). The pharmacology of danazol is best understood by reviewing its molecular actions.[20] Most drugs work by binding to specific receptors. Danazol is capable of binding to intracellular androgen, progesterone and glucocorticoid receptors (Table 37.1). Danazol also interacts with enzymes of steroidogenesis and circulating steroid binding proteins. By binding to these receptors and enzyme systems, danazol suppresses pituitary gonadotropin secretion, ovarian follicular activity and estradiol and progesterone secretion, resulting in an anovulatory and amenorrheic state. In addition, danazol directly binds to intracellular androgen and progesterone receptors in endometriosis lesions, thereby blocking cell growth and inducing atrophy.

Most natural steroid hormones bind to only one class of intracellular steroid receptors. For example, estradiol binds with affinity to estradiol receptors but does not bind to androgen or progesterone receptors. In contrast, many synthetic steroids bind to multiple classes of steroid receptors.[24]

Danazol binds with high affinity to the intracellular androgen receptor, and in most experimental systems danazol is an androgen agonist. For example, danazol binds to the liver androgen receptor and decreases the production of high density lipoprotein cholesterol. It binds with only modest affinity to the progesterone and glucocorticoid receptors. In most experimental model systems, danazol appears to be a glucocorticoid agonist. In lymphocytes, danazol suppresses mitogen induced cell proliferation, probably by acting through the lymphocyte glucocorticoid receptors.[25] Interestingly, danazol is effective in the treatment of a number of autoimmune diseases, including idiopathic thrombocytopenic purpura.[26] This effect of danazol is probably mediated by glucocorticoid receptors in immune cells. Danazol binds to the progesterone receptor with modest affinity and has been demonstrated to be both a progestogen agonist and antagonist. It is not unusual for some synthetic steroids to display both antagonistic and agonist properties. (For example, tamoxifen is an estrogen agonist in the liver, uterus and bone, but is an estrogen antagonist in the breast.)

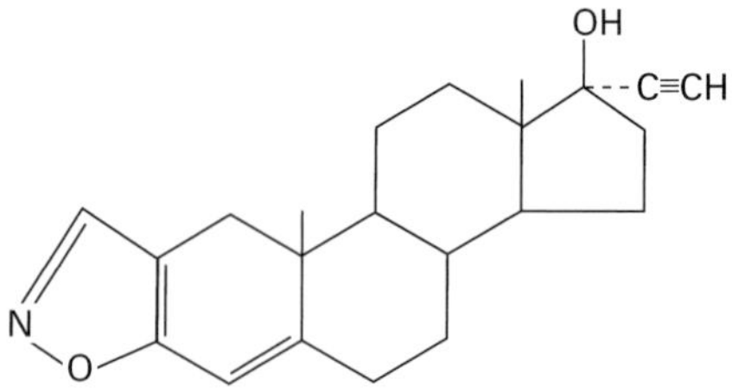

Fig. 37.2 The chemical structure of danazol.

Danazol binds to multiple enzymes of steroidogenesis[27] and suppresses estradiol and progesterone production by a direct action on the ovary. In addition, it binds to the circulating steroid carrier protein, sex hormone-binding globulin (SHBG) and increases the concentration of free testosterone by displacing testosterone from SHBG.[28]

From a clinical perspective the endocrine pharmacology of danazol is best understood by examining its effects on the hypothalamus and pituitary, the ovary and the endometrium. At doses of 400–800 mg daily danazol produces anovulation and amenorrhea in most women. It causes anovulation by suppressing gonadotropin secretion. However, danazol produces far less suppression of pituitary gonadotropin secretion than the GnRH agonists or combination oral

Table 37.1 Danazol binds to intracellular androgen, progesterone and glucocorticoid receptors; it does not bind to estrogen receptors.

Receptor class	Danazol affinity for receptor	Apparent inhibition constant (μM)	Biologic activity
Androgen	High	0.09	Agonist
Progesterone	Moderate	6	Mixed agonist–antagonist
Glucocorticoid	Moderate	7	Agonist
Estradiol	Low	80	No activity

contraceptives. Sakata and colleagues[29] studied the effects of the GnRH agonist depot-leuprolide and danazol on estradiol concentration, immunoreactive and bioactive LH concentration, LH pulse frequency and LH response to GnRH stimulation in women with endometriosis. The GnRH agonist suppressed circulating estradiol to the castrate range. The GnRH agonist also produced a profound suppression of circulating immunoreactive and bioactive LH, LH pulse frequency and LH response to GnRH stimulation. In contrast, danazol therapy suppressed circulating estradiol into the range seen in the early follicular phase of the menstrual cycle. Danazol produced only a modest suppression in bioactive LH and it did not suppress LH response to GnRH stimulation. This finding is supported by observations in laboratory animals.[30] These results demonstrate that danazol produces less suppression of gonadotropin secretion than the GnRH agonists.

Danazol directly inhibits multiple enzymes of steroidogenesis in the ovary. This inhibitory effect is modest but can be clearly demonstrated in both laboratory animals and humans.[31] Danazol has direct actions on the endometrium, and these effects are important to an understanding of the full clinical pharmacology of danazol. Androgens have recently been demonstrated to be potent anti-estrogens in human endometrium.[10] Surrey and Halme[8] studied the effects of estradiol, medroxyprogesterone acetate and danazol on cell proliferation in human endometrial cell cultures. Cell proliferation was monitored by measuring thymidine incorporation into endometrial cell DNA. Estradiol stimulated DNA replication and cell division. Both medroxyprogesterone acetate and danazol inhibited estradiol induced cell proliferation. Since danazol also suppresses ovarian estradiol production, it works to suppress endometrial proliferation by both a direct effect on the endometrium and an indirect effect on ovarian estrogen production. In a recent study of the effects of danazol on the ultrastructure of the endometrium, Fedele and colleagues[32] reported that danazol caused marked atrophy of the endometrial glands and a 'progestational' effect in the endometrial stroma. These studies demonstrate the importance of the direct effects of danazol on endometriosis lesions.

Danazol has been demonstrated to have significant effects on general metabolism. It causes insulin resistance and an increase in circulating insulin concentrations. Golland and colleagues[33] studied the effects of danazol and a GnRH agonist, goserelin, on insulin and glucagon metabolism in nonobese women with endometriosis. The women treated with danazol had an increase in insulin and glucagon response to oral glucose compared to women treated with goserelin. These results have been confirmed by Bruce and colleagues,[34] who reported that danazol treatment resulted in a 55% decrease in insulin sensitivity. For most women, these biochemical changes are probably of little clinical significance. Clinicians should be aware that there are a few reports of the new onset of diabetes associated with the initiation of danazol therapy.[35] In one case, the diabetes resolved after danazol therapy was discontinued.[35]

Danazol produces an increase in body mass and changes in body composition.[36] In women taking 800 mg of danazol daily, the increase in body mass is approximately 4 kg. Most of this increase is in lean body mass (muscle and bone). Body fat actually decreases in the upper body segment during danazol treatment. Occasional patients have reported that their strength in the upper body increased significantly during danazol therapy. This increase in strength was demonstrable by improved performance in certain sports such as the serve in tennis.

Danazol therapy results in major changes in circulating lipids.[37] Danazol produces a rapid reduction in high density lipoprotein cholesterol and in the HDL2 subfraction. In addition, it produces a significant increase in the atherogenic low density lipoprotein fraction. These detrimental effects are probably partially counterbalanced by a decrease in the atherogenic lipoprotein a subfraction.

In the next section, the effects of danazol and the GnRH agonists on bone density in women with endometriosis will be reviewed. Numerous studies suggest that danazol and the GnRH agonists have markedly divergent effects on bone density. Danazol increases bone mineral density and the GnRH agonists are associated with marked decreases in bone mineral density.[38,39]

Clinical applications of danazol

Danazol has been demonstrated to be effective in the treatment of endometriosis in open clinical trials and in randomized prospective studies comparing danazol to GnRH agonists. End points that have been studied include, dysmenorrhea, dyspareunia and noncyclic pelvic pain. Additional end points include 'quality of life' and regression of endometriosis lesions as demonstrated by pre- and post-therapy surgical staging. In open clinical trials of danazol, most studies demonstrate that between 72–100% of women have a decrease in dysmenorrhea, pelvic pain and dyspareunia. Approximately 85–95% of women have a decrease in their endometriosis lesions as demonstrated by surgical staging before and after surgery.[20]

The efficacy of danazol in the treatment of pelvic pain is essentially equivalent to the GnRH agonists. The major difference between the two treatments is in their profiles of side effects. Danazol produces weight gain, bloating, acne, decreased HDL-cholesterol, increased LDL-cholesterol and increased bone mineral density. In contrast, the GnRH agonists are associated with hot flashes, headache, dry vagina, decreased libido and decreased bone mineral density.[40]

Most clinicians agree that patients with a suspected diagnosis of endometriosis must have confirmation of the diagnosis by laparoscopy prior to initiation of hormonal therapy. Danazol should only be administered to women who are not pregnant and who are willing to use a barrier contraceptive. To decrease the risk of prescribing danazol to a pregnant woman, most clinicians initiate danazol therapy after the onset of a normal menses. As an androgen that crosses the placenta, danazol is a known teratogen and can cause virilization of the external genitalia in a female fetus. Brunskill[41] studied 129 women who were exposed to danazol during early pregnancy. Of the 129 women, 12 miscarried and 23 terminated their pregnancy. Ninety four births occurred including 37 males and 56 females. Of the 56 females, 34 were not virilized and 22 were virilized. In the virilized females the most common abnormalities were clitoromegaly, labioscrotal fusion and an abnormal course of the urethra. Virilization was most common at doses of danazol of 800 mg daily, but also occurred at doses as low as 200 mg daily. Virilization was uncommon when danazol was discontinued prior to eight weeks from the last menstrual period. Care should be taken to avoid prescribing danazol to pregnant women due to its potent teratogenic effects.

Danazol is effective in the treatment of endometriosis in doses ranging from 50–800 mg daily. Dmowski and colleagues[42] randomized 27 women to receive one of four different doses of danazol: 100 mg, 200 mg, 400 mg or 600 mg daily for six months. All study subjects had a pre- and post-therapy laparoscopy with surgical staging of their endometriosis. The women receiving 100 or 200 mg of danazol had a 40% improvement in their endometriosis surgical scoring. The women receiving 400 or 600 mg of danazol had a 74% improvement in their endometriosis scores. Similar observations have been made by Rock and colleagues.[43] Based on these findings, and the observation that many women receiving danazol at doses less than 400 mg daily ovulate, we prescribe 400 mg of danazol daily for women with Stage I or II endometriosis. For women with Stage III or IV endometriosis, danazol is initiated at a dose of 600 or 800 mg daily and after a good clinical response has occurred, the dose is tapered to 400 mg daily.

Vercellini[44] studied the effects of very low dose danazol, 50 mg daily, on pelvic pain. Forty two women with endometriosis were randomized to receive either danazol 50 mg daily for 9 months or the GnRH agonist, leuprolide depot, 3.75 mg every four weeks for 12 weeks, followed by danazol 50 mg daily for six months. Significant improvement occurred in dysmenorrhea, deep dyspareunia and nonmenstrual pelvic pain in both groups. Also, menstrual blood loss was significantly reduced in both groups. These studies suggest that a wide range of doses of danazol may be effective in the treatment of pain associated with endometriosis. At doses of less than 400 mg daily, ovulation is not reliably inhibited. Clinicians who utilize low doses of danazol should ensure that the patient does not become pregnant during treatment.

Most clinical trials of danazol have evaluated a six month course of treatment. In individualized cases, the treatment interval may be tailored to be as short as three months or as long as 24 months. For women who use danazol for more than six months, liver function tests should be monitored to ensure that hepatocellular changes have not occurred during treatment. Long-term, high-dose danazol therapy has been associated with the development of two liver diseases, peliosis hepatitis and liver adenomas.[45] There are few contraindications to danazol therapy other than pregnancy and active liver disease.

Danazol therapy is not effective in increasing fecundity in women with infertility and endometriosis. Bayer[46] and Seibel[13] have reported that danazol treatment does not result in improvement in subsequent fecundity in women with minimal endometriosis. Seibel and colleagues[13,46] randomized women with infertility and minimal endometriosis to receive either danazol or no hormone treatment. After 12 months of follow-up, 35% of the danazol treated and 47% of the no treatment subjects became pregnant; while this difference was not statistically different (Fig. 37.3), the trend is against danazol use. That suppressive hormone treatment of infertility associated with endometriosis is not effective was also demonstrated in two studies that assessed monthly fecundity following danazol (0.035) and in controls (0.051);[46] and following buserelin (0.04) compared with controls (0.04).[14]

A major problem in the hormone treatment of pelvic pain associated with endometriosis is that the

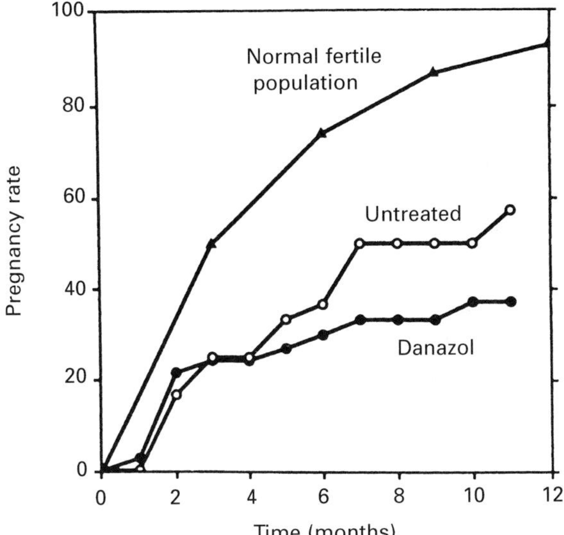

Fig. 37.3 Women with early stage endometriosis and infertility were randomized to receive six months of danazol or no hormonal treatment. Fecundity was similar in both groups during months of follow-up.[46]

disease tends to recur. Following a course of danazol therapy the recurrence of pain tends to occur in up to 50% of women during the first year of follow-up. In order to reduce the rate of recurrence, some clinicians are exploring the use of combination estrogen–progestogen contraceptives as follow up to danazol treatment.

During the early 1980s danazol was among the most commonly used hormone treatments for endometriosis. However, the side effects of this attenuated androgen, including weight gain and hirsutism, have resulted in a gradual decrease in the use of the drug and an increase in the use of the GnRH agonists.

GnRH agonists

The pulsatile release of the native decapeptide GnRH by the hypothalamus is absolutely necessary for normal ovulatory menstrual cyclicity.[47] Continuous infusion of native pituitary GnRH results in down regulation and desensitization of the pituitary GnRH receptor, resulting in the paradoxical and chronic suppression of LH and FSH release. Long acting agonists of GnRH can be produced by changing one or more of the amino acids in the native decapeptide, thereby reducing the metabolic clearance rate of the synthetic analog. The administration of long acting GnRH agonists results in an initial increase in gonadotropin secretion (the agonist phase) followed by a profound suppression of gonadotropin secretion, cessation of ovarian follicular development and a decrease in circulating estradiol to the castrate range (10–15 pg/ml). The GnRH agonists probably suppress gonadotropin secretion by desensitizing and down regulating the pituitary GnRH receptor. The clinical efficacy of all the GnRH agonists is due to their ability to create a reversible medical 'menopause'. This review will focus on three of the most widely used GnRH analogs: leuprolide, nafarelin and goserelin.

Many randomized prospective clinical trials have directly compared the efficacy of the GnRH agonists versus danazol in the treatment of endometriosis. Essentially all the studies demonstrate that danazol and the GnRH agonists have similar efficacy.[21,48] Henzl and colleagues[21] were the first investigators to compare the efficacy of danazol and the GnRH agonist nafarelin in a large randomized, double-blind clinical trial. The study followed self-reporting of pelvic pain symptoms and assessed the status of endometriosis lesions with pre- and post-treatment laparoscopy. Approximately 90% of subjects in each group reported an improvement in pelvic pain. Laparoscopy demonstrated a 43% improvement in the surgical staging score for endometriosis in both the danazol and nafarelin treated subjects. The women treated with danazol reported weight gain, edema and myalgia. The women treated with nafarelin reported hot flashes, decreased libido and vaginal dryness. Similar findings have been reported in a comparison of danazol versus leuprolide[49,50] and danazol versus goserelin.[51,52]

The major problem with the GnRH agonists is the severe hypoestrogenism they produce. In women receiving 3.75 mg of leuprolide or goserelin the estradiol concentration is in the region of 15 pg/ml. This concentration of estradiol is associated with hot flashes, dry vagina, headache and a decrease in bone density. The magnitude of the decrease in bone density caused by GnRH agonist treatment has been the focus of numerous studies. Orwoll and colleagues[53] used dual photon absorptiometry to study the effects of nafarelin treatment on vertebral body bone density. Bone mineral density declined at spinal and femoral sites after both three and six months of treatment. There was a partial, but incomplete return of bone mass towards pretreatment baseline 12 months after completing treatment. These results are similar to those observed by Dawood and colleagues[38] and others.[54]

Dawood[38] randomized 12 women with endometriosis to receive either leuprolide acetate 3.75 mg i.m. every 4 weeks or danazol 800 mg daily. Quantitative computerized tomography was utilized to measure vertebral body trabecular bone density after 24 weeks of treatment and six and 12 months after the completion of hormone therapy. The women who received leuprolide had a 14% decrease in vertebral body bone density after 24 weeks of treatment. The bone density returned toward baseline after therapy was discontinued. Twelve months after completing treatment, bone density was only 3% below pretreatment levels. In contrast, danazol increased bone density by 5% after 24 weeks of treatment. These studies demonstrate the bone loss induced by the GnRH agonists and contrasts this effect with the gain in bone density observed with danazol. Many recent studies have focused on trying to minimize the hypoestrogenic effects of the GnRH agonists without reducing their efficacy in treating pelvic pain caused by endometriosis.

Estradiol response hierarchy

An important concept is that tissues vary in their sensitivity to estradiol. In some tissues, maximal response to estradiol occurs in the region of 60 pg/ml, in other tissues estradiol must be greater than 100 pg/ml to produce a maximal stimulatory effect. Chetkowski and colleagues[55] reported the response of various estrogen responsive tissues to low and high concentrations of estradiol. Chetkowski randomized menopausal women to receive four different doses of transdermal estradiol: 25 µg/day, 50 µg/day, 100 µg/day or 200 µg/day. Before estradiol replacement was instituted, the circulating concentration of estradiol was approximately 10 pg/ml, and the subjects were noted to have elevated urinary calcium excretion, elevated serum gonadotropins, decreased vaginal superficial epithelial cells and elevated low density lipoprotein cholesterol. Transdermal estradiol therapy resulted in a dose dependent increase in circulating estradiol. At replacement doses of 25, 50, 100 and 200 µg/day, the circulating estradiol levels were 28 pg/ml, 25 pg/ml, 65 pg/ml and 110 pg/ml respectively. At the low estradiol replacement dose, 25 µg/day, there was a significant decrease in urinary calcium excretion and FSH concentration. At this dose of estradiol replacement, there was no significant change in LH concentration, vaginal superficial epithelial cells or circulating lipids. This suggests that components of calcium metabolism could be very sensitive to small changes in circulating estradiol, while LH secretion, vaginal epithelial responses and lipids may require larger changes in estradiol concentration. This conclusion is supported by the observation that at estradiol replacement doses of 100 µg/day, LH secretion was significantly suppressed and vaginal superficial epithelial cells demonstrated a significant increase.

These observations demonstrate that there is a hierarchy of responsiveness of different organs to estradiol,[56] (Fig. 37.4). The studies of Chetkowski suggest that the hierarchy of most sensitive to least sensitive estrogen dependent processes is as follows:

1. Urinary calcium excretion
2. Gonadotropin secretion
3. Vaginal epithelial growth
4. Lipid production
5. Liver sex hormone-binding globulin secretion.

The estradiol therapeutic window

The demonstration of an estradiol response hierarchy suggests that an estradiol therapeutic window might exist. At estradiol concentrations of less than 20 pg/ml, endometriosis lesions will atrophy, but bone loss will be substantial. At estradiol concentrations greater than 100 pg/ml, endometriosis lesions will grow, but bone mineral loss will not occur. Perhaps a concentration of estradiol can be found where bone loss is minimal and endometriosis lesions will tend to become atrophic. This estradiol target could be in the range of 30–60 pg/ml[57] (Fig. 37.5).

An estradiol target of 30–60 pg/ml can be achieved in many different ways. One method is to adjust the dose of GnRH agonist utilized. It is difficult to adjust the dose of a parenteral GnRH agonist, but dose adjustment is possible with intranasal drug administration. Hull and Barbieri[58] reported that the dose of nasal nafarelin could be adjusted to achieve a circulating estradiol concentration in the range of 30 pg/ml. Women with endometriosis were started on nasal nafarelin 400 µg daily. After achieving amenorrhea and improvement in pelvic pain, the nafarelin dose was tapered to 200 µg daily on the odd days of the month and 400 µg on the even days. If amenorrhea persisted, the dose was then tapered to 200 µg daily. Using this regimen, many women achieved amenorrhea, a decrease in pelvic pain and a circulating estradiol concentration in the region of 30 pg/ml.

In a study of the effects of low doses of nafarelin, Jacobson[59] observed that doses of nafarelin of 200 µg daily produced no significant loss of bone mineral

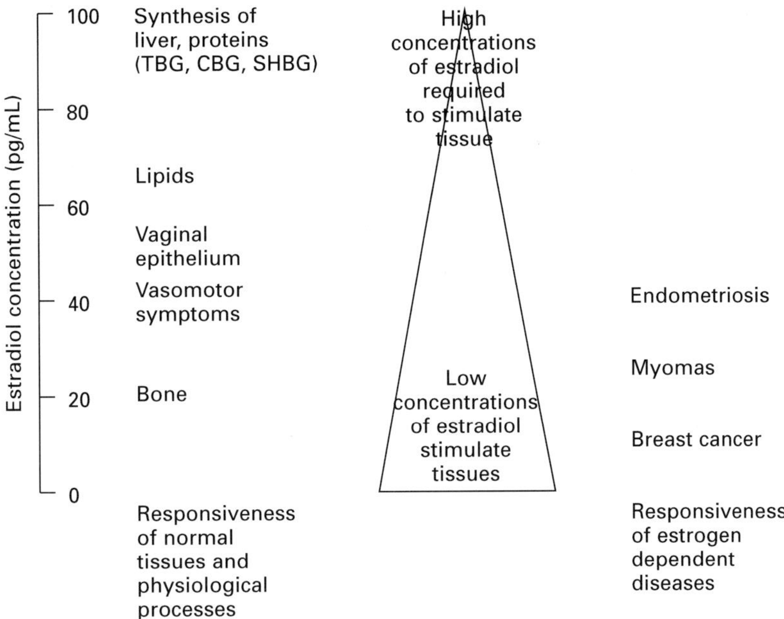

Fig. 37.4 Estrogen response hierarchy. Urinary calcium excretion may be more sensitive to estradiol than vaginal epithelium and lipid concentrations. (From Barbieri RL 1992 Hormonal therapy of endometriosis. Infertility and Reproductive Medicine Clinics of North America 3: 187–200.)

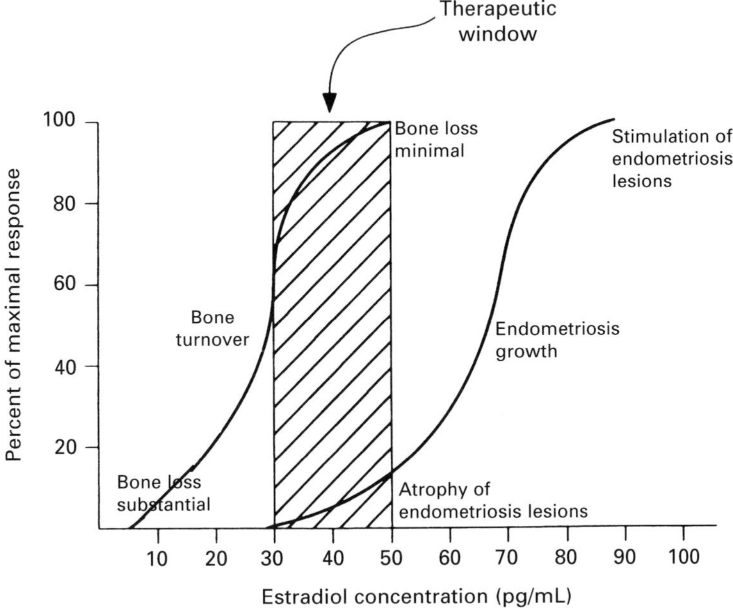

Fig. 37.5 Estradiol therapeutic window. The concentration of estradiol required to cause growth of endometriosis lesions may be greater than the concentration required to stabilize bone mineral density. (From Barbieri RL 1992 Hormonal therapy of endometriosis. Infertility and Reproductive Medicine Clinics of North America 3: 187–200.)

density. In an open study of low doses of nafarelin, Jacobson and colleagues[60] treated 25 women with endometriosis using nafarelin 200 μg daily. At the end of treatment, circulating estradiol was in the range of 25 pg/ml, pelvic pain improved, the surgical endometriosis score improved and bone loss was insignificant.

An alternative to using lower doses of the GnRH agonist is to shorten the length of therapy so that bone loss is minimized. Hornstein and colleagues[61] determined the comparative efficacy of three versus six months of nafarelin therapy in the treatment of pelvic pain caused by endometriosis. The women were randomized to three months (n = 91) or six months (n = 88) of nafarelin 400 μg daily. The reduction in pain scores was similar in both groups, but the loss of bone density was greater in the group treated for six months. Unfortunately, after discontinuation of treatment, symptoms tended to recur.

Estradiol and progestogen replacement

An alternative strategy to achieving the estradiol target is to fully suppress ovarian estradiol secretion with a GnRH agonist and then to replace estradiol using exogenously administered estrogens. This strategy has been studied by Howell and colleagues.[62] Fifty women with surgically proven endometriosis were randomized to receive goserelin 3.6 mg s.c. depot every 4 weeks for 24 weeks, or goserelin for 24 weeks plus 25 μg of transdermal estradiol with 5 mg of medroxyprogesterone daily for 20 weeks, beginning with the second goserelin injection. Both groups had a significant decrease in dysmenorrhea, dyspareunia and pelvic pain scores. Both groups also had a significant decrease in endometriosis score as determined by surgical staging. The bone mineral loss was significantly greater in the group that received only goserelin. Addition of the estradiol–progestogen reduced the magnitude of bone loss, but did not prevent it completely. These findings support the concept of an estradiol therapeutic window, and suggests that the estradiol replacement dose might need to be slightly greater than 25 μg/day.

An alternative approach to GnRH agonist plus estrogen and progestogen replacement is to combine a GnRH agonist with a progestogen alone. The theoretical advantage of this approach is that the endometriosis lesions will not be stimulated by the exogenously replaced estradiol. A theoretical disadvantage of this approach is that progestogens alone do not tend to protect bone mineral density as well as estrogen. Surrey and Judd[63] randomized 20 women with endometriosis to receive either leuprolide 3.75 mg i.m. every four weeks, or leuprolide plus norethindrone, up to 10 mg daily. Both regimens resulted in complete suppression of ovarian estradiol production. In both groups there was a significant decrease in pelvic pain scores and in the extent of the endometriosis lesions as determined by pre- and post-treatment surgical staging. The women receiving combination therapy experienced less severe vasomotor symptoms and vaginal symptoms than the women receiving the GnRH agonist alone. Bone mineral density was decreased in both groups, but the decrease was less marked and more completely reversible at the end of treatment in the group that received both the GnRH agonist and norethindrone. One disadvantage to the norethindrone treatment was a major decrease in high density lipoprotein cholesterol. Similar results have been observed utilizing other GnRH agonists and synthetic progestogens.[64,65] However, in one small study, combined treatment with a GnRH agonist plus medroxyprogesterone acetate did not result in clear improvement in the endometriosis lesions nor in pelvic pain scores.[66] These findings suggest that in regimens utilizing combination GnRH agonist plus progestogens it could be advantageous to utilize 'androgenic' progestogens such as the 19-nor-progestogens rather than medroxyprogesterone acetate.

An alternative approach to GnRH agonist plus steroid replacement therapy is to combine long-term GnRH agonist treatment with a bisphosphonate in an attempt to reduce bone mineral loss. Surrey and colleagues[67] randomized 19 women with endometriosis to one of two combination treatment regimens. Group I received leuprolide acetate, 3.75 mg i.m. every 4 weeks plus norethindrone 2.5 mg daily plus cycles of bisphosphonate treatment with etidronate and calcium supplementation for 48 weeks. Group II received leuprolide plus high dose norethindrone, 10 mg daily. Pelvic pain symptoms and endometriosis lesions were decreased by both treatment regimens. No changes in bone mineral density were noted in either treatment group. In the group that received the high dose norethindrone treatment, there was a significant decrease in high density lipoprotein cholesterol. The investigators concluded that the combination of etidronate with low dose norethindrone decreased the side effects of long term GnRH agonist treatment without adversely affecting clinical efficacy.

Progestogen-only regimens

Many progestogens have been utilized to treat endometriosis, including norethindrone, norethindrone acetate, gestrinone, medroxyprogesterone acetate, megestrol acetate and lynestrenol. From a theoretical perspective the progestogens are probably effective in the treatment of endometriosis because they both decrease ovarian estradiol production, by suppressing pituitary gonadotropin secretion, and have a direct effect on the endometriosis lesions, blocking estrogen action in the lesions and inducing terminal differentiation of the cells ('pseudodecidualization'). Synthetic progestogens can be conveniently divided into two broad classes, the androgenic first generation C-19 progestogens and the less androgenic C-21 progestogens, such as medroxyprogesterone acetate. Both classes of agents appear to be effective in the treatment of endometriosis if used at appropriate doses.

Few prospective randomized clinical trials have been reported using these agents. Most reports used open clinical treatment protocols. Luciano and colleagues[68] reported one of the most thorough clinical studies of the effects of medroxyprogesterone acetate (MPA) in the treatment of endometriosis. Twenty one women with endometriosis were treated with oral MPA, 50 mg daily for four months. Symptoms were monitored with questionnaires and endometriosis lesions were surgically staged before and after treatment. Pre- and post-treatment laparoscopy demonstrated a 68% decrease in endometriosis surgical scores. Pelvic pain symptoms improved in 80% of the treated women. The major side effect of treatment was irregular uterine bleeding, which was reported by 20% of the women. At the post-treatment laparoscopy, the endometriosis lesions were biopsied. Histologic analysis demonstrated that MPA treatment induced atrophy and pseudodecidual change in the endometriosis lesions. The major problem with this study is that it lacked a control group; nevertheless, the study suggests that MPA is effective in the treatment of endometriosis.

Schlaff and colleagues[69] studied the effects of megestrol acetate on the pelvic pain caused by endometriosis. Treatment consisted of megestrol acetate 40 mg daily for up to 24 months. Dysmenorrhea, dyspareunia and noncyclic pelvic pain decreased in 86% of women who completed an adequate course of therapy. Treatment was discontinued by 28% of the women, due to irregular uterine bleeding, weight gain and bloating.

The effects of gestrinone, a C-19 progestogen, on endometriosis was investigated by Hornstein and colleagues.[70] Women with Stage II or III endometriosis were randomized to receive 1.25 mg or 2.5 mg of gestrinone twice weekly. In both groups, pre- and post-treatment laparoscopy demonstrated a decrease in endometriosis surgical scores of 52% and 63% in the two groups. Both groups had a decrease in pelvic pain symptoms. The major side effects were weight gain (mean 2.1 kg), headache, palpitations, hirsutism and irregular uterine bleeding. Fedele and colleagues[71] examined the effects of gestrinone on the endometrium in women with pelvic pain and endometriosis. In the women who became amenorrheic on gestrinone, the endometrial glands were atrophic and the stroma demonstrated decidual changes. In women who did not become amenorrheic on gestrinone, the endometrium had areas with only modest involution and areas where the surface epithelium was lost.

Overton and colleagues[72] have recently reported that the pelvic pain associated with endometriosis can be treated with a progestogen, dydrogesterone, administered only in the luteal phase of the cycle. Women with endometriosis were randomized to receive either 40 mg or 60 mg of dydrogesterone or a placebo for 12 days during the luteal phase of the menstrual cycle. Treatment was initiated two days after the LH surge. The investigators noted that pain was significantly reduced in the women who received 60 mg but not 40 mg of dydrogesterone, and the effect persisted six months after discontinuing treatment.

A major advantage of progestogen-only hormone treatment regimens is that they are substantially less expensive than any available GnRH agonist. In addition, unlike the GnRH agonists, long-term therapy is probably associated with few significant side effects.

Combined estrogen–progestogen regimens

In 1959, Kistner[18] reported that combined estrogen–progestogen contraceptives were effective in the treatment of pelvic pain caused by endometriosis. Kistner proposed using the combined agents in a continuous, not a cyclic, manner. He coined the term 'pseudopregnancy' to describe the intent to use relatively high doses of both estrogen and progestogen over a prolonged period of time in an acyclic manner. Long-term administration of a combination of estrogen and progestogen results in a decrease in ovarian estradiol production by suppressing gonadotropin secretion and decidualization of the endometrium. Most synthetic progestogens have substantial anti-estrogenic properties and produce terminal differentiation (pseudodecidualization) and atrophy in the endometriosis lesions.

There are few prospective randomized trials of pseudopregnancy regimens in the treatment of endometriosis. Noble and Lechtworth[73] reported a small randomized clinical trial comparing the efficacy of pseudopregnancy (mestranol plus norethynodrel) versus danazol in the treatment of pelvic pain caused by endometriosis. Pelvic pain improved in 30% of the women treated with pseudopregnancy and 84% of the danazol treated women. Due to side effects, including irregular uterine bleeding, nausea and bloating, 41% of the women in the pseudopregnancy group discontinued treatment. In a recent randomized trial comparing pseudopregnancy to GnRH agonist treatment, Fedele[74] reported that both treatments were equally effective in reducing dysmenorrhea, but that GnRH agonist treatment was more effective in decreasing the severity of dyspareunia. More randomized trials of combined estrogen–progestogen treatment are necessary to fully delineate the role of this treatment in the management of pelvic pain caused by endometriosis.

Young women with dysmenorrhea and minimal or mild endometriosis could be especially suitable for treatment with combined estrogen–progestogen. In our practice we have used 'mini-pseudopregnancy' treatment with 15 weeks of continuous estrogen–progestogen treatment (five packs of active birth control pills) followed by one week withdrawal of hormone therapy. After the week of withdrawal, 15 weeks of continuous estrogen–progestogen treatment is reinstituted. Using this regimen, many young women with 13 painful menses per year prior to treatment have reported marked improvement and experience only three menses per year after instituting treatment.

Antiprogestogens

Recent studies suggest that the antiprogestogen RU-486 (mefipristone) may be effective in the treatment of pelvic pain due to endometriosis. Kettel and colleagues[75] treated six women with endometriosis using mefipristone, 100 mg daily for three months. All women became amenorrheic and anovulatory. All women had improvement in pain symptomatology, but no significant change in surgical endometriosis scores were observed in this small series. A careful examination of the effects of mefipristone on the endometrium[76] demonstrated a dense cellular stroma with frequent mitotic figures. The glands were irregular in size and shape and demonstrated a weak progestational effect. An advantageous feature of mefipristone treatment is that circulating estradiol levels are in the range of 40 pg/ml when a dose of mefipristone, 50 mg daily is utilized. This concentration of estradiol will probably result in minimal bone loss during chronic treatment. Additional randomized trials are necessary to confirm these preliminary observations, but it is likely that the antiprogestogens will become an important part of our armamentarium to treat endometriosis.

ADENOMYOSIS

Adenomyosis is the presence of intramyometrial aggregates of endometrial glands and stromal cells. In many cases of adenomyosis, the surrounding myometrial cells demonstrate hypertrophic smooth muscle cells. Most women with adenomyosis have dysmenorrhea, noncyclic pelvic pain and menorrhagia. The most common gynecologic conditions requiring hysterectomy are leiomyomata, endometriosis and adenomyosis. Of these three diseases, adenomyosis remains the most difficult to diagnose and the least understood.

A major problem with the study of adenomyosis is that the diagnosis is often difficult to make definitively prior to hysterectomy. In studies of the prevalence of adenomyosis in hysterectomy specimens, investigators have found that between 15–55% of hysterectomy specimens contain adenomyosis.[77–80] Women with adenomyosis often are parous and in the fourth or fifth decades of life.[78] Vercellini and colleagues[80] reported that the risk of adenomyosis was increased 1.5 fold in women with two children compared to women without children. The pathologic diagnosis of adenomyosis often occurs in association with endometrial hyperplasia, leimyoma uteri, endometriosis and endometrial carcinoma. However, these associations could be due to the statistical likelihood that two common diseases would be expected to be frequently found together.

The cause of adenomyosis is unknown. Recently, Pandis and colleagues[81] reported three cases of adenomyosis in which a clonal cytogenetic abnormality, del (7) (q21.2 q31.2), was identified. This cytogenetic abnormality has been observed frequently in uterine myomas. If follow-up studies suggest that adenomyosis lesions are clonal and cytogenetically abnormal, it is likely that the disease is caused by a somatic mutation in a gene that regulates growth and differentiation.

Advances in the treatment of adenomyosis will only be possible if nonhysterectomy techniques are developed to diagnose the disease prior to removal of the uterus. Progress has been made in the development of transmyometrial biopsy, sonography and magnetic resonance imaging techniques to diagnose adenomyosis prior to hysterectomy. Attempts have been made to develop hysteroscopic myometrial biopsy techniques to diagnose adenomyosis.[82–84] An advantage of the hysteroscopic technique is that many women with adenomyosis have menorrhagia, and hysteroscopy is commonly performed as a diagnostic modality in these patients. McCausland[82] studied 90 women with menorrhagia. All the women had hysteroscopic myometrial biopsies. Of the 90 women, 50 had normal uterine cavities by hysteroscopy. Of these 50 women, 33 had endometrial glands and stroma more than 1 mm from the endometrial lumen. McCausland observed a statistically significant correlation between the depth of invasion of the adenomyosis lesions and the severity of the menorrhagia. McCausland treated the women with superficial adenomyosis with hysteroscopic resection, and deep adenomyosis with hysterectomy. Popp and colleagues[83] examined the sensitivity and specificity of automatic cutting needle sampling of the myometrium to diagnose adenomyosis. Although the specificity was 100%, the sensitivity of the technique was low, with a single biopsy having a sensitivity less than 20%. The high specificity and low sensitivity of myometrial biopsy to diagnose adenomyosis was confirmed by Brosens and Barker.[84]

In contrast, vaginal sonography has a high sensitivity but low specificity in the diagnosis of adenomyosis.[85,86] Brosens and colleagues[85] studied 56 women with menorrhagia and dysmenorrhea. In these 56 women, the diagnosis of adenomyosis was made by hysterectomy (n = 34) or magnetic resonance imaging (n = 22). Endovaginal sonography had specificity of 50% and a sensitivity of 86% to diagnose endometriosis by examining uterine body morphometry and myometrial echogenicity. Fedele and colleagues[86] observed similar results. Fedele and colleagues reported that transvaginal sonography had a specificity of 74% and a sensitivity of 80% in the diagnosis of adenomyosis.

Magnetic resonance imaging (MRI) appears to be useful in the diagnosis of adenomyosis. The endometrial glands that are deep in the myometrium have highly specific signal characteristics. MRI is probably the best noninvasive method currently available for diagnosis of this condition.[87,88]

Adenomyosis lesions are sensitive to both estradiol and progesterone, and contain both classes of receptor. Peng and colleagues[89] studied the levels of estrogen and progesterone receptors in 18 cases of ovarian endometriosis and 13 cases of adenomyosis. ER and PR were identified in most samples of adenomyosis lesions. The concentrations of ER and PR were lower in endometriosis and adenomyosis lesions than in matched endometrium. It is likely that the agents that have been successful in the treatment of endometriosis will also be effective in the treatment of adenomyosis.

Unfortunately, there are no randomized, controlled, prospective clinical trials of hormone therapy to treat adenomyosis. To date, the available data consist of case reports and small case series. The GnRH agonists appear to be effective in treating the dysmenorrhea and menorrhagia caused by adenomyosis.[90–93] In the case series reported to date, medical treatment was usually chosen because the patient desired to preserve child bearing potential and refused hysterectomy. GnRH agonist treatment has been associated with a reduction in the size of the uterus, amenorrhea and improvement in pelvic pain.

Danazol has also been demonstrated to be effective in the treatment of adenomyosis in a small case series.[97] Igarashi[94] studied the effects of intravaginal danazol on adenomyosis. Although the intravaginal danazol treatment did not reliably suppress ovulation, it did cause a reduction in the size of the uterus and decreased the severity of the reported dysmenorrhea.

Tamoxifen therapy is now widely utilized in the treatment of postmenopausal breast cancer. Recent case reports suggest that chronic tamoxifen treatment could cause the development of adenomyosis. Cohen and colleagues[95] studied 173 postmenopausal breast cancer patients being treated with tamoxifen. During a five year follow-up period, 14 of these women had a hysterectomy for various indications. Eight women (57%) were found to have adenomyosis. This is a relatively high rate of adenomyosis compared to other reviews.[77–80] A similar observation has been reported by Ugwumadu and colleagues.[96] The estrogen agonist properties of tamoxifen on the uterus might account for this finding.

Conclusion

During the past 50 years there has been a remarkable evolution in the hormonal treatment of endometriosis. Many effective hormonal treatments are now available for the nonsurgical treatment of this common disease. In contrast, no clinical trials of hormonal treatment of adenomyosis have been reported. Much work remains to be done before hormonal treatments for adenomyosis are available.

REFERENCES

1. Hornstein MD, Barbieri RL 1995 Endometriosis. In: Ryan KJ, Berkowitz RS, Barbieri RL (eds) Kistner's gynecology: principles and practice. Mosby, St Louis, pp 251–277
2. Olive DL, Silverberg KM 1993 Endometriosis and adenomyosis. In: Copeland LJ (ed) Textbook of gynecology. WB Saunders Co., Philadelphia, pp 481–504
3. Barbieri RL, Ryan KJ 1986 Medical therapy for endometriosis: endocrine pharmacology. Seminars in Reproductive Endocrinology 3: 339–352
4. Barbieri RL 1992 Hormonal therapy of endometriosis. Infertility and Reproductive Medicine Clinics of North America 3: 187–200
5. Nisolle M, Casanas-Roux F, Wyns C, deMenten Y, Mathieu PE, Donnez J 1994 Immunohistochemical analysis of estrogen and progesterone receptors in endometrium and peritoneal endometriosis: a new quantitative method. Fertility and Sterility 62: 751–759
6. Bergqvist A, Ferno M 1993 Estrogen and progesterone receptors in endometriotic tissue and endometrium: comparison according to localization and recurrence. Fertility and Sterility 60: 63–68
7. Tamaya T, Motoyama T, Ohono Y 1979 Steroid receptor levels and histology of endometriosis and adenomyosis. Fertility and Sterility 31: 396
8. Surrey ES, Halme J 1992 Direct effects of medroxyprogesterone acetate, danazol, and leuprolide acetate on endometrial stromal cell proliferation in vitro. Fertility and Sterility 58: 273–278
9. Mellor SJ, Thomas EJ 1994 The actions of estradiol and epidermal growth factor in endometrial and endometriotic stroma in vitro. Fertility and Sterility 62: 507–513
10. Neulen J, Wagner B, Runge M, Breckwoldt M 1987 Effect of progestins, androgens, estrogens and antiestrogens on 3H-thymidine uptake by human endometrial and endosalpinx cells in vitro. Archives of Gynecology 240: 225–232
11. Barbieri RL 1991 Infertility aspects of endometriosis. In: Droegemueller W, Sciarra JJ (eds) Gynecology and obstetrics, vol. V. Lippincott, Philadelphia, ch 59, pp 1–17
12. Wright S, Valdes CT, Dunn RC, Franklin RR 1995 Short-term Lupron or danazol therapy for pelvic endometriosis. Fertility and Sterility 63: 504–507
13. Seibel MM, Berger MJ, Weinstein FG 1982 The effectiveness of danazol on subsequent fertility in minimal endometriosis. Fertility and Sterility 38: 534
14. Fedele L, Parazzini F, Radici E, Bocciolone L, Bianchi S, Bianchi C, Candianai GB 1992 Buserelin acetate versus expectant management in the treatment of infertility associated with minimal or mild endometriosis: a randomized clinical trial. American Journal of Obstetrics and Gynecology 166: 1345
15. Hughes EG, Fedorkow DM, Collins JA 1993 A quantitative overview of controlled trials in endometriosis associated infertility. Fertility and Sterility 59: 963
16. Preston SN, Campbell HB 1953 Pelvic endometriosis, treatment with methyl testosterone. Obstetrics and Gynecology 2: 152
17. Karnaky KJ 1948 The use of stilbestrol for endometriosis. Southern Medical Journal 41: 1109–1110
18. Kistner RW 1958 The use of newer progestins in the treatment of endometriosis. American Journal of Obstetric Gynecology 75: 264–278
19. Kistner RW 1959 The treatment of endometriosis by inducing pseudopregnancy with ovarian hormones: a report of 58 cases. Fertility and Sterility 10: 539
20. Barbieri RL, Ryan KJ 1981 Danazol: endocrine pharmacology and therapeutic applications. American Journal of Obstetrics and Gynecology 141: 453–463
21. Henzl MR, Corson SL, Moghissi K et al 1988 Administration of nasal nafarelin as compared with oral danazol for endometriosis. A multicenter double-blind comparative trial. New England Journal of Medicine 318: 485
22. Shaw RW 1988 GnRH agonists-antagonists — clinical applications. European Journal of Obstetrics and Reproductive Biology 28: 109–116
23. Kettel LM, Murphy AA, Morales AJ, Yen SS 1994 Clinical efficacy of the antiprogesterone RU486 in the treatment of endometriosis and uterine fibroids. Human Reproduction 9(suppl)1: 116–120
24. Barbieri RL, Lee H, Ryan KJ 1979 Danazol binding to rat androgen glucocorticoid, progesterone and estrogen receptors; correlation with biologic activity. Fertility and Sterility 31: 182–186
25. Hill JA, Barbieri RL, Anderson DJ 1987 Immunosuppressive effects of danazol in vitro. Fertility and Sterility 48: 414–418
26. Wattel E, Cambier N, Caulier MT, Sautiere D, Bauters F, Fenaux P 1994 Androgen therapy in myelodysplastic syndromes with thrombocytopenia: a report on 20 cases. British Journal of Haematology 87: 205–208
27. Barbieri RL, Canick JA, Makris A, Todd RB, Davies IJ, Ryan KJ 1977 Danazol inhibits steroidogenesis. Fertility and Sterility 28: 809–813
28. Nilsson B, Sodergard R, Damber MG et al 1983 Free testosterone levels during danazol therapy. Fertility and Sterility 39: 505–509
29. Sakata M, Ohtsuka S, Kurachi H, Miyake A, Terakawa N, Tanizawa O 1994 The hypothalamic-pituitary-ovarian axis in patients with endometriosis is suppressed by leuprolide acetate but not by danazol. Fertility and Sterility 61: 432–437
30. Shane JM, Kates J, Barbieri RL, Todd RB, Davies IJ 1978 Pituitary gonadotropin responsiveness with danazol. Fertility and Sterility 29: 637–639
31. Steingold KA, Lu JKH, Judd HL 1986 Danazol inhibits steroidogenesis by the human ovary in vivo. Fertility and Sterility 45: 649
32. Fedele L, Marchini M, Bianchi S, Baglioni A, Bocciolone L, Nava S 1990 Endometrial patterns during danazol and buserelin therapy for endometriosis: comparative structural and ultrastructural study. Obstetrics and Gynecology 76: 79–84
33. Golland IM, Vaughan-Williams CA, Shalet SM, Laing I, Elstein M 1990 Influence of danazol and goserelin on insulin and glucagon in non-obese women with endometriosis. Acta Endocrinologica (Copenhagen) 123: 405–410
34. Bruce R, Godsland I, Stevenson J, Devenport M, Borth F, Crook D, Ghatei M, Whitehead M, Wynn V 1992 Danazol induces resistance to both insulin and glucagon in young women. Clinical Science (Colch) 82: 211–217

35. Seifer DB, Freedman LN, Cavender JR, Baker RA 1990 Insulin-dependent diabetes mellitus associated with danazol. American Journal of Obstetrics and Gynecology 162: 474–475
36. Bruce R, Lees B, Whitcroft SI, McSweeney G, Shaw RW, Stevenson JC 1991 Changes in body composition with danazol therapy. Fertility and Sterility 56: 574–576
37. Packard CJ, Shepherd J 1994 Action of danazol on plasma lipids and lipoprotein metabolism. Acta Obstetrica Gynecologica Scandinavica 159 (Suppl): 35–40
38. Dawood MY, Ramos J, Khan-Dawood FS 1995 Depot leuprolide acetate versus danazol for treatment of pelvic endometriosis: changes in vertebral bone mass and serum estradiol and calcitonin. Fertility and Sterility 63: 1177–1183
39. Dodin S, Lemay A, Maheux R, Dumont M, Turcot-Lemay L 1991 Bone mass in endometriosis patients treated with GnRH agonist implant or danazol. Obstetrics and Gynecology 77: 410–415
40. Burry KA 1992 Nafarelin in the management of endometriosis: quality of life assessment. American Journal of Obstetrics and Gynecology 166: 735–739
41. Brunskill PJ 1992 The effects of fetal exposure to danazol. British Journal of Obstetrics and Gynaecology 99: 212–215
42. Dmowski WP, Kaperawakis E, Scommegna A 1982 Variable effects of danazol on endometriosis at four low-dose levels. Obstetrics and Gynecology 59: 408
43. Moore EE, Harger JN, Rock JA et al 1981 Management of pelvic endometriosis with low dose danazol. Fertility and Sterility 36: 15
44. Vercellini P, Trespidi L, Panazza S, Bramante T, Mauro F, Crosignani PG 1994 Very low dose danazol for relief of endometriosis-associated pelvic pain: a pilot study. Fertility and Sterility 62: 1136–1142
45. Makdisi WJ, Cherian R, Vanveldhuizen PJ, Talley RL, Stark SP, Dixon AY 1995 Fatal peliosis of the liver and spleen in a patient with angiogenic-myeloid metaplasia treated with danazol. American Journal of Gastroenterology 90: 317–318
46. Bayer SR, Seibel MM, Saffan DS et al 1988 Efficacy of danazol treatment for minimal endometriosis in infertile women: a prospective randomized study. Journal of Reproductive Medicine 33: 179
47. Knobil E 1980 The neuroendocrine control of the menstrual cycle. Recent Progress in Hormone Research 36: 53
48. Barbieri RL 1990 Comparison of the pharmacology of nafarelin and danazol. American Journal of Obstetrics and Gynecology 162: 581–585
49. Wheeler JM, Knittle JD, Miller JD 1993 Depot leuprolide acetate versus danazol in the treatment of women with symptomatic endometriosis: a multicenter, double-blind randomized clinical trial II. Assessment of safety. The Lupron Endometriosis Study Group. American Journal of Obstetrics and Gynecology 169: 26–33
50. Wheeler JM, Knittle JD, Miller JD 1992 Depot leuprolide versus danazol in treatment of women with symptomatic endometriosis I. Efficacy results. American Journal of Obstetrics and Gynecology 167: 1367–1371
51. Shaw RW 1992 An open randomized comparative study of the effect of goserelin depot and danazol in the treatment of endometriosis. The Zoladex Endometriosis Study Team. Fertility and Sterility 58: 265–272
52. Rock JA, Truglia JA, Caplan RJ 1993 Zoladex (goserelin acetate implant) in the treatment of endometriosis: a randomized comparison with danazol. The Zoladex Endometriosis Study Group. Obstetrics and Gynecology 82: 198–205
53. Orwoll ES, Yuzpe AA, Burry KA, Heinrichs L, Buttram VC Jr, Hornstein MD 1994 Nafarelin therapy in endometriosis: long-term effects on bone mineral density. American Journal of Obstetrics and Gynecology 171: 1221–1225
54. Damewood MD, Schlaff WD, Hesla JS, Rock JA 1989 Interval bone mineral density with long-term gonadotropin-releasing hormone agonist suppression. Fertility and Sterility 52: 596–599
55. Chetkowski RJ, Meldrum DR, Steingold KA et al 1986 Biologic effects of transdermal estradiol. Journal of Clinical Endocrinology and Metabolism 314: 1615
56. Barbieri RL 1991 Gonadotropin-releasing hormone agonist and estrogen–progestogen replacement therapy. American Journal of Obstetrics and Gynecology 165: 1156–1157
57. Barbieri RL, Gordon AMC 1991 Hormonal therapy of endometriosis: the estradiol target. Fertility and Sterility 56: 820–822
58. Hull ME, Barbieri, RL 1994 Nafarelin in the treatment of endometriosis: dosage management. Gynecological and Obstetrical Investigation 37: 263–264
59. Jacobson JB 1990 Effects of nafarelin on bone density. American Journal of Obstetrics and Gynecology 162: 591–592
60. Jacobson J, Harris SR, Bullingham RE 1994 Low dose intranasal nafarelin for the treatment of endometriosis. Acta Obstetrica Gynecologica Scandinavica 73: 144–150
61. Hornstein MD, Yuzpe AA, Burry KA, Heinrichs LR, Buttram VL Jr, Orwoll ES 1995 Prospective randomized double-blind trial of 3 versus 6 months of nafarelin therapy for endometriosis-associated pelvic pain. Fertility and Sterility 63: 955–962
62. Howell R, Edmonds DK, Dowsett M, Crook D, Lees B, Stevenson JC 1995 Gonadotropin-releasing hormone analogue (goserelin) plus hormone replacement therapy for the treatment of endometriosis: a randomized controlled trial. Fertility and Sterility 64: 474–481
63. Surrey ES, Judd HL 1992 Reduction of vasomotor symptoms and bone mineral density loss with combined norethindrone and long-acting gonadotropin-releasing hormone agonist therapy of symptomatic endometriosis: a prospective randomized trial. Journal of Clinical Endocrinology and Metabolism 75: 558–563
64. Surrey ES, Gambone JC, Lu JK, Judd HL 1990 The effects of combining norethindrone with a gonadotropin-releasing hormone agonist in the treatment of symptomatic endometriosis. Fertility and Sterility 53: 620–626
65. Riis BJ, Christiansen C, Johansen JS, Jacobson J 1990 Is it possible to prevent bone loss in young women treated with luteinizing hormone-releasing hormone agonists? Journal of Clinical Endocrinology and Metabolism 70: 920–924
66. Cedard MI, Lu JK, Meldrum DR, Judd HL 1990 Treatment of endometriosis with a long-acting gonadotropin-releasing hormone agonist plus medroxyprogesterone acetate. Obstetrics and Gynecology 75: 641–645

67. Surrey ES, Voigt B, Fournet N, Judd HL 1995 Prolonged gonadotropin-releasing hormone agonist treatment of symptomatic endometriosis: the role of cyclic sodium etidronate and low-dose norethindrone 'add-back' therapy. Fertility and Sterility 63: 747–755
68. Luciano AA, Turksoy RN, Carleo J 1988 Evaluation of oral medroxyprogesterone acetate in the treatment of endometriosis. Obstetrics and Gynecology 72: 323
69. Schlaff WD, Dugoff L, Damewood MD, Rock JA 1990 Megestrol acetate for treatment of endometriosis. Obstetrics and Gynecology 75: 646–648
70. Hornstein MD, Gleason RE, Barbieri RL 1990 A randomized double-blind prospective trial of two doses of gestrinone in the treatment of endometriosis. Fertility and Sterility 53: 237–241
71. Fedele L, Marchini M, Baglioni A, Dell'Antonio G, Motta T 1990 Evaluation of histological and ultrastructural aspects of endometrium during treatment with gestrinone in women with amenorrhea or spotting. Acta Obstetrica Gynecologica Scandinavica 69: 143–146
72. Overton CE, Lindsay PC, Johal B, Collins SA, Siddle NC, Shaw RW, Barlow DH 1994 A randomized, double-blind, placebo-controlled study of luteal phase dydrogesterone (Duphaston) in women with minimal to mild endometriosis. Fertility and Sterility 62: 701–707
73. Noble AD, Letchworth AT 1979 Medical treatment of endometriosis: a comparative trial. Postgraduate Medical Journal 55 (Suppl 5): 37
74. Vercellini P, Trespidi L, Colombo A, Vendola N, Marchini M, Crosignani PG 1993 A gonadotropin-releasing hormone agonist versus a low-dose oral contraceptive for pelvic pain associated with endometriosis. Fertility and Sterility 60(1): 75–79
75. Kettel LM, Murphy AA, Mortola JF, Liu JH, Ulmann A, Yen SS 1991 Endocrine responses to long-term administration of the antiprogesterone RU486 in patients with pelvic endometriosis. Fertility and Sterility 56: 402–407
76. Murphy AA, Kettel LM, Morales AJ, Roberts V, Parmley T, Yen SS 1995 Endometrial effects of long-term low-dose administration of RU486. Fertility and Sterility 63: 761–766
77. Chrysostomou M, Akalestos G, Kallistros S, Papadimitriou V, Nazar S, Chronis G 1991 Incidence of adenomyosis uteri in a Greek population. Acta Obstetrica Gynecologica Scandinavica 70: 441–444
78. Shaikh H, Khan KS 1990 Adenomyosis in Pakistani women: four year experience at the Aga Khan University Medical Centre, Karachi. Journal of Clinical Pathology 43: 817–819
79. Bocker J, Tadmor OP, Gal M, Diamant YZ 1994 The prevalence of adenomyosis and endometriosis in an ultra-religious Jewish population. Asia and Oceania Journal of Obstetrics and Gynaecology 20: 125–129
80. Vercellini P, Parazzini F, Oldani S, Panazza S, Bramante T, Crosignani PG 1995 Adenomyosis at hysterectomy: a study on frequency distribution and patient characteristics. Human Reproduction 10: 1160–1162
81. Pandis N, Karaiskos C, Bardi G, Sfikas K, Tserkezoglou A, Fotiou S, Heim S 1995 Chromosome analysis of uterine adenomyosis. Detection of the leiomyoma-associated del(7q) in three cases. Cancer Genetics and Cytogenetics 80: 118–120
82. McCausland AM 1992 Hysteroscopic myometrial biopsy: its use in diagnosing adenomyosis and its clinical application. American Journal of Obstetrics and Gynecology 166: 1619–1628
83. Popp LW, Schwiedessen JP, Gaetje R 1993 Myometrial biopsy in the diagnosis of adenomyosis uteri. American Journal of Obstetrics and Gynecology 169: 546–549
84. Brosens JJ, Barker FG 1995 The role of myometrial biopsies in the diagnosis of adenomyosis. Fertility and Sterility 63: 1347–1349
85. Brosens JJ, de Souza NM, Barker FG, Paraschos T, Winston RM 1995 Endovaginal ultrasonography in the diagnosis of adenomyosis uteri: identifying the predictive characteristics. British Journal of Obstetrics and Gynaecology 102: 471–474
86. Fedele L, Bianchi S, Dorta M, Arcaini L, Zanotti F, Carinelli S 1992 Transvaginal ultrasonography in the diagnosis of diffuse adenomyosis. Fertility and Sterility 58: 94–97
87. Arnold LL, Ascher SM, Simon JA 1994 Familial adenomyosis: a case report. Fertility and Sterility 61: 1165–1167
88. Arnold LL, Ascher SM, Schruefer JJ, Simon JA 1995 The nonsurgical diagnosis of adenomyosis. Obstetrics and Gynecology 86: 461–465
89. Peng Z, Liu S, He B, Xi M, Cao Z 1993 [Study on estrogen and progesterone receptors in endometriosis and adenomyosis]. Hua Hsi I Ko Ta Hsueh Hsueh Pao 24: 290–292
90. Silva PD, Perkins HE, Schauberger CW 1994 Live birth after treatment of severe adenomyosis with a gonadotropin-releasing hormone agonist. Fertility and Sterility 61: 171–172
91. Hirata JD, Moghissi KS, Ginsburg KA 1993 Pregnancy after medical therapy of adenomyosis with a gonadotropin-releasing hormone agonist. Fertility and Sterility 59: 444–445
92. Nelson JR, Corson SL 1993 Long-term management of adenomyosis with a gonadotropin-releasing hormone agonist: a case report. Fertility and Sterility 59: 441–443
93. Grow DR, Filer RB 1991 Treatment of adenomyosis with long-term GnRH analogues: a case report. Obstetrics and Gynecology 78: 538–539
94. Igarashi M 1990 A new therapy for pelvic endometriosis and uterine adenomyosis: local effect of vaginal and intrauterine danazol application. Asia and Oceania Journal of Obstetrics and Gynaecology 16: 1–12
95. Cohen I, Beyth Y, Tepper R, Figer A, Shapira J, Cordoba M, Yigael D, Altaras MM 1995 Adenomyosis in postmenopausal breast cancer patients treated with tamoxifen: a new entity? Gynecological Oncology 58: 86–91
96. Ugwumadu AH, Bower D, Ho PK 1993 Tamoxifen induced adenomyosis and adenomyomatous endometrial polyp. British Journal of Obstetrics and Gynaecology 100: 386–388

38. Leiomyomata

Beverley J. Vollenhoven David L. Healy

Introduction

Uterine leiomyomata ('fibroids' — a patent misnomer) are the commonest solid tumors in women. They are neoplasms of the smooth muscle of the uterus, but they also contain varying amounts of fibrous tissue. They are said to occur in 20–25% of females over the age of 30 years. However, this figure is probably an underestimate and they are more likely to occur in about 50% of women.[1]

CLINICAL FEATURES

The clinical features of uterine fibroids are variable. In fact, 50% of women with fibroids are thought to be asymptomatic and these tumors are then diagnosed on routine pelvic examination or at an antenatal examination.[2] If symptoms are present, their nature and severity usually depend on the size, site and the number of fibroids present.

Fibroids are classified according to their position in the uterus, being submucous, intramural or subserosal. Subserosal fibroids may become pedunculated and submucous fibroids may become polypoidal. However, multiple tumors are often present, which may cause considerable uterine enlargement and both cavity and outer contour distortion (Figs 38.1, 38.2).

Menstrual abnormalities

Approximately 30% of women with fibroids have been reported to have menstrual abnormalities, most often menorrhagia.[2] This figure may be controversial as 50% of women who complain of menorrhagia do not have excessive menstrual loss (>80 mL/period) when this is measured objectively.[3] Nevertheless, when menorrhagia truly exists in a patient with fibroids it can be torrential, causing a rapid fall in hemoglobin (Hb). When this occurs on a monthly basis not only are the medical consequences severe, but the social effects may also be of great concern.

Menorrhagia can occur when the uterine cavity surface area is expanded and distorted by submucous fibroids. However, in over 50% of cases, submucous fibroids are not present but excessive uterine bleeding occurs. It is now thought that menorrhagia can be

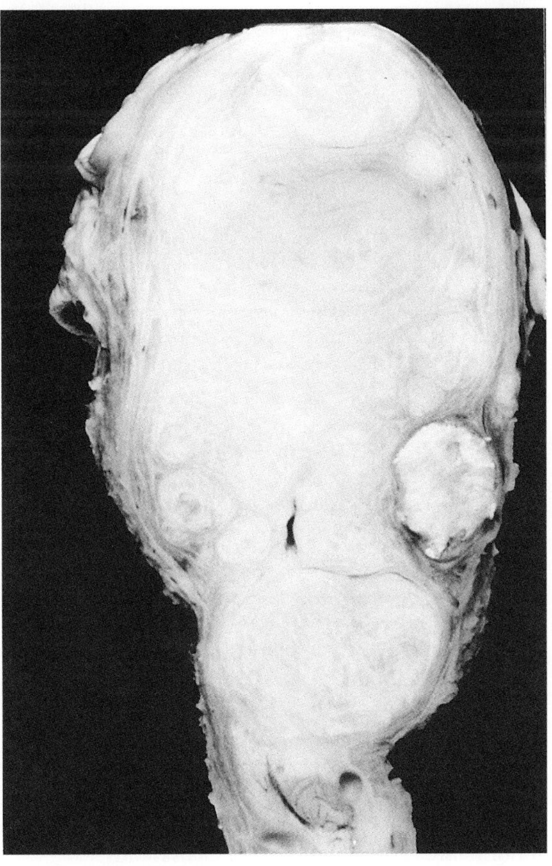

Fig. 38.1 An enlarged uterus showing multiple fibroids. The fibroids are submucosal (causing cavity distortion), intramural and subserosal. The subserosal fibroid has undergone degeneration. (See color plate p3.)

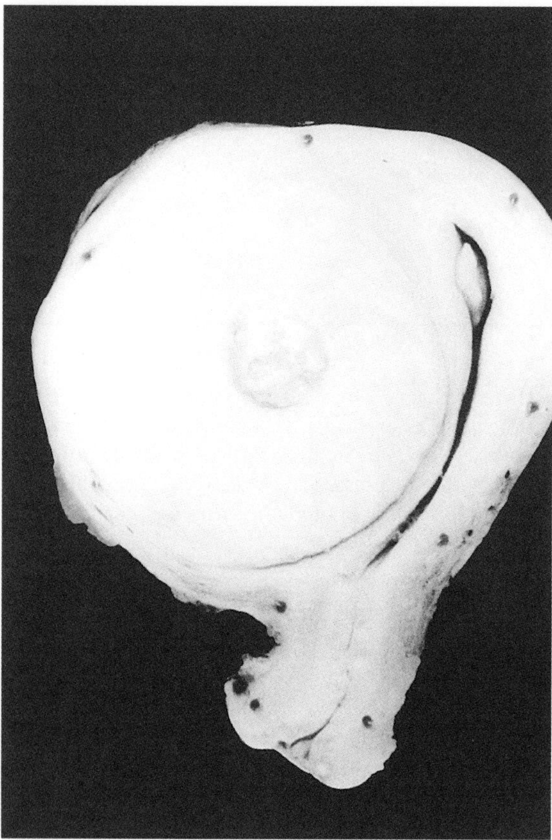

Fig. 38.2 A large intramural fibroid with central degeneration and a single polypoid submucous fibroid. (See color plate p3.)

associated with fibroids no matter their location in the uterus.[4]

Unsubstantiated theories for the increased bleeding are: increased vascularity of the uterus, anovulatory cycles and abnormal myometrial contraction.[2] By radiographic methods, Farrer-Brown and associates[5,6] showed that fibroids arising at various sites in the uterus could cause congestion and dilation of endometrial venous plexuses by impinging upon and obstructing veins of the myometrium. The resultant obstruction could then cause endometrial venule ectasia which could play a role in enhanced uterine bleeding. Alternatively, it has been suggested that fibroid-associated menorrhagia can be caused by an abnormality in locally produced eicosanoids.

Pain and pressure effects

Chronic dull backache may be present when the fibroid is of moderate size in a retroverted uterus. Dysmenorrhea is also common. Acute pain may be present with red degeneration, necrosis or with torsion of a pedunculated fibroid. Acute pain has also been noted in association with the use of the combined birth control pill (BCP), most probably due to haemorrhage within these tumors.[7] There has also been a case report of three women who developed severe abdominal pain while taking gonadotropin-releasing hormone agonists (GnRHa) for fibroid shrinkage. The pain suffered by these patients was thought due to acute necrosis of their fibroids secondary to the hypoestrogenism induced by the GnRHa.[8]

Pressure symptoms depend on the area of impingement of the fibroid, its size and its position within the uterus, i.e. anterior, posterior or inferior near the cervix. There may be bladder, bowel, renal or rarely vascular symptoms. The most common pressure symptom is frequency of micturition due to pressure on the bladder from an anteriorly placed fibroid.

Fibroids and infertility

The role of fibroids as a causal factor in infertility remains controversial. It is obvious that obstruction of both fallopian tubes by fibroids or gross uterine cavity distortion could contribute to infertility. However, these tumors are common and occur in both apparently normally fertile and also infertile women. There is no clear evidence that the mere presence of fibroids is causally linked to infertility, especially when small and not impinging on the uterine cavity. A review by Buttram and Reiter[2] of 677 patients undergoing major operations for preservation or enhancement of fertility revealed that in only 2% of patients undergoing myomectomy could no other cause for infertility be found. This suggests that uterine fibroids alone are an infrequent cause of infertility. These authors also showed that the size of the fibroid at myomectomy was the most important prognostic factor for subsequent fertility.

Once again, a number of unsubstantiated theories have been presented to explain infertility in women with fibroids. These are: distortion of the endometrial cavity, greater distance for sperm travel, impairment of blood supply to the endometrium causing atrophy and ulceration of the endometrium, thereby preventing implantation.[9]

Fibroids have also been associated with a higher rate of miscarriage, particularly if implantation occurs in relation to a submucous fibroid. Buttram and Reiter,[2] in their review of myomectomies, reported a

41% miscarriage rate preoperatively and a 19% rate postoperatively.

Fibroids and pregnancy

An overall view of the importance of fibroids in association with pregnancy was reported by Hasan and associates.[10] In a review of obstetric records spanning 10 years, they showed that the incidence of uterine fibroids in pregnancy was 0.1%, that a significant number of these women (43%) had had a history of infertility prior to pregnancy, that the most common antenatal complication was malpresentation, that the red degeneration rate was 10%, and that the caesarian section rate was 73%. The most common reason for this type of delivery was due to obstructed labor secondary to lower uterine/cervical fibroids.

It has been axiomatic that fibroids enlarge in pregnancy. This has now been disputed by two prospective ultrasound studies, both of which showed that 70–80% of tumors did not enlarge.[11,12] However, in the first study, 70% of women suffered mild abdominal pain, 10% required admission to hospital for severe pain, 10% of pregnancies were complicated by preterm labor and 21% ended in cesarian section.[11] A number of other ultrasound studies have shown that the location of a fibroid in relation to the site of the placenta is probably more important in predicting pregnancy outcome than the actual size of the fibroid alone.[13–15] Conversely, Davis and others[16] in another prospective ultrasound study reported that size, number or location of the fibroid(s) had no influence on outcome. Nevertheless, they reported a 37% incidence of obstetric complications.

ETIOLOGY

Fibroids are only known to occur during the reproductive years and to regress after menopause — whether this is a natural event or induced by surgery, radiation or mimicked by repetitive administration of GnRHa. This circumstantial evidence suggests that estrogen (E) plays a part in fibroid growth.

Risk factors for fibroid growth

Nulliparity

There is a strong association between nulliparity and the incidence of fibroids. The relative risk of fibroids has been shown to decrease with each additional term pregnancy, the risk being reduced to one fifth with five term pregnancies compared with the nulliparous woman.[17] It is an increased number of menstrual cycles rather than an increase in serum estradiol (E_2) per cycle that is the risk factor because it has been shown that women with fibroids have similar circulating E_2 levels to women who do not.[18]

Obesity

Obesity increases the risk of fibroid development by 21% with each 10 kg weight gain.[17] There may be two reasons for this. First, there is peripheral conversion by fat aromatase of circulating androgens to oestrone. Secondly, in the obese, there is a decrease in the hepatic production of sex hormone-binding globulin (SHBG) — a carrier for E_2.[19] This lowered concentration of SHBG may result in higher levels of 'free' physiologically active E_2. Therefore, obesity confers a relative hyperestrogenic state which may predispose to fibroid growth.

Race

Epidemiological surveys in the USA have shown that fibroids are 2–9 times more common in blacks than in whites.[17,20] This may be due to genetic factors because, anecdotally, there is often a positive family history in women who develop fibroids. Alternatively, it has been suggested that the uterine environment in these black women may be different so as to predispose them to fibroid growth.

Protective factors against fibroid growth

Cigarette smoking

Women who smoke 10 cigarettes per day have an 18% lowered risk of fibroid development compared with nonsmokers.[17] Smoking is antiestrogenic and smokers undergo menopause on average 3 years earlier than nonsmokers.

The birth control pill (BCP)

The combined BCP reduces the risk of fibroids by approximately 17% with each five years of usage. It is thought that this mechanism of protection acts through the progestogenic component.[17]

Steroid factors

Estrogen has been implicated in the growth of fibroids, because:

1. Fibroids only grow in the reproductive years
2. Fibroids regress after the menopause

3. Estrogen and/or progesterone receptor (ER, PR) concentrations (both cytosolic and nuclear) have been shown to be greater in fibroids than in surrounding myometrium (reviewed by Vollenhoven et al 1994[21])
4. Immunohistochemistry has shown a greater staining intensity and a greater ER:PR ratio in fibroids than myometrium.[22]

In contrast to the reports that have shown an increase in ER and/or PR concentration in fibroids compared with myometrium, there have been others that have contradicted these findings (reviewed by Vollenhoven et al 1994[21]). The reason for these contradictory findings may have been recently established. Two forms of the nuclear PR have been described in fibroids and myometrium. Receptor A is 94 kDa and receptor B is 120 kDa. They both result from the same gene by transcription from different promoters which are regulated independently *in vitro*. In the presence of P the two forms activate transcription but are functionally different. In the presence of a P antagonist, the B form activates transcription inappropriately so that the antagonist behaves as a partial agonist. Estrogen responsiveness is conferred on the part of the gene from which the A form is produced and therefore it is probable that there will be consequences for the regulation of PR by E.[23]

Receptor binding studies in GnRHa treated women

Pasqualini and associates[24] showed a significant decrease in PR content in both fibroids and myometrium after treatment with these agents. However, Rein and colleagues[25] showed that the PR content was unchanged and that the fibroid ER content (no change in myometrial content) was six times greater than in the fibroids from untreated women. They explained the increased ER content in pretreated fibroids as possibly being due to an altered receptor metabolism causing an increased sensitivity of fibroids to low levels of E. This, acting in conjunction with the low P levels in GnRHa pretreated women, may then result in overexpression of the ER. Lumsden and coworkers[26] confirmed increased ER levels in women pretreated with GnRHa but showed that the PR content was decreased. Vollenhoven and associates[21] showed that there was no difference in ER or PR binding between treated and untreated fibroids and that there was also no difference in the mRNA expression of either of the receptors in these tissues. They postulated that fibroids shrink when these agents are administered because of a decrease in the ligand concentration (E_2 and P) available to react with their respective receptors.

Peptide growth factors

Insulin-like growth factors (IGF)

Serum IGF-I levels in women with myomata have been found to be similar to the levels in myoma-free women.[27] Straum and others[28] have shown that IGF-I (10 ng/mL and 100 ng/mL), but not IGF-II, preferentially stimulates myoma cells in monolayer culture. These results appear to confirm a paracrine or autocrine role for this factor in the growth of myomata.

The mRNA expression of IGF-I and IGF-II in fibroids and myometrium have been investigated by Hoppener and others,[29] Boehm and associates[30] and Vollenhoven and colleagues.[31] The first two studies found that IGF-I and IGF-II mRNA expression were greater in myomata than in myometrium. However, both these studies were limited by small numbers of patients and neither addressed the very important issue of the expression of the insulin-like growth factor binding proteins (IGFBPs) which are known to modulate IGF action, at least *in vitro*. Vollenhoven et al[31] investigated the mRNA expression of IGF-I, IGF-II and IGFBP1–3 in myomata, corresponding myometrium and in GnRHa pretreated samples. They showed that in fibroids compared with myometrium from 20 untreated women:

1. The IGF-I mRNA expression was no different
2. There was a 12 fold increase in IGF-II mRNA abundance in fibroids compared with myometrium
3. IGFBP-1 mRNA was not detected in fibroids or myometrium
4. There was no difference in the relative abundance for IGFBP-2 mRNA
5. There was a two fold decrease in IGFBP-3 mRNA abundance in fibroids compared with myometrium, although protein levels appeared to be similar (IGFBP-2 and IGFBP-3).

These findings led them to postulate that the differential expression of IGF-II and IGFBP-3 mRNA expression between myomata and myometrium leads to an increase in the bioavailability of IGF-II in these tissues, thereby leading to fibroid growth. When IGFBP-2 mRNA was investigated, because of the differential expression of IGF-II between fibroids and myometrium, this would further lead to an increase in the bioavailability of IGF-II in these tissues. Unpublished findings by Vollenhoven and others also show that growth hormone (GH) is probably not the regulatory factor of IGF-I and IGFBP-3 in these tissues as the mRNA for its receptor (examined by Northern blot analysis) was not present in these sites.

Receptor studies have shown that IGF-I receptor (type I) numbers, but not IGF-II receptor (type II) numbers, have been found to be greater in fibroids compared with myometrium.[32,33] It can be presumed that the increased amount of IGF-II in fibroids[31] may interact with the type I and/or the type II receptors leading to a greater growth promoting effect in fibroids compared with the myometrium. The same may also apply to IGF-I given the increased receptor numbers in fibroids as compared with myometrium. In fact, Jones and Clemmons[34] have suggested that most of the actions of IGF-I and IGF-II are mediated by the type I receptor while the type II receptor may be involved in the uptake and degradation of IGF-II.

Epidermal growth factor (EGF) and transforming growth factor alpha and beta (TGFα and β)

EGF binding was first demonstrated in human endometrium, myometrium and fibroids by Hofmann and others.[35] They showed the presence of high affinity binding sites for EGF with no significant variation in EGF binding between the phases of the cycle, the smooth muscle content of the tissue, or between myometrium and fibroid. This was confirmed by Lumsden and colleagues.[36] Conversely, Tommola and associates[32] and Fayed and coworkers[37] showed a decreased binding of EGF, due to decreased receptor concentration, in fibroid membranes compared with normal myometrial membranes. In women pretreated with GnRHa, binding of EGF to fibroid cell membranes has been shown to be lower when compared with fibroids from untreated patients. However, EGF binding to the myometrium was found to be unchanged.[36] Part of the role of E_2 in fibroid growth may be mediated by EGF.[36]

Using immunohistochemistry, Leone and others[38] showed EGF receptor localization to be mainly in endothelial cell membranes in both fibroids and myometrium. They also showed, in women pretreated with GnRHa, that there was a decrease in fibroid EGF binding. They concluded, therefore, that the reduction in fibroid size in GnRHa pretreated women may be related to a decrease in the blood supply in these tumors and that this may be EGF-mediated. Matta and others[39] demonstrated, by Doppler ultrasound, that hypo-estrogenism leads to a decrease in uterine arterial blood flow.

By quantitative RT-PCR it has been shown that EGF mRNA expression in fibroids was greater than that in myometrium but only in the secretory phase. This raises the possibility that P may also be an important mediator in fibroid growth.[40]

Platelet derived growth factor (PDGF)

PDGF binding sites have been found in greater numbers in fibroid as compared with normal myometrium but the receptor affinity was found to be greater in myometrium than fibroids.[37] These findings led Fayed et al to conclude that this factor may not be important in fibroid growth. The mRNA expression of PDGF has been found to be the same in fibroid and myometrium.[30] Vollenhoven et al (unpublished) have also concluded that PDGF is probably not important in fibroid growth as the mRNA expression in these tissues is present only at very low levels.

Connective tissue factors

The extracellular matrix proteins — collagen type I and III and fibronectin — have been investigated in fibroids and adjacent myometrium. It was shown that both collagen type I and III mRNA expression are increased in fibroids as compared with myometrium in patients in the proliferative phase, not the secretory phase, of the cycle. There was no change in fibronectin mRNA expression between fibroids and myometrium. Immunohistochemistry localized fibronectin around individual smooth muscle cells, collagen type I across the extracellular matrix and in the cytoplasm of smooth muscle cells and collagen type III in the extracellular matrix.[41] Oestrogen has been found to stimulate collagen type I and III mRNA expression as well as the mRNA expression of the gap junction protein connexin 43.[42]

Chromosomal features of fibroids

The cytogenetic analysis of fibroids has revealed normal karyotypes in about 50% of cases, as well as a variety of chromosomal aberrations such as deletions, trisomies and translocations.[43] The cytogenetic changes are dissimilar to those reported in leiomyosarcomas, but are similar to those reported in lipomas.[44] Recent molecular endocrinology has concentrated on the chromosomal abnormalities involving chromosome 12, in particular 12q13–15. Sequencing of clones from a 40 kb section of the abnormal region has led to the identification of a candidate gene which may be related to the genesis of fibroids.[45]

INVESTIGATIONS AND DIAGNOSIS

The diagnosis of fibroids has traditionally been undertaken by palpation of a pelvic mass in a woman who presents with symptoms suggesting this condition. The most important differential diagnosis of this condition is an ovarian mass.

Imaging techniques

Ultrasound (US)

Pelvic US is the major imaging technique for the diagnosis of fibroids. The typical US appearance of a fibroid is a homogeneous, hypoechoic area within the uterine wall causing deformity of the uterine contour. However, if on the posterior or lateral uterine walls, it may be indistinguishable from an adnexal or pouch of Douglas mass. If multiple small fibroids are present the appearance may be only of globular uterine enlargement. Submucous fibroids may distort the linear central endometrial echo. The sonographic texture on US depends on the relative ratio of fibrous tissue to smooth muscle and to the presence or absence of degeneration[46] (Fig. 38.3).

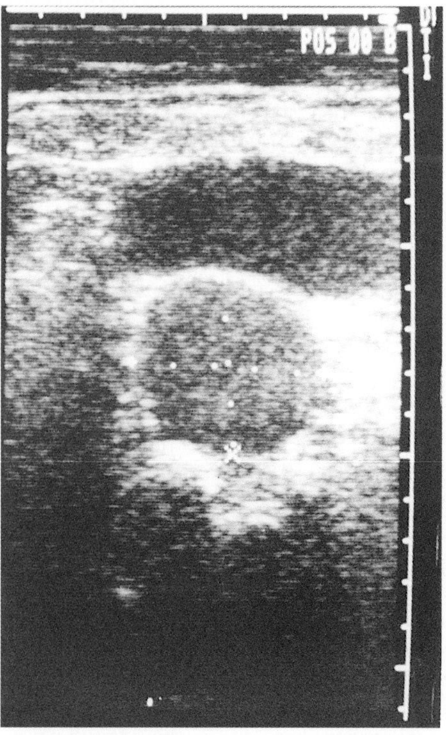

Fig. 38.3 The typical appearance of a fibroid on transabdominal ultrasound. (See also color plate p4.)

Hysterosalpingography (HSG)

In the past this was the gold standard for the identification of a submucous leiomyoma. On HSG, fibroids are seen as smooth or irregular, single or multiple, filling defects with or without gross distortion of the uterine cavity. A subserous fibroid has no definitive sign, but may be seen as a soft tissue mass compressing, displacing or occluding the fallopian tube.[46] Hysterosalpingography has now largely been replaced by hysteroscopy (Fig. 38.4) as it allows histopathological diagnosis and treatment in one procedure.

CT scan

This is not the primary modality for the detection of these tumors. Usually, the fibroid is found by chance when the patient is having this procedure for another reason. The common findings on CT examination are a deformed uterine contour and an enlarged uterus. The fibroid may be seen as a solid or heterogeneous mass if degeneration has occurred. The finding of calcification is the most specific sign of fibroid presence on CT scanning.[46]

Magnetic resonance imaging (MRI)

MRI provides excellent visualization and localization of tumors. If large or multiple neoplasms are present,

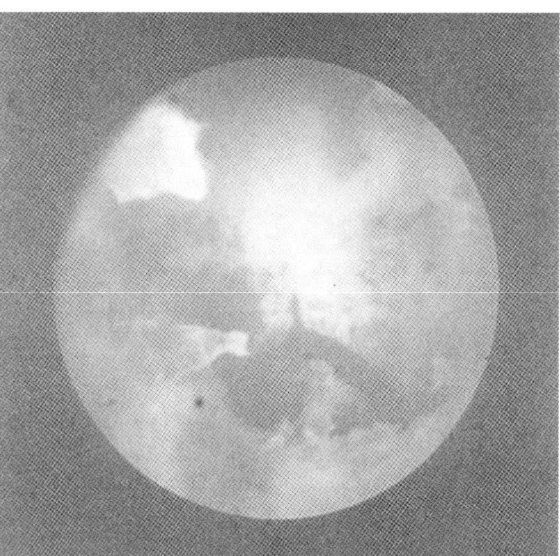

Fig. 38.4 The typical appearance of a fibroid on diagnostic hysteroscopy. (See also color plate p4.)

MRI with its multiplanar capability is often the best way to delineate precisely the exact location of each mass. It is ideal to show the proximity of the tumor to the bright endometrial cavity.[46] Because of access and cost MRI cannot usually be used as the primary diagnostic modality.

MEDICAL MANAGEMENT

Traditionally, the treatment of fibroids has been surgical. Where once a woman had no choice other than hysterectomy, particularly if the fibroids were symptomatic, recent medical advances using GnRHa and the surgical techniques of laser and hysteroscopic resection, with pretreatment using GnRHa, are becoming increasingly common in the management of these patients. These advances have been paralleled by increasing demands of women for alternatives to hysterectomy.

Gonadotropin-releasing hormone agonists (GnRHa)

GnRHa are a group of drugs which are derivatives of natural hypothalamic GnRH. Peptide substitutions in the amino acid structure make them 40–200 times more potent than native GnRH. The peptide modifications cause both an increase in binding affinity to pituitary GnRH receptors and an increase in resistance to proteolytic degradation.[47]

On initial exposure to the drugs there is elevation of serum gonadotropin levels and subsequently plasma sex steroid levels, which may last for several hours or days. However, with continuous administration there is suppression of the pituitary-ovarian axis with the induction of a state of E_2 deficiency which is readily reversible on cessation of the medication. The mechanism of this suppression is thought due to down regulation of pituitary GnRH binding sites.[47]

The agonists cannot be administered orally because of inactivation by gastric peptidases. They may be given by nasal spray, subcutaneous injection and in slow release preparations such as microcapsules or implants. The timing of administration of GnRHa in relation to the menstrual cycle is an important consideration. When the drug is begun during the first half of the cycle, ideally day 2–4, there will often be an E_2 withdrawal bleed 10–14 days later, as well as the normal period at the expected time. This time of commencement rules out the possibility of accidental administration during pregnancy. Its disadvantage is the unopposed increase in serum E_2 which presumably would predispose to further myoma growth. When begun in the second phase of the menstrual cycle, around day 21 if possible, the elevation of gonadotropins and sex steroids is restricted to this phase and normal menstruation occurs at the expected time without a subsequent withdrawal bleed in the following cycle.[47,48] This is advantageous in a woman who suffers from heavy menstrual loss because of fibroids.

Side effects

The side effects of prolonged GnRHa administration are due mainly to E_2 deficiency. All patients suffer from hot flashes. Mood changes, headaches, vaginal dryness, arthralgias and decreased libido are reported by 12–32% of patients.[49] Rare, idiosyncratic reactions reported are paraesthesias, palpitations, chloasma, skin rash, lactation and breast engorgement.[50]

The more worrying sequel to hypo-estrogenism is the potential development of osteoporosis. Reported studies have shown a significant bone loss (6%) in trabecular bone of the lumbar vertebrae, when measured by computerized tomography, after six months of treatment. This loss, however, has been shown to be partially reversible within six months of the cessation of treatment.[51] Others have confirmed incomplete recovery in bone density even over longer periods after these drugs are ceased.[52,53] Biochemical markers of bone catabolism, such as alkaline phosphatase and hydroxyproline, have also been shown to be significantly increased during therapy and to be reversible following therapy cessation.[54] The side effect of loss of bone density is the limiting factor to the long term usage of GnRHa. The other group of side effects are those due to the delivery system of the agonist. Rhinorrhoea occasionally occurs (4.8%) with intranasal preparations[49] and up to 10% of patients manifest a local allergic reaction to the depot preparations.[55]

Rationale for use

The rationale behind the usage of GnRHa in fibroids is that the smaller and less vascular the fibroid the less likely it is to cause symptoms and the less the blood loss at myomectomy or hysterectomy. Since the first case report was published showing successful treatment of fibroids with GnRHa,[56] there have been multiple studies, including randomized, double-blind, placebo-controlled trials, that have attested to the potential use of GnRHa, not only as an option initially, but also as an adjunct to surgical management. There has been regression of fibroids typically to 50% of their initial volume, complete regression only occurring with smaller tumors (<2 cm diameter). Women with the greatest initial fibroid volume are most likely to experience the greatest shrinkage of their tumors. This usually occurs during the first 12 weeks of therapy with further significant reductions being unlikely with continuing treatment.[49] The reduction in total fibroid/uterine volume seems to be dependent on the level of E_2 suppression.[57–60] Moreover, Friedman and others[61] have shown a statistically significant negative correlation between the percent reduction in uterine volume and the serum E_2 concentration at week 12. They also showed a significant negative correlation between the percent reduction in uterine volume and the pretreatment weight of the patient.

One of the major advantages of the E_2 deficient state induced by GnRHa is that menstrual bleeding may cease completely or become scant. This usually allows restoration of normal hemoglobin levels and allows the possibility of blood collection for autologous transfusion. Invariably, however, after therapy is stopped there is regrowth of the fibroids.[48,49,54–60,62,63] Long-term follow-up studies have shown regrowth in all cases with symptom recurrence in a smaller percentage of women.[64,65] The regrowth usually occurs within the first year after treatment has ceased.[66]

Presurgical therapy

Since these tumors will regrow after therapy cessation, the major therapeutic situation for the use of GnRHa at present is prior to surgery, either hysterectomy or myomectomy. Studies have concluded that pretreatment prior to hysterectomy results in reduced blood loss, easier operations more often performed through transverse abdominal incisions or vaginally (especially if the pretreatment intra-uterine size was 14–18 weeks) than abdominally.[67–69] This final consequence is an advantage for the patient as vaginal hysterectomy is associated with a lower morbidity compared with abdominal hysterectomy — 24.5% versus 42.8%.[70] The preoperative Hb is also usually higher in the GnRHa treated women so that if considerable blood loss occurs it is better tolerated and less likely to result in transfusion.[67–69]

Myomectomy is considered a 'bloody' operation. Pretreatment with GnRHa also seems to confer benefits to the patient and the surgeon in terms of ease of operation, reduced blood loss, especially with large fibroid uteri (>10 weeks gestational size) and consequently less postoperative pelvic adhesion formation (reviewed by Benagiano et al[71]). It has been shown that the size of the fibroid prior to myomectomy is an important prognostic factor in subsequent fertility.[2] Therefore, if the fibroid is shrunk prior to surgery, theoretically, there should be an improved postoperative pregnancy rate. Abramovici and others[72] and Vollenhoven and associates[73] reported a 50% postmyomectomy pregnancy rate in infertile women whose sole cause for infertility was fibroids. These women had been pretreated with GnRHa and then underwent myomectomy. This figure for postmyomectomy pregnancy rate is consistent with other reported series in which women had no pretreatment (reviewed by Vollenhoven et al[73]). The only method of rigorously investigating if GnRHa has any effect on the postmyomectomy pregnancy rate is to perform a randomized trial (treatment versus no treatment) in women whose only cause for infertility is the presence of fibroids. This has never been reported.

One disadvantage of pretreatment with GnRHa has also been reported. Fedele and others[74] reported that six months after myomectomy significantly more women who had been pretreated, compared with untreated women, had small fibroids, less than 1.5 cm, when examined by transvaginal US. This may occur because the smaller fibroids shrink to such an extent prior to surgery that they are missed at operation. As the effect of the GnRHa reverses, these small fibroids regrow. It may be that women with small fibroids should be treated for a shorter time-period if the ultimate aim is to remove all fibroids at surgery. However, this finding has been disputed by another study which showed that GnRHa pretreatment made no difference to the postoperative recurrence rate of fibroids.[75]

'Add-back' therapy

Fibroid recurrence after GnRHa treatment is inevitable and long-term therapy (two years or more) with these drugs is not possible because of the risk of loss of bone density. Therefore, to overcome the side effects associated with the long-term use of GnRHa, several studies have added P and/or E at the same time as GnRHa treatment or after three months of therapy and once fibroid shrinkage has occurred. This is called sex hormone 'add-back' therapy. It may be the answer to long-term GnRHa treatment, especially in a woman who has a contraindication to surgery.[76]

The studies using a progestogen beginning at the same time as GnRHa treatment have shown that fibroid shrinkage does not occur.[77,78] However, if the progestogen is begun three months after the agonist treatment has started, and once fibroid shrinkage has occurred, there are fewer hypo-estrogenic side effects and this sequential therapy also seems to be successful in preventing fibroid regrowth for longer.[78,79] It is thought that this therapy combination is successful because once E_2 levels are suppressed after three months of agonist treatment alone, the introduction of a progestogen results in decreased P binding to its receptor. Estrogen is known to cause production of the PR. If a hypoestrogenic state exists, then the PR numbers will also be low. When a progestogen is introduced at the same time as the GnRHa, the initial E_2 surge due to the GnRHa causes production of PR; with the introduction of a progestogen the P/PR binding probably prevents fibroid shrinkage.[78] It has previously been shown that there is increased PR binding in fibroids compared with myometrium (reviewed by Vollenhoven et al[21]). However, a recent study using progestogen alone as add-back therapy showed that it was not as effective when compared with hormone replacement therapy (HRT) add-back treatment in maintaining fibroid shrinkage and the former may also cause a detrimental effect on lipid profiles.[80]

Combined E and P treatment or HRT, begun after fibroid shrinkage has occurred and continuing with the GnRHa, is successful in maintaining shrinkage, relieving the hypo-estrogenic side effects and, importantly, maintaining bone density.[81,82] The protocols of initial GnRHa therapy with the addition of HRT or progestogen treatment alone once fibroid shrinkage has occurred may be the answer to long-term agonist use.

Why do fibroids shrink on GnRHa treatment?

Studies by Vollenhoven et al[21,31] suggest that these drugs do not cause fibroid shrinkage by acting through the peptide growth factors or through changes in ER or PR binding. Rather, fibroids may shrink because there is a decrease in the circulating E_2 and P concentration leading to less available ligand for binding with the ER and PR.

Treatment with these drugs has also been shown to decrease the mitotic activity of fibroids[83] and they may also affect the extracellular matrix to cause a reduction in these components.

Other medical management

Mifepristone (RU 486)

RU486 is a synthetic steroid analog with antiprogestational and antiglucocorticoid properties.[84] It has been used, in a dose of 50 mg daily for three months, with success to shrink fibroids with few side effects (mild hot flashes).[85] Its mode of action in shrinking fibroids is thought to occur via a decrease in blood flow to the uterus. It has been shown that this reduction is about 40% and is greater than the reduction that occurs on GnRHa.[86] Widespread availability of Mifepristone is urgently needed to confirm and extend these early reports.

Progestogens

In an older study, Goldzieher and others[87] treated 46 women with 25 mg medrogestone and reported fibroid shrinkage after just 14 days of treatment. They showed that marked degenerative changes similar to 'red degeneration' of pregnancy were induced in the fibroids. It was thought that progestogens had the potential to decrease the size of uterine fibroids, but this not been further substantiated.

Gestrinone

Gestrinone is a synthetic trienic 19 norsteroid which has mild androgenic side effects. It too has been reported to shrink fibroids.[88]

SURGICAL MANAGEMENT

Traditional surgical methods

As stated previously, fibroids have traditionally been treated surgically. Myomectomy has been the operation of choice for the woman with fibroids who wants to maintain her fertility. In most cases it is a safe operation which carries a low morbidity.[89] Minimization of blood loss and prevention of postoperative adhesions are the two main concerns during myomectomy because, if adhesions occur, myomectomy may actually decrease rather than enhance fertility.[2,90]

A number of techniques have been used to minimize blood loss, including clamps and rubber tourniquets which, when applied across the base of the uterus at its junction with the cervix, occlude the uterine arteries. A blend of cutting/coagulation cautery rather than scalpel dissection can also be used for myomectomy. Pharmacological methods such as injection of vasopressin have also been advocated. A study comparing diluted vasopressin (20 U in 20 mL of normal saline) with mechanical obstruction of blood flow showed no difference in efficacy as far as blood loss was concerned. This study also reported that the amount of blood lost correlated with uterine size and fibroid weight.[91] Vasopressin has also been shown to be effective in reducing blood loss at myomectomy and preventing a fall in the Hb when compared with a control group.[92] If blood loss is minimized, the risk of postoperative adhesion formation is also decreased. Instillation of dextran, hyscon and normal saline, prior to closure of the peritoneum, all aim to achieve a 'flotation' effect and minimize the development of adhesions.

Laparoscopic myomectomy

The recent advances in operative laparoscopy can now be applied to myomectomy performed for subserosal or superficial intramural fibroids. However, considerable technical skill is involved and the procedure should only be undertaken after adequate training. There are two major concerns with this procedure. First, the concern of uterine rupture in a subsequent pregnancy if the uterine incision is inadequately sutured or not sutured at laparoscopy. Secondly, the concern regarding adhesion formation when the myomectomy site is sutured compared with leaving it unsutured.[93,94] Nevertheless, the studies so far performed show laparoscopic myomectomy to be a safe procedure in skilled hands. The added advantages of this procedure are: shortened hospital stay — 1–3 days on average, and less postoperative pain when compared with an open myomectomy.[95] Surgery may be facilitated with GnRHa pretreatment[93,95] with laparoscopic diathermy of the tumours causing coagulative necrosis of the fibroid as an alternative to myomectomy.

Resectoscopic surgery

The recent development of hysteroscopic surgical techniques has added a new dimension to myomectomy. The available data on hysteroscopic resection of small submucous fibroids and polyps, using electrocautery, indicates that the use of the resectoscope to remove these lesions is safe and effective in skilled hands.[96,97] With concomitant use of laparoscopy to detect uterine perforation and keep bowel out of the pelvis, the potential risk of bowel trauma following uterine perforation with the resectoscope is minimized. This technique has the distinct advantage of avoiding major abdominal surgery and appears to be associated with a lower morbidity than abdominal myomectomy. In patients who have symptomatic menorrhagia and who have completed childbearing, fibroid resection may be combined with endometrial ablation to improve results further.

Fibroids which are pedunculated or smaller than 4 cm can be resected using the standard hysteroscopic scissors, whereas those greater than 4 cm, or sessile myomas, can be shaved away using the resectoscope. The portion of the tumor within the myometrium is left behind. Ideally, greater than 50% of the fibroid should be submucous for hysteroscopic resection success.[98] Michlewitz and Reindollar[99] performed resectoscopic surgery on 10 patients with submucous fibroids and intractable menorrhagia; eight patients were successfully treated and two required a transabdominal myomectomy. Of the five infertile patients in their series, four became pregnant. They conclude that this form of surgery is useful for submucous fibroids, thereby avoiding peritoneal adhesion formation that may occur with a transabdominal approach. Similarly, Loffer[100] successfully treated 43 women with submucous fibroids using the resectoscope. Of the 12 infertile women in his series seven subsequently delivered live born infants. A large series of patients (92) reported by Corson and Brooks[101] also attested to the success of hysteroscopic resection of submucous myomas. In their series, dysmenorrhoea was alleviated in 24 of 28 women, menorrhagia in 65 of 80 and pregnancy was achieved in 10 of 13 infertile women. Pretreatment with either danazol or depot leuprolide was used only if the fibroid was greater than 4 cm in diameter.

The long-term effectiveness of hysteroscopic resection of submucous fibroids has been reviewed by Derman et al.[102] They performed a follow-up study of 94 women who had had this procedure performed between the years 1973–88. They found that 24.5% of these women reported late postoperative complications. Of these women 87% had the problem of recurrent abnormal bleeding, 4% the problem of persistent submucous myoma, 4% had increasing pelvic pain due to fibroids and 4% had a uterine rupture in a subsequent pregnancy. Fifteen of the 23 symptomatic women ultimately required reoperation — either hysteroscopically or abdominally. They concluded that hysteroscopic management of submucous fibroids proved a reasonable alternative to an abdominal procedure.

Laser surgery

Laser myomectomy is another option. Its potential advantages over conventional methods include: decreased adhesion formation, better hemostasis, direct vaporization of smaller fibroids, increased precision in destroying abnormal tissue with decreased tissue injury and, therefore, theoretically improved reproductive performance.[90,103] The reported pregnancy rates after CO_2 laser abdominal myomectomy range from 59–70%.[90,103,104] Extensive published studies by Donnez and others[105,106] show that hysteroscopic myomectomy, using the Nd-YAG laser as a one or two step procedure, is universally successful. Pretreatment with a GnRHa, apart from decreasing fibroid size, is also advantageous in that fluid absorption during the procedure is decreased and a normal Hb concentration is restored preoperatively in women who are anemic. In women who desired pregnancy, the reported postmyomectomy pregnancy rate was 66%.

Myoma recurrence

The risk of fibroid recurrence postmyomectomy has been addressed. A follow-up analysis of over 600 women who had myomectomies performed between 1970–84 reported that the cumulative 10 year recurrence rate was 27% and that this rate increased steadily. The recurrence rate was independent of the age of the woman or the site of the tumor. Women with a single fibroid tended to have a lower recurrence rate. The single greatest protection against recurrence was the birth of a child after myomectomy.[107] These recurrence figures are comparable to other reported sources.[2] Pregnancy may be protective against fibroid recurrence because of an inhibition of fibroid growth during this time or, more likely, in the lactational period, or because of the BCP which is often used by parous women. This medication decreases the risk of fibroid growth.[17]

Conclusion

Gonadotropin-releasing hormone agonists are the first effective medical treatment for fibroids. However, regrowth occurs with cessation of treatment. They are sometimes invaluable as a preoperative treatment for myomectomy and hysterectomy, especially when combined with laparoscopic and resectoscopic procedures and in combination with open microsurgical techniques. The size of the myoma preoperatively is an important prognostic indicator of future reproductive ability. If GnRHa can decrease the size of a fibroid preoperatively then the chance of an infertile woman regaining her fertility postoperatively is increased. In the future, RU 486 may complement GnRHa in the medical management of fibroids by an antiprogesterone action.

If a woman presents with symptoms suggestive of a fibroid or a mass suggestive of fibroids the primary imaging technique should be a vaginal US performed by an appropriate specialist. If this suggests fibroids the line of management depends on the age of the patient and her desire for children. If a woman has completed child bearing then the options depend on the size of the fibroids and their number. If multiple, large, subserosal or intramural tumors are present, the best option is still hysterectomy. If the fibroids are submucosal then the therapeutic option of choice is a hysteroscopic myoma and endometrial resection following pretreatment with GnRHa.

If the patient desires children, then the treatment of choice is a myomectomy, ideally with GnRHa pretreatment. The myomectomy technique — via laparotomy, the laparoscope or the hysteroscope — will depend on the number of fibroids, their size and their site.

REFERENCES

1. Thompson JD, Rock JA (ed) 1992 Te Linde's operative gynecology, 7th edn. Lippincott, London, pp 647–662
2. Buttram VC, Reiter RC 1981 Uterine leiomyomata: etiology, symptomatology and management. Fertility and Sterility 36: 433–445
3. Fraser I, McCarr G, Markham R et al 1987 Measured menstrual blood loss in women with menorrhagia associated with pelvic disease or coagulation disorder. Obstetrics and Gynecology 69: 630–633
4. Candiani GB, Vercellini P, Fedele L, Arcaini L, Bianchi S, Candiani M 1990 Use of Goserelin depot, a gonadotropin-releasing hormone agonist, for the treatment of menorrhagia and severe anaemia in women with leiomyomata uteri. Acta Obstetrica Gynecologica Scandinavica 69: 413–415
5. Farrer-Brown G, Beilby JOW, Tarbit MH 1970 The vascular patterns in myomatous uteri. Journal of Obstetrics and Gynaecology of the British Commonwealth 77: 967–970
6. Farrer-Brown G, Beilby JOW, Tarbit MH 1971 Venous changes in the endometrium of myomatous uteri. Obstetrics and Gynecology 38: 743–751
7. Myles JL, Hart WR 1985 Apoplectic leiomyomas of the uterus. A clinico-pathologic study of five distinctive haemorrhagic leiomyomas associated with oral contraceptive usage. American Journal of Surgical Pathology 17: 548–549
8. Chipato T, Healy DL, Vollenhoven BJ, Buckler HM 1991 Pelvic pain complicating LHRH analogue treatment of fibroids. Australian and New Zealand Journal of Obstetrics and Gynaecology 31: 383–384
9. Hunt JE, Wallach EE 1974 Uterine factors in infertility — an overview. Clinical Obstetrics and Gynaecology 17: 44–64
10. Hasan F, Arumugam K, Sivanesaratnam V 1990 Uterine leiomyomata in pregnancy. International Journal of Gynecology and Obstetrics 34: 45–48

11. Aharoni A, Reiter A, Golan D, Paltiely Y, Sharf M 1988 Patterns of growth of uterine leiomyomas during pregnancy: a prospective longitudinal study. British Journal of Obstetrics and Gynaecology 95: 510–513
12. Rosati P, Exacoustos C, Mancuso S 1992 Longitudinal evaluation of uterine myoma growth during pregnancy. A sonographic study. Journal of Ultrasound in Medicine 1: 511–515
13. Muram D, Gillieson M, Walters JH 1980 Myomas of the uterus in pregnancy, ultrasonographic follow-up. American Journal of Obstetrics and Gynecology 138: 16–19
14. Rice JP, Kay HH, Mahony BS 1989 The clinical significance of uterine leiomyomas in pregnancy. American Journal of Obstetrics and Gynecology 160: 1212–1216
15. Rosati P, Bellati U, Exacoustos C, Angelozzi P, Mancuso S 1989 Uterine myoma in pregnancy: ultrasound study. International Journal of Gynecology and Obstetrics 28: 109–117
16. Davis JL, Ray-Mazumder S, Hobel CJ, Baley K, Sassoon D 1990 Uterine leiomyomas in pregnancy: a prospective study. Obstetrics and Gynecology 75: 41–44
17. Ross RK, Pike MC, Vessey MP, Bull D, Yeates D, Casagrande JT 1986 Risk factors for uterine fibroids: reduced risk associated with oral contraceptives. British Medical Journal 293: 359–363
18. Spellacy WN, Le Maire WJ, Buhi WC, Birk SA, Bradley BA 1972 Plasma growth hormone and estradiol levels in women with uterine myomas. Obstetrics and Gynecology 40: 829–834
19. Plymate SR, Fariss BL, Bassett ML, Matej L 1981 Obesity and its role in polycystic ovary syndrome. Journal of Clinical Endocrinology and Metabolism 52: 1246–1251
20. Kjerulffel KH, Guzinski GM, Langenberg PW, Stolley PD, Moye NE, Kazandjian VA 1993 Hysterectomy and race. Obstetrics and Gynecology 82: 757–764
21. Vollenhoven BJ, Pearce P, Herington AC, Healy DL 1994 Steroid receptor binding and messenger RNA expression in fibroids from untreated and luteinizing hormone-releasing hormone agonist pre-treated women. Clinical Endocrinology 40: 537–544
22. Kawaguchi K, Fujii S, Konishi I et al 1991 Immunohistochemical analysis of oestrogen receptors, progesterone receptors and Ki-67 in leiomyoma and myometrium during the menstrual cycle and pregnancy. Virchows Archives A Pathology Anatomy 419: 309–315
23. Viville B, Charnock-Jones DS, Sharkey YAM, Smith SK 1995 Progesterone A and B receptors in fibroids and normal myometrium. Abstracts of the 11th Annual Meeting of ESHRE, Hamburg, Abstract 349
24. Pasqualini JR, Vella C, Cornier E, Schatz B, Grenier J, Netter A 1990 Effect of Decapeptyl, an agonist analog of gonadotropin-releasing hormone on estrogens, estrogen sulfates and progesterone receptors in leiomyoma and myometrium. Fertility and Sterility 53: 1012–1017
25. Rein MS, Friedman AJ, Stuart J, MacLaughlin DT 1990 Fibroid and myometrial steroid receptors in women treated with a gonadotropin-releasing hormone agonist leuprolide acetate. Fertility and Sterility 53: 1018–1023
26. Lumsden MA, West CP, Hawkins RA, Bramley TA, Rumgay L, Baird DT 1989 The binding of steroids to myometrium and leiomyomata (fibroids) in women treated with the gonadotrophin releasing hormone agonist Zoladex (ICI 118630) Journal of Endocrinology 121: 389–396
27. Dawood MY, Khan-Dawood FS 1991 Plasma insulin like growth factor-I (IGF I), CA 125, estrogen and progesterone in women with leiomyomas. Abstracts of the 47th Annual Meeting of the American Fertility Society, Abstract P-205
28. Strawm EY, Novy MJ, Burry KA, Bethea CL 1995 Insulin-like growth factor I promotes leiomyoma cell growth in vitro. American Journal of Obstetrics and Gynecology 172: 1837–1844
29. Hoppener JWM, Mosselman S, Roholl PJM et al 1988 Expression of insulin-like growth factors I and II genes in human smooth muscle tumours. EMBO 7: 1379–1385
30. Boehm KD, Daimon M, Gorodeski IG, Sheean LA, Utian WH, Ilan J 1990 Expression of insulin-like and platelet derived growth factor genes in human uterine tissues. Molecular Reproduction Development 27: 93–101
31. Vollenhoven BJ, Herington AC, Healy DL 1993 Messenger ribonucleic acid expression of the insulin-like growth factors and their binding proteins in uterine fibroids and myometrium. Journal of Clinical Endocrinology and Metabolism 76: 1106–1110
32. Tommola P, Pekonen F, Rutanen E 1989 Binding of epidermal growth factor, insulin-like growth factor I in human myometrium and leiomyomata. Obstetrics and Gynecology 74: 658–662
33. Chandrasekhar Y, Heiner J, Osuamkpe C, Nagamani M 1992 Insulin-like growth factor I and II binding in human myometrium and leiomyomas. American Journal of Obstetrics and Gynecology 166: 64–69
34. Jones JI, Clemmons DR 1995 Insulin-like growth factors and their binding proteins: biological actions. Endocrine Reviews 16: 3–34
35. Hofmann GE, Rao V, Barrows GH, Schultz GS, Sanfilippo JS 1984 Binding sites for epidermal growth factors in human uterine tissues and leiomyomas. Journal of Clinical Endocrinology and Metabolism 58: 880–883
36. Lumsden MA, West CP, Bromley J, Rumgay L, Baird DT 1988 The binding of epidermal growth factor to the human uterus and leiomyomata in women rendered hypo-oestrogenic by continuous administration of an LHRH-agonist. British Journal of Obstetrics and Gynaecology 95: 1299–1304
37. Fayed YM, Tsibris JCM, Langenberg PW, Robertson AL. Human leiomyoma cells: binding and growth responses to epidermal growth factor, platelet derived growth factor and insulin. Laboratory Investigation 60: 30–37
38. Leone M, Cucuccio S, Venturini PL, Valenzano U, Menada M, DeCecco L 1991 Immunohistochemical localization of epidermal growth factor receptor in leiomyomas from women treated with Goserelin depot. Hormone and Metabolism Research 23: 442–445

39. Matta WHM, Stabile I, Shaw RW, Campbell S 1988 Doppler assessment of uterine blood flow changes in patients with fibroids receiving the gonadotrophin releasing hormone agonist buserelin. Fertility and Sterility 49: 1083–1085
40. Harrison-Woolrych ML, Charnock-Jones DS, Smith SK 1994 Quantification of messenger ribonucleic acid for epidermal growth factor in human myometrium and leiomyomata using reverse transcriptase polymerase chain reaction. Journal of Clinical Endocrinology and Metabolism 78: 1179–1184
41. Stewart EA, Friedman AJ, Peck K, Nowak RA 1994 Relative overexpression of collagen type I and collagen type III messenger ribonucleic acids by uterine leiomyomas during the proliferative phase of the menstrual cycle. Journal of Clinical Endocrinology and Metabolism 79: 900–906
42. Anderson J, Grine E, Eng CLY, et al 1993 Expression of connexin 43 in human myometrium and leiomyoma. American Journal of Obstetrics and Gynecology 169: 1266–1276
43. Meloni AM, Surti U, Contento AM, Davare J, Sandberg AA 1992 Uterine leiomyomas: cytogenetic and histologic profile. Obstetrics and Gynecology 80: 209–217
44. Koutsilieris M 1992 Pathophysiology of uterine leiomyoma. Biochemistry Cell Biology 70: 273–278
45. Bullerdiek J, Hennig Y, Deichert U et al 1995 A common molecular basis of leiomyomas and endometrial polyps. Abstracts of the 11th Annual Meeting of ESHRE, Hamburg, Abstract 077
46. Karasick S, Lev-Toaff AS, Toaff ME 1992 Imaging of uterine leiomyomas. American Journal of Radiology 158: 799–805
47. McLachlan RI, Healy DL, Burger HG 1986 Clinical aspects of LHRH analogues in gynaecology: a review. British Journal of Obstetrics and Gynaecology 99: 431–454
48. Healy D, Lawson S, Abbott M, Baird DT, Fraser HM 1986 Toward removing uterine fibroids without surgery: subcutaneous infusion of a luteinizing hormone releasing hormone agonist commencing in the luteal phase. Journal of Clinical Endocrinology and Metabolism 63: 619–625
49. Vollenhoven BJ, Shekleton P, McDonald J, Healy DL 1990 Clinical predictors of buserelin acetate treatment of uterine fibroids: a prospective study of 40 women. Fertility and Sterility 54: 1032–1038
50. Penzias AS, Gutmann JN, Seifer DB, De Cherney AH 1991 Facial and neck paresthesia associated with Naferelin administration. Fertility and Sterility 56: 357–358
51. Matta WH, Shaw RW, Hesp R, Katz D 1987 Hypogonadism induced by luteinizing hormone releasing hormone analogues: effects on bone density in premenopausal women. British Medical Journal 294: 1523–1524
52. Surrey ES, Judd HL 1992 Reduction of vasomotor symptoms and bone mineral density loss with combined norethindrone and long-acting gonadotropin-releasing hormone agonist therapy of symptomatic endometriosis: a prospective randomized trial. Journal of Clinical Endocrinology and Metabolism 75: 558–563
53. Orwoll ES, Yuzpe AA, Burry KA, Heinrichs L, Buttram VC, Hornstein MD 1994 Nafarelin therapy in endometriosis: long-term effects on bone mineral density. American Journal of Obstetrics and Gynecology 171: 1221–1225
54. Eckstein N, Foldes J, Feinstein Y et al 1992 Calcium homeostasis, bone metabolism and safety aspects during long-term treatment with a GnRH agonist. Maturitas 15: 25–32
55. Letterie GS, Stevenson D, Shah A 1991 Recurrent anaphylaxis to a depot form of GnRH analogue. Obstetrics and Gynecology 78: 943–946
56. Filicori M, Hall DA, Loughlin JS, Rivier J, Vale W, Crowley W 1983 A conservative approach to the management of uterine leiomyoma: pituitary desensitization by a luteinizing hormone-releasing hormone analog. American Journal of Obstetrics and Gynecology 147: 7267–7270
57. Coddington CC, Collins RL, Shawker TH, Anderson R, Loriaux DL, Winkel CA 1986 Long acting gonadotrophin hormone releasing hormone analog used to treat leiomyomata uteri. Fertility and Sterility 45: 624–629
58. Maheux R, Lemay A, Merat P 1987 Use of intranasal luteinizing hormone releasing hormone agonist in uterine leiomyomas. Fertility and Sterility 43: 229–233
59. West CP, Lumsden MA, Lawson S, Williamson J, Baird DT 1987 Shrinkage of uterine fibroids during therapy with goserelin: a luteinizing hormone releasing hormone agonist administered as a monthly subcutaneous depot. Fertility and Sterility 48: 45–51
60. Friedman AJ, Hoffman DI, Comite F, Browneller RW, Miller JD 1991 Treatment of leiomyomata uteri with leuprolide acetate depot: a double-blind placebo-controlled multicenter study. Obstetrics and Gynecology 77: 720–725
61. Friedman AJ, Daly M, Juneau-Norcross M, Rein MS 1992 Predictors of uterine volume reduction in women with myomas treated with a gonadotropin-releasing hormone agonist. Fertility and Sterility 58: 413–415
62. Kessel B, Liu J, Mortola J, Berga S, Yen SSC 1988 Treatment of uterine fibroids with agonist analogs of gonadotrophin releasing hormone. Fertility and Sterility 49: 538–541
63. Franssen AMHW, Willemsen WNP, Corbey RS et al 1991 Subcutaneous injection of gonadotrophin releasing-hormone agonist buserelin in the treatment of enlarged uteri harbouring leiomyomata. European Journal of Obstetrics and Gynecology 40: 221–228
64. Letterie GS, Shawker TH, Coddington CC, Loriaux DL, Winkel CA, Collins RL 1989 Efficacy of a gonadotropin-releasing hormone agonist in the treatment of uterine leiomyomata: long-term follow-up. Fertility and Sterility 51: 951–956
65. Matta WHM, Shaw RW, Nye M 1989 Long-term follow-up of patients with uterine fibroids after treatment with the LHRH agonist buserelin. British Journal of Obstetrics and Gynaecology 96: 200–206
66. Van Leusden HAIM 1992 Symptom-free interval after triptorelin treatment of uterine fibroids: long term results. Gynecological Endocrinology 6: 189–198

67. Schneider D, Golan A, Bukovsky I, Pansky M, Caspi E 1991 GnRH analog-induced uterine shrinkage enabling a vaginal hysterectomy and repair in large leiomyomatous uteri. Obstetrics and Gynecology 78: 540–541
68. Stovall TG, Ling FW, Henry LC, Woodruff MR 1991 A randomized trial evaluating leuprolide acetate before hysterectomy as treatment for leiomyomas. American Journal of Obstetrics and Gynecology 164: 1420–1425
69. Lumsden MA, West CP, Thomas E et al 1994 Treatment with the gonadotrophin releasing hormone agonist goserelin before hysterectomy for uterine fibroids. British Journal of Obstetrics and Gynaecology 101: 438–442
70. Dicker RC, Greenspan JR, Strauss LT et al 1982 Complications of abdominal and vaginal hysterectomy among women of reproductive age in the United States. American Journal of Obstetrics and Gynecology 144: 841–848
71. Benagiano G, Morini A, Primiero FM 1992 Fibroids: overview of current and future treatment. British Journal of Obstetrics and Gynaecology 99(Suppl 7): 18–22
72. Abramovici H, Dirnfeld M, Auslender R, Sorokin Y, Blumenfeld Z 1990 Pregnancies following treatment by GnRHa (D-TRP-6) and myomectomy in infertile women caused by uterine leiomyomata. Gynecological Endocrinology 4(Suppl 2): Abstract 041
73. Vollenhoven BJ, McCloud P, Shekleton P, McDonald J, Healy DL 1993 An open study of luteinizing hormone-releasing agonists (LHRHa) in infertile women with uterine fibroids. Gynecological Endocrinology 7: 57–61
74. Fedele L, Vercellini P, Bianchi S, Arcaini L, Marchini M, Bocciolone L 1990 Treatment with GnRH agonists before myomectomy and the risk of short-term myoma recurrence. British Journal of Obstetrics and Gynaecology 97: 393–396
75. Friedman AJ, Daly M, Juneau-Norcross M, Fine C, Rein MS 1992 Recurrence of myomas after myomectomy in women pre-treated with leuprolide acetate depot or placebo. Fertility and Sterility 58: 205–208
76. Barbieri RL 1990 Gonadotropin-releasing hormone agonists and estrogen-progesterone replacement therapy. American Journal of Obstetrics and Gynecology 162: 593–595
77. Friedman AJ, Barbieri RL, Doubilet PM, Fine C, Schiff I 1988 A randomized double blind trial of a gonadotrophin releasing hormone agonist (leuprolide) with or without medroxy progesterone acetate in the treatment of leiomyomata uteri. Fertility and Sterility 49: 404–409
78. West CP, Lumsden MA, Hillier H, Sweeting V, Baird DT 1992 Potential role for medroxyprogesterone acetate as an adjunct to goserelin (Zoladex) in the medical management of uterine fibroids. Human Reproduction 7: 328–332
79. Benagiano G, Morini A, Aleadri V et al 1990 Sequential Gn-RH superagonist and medroxyprogesterone acetate treatment of uterine leiomyomata. International Journal of Obstetrics and Gynecology 33: 333–343
80. Friedman AJ, Daly M, Juneau-Norcross M et al 1993 A prospective, randomized trial of gonadotropin-releasing hormone agonist plus estrogen-progestin or progestin 'add-back' regimens for women with leiomyomata uteri. Journal of Clinical Endocrinology and Metabolism 76: 1439–1445
81. Maheux R, Lemay A, Blanchet P, Friede J, Pratt J 1991 Maintained reduction of uterine leiomyoma following addition of hormonal replacement therapy to a monthly luteinizing hormone-releasing hormone agonist implant: a pilot study. Human Reproduction 6: 500–505
82. Friedman AJ 1989 Treatment of leiomyomata uteri with short-term leuprolide followed by estrogen-progestin hormone replacement therapy for two years: a pilot study. Fertility and Sterility 51: 526–528
83. Barbieri RL, Dilena M, Chumas J, Rein MS, Friedmen AJ 1993 Leuprolide acetate depot decreases the number of nucleolar organizer regions in uterine leiomyomata. Fertility and Sterility 60: 569–570
84. Herrmann WL, Schindler AM, Wyss R et al 1985 Effects of the anti progesterone RU486 in early pregnancy and during the menstrual cycle. In: Baillieu EE, Segal SJ (eds). The anti progestin steroid RU486 in human fertility control. Plenum Press, New York, pp 179–198
85. Murphy AA, Kettel LM, Morales AJ, Roberts VJ, Yen SSC 1993 Regression of uterine leiomyomata in response to the antiprogesterone RU486. Journal of Clinical Endocrinology and Metabolism 76: 513–517
86. Reinsch RC, Murphy AA, Morales AJ, Yen SSC 1994 The effects of RU486 and leuprolide acetate on uterine artery blood flow in the fibroid uterus: a prospective randomized study. American Journal of Obstetrics and Gynecology 170: 1623–1628
87. Goldzieher JW, Maqueo M, Ricaud L, Aguilar A, Canales E 1966 Induction of degenerative changes in uterine myomas by high dose progestin therapy. American Journal of Obstetrics and Gynecology 96: 1078–1087
88. Coutinho EM, Goncalves MT 1989 Long-term treatment of leiomyomas with gestrinone. Fertility and Sterility 51: 939–946
89. La Morte AI, Lalwani S, Diamond MP 1993 Morbidity associated with abdominal myomectomy. Obstetrics and Gynecology 82: 897–900
90. Starks GC 1988 CO_2 laser myomectomy in an infertile population. Journal of Reproductive Medicine 33: 184–186
91. Ginsburg ES, Benson CB, Garfield JM, Gleason RE, Friedman AJ 1993 The effect of operative technique and uterine size on blood loss during myomectomy: a prospective randomized study. Fertility and Sterility 60: 956–962
92. Frederick J, Fletcher H, Simeon D, Mullings A, Hardie M 1994 Intra myometrial vasopressin as a haemostatic agent during myomectomy. British Journal of Obstetrics and Gynaecology 104: 435–437
93. Nezhet C, Nezhat F, Silfen SL, Schaffer N, Evans D 1991 Laparoscopic myomectomy. International Journal of Fertility 36: 275–280
94. Harris WJ 1992 Uterine dehiscence following laparoscopic myomectomy. Obstetrics and Gynecology 80: 545–546

95. Dubuisson JB, Lecru F, Foulot H, Mandelbrot L, Aubriot FX, Mooly M 1991 Myomectomy by laparoscopy: a preliminary report of 43 cases. Fertility and Sterility 56: 827–830
96. Loffer FD 1987 Hysteroscopic endometrial ablation with the Nd-YAG laser using a non-touch technique. Obstetrics and Gynecology 69: 679–682
97. Loffer FD 1989 Hysteroscopic management of menorrhagia. Acta Europa Fertilis 17: 463–467
98. Wamsteker K, Emanuel MH, de Kruif JH 1993 Transcervical hysteroscopic resection of submucous fibroids for abnormal uterine bleeding: results regarding the degree of intramural extension. Obstetrics and Gynecology 82: 736–740
99. Michlewitz H, Reindollar RH 1988 Hysteroscopic myomectomy using hysteroscopic guidance. Abstracts of XII World Congress of Gynecology and Obstetrics, No. 661
100. Loffer FD 1990 Removal of large symptomatic intrauterine growths by the hysteroscopic resectoscope. Obstetrics and Gynecology 76: 836–840
101. Corson SL, Brooks PG 1991 Resectoscopic myomectomy. Fertility and Sterility 55: 1041–1044
102. Derman SG, Rehnstrom J, Neuwirth RS 1991 The long-term effectiveness of hysteroscopic treatment of menorrhagia and leiomyomas. Obstetrics and Gynecology 77: 591–594
103. McLaughlin DS 1985 Metroplasty and myomectomy with the CO_2 laser for maximizing the preservation of normal tissue and minimizing blood loss. Journal of Reproductive Medicine 30: 1–9
104. Reyniak JV, Corenthal L 1987 Microsurgical laser technique for abdominal myomectomy. Microsurgery 8: 92–98
105. Donnez J, Gillerot S, Bourgonjon D, Clerckx F, Nisolle M 1990 Neodymiuim: YAG laser hysteroscopy in large submucous fibroids. Fertility and Sterility 54: 999–1003
106. Donnez J, Nisollen M, Grandjean P, Gillerot S, Clerckx F 1992 The place of GnRH agonists in the treatment of endometriosis and leiomyomas by advanced endoscopic techniques. British Journal of Obstetrics and Gynaecology 99(Suppl 7): 31–33
107. Candiani GB, Fedele L, Parazcini F, Villa L 1991 Risk of recurrence after myomectomy. British Journal of Obstetrics and Gynaecology 98: 385–389

39. The pathophysiology and therapy of benign breast disease

Ian S. Fentiman

Introduction

The chaos in classification and understanding of benign breast disease is not new. In 1905 J. Collins Warren wrote 'As an instance of the confusion in nomenclature, I might here state that in 199 cases of benign disease of the breast occurring in the Massachusetts General Hospital in ten years, 70 different pathological diagnoses appeared on the record books.'[1] The overriding problem is that the major disease which affects the breast is cancer, this is a source of great fear in patients and is the subject of greatest interest to surgeons and pathologists dealing with breast diseases. Thus all other conditions have been regarded as subservient and consigned to the catch-all category 'benign breast disease'. This etymological dustbin comprises some disease states but also a substantial number of normal variations.

Historical background

Many surgeons and pathologists have attempted to shed light on benign breast diseases by introducing their own terminology but unfortunately this has often led to further confusion with such terms as Bloodgood's cysts, Reclus' disease, chronic mastitis, fibroadenosis, benign mammary dysplasia and mastodynia.

As a specific example, the term 'dysplasia' is often used by surgeons, pathologists and radiologists and has different meanings for each group. A surgeon may refer to a nodular breast as being dysplastic, a pathologist might have described borderline histological changes as being dysplastic and a radiologist may call a dense breast dysplastic. All of these situations serve to cloak an unknown variable in a discrete but meaningless term.

A further concern is that some benign changes may be forerunners of malignancy. If imprecise terms are used to describe benign breast changes those at risk may not be properly identified and others who are not at increased risk of breast cancer may be needlessly worried.

Work carried out by Page et al has delineated the histological risk factors for breast cancer.[2] After a histological review and follow-up for more than 15 years it was found that atypical epithelial hyperplasia led to a doubling in risk of breast cancer. Cysts, sclerosing adenosis, fibrosis and other nonproliferative lesions did not lead to any increase in risk. A subsequent study from the same group found a 4–5 fold increase in risk for women with atypical lobular hyperplasia (ALH) and atypical ductal hyperplasia (ADH), with this risk being doubled further in those with a first degree family history of breast cancer.[3]

These findings have now been confirmed by several other groups as shown in Table 39.1.[3–6] Thus it is only those patients who have histologically confirmed atypical lobular or ductal hyperplasia who are at increased risk and could therefore be considered as candidates for endocrine studies to try and reduce their subsequent risk of breast cancer.

ANDI classification

Many classifications have been proposed for benign breast conditions but these did not take into account the extremes of normality which needed to be included to render the system all-encompassing. This problem was overcome in the classification proposed by the Cardiff group.[5] This was dubbed ANDI (Aberrations of Normal Development and Involution), and the outline of this is given in Table 39.2. The classification describes the four phases of breast existence: development, cyclical changes, pregnancy and lactation and finally postmenopausal involution. As an example, a simple fibroadenoma can be described as an aberration of lobular development which only becomes a disease state when there is massive increase in size associated with pain (giant fibroadenoma).

Table 39.1 Risk of breast cancer in patients with atypical epithelial hyperplasia.

Author	*n*	Follow-up	Type	Relative risk
Page 1985[3]	10 542	17 years	ADH	4.7
			FH–	3.9
			FH+	9.7
Tavassoli 1990[4]	199	13 years	ADH	3.8
			FH–	0.8
			FH+	2.2
London 1992[5]	609	8 years	AH (Pre)	5.9
			AH (Post)	2.3
			FH–	3.7
			FH+	7.3
Dupont 1993[6]	15 161	10 years	AH	4.3
			FH–	1.4
			FH+	22

ADH = Atypical ductal hyperplasia; AH = Atypical hyperplasia; FH– = No family history; FH+ = Positive family history; Pre = Premenopausal; Post = Postmenopausal

Table 39.2 Benign breast conditions and diseases in the ANDI classification.

Phase	Normal	Problem	Disease
Development	Ducts	Nipple inversion	Mammillary fistula
	Lobules	Fibroadenoma	Giant fibroadenoma
Cyclical change	Epithelial hyperplasia	Mastalgia Focal nodularity Diffuse nodularity Duct papilloma	Severe mastalgia
Pregnancy/ lactation	Epithelial hyperplasia	Bloody nipple discharge Galactocele	Abscess
Involution	Ducts	Duct ectasia	Abscess
	Lobules	Cysts Sclerosing adenosis	
	Hyperplasia	Simple hyperplasia	ADH/ALH

Mastalgia can be a normal association with menstrual breast changes but becomes pathological when it interferes with the patient's family, sexual and social life.

ENDOCRINOLOGY

The majority of benign breast conditions occur in premenopausal women and cease after the menopause or at the time of stopping hormone replacement therapy (HRT). Thus there is strong indirect evidence of ovarian/pituitary axis involvement in many benign breast problems. However that is not the same as saying that oestrogens/progesterone are the cause of benign breast diseases. A substantial amount of work has been conducted to try and find endocrine abnormalities in women with benign breast problems and this has been largely negative, i.e., no excess or lack of hormones could be identified. Unfortunately most of these studies reflected the lack of clinical precision in describing benign breast conditions and lumped together results from patients with fibroadenomata, localized and diffuse nodularity (fibroadenosis), gross cystic disease and cyclical mastalgia. Therefore it is not surprising that few significant findings emerged.

Localized and diffuse nodularity (fibrocystic change)

Several studies have measured urinary and plasma estrogens in patients with localized and diffuse nodularity (fibrocystic disease). The majority have reported normal estradiol (E_2) levels,[7–12] but in one study there were elevated E_2 levels in the luteal phase.[13] Low levels of estradiol have not been reported.

When the concept of 'luteal phase insufficiency' was suggested by Sherman and Korenman in an attempt to explain the endocrine basis of breast cancer this was also used as a hypothesis for development of benign breast disease.[14] Mauvais-Jarvis and colleagues reported subnormal synthesis of progesterone in the luteal phase of women with fibrocystic change[15] and support for this also came from other studies.[11,12,13,16,17] However other studies have found normal or elevated luteal phase progesterone levels in blood from cases of biopsied nodularity.[8,18,19] Urinary androgens have been reported as elevated in patients with biopsy proven epithelial hyperplasia[20] but plasma levels of testosterone have been consistently reported as normal in women with nodularity.[10,20,21,22] Studies which have examined plasma prolactin levels in patients with this condition have found no abnormality.[23–26]

Gross cystic disease

Cysts may present as a sudden onset tender breast lump, usually in premenopausal women aged 40 years or more and at a age when the patient will be very concerned that the lump is malignant. They occur in approximately 7% of this age group as clinical lumps but may be detected by mammograms or ultrasound in up to one third. Treatment is by aspiration and provided that the lump disappears and the aspirate is not blood-stained no cytological investigation of the fluid is necessary.[27]

Although breast cysts without atypia do not place patients at increased risk of subsequent malignancy, nevertheless follow-up studies of patients with aspirated cysts show an approximate doubling of risk.[28] This increased risk is carried by a subset and these appear to be patients who have cysts lined by apocrine epithelium rather than flattened epithelial cells.[29] The characteristics of these different cyst types are shown in Table 39.3. The cyst fluid itself may be distinguished by the ratio of Na/K and by levels of the androgen dehydroxyepiandrosterone (DHA) sulphate.[29] Apocrine cysts are more likely to contain apocrine cells in the cyst fluid, to recur, be multiple or bilateral and to be associated with histological evidence of atypia if they are excised.[30]

Table 39.3 Comparison of the features of apocrine and flattened cysts.

Feature	Apocrine	Flattened
Proportion[30]	60%	40%
Na/K ratio[29]	High K	High Na
DHA sulphate[29]	High	Low
pH[31]	<7	>7
Apocrine cells in cyst fluid[30]	>50%	<50%
Associated atypia on histology[30]	15%	0%
Multiple[30]	70%	20%
Bilateral[30]	18%	14%
Recurrent[30]	25%	8%

Additionally, apocrine cyst fluid is more likely to have a pH less than 7.[31] Levels of epidermal growth factor (EGF) and insulin-like growth factor-1 (IGF-1) have been measured in breast cyst fluid and found to be elevated in that from cysts of apocrine type.[32] In contrast cell adhesion molecules VCAM-1 (vascular cell adhesion molecule-1) and sE-selection (soluble e selectin) were elevated in fluid drawn from flattened cysts.[33] The relation between elevated expression of adhesion molecules and reduced risk of malignancy is unclear. Despite these interesting findings, which may help to elucidate the etiology of cyst formation, patients with single cysts of apocrine or flattened type are not regarded as being at such a high risk of malignancy that they merit close surveillance and biochemical analysis is not used in routine clinical practice.

Cyclical mastalgia

The commonest breast symptom for which women consult their general practitioners is pain, with or without lumpiness.[34] In the majority of cases the condition is an exaggeration of the physiological premenstrual breast fullness and resolves spontaneously within 2–3 months. Sometimes, noncyclical pain arises not from the breast tissue itself but from the underlying rib cage and is musculoskeletal in origin and responds to reassurance and nonsteroidal anti-inflammatory drugs (NSAIDs).

However there is a small proportion (5%) of women with breast pain who have incapacitating symptoms which render their life a misery. It is these cases, who have moderate or severe symptoms which have been present for six months or more, who have a disease state for which treatment is required. Even after this time there is a tendency for the disease to remit and up to 60% of cases who have had symptoms for more than six months will not require treatment when seen again after a full history and examination have been carried out followed by a sympathetic explanation of the problem.[35]

The pathophysiology of cyclical mastalgia is unknown. These patients do not produce abnormal amounts of ovarian or adrenal steroids.[28] There are no recognized histopathological findings in patients with fibrocystic disease and pain compared with those who are pain-free.[36] Baseline levels of prolactin are normal in women with severe mastalgia but there is an increase in prolactin storage as evidenced by a significantly elevated prolactin level after domperidone stimulation.[37] The significance of this finding is not known but the increased storage of prolactin may be a reflection of the chronic stress to which these patients are exposed.

Patients with severe mastalgia do differ from age matched women including those with mild mastalgia. They are more likely to be divorced or separated, to have had more than one termination, and to have had a hysterectomy.[38] However, these risk factors are social rather than biological. The psychosocial adjustment of patients with mastalgia seen at Guy's Hospital Breast Unit has been assessed in 33 with severe pain and 21 with nonsevere pain for which no treatment was required.[39] Mood disturbance was measured using the Hospital Anxiety and Depression Scale (HADS) and social functioning by the Psychosocial Adjustment to Illness Scale (PAIS). The levels of anxiety and depression in the patients with severe mastalgia were similar to those experienced by breast cancer patients on the morning of their operation. For those whose pain was not relieved by treatment there was no improvement in depression or social functioning. However there were significant improvements in both measures among those whose pain was reduced or disappeared.

THERAPY

Which conditions require treatment?

It is important that patients are not subjected to surgery or drug treatment because they have been labeled as having benign breast disease. Many symptoms are within normal limits and will remit spontaneously. Localized nodularity is not necessarily an indication for a biopsy and some patients with discrete lumps may be managed safely without surgery. The mislabeling of normal women as having a disease reached such a state that Love et al wrote a paper 'Fibrocystic disease of the breast: a non-disease.'[40]

Customary teaching has been that all discrete breast lumps should be excised irrespective of the age of the patient. This would mean that many young women may have unnecessary operations. A discrete mobile painless lump in a nonlactating young woman is likely to be a fibroadenoma. Provided that this is the clinical diagnosis, backed up by fine needle aspiration cytology (FNAC) showing benign epithelial cells and an ultrasound scan confirming a well defined echogenic mass, the lump does not need to be removed, provided that the situation has been explained to the patient and she is happy with this course of action.

Should the lump become painful, increase in size or the patient changes her mind, surgery can then be carried out. Adopting a strategy of watch and wait, approximately 50% of women with presumed fibroadenomata will eventually come to excision biopsy.[41]

Localized nodularity (fibrocystic change)

Localized nodularity does not necessarily need to be biopsied provided that a good FNAC specimen is benign. A dry tap (acellular specimen) or the presence of atypical cells are indications for biopsy. Ultrasound is a useful test for distinguishing between a solid lump and a cyst but is not a screening test for cancer. An equivocal ultrasound report on a lump or region of localized nodularity are reasons for at least performing FNAC and possibly open biopsy. The majority of women with putative benign problems will be premenopausal and in this age group bilateral mammography may not be indicated unless carcinoma is definitely suspected.

A normal mammogram in the presence of a lump is an indication for cytological or histological investigation. Most centers do not carry out mammography in patients with clinically normal or nodular breasts if they are less than 35 years of age and many have a lower age limit of 40, some not carrying out 'screening' x-rays on women under 50.

A few women who have nipple discharge will require intervention. The majority who have a milky discharge from both breasts have incomplete involution after lactation. Provided that there is no menstrual disturbance it is very unlikely that the galactorrhea results from hyperprolactinemia and blood tests are not necessary. Others with bilateral yellow discharge have duct ectasia and can be reassured. The only cases who need investigation are those with a unilateral discharge from a single duct which on testing is shown to contain hemoglobin. Such patients need a microdochectomy which will deal with the problem and give a histological diagnosis, usually intraduct papilloma or duct ectasia and only rarely an intraductal or invasive carcinoma.[42]

Gross cysts

The standard treatment for a lump which is suspected to be a cyst is to attempt aspiration. This can serve as both treatment and diagnosis. Excision of cysts is unnecessary unless the lump does not disappear or if blood is aspirated. Although a simple and relatively painless form of treatment, some patients find breast aspiration unpleasant and even when they have had multiple cysts will still be anxious that the lump will turn out to be malignant. To try and reduce the need for repeated aspirations in women with multiple cysts Hinton et al examined the value of the impeded androgen danazol in a randomized clinical trial.[43]

Patients with recurrent cysts were given either danazol 100 mg three times daily for three months or no treatment. There was a significant reduction in subsequent cyst formation in the danazol-treated group. After 36 months follow-up, 38% of the treated cases had developed new cysts compared with 91% of the control group.[44] Thus a relatively short course of therapy can lead to a long-term reduction in need for cyst aspiration.

Cyclical mastalgia

The majority of patients with cyclical breast pain do not need treatment, other than reassurance. There is a natural tendency for mastalgia to remit spontaneously, even when it has been present for more than six months. Thus alleged effective treatments may exert a profound placebo effect and only those therapies which have confirmed efficacy in randomized controlled trials should be used.

Goodwin et al reviewed critically the available treatments for mastalgia and identified certain effective treatments, together with others such as bellergal and norethisterone which were ineffective, together with diuretics, vitamin E and methylxanthine reduction which had been inadequately evaluated.[45] More recent studies have shown the inefficacy of progesterone cream[46] and medroxyprogesterone acetate.[47]

Effective therapies for cyclical mastalgia

Bromocriptine is a dopaminergic agonist which inhibits prolactin release from the pituitary. Although baseline prolactin levels are not elevated in patients with cyclical mastalgia nevertheless administration of bromocriptine can relieve breast pain, as shown in Table 39.4.[48–51] However, in a trial which compared bromocriptine, danazol and placebo, danazol proved to be more effective.[49] The largest trial of bromocriptine was a multicenter European study.[51]

Table 39.4 Effective treatments for cyclical mastalgia.

Therapy	Author	*n*	Dose	Effect
Bromocriptine	Mansel[48]	29	5 mg	67% pain relief
	Hinton[49]	47	5 mg	Worse than danazol
	Blichert-Toft[50]	8	5 mg	88% pain relief
	Durning[51]	38	5 mg	Better than placebo
	Mansel[52]	272	5 mg	Better than placebo
Danazol	Mansel[53]	28	200 mg	Better than placebo
	Doberl[54]	30	200 mg	Better than placebo
	Gorins[55]	38	400 mg	84% pain relief
	Hinton[49]	47	300 mg	Better than bromocriptine
Tamoxifen	Fentiman[35]	60	20 mg	75% pain relief
	Powles[56]	50	20 mg	Tamoxifen better than danazol
	Messinis[57]	34	10 mg	89% pain relief
	Sandrucci[58]	40	10 mg	90% pain relief
	Fentiman[59]	60	10/20 mg	Equal efficacy
Evening primrose oil	Preece[60]	103	3 g	Better than placebo
	Campbell[61]	49	4 g	EPO = placebo
Goserelin	Hamed[62]	21	3.4 mg	81% pain relief

This placebo-controlled trial confirmed the efficacy of bromocriptine but substantial numbers of cases (36%) dropped out because of side effects, nausea and dizziness or because of symptom improvement or desire to start a different therapy.

The other main agent licensed for treating mastalgia is danazol, an antigonadotrophin which acts as an impeded androgen. Many studies have confirmed its efficacy,[49,52–55] but this is at the expense of side effects including headaches, weight gain and nausea.

Tamoxifen, which is an estrogen antagonist and partial agonist, has been used for many years in the treatment of breast cancer, with a low profile of side effects. Various studies have now shown that the agent is effective in treating cyclical mastalgia,[35,56–59] and at a dose of 10 mg daily carries a very low incidence of side effects.[59] In a direct comparison of tamoxifen and danazol there was a higher response rate in those given tamoxifen (88% versus 80%), but substantially fewer side effects.[56] The drug is not licensed for this indication but can be safely prescribed for short courses by breast clinics after patients have been fully evaluated.

A different approach is the use of evening primrose oil. This is not a drug but is a normal dietary constituent, gamma linolenic acid (GLA), which is almost devoid of side effects but can relieve breast pain if given for fairly protracted courses (three months or more), although it is not as effective as bromocriptine, danazol or tamoxifen. Many doctors now prescribe evening primrose oil capsules for mastalgia at the time of first onset, since it is so nontoxic. It is probably better to wait for six months since so many of these patients will have a spontaneous remission of their symptoms.

One of the major problems in managing women with protracted severe mastalgia is the duration of treatment which needs to be given. Even after effective therapy, a substantial proportion of these cases will get a recurrence of pain. This is not affected by prolonging the course of treatment from three months to six.[56] In an attempt to produce a major endocrine upheaval which might produce a more permanent relief of pain, a study was conducted at Guy's Hospital using the GnRH agonist goserelin to produce reversible ovarian suppression which lasted for six months.[60] The agent proved to be effective, relieving pain in more than 80% of cases, but the majority had recurred within six months of stopping treatment. Apart from this there were substantial menopausal side effects including hot flashes, headaches, vaginal dryness and joint pains. When bone density was measured there was a substantial reduction, which had not returned to normal one year after stopping treatment.[61] Thus the use of a GnRH agonist should not be contemplated as therapy for cyclical mastalgia.

Premalignant conditions

Patients with biopsy proven hyperplasia, or with recurrent breast cysts, are not usually kept under surveillance because they are not at substantially increased risk of malignancy. The group who do need follow-up are those with epithelial atypical hyperplasia, or lobular carcinoma *in situ* (lobular neoplasia). Such cases are at increased risk. It is usual for them to have six-monthly clinical check-ups and biennial mammograms. Whether such a system leads to earlier diagnosis and better prognosis is as yet unproven.

These patients are eligible for the IBIS study. This is the International Breast Cancer Intervention Study which is seeking to determine the value of tamoxifen in women at increased risk of breast cancer.[62] Eligible volunteers who have either a strong family history of breast cancer, or have histological confirmation of premalignancy, are randomized to receive either tamoxifen 20 mg daily, or placebo for 5 years, while remaining under close clinical and radiological follow-up.

Conclusion

A substantial number of women labeled as having benign breast disease do not have anything wrong with them and can be reassured and not kept under surveillance. So strong has been the reaction against 'fibroadenosis' in the USA that there is a denial that any women with painful lumpy breasts need treatment. Of course, the majority do not. Nevertheless European studies have indicated the extent of the problem, and effective therapies which are available. Future work will focus on making treatments less toxic and refining risk so that appropriate patients can be considered for surveillance and possible intervention.

REFERENCES

1. Warren JC 1905 The surgeon and the pathologist. A plea for reciprocity as illustrated by the considerations of the classification and treatment of benign tumors of the breast. Journal of the American Medical Association 45: 149–165
2. Page DL, Vander Zwaag R, Rogers LW, Williams LT, Walker WE, Hartmann WH 1978 Relation between component parts of fibrocystic disease complex and breast cancer. Journal of the National Cancer Institute 61: 1055–1063
3. Page DL, Dupont WD, Rogers LW, Rados MS 1985 Atypical hyperplastic lesions of the female breast. Cancer 55: 2698–2708
4. Tavassoli FA, Norris HJ 1990 A comparison of the results of long-term follow-up for atypical intraductal hyperplasia and intraductal hyperplasia of the breast. Cancer 65: 518–529
5. London SJ, Connolly JL, Schnitt SJ, Colditz GA 1992 A prospective study of benign breast disease and the risk of breast cancer. Journal of the American Medical Association 267: 941–944
6. Dupont WD, Parl FF, Hartmann WH, Brinton LA, Winfield AC, Worrell JA, Schuyler PA, Plummer WD 1993 Breast cancer risk associated with proliferative breast disease and atypical hyperplasia. Cancer 71: 1258–1265
7. Hughes LE, Mansel RE, Webster DJT 1987 Aberrations of normal development and involution (ANDI): a new perspective on pathogenesis and nomenclature of benign breast disorders. Lancet ii: 1316–1319
8. Swain MC, Hayward JL, Bulbrook RD 1973 Plasma oestradiol and progesterone in benign breast disease. European Journal of Cancer 9: 553–556
9. Sitruk-Ware LR, Sterkers N, Mowszowicz I, Mauvais-Jarvis P 1977 Inadequate corpus luteum function in women with benign breast disease. Journal of Clinical Endocrinology Metabolism 44: 771–774
10. Golinger RC, Krebs J, Fisher ER, Danowski TS 1978 Hormones and the pathophysiology of fibrocystic mastopathy: elevated luteinizing hormone levels. Surgery 84: 212–215
11. DeBoever J, Vanderkerckhove D 1982 Benign breast disease: steroid concentrations. Journal of Steroid Biochemistry 17: cxiii
12. Marchesoni D, Gangemi M, Mozzanega B, Paternoster D, Grazziotin A, Maggino T 1981 Inadequate luteal phase and benign breast disease. Clinical Endocrinology Obstetrics and Gynecology 8: 160–163
13. England PC, Skinner LG, Cottrell KM, Sellwood RA 1976 Serum oestradiol-17beta in women with benign and malignant breast disease. British Journal of Cancer 30: 571–576
14. Sherman BM, Korenman SG 1974 Inadequate corpus luteum function: a pathophysiological interpretation of human breast cancer epidemiology. Cancer 33: 1306–1312
15. Mauvais-Jarvis P, Sitruk-Ware R, Kuttenn F, Sterkers N 1976 Luteal phase insufficiency: a common pathophysiologic factor in development of benign and malignant breast diseases. Commentaries on Research in Breast Diseases 1: 25–29
16. Balbi C, Candido R, D'Ajello M 1978 Tassi ematici dell'estradiolo e del'progesterone nelle mastopatie benigne. Archives of Obstetrics and Gynecology 83: 93–97
17. Rolland PH, Martin PM, Bourry M, Rolland AM, Serment H 1980 Human benign breast disease: relationships between prostaglandin E2, steroid hormones and thermographic effects of the inhibitors of prostaglandin biosynthesis. Advances in Prostaglandin Thromboxane Research 6: 581–584
18. Walsh PV, Wang DY, McDicken I, Stell PM, Bulbrook RD, George WD 1984 Serum progesterone concentration during the luteal phase in women with benign breast disease. European Journal of Cancer and Clinical Oncology 20: 1339–1343
19. Geller S, Grenier J, Nahoul K, Scholler R 1979 Insuffisance luteale et mastopathies benignes. Annals of Endocrinology (Paris) 40: 45–46
20. Wang DY, Hayward JL, Bulbrook RD 1981 Testosterone levels in the plasma of normal women and patients with benign breast disease or breast cancer. European Journal of Cancer 2: 373–376
21. England PC, Sellwood RA, Knyba RE, Irvine JDB 1981 Serum androgen levels and the menstrual cycle in women with benign or malignant breast disease. Clinical Oncology 7: 213–219
22. Jones MK, Dyer GI, Ramsay ID, Collins WP 1981 Studies on apparent free cortisol and testosterone in plasma from patients with breast tumours. Postgraduate Medical Journal 57: 89–94
23. Boyns AR, Cole EN, Griffiths K, Roberts MM, Buchan R, Wilson RG, Forrest APM 1973 Plasma prolactin in breast cancer. European Journal of Cancer 9: 99–102
24. Sheth NA, Ranadive KJ, Suraiya JN, Sheth AR 1975 Circulating levels of prolactin in human breast cancer. British Journal of Cancer 32: 160–167
25. Franchimont P, Dourcy C, Legros JJ, Reuter A, Vrindts-Gevaert Y, Van Cauwenberge JR, Remacle P, Gaspard U, Colin C 1976 Dosage de la prolactine dans les conditions normales et pathologiques. Annals of Endocrinology (Paris) 37: 127–156
26. Bischoff J, Rebhan EM, Prestele H, Becker H 1980 Serum prolaktin und Anamnesevergleich bei Mammazysten und zysticher Mastopathie. Geburtsh Frauenheilk 40: 65–71
27. Hamed HH, Cody A, Chaudary MA, Fentiman IS 1989 Follow-up of patients with aspirated breast cysts: is it necessary? Archives of Surgery 21: 253–259
28. Wang DY, Fentiman IS 1985 Epidemiology and endocrinology of benign breast disease. Breast Cancer Research and Treatment 6: 5–36
29. Leis HP 1993 Gross breast cysts: significance of apocrine type, identification by cyst fluid analysis. Breast Disease 6: 185–194
30. Miller WR, Dixon JM, Scott WN, Forrest APM 1983 Classification of human breast cysts according to electrolyte and androgen conjugate composition. Clinical Oncology 9: 227–232
31. Dixon JM, Miller WA, Scott WN 1984 pH of human breast cyst fluids. Clinical Oncology 10: 221–224
32. Hamed H, Wang DY, Moore JW, Clark GMG, Fentiman IS 1990 Growth factor and electrolyte concentration in human breast cyst fluid. European Journal of Cancer 26: 479–480

33. Lai LC, Siraj AK, Kadory S, Lennard TWJ 1995 Concentrations of soluble vascular adhesion molecule-1 and E-selectin in breast cyst fluid and their relation with cyst type. British Journal of Cancer 82: 83–85
34. Nichols S, Waters WE, Wheeler MJ 1980 Management of female breast disease by Southampton general practitioners. British Medical Journal 281: 1450–1453
35. Fentiman IS, Caleffi M, Brame K, Chaudary MA, Hayward JL 1986 Double-blind controlled trial of tamoxifen therapy for mastalgia. Lancet i: 287–288
36. Watt-Boolsen S, Emus HC, Junge J 1982 Fibrocystic disease and mastalgia: a histological and enzyme-histochemical study. Danish Medical Bulletin 29: 252–254
37. Kumar S, Mansel RE, Hughes LE, Woodhead JS, Edwards CA, Scanlon MF, Newcombe RG 1984 Prolactin response to thyrotropin hormone stimulation and dopaminergic inhibition in benign breast disease. Cancer 53: 1311–1315
38. Fentiman IS 1992 Mastalgia mostly merits masterly inactivity. British Journal of Clinical Practice 46: 158
39. Ramirez AJ, Jarrett SR, Hamed H, Smith P, Fentiman IS 1995 Psychosocial adjustment of women with mastalgia. The Breast 4: 48–51
40. Love SM, Gelman RS, Silen W 1982 Fibrocystic disease of the breast: a non-disease. New England Journal of Medicine 307: 1010–1014
41. Cant PJ, Madden MV, Close PM, Learmonth GG, Hacking EA, Dent D 1987 Case for conservative management of selected fibroadenomas of the breast. British Journal of Surgery 74: 857–859
42. Chaudary MA, Millis RR, Davies GC, Hayward JL 1982 Nipple discharge. The diagnostic value of testing for occult blood. Annals of Surgery 196: 651–655
43. Hinton CP, Williams MR, Roebuck EJ, Blamey RW 1986 A controlled trial of danazol in treatment of multiple recurrent breast cysts. British Journal of Clinical Practice 40: 3–5
44. Locker AP, Hinton CP, Roebuck EJ, Blamey RW 1989 Long-term follow-up of patients treated with a single course of danazol for recurrent breast cysts. British Journal of Clinical Practice 68 (Suppl): 100–101
45. Goodwin PJ, Neelam M, Boyd NF 1988 Cyclical mastopathy: a critical review of therapy. British Journal of Surgery 75: 837–844
46. McFadyen IJ, Raab GM, Macintyre CCA, Forrest APM 1989 Progesterone cream for cyclic breast pain. British Medical Journal 298: 931
47. Maddox PR, Mansel RE, Harrison BJ, Horobin JM, Preece PE, Walker K, Nicholson RI 1990 A randomised controlled trial of medroxyprogesterone acetate in mastalgia. Annals of the Royal College of Surgeons of England 72: 71–76
48. Mansel RE, Preece PE, Hughes LE 1978 A double blind trial of the prolactin inhibitor bromocriptine in painful benign breast disease. British Journal of Surgery 65: 724–727
49. Hinton CP, Bishop HM, Holliday HW, Doyle PJ, Blamey RW 1986 A double-blind controlled trial of danazol and bromocriptine in the management of severe cyclical breast pain. British Journal of Clinical Practice 40: 326–330
50. Blichert-Toft M, Andersen AN, Henriksen OB, Mygind T 1979 Treatment of mastalgia with bromocriptine: a double-blind cross-over study. British Medical Journal i: 237
51. Durning P, Sellwood RA 1982 Bromocriptine in severe cyclical breast pain. British Journal of Surgery 69: 248–250
52. Mansel RE, Dogliotti L 1990 European multicentre trial of bromocriptine in cyclical mastalgia. Lancet 335: 190–193
53. Mansel RE, Wisbey JR, Hughes LE 1979 Controlled trial of the anti-gonadotrophin danazol in painful benign breast disease. Lancet i: 928–930
54. Doberl A, Tobiassen T, Rasmussen T 1984 Treatment of recurrent cyclical mastodynia in patients with fibrocystic breast disease. Acta Obstetrica Gynecologica Scandinavica 123(suppl): 177–184
55. Gorins A, Perret F, Tournant B, Rogier C, Lipszyc J 1984 A French double-blind crossover study (danazol versus placebo) in the treatment of severe fibrocystic breast disease. European Journal of Gynecological Oncology 2: 85–89
56. Powles TJ, Ford HT, Gazet J-C 1987 A randomised clinical trial to compare tamoxifen with danazol for treatment of benign mammary dysplasia. Senologia 2: 1–5
57. Messinis IE, Lolis D 1988 Treatment of premenstrual mastalgia with tamoxifen. Acta Obstetrica Gynecologica Scandinavica 67: 307–308
58. Sandrucci S, Mussa A, Festa A, Borre A, Grosso M, Dogliotti L 1986 Comparison of tamoxifen and bromocriptine in management of fibrocystic breast disease: a randomized blind study. Annals of the New York Academy of Science 464: 626–628
59. Fentiman IS, Caleffi M, Hamed H, Chaudary MA 1988 Dosage and duration of tamoxifen treatment for mastalgia: a controlled trial. British Journal of Surgery 75: 845–846
60. Hamed H, Chaudary MA, Caleffi M, Fentiman IS 1990 LHRH analogue for treatment of recurrent and refractory mastalgia. Annals of the Royal College of Surgeons of England 72: 221–224
61. Hamed H, Fogelman I, Smith P, Gregory W, Fentiman IS 1993 Effect of a GnRH analogue on bone mass in premenopausal patients with mastalgia. The Breast 2: 79–82
62. Fentiman IS 1990 The role of tamoxifen in the prevention of breast cancer. European Journal of Cancer 26: 655–656

40. Precocious puberty

M. T. Dattani C. G. D. Brook

Introduction

Puberty is the process by which reproductive capability is attained. It is the transitional period between childhood and adulthood during which profound physical and psychological changes occur and is characterized by the adolescent growth spurt, the development of secondary sexual characteristics, the attainment of fertility and the establishment of an individual's identity.

The timing of these events is extremely variable in individuals. Underlying this variation is a secular trend, whereby the age of menarche in developed countries has decreased by approximately 2–3 months per decade over the last 100–150 years.[1,2] This positive secular trend is thought to be due to an improvement is socioeconomic conditions, nutritional status and general health and well-being, and has now ceased in the USA, where the age of menarche is 12.8 years.[3]

Genetic factors play an important role in determining the onset of puberty, as evidenced by twin studies which have shown that identical twin sisters growing up together under identical circumstances in developed West European countries achieved menarche an average of two months apart.[4] Nonidentical twins, on the other hand, achieved menarche an average of 10 months apart. Additionally, secondary sexual development occurs earlier in girls from an Asian and Afro-Caribbean background than in white girls.

In girls, the first external sign of pubertal development is breast growth. This is the result of the secretion of estrogen by the ovaries, whereas the development of pubic and axillary hair is the result of the secretion of androgens by the adrenal gland.[5] With careful observation, it is clear that an increase in height velocity predates breast development as the first sign of puberty in girls.[6]

Breast and pubic hair development are staged according to Tanner (1962),[4] where stage 1 represents the pre-adolescent appearance and stage 5 the adult appearance (Figs 40.1, 40.2). Since the different components of puberty are due to different underlying endocrine mechanisms, an overall stage of puberty cannot be applied, and so each component should be staged separately. Preceding the external changes, the ovaries undergo a major transformation controlled by the secretion of the gonadotropins, luteinizing hormone (LH) and follicle stimulating hormone

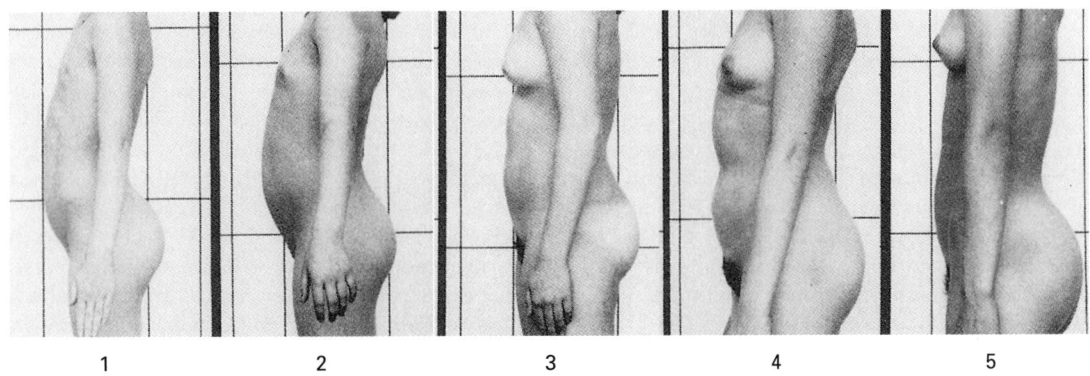

Fig. 40.1 Stages of breast development according to Marshall and Tanner[5] during normal puberty.

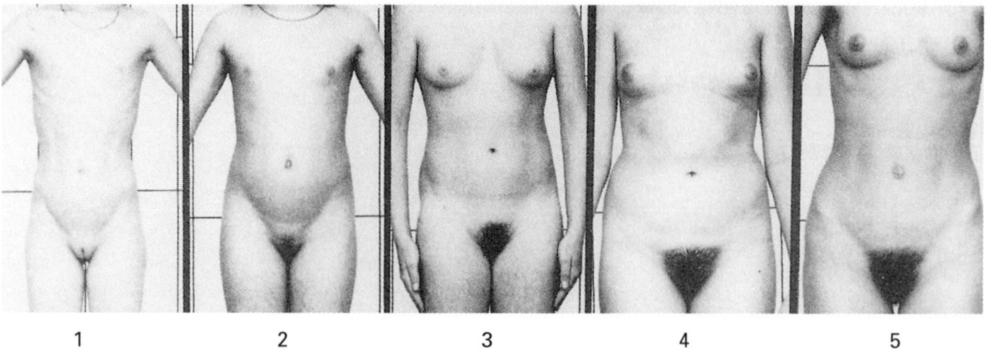

Fig. 40.2 Stages of pubic hair development according to Marshall and Tanner[5] during normal puberty.

(FSH), by the anterior pituitary gland. At puberty, the nocturnal pulsatile secretion of these gonadotropins results in the development of several follicles which give the ovary its multicystic appearance. This phase of development is characteristic of the pattern of gonadotropin secretion in early puberty, prior to the onset of positive feedback.[7]

The pubertal growth spurt represents the fastest rate of growth achieved by an individual after the rapid growth of infancy. The growth spurt in girls is dependent upon a combination of human growth hormone and sex steroids in the form of estradiol produced by the ovaries. The growth rate doubles to about 9 cm/year during this phase, which usually coincides with breast stages 2–3. A rise in pulsatile growth hormone (GH) secretion must occur for this increase in growth rate to be manifest.[8,9,10] The change in GH secretion is brought about by an increase in pulse amplitude rather than frequency.[11,12] Both GH and sex steroids will lead to the increased production of insulin-like growth factor (IGF-1) which is responsible for linear growth.[13]

The duration of puberty, as defined by the time interval between the first sign of puberty and the attainment of complete maturity as defined by menarche, ranges from 18 months to six years with a mean of 2.34 years (SD 1.03).[5] The progression of puberty from breast stage 2 to 5 takes on average four years, with 5% progressing within 1.5 years and 5% taking up to nine years to achieve stage 5. 75% of girls will have achieved their peak height velocity before reaching breast stage 4. Once menarche has been achieved, a girl will usually only grow by a further 5 cm.

ENDOCRINE REGULATION OF PUBERTY

Gonadotropin-releasing hormone present in GnRH neurons in the arcuate nucleus of the mediobasal hypothalamus is released in a pulsatile fashion. Its secretion is regulated by catecholamines, which release GnRH, and by dopamine, serotonin and opioids which decrease GnRH release. GnRH migrates down the hypothalamo-hypophyseal tracts to the anterior pituitary gland. It then binds to cell surface receptors on gonadotrophs[14,15] and stimulates the production and secretion of luteinizing hormone (LH) and follicle stimulating hormone (FSH) from the gonadotrophs,[16] which then stimulate the gonads. LH initiates steroidogenesis in theca interna cells surrounding ovarian follicles, with the resultant production of ovarian androgens, and FSH increases the proliferation of granulosa cells, inducing an aromatizing enzyme which then converts testosterone to estradiol and androstenedione to estrone. Estrogens stimulate granulosa cells locally and influence higher centers, the hypothalamus and pituitary to modulate gonadotropin secretion.

The human fetal hypothalamus contains GnRH-containing neurons by 14 weeks of gestation. The fetal pituitary gland can synthesize and store FSH and LH by 20 weeks of gestation and secretes these hormones in response to GnRH.[17] In midgestation, peak serum levels of FSH and LH reach adult castrate levels. Levels subsequently decline and remain low until term, in response to the high concentrations of estrogen in pregnancy. Following birth, a fall in the estrogen concentration leads to a rapid increase in gonadotropin secretion. Levels of FSH and LH fluctuate widely in the first months of life, and the overall effect is to increase serum estradiol concentrations, although levels of both estradiol and gonadotropins are lower than those in the fetus and the pubertal child. Between the ages of 12–18 months, the concentrations of gonadotropins decrease, and during childhood, the secretion of GnRH, and hence FSH and LH, is quiescent, reaching a nadir at 7–7.5 years.[18] The inhibition of gonadotropin secretion during the juvenile phase is probably centrally mediated.

In the peripubertal period, gonadotropin levels increase, initially at night.[19] An increase in both baseline and peak LH levels occurs in early puberty.[18] In early and midpuberty, the secretion of LH is predominantly sleep-related and is pulsatile in nature. Later in puberty, the pulsatile secretion of LH is observed during the daytime, as well as at night. In adults, discrete pulses of LH occur at 90 minute intervals during the follicular and early luteal phases. Superimposed upon this pulsatile secretion of gonadotropins is a cyclical pattern, which is dependent upon the positive feedback effect of estradiol secreted in the follicular phase on gonadotropin secretion by the anterior pituitary. This effect, which is established later in puberty in females,[20] results in the midcycle surge of FSH and LH, and hence ovulation. The LH surge lasts for 24–36 hours and the pulsatility of LH over 24 hours is essential for ovulation.

During the peripubertal period, the response of pituitary gonadotrophs to exogenous GnRH changes, such that prepubertally, the release of LH in response to GnRH is minimal beyond infancy. This response increases strikingly during puberty, and this response is maintained in adults.[21] The prepubertal pattern of gonadotropin secretion can be converted to the pubertal pattern by the administration of GnRH in low dose boluses at 60–120 minute intervals over a five day period.[22] Recent development of immunochemiluminescent assays for LH and FSH have underlined the value of using stimulated LH values in the diagnosis of precocious puberty.[23] On the other hand, stimulated FSH levels cannot discriminate adequately between normal prepubertal controls and girls with precocious puberty.[24] Interestingly, using this highly sensitive assay, basal levels of both LH and FSH were highly sensitive and specific for the diagnosis of gonadotropin-dependent precocious puberty, and this may be a useful method for monitoring the adequacy of treatment in suppressing gonadotropin secretion in this group of patients.

In addition to the hypothalamo-pituitary-gonadal axis, a significant increase in adrenal androgen secretion is observed by the age of eight years.[25] The androgens dehydroepiandrosterone and androstenedione are produced by the zona reticularis in the adrenal gland under the control of ACTH, with suppression by dexamethasone. The exact underlying mechanism for this process, which is known as adrenarche, remains unknown. It is essential for the normal development of pubic hair in females.

There is considerable evidence to suggest that adrenarche and gonadarche are independent events. Adrenarche is not essential for the process of gonadarche, since children with Addison's disease enter puberty at the normal time. Additionally, children with premature adrenarche achieve gonadarche at the appropriate age.

PRECOCIOUS PUBERTY—DEFINITION AND CLASSIFICATION

Precocious puberty is defined by the onset of secondary sexual characteristics before the age of eight years (mean pubertal age –3 standard deviations from the mean) in girls. If the sexual precocity is consonant, the temporal relationship of the various events is maintained, i.e. breast development precedes the appearance of pubic hair development, with the growth spurt occurring at breast stage 2–3. Menarche is a late event, occurring at breast stage 4–5. Lack of consonance of puberty is defined by the isolated early development of breast tissue (premature thelarche, thelarche variant) or pubic and axillary hair (premature adrenarche, late-onset congenital adrenal hyperplasia). The classification of precocious puberty is based upon the activation of the hypothalamo-pituitary-gonadal axis (central or gonadotropin-dependent precocious puberty) or the activation of the ovaries independently of gonadotropin secretion (gonadotropin-independent precocious puberty). Other variants include thelarche, thelarche-variant and the virilization associated with adrenarche, congenital adrenal hyperplasia and adrenal tumours. The causes of precocious puberty are described in Table 40.1. In a retrospective study of 197 girls with precocious sexual maturation, the commonest underlying etiology was idiopathic gonadotropin-dependent precocious puberty (Fig. 40.3).

Gonadotropin-dependent precocious puberty

In central or gonadotropin-dependent precocious puberty, the hypothalamo-pituitary-gonadal axis is prematurely activated, the pattern of endocrine changes is the same as in normal puberty and the pubertal development is consonant.

Etiology

The cause of the premature activation of the hypothalamo-pituitary-gonadal axis is unknown in a large majority of girls with precocious puberty, and may be due to the removal of the inhibitory CNS

Table 40.1 Causes of precocious puberty.

I. Gonadotropin-dependent precocious puberty
 Idiopathic—commonest cause in females
 Secondary
 — congenital anomalies
 — brain neoplasms
 — cysts
 — hydrocephalus
 — post-infection
 — post-trauma
 — post-cranial radiotherapy
 — neurofibromatosis
 HCG-producing neoplasms

II. Gonadotropin-independent precocious puberty
 Ovarian cysts
 McCune-Albright syndrome

III. Abnormal patterns of gonadotropin secretion
 Premature thelarche
 Thelarche variant
 Hypothyroidism

IV. Virilization
 Adrenarche
 Congenital adrenal hyperplasia
 Cushing's syndrome
 Adrenal tumour

V. Exogenous sex steroids

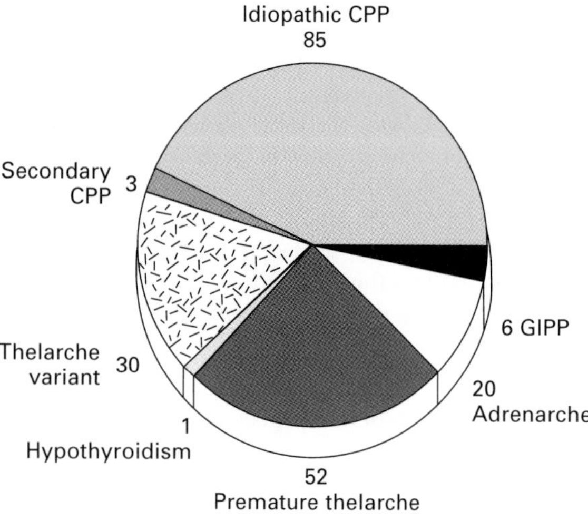

Fig. 40.3 Etiology of precocious puberty in 197 girls presenting at the Middlesex Hospital with sexual precocity over a 15 year period (GIPP: gonadotropin independent precocious puberty; CPP: central precocious puberty). (From Bridges NA, Christopher IA, Hindmarch PC 1994 Archives of Diseases in Childhood 70: 116–118. Reproduced with permission.)

regulation of the axis. Gonadotropin-dependent precocious puberty can be secondary to a number of causes. These include tumors (optic nerve glioma and pineal tumor), hamartomata, hydrocephalus, trauma and neurofibromatosis.[26,27,28] Girls who have received cranial radiotherapy for brain tumors or prophylactically for leukemia have a greater incidence of precocious puberty.[29] Other causes of precocious puberty include adoption of girls from developing countries, and children who have been sexually abused.[30,31]

Clinical features

Breast development is usually the first sign, with the later development of pubic and axillary hair, and menarche. The child is usually tall, with a rapid height velocity. However, as an adult, the child will be disproportionately short with an increased trunk to limb length ratio. Other features include abnormal neurological signs in girls with brain tumors and hydrocephalus, cutaneous features of neurofibromatosis, etc.

Investigations

A pelvic ultrasound scan will reveal multicystic ovaries with a change in the shape of the uterus to an adult configuration. An endometrial echo is also visible. Bone age is advanced given the chronological age. Gonadotropins and sex steroids are secreted in a pulsatile fashion, and there is a circadian variation, with concentrations of gonadotropins greatest at night and sex steroids highest in the early morning. Single samples of blood are useless, and an overnight profile of gonadotropin secretion may yield more information, although this procedure entails sampling of blood at 20 minute intervals. This is time-consuming and expensive, and so, in practice, the gonadotropin response to GnRH stimulation is used. In normal prepubertal girls, an increment of 3–4 IU/L in LH values and 2–3 IU/L in FSH values is observed in response to 100 μg administered intravenously, whereas the response is much more dramatic in pubertal girls, particularly for LH.[32] It has been suggested that a single LH measurement 30 minutes after GnRH administration is diagnostic in gonadotropin-dependent precocious puberty.[33] An early morning measurement of serum estradiol concentration would be elevated.

Although in boys sexual precocity is almost never idiopathic and an MRI scan of the brain is mandatory, gonadotropin-dependent precocious puberty is often idiopathic in girls, and neuroradiological imaging need probably only be performed if neurological signs and symptoms are present. In a study of 62 children (51 girls, 11 boys) with gonadotropin-dependent precocious puberty, 18 (11 girls, 7 boys) showed intracranial pathology.[34] In our practice, we have never seen a girl develop neurological signs or symptoms after presenting solely with precocious puberty.

A transabdominal pelvic ultrasound scan, performed in the right hands, is essential in all girls with precocious puberty.[35] With a full bladder, the uterus and ovaries can be visualized and appropriate measurements of the length, fundal and cervical diameter of the uterus, and endometrial thickness can be made. Ovarian volume can also be calculated. In girls with pubertal levels of gonadotropins, the ovaries become multicystic, defined as more than six follicles with a diameter of more than 4 mm.[36] The prepubertal uterus is tubular in shape, and becomes pear-shaped in puberty. In response to adequate secretion of estrogen, the endometrium thickens and an endometrial thickness of 5 mm or more indicates that menarche is imminent. In a recent study of 67 girls with sexual precocity, pelvic ultrasound scans performed at initial presentation showed significantly increased uterine lengths and ovarian volumes compared with the normal population, with a significantly increased fundal-cervical ratio.[37] The ultrasound findings which were the most sensitive predictors of sexual precocity included the presence of a midline endometrial echo and a uterine length above the 97th centile for age.

Treatment

In children with sexual precocity secondary to underlying brain tumors, cysts and hydrocephalus, treatment of the primary lesion should be undertaken in the first instance. In children with idiopathic precocious puberty, the decision to treat should be based upon the age of the child, and the effect of early menses upon the psyche of the child.[38] A further consideration is the effect on final height of early puberty. Children with precocious puberty have a truncated period of childhood growth, and short stature is therefore a feature of untreated precocious puberty since the pubertal growth spurt occurs at an age when insufficient growth has occurred in childhood. Treatment of precocious puberty will revert the growth rate to a suboptimal childhood rate, and there is little evidence to support an increase in final height as a result of the suppression of puberty, since lost growth potential is not retrieved.[39] The social and psychological consequences of early puberty are profound, particularly if menarche has been achieved. These psychosocial effects are the main indications for treatment of early puberty. Early puberty will have maximum effects on final height and psyche on the youngest children, and it is this group who will benefit the most from treatment. In particular, if menses are imminent as determined by pelvic ultrasound scan, then treatment may be indicated in order to postpone this event.

In gonadotropin-dependent precocious puberty, the first line of treatment is the use of gonadotropin-releasing hormone analogs.[40] High doses of the analogs will initially lead to stimulatory effects, but subsequently, the receptors on gonadotrophs undergo down-regulation, and gonadotropin secretion ceases.[41] Hence, initial stimulatory effects of gonadotropins on the ovaries lead to secretion of estradiol and further progression of pubertal signs until down-regulation of the receptors on gonadotrophs leads to a decrease in gonadotropin levels, with a reduction in estradiol levels. The effectiveness of treatment can be sensitively and reliably monitored by measurement of early morning urine estrone-3-glucuronide levels, which are suppressed by the treatment.[42] Regression of breast development and suppression of menses is observed. The shape of the uterus does not revert to the prepubertal form. However, follow-up with regular pelvic ultrasound scans reveals that the endometrium remains thin, and the ovaries remain quiescent.

Synthetic depot preparations of GnRH analogs are now available with enhanced activity and a longer half-life than natural GnRH. These are administered subcutaneously on a once-monthly basis.[43] Gonadal suppression is observed in most children with this regimen.[44] Studies have suggested that the depot preparations are more efficacious in suppressing the height velocity and bone maturation than the intranasal preparations, which need to be administered daily.[45] Initial stimulatory effects can be prevented by the use of cyproterone acetate in conjunction with the GnRH analog over the first 4–6 weeks. Vaginal bleeding may occur at the start of treatment due to estrogen withdrawal, and can usually (but not always) be prevented by the administration of cyproterone.

The effect of GnRH analog is to suppress gonadotropin secretion. This leads to a fall in estradiol concentration and a fall in GH secretion and IGF-1 levels since sex steroids stimulate GH secretion via an action on the hypothalamus.[46,47] This translates to a reduction in the height velocity,[48] and this is most dramatic in those children with the most advanced bone age.[49]

Although it has been suggested that treatment with GnRH analogs improves predicted height,[50] a similar improvement has also been observed with time in untreated precocious puberty.[51] Data on actual final height suggest that treatment with GnRH analogs and cyproterone acetate cannot recover lost height potential, and children cannot attain their target midparental height,[52,53,54] although more recently, it has been suggested that an intranasal GnRH analog improves the initially impaired height prognosis.[55] Girls who have a poor height prediction at the start of treatment may well benefit to a greater extent from GnRH treatment compared with girls who have an initial predicted height which is not dissimilar to their target height.[56] Additionally, the benefit of GnRH treatment on final height may be more clear-cut in younger children with sexual precocity.[57]

It has been suggested that a combination of GH and GnRH analogs may result in an increase in final height in GH-insufficient children,[58,59] but although the combination treatment leads to an increase in height standard deviation score (SDS) for bone age and in predicted adult height in girls with precocious puberty, there are limited data to support a similar increase in final height.[60] We have recently followed 10 girls with idiopathic gonadotropin-dependent precocious puberty who received a combination of GnRH analog and hGH to final height. Our data show no increment in final height over the predicted height at the start of treatment (Bridges NA, Hindmarsh PC, Brook CGD; personal communication submitted for publication). Additionally, such a treatment is likely to lead to polycystic ovarian disease, with its attendant problems such as obesity, menstrual irregularities and hyperandrogenism (see ch. 34), and should not be embarked upon without careful consideration.[61]

Treatment should be stopped once the child has reached an age where puberty is acceptable. Pubertal development is then recommenced at an advanced stage approximately three months later.[62] Gonadotropin secretion recommences approximately four months after cessation of depot GnRH analogs, and most girls menstruate within a year of stopping treatment.[48,63] Normal fertility has been documented in girls with both treated and untreated gonadotropin-dependent precocious puberty.[64,65,66]

Gonadotropin-independent precocious puberty

This condition is characterized by the secretion of estradiol by the ovaries, independent of the secretion of gonadotropins from the pituitary gland, which remain at low levels.[67] There is often a lack of consonance in pubertal development, and menses may be observed with minimal breast development. Girls with this condition usually have the McCune-Albright syndrome (MAS), which is characterized by large irregular café-au-lait pigmented areas (Fig. 40.4), polyostotic fibrous dysplasia and a variety of endocrinopathies. This condition occurs in both males and females with an equal sex incidence, and is due to a somatic activating missense mutation in the gene for the α-subunit of the G-protein ($G_{s\alpha}$) which stimulates cAMP formation.[68] The mutation is found in variable abundance in different affected endocrine and nonendocrine tissues, consistent with the mosaic distribution of abnormal cells generated by a somatic cell mutation early in embryogenesis.[69] Excessive cAMP production leads to various clinical features. For instance, G-proteins associated with the gonadotropin receptor are vital signal transducing messenger proteins, leading to a rise in the intracellular concentration of cAMP. In normal individuals, activation occurs for a limited time period. However, in patients with MAS, mutations in the α-subunit of the G-protein lead to constitutive activation of the receptor, with excessive secretion of estradiol by large ovarian cysts.

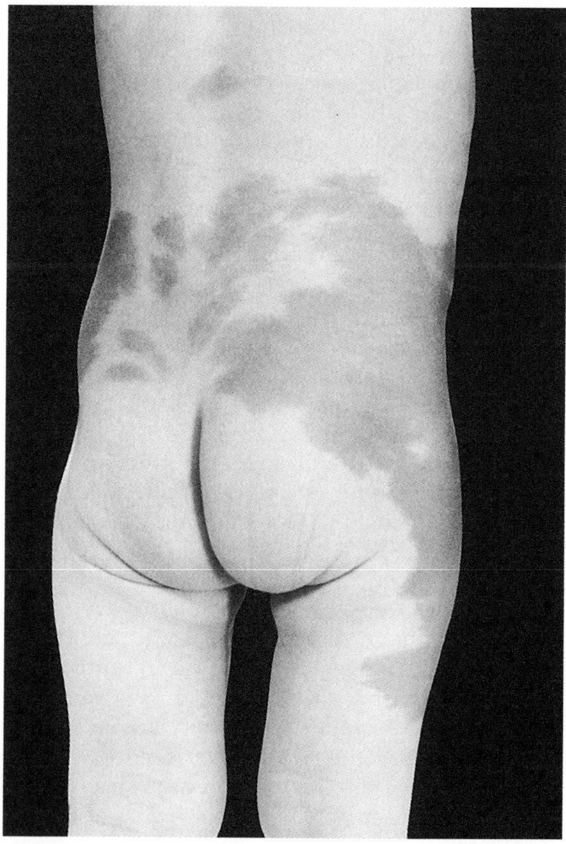

Fig. 40.4 Irregular café-au-lait pigmentation in McCune-Albright syndrome.

Clinical features

Sexual precocity is one of the commonest clinical features of the condition. For instance, in a study of 13 females with the condition, sexual precocity (age of onset 0.3–8.5 years) was observed in all of the patients.[70] In three of these patients, the first sign of sexual precocity was menarche, whilst in two patients, the first sign was the development of pubic hair. The large ovarian cysts may lead to the presence of palpable ovaries. Other features include polyostotic fibrous dysplasia, large irregular café-au-lait patches of skin hyperpigmentation which are unilateral in 50% of cases, thyrotoxicosis, Cushing's syndrome, pituitary gigantism, cardiac disease and hepatobiliary disease.

Investigations

Investigation of the precocious puberty should include a pelvic ultrasound scan, a bone age and an GnRH test. The pelvic USS may show large ovarian cysts, with uterine development and endometrial thickening. The bone age is generally advanced. The gonadotropin response to exogenous GnRH is absent, since the sexual precocity is gonadotropin-independent. Serum estradiol levels are usually raised.

Other investigations include a skeletal survey and a bone scan, which may show evidence of polyostotic fibrous dysplasia, an echocardiogram, liver function tests, 24-hour urinary free cortisol levels, thyroid function tests and assessment of GH secretion.

Treatment

Since the sexual precocity is independent of gonadotropin secretion, GnRH analogs cannot be used to treat this condition. Other options available are the use of cyproterone acetate and medroxyprogesterone. Cyproterone acetate is an anti-androgen with progestogenic properties.[71] Its effect on sexual precocity is partly due to its progestational action, and partly due to its anti-androgenic effects. One drawback of cyproterone lies in its effect on adrenal function, which is suppressed by this drug.[72] However, it remains the drug of first choice for the treatment of gonadotropin-independent precocious puberty.[73] Medroxyprogesterone is a progestogen which has a similar mode of action to cyproterone and is also used in the treatment of gonadotropin-independent precocious puberty, when it is administered parenterally.[74]

Ketoconazole is an inhibitor of steroid biosynthesis, and acts via the inhibition of cytochrome P450 enzymes.[75] High doses are effective in the treatment of precocious puberty,[76] but side-effects include adrenal suppression and hepatic dysfunction. Testolactone inhibits the aromatization of testosterone to estradiol and therefore estradiol levels are decreased and pubertal progression arrested. It has been used in the treatment of gonadotropin-independent precocious puberty.[77] Ketoconazole and testolactone are used in the event of failure of cyproterone acetate treatment.

Prognosis

Girls with gonadotropin-independent precocious puberty usually experience normal gonadotropin-dependent precocious puberty at the appropriate time,[78] but abnormal ovarian function continues into adult life, with development of ovarian cysts and menstrual irregularities. The prognosis for height is better in girls with the MAS than in girls with gonadotropin-dependent precocious puberty.[51] The long-term outlook is determined by the presence of nonendocrine manifestations such as cardiomyopathy and hepatic abnormalities.

Premature thelarche/thelarche variant

Clinical features

Thelarche describes the phenomenon of isolated breast development. It is not generally accompanied by other signs of puberty. Growth velocity is normal and the bone age is not advanced. Premature thelarche is often present from infancy. The degree of development may fluctuate.

Thelarche variant describes the isolated development of breast tissue in girls with an advanced bone age and an increase in the growth velocity.

Investigations

In thelarche, measurement of gonadotropins reveals a pulsatile pattern of FSH secretion, with no increase in LH values.[79] On administration of GnRH, the LH values remain low, but the FSH levels increase. A pelvic ultrasound scan may reveal an increase in ovarian volume with the formation of cysts, which can fluctuate in size.[35,80] However, these appearances are by no means invariable, and the pelvic ultrasound scan appearances of premature thelarche may not differ from those of age-matched controls.[81] The bone age is not advanced, and this, together with the predominant FSH response to GnRH, is characteristic of premature thelarche.[82]

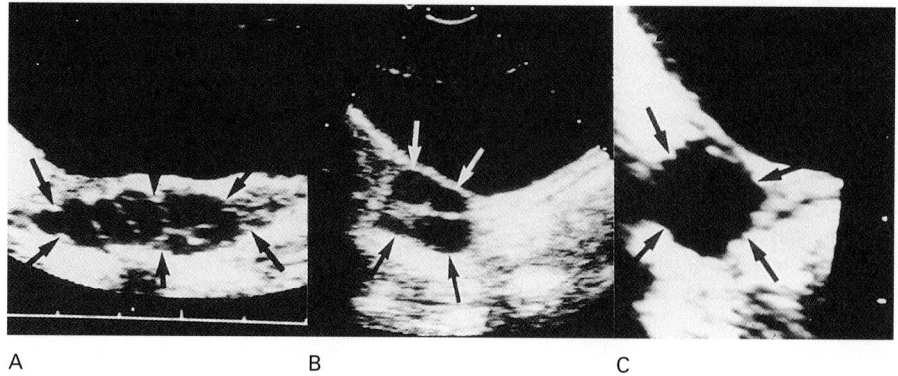

Fig. 40.5 Pelvic ultrasound scan appearances of the ovary in precocious puberty (**A**), thelarche variant (**B**) and premature thelarche (**C**).

In thelarche variant, the gonadotropin secretion shows a dominant FSH pulsatility, and pelvic ultrasound appearances are midway between those of thelarche and gonadotropin-dependent precocious puberty[83] (Fig. 40.5). The skeletal age is usually advanced.

Treatment

No treatment is required for either thelarche or for thelarche variant, apart from reassurance. Recently, in a retrospective study of 100 girls with premature thelarche, 14 progressed to early gonadotropin dependent puberty.[84] Final height is reported to be unaffected in both thelarche and thelarche variant.

Primary hypothyroidism

In some girls with primary hypothyroidism, in addition to an elevated TSH concentration, FSH levels are also increased. Additionally, recent *in vitro* studies have demonstrated that TSH has weak agonist properties at the human FSH receptor.[85] Stimulation of the ovaries results, with consequent secretion of estradiol. This in turn leads to isolated breast development.[86,87] There is, however, no pubertal progression in the majority of cases. Nevertheless, in certain cases, normal gonadotropin-dependent puberty occurs at an inappropriately early age.

The diagnosis of hypothyroidism must be considered in all girls with isolated breast development, a delayed bone age and an increased growth rate. The diagnosis is confirmed on analysis of thyroid function, when the free thyroxine level will be low and the TSH level high. Treatment in the form of thyroxine administered orally is commenced cautiously. The prognosis is excellent, but the final height may be affected if the diagnosis is delayed, or if normal puberty occurs at an early age.

Virilization of females

Virilization is normally due to excessive secretion of adrenal androgens. The following are the principal causes of virilization in females.

Adrenarche

Between the ages of 5–8 years, the zona reticularis of the adrenal cortex matures and secretes adrenal androgens. These can cause an increase in the height velocity, excessive secretion of sweat, the development of pubic and axillary hair and an advanced bone age. The condition is commoner in girls from an Asian or Afro-Caribbean background, and is benign in that final height is unaffected.

Congenital adrenal hyperplasia

The classical form of this condition may present with salt loss and clitoromegaly in the neonatal period. However, the 'late-onset' or 'simple virilizing' form of the condition may present with tall stature, an increased height velocity, an advanced bone age, clitoromegaly and the development of pubic and axillary hair. The diagnosis is usually based upon a raised 17 hydroxyprogesterone (17-OHP) level, and an exaggerated 17-OHP response to exogenous ACTH, with a blunted cortisol response. The urinary steroid profile confirms the diagnosis. Treatment should be instigated with hydrocortisone and, if the plasma renin activity is elevated, 9-α fludrocortisone.

Gonadotropin-dependent precocious puberty and the polycystic ovary syndrome are common sequelae.[88] The final height is usually compromised.

Adrenal tumors

The characteristic picture is that of a short history of virilization, with an accelerated growth rate and an advanced bone age. The diagnosis can only be revealed by careful analysis of urine, looking at the pattern of steroid metabolites. Imaging of the adrenal glands should be performed. Treatment involves surgical resection of the tumor, with the option of adjuvant chemotherapy. The prognosis is usually guarded, and careful monitoring of the growth velocity and the urinary steroid profile is warranted.

Conclusion

Recent research has revealed that precocious puberty can no longer be regarded as a single entity. It follows that the treatment of the different forms of precocious puberty will vary. At present, treatment has little effect on the final height of children with gonadotropin-dependent precocious puberty, and the main indication for treatment is to avoid the psychological consequences of early menarche.

Data from long-term studies should help optimize the management of this difficult group of conditions in the future. Additionally, ongoing research at the cellular and molecular levels should aid us in understanding the pathophysiology of these conditions and, in particular, the complex inter-relationship between growth and puberty.

REFERENCES

1. Tanner JM 1973 Trend toward earlier menarche in London, Oslo, Copenhagen, The Netherlands and Hungary. Nature 243: 95–97
2. MacMahon B 1973 Age at menarche. In: National Survey DHEW Publication, No. 133 (HRA), Series 11, Bethesda, MD, pl
3. Zacharias LM, Rand M, Wurtman R 1976 A prospective study of sexual development in American girls: the statistics of menarche. Obstetrics and Gynecology Survey 31: 325–337
4. Tanner JM 1962 Growth at Adolescence, 2nd edn. Blackwell Scientific Publications, Oxford,
5. Marshall WA, Tanner JM 1969 Variations in pattern of pubertal changes in girls. Archives of Diseases in Childhood 44: 291–303
6. Tanner JM, Whitehouse RH, Marubini E, Resele LF 1976 The adolescent growth spurt of boys and girls of the Harpenden Growth Study. Annals of Human Biology 3: 109–126
7. Stanhope R, Adams RJ, Jacobs HS, Brook CGD 1985 Ovarian ultrasound assessment in normal children, idiopathic precocious puberty, and during low dose pulsatile gonadotrophin releasing hormone treatment of hypogonadotrophic hypogonadism. Archives of Diseases in Childhood 60: 116–119
8. Dunger DB, Matthews DR, Edge JA, Jones J, Preece MA 1991 Evidence for temporal coupling of growth hormone, prolactin, LH and FSH pulsatility overnight during normal puberty. Journal of Endocrinology 130: 141–149
9. Finkelstein JW, Roffwarg HP, Boyar RM, Kream J, Hellman L 1972 Age-related change in the twenty-four hour spontaneous secretion of growth hormone. Journal of Clinical Endocrinology and Metabolism 35: 665–670
10. Miller JD, Tannenbaum GS, Colle E, Guyda J 1982 Daytime pulsatile growth hormone secretion during childhood and adolescence. Journal of Clinical Endocrinology and Metabolism 55: 989–994
11. Hindmarsh PC, Matthews DR, Brook CGD 1988 Growth hormone secretion in children determined by time series analysis. Clinical Endocrinology 29: 35–44
12. Mauras N, Blizzard RM, Link K, Johnson ML, Rogol AD, Veldhuis JD 1987 Augmentation of growth hormone secretion during puberty: evidence for a pulse amplitude modulated phenomenon. Journal of Clinical Endocrinology and Metabolism 64: 596–601
13. Harris DA, Van Vliet G, Egli CA, Grumbach MM, Kaplan SL, Styne DM, Vainsel M 1985 Somatomedin-C in normal puberty and in true precocious puberty before and after treatment with a potent luteinizing hormone-releasing hormone agonist. Journal of Clinical Endocrinology and Metabolism 61: 152–159
14. Huckle W, Conn PM 1988 Molecular mechanism of gonadotrophin-releasing hormone action II. The effector system. Endocrine Reviews 9: 387–395
15. Hazum E, Conn PM 1988 Molecular mechanism of gonadotrophin releasing hormone (GnRH) action. The GnRH receptor. Endocrine Reviews 9: 379–386
16. Crowley WF, Filicori M, Spratt DI, Santoro NF 1985 The physiology of gonadotrophin-releasing hormone (GnRH) secretion in men and women. Recent Progress in Hormone Research 41: 473–526
17. Gluckman PD, Grumbach MM, Kaplan SL 1981 The neuroendocrine regulation and function of growth hormone and prolactin in the mammalian fetus. Endocine Reviews 2: 363–395
18. Bridges NA, Matthews DR, Hindmarsh PC, Brook CGD 1994 Changes in gonadotropin secretion during childhood and puberty. Journal of Endocrinology 141: 169–176
19. Boyar R, Finkelstein J, Roffwarg H, Kapen S, Weitzman ED, Hellman L 1972 Synchronization of augmented luteinizing hormone secretion with sleep during puberty. New England Journal of Medicine 287: 582–586
20. Reiter EO, Kulin HE, Hamwood SM 1974 The absence of positive feedback between estrogen and luteinizing hormone in sexually immature girls. Pediatric Research 8: 740–745
21. Roth JC, Grumbach MM, Kaplan SL 1973 Effect of synthetic luteinizing hormone-releasing factor on serum testosterone and gonadotrophins in prepubertal, pubertal, and adult males. Journal of Clinical Endocrinology and Metabolism 37: 680–686

22. Corley KP, Valk TW, Kelch RP, Marshall JC 1981 Estimation of GnRH pulse amplitude during pubertal development. Pediatric Research 15: 157–162
23. Neely EK, Hintz RL, Wilson DM, Lee PA, Gautier T, Argente J, Stene M 1995 Normal ranges for immunochemiluminometric gonadotrophin assays. Journal of Paediatrics 127(1): 40–46
24. Neely EK, Wilson DM, Lee PA, Stene M, Hintz RL 1995 Spontaneous serum gonadotrophin concentrations in the evaluation of precocious puberty. Journal of Paediatrics 127: 47–52
25. Grumbach MM, Richards GE, Conte FA, Kaplan SL 1977 Clinical disorders of adrenal function and puberty; an assessment of the role of the adrenal cortex in normal and abnormal puberty in man and evidence for an ACTH-like pituitary adrenal androgen stimulating hormone. In: Serio M (ed) The endocrine function of the human adrenal cortex. Serono Symposium. Academic Press, New York, pp 583–612
26. Boyko OB, Curnes JT, Oakes WJ, Burger PC 1991 Hamartomas of the tuber cinereum: CT, MR and pathologic findings. American Journal of Neuroradiology 12: 309–314
27. Junier MP, Wolff A, Hoffman G, Ma YJ, Ojeda SR 1992 Effect of hypothalamic lesions that induce precocious puberty on the morphological and functional maturation of the luteinizing hormone releasing hormone neuronal system. Endocrinology 131: 787–798
28. Reith KG, Comite F, Dwyer AJ, Nelson MJ, Pescovitz O, Shawker TH, Cutler GB, Loriaux DL 1987 CT of cerebral abnormalities in precocious puberty. American Journal of Roentgenology 148: 1231–1238
29. Shalet SM, Crowne EC, Didi MA, Ogilvy-Stuart AL, Wallace WH 1992 Irradiation induced growth failure. Ballières Clinics in Endocrinology and Metabolism 6: 513–526
30. Proos LA, Hofvander Y, Tuvemo T 1991 Menarcheal age and growth pattern of Indian girls adopted in Sweden I. Menarcheal age. Acta Paediatrica Scandinavica 80 (Suppl.): 852–858
31. Herman ME, Giddens AD, Sandler NE, Freidman NE 1988 Sexual precocity in girls: an association with sexual abuse? American Journal of Diseases in Childhood 142: 431–433
32. Hughes IA 1986 Handbook of endocrine investigations in children. Wright, London,
33. Cavallo A, Richards GE, Busey S, Michaels SE 1995 A simplified gonadotrophin-releasing hormone test for precocious puberty. Clinical Endocrinology (Oxford) 42(6): 641–646
34. Kornreich L, Horev G, Blaser S, Daneman D, Kauli R, Grunebaum M 1995 Central precocious puberty: evaluation by neuroimaging. Pediatric Radiology 25(1): 7–11
35. Salardi S, Orsini L, Cacciari E, Partesotti S, Brondelli L, Cicognani A, Frejaville E, Pluchinotta V, Tonioli S, Boricelli L 1988 Pelvic ultrasonography in girls with precocious puberty, congenital adrenal hyperplasia, obesity or hirsutism. Journal of Paediatrics 112: 880–887
36. Stanhope R, Adams J, Jacobs HS, Brook CGD 1985 Ovarian ultrasound assessment in normal children, idiopathic precocious puberty and during low dose pulsatile GnRH treatment of hypogonadotrophic hypogonadism. Archives of Diseases in Childhood 60: 116–119
37. Griffin IJ, Cole TJ, Duncan KA, Hollman AS, Donaldson MD 1995 Pelvic ultrasound findings in different forms of sexual precocity. Acta Paediatrica 84(5): 544–549
38. Ehrhardt AA, Meyer-Bahlburg HF 1994 Psychosocial aspects of precocious puberty. Hormone Research 41(Suppl. 2): 30–35
39. Kletter GB, Kelch RP 1994 Effects of gonadotropin-releasing hormone analog therapy on adult stature in precocious puberty. Journal of Clinical Endocrinology and Metabolism 79: 331–334
40. Breyer P, Haider A, Pescovitz OH 1993 Gonadotrophin-releasing hormone agonists in the treatment of girls with central precocious puberty. Clinics in Obstetrics and Gynaecology 36(3): 764–772
41. Conn PM 1986 The molecular basis of gonadotrophin-releasing hormone action. Endocrine Reviews 7: 3–10
42. Bassi F, Bartolini O, Neri AS, Gheri RG, Magini A, Bucciantini S, Bruni V 1995 Usefulness of early morning urine estrone-3-glucuronide assay in the monitoring of ovarian secretory function in precocious puberty. Journal of Endocrinological Investigation 18(2): 98–103
43. Parker KL, Lee PA 1989 Depot Leuprolide acetate for treatment of precocious puberty. Journal of Clinical Endocrinology and Metabolism 69: 689–691
44. Carel JC, Lahlou N, Guazzarotti L, Joubert-Collin M, Roger M, Colle M, Chaussain JL 1995 Treatment of central precocious puberty with depot leuprorelin. European Journal of Endocrinology 132(6): 699–704
45. Partsch CJ, Hummelink R, Sippell WG, Oostdijk W, Odink RJ, Drop SL 1993 Comparison between complete and incomplete suppression of the hypophyseal-gonadal axis in girls with central precocious puberty: effect on growth and prospective final height. Monatsschr-Kinderheilkd 141(12): 935–939
46. Moll GW, Rosenfeld RL, Fang VS 1986 Administration of low dose estrogen rapidly and directly stimulates GH production. American Journal of Diseases in Childhood 140: 124–127
47. DiMartino-Nardi J, Wu R, Varner R, Wong WL, Saenger P 1994 The effect of luteinizing hormone-releasing hormone analogue for central precocious puberty on growth hormone (GH) and GH-binding protein. Journal of Clinical Endocrinology and Metabolism 78(3): 664–668
48. Boepple PA, Mansfield MJ, Link K, Crawford JD, Crigler JF Jr, Kushner DC, Blizzard RM, Crowley WF Jr 1988 Impact of sex steroids and their suppression on skeletal growth and maturation. American Journal of Physiology 255: E559–566
49. Boepple PA, Mansfield MJ, Crawford JD, Crigler JF, Blizzard RM, Crowley WF 1990 Gonadotrophin releasing hormone agonist treatment of central precocious puberty: an analysis of growth data in a developmental context. Acta Paediatrica Scandinavica Suppl. 367: 38–43
50. Lee PA, Page JG 1989 The Leuprolide study group. Effects of Leuprolide in the treatment of central precocious puberty. Journal of Paediatrics 114: 321–324

51. Werder EA, Murset G, Zachmann M, Brook CGD, Prader A 1974 Treatment of precocious puberty with cyproterone acetate. Pediatric Research 8: 248–256
52. Kauli R, Kornreich L, Laron Z 1990 Pubertal development, growth and final height in girls with sexual precocity treated with the GnRH analogue D-TRP-6-LHRH. Hormone Research 33: 11–17
53. Oerter KE, Manasco P, Barnes KM, Jones J, Hill S, Cutler GB 1991 Adult height after long term treatment with deslorelin. Journal of Clinical Endocrinology and Metabolism 73: 1235–1240
54. Sorgo W, Kiraly E, Homoki J, Heinze E, Teller WM, Bierich JR, Moeller H, Ranke MB, Butenandt O, Knorr D 1987 The effects of cyproterone acetate on statural growth in children with precocious puberty. Acta Endocrinologica 115: 44–56
55. Stasiowska B, Vannelli S, Benso L 1994 Final height in sexually precocious girls after therapy with an intranasal analogue of gonadotrophin-releasing hormone (buserelin). Hormone Research 42(3): 81–85
56. Brauner R, Adan L, Malandry F, Zantleifer D 1994 Adult height in girls with idiopathic true precocious puberty. Journal of Clinical Endocrinology and Metabolism 79(2): 415–420
57. Paul D, Conte FA, Grumbach MM, Kaplan SL 1995 Long-term effect of gonadotrophin-releasing hormone agonist therapy on final and near-final height in 26 children with true precocious puberty treated at a median age of less than 5 years. Journal of Clinical Endocrinology and Metabolism 80(2): 546–551
58. Cara JF, Kreiter ML, Rosenfeld RL 1992 Height prognosis of children with true precocious puberty and growth hormone deficiency: effect of combination therapy with gonadotrophin-releasing hormone agonist and growth hormone. Journal of Paediatrics 120: 709–715
59. Hibi I, Tanaka T, Tanae A, Kagawa J, Hashimoto N, Yoshizawa A, Shizume K 1989 The influence of gonadal function and the effect of gonadal suppression treatment on final height in growth hormone treated growth hormone deficient children. Journal of Clinical Endocrinology and Metabolism 69: 221–226
60. Saggese G, Pasquino AM, Bertelloni S, Baroncelli GI, Battini R, Pucarelli I, Segni M, Franchi G 1995 Effect of combined treatment with gonadotrophin releasing hormone analogue and growth hormone in patients with central precocious puberty who had subnormal growth velocity and impaired height prognosis. Acta Paediatrica 84(3): 299–304
61. Bridges NA, Cooke A, Healy MJR, Hindmarsh PC, Brook CGD 1995 Ovaries in sexual precocity. Clinical Endocrinology 42: 135–140
62. Boucekkine C, Blumberg TJ, Roger M, Thomas F, Chaussain JL 1994 Treatment of central precocious puberty with sustained-release triptorelin. Archives of Paediatrics 1(12): 1127–1137
63. Schroor EJ, Van Weissenbruch MM, Delemarre-van-de-Waal HA 1995 Long term GnRH-agonist treatment does not postpone central development of the GnRH pulse generator in girls with idiopathic precocious puberty. Journal of Clinical Endocrinology and Metabolism 80(5): 1696–1701
64. Murram D, Dewhurst J, Grant DB 1984 Precocious puberty: a follow-up study. Archives of Diseases in Childhood 59: 77–78
65. Jay N, Mansfield MJ, Blizzard RM, Crowley WF Jr, Schoenfield D, Rhubin L, Boepple PA 1992 Ovulation and menstrual function of adolescent girls with central precocious puberty after therapy with gonadotrophin releasing hormone agonists. Journal of Clinical Endocrinology and Metabolism 75: 890–894
66. Cisternino M, Pasquino A, Bozzola M, Balducci R, Lorini R, Pucarelli I, Segni M, Severi F 1992 Final height attainment and gonadal function in girls with precocious puberty treated with cyproterone acetate. Hormone Research 37: 86–90
67. Holland FJ 1991 Gonadotrophin independent precocious puberty. Endocrinology and Metabolic Clinics of North America 20: 191–210
68. Weinstein LS, Shenker A, Gejman PV, Merino MJ, Friedman E, Speigel AM 1991 Activating mutations of the stimulatory G protein in the McCune-Albright syndrome. New England Journal of Medicine 325: 1688–1695
69. Landis CA, Masters SB, Spada A, Pace AM, Bourne HR, Vallar L 1989 GTPase inhibiting mutations activate the α chain of Gs and stimulate adenylyl cyclase in human pituitary tumours. Nature 340: 692–696
70. Lee PA, Van Dop C, Migeon CJ 1986 McCune-Albright syndrome — long term follow-up. Journal of the American Medical Association 256: 2980–2984
71. Stanhope R, Pringle J, Adams J, Jeffcoate SC, Brook CGD 1985 Spontaneous gonadotrophin pulsatility in girls with central precocious puberty treated with cyproterone acetate. Clinical Endocrinology 23: 547–553
72. Savage DCL, Swift PGF 1981 Effect of cyproterone acetate on adrenocortical function in children with precocious puberty. Archives of Disease in Childhood 56: 218–222
73. Foster CM, Comite F, Pescovitz OH, Ross JL, Loriaux DL, Cutler GB 1984 Variable response to a long acting agonist of LHRH in girls with McCune-Albright syndrome. Journal of Clinical Endocrinology and Metabolism 59: 801–805
74. Lee PA 1981 Medroxyprogesterone therapy for sexual precocity in girls. American Journal of Diseases in Childhood 135: 443–445
75. Sonino N 1987 The use of ketoconazole as an inhibitor of steroid production. New England Journal of Medicine 317: 812–818
76. Holland FJ, Fishman L, Bailey JD, Fazekas ATA 1985 Ketoconazole in the treatment of precocious puberty not responsive to LHRH analogue therapy. New England Journal of Medicine 312: 1023–1028
77. Feuillan PP, Foster CM, Pescovitz OH, Hench KD, Showker T, Dwyer A, Molley JD, Banes K, Loriaux DL, Cutler GB 1986 Treatment of precocious puberty in the McCune-Albright syndrome with the aromatase inhibitor testolactone. New England Journal of Medicine 315: 1115–1119
78. Boepple PA, Frisch LS, Weirman ME, Hoffman WH, Crowley WF 1992 The natural history of autonomous gonadal function, adrenarche and central puberty in gonadotrophin independent precocious puberty. Journal of Clinical Endocrinology and Metabolism 75: 1550–1555

79. Stanhope R, Abdulwahid NA, Adams J, Brook CGD 1986 Studies of gonadotrophin pulsatility and pelvic ultrasound examinations distinguish between isolated premature thelarche and central precocious puberty. European Journal of Paediatrics 145: 190–194
80. Freedman SM, Krietzer PM, Elkovitz SS, Saberman N, Leonidas JC 1993 Ovarian microcysts in girls with isolated premature thelarche. Pediatrics 122: 246–249
81. Haber HP, Wollmann HA, Ranke MB 1995 Pelvic ultrasonography: early differentiation between isolated premature thelarche and central precocious puberty. European Journal of Paediatrics 154(3): 182–186
82. Pohlenz J, Habermehl P, Wemme H, Grimm W, Schonberger W 1994 The differentiation between premature thelarche and pubertas praecox on the basis of clinical, hormonal and radiological findings. Dtsch Med Wochenschr. 119(39): 1301–1306
83. Stanhope R, Brook CGD 1990 Thelarche variant: a new syndrome of precocious sexual development? Acta Endocrinologica 123: 481–486
84. Pasquino AM, Pucarelli I, Passeri F, Segni M, Mancini MA, Municchi G 1995 Progression of premature thelarche to central precocious puberty. Journal of Pediatrics 126: 11–14
85. Anasti JN, Flack MR, Froehlich J, Nelson LM, Nisula BC 1995 A potential novel mechanism for precocious puberty in juvenile hypothyroidism. Journal of Clinical Endocrinology and Metabolism 80(1): 276–279
86. Pringle PJ, Stanhope R, Hindmarsh PC, Brook CGD 1988 Abnormal pubertal development in primary hypothyroidism. Clinical Endocrinology 28: 479–486
87. Buchanan C, Stanhope R, Jones J, Grant DB, Preece MA 1988 Gonadotrophin, GH and prolactin secretion in children with primary hypothyroidism. Clinical Endocrinology 29: 427–436
88. Pescovitz OH, Comite F, Cassorla F, Dwyer AJ, Poth MA, Sperling MA, Hench K, McNemar A, Skerda M, Loriaux DL, Cutler GB 1984 True precocious puberty complicating congenital adrenal hyperplasia: treatment with a LHRH analogue. Journal of Clinical Endocrinology and Metabolism 58: 857–861

41. Assisted reproductive technologies

Rogerio A. Lobo

Introduction

The practice of assisted reproductive technologies (ART) results in many changes in circulating levels of estrogen and progesterone. Although these fluctuations are wide and generally above the range of values expected in normal premenopausal women, the intent is to mimic the pattern of the normal menstrual cycle. Only in the area of oocyte donation is estrogen and progesterone actually administered to simulate more closely the ovulatory menstrual cycle. This chapter will begin with an overview of ART procedures which includes induction of ovulation and which, in a less aggressive mode, is used in patients who are amenorrheic or anovulatory. This review of ART will not be exhaustive but will stress changes in estrogen and progesterone and their supplemental use in the case of oocyte donation.

Definitions

ART includes *in vitro* fertilization (IVF) and uterine embryo transfer (ET) as well as other manipulations of the cycle as will be described below. The word 'assisted' is sometimes used interchangeably with 'advanced.' 'Controlled' ovarian hyperstimulation (COH) or 'superovulation' employs large doses of injected gonadotropins and is intended to stimulate as many oocytes as possible for the purpose of IVF-ET. This is a common feature of most of the other ART procedures listed below. Strictly speaking, however, COH can be used without IVF and ET. Here 'superovulation' *in vivo* is induced to increase fecundibility (ability to achieve pregnancy) in a given cycle; in practise it is most frequently combined with intrauterine insemination (IUI). On the other hand, ART also includes natural cycle or 'unstimulated' IVF-ET, which is carried out without COH but requires the *in vitro* manipulation of gametes (sperm and oocyte).

Other ART procedures include GIFT (gamete intrafallopian transfer), ZIFT (zygote intrafallopian transfer), PROST (pronuclear stage tubal transfer) and TET (tubal embryo transfer). Other manipulations have also been used but are less common, and therefore will not be discussed.

CONTROLLED OVARIAN STIMULATION/SUPEROVULATION

IVF was first attempted by inducing superovulation with human menopausal gonadotropin (hMG). Human chorionic gonadotropin (hCG), whose biologic activity mimics that of luteinizing hormone (LH), was used to time ovulation.[1] This procedure led to the first human pregnancy, but was an ectopic gestation.[2] Limited success led Steptoe and Edwards to return to the spontaneous cycle with monitoring of the spontaneous LH surge. This resulted in the first successful human birth.[3] However, almost universally, ovarian hyperstimulation is now used as a more efficient way to increase the number of oocytes and subsequently embryos available for transfer. Pregnancy rates correlate best with the number of embryos replaced.[4,5] The procedures are similar but more aggressive than routine induction of ovulation in anovulatory or amenorrheic women, where fertilization occurs *in vivo*.

Various hyperstimulation regimens have been used successfully to achieve pregnancies by IVF.[5] By the late 1980s the most common regimens in the United States utilized hMG alone or hMG combined with GnRH agonists. During the early years of IVF, clomiphene citrate alone or in combination with hMG was commonly used because it helped reduce the total gonadotropin dose and thus the cost of the stimulation. However, the number of oocytes obtained was less than that obtained with hMG alone. To maximize oocyte yield, ovarian superovulation regimens were begun prior to the selection of a dominant follicle, during the phase of follicle recruitment. The ovarian response was monitored and the subsequent medication dose adjusted to the response.

In the late 1980s many programs started using gonadotropin-releasing hormone (GnRH) agonists for pituitary down-regulation prior to the initiation of gonadotropins.[6] This approach ensured that the ovary was in a resting phase prior to the onset of superovulation, thus minimizing the likelihood of the development of a single dominant follicle. In addition, the agonist prevented the occurrence of a premature LH surge and ovulation, which had previously resulted in the cancellation of approximately 15–20% of IVF cycles. The addition of the GnRH agonist also appeared to increase the number of oocytes obtained at the time of follicle aspiration, leading to an increased number of embryos available for transfer and cryopreservation.[7] Nevertheless, this required a larger total dose of gonadotropins. A meta-analysis of randomized clinical trials showed an increase in the probability of pregnancy with this concomitant use of a GnRH agonist.[8] By giving the clinician the ability to adjust the time of initiation of hMG, use of the GnRH agonist increased the flexibility in scheduling the time for follicular aspiration. As a result, routine use of the agonists has been advocated.[9,10] Despite the added expense of more injected gonadotropins, the advantages of using GnRH agonists outweigh the disadvantages, and this combination represents the most commonly used method of controlled ovarian hyperstimulation for ART.

Down-regulation is achieved most easily when GnRH agonist treatment is initiated in the mid-luteal phase.[11] Leuprolide acetate (Lupron, TAP Pharmaceuticals, North Chicago, IL) is the most commonly used GnRH agonist in the United States but nafarelin acetate, buserelin and goserelin have all been used widely. All GnRH agonists act by the same physiologic principle and pregnancy success is obtainable with the use of any of them.[12,13] When the GnRH agonist is initiated during the luteal phase of the cycle, down-regulation is achieved approximately 10–14 days after the agonist is begun. Attainment of pituitary down-regulation is confirmed by ultrasonographic visualization of quiescent ovaries and a thin endometrial echo complex, along with low serum E_2 levels (<30 pg/mL; <100 pmol/L).

Once down-regulation has occurred, ovarian hyperstimulation with hMG can be initiated. The GnRH agonist is continued during the stimulation phase to prevent a premature LH surge. The dose required is less than that needed for the initial down-regulation and the dose of leuprolide acetate, given subcutaneously, is usually decreased. With some longer acting (depot) agonists, one administration may be used for an entire cycle. The initial dose of gonadotropins (hMG or FSH) is usually in the range of 225–300 IU/day. Patients with polycystic ovary syndrome and those who previously demonstrated exaggerated responses to gonadotropins are given a lower initial dose (150 IU/day). Even lower doses are often used for routine ovulation induction. The dose is subsequently adjusted according to follicular growth and serum levels of E_2. Two studies[14,15] compared hMG and FSH and found no difference in outcome. A recent meta-analysis suggested a higher probability of pregnancy with pure FSH over hMG but the effect appeared to be due to the inclusion of studies that did not use a GnRH agonist.[16] Most recently recombinant human FSH has been made available for use by subcutaneous injection.

Patients who respond poorly to the GnRH agonist-gonadotropin protocol can be treated with a shortened GnRH agonist protocol that utilizes the initial agonistic phase of the pituitary response to augment ovarian stimulation. In such a 'flare' protocol, the agonist is started on day 2 of the cycle. Stimulation with gonadotropins is begun on cycle day 3 or 4. In a recent modification of this approach, a low dose of the agonist is used throughout the follicular phase without down-regulation taking place.[17] The adjunctive use of growth hormone in pharmacologic doses initially was reported to enhance the ovarian responses of women who were relatively resistant to menotropin therapy;[18] however, subsequent controlled studies have been unable to document any beneficial impact of exogenous growth hormone treatment in poor responders undergoing IVF.[19]

A more convenient formulation of the GnRH analogs is the antagonist, which blocks pituitary gonadotropin secretion without the initial agonistic response. However, the development of GnRH antagonists for clinical use has been slow because of side effects from histamine release. Preliminary data on the use of second and third generation antagonists have now been obtained. The simplest regimen utilizes the antagonist in the midfollicular phase when the serum E_2 level or the follicular diameter has reached a certain value. In one study, the majority of patients required only a single dose of antagonist[20] and outcomes were similar to the use of the GnRH agonist. The advantage to the patient is a shorter course of treatment and, potentially, a lower total dose of gonadotropins and lower cost. Another approach has been to give the antagonist intermittently, first at the onset of menses for a variable time, then again late in follicular development.[21] This approach allows for the control of the time of oocyte retrieval. GnRH antagonists have also been used in natural-cycle IVF to suppress the LH surge in the spontaneous cycle.[22,23]

MONITORING THE FOLLICULAR RESPONSE

Since the success of IVF depends on adequate follicular development,[24] gonadotropin doses and the timing of hCG administration have to be carefully assessed. Monitoring of follicular growth is achieved by transvaginal ultrasound measurements of the size of the developing follicles and the measurement of serum E_2. Ovulation is induced with doses of hCG in the range of 5000–10 000 IU intramuscularly, when follicle maturity is obtained. Newer approaches employ the use of native GnRH or an agonist. Recombinant LH can also be used but the doses required add substantially to the expense of the procedure. Maturity criteria are based on both follicle size and serum E_2 levels and vary from regimen to regimen (Tables 41.1 and 41.2). If hCG is given prematurely, immature oocytes will be obtained; if it is given too late, a premature LH surge can occur, unless a GnRH agonist is used, or the oocytes may be 'postmature'. At the time of hCG administration, the endometrial thickness should be in the region of 8 mm as measured in the anteroposterior direction by transvaginal ultrasonography. Some evidence suggests that a thinner endometrium is associated with decreased pregnancy rates.[25]

The measurement of serum progesterone on the day of hCG is controversial. Some reports[26,27] suggested that elevated progesterone levels are associated with decreased pregnancy rates, whereas others[28] have not confirmed this finding. Elevated progesterone levels could be associated with altered endometrial receptivity[29] rather than with poor oocyte quality.[30]

Cancellation of the cycle and avoidance of hCG administration might be considered if the ovaries are markedly hyperstimulated (> 25 follicles) or the E_2 level is higher than 5000 pg/mL (>15 000 pmol/L), to avoid the risk of ovarian hyperstimulation syndrome.[31] Aspiration of the follicles does not protect against the

Table 41.1 Gonadotropin stimulation regimen.*

Start	Day 2 (baseline ultrasound scan)
Initial hMG dose	225 IU (3 ampules) daily for 4 days
Serial monitoring	Day 6 (day 5 of gonadotropin) — day of hCG
Adjust hMG dose	Increase/decrease dose after 4 days of stimulation
Completion of stimulation	hCG, 10 000 IU intramuscularly at follicle maturity
Follicle maturity criteria	Follicle diameter = 16 mm E_2 = 200 pg/mL/codominant follicle

*Adapted from experience at The University of Southern California. Lobo RA, Mishell DR, Paulson RJ, Shoupe D (eds) 1997 Mishell's textbook of infertility, contraception, and reproductive endocrinology, 4th edn. Blackwell Scientific Publications, Malden, Massachusetts

Table 41.2 Gonadotropin-releasing hormone agonist (GnRHa)-gonadotropin stimulation protocol.*

GnRHa start	Midluteal phase[a]
Initial GnRHa dose	1 mg subcutaneously daily
Start gonadotropin	After 2 weeks of GnRHa, when $E_2 \leq 30$ pg/mL
Initial gonadotropin	225 IU daily (decrease daily GnRHa dose to 0.5 mg when starting hMG)
Adjust gonadotropin	Increase/decrease dose after 4 days of stimulation
Completion of stimulation	hCG, 10 000 IU at follicle maturity
Follicle maturity criteria	Follicle diameter = 18 mm E_2 = 200 pg/mL/codominant follicle

[a]If anovulatory, or if the serum progesterone level is ≤ 3 ng/mL, add norethindrone, 5 mg orally twice daily for 10 days starting 3 days before leuprolide acetate.
*Adapted from experience at The University of Southern California. Lobo RA, Mishell DR, Paulson RJ, Shoupe D (eds) 1997: Mishell's textbook of infertility, contraception, and reproductive endocrinology, 4th edn. Blackwell Scientific Publications, Malden, Massachusetts

development of ovarian hyperstimulation.[32] The avoidance of pregnancy by cryopreservation of all embryos can substantially decrease the risk of severe hyperstimulation in otherwise high-risk patients. Use of intravenous albumin at the time of hCG or oocyte aspiration to reduce the risk of hyperstimulation has been suggested, but has not been supported in all studies.

FERTILIZATION IN VITRO

To achieve fertilization, recovered oocytes are combined with spermatozoa in a solution of culture medium. Most programs use one of several standard commercially available culture media, such as Hams F-10[34] or artificial human tubal fluid,[35] although other substances, notably amniotic fluid,[36] and pure serum,[37] have been used. Culture media are routinely supplemented with the patient's serum in a concentration of 10–20%, with the intent of providing protein to help satisfy the metabolic requirements of the gametes and embryos. More recently, synthetic protein sources have been introduced.

There is a large range of sperm concentrations used for ART. As few as 2500 spermatozoa have been used during GIFT without a decrease in pregnancy rates.[38] Most programs, however, use a concentration range of 50 000–500 000 motile sperm per milliliter of culture medium for IVF, with higher concentrations used for patients with male factor infertility.[39] However, all of the techniques of sperm enhancement[40] have now been overshadowed by the use of sperm micromanipulation.[41] These micromanipulation techniques include the opening of a 'window' in the zona pellucida to allow ingress of sperm (partial zona dissection, or PZD), and injection of sperm into the perivitelline space (subzonal insemination, or SUZI) or directly into the cytoplasm of the egg (intracytoplasmic sperm injection, or ICSI). Van Steirteghem pioneered the technique for ICSI[42] and demonstrated fertilization rates in excess of those obtained with SUZI. According to one of their reports, 53% of oocytes with a single sperm injected into the cytoplasm fertilized, compared to only 17% with SUZI.[43] Furthermore, the clinical pregnancy rate with ICSI has been reported to be in the region of 26% per cycle. The method of ICSI has rapidly gained acceptance and has been adopted by virtually all programs around the world.[44] Recently, success has been achieved with sperm obtained from the epididymis and is called MESA or microsurgical epididymal sperm aspiration[45] or directly from the testis.[44,46] These techniques are still new and there remains some controversy regarding the follow-up of births with some suggestion that there may be a small increase in abnormal karotypes and other reports showing no change.

GAMETE AND EMBRYO CULTURE IN VITRO

Gametes and embryos are typically maintained in individual culture vessels (tubes or dishes) containing 1–2 mL of culture medium. Maintenance of physiologic temperature and pH is critical to the success of IVF. Culture vessels are therefore kept in an incubator at 37°C in an atmosphere containing 5% carbon dioxide (CO_2), which produces a pH of 7.4 within the culture media. Gametes and embryos can also be kept in small droplets of media (20–50 μL) that are covered with mineral oil to protect the small volume of medium from sudden changes in temperature or CO_2. Several studies[47–49] addressed the possibility of maintaining gametes and embryos in coculture with other cells. However, whereas the concept is attractive, the technique has not been proved to be of definitive value.[50]

Sperm are added to the oocytes approximately 6 hours after oocyte collection. Fertilization is confirmed by visualization with a dissecting microscope of two pronuclei (2 PN) in the fertilized zygotes 16–20 hours later. Polynuclear zygotes are the result of polyspermic fertilization. Although these embryos generally undergo cleavage, they are aneuploid and are not transferred.

After fertilization, embryos are maintained in culture for a variable period of time. Pregnancy can be attained after the transfer of embryos at any stage of development from the 2 PN to blastocyst stages; however, most programs at present transfer embryos to the uterus about 48–72 hours after follicle aspiration. Potentially, if there was a high efficiency of embryos in culture reaching the blastocyst stage, then transferring a limited number of blastocysts should result in higher implantation rates.

Oocyte aspiration and embryo transfer

The purely technical aspects of oocyte recovery by ultrasound and embryo transfer will not be discussed here. It is sufficient to say that recent advances in techniques have allowed a less invasive and purely outpatient procedure to be carried out, which requires only minimal analgesia (so called 'conscious sedation').

THE LUTEAL PHASE

There is little doubt that endometrial receptivity plays a major role in the success or failure of embryo implantation after IVF.[51,52] In an effort to enhance endometrial receptivity, it is common to supplement the luteal phase with progesterone.[53] Edwards et al[1] were the first to postulate luteal phase inadequacy resulting from ovarian hyperstimulation prior to follicle aspiration as a cause of failure of IVF. In addition, the mechanical trauma to the follicle and the physical removal of granulosa cells was suggested to result in decreased progesterone secretion and luteal phase disruption.[54] This latter effect was demonstrated in the primate model.[55] Several randomized studies[56–58] however have failed to show a benefit of progesterone supplementation during cycles stimulated with the combination of clomiphene citrate and hMG. However, when GnRH agonists are used, the pituitary remains down-regulated during the ensuing luteal phase. There is little controversy that these cycles require progesterone (or hCG) supplementation.[59] Because of the concern over ovarian hyperstimulation, progesterone is the preferred agent. Progesterone administration is initiated at the time of ET and is given either intramuscularly in a dose of 25 mg once or twice daily, by vaginal suppositories or capsules, 100 mg twice daily or by a progesterone gel. The initial quantitative β-hCG level may be determined 9 and 12 days after ET. These levels establish the success or failure of implantation and provide prognostic information. Progesterone supplementation is discontinued at approximately 10 weeks' gestational age or when the second hCG level is negative.

NATURAL-CYCLE IN VITRO FERTILIZATION

In the late 1980s, several groups[60–62] began investigating the feasibility of IVF without the use of exogenous gonadotropins to induce multiple follicles. The 'spontaneous' cycle is supplemented by a midcycle dose of hCG to 'trigger' ovulation, and has been referred to as natural-cycle or unstimulated IVF.

All patients who are potential candidates for IVF in stimulated cycles may be considered for unstimulated IVF except those in whom a dominant follicle does not form without some exogenous augmentation of follicular development.[63] Patients with male factor infertility resulting in reduced fertilization rates are best served by IVF with controlled ovarian hyperstimulation, as a larger number of oocytes can maximize the likelihood of obtaining at least one fertilized egg. Patients over the age of 40 whose potential for multiple follicular development is limited can benefit from the additional stimulation of controlled ovarian hyperstimulation to increase the number of potentially healthy oocytes. Most reported series[62,64–66] excluded patients over the age of 40.

The key difference between the current practice of IVF in unstimulated cycles as compared with purely spontaneous cycles lies in the administration of hCG during the midcycle to trigger ovulation. This relatively small but important addition to the spontaneous cycle ensures a predictable duration of LH-like stimulation to the preovulatory follicle and allows follicle aspiration to be scheduled for a convenient time of day. However, accurate timing of hCG administration, as in cycles utilizing controlled ovarian hyperstimulation, requires careful cycle monitoring. Both transvaginal ultrasonography and serum E_2 measurements are useful for estimating the optimal time for hCG administration, though the E_2 measurement could be more important.[63] Guidelines have been developed by Paulson that utilize both measurements as a guide (Table 41.3).

Either serum or urine measurements of LH can be used to detect the LH surge. Serum E_2 measurements on the day after hCG administration help to confirm premature ovulation if the level is noted to decrease by more than 20% from the previous day, but it does not appear to be useful in timing hCG administration. Follicular aspiration and ET procedures do not deviate appreciably from those used for standard stimulated cycles. All successfully recovered oocytes, except those containing an obvious germinal vesicle, are inseminated on the day of follicle aspiration. Oocytes that at the time of recovery appear to contain a germinal vesicle are allowed to mature *in vitro* in 50% follicular fluid for up to 72 hours prior to insemination. Sperm are introduced only after the first polar body is extruded. If fertilization occurs in an oocyte successfully matured *in vitro*, the resulting zygote is cryopreserved for transfer in a subsequent cycle.[63]

In the original series by Edwards and Steptoe with natural cycle IVF, four clinical pregnancies and two live births resulted after 68 laparoscopies and 32 ETs.[1] Essentially no data on unstimulated cycles were generated between the early attempts and the more

Table 41.3 Criteria for human chorionic gonadotropin administration in unstimulated cycles based on follicle size and serum estradiol.*

Maximum follicle size (mm)	Serum estradiol level (pg/mL)
> 15	> 300
> 18	> 250
> 20	> 200

*Adapted from Paulson RJ, Sauer MV, Francis MM et al 1990[65]

Table 41.4 Pregnancy and embryo implantation rates in unstimulated compared with stimulated IVF cycles.*

Type of IVF cycle	No. of pregnancies (%) per cycle	No. of implantations (%) per cycle
Unstimulated	14%	13%
Stimulated	28%	9%

*Adapted from Paulson et al in Lobo RA, Mishell DR, Paulson RJ, Shoupe D (eds) 1997 Mishell's textbook of infertility, contraception, and reproductive endocrinology, 4th edn. Blackwell Scientific Publications, Malden, Massachusetts

recent era of unstimulated cycle IVF. Foulot et al[64] reported clinical pregnancies in 22.5% cycles and ongoing pregnancies in 17.5% cycles. Paulson et al[61,63,65,66] have observed a pregnancy rate of 17% and an ongoing rate of 13% per aspiration.

The per embryo implantation rate is higher in unstimulated compared with stimulated cycles (13% versus 9%). Because pregnancy rates are higher in stimulated cycles with multiple embryos transferred, the benefit of multiple ETs outweighs the benefit of the more natural uterine environment, at least on a per cycle basis (Table 41.4). A life-table analysis of repeat cycles indicated that pregnancy rates for unstimulated cycle IVF did not decrease for at least three cycles. Based on these data, two cycles of unstimulated IVF would be expected to yield the same likelihood of pregnancy as a single cycle with controlled ovarian hyperstimulation.[66] These data have made it possible to counsel patients on an individual basis as to whether the cost, convenience and other patient concerns would favor one stimulated or two unstimulated cycles.

OUTCOME AND PREGNANCY SUCCESS AFTER IN VITRO FERTILIZATION

On a per cycle basis, IVF results are similar to the fecundibility of natural conception cycles in the general population. Additionally, life-table analysis showed the per cycle pregnancy rate to be relatively constant for at least six cycles.[67,68] Therefore, IVF can be attempted on a repetitive basis and a considerably higher cumulative success rate can be achieved.

Unfortunately, 4–5% of all pregnancies achieved with IVF are tubal pregnancies, emphasizing the need for early surveillance of hCG titers and close ultrasonographic monitoring. This risk of ectopic pregnancy could be due to tubal disease, which may cause embryos that migrate into the tube after replacement into the uterine cavity to remain in the tube. It has also been suggested that controlled ovarian hyperstimulation utilized in stimulated IVF cycles could present an independent risk factor for ectopic pregnancy.[69] The multiple pregnancy rate following IVF is approximately 30%, with the majority of these being twins (25%) and 5% being triplets or higher order pregnancies.[33,70,71] Approximately 20% of all clinical pregnancies result in spontaneous abortion. This rate is consistent with the rate of miscarriage in the general population after spontaneous conception and increases as a function of age. Heterotopic pregnancy occurs in approximately 1 in every 100 IVF pregnancies as compared to 1 in every 30 000 spontaneous pregnancies.[72] An abdominal pregnancy has also been reported.[73]

The optimal number of embryos to be transferred has not been established. Although the chance of pregnancy generally increases as the number of embryos transferred increases, this additional benefit must be weighed against the increased risk of multiple gestation. While some clinics in the USA transfer up to nine embryos at one time, the Society for Assisted Reproductive Technology (SART) Registry data do not indicate any additional increase in live birth rates when more than four embryos are transferred.[81] For this reason, most clinics limit the maximum number of embryos transferred to four or five. In other countries, the maximum limit may be as low as two per transfer. The remaining embryos are usually cryopreserved and replaced in later cycles. The concern over the consequences of multiple births is significant and has led to a debate over tighter regulation of ART.

As a potential choice for the woman who becomes pregnant with triplets or more fetuses, selective reduction of fetuses can be carried out and is technically highly successful; it is carried out by ultrasound guidance, either vaginally or abdominally.

OOCYTE AND EMBRYO DONATION

Oocyte donation was introduced for the treatment of human infertility in 1984.[74] Originally, the method was applied to three groups of women:

1. Those with premature menopause
2. Patients afflicted with a genetic disease intent on having offspring without passing on the disease
3. Women with surgically inaccessible ovaries.

Today, donated oocytes are utilized in the management of women with a variety of reproductive disorders.[75–77] More than 2500 donation procedures are performed annually in the United States. The clinic-specific data submitted to the American Society of Reproductive Medicine (ASRM) reflect the increasing use of oocyte donation in the past few years (Table 41.5).[78–80]

Animal experimentation led to attempts at both oocyte and embryo donation in humans. In Australia, Trounson et al[82] reported the first human pregnancy achieved using oocyte donation. Interestingly, the recipient was ovulatory and her embryo transfer occurred during the early part of the luteal phase of a natural cycle. The transferred embryo was supported by the recipient's own corpus luteum and no exogenous hormones were prescribed. Unfortunately, the pregnancy ended in spontaneous abortion.

The first pregnancy in a woman with ovarian failure occurred in 1984 when a single donated, fertilized oocyte was given to a patient prescribed estrogen and progesterone.[74] Hormones were administered in a manner that mimicked the natural ovulatory cycle. Following conception, hormones were continued through the first trimester to support the developing pregnancy. The patient delivered a normal infant at term.

During the next few years refinements in oocyte donation continued. Several important reports further substantiated clinical efficacy using different transfer methods.[83–86] Improvements included:

1. Transition of *in vitro* fertilization from a surgical to a nonsurgical procedure
2. Use of gonadotropin-releasing hormone agonists to facilitate synchronization of donors and recipients while minimizing cancellations in stimulated cycles due to LH surges
3. Recruitment of designated known oocyte donors, which enhanced the quality, quantity and availability of gametes obtained for use in the procedure.

A major clinical breakthrough occurred in 1989 when oocyte donation was used to treat age-related infertility.[87,88] Women of advanced reproductive age (> 40 years) were previously thought to have a poor prognosis and were denied access to care due to concerns over the effect of age on uterine receptivity.

Table 41.5 Data adapted from the Report of Experience of Oocyte Donation in the United States by the Society for Assisted Reproductive Technology, The American Fertility Society.

Year	Clinics reporting	No. of clinical pregnancies (%)	No. of deliveries (%)
1987	17	20	18
1990	67	29	22
1994	163	51	34

Studies in hamsters, mice and rabbits implied that the uterus was responsible for much of the decreased fecundity and increased pregnancy wastage associated with aging.[89–91] However, in patients undergoing traditional care, the relative contributions of the oocyte and the uterus to success or failure could not be discerned, as both are inherent components in attempts to use autologous gametes. Yet, reports profiling women in their 40s receiving donated oocytes from younger women failed to demonstrate a change in efficacy related to age, with clinical pregnancy rates as high as 40%.[87,92–95] Regimens for hormone replacement similar to that used by Hodgen in monkeys[11] and later by Trounson et al[12] in humans maintained uterine receptivity despite advancing age. Most importantly, pregnancy rates were no different in the older recipient when oocytes were obtained from young donors. Recently, preliminary reports of menopausal women in their 50s who received embryos following oocyte donation demonstrated high success rates for pregnancy (Table 41.6).[96–98] Older patients, once considered hopelessly infertile, have experienced rates as high or higher than those normally seen in younger individuals undergoing assisted reproduction.

CURRENT METHODOLOGY FOR OOCYTE DONATION

Oocyte donation is performed by synchronizing the menstrual cycle of an infertile woman to the

Table 41.6 Pregnancies following oocyte donation to women over the age of 50 years.*

Investigators	No. of patients	No. of embryo transfers	Implantation rate (%)	Clinical pregnancy rate
Sauer et al[96]	14	21	19	38%
Antinori et al[97]	11	11	11	36%
Borini et al[98]	34	55	18	33%

*Adapted from Sauer et al in Lobo RA, Mishell DR, Paulson RJ, Shoupe D (eds) 1997 Mishell's textbook of infertility, contraception, and reproductive endocrinology, 4th edn. Blackwell Scientific Publications, Malden, Massachusetts

hyperstimulated cycle of a donor. The donor undergoes:

1. Ovarian hyperstimulation with gonadotropins
2. Monitoring and surveillance of the follicular response, usually by serial serum sampling and ultrasonographic visualization
3. Oocyte recovery, most commonly performed by transvaginal ultrasound-guided needle aspiration.

The risks are similar to those experienced traditionally by infertile women undergoing the same technique, and include anesthetic accidents, hemorrhage, infections and the development of ovarian hyperstimulation syndrome. Since complications are rare, the method is considered acceptable to young women who stand to gain nothing directly from participating, outside of financial remuneration.

The recipient's cycle is synchronized to the donor's cycle using hormone replacement therapy. Most often this consists of micronized oral estradiol and intramuscular progesterone prescribed prior to embryo transfer (Fig. 41.1).[88,99] Other formulations and routes of delivery include transdermal and vaginal administration. The different regimens for hormone replacement demonstrate similar success rates.[100] Use of any of these medications presents minimal risks to the mother and child, and no untoward side effects have been reported.

Reported complications in recipients include a tubo-ovarian abscess following embryo transfer,

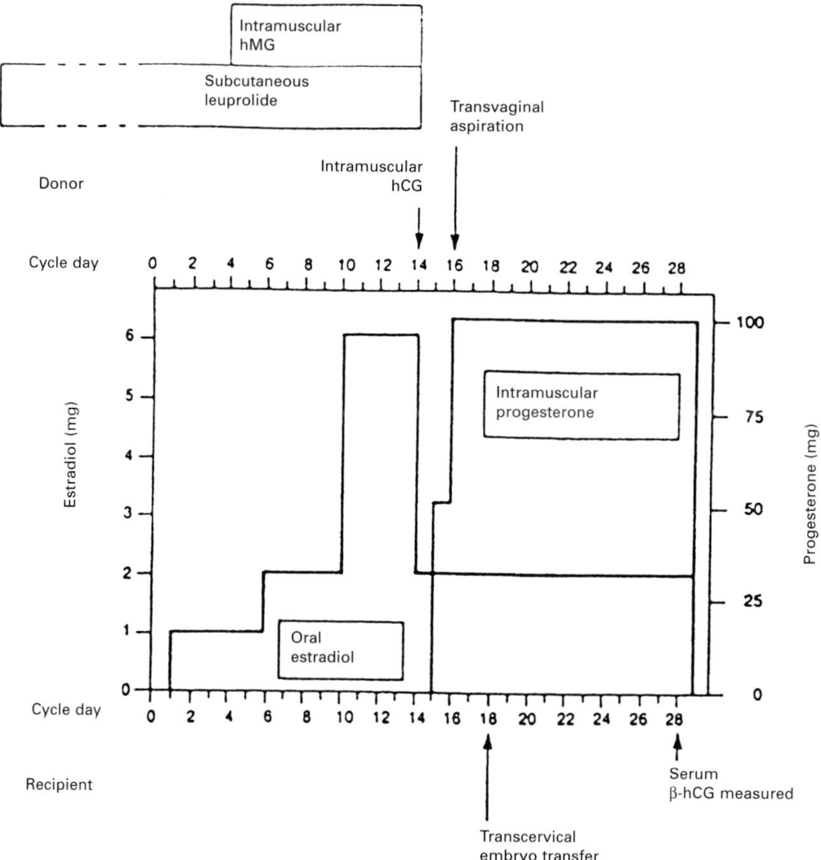

Fig. 41.1 Scheme used for synchronizing oocyte donors and recipients. Most often an incrementally increasing dose of oral estradiol has been used to prepare the endometrium for implantation. (Reprinted by permission of the New England Journal of Medicine.[88])

ectopic pregnancy, chromosomally abnormal babies and a third-trimester maternal death following a cerebral vascular accident.[101,102] Although all untoward events are unfortunate, such complications occur following both *in vitro* fertilization procedures and spontaneous pregnancies and are not unique to oocyte donation.

Indications for donor oocytes

Early attempts at oocyte donation were performed mostly in women with premature ovarian failure. Most recently, care has been provided to women with a variety of other disorders including individuals with gonadal dysgenesis, patients treated with chemotherapy and radiation, and women whose ovaries were surgically removed.[103]

Occasionally, individuals with inheritable disorders choose oocyte donation to avoid passing on their illness. This includes women with histories of balanced chromosomal translocations, Robertsonian translocations, X-linked disorders, autosomal recessive and dominant disorders and idiopathic recurrent abortion.[104] In general, pregnancy rates in these patients appear to be no different to those reported in women with ovarian failure.

Using oocyte donation to treat age-related infertility has greatly increased the demand on services. The aging of the population of the United States, the large percentage of women deferring childbearing to fulfill educational and career goals, and the increased prevalence of divorce and later marriage have contributed to the increasing number of women in their 40s and 50s who desire pregnancy. Often, oocyte donation represents the only reasonably successful method of treatment available for older patients.

Recipient age and treatment efficacy

It seems fair to assume that uterine receptivity can be extended 10–20 years beyond menopause. Morphometric analyses of endometria taken from functionally agonadal women aged 25–60 years receiving hormone replacement prior to attempted embryo transfer reveal strikingly similar findings.[105]

Intense controversy has surrounded the use of donated oocytes to extend the reproductive life span of women.[106–108] Accusations ranging from misuse of the technology to exploitation and dangerous medical practice have been lodged against investigators by both the scientific and the lay community. However, clinical research has failed to demonstrate any harmful effects, and in fact women of very advanced reproductive ages have been as successful as their younger counterparts in both conceiving and delivering babies.[109–111] Traditionally, fertility care has been offered to older men with reproductive disorders. Nevertheless, given the physiologic effects and known risks of pregnancy in women of advanced reproductive age, it is advisable to thoroughly examine all aspects of the prospective recipient's medical and psychological health. This should include a thorough screening of the cardiovascular and endocrine systems. Consultation with specialists in internal medicine and fetal-maternal medicine can be prudent before pregnancy is attempted.

PREGNANCY RATES AND OBSTETRICAL OUTCOMES

Considering the high rate of success using oocyte donation, it is reasonable to assume that the majority of patients will eventually deliver babies. Life-table analysis performed on the first 500 cycles at the University of Southern California (USC) in the US has demonstrated that more than half of recipients achieve a viable pregnancy by the third transfer (Fig. 41.2).[112] Patients are commonly older than 35 years, and most pregnancies in these women should be considered high risk. Additionally, multiple gestations often occur, which further complicates obstetric care. This hazard can be minimized by intentionally restricting the number of embryos transferred.

The most frequent complication of pregnancy appears to be first trimester uterine bleeding. This usually follows the collapse and abortion of nonviable supernumerary implantations.[113] These events occur in up to two thirds of pregnant patients undergoing oocyte donation. Bleeding is self-limiting and rarely leads to pregnancy loss.

Gestational hypertension has also been frequently noted in women over the age of 40 years.[109–111,114] This has been associated with intrauterine fetal growth retardation and can necessitate early delivery. Cesarean section rates are elevated, occurring in 50–75% of deliveries, and many cesarean sections have been performed electively. Indications for surgical intervention are liberally applied given the special circumstances surrounding these pregnancies.

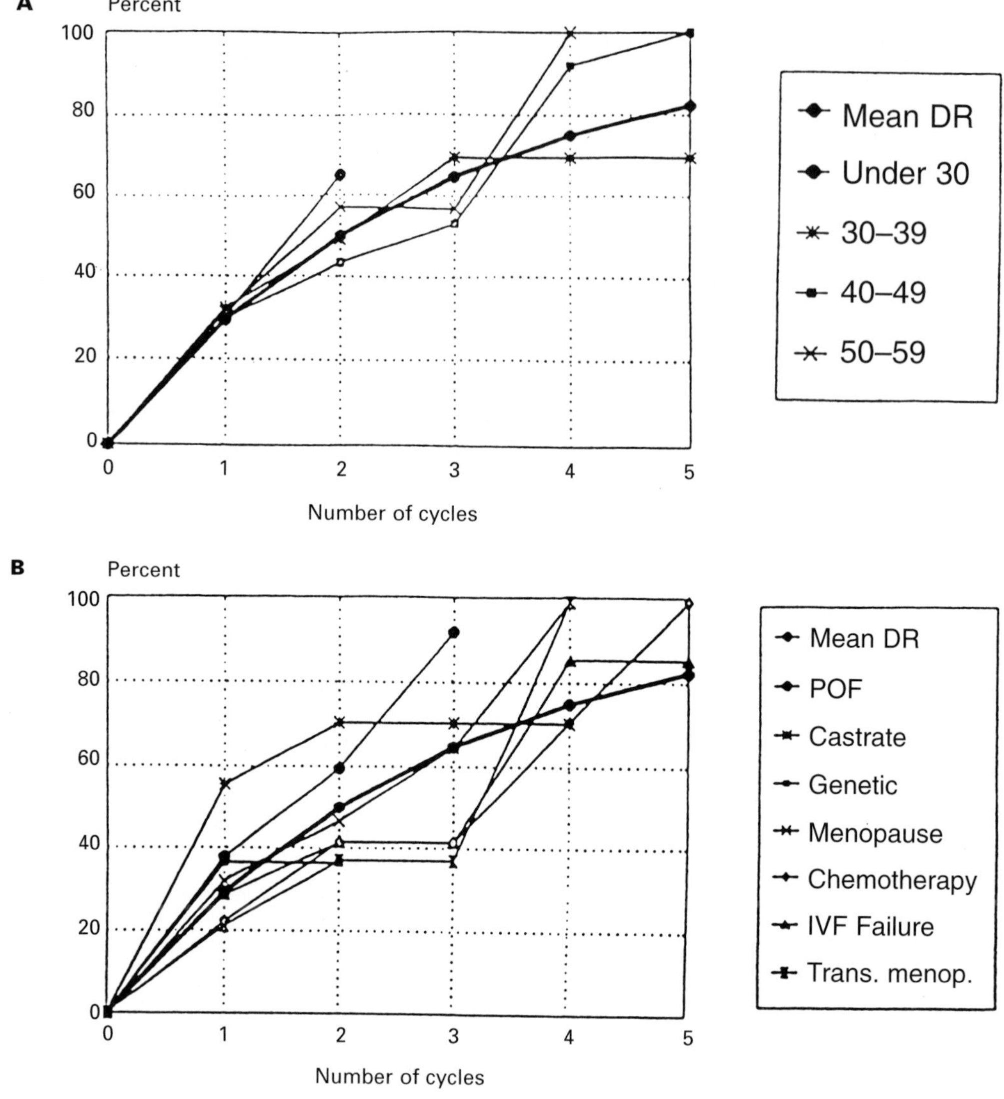

Fig. 41.2 Life-table analysis determined from 500 consecutive cases of oocyte donation to women with varying age (**A**) and diagnosis (**B**). No discernible effects are noted between subgroups. (DR: delivery rate; PR: pregnancy rate; POF: premature ovarian failure; Trans. Menop.: transitional menopause (perimenopause)).

REFERENCES

1. Edwards RG, Steptoe PC, Purdy JM 1980 Establishing full-term human pregnancies using cleaving embryos grown in vitro. British Journal of Obstetrics and Gynaecology 87: 737–756
2. Steptoe PC, Edwards RG 1976 Reimplantation of a human embryo with subsequent tubal pregnancy. Lancet 1: 880–882
3. Steptoe PC, Edwards RG 1978 Birth after the reimplantation of a human embryo. Lancet 2: 366
4. National IVF-ET Registry 1989 In vitro fertilization/embryo transfer in the United States: 1987 results from the National IVF-ET Registry. Fertility and Sterility 51: 13–19
5. Paulson RJ, Marrs RP 1986 Ovulation stimulation and monitoring for in vitro fertilization. Current Problems in Obstetrics, Gynecology and Infertility 10: 497–526

6. de Ziegler D, Cedars MI, Randle D et al 1987 Suppression of the ovary using a gonadotropin-releasing hormone agonist prior to stimulation for oocyte retrieval. Fertility and Sterility 48: 807–810
7. Rutherford AJ, Subak-Sharpe RJ, Dawson KJ et al 1988 Improvement of in vitro fertilization after treatment with buserelin, an agonist of luteinizing hormone releasing hormone. British Medical Journal 296: 1765–1768
8. Hughes EG, Fedorkow DM, Daya S et al 1992 The routine use of gonadotropin-releasing hormone agonists prior to in vitro fertilization and gametes intrafallopian transfer: a meta-analysis of randomized controlled trials. Fertility and Sterility 58: 888–896
9. Anderson RE, Paulson RJ, Sauer MV, Lobo RA 1988 Evidence supporting the routine use of a GnRH agonist (GnRH agonist) during ovarian stimulation for in vitro fertilization. Presented at the 44th Annual Meeting of The American Fertility Society, Atlanta, GA, October 10–13, 1988. Abstract P–149
10. Meldrum DR, Wisot A, Hamilton F et al 1989 Routine pituitary suppression with leuprolide before ovarian stimulation for oocyte retrieval. Fertility and Sterility 51: 455–459
11. Meldrum DR, Wisot A, Hamilton F et al 1988 Timing of initiation and dose schedule of leuprolide influences the time course of ovarian suppression. Fertility and Sterility 50: 400–402
12. Urbancsek J, Witthaus E 1996 Midluteal buserelin is superior to early follicular phase buserelin in combined gonadotropin-releasing hormone analog and gonadotropin stimulation in in vitro fertilization. Fertility and Sterility 65: 966–971
13. Martin MC, Givens CR, Schriock ED et al 1994 The choice of gonadotropin-releasing hormone analog influences outcome of in vitro fertilization treatment. American Journal of Obstetrics and Gynecology 170: 1629–1634
14. Edelstein MC, Brzyski RG, Jones GS et al 1990 Equivalency of human menopausal gonadotropin and follicle-stimulating hormone stimulation after gonadotropin-releasing hormone agonist suppression. Fertility and Sterility 53: 103–106
15. Bentick B, Shaw RW, Iffland CA et al 1988 A randomized comparative study of purified follicle stimulating hormone and human menopausal gonadotropin after pituitary desensitization with buserelin for superovulation and in vitro fertilization. Fertility and Sterility 50: 79–84
16. Daya S, Gunby J, Hughes EG et al 1995 Follicle-stimulating hormone versus human menopausal gonadotropin for in vitro fertilization cycles: a meta analysis. Fertility and Sterility 64: 347–354
17. Scott RT, Navot D 1994 Enhancement of ovarian responsiveness with microdoses of gonadotropin-releasing hormone agonist during ovulation induction for in vitro fertilization. Fertility and Sterility 61: 880–885
18. Homburg R, Eshel A, Abdalla HI, Jacobs HS 1988 Growth hormone facilitates ovulation induction by gonadotropins. Clinical Endocrinology (Oxford) 29: 113–117
19. Shaker AG, Fleming R, Jamiteson ME, Yates RW 1992 Absence of effect of adjuvant growth hormone therapy on follicular responses to exogenous gonadotropins in women: normal and poor responders. Fertility and Sterility 58: 919–923
20. Olivennes F, Fanchin R, Bouchard P et al 1995 Scheduled administration of a gonadotropin releasing hormone antagonist (Cetrorelix) on day 8 of in vitro fertilization cycles: a pilot study. Human Reproduction 10: 1382–1386
21. Cassidenti DL, Sauer MV, Paulson RJ et al 1991 Comparison of intermittent and continuous use of a gonadotropin-releasing hormone antagonist (Nal-Glu) in in vitro fertilization cycles: a preliminary report. American Journal of Obstetrics and Gynecology 165: 1806–1810
22. Paulson RJ, Sauer MV, Lobo RA 1994 Addition of a gonadotropin releasing hormone (GnRH) antagonist and exogenous gonadotropins to unstimulated in vitro fertilization (IVF) cycles: physiologic observations and preliminary experience. Journal of Assisted Reproduction and Genetics 11: 28–32
23. Meldrum DR, Rivier J, Garzo G et al 1994 Successful pregnancies with unstimulated cycle oocyte donation using an antagonist of gonadotropin-releasing hormone. Fertility and Sterility 61: 556–557
24. Jones HW Jr, Acosta A, Andrew MC et al 1983 The importance of the follicular phase to success and failure in in vitro fertilization. Fertility and Sterility 40: 317–321
25. Gonen Y, Casper RF 1990 Prediction of implantation by the sonographic appearance of the endometrium during controlled ovarian stimulation for in vitro fertilization (IVF). Journal of In Vitro Fertilisation and Embryo Transfer 7: 146–152
26. Silverberg KM, Burns WN, Olive DL et al 1991 Serum progesterone levels predict success of in vitro fertilization/embryo transfer in patients stimulated with leuprolide acetate and human menopausal gonadotropins. Journal of Clinical Endocrinology and Metabolism 73: 797–803
27. Schoolcraft W, Sinton E, Schlenker T et al 1991 Lower pregnancy rate with premature luteinization during pituitary suppression with leuprolide acetate. Fertility and Sterility 55: 563–566
28. Givins CR, Schriock ED, Dandekar PV, Martin MC 1994 Elevated serum progesterone levels on the day of human chorionic gonadotropin administration do not predict outcome in assisted reproduction cycles. Fertility and Sterility 62: 1011–1017
29. Kolb BA, Paulson RJ 1997 The luteal phase of cycles utilizing controlled ovarian hyperstimulation and its possible impact on embryo implantation. American Journal of Obstetrics and Gynecology 176: 1262–1267
30. Legro RS, Ary BA, Paulson RJ et al 1993 Premature luteinization as detected by elevated serum progesterone is associated with a higher pregnancy rate in donor oocyte in-vitro fertilization. Human Reproduction 8: 1506–1511
31. Morris RS, Paulson RJ 1994 Ovarian hyperstimulation syndrome: classification and management. Contemporary Obstetrics and Gynecology 39: 43–54
32. Aboulghar MA, Mansour RT, Serour GI, Elattar I 1992 Follicular aspiration does not protect against the development of ovarian hyperstimulation syndrome. Journal of Assisted Reproduction and Genetics 9: 238–243

33. Society for Assisted Reproductive Technology, The American Society for Reproductive Medicine 1995 Assisted reproductive technology in the United States and Canada: 1993 results generated from The American Society for Reproductive Medicine/Society for Assisted Reproductive Technology Registry. Fertility and Sterility 64: 13–21
34. Weatherbee PS, Francis MM, Macaso TM et al 1995 A new long shelf life formulation of modified Hams F-10 medium: biochemical and clinical evaluation. Journal of Assisted Reproduction and Genetics 12: 175–179
35. Quinn P, Kerin JF, Warnes GM 1985 Improved pregnancy rate in human in vitro fertilization with the use of a medium based on the composition of human tubal fluid. Fertility and Sterility 44: 493–498
36. Gianaroli L, Seracchioli R, Ferraretti AP et al 1986 The successful use of human amniotic fluid for mouse embryo culture and human in vitro fertilization, embryo culture, and transfer. Fertility and Sterility 46: 907–913
37. Kemeter P, Feichtinger W 1984 Pregnancy following in vitro fertilization and embryo transfer using pure human serum as culture and transfer medium. Fertility and Sterility 41: 936–937
38. Khan I, Camus M, Staessen C et al 1988 Success rate in gamete intrafallopian transfer using low and high concentrations of washed spermatozoa. Fertility and Sterility 50: 922–927
39. Wolf DP, Byrd W, Dandekar P, Quigley MM 1984 Sperm concentration and the fertilization of human eggs in vitro. Biology of Reproduction 31: 837–848
40. Rajah SV, Parslow JM, Howell RJ, Hendry WF 1993 The effects on in-vitro fertilization of autoantibodies to spermatozoa in subfertile men. Human Reproduction 8: 1079–1082
41. Cohen J, Adler A, Alikani M et al 1993 Assisted fertilization and abnormal sperm function. Seminars in Reproduction Endocrinology 11: 83–94
42. Pelermo G, Joris H, Devroey P, Van Steirteghem AC 1992 Pregnancies after intracytoplasmic injection of a single spermatozoon into an oocyte. Lancet 340: 17–18
43. Van Steirteghem A, Liu J, Nagy Z et al 1993 Use of assisted fertilization. Human Reproduction 8: 1784–1785
44. Filicori M, Flamigni C, Seracchioli R et al 1996 Intracytoplasmic sperm injection and related techniques: 1996 clinical update. Assisted Reproduction Reviews 6: 100–105
45. Nagy Z, Liu J, Janssenwillen C et al 1995 Using ejaculated, fresh, and frozen-thawed epididymal and testicular spermatozoa gives rise to comparable results after intracytoplasmic sperm injection. Fertility and Sterility 63: 808–815
46. Silber SJ, Van Steirteghem AC, Liu J et al 1995 High fertilization and pregnancy rates after intracytoplasmic sperm injection with spermatozoa obtained from testicular biopsy. Human Reproduction 10: 148–152
47. Quinn P, Margalit R 1996 Beneficial effects of coculture with cumulus cells on blastocyst formation in a prospective trial with supernumerary human embryos. Journal of Assisted Reproduction and Genetics 13: 9–14
48. Wiemer KE, Cohen J, Amborski GF et al 1989 In vitro development and implantation of human embryos following culture on fetal bovine uterine fibroblast cells. Human Reproduction 4: 595–600
49. Thibodeaux JK, Godke RA 1995 Potential use of embryo coculture with human in vitro fertilization procedures. Journal of Assisted Reproduction and Genetics 12: 665–677
50. Bavister BD 1992 Co-culture for embryo development: is it really necessary? Human Reproduction 7: 1339–1341
51. Paulson RJ, Sauer MV, Lobo RA 1990 Embryo implantation after human in vitro fertilization: importance of endometrial receptivity. Fertility and Sterility 53: 870–874
52. Paulson RJ, Sauer MV, Lobo RA 1990 Factors affecting embryo implantation after human in vitro fertilization: a hypothesis. American Journal of Obstetrics and Gynecology 163: 2020–2023
53. Pados G, Devroey P 1992 Luteal phase support. Assisted Reproduction Reviews 2: 148–153
54. Garcia J, Jones GS, Acosta AA, Wright GL Jr 1981 Corpus luteum function after follicle aspiration for oocyte retrieval. Fertility and Sterility 36: 565–572
55. Kreitman O, Nixon WE, Hodgen GD 1981 Induced corpus luteum dysfunction after aspiration of the preovulatory follicle in monkeys. Fertility and Sterility 35: 671–675
56. Leeton J, Trounson A, Jessup D 1985 Support of the luteal phase in in vitro fertilization programs: results of a controlled trial with intramuscular Proluton. Journal of In Vitro Fertilisation and Embryo Transfer 2: 166–169
57. Van Steirteghem AC, Smith J, Camus M et al 1988 The luteal phase after in vitro fertilization and related procedures. Human Reproduction 3: 161–164
58. Trounson A, Howlett D, Rogers P, Hoppen HO 1986 The effect of progesterone supplementation around the time of oocyte recovery in patients superovulated for in vitro fertilization. Fertility and Sterility 45: 532–535
59. Smith E, Anthony FW, Gadd SC, Masson GM 1989 Trial of support treatment with human chorionic gonadotropin in the luteal phase after treatment with buserelin and human menopausal gonadotrophin in women taking part in an in vitro fertilization programme. MBJ 298: 1483–1486
60. Ranoux C, Foulot H, Dubuisson JB et al 1988 Returning to spontaneous cycles in in vitro fertilization. Journal of In Vitro Fertilisation and Embryo Transfer 5: 304–305
61. Paulson RJ, Sauer MV, Lobo RA 1989 In vitro fertilization in unstimulated cycles: a new application. Fertility and Sterility 51: 1059–1060
62. Patton PE 1992 IVF in the unstimulated cycle. Contemporary Obstetrics and Gynecology 37: 67–74
63. Paulson RJ, Sauer MV, Francis MM et al 1994 Factors affecting pregnancy success of human in-vitro fertilization in unstimulated cycles. Human Reproduction 9: 1571–1575
64. Foulot H, Ranoux C, Dubuisson JB et al 1989 In vitro fertilization without ovarian stimulation: a simplified protocol applied in 80 cycles. Fertility and Sterility 52: 617–621

65. Paulson RJ, Sauer MV, Francis MM et al 1990 In vitro fertilization in unstimulated cycles: a clinical trial using hCG for timing of follicle aspiration. Obstetrics and Gynecology 76: 788–791
66. Paulson RJ, Sauer MV, Francis MM et al 1992 In vitro fertilization in unstimulated cycles: the University of Southern California experience. Fertility and Sterility 57: 290–293
67. Guzick DS, Wilkes C, Jones HW Jr 1986 Cumulative pregnancy rates for in vitro fertilization. Fertility and Sterility 46: 663–667
68. Kovacs GT, Rogers P, Leeton JF et al 1986 In vitro fertilization and embryo transfer: prospects of pregnancy by life-table analysis. Medical Journal of Australia 144: 682–683
69. Fernandez H, Coste J, Job-Spira N 1991 Controlled ovarian hyperstimulation as a risk factor for ectopic pregnancy. Obstetrics and Gynecology 78: 656–659
70. Society for Assisted Reproductive Technology, The American Fertility Society 1993 Assisted Reproductive Technology in the United States and Canada: 1991 results from the Society for Assisted Reproductive Technology generated from the American Fertility Society Registry. Fertility and Sterility 59: 956–962
71. Society for Assisted Reproductive Technology, The American Fertility Society 1994 Assisted Reproductive Technology in the US and Canada: 1992 results from the Society for Assisted Reproductive Tech. generated from the American Fertility Society Registry. Fertility and Sterility 62: 1121–1128
72. Snyder T, del Castillo J, Graff J et al 1988 Heterotopic pregnancy after in vitro fertilization and ovulatory drugs. Annals of Emergency Medicine 17: 846–849
73. Oehninger S, Kreiner D, Bass MJ, Rosenwaks Z 1988 Abdominal pregnancy after in vitro fertilization and embryo transfer. Obstetrics and Gynecology 72: 499–502
74. Lutjen P, Trounson A, Leeton J et al 1989 The establishment and maintenance of pregnancy using in vitro fertilization and embryo donation in a patient with primary ovarian failure. Nature 307: 174–175
75. Meldrum DR 1993 Oocyte donation. Infertility and Reproductive Medicine Clinics of North America 4: 761–768
76. Sauer MV 1995 Oocyte donation; reviewing a decade of growth and development. Seminars in Reproductive Endocrinology 13: 79–84
77. Morris RA, Sauer MV 1993 Oocyte donation in the 1990s and beyond. Assisted Reproductive Review 3: 211–217
78. Society for Assisted Reproductive Technology, Medical Research International 1989 In vitro fertilization/embryo transfer in the United States: 1987 results from the National IVF/ET Registry. Fertility and Sterility 51: 13–19
79. Medical Research International, The American Fertility Society Special Interest Group 1992 In vitro fertilization/embryo transfer in the United States: 1990 results from the National IVF/ET Registry. Fertility and Sterility 57: 15–24
80. Society for Assisted Reproductive Technology, The American Society for Reproductive Medicine 1996 Assisted Reproductive Technology in the US and Canada: 1994 results from the Society for Assisted Reproductive Tech. generated from The American Fertility Society Registry. Fertility and Sterility 66: 697–705
81. Hodgen GD 1983 Surrogate embryo transfer combined with estrogen-progesterone therapy in monkeys. Implantation, gestation, and delivery without ovaries. Journal of the American Medical Association 250: 2167–2171
82. Trounson A, Leeton J, Besanko M et al 1983 Pregnancy established in an infertile patient after transfer of a donated embryo fertilized in vitro. British Medical Journal 286: 835–838
83. Sauer MV, Bustillo M, Gorrill MJ et al 1988 An instrument for the recovery of preimplantation uterine ova. Obstetrics and Gynecology 71: 804–806
84. Sauer MV, Paulson RJ 1990 Human oocyte and preembryo donation: an evolving method for the treatment of infertility. American Journal of Obstetrics and Gynecology 163: 1421–1424
85. Borrero C, Remohi J, Ord T et al 1989 A program of oocyte donation and gamete intrafallopian transfer. Human Reproduction 4: 275–279
86. Balmaceda JP, Alam V, Roszjtein D et al 1992 Embryo implantation rates in oocyte donation: a prospective comparison of tubal versus uterine transfers. Fertility and Sterility 57: 362–365
87. Serhal PF, Craft IL 1989 Oocyte donation in 61 patients. Lancet 1: 1185–1197
88. Sauer MV, Paulson RJ, Lobo RA 1990 A preliminary report on oocyte donation extending reproductive potential to women over forty. New England Journal of Medicine 323: 1157–1160
89. Thorneycroft IH, Soderwall AL 1969 The nature of the litter size loss in senescent hamsters. Anatomical Record 165: 343
90. Harman SM, Talbert GB 1970 The effect of maternal age on ovulation, corpora lutea of pregnancy and implantation failure in mice. Journal of Reproduction and Fertility 23: 33–39
91. Maibenco HC, Krehbiel RH 1973 Reproductive decline in aged female rats. Journal of Reproduction and Fertility 32: 121–123
92. Navot D, Drews MR, Bergh PA et al 1994 Age-related decline in female fertility is not due to diminished capacity of the uterus to sustain embryo implantation. Fertility and Sterility 61: 97–101
93. Pantos K, Meimeti-Damianaki T, Vaxevanoglou T, Kapetanakis E 1993 Oocyte donation in menopausal women aged over 40. Human Reproduction 8: 488–491
94. Balmaceda JP, Bernardini L, Ciuffardi I et al 1994 Oocyte donation in humans: a model to study the effect of age on embryo implantation rate. Human Reproduction 9: 2160–2163
95. Sauer MV, Paulson RJ, Lobo RA 1992 Reversing the natural decline in human fertility. An extended clinical trial of oocyte donation to women of advanced reproductive age. Journal of the American Medical Association 268: 1275–1279
96. Sauer MV, Paulson RJ, Lobo RA 1993 Pregnancy after age 50: application of oocyte donation to women after natural menopause. Lancet 341: 321–323
97. Antinori S, Versaci C, Gholami GH et al 1993 Oocyte donation in menopausal women. Human Reproduction 8: 1487–1490

98. Borini A, Bafaro G, Violini F et al 1995 Pregnancies in postmenopausal women over 50 years old in an oocyte donation program. Fertility and Sterility 63: 258–261
99. Sauer MV, Paulson RJ, Macaso TM et al 1989 Establishment of a non-anonymous donor oocyte program: preliminary experience at the University of Southern California. Fertility and Sterility 52: 433–436
100. Sauer MV 1991 Hormone replacement prior to embryo donation to women with ovarian failure. Female Patient 16: 15–20
101. Sauer MV, Paulson RJ 1992 Pelvic abscess complicating transcervical embryo transfer. American Journal of Obstetrics and Gynecology 166: 148–149
102. Bewley S, Wright JT 1991 Maternal death associated with ovum donation twin pregnancy. Human Reproduction 6: 898–899
103. Sauer MV, Paulson RJ, Ary BA, Lobo RA 1994 Three hundred cycles of oocyte donation at the University of Southern California: assessing the effect of age and diagnosis on pregnancy and implantation rates. Journal of Assisted Reproduction and Genetics 11: 92–96
104. Hens L, Devroey P, Van Waesberghe L et al 1989 Chromosome studies and fertility treatment in women with ovarian failure. Clinical Genetics 36: 81–91
105. Sauer MV, Miles RA, Damoush L et al 1993 Evaluating the effect of age on endometrial responsiveness to hormone replacement therapy: a histologic, ultrasonographic, and tissue receptor analysis. Journal of Assisted Reproduction Genetics 10: 47–52
106. Paulson RJ, Sauer MV 1994 Regulation of oocyte donation to women over the age of 50: a question of reproductive choice. Journal of Assisted Reproduction Genetics 11: 177–182
107. Taylor PJ, Gomel V 1992 Abraham laughed. International Journal of Fertility 37: 202–203
108. Editorial Office 1993 Too old to have a baby? Lancet 341: 344–345
109. Sauer MV, Paulson RJ, Lobo RA 1995 Pregnancy after 50: results of 22 consecutive pregnancies following oocyte donation. Fertility and Sterility 64: 111–115
110. Shaw K, Sauer MV 1995 Obstetrical care of oocyte donation recipients and surrogates. Seminars in Reproductive Endocrinology 13: 231–236
111. Pados G, Camus M, Van Steirteghem A et al 1994 The evolution and outcome of pregnancies from oocyte donation. Human Reproduction 9: 538–542
112. Paulson RJ, Hatch IE, Lobo RA, Sauer MV 1995 Cumulative success rates after oocyte donation: life table analysis. Abstract presented at the IXth World Congress on In Vitro Fertilization and Assisted Reproduction, Vienna, Austria, April 1995
113. Legro RS, Wong IL, Paulson RS et al 1993 Multiple implantation following oocyte donation: a frequent but inefficient event. Fertility and Sterility 63: 849–853
114. Blanchette H 1993 Obstetric performance of patients after oocyte donation. American Journal of Obstetrics and Gynecology 168: 1803–1809

42. Use of therapeutic steroids in pregnancy

Phillip L. Matson John L. Yovich

Introduction

Human reproduction, on the face of it, is inefficient, with at best only one in three cycles in the fertile population resulting in pregnancy, and up to one third of these pregnancies aborting spontaneously.[1] The question of whether ovarian steroids generally, and progestogens in particular, can help maintain a threatened pregnancy has been posed for many years without a conclusive answer being forthcoming. Indeed, the clinical application of progestogen support was described back in the 1930s,[2] and yet the effectiveness of exogenous progesterone in preventing miscarriage is still the source of debate some 60 years later.[3] It appears that there are three broad difficulties in reviewing the extensive literature base to arrive at some consensus, namely:

1. The difficulty of patient selection. It is likely that certain subgroups of patients will benefit from ovarian steroid support more than others, but their identification is not easy
2. The choice of appropriate control subjects with which to compare the outcome of treatment is of paramount importance
3. There is a lack of agreement regarding the pharmaceutical preparation of choice, and the most effective dose and the schedule of administration.

Prospective, randomized, controlled trials are the only way to arrive at clear answers. Meta-analysis of controlled trials for women with recurrent miscarriage[4] or at-risk pregnancies[5] have been done, but the small number of trials worth including has prevented a definitive conclusion.

In the absence of large trials, the retrospective gathering of cases by individual clinics can be inconclusive, open to misinterpretation and possibly misleading. This is illustrated in Table 42.1 by the unpublished data gathered at PIVET Medical Centre during an audit of the practice of the clinic. The outcome of pregnancies following infertility treatment is given according to whether obstetric progestogen support was used, progestogens being administered in high risk patients presenting with either vaginal bleeding or low serum progesterone concentrations. At first sight there appears to be no statistically significant difference in the proportion of pregnancies that are on-going. But how should the data be viewed and how should the clinic decide upon future medical practice? Was the support ineffective, or had the progestogens been effective in rescuing pregnancies to a level seen in uncomplicated cases?

Table 42.1 The proportion of pregnancies achieved at PIVET Medical Centre in 1995 that were on-going (unpublished data).

	'Obstetric support'*	
Infertility treatment	Nil	Progestogen
Intra-uterine insemination	43/65 (66%)	34/50 (68%)
Frozen embryo transfer	22/30 (73%)	14/28 (50%)
In vitro fertilization	48/85 (56%)	34/71 (48%)
Total	113/180 (63%)	82/149 (55%)

*Oral medroxyprogesterone acetate and intramuscular progesterone given to cases with threatened pregnancy, and no support given to those progressing uneventfully.

Notwithstanding the paucity of good data on which to base a clinical decision, the clinician will still be faced with cases of threatened pregnancy in which the use of steroid support might seem attractive, based upon clinical pressures and the available information. Large, prospective, multi-centre studies take a long time, with the framing of the question and the drafting of the protocol requiring much effort, and there are few in existence. It is important, therefore, for the information we do have to be analyzed comprehensively and critically: it is our only current source of guidance in deciding what is and what is not useful.

ADMINISTRATION OF EXOGENOUS STEROIDS IN PREGNANCY

Rationale

The rationale for administering progesterone during early pregnancy, at its simplest level, is that progesterone is vital for the maintenance of the pregnancy. It is now clear that the corpus luteum in the human is indispensable during the first seven weeks of pregnancy, but that pregnancy can be maintained by exogenous progesterone after surgical removal of the corpus luteum.[6,7] Accordingly, many studies have tried to identify the women who are at risk of miscarriage due to progesterone deficiency. Progesterone status in these studies has been assessed by the examination of cervical mucus[8] and vaginal cytology,[9–12] the measurement of urinary metabolite excretion[13] and estimations of serum progesterone concentrations.[14]

The administration of progestogens later in pregnancy seems to revolve around several observations: that a drop in circulating progesterone is associated with the onset of labor[15] (although this is not universally recognized); that low progesterone concentrations are often seen in cases of premature labor in which there are no clear clinical complications;[16] and that progesterone and progestogens can have a tocolytic effect[17,18] (by the direct suppression of uterine contractions[19–20]). The administration of exogenous progesterone and related compounds might therefore reduce uterine contractions and help prevent premature labor.

It is also recognized that reduced circulating concentrations of progesterone are often seen in cases of early pregnancy failure around eight weeks,[21] possibly due to an inadequacy of the placenta in taking over steroid production as corpus luteum progesterone production falls (referred to as the 'luteo-placental shift' of progesterone production), but it is unclear whether this lower level of circulating progesterone is cause or effect of the failing trophoblast and therefore whether progesterone supplementation could be of value.

The requirement for estrogen in early pregnancy is much less clear, with its need beyond the proliferative phase of endometrial development having been questioned.[22] Supplementation with estrogen after surgical removal of the corpus luteum in the human, unlike progesterone supplementation, does not enable the pregnancy to continue.[23] Primate studies have also shown the relative unimportance of estrogen in maintaining an established pregnancy.[24] This lack of effect of estrogens in preventing pregnancy loss, coupled with adverse side effects (see below), has resulted in a general withdrawal from use of estrogens for these indications.

Adverse effects

Before exogenous steroids can be used during pregnancy one must be confident that the benefits are not outweighed by adverse effects. It appears that there are two main areas of concern: the effect of the compounds upon endogenous steroid production in the mother and the general outcome for the mothers and children.

The administration of exogenous progestogens in the luteal phase of an ovarian cycle, that is around the time of implantation, can have a marked inhibitory effect upon progesterone production by the corpus luteum.[25–27] On the other hand, despite medroxyprogesterone acetate given intramuscularly in the third trimester having been associated with a decreased pregnanediol excretion,[28] progestogen administration after the pregnancy has become established does not generally seem to have a detrimental effect upon circulating progesterone concentrations[29] or the profile of progesterone's urinary metabolites.[30] Interestingly, the current use of specific immunoassays to measure progesterone usually means that the synthetic progestogens such as medroxyprogesterone acetate are not recognized by the assay, presenting both an advantage and a disadvantage: the concentration of progesterone can be measured without interference from the cross-reacting substance but, by the same token, the progesterone assays in routine use cannot be used to monitor the absorption and circulating levels of the exogenous synthetic progestogen.

An evaluation of the safety of ovarian steroids given in pregnancy in relation to teratogenicity[31–43] is made in chapter 43. In summary, there appears to be no increase in pregnancy loss in these patients or abnormality of their off-spring following brief exposure to ovarian steroids as contraceptive agents. The potential adverse effect of progestogens with androgenic properties has been noted. The use of neither medroxyprogesterone acetate nor progesterone appears to be associated with an increased incidence of fetal abnormality.

Pregnancies at risk of loss or prematurity

The present review will concentrate on the use of ovarian steroids to support pregnancies in women with no ovarian function; on the administration of steroids, predominantly progestogens, in cases of threatened and habitual abortion and premature delivery; and in certain other clinical situations.

Choice of steroid preparation

The safe progestogens (those without androgenic properties) available to the prescribing clinician consist of progesterone, 17α-hydroxyprogesterone caproate (also known as 17α-hydroxyprogesterone hexanoate) and medroxyprogesterone acetate. Medroxyprogesterone acetate has strong progestational activity because of its methylation at carbon position 6,[44] and has been shown capable of supporting pregnancy totally in castrated rabbits.[45] The structural relationship of 17α-hydroxyprogesterone caproate and medroxyprogesterone acetate to progesterone is shown in Fig. 42.1.

There appears to be wide variation in the progestogen prescribing practice of clinicians in pregnancy in various parts of the world. Data from 1979 showed that 28% of the progestogens prescribed in Italy were for threatened abortion, whereas only 3% of the progestogens prescribed in the UK were for the this purpose.[46] Details of the drugs available presently in Australia, together with their route of administration and price, is given in Table 42.2. The cost of the different preparations varies enormously, with intramuscular progesterone being by far the most expensive: typical weekly costs of the various progestogens to support threatened pregnancies based on regimens described previously shows progesterone in oil to be about 30 times more expensive than medroxyprogesterone acetate and eight times the cost of 17α-hydroxyprogesterone caproate.

The main current use of estrogens is in the support of pregnancies in women without gonadal function having embryos transferred in an IVF program (see below) and the cost of the oral preparation is minimal in comparison.

THREATENED ABORTION

Definition and prognosis

A common definition of a threatened abortion is that of painless vaginal bleeding with a closed cervix during the first 20–28 weeks of pregnancy, and this occurs in approximately 16% of pregnancies.[2] The outcome of so-called threatened pregnancies without medical intervention must first be considered before the effectiveness of supportive medication can be fully

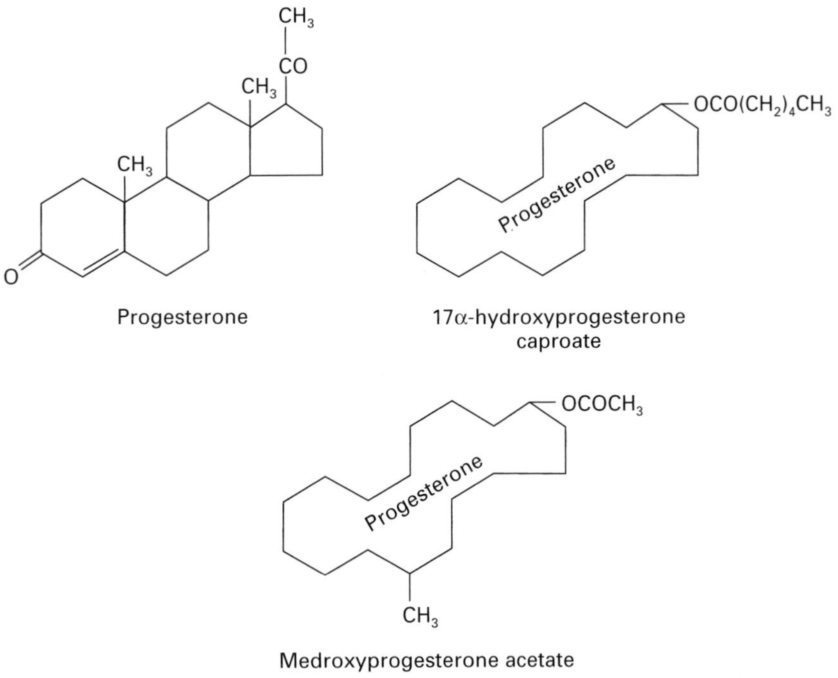

Fig. 42.1 The chemical relationship of 17α-hydroxyprogesterone caproate and medroxyprogesterone acetate to progesterone.

Table 42.2 Progestogens and estrogens currently available in Australia, and projected cost if used during pregnancy.

Preparation	Progestogen/ estrogen	Company	Route	Cost/100 mg	Approx. weekly cost	Reference
Depo-Provera	MPA	Upjohn	i.m.	Aus$10.10	Aus$10.10	Turner et al (1966)[28]
Depo-Ralovera	MPA	Kenral	i.m.	Aus$7.89	Aus$7.89	Turner et al (1966)[28]
Proluton	Progesterone	Schering	i.m.	Aus$90.44	Aus$1266	Fuchs and Stakemann (1960)[99]
Proluton depot	17-OHP-C	Schering	i.m.	Aus$16.65	Aus$167	Hauth et al (1983)[105]
Provera	MPA	Upjohn	Oral	Aus$4.86	Aus$41	Yovich et al (1988)[37]
Ralovera	MPA	Kenral	Oral	Aus$4.52	Aus$38	Yovich et al (1988)[37]
Primogyn depot	Estradiol valerate	Schering	i.m.	Aus$271.50	Aus$38	Leeton et al (1989)[91]
Progynova	Estradiol valerate	Schering	Oral	Aus$19.70	Aus$3	Leeton et al (1989)[91]

MPA = medroxyprogesterone acetate; 17-OHP-C = 17α-hydroxyprogesterone caproate

appreciated, and a succinct summary of the consequences of vaginal bleeding in early pregnancy has already been made.[47] It appears that about 50% of cases presenting with vaginal bleeding in early pregnancy will miscarry[48–50] and that half of these demonstrate a significant chromosomal abnormality of the fetus.[51–53] Furthermore, those pregnancies that do not abort can show an increased prevalence of premature delivery[49,54,55] and congenital anomalies.[54,56,57] Surprisingly, there does not seem to be an additional increase in risk of miscarriage if subchorionic bleeding[58] or the presence of a large intrauterine hematoma[59,60] is identified using ultrasound after a normally beating fetal heart has been detected.

Treatment

Overall, pregnancies complicated by early bleeding can have a poor outcome and so an attempt at rescuing the pregnancy might seem prudent. The choice of treatments is limited, with rest in bed appearing a first line choice among general practitioners in the UK, despite a relative lack of confidence in its effectiveness.[61] In that series, only 13% of responding practitioners used progestogens and this was usually on the advice of local specialists. Nevertheless, the treatment of threatened abortion remains the main use of steroids given during pregnancy.

The beneficial use of progestogens in cases at risk of threatened abortion has been claimed on many occasions,[8,9,10,62] although the reports are often the collection of data using a range of different regimens. A summary of the main studies examining systematically the effectiveness of progestogens in threatened abortion compared to controls is given in Table 42.3. The most encouraging historical data came from the use of intramuscular progesterone in women chosen by virtue of a reduced urinary pregnanediol excretion,[13] although this benefit was not seen by the other groups using vaginal progesterone,[63] oral medroxyprogesterone acetate[64] or intramuscular 17α-hydroxyprogesterone caproate[46] in women chosen because of vaginal bleeding but without evidence of progesterone deficiency. The widespread administration of progestogens is therefore unlikely to be helpful to all patients, but the most effective results will probably be achieved in women selected because of a definite hormonal deficiency.

RECURRENT MISCARRIAGE

Recurrent miscarriage, defined as three or more consecutive miscarriages, occurs in up to 2% of couples during their reproductive life.[65] It can occur through a number of mechanisms,[66] although there is not an increased prevalence of chromosomal

Table 42.3 Use of progestogens in threatened abortion.

Reference	Progestogen	Maximum dose	Route	Time given	Live births	
					Control	Progestogen
Morgan et al (1960)[13]	Progesterone	250 mg	i.m.	'Early'	11/40 (28%)	87/100 (87%)
Moller and Fuchs (1965)[64]	MPA	80 mg/day	Oral	≥8 weeks	26/46 (57%)	25/38 (66%)
Tognoni et al (1980)[46]	17-OHP-C	25 mg/5 days	i.m.	≤14 weeks	47/51 (66%)	45/74 (61%)
Gerhard et al (1987)[63]	Progesterone	25 mg	Vaginal	1st trimester	21/26 (81%)	23/26 (88%)

abnormalities over and above those abortuses from cases with no history of recurrent loss.[67] An expectation that ovarian steroid support might solve all problems is clearly naive. Numerous therapies such as immunotherapy[68] have been proposed[69] based upon different principles. Many of the studies using progestogens have attempted to focus on those cases with luteal deficiency[70] and progesterone deficiency in early pregnancy.[11,12,71]

The meta-analysis of controlled trials in cases of recurrent miscarriage has suggested a benefit of progestogen given in early pregnancy.[4] However, it should be noted that only three studies satisfied the criteria for inclusion in this analysis,[72–74] and none of these had sufficient statistical power to detect a benefit. Many other authors have reported on the use of progestogens in women with recurrent miscarriage, and a summary of the major studies is given in Table 42.4. The main choice of progestogen seems to have been between 17α-hydroxyprogesterone caproate (either 250 mg or 500 mg given once per week) or progesterone given as an implant or vaginally. Curiously, the often cited study of Shearman and Garrett[75] could not be detailed fully because the report was preliminary, appeared before the code of the double-blind study was broken and had data for treatments A and B without revealing which was placebo and which was progestogen; a Type II statistical error could thus not be excluded. In reviewing the relative success of the progestogens, various studies had the difficulty that there was either no control group,[71,76,77] the outcome of the patients' own previous pregnancies were used for comparison[78] (introducing the methodological hazard of regression towards the mean), or the definition of recurrent miscarriage was tenuous, with a history of only one miscarriage being sufficient for entry into the study.[79]

Overall, an obvious improvement in outcome following the administration of progestogen in early pregnancy was not readily apparent. However, one major difficulty might well have been the surprisingly good outcome observed in the control groups in some

Table 42.4 Use of progestogens in recurrent miscarriage.

Reference	Progestogen	Dose	Route	Time given	Term deliveries	
					Control	Progestogen
Bishop et al (1950)[76]	Progesterone	6 × 25 mg	i.m.	<10 weeks	–	38/45 (84%)
Swyer and Daley (1953)[74]	Progesterone	6 × 25 mg	i.m.	< 10 weeks	40/53 (75%)	48/60 (80%)
Shearman and Garrett (1963)[75]	17-OHP-C	250 mg/wk	i.m.	7–24 weeks	–*	–*
Banks et al (1964)[77]	Dimethisterone	25 mg/day	Oral	2–38 weeks	–	44/52 (85%)
Goldzieher et al (1964)[72]	MPA	10 mg/day	Oral	≥8 weeks	13/18 (72%)	12/14 (86%)
Le Vine (1964)[73]	17-OHP-C	500 mg/wk	i.m.	16–36 weeks	7/15 (46%)	11/15 (73%)
Cope and Emelife (1965)[78]	17-OHP-C	250 mg/wk	i.m.	6–30 weeks	55/193 (28%)**	48/55 (87%)
Klopper and MacNaughton (1965)[80]	Enol Luteovis	100 mg/day	Oral	5–18 weeks	10/15 (67%)	10/18 (56%)
Check et al (1987)[79]	Progesterone	50 mg/day	Vaginal		14/24 (58%)	120/132 (91%)
Daya et al (1988)[71]	17-OHP-C	250 mg/week	i.m.	4–12 weeks	–	13/16 (81%)***

*Control and treatment groups not identified; **Trial subjects' own pregnancy history; ***Progress to 13 weeks only noted of the studies,[72,74,80] emphasizing the need for great care in the classification of a patient with genuine recurrent miscarriage. Sadly, despite many years of trials evaluating the use of progestogens in cases of recurrent miscarriage, there is still no definitive answer as to whether there is an identifiable subgroup of patients with a real and primary deficiency of progesterone in whom supplementation would make a critical difference.

OVARIAN STEROID REPLACEMENT THERAPY AND THE TRANSFER OF EMBRYOS

Indications and use

The freezing of embryos for *in vitro* fertilization patients is a valuable method of increasing the chance of pregnancy per oocyte collection by enabling the repeated transfer of thawed embryos. In women with regular menstrual cycles, thawed embryos can be transferred in a natural cycle with the replacement timed relative to the onset of the endogenous LH surge or after the use of exogenous steroid hormones, whilst those with disordered ovulatory cycles or anovulation can use exogenous steroids in a cyclical estrogen then added progestogen regimen to stimulate the endometrium.[81] The exogenous steroids are given in a fixed schedule and have the benefit of the embryo transfer being arranged well in advance, usually on the 17th or 18th day of the cyclical regimen.[82] This convenience occasionally makes the use of exogenous ovarian steroids the first choice for some women even though they have regular ovulatory cycles. There are many reports in the literature of pregnancy rates achieved with such cyclical regimens, with the results of embryo transfers performed during 1995 at PIVET Medical Centre being shown in Table 42.5. The ongoing pregnancy rate with the steroid regimens compares favourably with that for natural cycles and, interestingly, with the transfer of fresh embryos in the IVF program over the same period (44/239; 18%).

The administration of exogenous steroids to stimulate the endometrium in readiness for the transfer of embryos is the only option for recipients of donated oocytes and embryos who have no endogenous ovarian activity.[83–85] The first report of pregnancy following the transfer of donated embryos was into an ovulatory recipient and timed relative to her endogenous LH surge, but she miscarried at 10 weeks of pregnancy.[86] However, a viable pregnancy was then achieved in a woman with primary ovarian failure using such cyclical steroid support,[87] and there have been many more such cases.

Table 42.5 The pregnancy rates achieved by the transfer of frozen-thawed embryos at PIVET Medical Centre in 1995 (unpublished data).

Replacement cycle*	Embryo transfers	Positive pregnancy tests	Viable pregnancies
Natural	46	12 (26%)	9 (20%)
Hormone replacement	80	19 (24%)	14 (18%)
FSH stimulated	5	1 (20%)	1 (20%)
Total	131	31 (24%)	24 (18%)

*Natural cycles had embryo transfer timed relative to the endogenous LH surge; Cyclical steroid therapy comprised oral estradiol valerate and intravaginal/intramuscular progesterone; FSH stimulated cycles used human menopausal gonadotropin and the transfer was relative to an ovulatory dose of chorionic gonadotropin.

In vitro fertilization programs

The first successful cyclical steroid regimen[87] used increasing daily doses of oral estradiol valerate to stimulate the proliferative stage of endometrial development, from 1–6 mg per day, followed by intramuscular injections of progesterone (50 mg per day) and intravaginal progesterone pessaries (25–100 mg per day) to cause the secretory transformation of the endometrium. These medications are usually prescribed until the placental function is sufficiently established, at around 8–10 weeks of pregnancy.[88–90]

Efforts have been made to simplify the protocols by giving low dose oral estrogen[91] or estrogen given using transdermal patches.[92] Progesterone can be given wholly intravaginally. Oral progesterone is not recommended because of its substantial metabolic degradation during absorption, before it can reach and exert an effect on the target tissue.[93]

Inadvertent withdrawal of exogenous ovarian steroids

When there is ovarian failure, exogenous ovarian steroids are crucial in the maintenance of pregnancy until the placenta takes over with endogenous steroid production. Before then, the time for which the drugs can be withheld before the pregnancy is compromised is not known. There have been isolated case reports in the literature in which the medication has been stopped inadvertently but the pregnancy has continued. The most dramatic cases involve the stopping of steroid support because of a negative

Table 42.6 The events and outcome of two frozen embryo pregnancies in which the hormone replacement therapy (HRT) was inadvertently stopped.

	Case	
	1	2
Estrogen:		
Progynova	3 mg t.d.s., every day	2 mg t.d.s., every day
Premarin	25 mg on d11, d12, d13	–
Progestogen:		
Proluton	50 mg/day from d14	50 mg/day from d14
Embryos replaced on d18	3	3
Serum hCG on d32	190 IU/L	340 IU/L
Day treatment stopped	d32	d32
Day treatment resumed	d36	d35
Scan at 7 weeks	No sac	No sac
Outcome	Missed abortion	Missed abortion

Days (d) are relative to the commencement of cyclical steroid replacement therapy.

pregnancy test result. One such case was an ectopic pregnancy in which the medication was stopped,[94] but 20 days later the patient presented with abdominal pain, a serum hCG value of 3660 mIU/ml and a progesterone concentration of 0.4 ng/ml. Laparoscopic assessment confirmed no ovarian activity but a tubal pregnancy. Similarly, another patient stopped medication after a negative pregnancy test, had sustained amenorrhea and then presented eight weeks later with a viable intra-uterine 11-week pregnancy.[95] Despite these reports, one should be careful about drawing firm conclusions about the lack of need for continued steroid administration once the pregnancy has been initiated, as the submission of these reports for publication might have been encouraged by their positive message without a full representation of cases with a different outcome; the only two cases at PIVET Medical Centre in which the steroid therapy was stopped inadvertently for just a few days before being resumed both ended in miscarriage, as summarized in Table 42.6.

PREVENTION OF PREMATURE LABOR

The nonsteroidal estrogen, diethylstilbestrol, was once used in late pregnancy to help reduce problems such as prematurity, toxemia and fetal loss.[39] Its relative ineffectiveness and notorious side effects in early pregnancy have ensured that it is no longer used.

The effect of medroxyprogesterone acetate upon the course of normal pregnancies after 36 weeks has been studied,[97] and it appears that in these cases the progestogen does not result in a delay in delivery. However, 17α-hydroxyprogesterone caproate did seem to have a beneficial effect when given in cases with an incompetent cervix,[98] shown in Table 42.7, with the authors believing that the effect in delaying delivery was due to the relaxing action upon the uterus, easing pressure on the cervix.

A number of other studies have examined systematically the role of exogenous progestogens in preventing premature delivery of singleton pregnancies, and these are summarized in Table 42.7. An early report[99] on the use of progesterone in patients presenting with symptoms such as ruptured membranes and uterine pain showed no effect, suggesting hormonal support to be of limited value once the symptoms had commenced, although the high rate of term deliveries in the control group was surprising. This contrasts with the work of Erny et al[100] who gave oral progesterone when women were admitted with symptoms, and showed an increase in the rate of term deliveries. Once women were selected early in the pregnancy before uterine contractions began, using criteria such as low blood concentrations of progesterone[14] or a past history of pregnancy loss and prematurity,[101] improvements in pregnancy outcome were seen. The report by Yemini et al[102] also confirmed fewer premature deliveries after the administration of 17α-hydroxyprogesterone caproate, but there was a higher incidence of miscarriage in the treated group, resulting in a similar proportion of women having term deliveries in the treated and control groups.

Table 42.7 Use of progestogens in premature labour.

Reference	Progestogen	Max. dose	Route	Time started	Clinical end-point	Clinical improvement	
						Control	Progestogen
Fuchs and Stakeman (1960)[99]	Progesterone	200 mg/day	i.m.	20 wks	Term delivery	32/36 (89%)	31/32 (97%)
Sherman (1966)[98]	17-OHP-C	1000 mg twice/wk	i.m.	25 wks	Term delivery	104/414 (25%)	68/74 (92%)
Johnson et al (1975)[101]	17-OHP-C	250 mg/wk	i.m.	29 wks	Term delivery	9/22 (41%)	14/14 (100%)
Sondergaard et al (1985)[14]	Progesterone	200 mg/day	Vaginal	<11 wks	Term delivery	2/19 (11%)	6/23 (26%)
Yemini et al (1985)[102]	17-OHP-C	250 mg/wk	i.m.	8 wks	Term delivery	23/40 (58%)	26/39 (67%)
Erny et al (1986)[100]	Progesterone	400 mg/8 h	Oral	30 wks	Contractions	12/28 (43%)	22/29 (76%)

Table 42.8 Use of progestogens in other circumstances during pregnancy.

Reference	Progestogen	Max. dose	Route	Time given	Clinical indication	Term deliveries	
						Control	Progestogen
Dalton (1960)[108]	Progesterone	100 mg/day	i.m.	16–40 wks	Pre-eclampsia	63/66 (96%)	61/63 (97%)
Hill et al (1975)[104]	17-OHP-C	250 mg/wk	i.m.	Mean 13 wks	Abdominal surgery	29/35 (83%)	30/35 (86%)
Hartikainen-Sorri et al (1980)[107]	17-OHP-C	250 mg/wk	i.m.	28–37 wks	Twins	27/38 (71%)	27/39 (69%)
Hauth et al (1983)[105]	17-OHP-C	1000 mg/wk	i.m.	16–36 wks	Military service	85/88 (97%)	77/80 (96%)
Prietl et al (1992)[103]	17-OHP-C	500 mg twice/wk	i.m.	4–12 wks	IVF patients	38/65 (59%)	48/55 (87%)

Progestogens have been used in an attempt to prevent the onset of labor in several other clinical situations, and these are summarized in Table 42.8. The most beneficial effect seems to be in IVF patients,[103] although such a use is not widespread among IVF units. The prophylactic use of 17α-hydroxyprogesterone caproate to try and help prevent disruption of the pregnancy in situations such as abdominal surgery[104] and active military service [105] did not seem to be particularly useful; the favorable outcome of the control groups, however, made the evaluations of reduced statistical sensitivity. The management of twin pregnancies is often complicated by prematurity: the insertion of cervical sutures does not appear of significant value[106] and neither does the administration of 17α-hydroxyprogesterone caproate.[107]

Conclusion

The general administration to unselected patients of progestogens as an obstetric support in threatened pregnancies, whether in early or late pregnancy, is of no proven general value, with beneficial effects only seen in cases in which progesterone deficiency is a major contributory factor. The lack of physiological importance of estrogen during pregnancy means that its use as a support is not justified.

Exogenous steroids can be used successfully to support totally pregnancies in cases in which the ovaries are not functional. Such examples include IVF patients having frozen embryos transferred in subsequent cycles in which the uterus is stimulated by hormone replacement therapy, and women receiving donated oocytes or embryos.

REFERENCES

1. Zinaman MJ, Clegg ED, Brown CC, O'Connor J, Selevan SG 1996 Estimates of human fertility and pregnancy loss. Fertility and Sterility 65(3): 503–509
2. Hertig A, Livingstone R 1944 Spontaneous, threatened and habitual abortion: their pathogenesis and treatment. New England Journal of Medicine 230: 797–806
3. Macdonald R 1989 Does treatment with progesterone prevent miscarriage? British Journal of Obstetrics and Gynaecology 96: 257–260
4. Daya S 1989 Efficacy of progesterone support for pregnancy in women with recurrent miscarriage. A meta-analysis of controlled trials. British Journal of Obstetrics and Gynaecology 96: 275–280
5. Goldstein P, Berrier J, Rosen S, Sacks H, Chalmers T 1989 A meta-analysis of randomized control trials of progestational agents in pregnancy. British Journal of Obstetrics and Gynaecology 96: 265–274
6. Csapo A, Pulkkinen M, Wiest W 1973 Effects of luteectomy and progesterone replacement therapy in early pregnant patients. American Journal of Obstetrics and Gynaecology 115: 759–765
7. Csapo A, Pulkkinen M 1978 Indispensability of human corpus luteum in the maintenance of early pregnancy; luteectomy evidence. Obstetrical and Gynecological Survey 33: 69–81
8. Jacobson B 1965 Abortion: its prediction and management. Use of progestins in patients with arborization of cervical mucus smears. Fertility and Sterility 16: 604–612
9. MacRae D 1965 Vaginal cytology and the use of progestational agents. Journal of Obstetrics and Gynaecology of the British Commonwealth 72: 1038–1039
10. Skipper J 1964 Vaginal cytology in the management of threatened abortion. Medical Journal of Australia 2: 492–496
11. Osmond-Clarke F, Murray M 1963 Vaginal cytology and recurrent abortion. British Medical Journal ii: 1172–1174
12. Hochstaedt B, Lange W, Spira W 1960 Vaginal cytology as a guide to treatment of habitual abortion. Journal of Obstetrics and Gynaecology of the British Empire 67: 102–103
13. Morgan J, Hackett W, Hunt T 1960 The place of progesterone in the treatment of abortion. Journal of Obstetrics and Gynaecology of the British Empire 67: 323–324
14. Sondergaard F, Ottesen B, Detlefsen G, Schierup L, Pederson S, Lebech P 1985 Traitement par la progesterone des menaces d'accouchement premature avec taux bas de progesterone plasmatique. Contraception-Fertilite-Sexualite 13: 1227–1231
15. Turnbull A, Patten P, Flint A, Keirse M, Jeremy J, Anderson A 1974 Significant fall in progesterone and rise in oestradiol levels in human peripheral plasma before onset of labour. Lancet i: 101–104
16. Csapo A, Pohanka O, Kaihola H 1974 Progesterone deficiency and premature labour. British Medical Journal i: 137–140
17. Ferre F, Uzan M, Janssens Y 1985 Oral administration of micronized natural progesterone in late human pregnancy: effects on progesterone and estrogen concentrations in the plasma, placenta and myometrium. American Journal of Obstetrics and Gynecology 148: 26–34
18. Garfield R, Puri C, Csapo A 1982 Endocrine, structural, and functional changes in the uterus during premature labour. American Journal of Obstetrics and Gynecology 142: 21–27
19. Lye S, Porter D 1978 Demonstration that progesterone blocks uterine activity in the ewe in vivo by a direct action on the endometrium. Journal of Reproduction and Fertility 52: 87–94
20. Csapo A 1976 Effects of progesterone, prostaglandin F2α and its analogue ICI 81008 on the excitability and threshold of the uterus. American Journal of Obstetrics and Gynecology 124: 367–378
21. Whittaker P, Stewart M, Taylor A, Lind T 1989 Some endocrinological events associated with early pregnancy failure. British Journal of Obstetrics and Gynaecology 96: 1207–1214
22. Trounson A 1992 Development of the technique of oocyte donation and hormonal replacement therapy: is oestrogen really necessary for the establishment and maintenance of pregnancy? Reproduction, Fertility and Development 4: 671–679
23. Csapo A, Pulkkinen M, Kaihola H 1973 The effect of estradiol replacement therapy on early pregnant luteectomized patients. American Journal of Obstetrics and Gynecology 217: 987–990
24. Ghosh D, De P, Sengupta J 1994 Luteal phase ovarian oestrogen is not essential for implantation and maintenance of pregnancy from surrogate embryo transfer in the rhesus monkey. Human Reproduction 9: 629–637
25. Johansson EDB 1971 Depression of progesterone levels in women treated with synthetic gestagens after ovulation. Acta Endocrinologica 68: 779–792
26. Shinada T, Yokota Y, Igarashi M 1978 Inhibitory effect of various gestogens upon the pregnenolone 3b-ol-dehydrogenase-delta5-4-isomerase system in the human corpora lutea of menstrual cycles. Fertility and Sterility 29: 84–87
27. Yovich JL, Stanger JD, Yovich JM, Tuvik A 1984 Assessment and hormonal treatment of the luteal phase of in vitro fertilization cycles. Australian and New Zealand Journal of Obstetrics and Gynaecology 24: 125–130
28. Turner S, Mizock G, Feldman G 1966 Prolonged gynecologic and endocrine manifestations subsequent to administration of medroxyprogesterone acetate during pregnancy. American Journal of Obstetrics and Gynecology 95: 222–227
29. Nygren K, Johansson E 1975 The effect of norethisterone and some other synthetic gestagens upon the peripheral plasma levels of progesterone and estradiol during early human pregnancy. Acta Obstetrica Gynecologica Scandinavica 54: 57–63
30. Yovich JL, Willcox DL, Wilkinson SP, Polletti PM, Hahnel RA 1985 Medroxyprogesterone acetate does not perturb the profile of steroid metabolites in urine during pregnancy. Journal of Endocrinology 104: 453–459

31. Vessey M, Meisler L, Flavel R, Yeates D 1979 Outcome of pregnancy in women using different methods of contraception. British Journal of Obstetrics and Gynaecology 86: 548–556
32. Harlap S, Shiona P, Ramcharan S 1980 Spontaneous fetal losses in women using different contraceptives around the time of conception. International Journal of Epidemiology 9: 49–56
33. Harlap S, Shiono P, Ramcharan S 1985 Congenital abnormalities in the off-spring of women who used oral and other contraceptives around the time of conception. International Journal of Fertility 30: 39–47
34. Burstein R, Wasserman HC 1964 The effect of Provera on the fetus. Obstetrics and Gynecology 23: 931–934
35. Aarskog D 1979 Maternal progestins as a possible cause of hypospadias. New England Journal of Medicine 300: 75–78
36. Wilkins L 1960 Masculinization of female fetus due to use of orally given progestins. Journal of the American Medical Association 118: 1028–1032
37. Yovich JL, Turner SR, Draper R 1988 Medroxyprogesterone acetate therapy in early pregnancy has no apparent fetal effects. Teratology 38: 135–144
38. Katz Z, Lancet M, Skornik J, Chemke J, Mogilner B, Klimberg M 1985 Teratogenicity of progestogens given during the first trimester of pregnancy. Obsterics and Gynecology 65: 775–780
39. Check J, Rankin A, Teichman M 1986 The risk of fetal anomalies as a result of progesterone therapy during pregnancy. Fertility and Sterility 45: 575–577
40. Smith O, Smith G 1949 The influence of diethylstilbestrol on the progress and outcome of pregnancy as based on a comparison of treated with untreated primigravidas. American Journal of Obstetrics and Gynecology 58: 994–1009
41. Meara J, Vessey M, Fairweather D 1989 A randomized double-blind controlled trial of the value of diethylstilboestrol therapy in pregnancy: 35-year follow-up of mothers and their off-spring. British Journal of Obstetrics and Gynaecology 96: 620–622
42. Gill W, Schumacher G, Bibbo M 1977 Pathological semen and anatomical abnormalities of the genital tract in human male subjects exposed to diethylstilboestrol *in utero*. Journal of Urology 117: 477–480
43. Melnick S, Cole P, Anderson D, Herbst A 1987 Rates and risks of diethylstilboestrol-related clear cell adenocarcinoma of the vagina and cervix. New England Journal of Medicine 316: 514–516
44. Greenblatt R, Barfield W 1959 The progestational activity of 6-methyl-17-acetoxyprogesterone. Southern Medical Journal 52: 345–351
45. Wu D 1961 Maintenance of pregnancy in castrated rabbits by an orally active progestational agent 6-methyl 17-hydroxyprogesterone acetate. Fertility and Sterility 12: 236–244
46. Tognoni G, Ferrario L, Inzalaco M, Crosignani P 1980 Progestogens in threatened abortion. Lancet 2: 1242–1243
47. Anon 1980 Vaginal bleeding in early pregnancy. British Medical Journal 281: 470
48. Stabile I, Campbell S, Grudzinskas JG 1987 Ultrasonic assessment of complications during first trimester of pregnancy. Lancet ii: 1237–1240
49. Johannsen A 1970 The prognosis of threatened abortion. Acta Obstetrica Gynecologica Scandinavica 49: 89–93
50. Jouppila P, Huitaniemi I, Tapaneinen J 1980 Early pregnancy failure: a study by ultrasonic and hormonal methods. Obstetrics and Gynecology 55: 42–47
51. Geisler M, Kleinebrecht J 1978 Cytogenetic and histologic analyses of spontaneous abortions. Human Genetics 45: 239–251
52. Boue J, Boue A, Lazar P 1975 Retrospective and prospective epidemiological studies of 1500 karyotyped spontaneous human abortions. Teratology 12: 11–26
53. Lauritsen J 1976 Aetiology of spontaneous abortion. A cytogenetic and epidemiological study of 288 abortuses and their parents. Acta Obstetrica Gynecologica Scandinavica 52(Suppl): 1–28
54. South J, Naldrett J 1973 The effect of vaginal bleeding on the infant born after the 28th week of pregnancy. Journal of Obstetrics and Gynaecology of the British Commonwealth 80: 236–239
55. Funderburk S, Guthrie D, Meldrum D 1980 Outcome of pregnancies complicated by early vaginal bleeding. British Journal of Obstetrics and Gynecology 87: 100–105
56. Ornoy A, Benady S, Kohen-Raz R, Russell A 1976 Association between maternal bleeding during gestation and congenital anomalies in the offspring. American Journal of Obstetrics and Gynecology 124: 474–478
57. Peckham C 1970 Uterine bleeding during pregnancy 1. When not followed by immediate termination of pregnancy. Obstetrics and Gynecology 35: 937–941
58. Goldstein S, Subramanyan B, Raghavendra B, Horii S, Hilton S 1983 Subchorionic bleeding in threatened abortion. American Journal of Roentgenology 141: 975–978
59. Pedersen J, Mantoni M 1990 Large intra-uterine haematoma in threatened miscarriage. Frequency and clinical consequences. British Journal of Obstetrics and Gynaecology 97: 75–77
60. Jouppila P 1983 Clinical consequences after ultrasonic diagnosis of intra-uterine haematoma in threatened abortion. Journal of Clinical Ultrasound 13: 107–111
61. Everett C, Ashurst H, Chalmers I 1987 The management of threatened miscarriage by general practitioners in Wessex. British Medical Journal 295: 583–586
62. Randall C, Baetz R, Hall D, Birtch P 1955 Pregnancies observed in the likely-to-abort patient with or without hormone therapy before or after conception. American Journal of Obstetrics and Gynaecology 69: 643–656
63. Gerhard I, Gwinner B, Eggert-Kruse W, Runnenbaum B 1987 Double-blind controlled trial of progesterone substitution in threatened abortion. Biological Research in Pregnancy and Perinatology 8: 26–34
64. Moller K, Fuchs F 1965 Double-blind controlled trial of 6-methyl,17-hydroxyprogesterone in threatened abortion. Journal of Obstetrics and Gynaecology of the British Commonwealth 72: 1042–1044

65. Coulam C 1991 Epidemiology of recurrent spontaneous abortion. American Journal of Reproductive Immunology 26: 23–27
66. Cook CL, Pridham DD 1995 Recurrent pregnancy loss. Current Opinion in Obstetrics and Gynecology 7(5): 357–366
67. Stern JJ, Dorfmann AD, Gutierreznajar AJ, Cerrillo M, Coulam CB 1996 Frequency of abnormal karyotypes among abortuses from women with and without a history of recurrent spontaneous abortion. Fertility and Sterility 65(2): 250–253
68. Mowbray JF, Gibbings C, Liddell H, Reginald PW, Underwood JL, Beard RW 1985 Controlled trial of treatment of recurrent spontaneous abortion by immunisation with paternal cells. Lancet i: 941–943
69. Cowchock S 1991 What's a Mother to Do? Analysis of trials evaluating new treatments for unexplained recurrent miscarriages and other complaints. American Journal of Reproductive Immunology and Microbiology 126(4): 156–159
70. Horta J, Fernandez J, De Soto L 1977 Direct evidence of luteal insufficiency in women with habitual abortion. Obstetrics and Gynecology 49: 705–708
71. Daya S, Ward S, Burrows E 1988 Progesterone profile in luteal phase defect cycles and outcome of progesterone treatment in patients with recurrent spontaneous abortion. American Journal of Obstetrics and Gynecology 158: 225–232
72. Goldzieher J 1964 Double-blind trial of a progestin in habitual abortion. Journal of the American Medical Association 188: 651–654
73. Le Vine L 1964 Habitual abortion: a controlled study of progestational therapy. Western Journal of Surgery, Obstetrics and Gynecology 72: 30–36
74. Swyer G, Daley D 1953 Progesterone implantation in habitual abortion. British Medical Journal 1: 1073–1086
75. Shearman RP, Garrett WJ 1963 Double-blind study of the effect of 17-hydroxyprogesterone caproate on abortion rate. British Medical Journal 1: 292–295
76. Bishop P, Richards N, Doll R 1950 Habitual abortion. Prophylactic value of progesterone pellet implant. British Medical Journal ii: 130–133
77. Banks A, Rutherford R, Coburn W 1964 The value and safety of progestin-like substances for the habitual aborter and the fertility patient. Fertility and Sterility 15: 94–96
78. Cope E, Emelife E 1965 Habitual abortion treated with 17-hydroxyprogesterone caproate. Journal of Obstetrics and Gynaecology of the British Commonwealth 72: 1035–1037
79. Check J, Chase J, Nowroozi K, Wu C, Adelson H 1987 Progesterone therapy to decrease first-trimester spontaneous abortions in previous aborters. International Journal of Fertility 32: 192–199
80. Klopper A, MacNaughton M 1965 Hormones in recurrent abortion. Journal of Obstetrics and Gynaecology of the British Commonwealth 72: 1022–1028
81. Schmidt CL, de Ziegler D, Gagliardi CL et al 1989 Transfer of cryopreserved-thawed embryos: the natural cycle versus controlled preparation of the endometrium with gonadotropin-releasing hormone agonist and exogenous estradiol and progesterone (GEEP). Fertility and Sterility 52: 609–616
82. Jaroudi K, Hamilton C, Willemson W, Sieck U, Roca G 1991 Artificial endometrial stimulation for frozen embryo replacement. Fertility and Sterility 55: 835–837
83. Formigli L, Roccio C, Belotti G, Stangalini A, Coglitore MGF 1989 Oocyte donation by gamete intra-fallopian transfer to amenorrheic and cycling patients given replacement steroids. Human Reproduction 4(7): 772–776
84. Meldrum DR, Wisot A, Hamilton F, Gutlay-Yeo AL, Marr B, Huynh D 1989 Artifical agonadism and hormone replacement for oocyte donation. Fertility and Sterility 52(3): 509–511
85. Abdalla H, Baber R, Kirkland A, Leonard T, Power M, Studd J 1990 A report on 100 cycles of oocyte donation; factors affecting the outcome. Human Reproduction 5: 1018–1022
86. Trounson A, Leeton J, Besanko M, Wood C, Conti A 1983 Pregnancy established in an infertile patient after transfer of a donated embryo fertilized in vitro. British Medical Journal 286: 835–839
87. Lütjen P, Trounson A, Leeton J, Findlay J, Wood C, Renou P 1984 The establishment and maintenance of pregnancy using in vitro fertilization and embryo donation in a patient with primary ovarian failure. Nature 307: 174–175
88. Leeton J, Cameron I, Burden J, Azuma K, Renou P 1992 Maintenance of pregnancy and obstetric outcome in donor egg pregnancies. Reproduction and Fertility Developments 4: 713–718
89. Devroey P, Camus M, Palermo G et al 1990 Placental production of estradiol and progesterone after oocyte donation in patients with primary ovarian failure. American Journal of Obstetrics and Gynecology 162: 66–70
90. Schneider MA, Davies MC, Honour JW 1993 The timing of placental competence in pregnancy after oocyte donation. Fertility and Sterility 59(5): 1059–1064
91. Leeton J, Rogers P, Cameron I, Caro C, Healy D 1989 Pregnancy results following embryo transfer in women receiving low dosage of variable estrogen therapy for premature ovarian failure. Journal of In Vitro Fertility and Embryo Transfer 6: 232–235
92. Droesch K, Navot D, Scott R, Kreiner D, Liu H, Rosenwaks Z 1988 Transdermal estrogen replacement in ovarian failure for ovum donation. Fertility and Sterility 50: 931–934
93. Devroey P, Palermo G, Bourgain C, Van Waesberghe L, Smitz J, Van Steirteghem A 1989 Progesterone administration in patients with absent ovaries. International Journal of Fertility 34: 188–193
94. Ben-Nun I, Ghetler Y, Kareti H, Wolfson L, Fejgin M, Beyth Y 1990 Tubal pregnancy without ovarian hormonal support. Fertility and Sterility 54: 351–352
95. Kapetanakis E, Pantos K 1990 Continuation of a donor oocyte pregnancy in menopause without early pregnancy support. Fertility and Sterility 54: 1171–1173
96. Ferguson J 1953 Effect of stilboestrol on pregnancy compared to the effect of a placebo. American Journal of Obstetrics and Gynecology 65: 592–601

97. Brenner W, Hendricks C 1962 Effect of medroxyprogesterone acetate upon the duration and characteristics of human gestation and labour. American Journal of Obstetrics and Gynecology 83: 1094–1098
98. Sherman A 1966 Hormonal therapy for control of the incompetent os of pregnancy. Obstetrics and Gynecology 28: 198–205
99. Fuchs F, Stakemann G 1960 Treatment of threatened premature labor with large doses of progesterone. American Journal of Obstetrics and Gynecology 79: 172–176
100. Erny R, Pigne A, Prouvost C et al 1986 The effects of oral administration of progesterone for premature labour. American Journal of Obstetrics and Gynecology 154: 525–529
101. Johnson J, Austin K, Jones G, Davis G, King T 1975 Efficacy of 17α-hydroxyprogesterone caproate in the prevention of premature labor. New England Journal of Medicine 293: 675–680
102. Yemini M, Borenstein R, Dreazen E et al 1985 Prevention of premature labor by 17α-hydroxyprogesterone caproate. American Journal of Obstetrics and Gynecology 151: 574–577
103. Prietl G, Diedrich K, Vanderven HH, Luckhaus J, Krebs D 1992 The effect of 17α-hydroxyprogesterone caproate/oestradiol valerate on the development and outcome of early pregnancies following in vitro fertilization and embryo transfer — a prospective and randomized controlled trial. Human Reproduction 7(Suppl 1): 1–5
104. Hill L, Johnson C, Lee R 1975 Prophylactic use of hydroxyprogesterone caproate in abdominal surgery during pregnancy. Obstetrics and Gynecology 46: 287–290
105. Hauth J, Gilstrap III L, Brekken A, Hauth J 1983 The effect of 17α-hydroxyprogesterone caproate on pregnancy outcome in an active-duty military population. American Journal of Obstetrics and Gynecology 146: 187–190
106. Dor J, Shalev J, Maschiach G, Blankstein J, Serr D 1982 Elective cervical suture of twin pregnancies diagnosed ultrasonically in the first trimester following induced ovulation. Gynaecological and Obstetrical Investigation 13: 55–60
107. Hartikainen-Sorri A, Kauppila A, Tuimala R 1980 Inefficacy of 17α-hydroxyprogesterone caproate in the prevention of prematurity in twin pregnancy. Obstetrics and Gynecology 56: 692–695

43. Fetal effects of estrogens, progestogens and diethylstilbestrol

Joe Leigh Simpson   Raymond H. Kaufman

Introduction

Progestogens and estrogens share with all drugs the ability to affect the fetus when given to its pregnant mother. Claims for teratogenic effects of progestogens in particular have been levied for over four decades. Even when scientific evidence is thin, a litigious environment exists. Thus, it is appropriate in this volume to consider both proven and alleged fetal effects of progestogen exposure. Excepting the well known circumstance of exposure to the synthetic compound diethylstilbestrol (DES), estrogen does not seem to be under serious consideration as a teratogen. We shall first restrict comments to progestogens, and then discuss stilbestrol. This contribution updates our earlier reviews.[1,2]

Limitations in determining teratogenesis

In evaluating claims of hormone teratogenicity, it would be preferable to stratify exposures by progestogens alone, estrogens alone and progestogens and estrogens in combination (e.g. oral contraceptives). Unfortunately, available data do not permit such an analysis — and such data probably never will be available, because progestogen exposure during pregnancy is now uncommon. For example, in 1978 Doering and Stewart[3] found that 65% of their study population were exposed to hormones. A decade later a trend toward decreased drug ingestion during pregnancy was identified in a United States population by Simpson et al.[4] A cohort of 729 women comprising insulin-dependent diabetics and non-diabetic controls were followed. Mean exposures to drugs of any sort (excluding insulin, iron and vitamins) for diabetic women during gestational weeks 1–10 was 0.72 (± 1.05 SD), and for control subjects 0.54 (± 1.05). Only two among the 729 were exposed to progestogens. This secular decrease in exposure among American women is consistent with trends identified by Wiseman in the United Kingdom.[5] That the frequency of birth defects has failed to decline despite decreasing exposure furnishes, incidentally, evidence that progestogens are not teratogenic.

Studies such as these necessarily pool outcomes following exposure to various sex hormones. Often progestogen exposure is combined with estrogen. However, it is implausible that progestogens could be teratogenic only in association with estrogens; thus, this approach is not unreasonable because the only estrogen implicated seriously as a teratogen is diethylstilbestrol, an agent not found in oral contraceptives. Pooling exposures to progestogens alone and exposures to oral contraceptives should yield useful information in evaluating risks of progestogens to the fetus.

The historical indications for receiving progestogens have been pregnancy diagnosis (intentional), pregnancy maintenance (intentional) and birth control (unintentional). Pooling exposures following these different indications poses the problem of dealing with differing doses. Selection biases could exist as well. However, in the absence of data from a single source — unlikely given infrequency of exposure — pooling of data is unavoidable.

In order to assess teratogenicity, various study designs have been utilized, each with its distinct pitfalls. *Cohort* (prospective) studies are expensive and laborious, and suffer from relatively few subjects being affected and thus being informative. Frequently there is lack of systematic surveillance for anomalies — a concern in cohort studies, given the incidence of anomalies being compared to the expected frequency of 2–3% in the general population. Too rigorous surveillance in a cohort will result in spurious positive findings; too lax surveillance will result in the converse. Ideally, both exposed and unexposed samples are derived from the population and assessed comparably.

Case-control (retrospective) studies suffer from different pitfalls. In these studies, subjects with a specified abnormal outcome (e.g. mother having an infant with a cardiac anomaly) are matched with control subjects who ideally differ only with respect to the variable being tested (e.g. drug exposure). Often years pass between the exposure and the study interview, producing memory bias. Women whose pregnancies result in an abnormal outcome may search harder for factors potentially responsible (recall bias). Case-control studies thus frequently yield spurious associations (i.e. false positives).

EFFECTS ON THE FETUS

Genital ambiguity and progestogens

Certain progestogens, especially 19-nortestosterone derivatives, unequivocally can masculinize the female fetus if given in high doses at susceptible times of embryogenesis. Labioscrotal fusion can occur if exposure occurs before the 12th week of gestation; clitoral or labial enlargement without labioscrotal fusion can occur if exposure occurs after the 12th week.

The incidence of fetal masculinization varies according to the drug and dosage. In 1984 Carson and Simpson[6] reviewed information on specific progestogens; principles and conclusions have remained largely unchanged. In general, C-21 progestogen derivatives (e.g. medroxyprogesterone) do not virilize even in high dose; 19-nortestosterone derivatives (e.g. norethindrone) generally virilize, but there are exceptions (e.g. norethynodrel). Jacobson[7] reported an 18% incidence of masculinization in female infants whose mothers were given norethindrone acetate for pregnancy maintenance, whereas virilization occurred in only 1% exposed to medroxyprogesterone acetate.[8] Doses of 19-nortestosterones required for virilization are 10–20 mg/day, far in excess of that associated with inadvertent contraceptive exposure during pregnancy. When progestogen therapy at such dosage is currently administered, the compound administered will almost certainly be progesterone, 17α-hydroxyprogesterone caproate or medroxyprogesterone. Genital ambiguity due to progestogen exposure of female fetuses is thus mostly a topic of historical concern.

The only currently utilized sex steroid that causes virilization when administered in usually administered doses is danazol, a derivative of 17α-ethinyl testosterone.[9,10] In Brunskill's study of adverse drug reports of pregnant women receiving danazol, 23 of 57 female infants were virilized; male offspring were ostensibly normal.[10] Genital virilization has resulted from doses as low as 200 mg daily, whereas 800 mg daily is the usual dose when danazol is used to treat endometriosis.

An agent that should be considered teratogenic is cyproterone acetate, an antiandrogen that blocks androgen receptors. This agent is available in Europe, Australia and elsewhere for treatment of hirsutism, but the Food and Drug Administration has not approved its usage in the United States. When cyproterone is given during the susceptible period of embryogenesis, genital virilization is impeded in male fetuses in rodents tested. If the dose is sufficiently high, a similar effect would be expected in humans.

Somatic anomalies and progestogens

A simplistic but often voiced question is whether exposure to hormones produces a general (nonspecific) increase in anomalies. Such a claim is implausible. Every known human teratogen produces a specific anomaly or spectrum of characteristic anomalies. It is not likely that a generalized increase in malformations would occur in the absence of an increase in any specific defect. Investigations claiming solely an overall increase in anomalies associated with any given agent should thus be considered more as hypothesis-generating studies, the denouement awaiting studies of specific anomalies.

These reservations notwithstanding, several case-control studies in the 1970s claimed generalized increased anomaly rates associated with oral contraceptive exposure. An example is the study of Greenberg et al;[11] however, the validity of this study can be questioned because only a small and possibly unrepresentative proportion of eligible women participated. More rigorous was the study of Pardthaisong et al,[12] who found a statistically significant increase in the rate of all major malformations among depo-medroxyprogesterone users, compared with the rate among oral contraception users; however, the latter rate was unexpectedly low, suggesting selection bias to the authors. In relation to oral contraceptive exposure, no significant associations between exposure and pill use were found in the case-control studies of Bracken et al[13] and Oakley et al.[14] The frequency of anomalies was also not increased in 541 pill failure pregnancies gathered by Harlap and Eldor.[15] Tables 43.1 and 43.2 provide the details of two well constructed and relatively recent case-control studies.

Far more powerful are cohort studies, of which 18 are summarized in Table 43.3. Only one reported an association between progestogens and an overall increased anomaly rate, namely one of the two studies

Table 43.1 No significant differences between any exposure groups and malformations, the authors attributing to chance odds ratios greater than 2.[13]

Malformation	Odds ratio		
	Use 12–3 months before conception	Use 2 months–1 week before conception	Use at conception during pregnancy
All malformations $n = 1370$	0.9	0.9	1.3
Anencephaly $n = 81$	1.4	0.8	3.0
Common truncus Tetralogy of Fallot $n = 53$	0.9	1.6	2.3
Ventricular/atrial septal defects $n = 200$	0.9	1.1	2.2
Tracheoesophageal fistula $n = 48$	1.1	0.7	2.4
Polysyndactyly $n = 47$	0.4	0.8	0.0
Down syndrome $n = 52$	1.1	0.9	2.2
Inguinal hernia $n = 154$	0.9	1.2	1.1
Cleft lip and palate $n = 38$	1.5	0.7	1.6
Pyloric stenosis $n = 70$	1.5	1.9	0.0
Musculoskeletal anomalies $n = 68$	0.8	0.7	0.0

Table 43.2 The case control study of Lammer and Cordero. First-trimester sex hormone study among 1091 malformed infants was associated with a statistically significant association only for esophageal atresia. Controls consisted of infants with other malformations.[48]

Malformation	n	Number exposed (%)	Odds ratio
All cases	1091	136 (12.5)	
Anencephaly	108	9 (12.2)	0.64
Spina bifida	181	22 (12.2)	1.02
Encephalocele	24	4 (16.7)	1.49
Down syndrome	176	22 (12.5)	1.06
Esophageal atresia	36	10 (25.6)	2.84
Limb reduction	98	14 (14.3)	1.26
Cleft lip	200	23 (11.5)	0.95
Small bowel atresia	51	4 (7.8)	0.62
Rectal-anal atresia	70	8 (11.4)	0.95
Diaphragmatic hernia	49	8 (18.3)	1.47

Table 43.3 Summary of 18 cohort studies evaluating effects of progestogen exposure during pregnancy. The clear consensus is that progestogens in the doses administered are not teratogenic. Updated from Simpson.[1]

Investigators	Description of sample (location)	Control	Anomalies in exposed and control subjects	Interpretation
Spira et al (1972)[29]	9566 women, interviewed in the 3rd month, who received hormones (mostly for pregnancy support or diagnosis) (France)		171/9566 (1.8%)	Anomalies equally frequent in exposed and unexposed pregnancies
		8387 not receiving hormones	168/8387 (2.0%)	
Harlap et al (1975)[16]	11 468 women, 432 receiving 'hormones' (Israel)		47/432 (10.9%) all anomalies, 21/432 (4.9%) major anomalies only	Small increase (25%) ($P < 0.02$) observed, but recall bias possible because interviews were months after exposure
		11 036 unexposed	925/11 036 (8.4%); 426/11 036 (3.9%), major only	
Kullander and Källen 1976[33]	6379 pregnancies from which 194 mothers had abnormal infants (Sweden)		5/194 exposed to progestogen (2.6%)	Exposure rates similar in both groups
		5002 women delivered normal infants	98/5002 exposed to progestogen (2.0%)	
Royal College of General Practitioners 1976[34]	136 pregnancies conceived during oral contraceptive therapy (United Kingdom)		2/136 (1.5%)	No differences among groups
		11 009 pregnancies in nonusers;	177/11 009 (1.6%)	
		5530 pregnancies in previous contraceptive users	86/5530 (1.6%)	
Goujard and Rumeau-Rouquette 1977[30]	12 895 mothers interviewed in the first trimester, of whom 1165 were exposed (France) (same population as Spira et al[27])		5/335 (1.5%) 'testosterone derivatives' 15/830 (1.8%) 'progesterone derivatives'	Chromosomal abnormalities excluded from analysis; no differences observed either overall or after separate analysis for cardiac and skeletal defects
		9822 nonexposed	160/9822 (1.6%)	
Heinonen et al 1977[23] (Reanalysis by Wiseman and Dodds-Smith)	Collaborative Perinatal Project (50 282 women) 1958–66, of whom 1042 were exposed to 'sex hormones' and 866 to progestogens only (United States)		19/1042 (1.8%) cardiac after any sex hormone exposure; 75/866 (8.7%) all anomalies after progestogen exposure alone	No significant differences for total anomalies but significantly increased for cardiac anomalies alone (relative risk 2.3, $P < 0.05$). However, some infants exposed only during 1st

Table 43.3 *Cont'd*

Investigators	Description of sample (location)	Control	Anomalies in exposed and control subjects	Interpretation
		49 240 not exposed to any sex hormones; 49 416 not to progestogens	385/49 240 (0.8%) cardiac; 3172/ 49 416 (6.5%) all anomalies	lunar month; others exposed during 4th lunar month. Table 44.2B shows that relative risk no longer increased when these and other factors taken into account. Hook[26] does not agree with reanalysis[26]
Nora et al 1978[21]	118 women who received hormones in 'first trimester' (United States)		16/118 (13.6%)	Not truly prospective for controls, with bias toward unrecognized exposure in controls. Exposure interval not well defined
		At time of delivery of exposed women, 'control infant without ... exposure ... selected'	4/118 (3.4%)	
Torfs et al 1981[37]	Over 18 000 women, 203 had 'hormonal pregnancy tests' (United States)		9/203 (4.4%)	No significant differences among groups
		689 with serum pregnancy tests; 332 with urine pregnancy tests; 17 057 with no pregnancy test	30/689 (4.4%) 9/332 (2.7%) 650/17 047 (3.8%)	
Goujard et al 1979[87]	3451 women, of whom 133 used progestogens (France)		5/133 (3.8%)	4 of 5 anomalies occurred in subset of 35 women who used testosterone derivatives
		3318 nonexposed	3318 (2.3%) overall	
Vessey 1979[36]	66 pregnancies conceived while on oral contraceptives (United Kingdom)	None	1/66 (1.5%)	
Savolainen et al 1981[31]	3002 mothers of malformed infants, of whom 38 conceived while receiving 'pills' (Finland)			Anomaly rates similar in sample and control, both for previous and concurrent contraceptive use
		3002 matched controls		
Varma and Morsman 1982[35]	150 pregnancies treated with hydroxyprogesterone lexonoate from 6–18 weeks gestation for repetitive abortions (United Kingdom)		1/150 (0.7%)	No significant difference between exposed and unexposed subjects

Table 43.3 *Cont'd*

Investigators	Description of sample (location)	Control	Anomalies in exposed and control subjects	Interpretation
Michaelis et al 1983[32]	13 643 pregnancies, about 10% of whom received hormones for diagnosis or support (West Germany)		4/320 (1.3%) progesterone alone; 11/160 (1.8%) progesterone and estradiol	No significant difference between exposed cases and their unexposed matched controls
		Matched controls within same population who were not exposed		
Katz et al 1985[39]	1608 pregnancies treated with progestogens for first trimester bleeding (Israel)		85/1608 (5.3%)	Anomalies equally frequent in exposed and unexposed pregnancies
		1146 pregnancies who had bleeding but were not treated with hormones	64/1146 (5.6%)	
Resseguie et al 1985[40]	988 exposed to progestogens, mostly progesterone and 17α-hydroxyprogesterone caproate (United States)		54/988 (5.5%)	No differences among groups
		1976 unexposed	88/1976 (4.5%)	
Harlap and Eldor 1980[15]	8522 women who had used oral contraceptives prior to conception (United States)		17.2/1000 (1.7%)	Relative risk 19.6 for coarctation of aorta. Relative risk 3.9 for valvular defects seen with *in utero* exposure.
		25 023 women who used other forms or no birth control	other: 15/1000 (1.5%) none: 20/1000 (2%)	No overall increase in anomalies. After corrections for multiple comparisons, no statistically significant associations for mutagenic effect
Check et al 1986[41]	475 women given 17α-hydroxyprogesterone or progesterone vaginal suppositories for recurrent abortions (United States)		5/382 (1.3%)	No control group but low absolute rate of anomalies
		None		
Yovich et al 1988[42]	508 infertility patients treated with medroxyprogesterone for recurrent pregnancy loss or threatened abortion in first trimester (Australia)		15/366 liveborn (4.1%)	High percentage of fetal wastage in both groups, but no significant difference in congenital malformation rate
		508 patients with recurrent pregnancy loss who were not treated		

conducted by Harlap et al,[16] which we discuss below. The other 17 prospective studies failed to show a general increase in anomalies. Wiseman[5] studied trends of sex hormone use in the United Kingdom over a 14 year period (1966–80). Sex hormone usage increased after its 1966 introduction, only to later decline sharply over the years 1976–80. Yet during the entire 1966–80 interval the major malformation rate remained stable.

Of further relevance to the hypothesis of a general effect on nonspecific birth defects are data on perinatal mortality gathered by Gray and Pardthaisong.[17] Neither perinatal mortality nor infant mortality were increased when 565 children of women who used oral contraceptives were compared to offspring of 2307 control women who were not exposed; an increase in mortality and low birth weight was observed in offspring of 1431 women who received injectable medroxyprogesterone, risks being highest for accidental pregnancies occurring within four weeks of a 150 mg injection. However, pregnancies associated with this method of contraception are rare; thus the attributable risk is low.

In conclusion, the evidence is considerable that orally ingested progestogens do not cause a general increase in birth defects.

Specific somatic anomalies and progestogens

Cardiac

Cardiac disorders occur in 0.1–0.5% liveborns, the range largely reflecting the number of years children are followed and the vigilance of detection at birth. Ninety percent of cardiac defects result from polygenic/multifactorial causes, conditions carrying a recurrence risk for a first degree relative of 1–4%; for second and third degree relatives, risks are 1% or less. Known teratogens are responsible for only 1% of cardiac defects; an additional 4% have a demonstrable chromosomal abnormality. The final 4% represent Mendelian mutations.[18]

Levy et al[19] were the first to claim that progestogens cause cardiac anomalies. In a 1973 case-control study, 7 of 76 mothers delivered of infants with transposition of the great vessel had received what they identified as 'hormones' during the first trimester; none of the 76 controls was exposed ($P < 0.007$). Similar findings were reported by Nora and Nora.[20] In the initial retrospective case-control study 20 of 224 (8.9%), mothers delivered of infants with cardiac abnormalities recollected receiving an estrogen and/or progesterone compound; only 4 of 262 controls ($P < 0.001$) had such recollection. In a follow-up prospective study, Nora et al[21] first reported no significant differences in hormone use between the 60 mothers of affected infants and their controls. A second prospective study was then undertaken, now with two controls per subject. This time, 31 of 176 mothers with affected offspring were said to have received hormones, compared with 21 of 352 control mothers ($P < 0.001$). Janerich et al[22] identified 104 infants with cardiac defects ascertained through birth certificates in New York State. Of the 104, 18 of their mothers had received hormones, 16 for pregnancy diagnosis and two inadvertently for contraception despite already being pregnant. Significantly fewer controls reported exposure.

The above studies are counterbalanced by several negative case-control studies. Among 1370 offspring with congenital malformations, Bracken et al[13] initially found that exposure to oral contraceptives 'around the time of conception' was associated with a two-fold relative risk for certain cardiac defects (tetralogy of Fallot, ventricular septal defect; and atrial septal defect); however, after corrections for multiple comparisons, no significant increase persisted for any cardiac malformations (Table 43.1). No association was observed when exposure was stratified by specific estrogen or progestogen.

The hypothesis of progestogen teratogenicity might not have been entertained beyond the 1970s were it not for the analysis of the US Collaborative Perinatal Project by Heinonen et al.[23,24] Of 1042 offspring said to be exposed to 'sex hormones', 19 had a cardiac defect (1.82%); 385 of 49 240 (0.78%) unexposed offspring were affected (relative risk 2.3, $P < 0.05$) (Table 43.4A). Analysis by specific hormones was not possible because of the relatively small number of cases, but inadvertent oral contraceptive use was inexplicably stated to carry greatest relative risk 2.4), despite having the lowest dose; exposure to progesterone only carried a lower but still significantly increased relative risk (1.8, $P < 0.05$); exposure to only estrogens carried a relative risk of 1.44.

Wiseman and Dodds-Smith[25] reported several shortcomings when reanalyzing the original data from the US Collaborative Perinatal Project (Table 43.4B). First, the *a priori* risk of anomalies proved dissimilar between subjects and controls, the frequency of affected relatives being higher in the former. In four of the 17 hormone-exposed cases, a previous pregnancy was characterized by a major malformation (ventricular septal defect, Down syndrome with a cardiac defect, neonatal death with serious malformations, a stillborn); only one subject in a control group of 100 (selected from among the 1023 who had a noncardiac

Table 43.4A US Collaborative Perinatal Project data on cardiovascular malformations and male sex hormone exposure.[23,24]

	Number of infants with cardiovascular malformations	Rate/1000	Relative risk
Not exposed *n* = 49 240	365	7.8	1.0
Exposed *n* = 142	19	18.2	2.3

Table 44.4B The Wiseman and Dodds-Smith reanalysis of the 19 exposed cases cited in Table 44.4A. Only 8 cases were actually exposed during the critical period.

Coding error Hormone exposure never occurred	2
Timing error Exposure 'too early' (before day 19) for biologic plausibility	2
Exposure 'too late' (after day 50) for biologic plausibility	5
**Misclassification* Down syndrome present (not isolated cardiac defect)	2
Exposure within critical interval and having correct diagnosis	8

*In two additional cases, the final diagnosis was a transient cardiac murmur and not a structural defect.

malformation and were exposed to progestogens) gave a history for a prior major anomaly. Thus, subject and control groups were not comparable. Second, two of the index (exposed) cases actually had no exposure (a coding error). Third, in the exposed group two infants with cardiac anomalies had Down syndrome, the cardiac anomaly thus almost certainly not being related to drug exposure. Fourth, timing of exposure was often incompatible with a teratogenic effect. Among the 19 progestogen-exposed infants with cardiac defects, two were exposed during the first lunar month (gestational weeks 1–4), a time when anomalies are not ordinarily induced (it is an all-or-none period); five other infants were exposed only in the fourth month, considerably later than completion of cardiac development (42 embryonic days or 56 gestational days). Wiseman and Dodds-Smith[25] ultimately concluded that no significant association existed between hormone use and cardiac defects in the US Collaborative Perinatal Project data. Hook[26] criticized the reanalysis of Wiseman and Dodds-Smith,[25] in particular taking exception to reclassifying and excluding the two cases with Down syndrome. Without this reclassification, Hook[26] calculated that the relative risk would 'no longer be of nominal statistical significance'. However, Wiseman[27] was not persuaded by the critique of Hook.[26]

The senior author has (J.L.S.) long believed that progestogens do not produce cardiac defects, a claim supported by no cohort studies other than the US Collaborative Perinatal Study showing an association with cardiac anomalies (Table 43.3). The only cohort study showing an association of any type was the 1975 study of Harlap et al,[16] who found a positive association between progestogens and the overall abnormal outcome mentioned in the previous section (Table 43.3). In that study, however, exposure considered causative for a teratogenic effect included that during the first lunar month, the same erroneous assumption made in the US Collaborative study. In a later study, Harlap et al[28] failed to find an association, although prior to corrections for multiple comparisons an association with coarctation of the aorta and heart valve defects was observed. Representative of the far more frequent negative studies is the French cohort of Spira et al.[29] Over 20 000 women were followed throughout gestation; half (n = 9566) received hormones, usually for pregnancy diagnosis or pregnancy maintenance. The anomaly rate was no different in exposed and unexposed subjects. When the same population was re-examined by Goujard and Rumeau-Rouquette[30] no significant differences in the rates of cardiac anomalies were observed between exposed

(43%) versus unexposed mothers (41%). Cohort studies in Finland,[31] Germany,[32] Sweden,[33] Great Britain[34–36] and USA[37] similarly revealed no increased incidence of cardiac defects (Table 43.2). Finally, Nishimura et al[38] failed to detect cardiac anomalies in 108 microdissected embryos exposed to hormones, despite several controls having cardiac defects.

Several other studies are of interest because exposed subjects received hormones for specific indications. Katz et al[39] prospectively followed women treated with hormones because of bleeding during the first trimester. One group (n = 1608) was treated with the progestogens (medroxyprogesterone acetate or 17α-hydroxyprogesterone caproate) beginning in the first trimester. Comparing outcomes with those of 1146 unexposed mothers, no significant differences were observed with respect to any malformation. Based on 988 Minnesota offspring exposed *in utero*, Resseguie et al[40] reported that 17α-hydroxyprogesterone caproate and progesterone exposures were not associated with increased risk for cardiovascular anomalies or other anomalies. Check et al[41] reported offspring of 382 women treated with either 17α-hydroxyprogesterone or progesterone vaginal suppositories for recurrent abortions. Of five anomalies observed, the two cardiac defects (ventricular septal defect; transposition of great vessels) occurred in patients exposed to progesterone suppositories. Yovich et al[42] reported the outcome of 449 Australian women and their 508 pregnancies: recurrent abortion was the indication for medroxyprogesterone treatment in 199, therapy beginning at five weeks gestation and continuing until 16 weeks; threatened abortion was the indication in 309. Pregnancy outcome was compared with that of a matched group of women conceiving after infertility treatments. Only one cardiac defect was noted in the exposed group, an individual with Noonan syndrome.

In a more recent study of 8816 births in Thailand, Pardthaisong et al[12] compared the incidence of cardiovascular anomalies among several groups: users of oral contraceptives either prior to conception or during gestation (n = 3038), users of injectable medroxyprogesterone (n = 1229) and women using no contraception (n = 4023). No significant differences were found among the three groups. Interestingly, the incidence of anomalies among oral contraceptive users was lower than the incidence in the general population.

We have already alluded to the secular trend data of Wiseman,[5] who compared patterns of progestogen usage to rates of cardiac anomalies in the United Kingdom for the years 1966–80. Recall that over the 14 year period surveyed progestogen use first increased sharply and then declined rapidly; however, no change occurred in the incidence of cardiac anomalies. Consistent also with the observations of Wiseman[5] was the finding of only two progestogen exposures among 729 women followed by Simpson et al.[4] The practical consequences are that little additional population-based data can be expected in the future.

Overall, the clear consensus is that progestogens are *not* cardiac teratogens. The United States Food and Drug Administration now accepts this conclusion as well.

Limb reduction defects

In limb reduction defects there exists shortening or absence of a limb, finger or toe. Like cardiac defects, limb reduction defects can result from polygenic/multifactorial factors. This deduction can be made on the basis of increased recurrence risks in siblings for terminal transverse upper limb deficiency.[43] Structural abnormalities of the uterus leading to deformations and vascular occlusive phenomena[44,45] have also been implicated. With the exception of thalidomide there is no evidence that drugs play a role. However, the enormous publicity surrounding thalidomide guarantees that teratogenic influences are ineluctably suspected whenever limb reduction defects occur.

To this end, an association between progestogens and limb reduction defects has inevitably been claimed. The first such claim was by Janerich et al.[46] Fifteen of 108 women with an affected infant received hormones (inadvertent oral contraceptive exposure, hormone pregnancy test, hormones for pregnancy maintenance). Only four of 108 controls were exposed ($P < 0.05$). The significance failed to persist when oral contraceptives were considered separately. Greenberg et al[11] also found an overall increase in anomalies following progestogen exposure, limb reduction defects contributing to this increase. A case-control study in Australia by Kricker et al[47] also claimed an association between oral contraceptive usage and limb reduction abnormalities. Eighteen of 155 affected children were exposed, compared with only one control (relative risk 16.6; $P < 0.05$). No association was found when analysis was restricted to progestogen use only, suggesting that the findings were spurious. The most serious methodologic shortcoming in this study is the potential for recall and memory bias, given that interviews had been conducted on average 4.5 years after birth of an affected child.

Far better designed case-control studies have found no association between limb anomalies and maternal hormonal exposure. In his study of 1370 Connecticut women, Bracken et al[13] showed no statistically significant association, as did Oakley et al[14] in a well designed case-control study in which the control group consisted of women delivered of offspring with chromosomal abnormalities. (Use of an abnormal control group obviates the potential for recall bias.) The case-control study of Lammer and Cordero[48] (Table 43.2) also found no significant association between hormone exposure and limb reduction defects in a sample of 1091 infants. Likewise, Pardthaisong et al[12] failed to observe an association between limb reduction defects and either injectable contraceptive medroxyprogesterone or oral contraceptives, prior to or during gestation.

Cohort studies have further failed to confirm an association (Table 43.3). Prospective studies ascertaining limb reduction defects carry unusual validity because missing digits or severe limb shortening should be obvious to even the casual observer. In Perth, Yovich et al[42] found no limb reduction defects among 508 exposed pregnancies, and in Japan Nishimura et al[38] failed to observe limb reduction deformities in 108 microdissected embryos recovered from progestogen-exposed Japanese mothers.

In summary, most retrospective studies and all cohort studies have shown no association between progestogen exposure and limb reduction defects.

Polydactyly and syndactyly

In their case-control study of 8816 newborns in Thailand, Pardthaisong et al[12] analyzed 1229 women who became pregnant despite their use of the injectable contraceptive depo-medroxyprogesterone (DMPA), 3038 who became pregnant after oral contraceptive use prior to conception or during pregnancy, and 4549 who used no contraceptive method prior to or after conception. The frequency of polydactyly and syndactyly was significantly increased when DMPA users (relative risk 4.9/1000) were compared with oral contraceptive users (1.2); however, no significant difference was observed in comparison to women receiving no contraception (1.7/1000). In only three cases were mothers of infants with polysyndactyly exposed during the biologically plausible period of limb organogenesis (days 28–52). Moreover, rates of polysyndactyly in the offspring of DMPA users were higher than those reported in other studies. For this reason the authors reasonably concluded that the association could be the result of a genetic predisposition in the population studied. Furthermore, no other case-control studies nor cohort studies (Table 44.3) have reported an association between progestogens and either polydactyly or syndactyly.

Neural tube defects and hydrocephalus

Neural tube defects (NTDs) and, to a lesser extent, hydrocephalus were once alleged to be associated with hormone exposure. This association has now been discounted.

The first claim of a relationship between NTD and progestogens was made by Gal et al[49] in a 1967 case-control study in which 19 of 100 women delivered of infants with myelomeningocele or hydrocephalus received hormones (estradiol plus ethisterone or norethisterone) for pregnancy diagnosis; only four of 100 controls recollected hormone exposure ($P < 0.01$). Greenberg et al[11] reported a possible relationship between NTD and hormone exposure on the basis of 25 of 93 infants with NTD having a history of hormone exposure. An important variable ignored by Gal et al[49] was prior reproductive history, especially relevant in the United Kingdom because of the high incidence of NTD at that time and, hence, high recurrence risk for first degree relatives (5%). The stage of embryogenesis at which exposure occurred was also not considered. Given that the neural tube closes at 28 embryonic days, hormones administered for pregnancy diagnosis probably would have been given before neural tube closure. Harlap et al[28] observed three infants with NTD among 850 women (0.35%) exposed to oral contraceptives *in utero*, an ostensible increase compared with only 27 affected infants among 32 695 (0.08%) unexposed women (relative risk 4.3). However, exposure was defined as any contraceptive use after the last menstrual period. In some cases, oral contraceptives might have been discontinued when the anticipated menstrual period failed to occur; if so, exposure would have occurred in the all-or-none period, rather than during organogenesis.

No cohort study has shown an association between progestogens and either NTD or hydrocephalus (Table 43.3). Nishimura et al[38] failed to detect NTD in 108 microdissected embryos exposed to progestogens. Case-control studies that have failed to show an association between NTD and progestogens include those of Laurence et al,[50] Bracken et al[13] and Lammer and Cordero.[48] In summary, progestogens are no longer seriously considered to be causes of neural tube defects or hydrocephalus.

Esophageal atresia

Esophageal atresia can occur as an isolated birth defect, in tandem with tracheoesophageal fistula, or as part of the VACTERL syndrome (see below). In the first two situations, recurrence risks are similar to those of other polygenic/multifactorial disorders, namely 1–2% for first degree relatives.

That esophageal atresia might be associated with progestogen teratogenicity was raised in a case-control study by Lammer and Cordero[48] (Table 44.2). When first trimester sex hormone exposure was studied in 1091 infants having at least one of 11 major types of malformations, esophageal atresia was the only anomaly for which the odds ratio was increased (odds ratio 2.8). However, Bracken et al[13] reported no association between progestogens and tracheoesophageal fistula, inguinal hernia, cleft lip and palate, pyloric stenosis, musculoskeletal anomalies or polysyndactyly. In a cohort study of 1608 newborns exposed to progestogens, Katz et al[39] specifically found no association with polydactyly, talipes equinovarus, genitourinary malformations, cleft lip and palate and tracheoesophageal fistula. The frequency of esophageal atresia has not been increased in any of the cohort studies.

Hypospadias

Hypospadias is the most common genital anomaly in males, occurring in perhaps one per 500 newborn boys. Although most cases are considered polygenic/multifactorial in etiology, the high recurrence risk for first degree relatives (6–14%)[51] suggests that in some families an autosomal recessive form exists. However, the recurrence risk increases as severity of the malformation increases,[51] as expected in polygenic/multifactorial etiology.

The first claim that antenatal exposure to progestogens (medroxyprogesterone in particular) caused penile or perineoscrotal hypospadias was by Aarskog.[52] Aarskog's study was observational only, but case-control studies were later conducted. The most persuasive data in favor of an association are the Latin American Collaborative Congenital Anomaly Study (Spanish abbreviation ECLAMC),[53] which found a 2.4 relative risk for progestogen exposure. Of 314 cases of hypospadias, 24 (7.6%) were exposed *in utero* to progestogens; 12 of 319 controls (3.8%) ($P < 0.05$) were exposed. However, the time of exposure could not be provided, and the incidence of hypospadias varied widely among the countries surveyed. Czeizel et al[54] found a similar association in Hungary: 28 of 294 (9.5%) mothers delivered of males with hypospadias received sex hormones, compared with 12 of an unspecified number of controls. Although this difference was significant, matching criteria for controls were uncertain. Moreover, the high prevalence of hypospadias in the subjects' male relatives suggests unwitting selection bias.

In contrast to these studies, many others have failed to show an association between progestogens and hypospadias.[13,38,55,56] Neither the US Collaborative Perinatal Project[23,24] nor the other cohort studies listed in Table 44.3 found an association. Katz et al[39] found no cases of pseudohermaphroditism among infants exposed to progestogens administered because of threatened miscarriage; the frequency of hypospadias and clitoromegaly was the same in exposed (n = 1605) and unexposed groups (n = 1146). Yovich et al[42] found only two infants with hypospadias among 508 (0.4%) exposed *in utero* to medroxyprogesterone, an incidence differing little from the general incidence in Western Australia (0.5%). In their cohort study of 988 offspring exposed *in utero* to exogenous progestogens, Resseguie et al[40] found no increased risk of hypospadias. Another study failed to find hypospadias in offspring of 382 women treated early in gestation with vaginal progesterone or 17 α-hydroxyprogesterone caproate.[41]

To us, *in utero* exposure to progestogens is unlikely to result in abnormal development of the male genitalia. Despite our belief that the issue has been adequately addressed, the US Food and Drug Administration still considers the topic in need of additional studies. The requisite warning brochure still cites hypospadias as a possible complication.

Multiple malformation syndromes

In theory, a teratogenic effect might exist not for a single defect, not for all anomalies, but only for a specific pattern of malformations. This pattern might not be appreciated if analysis was restricted solely to individual anomalies. Specifically, there have been claims that the VACTERL complex is associated with progestogen exposure. The VACTERL complex is diagnosed when three of the following organ systems are involved: vertebral, anal, cardiac, tracheal, esophageal, renal and limb. In 1978, Nora et al[21] found that 11 of 30 (36%) VACTERL probands had been exposed to progestogens, compared with five of 60 (8.3%) controls ($P < 0.001$). However, the sample size was small, and recall bias would likely be amplified in mothers whose infants had multiple malformations. Later studies[1,15,57–59] failed to confirm such an association. Nor has any cohort study found an association between hormone exposure and either the VACTERL complex or any of its individual components (e.g. the cardiac or limb abnormalities described earlier).

Diethylstilbestrol

The effects of *in utero* exposure to diethylstilbestrol are by now well known. The report of Herbst et al in 1971[60] first demonstrated the association of *in utero* exposure to diethylstibestrol (DES) to the development of clear cell adenocarcinoma of the vagina in DES exposed female offspring. In this case-control study, the authors reported eight cases of clear cell adenocarcinoma of the vagina matched to four controls for each reported case. Seven of the eight women with vaginal clear cell adenocarcinoma were born to mothers who had received estrogen during the relevant pregnancies. None of the 32 controls was exposed to diethylstilbestrol.

The manner by which stilbestrol leads to the development of these carcinomas is, as yet, not clearly understood. Walker and Kurth[61] have demonstrated multigenerational carcinogenesis from DES in mice. This study suggested that the prenatal exposure of the mouse to DES produced a maternal environment that increased the incidence of ovarian and uterine tumors in the offspring. Furthermore, they also noted that DES has a multigenerational effect that is transmitted through the blastocyst, an effect the authors felt to be consistent with a fetal germ cell mutation resulting from exposure to DES during pregnancy. In a preliminary study, Hajek et al[62] compared chromosomal alterations in biopsies taken from 19 DES exposed women to those noted in 19 controlled patients. Using fluorescent *in situ* hybridization (FISH) with centromeric probes for chromosomes 1, 7, 11 and 17, four of the 19 DES exposed women had a trisomy frequency (three signals) greater that 5%. In contrast, frequency of cells with three signals in the control patients was less than 1.5% for all probes.

Numerous studies subsequent to the 1971 report by Herbst et al have noted the relationship of *in utero* DES exposure to the presence of other changes in the offspring, including vaginal epithelial changes, and structural changes of the cervix and upper genital tract. Several reports have also noted the relationship of *in utero* DES exposure to minor structural abnormalities in the genital tracts of exposed males. This section will briefly review this subject.

Many of the early studies related to *in utero* DES exposure were conducted under the auspices of the national cooperative diethylstilbestrol adenosis (DESAD) project.[63] This multicenter study prospectively followed more than 4500 women. Subjects comprised women identified through review of their mothers' pregnancy records and determined to have been exposed to DES; another group of women had no such prenatal exposure; other women were referred by physicians or were self-referred for gynecologic examination and follow-up on the basis of documentation of *in utero* DES exposure. The largest and least biased group of women entered into the study (40%) fell into the record review category. The frequency of vaginal epithelial changes in the record review population is significantly less than that noted in the documented 'walk-in' and referral patients (Table 43.5).

Lower genital tract changes

Vaginal epithelial changes have provoked interest because of the frequent association between clear cell adenocarcinoma of the vagina and adenosis. However, the term vaginal epithelial changes (VEC) refers to any mucosal change observed on the basis of colposcopic examination and/or iodine staining, or as a microscopic change in the mucosa of the vaginal wall. Gross findings include columnar epithelium, glands, nabothian cysts, white epithelium, leukoplakia, mosaicism, punctation and areas that remain nonstaining with Lugol's solution. Microscopic changes include adenosis (columnar cells or their secretory products in the vagina) and squamous metaplasia. Table 43.5 demonstrates the frequency of these findings in the different study populations. Patients with vaginal epithelial changes were generally exposed *in utero* to a larger total dose of DES over a longer period of time and at an earlier date of gestation

Table 43.5 Greatest extent of colposcopically observed epithelial change.[63]

	Participant classification			
Most distal extent of change	Record reviews	Documented walk-ins	Documented referrals	Changes, no documentation
Vagina	435 (34%)	480 (59%)	473 (65%)	334 (84%)
Upper third	295 (23%)	319 (39%)	305 (42%)	213 (54%)
Mid third	117 (9%)	143 (18%)	134 (18%)	104 (26%)
Lower third	23 (2%)	18 (2%)	34 (5%)	17 (4%)
Total	1275 (100%)	815 (100%)	726 (100%)	396 (100%)

than were offspring without these changes. Of interest is that the frequency of vaginal epithelial changes appeared to diminish with age, occurring less frequently among women older than 26 years. An explanation was offered by Noller et al,[64] who noted a decrease in the frequency of vaginal epithelial changes as the study population was prospectively followed. A decrease in the extent of these changes occurred in 29.2% of the women followed.

When 3246 biopsy specimens taken during the initial examination of the 3339 DES-exposed women were evaluated, it was further observed that only 45% of women with vaginal epithelial changes who had undergone biopsy had adenosis. As already alluded, the relationship of the development of clear cell adenocarcinoma to adenosis is suggestive yet uncertain. Several reports have noted a relationship between clear cell adenocarcinoma and adenosis of the tubo-endometrial type, often in association with atypical adenosis.[65,66]

Various structural changes of the cervix and vagina have also been observed in DES-exposed female offspring (Table 43.6). The prevalence of structural changes was 25% in the record review participants but only 2% in the comparison population (Table 43.7). Structural abnormalities of the vagina were only rarely

Table 43.6 Structural defects.

Abnormalities of cervix and vaginal fornix	
Cockscomb	
Description:	Raised ridge, usually on anterior cervix
Synonym:	Hood, transverse ridge of cervix
Collar	
Description:	Flat rim involving part to all of circumference of cervix
Synonym:	Rim, hood, transverse ridge of cervix
Pseudopolyp	
Description:	Polypoid appearance of cervix resulting from circumferential constricting groove, thickening of stroma of anterior or posterior endocervical canal
Includes:	Endocervical stromal hyperplasia
Hypoplastic cervix	
Description:	Cervix smaller than 1.5 cm in diameter
Synonym:	Immature cervix
Altered fornix of vagina	
Includes:	Absence — complete or partial — of pars vaginalis; abnormality of fornices; fusion of cervix to vagina; partial or complete forniceal obliteration
Abnormalities of vagina exclusive of fornix	
Transverse septum, incomplete	
longitudinal septum, incomplete	

From Jefferies JA, Robboy SJ, O'Brien PC et al 1984 Structural anomalies of the cervix and vagina in women enrolled in the diethylstilbestrol adenosis (DESAD) project. American Journal of Obstetrics and Gynecology 148: 59

Table 43.7 Types and frequency of structural changes found on entry examination.

	Structural changes of cervix and vaginal fornix (%)						
Participant classification	Any structural changes	Any type	Cockscomb	Collar	Pseudopolyp	Abnormal fornix	Hypoplastic cervix
Record review (n = 1655)	25.3	24.8	9.1	13.4	3.4	3.1	3.2
Control (n = 963)	2.3†	2.1†	0.9†	0.8†	0.1†	0.3†	0.0†
Walk-in (n = 800)	42.6	42.1	14.0	24.5	1.9	7.0	9.1
Referral (n = 1089)	48.6	47.8	16.1	30.9	4.5	5.7	6.0

From Jeffries JA, Robboy SJ, O'Brien PC et al 1984 Structural anomalies of the cervix and vagina in women enrolled in the diethylstilbestrol adenosis (DESAD) project. American Journal of Obstetrics and Gynecology 148: 59. *Values are precentages of persons in each classification who had the indicated abnormalities. Some participants had more than one. †Significantly ($P < 0.01$) less than the record review group (chi-square test); †Two-sided P value = 0.059.

encountered and were limited to the presence of an incomplete transverse vaginal septum. As was noted with the vaginal epithelial changes, these findings are associated with the early onset of DES exposure and the total dose of DES administered.

The structural abnormalities most commonly seen include cervical collar (Fig. 43.1), pseudopolyp (Fig. 43.1), cockscomb (Fig. 43.2), abnormal fornix and hypoplastic cervix (Fig. 43.3). Because these patients were prospectively followed and examined on an annual basis, it could be observed that these structural changes often disappeared. Over a 1–5 year interval regression was noted in 41% of 361 women. The changes most often disappeared among women who had experienced pregnancy.

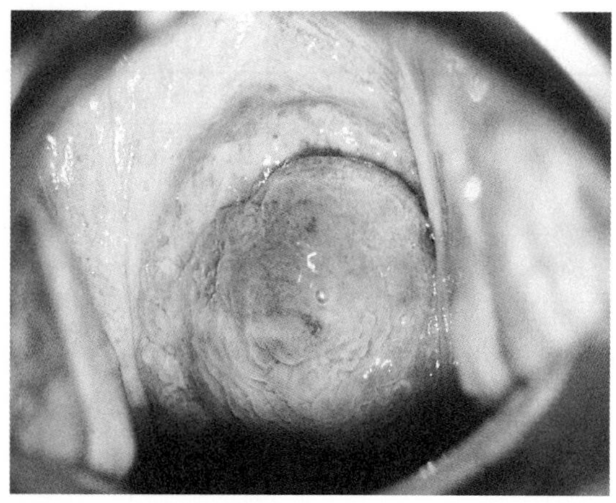

Fig. 43.1 A cervical collar is evident around a central area of ectropion having the appearance of a pseudopolyp. (From Kaufman RH, Noller K 1993 Consequences of *in utero* exposure to diethylstilbestrol. In: Copeland L (ed). Textbook of gynecology. WB Saunders, Philadelphia) 1993

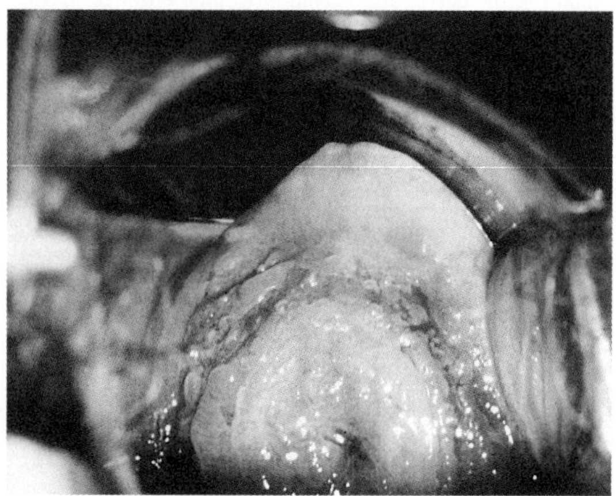

Fig. 43.2 Coxcomb on anterior cervix is visible (reference 73).

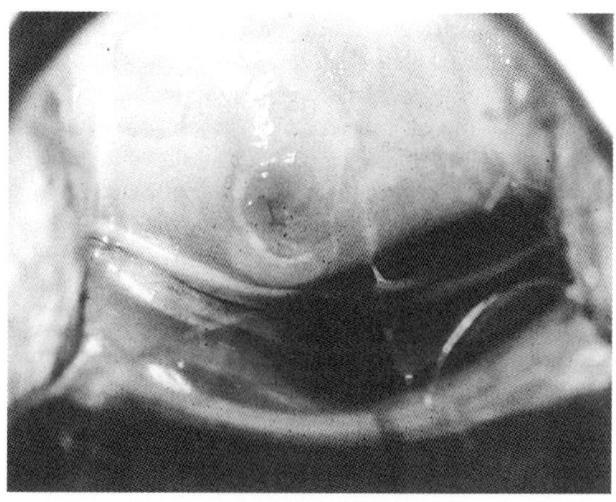

Fig. 43.3 Hypoplastic cervix is shown. The cervical portion is almost completely absent. (From Kaufman RH, Noller K 1993 Consequences of *in utero* exposure to diethylstilbestrol. In: Copeland L (ed) Textbook of gynecology. WB Saunders, Philadelphia)

Clear cell adenocarcinoma of the vagina and cervix

Following the 1971 report by Herbst et al[60] identifying the relationship between *in utero* DES exposure and the development of clear cell adenocarcinoma of the vagina, close monitoring of DES exposed individuals has in fact revealed a higher incidence of this type of carcinoma in the DES exposed as compared to the unexposed. Even so, the absolute risk is small, occurring in fewer than 1 in 1000 DES-exposed women. The Registry for Research on Hormonal Transplacental Carcinogenesis of the University of Chicago, established by Herbst, has now entered over 600 cases of clear cell adenocarcinoma of the vagina or cervix. Approximately 60% of these women were exposed to DES.[67] 12% of the women had been exposed to another hormone or to another unidentified medication during pregnancy, 23% of the patients had a history negative for hormone or other medication exposure during pregnancy, and in 5% of individuals the use of medication during pregnancy was not known. The peak incidence for the diagnosis of clear cell adenocarcinoma occurred in 1975. Since then there has been a steady decrease in the frequency of diagnoses. The median age of diagnosis of clear cell adenocarcinoma was 19 years. Clear cell carcinoma has been identified in DES exposed women in their early 40 s, although at present such late detections are relatively rare. It is uncertain whether or not there will be an increase in the occurrence of clear cell adenocarcinoma of the vagina and cervix as the DES exposed women approach those years in life when this type of carcinoma is most commonly seen (sixth decade and above). DeMars[68] reported two cases of non-clear cell mucinous adenocarcinoma of the vagina in older women having a history of *in utero* DES exposure. These cancers were more advanced than the clear cell adenocarcinoma associated with DES exposure. One woman was 34 and the other 41 years of age. However, lack of additional data suggest that these two reported cancers could have been chance occurrences.

Herbst et al[69] evaluated factors related to the development of clear cell adenocarcinoma in DES exposed women. They found that the relative risks for clear cell adenocarcinoma were greater in those women whose mothers began DES before the 12th week of pregnancy and as well when the pregnancies were conceived during the winter. Furthermore, a maternal history of at least one spontaneous abortion increased the risk for the development of adenocarcinoma. Another factor that appeared to predispose to the development of clear cell adenocarcinoma was premature birth of the infant. However, the number of such cases was small.

A recent study by Waggoner et al[70] detected p53 protein in tumors from 14 of 21 cases (67%) of clear cell adenocarcinoma. Further analysis of the tissue failed to identify p53 mutations in any of the cases, suggesting that the tumors contained only wild-type p53 alleles. The authors hypothesized that p53 overexpression in clear cell adenocarcinomas was a response to generalized DNA damage, rather than a result of p53 protein half life prolongation resulting from mutational inactivation. They speculated that the overexpression of wild-type p53 protein in these clear cell adenocarcinomas might connote a more favorable prognosis compared to other gynecologic tumors containing mutated p53.

Robboy et al[71] observed that the incidences for dysplasia and carcinoma *in situ* of the vagina and cervix were significantly higher in women exposed to DES than in the unexposed matched cohort (15.7 versus 7.9 cases for 1000 person years of follow-up). The matched cohorts were similar in all respects to the women with intraepithelial neoplasia except for the finding of a greater frequency of genital herpes in exposed as compared to unexposed women. Unfortunately, no new reliable data relative to this area have been published. The study does suggest that women exposed *in utero* to DES should be considered at high risk for the development of intraepithelial neoplasia of the vagina and cervix.

Upper genital tract changes

On the basis of hysterosalpingography, significant variations in the appearance of the uterus have been observed in DES-exposed women as compared to nonexposed women. These changes consist primarily of a T-shaped appearance of the uterus, constricting bands to the uterine cavity, a hypoplastic uterus, and often intra-uterine polypoid defects and synechiae (Figs 43.4 and 43.5). Table 43.8 presents hysterosalpingographic findings in 676 women in relationship to the shape of the uterine cavity. Of the DESAD record review patients studied, 42%

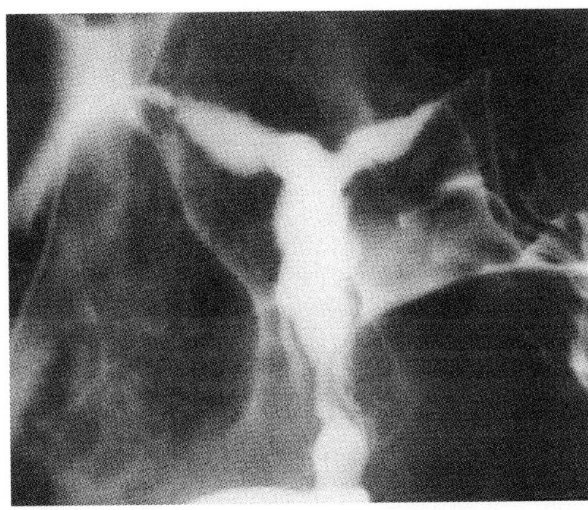

Fig. 43.4 T-shaped uterus with exaggerated horns. The borders of the uterine cavity are irregular. (From reference 73)

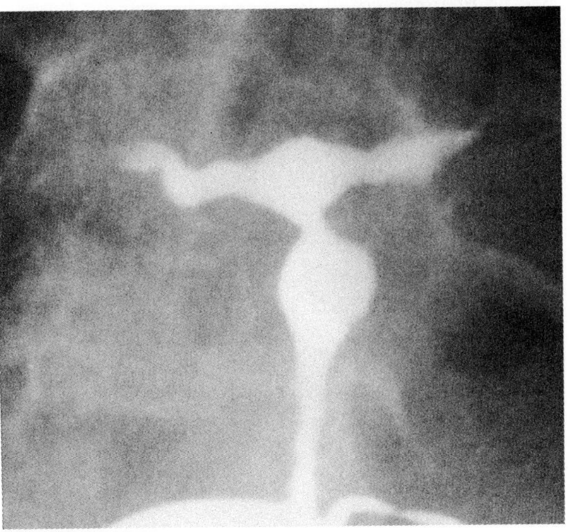

Fig. 43.5 T-shaped appearance of the uterus with pronounced stricture noted around the uterine fundus. (From reference 73).

Table 43.8 Hysterosalpingographic findings in 676 women: cavity shape.[74]

Cavity shape	Record reviews (%) (n = 291)	Walk-ins, referrals, others (%) (n = 385)
Normal	58.4*	39.0*
T-shape	29.9	46.5*
Constriction	30.2	59.2*
Wide lower segment	12.7	9.5
Arcuate	11.6	6.0*
Hypoplastic	6.5	20.0*
Bicornuate	1.4	1.6
Unicornuate	0.3	0.8
Other	2.4	2.1
No. of women examined	291	385

Modified from reference 77.
*Significance of difference between the cohorts: $P < 0.01$.

demonstrated some type of uterine abnormality. Intra-uterine defects (Table 43.9) were found in 35% of record review patients.

Barnes et al[72] had noted an increased risk of unfavorable pregnancy outcome in women exposed to DES, but at that time the authors could not present a reasonable explanation for this increased risk. Later, Kaufman et al[73,74] observed a relationship between upper genital tract abnormalities to pregnancy outcome in this population of women. The observation was made that although certain abnormalities were often associated with poor pregnancy outcome, no specific changes could be related to specific types of pregnancy failure. The most consistently poor pregnancy outcomes were preterm delivery and ectopic pregnancy (Table 43.10). When comparing outcomes of first pregnancies in the DESAD record review population to women with a normal hysterosalpingogram, an individual with an abnormal hysterosalpingogram was less likely to have a term live birth, more likely to give birth to a preterm infant, and more likely to have an ectopic pregnancy.

Table 43.9 Hysterosalpingographic findings in 676 women: intra-uterine defects.[74]

Type of irregularity	Record reviews (%) (n = 291)	Walk-ins, referrals, others (%) (n = 385)
Regular surface	64.9	50.6*
Irregular margins	28.2	39.7*
Filling defects	10.0	6.5
Ridge	3.8	9.6*
Diverticuli	4.1	7.5
Synechiae	2.7	6.5†
Other	3.1	2.6

*Significance of difference between the cohorts: $P < 0.05$;
†significance of difference between the cohorts: $P < 0.01$.

The anatomic basis for the abnormalities noted on hysterosalpingogram became evident when uteri from DES-exposed women were examined after hysterectomy. Isolated areas of myometrial thickening produced indentations into the endometrial cavity, explaining x-ray observations. Robboy et al[75] offered a possible explanation for the abnormal uterine changes based on studies of the fetal reproductive tracts in nude mice exposed to DES. The upper genital tract failed to develop normally: stunted growth of the upper mullerian ducts occurred and the inner and outer stromal layers of the uterine wall failed to segregate normally.

Fertility

The question of fertility in the DES exposed woman has still not been completely clarified. Given that most women who were exposed to DES as fetuses are now over 40 years old, it is arguable whether definitive information will be gathered. Barnes et al[72] reported that infertility, as measured by pregnancies achieved, did not differ between women exposed to DES and a control population. However, Herbst et al[76] reported increased infertility in DES exposed women. Kaufman et al[77] investigated the possible relationship of upper genital tract abnormalities to infertility and found that the presence of an abnormal hysterosalpingogram *per se* was not related to infertility. However, when data were stratified by specific HSG abnormalities, the presence of a constriction of the upper uterine cavity was associated with a 2.3 times greater likelihood that a woman would be unable to conceive. If a T-shaped uterus was found in association with a constriction of the upper uterine cavity, the odds ratio for being unable to conceive was 2.6.

Other diseases

Noller[78] reviewed medical and surgical diseases associated with *in utero* exposure to DES, reviewing data on more than 1200 different medical diseases reported by DESAD project participants. In only eight conditions were significant differences noted between exposed and control subjects (Table 43.11). However, the cases found in both exposed and unexposed groups were too few to draw definitive conclusions. When the

Table 43.10 Relationship of first pregnancy outcome to cavity shape.[74]

Cohort (%)	Cavity shape	No. of women	Outcome of pregnancy: Term live birth *n*	%	Preterm live birth *n*	%	Spontaneous abortion *n*	%	Ectopic pregnancy *n*	%	Stillbirth *n*	%	Any unfavorable outcome *n*
Record reviews													
25	Normal	99	74	75	8	8	15	15	1	1	1	1	25
49*	Abnormal	70	36	51 *	11	16 †	15	21	7	10 †	1	1	34
Walk-ins, referrals others													
56	Normal	63	28	44	15	24	14	22	6	9	0	0	35
66	Abnormal	95	32	34	26	27	19	20	14	15	4	4	63
All													
37	Normal	162	102	63	23	14	29	18	7	4	1	1	60
59*	Abnormal	165	68	41 *	37	22	34	21	21	13 *	5	3	97

*Significance of difference between abnormal and normal hysterosalpingography groups: $P < 0.01$; †significance of difference between abnormal and normal hysterosalpingography groups: $P < 0.05$.

Table 43.11 National cooperative diethylstillbestrol adenosis project: diseases reported by seven or more exposed women, 1984–88.[78]

Disease	Exposed ($n = 1765$)	Controls ($n = 957$)	*P* Value*
Candida infections	26.1†	13.6†	0.033
Otitis media	4.5	0.0	0.037
Mitral valve disorder	10.8	3.1	0.034
Kidney infections	5.1	13.6	0.018
Solitary cyst of breast	12.5	3.1	0.015
Diffuse cystic mastopathy	30.6	16.7	0.029
Cervical dysplasia	36.3	17.8	0.007
Female infertility	15.9	4.2	0.007

*Based on Chi-square statistic; †rate per 1000 participants.

differences in observed mitral valve disorders and breast cysts were studied in more detail, the ostensible difference furthermore became insignificant. Recall bias appeared to be a more logical explanation for the initially observed difference.

Psychologic impact and gender related behavior

Gufstavson et al[79] found an increased occurrence of eating disorders among DES-exposed women compared with unexposed controls. A significantly greater number of young DES-exposed women gave histories of bulimia and anorexia nervosa than did the unexposed controls.

Evidence in experimental animals suggests that mammalian brain development and differentiation of the central nervous system are influenced by prenatal exposure to sex hormones. Thus, changes in human behavioral patterns plausibly might be associated with prenatal exposure to estrogenic substances such as DES. Newbold[80] has studied gender-related behavior in women exposed prenatally to diethylstilbestrol, concluding that a vast number of biological and psychosocial factors interact to explain specific behavioral traits. To date, no clear cut differences have been reported between unexposed and DES-exposed women in gender related behavior. Newbold[80] felt that if both prenatal and postnatal influences such as social, economic and environmental factors are considered, individual variation is more apparent than differences between unexposed and DES-exposed women. In contrast to this conclusion was that of Meyer-Bahlburg et al,[81] who found that DES-exposed women were more likely than controls to be bisexual or homosexual.

Very little reproducible data relate to psychopathology and social functioning in individuals exposed *in utero* to diethylstilbestrol. Pillard et al[82] compared the psychiatric histories and social functioning in 27 *men* with a history of high-dose prenatal DES exposure and compared the findings to their unexposed brothers. The DES subjects had a greater frequency of major depressive disorders than their unexposed brothers, but this finding did not reach statistical significance. Unfortunately, many of the studies related to the psychological impact of ingestion of DES by the mothers and exposure to this drug *in utero* by offspring have been biased. Most of the psychologic studies performed were confined to assessment of reactions of individuals who already were informed that they were at risk for many of the problems associated with DES exposure.[83]

Breast cancer

The consensus is that there is no evidence to suggest the DES exposed offspring are at increased risk for the development of carcinoma of the breast. Reporting on the same population, Greenburg et al[84] and subsequently Colton et al[85] found the relative risk of breast cancer associated with DES exposure to be 1.35 in mothers who took diethylstibestrol during their pregnancies. In the Colton et al study, this risk did not appear to increase in women followed for 30 years or more following exposure.

DES effects on the male

Various anomalies of the lower genital tract have been reported in males. These consist of urethral meatal stenosis, epididymal cysts, varicocele, cryptorchidism, hypospadias, hypoplastic testes, hypoplastic penis and capsular induration of the testes. Wilcox et al[86] found that the risk of genital malformation is higher among men who were exposed relatively early in gestation to stilbestrol. This is not unexpected, given that the external genitalia are suspectible to the effect of teratogens through the ninth week of embryonic life. These authors also found that the DES exposed male had no apparent impairment of fertility. *In utero* DES exposure did not impair sexual function as measured by the frequency of intercourse or reported episodes of decreased libido.

There has been no conclusive evidence to suggest an increase of occurrence of testicular or prostatic cancer in DES exposed males.

Conclusion

Despite many cohort and case control studies, there still remains little reason to suspect that progestogen exposure *in utero* exerts a deleterious effect on fetal development. The sole exceptions are 19-nortestosterone derivatives, which in high doses (10–20 mg daily) can cause genital virilization. Danazol is also capable of virilizing female fetuses. Cyproterone acetate can impede virilization in male fetuses. To the contrary, cardiac anomalies, limb reduction defects, neural tube defects and anomalies in general have been excluded beyond reasonable medical certainty as being associated with progestogen exposure.

REFERENCES

1. Simpson JL 1985 Relationship between congenital anomalies and contraception. Advances in Contraception 1: 3–30
2. Simpson JL, Phillips OP 1990 Spermicides, hormonal contraception and congenital malformations. Advances in Contraception 6: 141–167
3. Doering PL, Stewart RB 1978 The extent and character of drug consumption in pregnancy. Journal of the American Medical Association 239: 843–846
4. Simpson JL, Mills JL, Morrey A, Metzger BE et al 1989 Drug ingestion during pregnancy: infrequent exposure in a contemporary United States sample. American Journal of Perinatology 6: 244–251
5. Wiseman RA 1996 Prevention of physical and mental congenital defects, part C: Basic and medical science, education and future strategies. Negative correlation between sex hormone usage and malformations. Alan R. Liss, Inc., pp 171–175
6. Carson SA, Simpson JL, Maheesh VB, Greenblatt RB (eds) 1984 Hirsutism and virilization. Virilization of female fetuses following maternal ingestion of progestional and androgenic steroids. PSG Publishing Co., Littleton, MA, pp 177–187
7. Jacobson BD 1962 Hazards of norethindrone therapy during pregnancy. American Journal of Obstetrics and Gynecology 84: 962–968
8. Burstein R, Wasserman HC 1964 The effects of Provera on the fetus. Obstetrics and Gynecology 23: 931–934
9. Kingsbury AC 1985 Danazol and fetal masculinization: a warning. Medical Journal of Australia 143: 410–411

10. Brunskill PJ 1992 The effects of fetal exposure to Danazol. British Journal of Obstetrics and Gynecology 99: 212–215
11. Greenberg G, Inman WHW, Weatherall JAC, Adelstein AM, Haskey JC 1977 Maternal drug histories and congenital abnormalities. British Medical Journal 2: 853–856
12. Pardthaisong T, Gray RH, McDaniel EB, Chandacham A 1988 Steroid contraceptive use and pregnancy outcome. Teratology 38: 51–58
13. Bracken MB, Holford TR, White C, Kelsey JL 1978 Role of oral contraception in congenital malformations of offspring. International Journal of Epidemiology 7: 309–317
14. Oakley GP, Flynn JW, Ealek A 1973 Hormonal pregnancy tests and congenital malformations. Lancet 25: 256–257
15. Harlap S, Eldor J 1980 Births following oral contraceptive failure. Obstetrics and Gynecology 55: 44–47
16. Harlap S, Prywes R, Davies AM 1975 Birth defects and estrogens and progesterones in pregnancy. Lancet 1: 682–683
17. Gray RH, Pardthaisong T 1991 In utero exposure to steroid contraceptives and survival during infancy. American Journal of Epidemiology 134: 804–811
18. Simpson JL, Golbus MS 1992 Genetics in obstetrics and gynecology, 2nd edn. WB Saunders, Philadelphia, p 1
19. Levy EP, Cohen A, Fraser FC 1973 Hormone treatment during pregnancy and congenital heart disease. Lancet 1: 611
20. Nora JJ, Nora AH 1973 Preliminary evidence for a possible association between oral contraceptives and birth defects. Teratology 7: 24 [Abstract]
21. Nora JJ, Nora AH, Blum J, Ingram J et al 1978 Exogenous progestogen and estrogen implicated in birth defects. Journal of the American Medical Association 240: 837–843
22. Janerich DT, Dugan JM, Standfast SJ, Strite L 1977 Congenital heart disease and prenatal exposure to exogenous sex hormones. Obstetrics and Gynecology Survey 32: 606–608
23. Heinonen OP, Slone D, Monson RR, Hook EB, Shapiro S 1977 Cardiovascular birth defects in antenatal exposure to female sex hormones. New England Journal of Medicine 296: 67–70
24. Heinonen OP, Slone D, Shapiro S 1996 Birth defects and drugs in pregnancy. Sciences Group, Littleton, MA
25. Wiseman RA, Dodds-Smith IC 1984 Cardiovascular birth defects and antenatal exposure to female sex hormones: a revaluation of some base data. Teratology 30: 359–370
26. Hook EB 1994 Cardiovascular birth defects and prenatal exposure to female hormones: a reevaluation of data reanalysis from a large prospective study. Teratology 49: 162–166
27. Wiseman RA 1994 Comments on 'Cardiovascular birth defects and prenatal exposure to female sex hormones'. Teratology 49: 172–173
28. Harlap S, Shiono PH, Ramcharan S 1985 Congenital abnormalities in the offspring of women who used oral and other contraceptives around the time of conception. International Journal of Fertility 30: 39–47
29. Spira N, Goujard J, Huel G, Rumeau-Roquette C 1972 Etude teratogene des hormones sexuelles. Premier resultats d'une enquete epidemiologique portant sur 20 000 femmes. Rev Red Fr 41: 2683
30. Goujard J, Rumeau-Rouquette C 1977 First trimester exposure to progestogen/estrogen and congenital malformations. Lancet 1: 482–483
31. Savolainen E, Saksela E, Saxen L 1981 Teratogenic hazards of oral contraceptives analyzed in a national malformation register. American Journal of Obstetrics and Gynecology 140: 521–524
32. Michaelis J, Michaelis H, Gluck E, Koller S 1983 Prospective study of suspected associations between certain drugs administered during early pregnancy and congenital malformations. Teratology 27: 57–64
33. Kullander S, Kallen B 1976 A prospective study of drugs and pregnancy. Acta Obstetrica Gynecologica Scandinavica 55: 287–295
34. Royal College of General Practitioners 1976 The outcome of pregnancy in former oral contraceptive users. British Journal of Obstetrics and Gynecology 83: 608–616
35. Varma TR, Morsman J 1982 Evaluation of the early use of proluton-depot (hydroxyprogesterone hexamoate) in early pregnancy. International Journal of Gynecology and Obstetrics 20: 13–17
36. Vessey MP 1979 Outcome of pregnancy in women using different methods of contraception. British Journal of Obstetrics and Gynecology 86: 548–556
37. Torfs CP, Milkovich L, Van Den Berg BJ 1981 The relationship between hormonal pregnancy tests and congenital abnormalities: a prospective study. American Journal of Epidemiology 113: 563–574
38. Nishimura H, Uwabe C, Semba R 1974 Examination of teratogenicity of progestogens and/or estrogens by observation of the induced abortuses. Teratology 10: 93
39. Katz Z, Lancet M, Skornik J, Chemke J, Mogilner BM, Klinberg M 1985 Teratogenicity of progestogens given during the first trimester of pregnancy. Obstetrics and Gynecology 65: 775–780
40. Resseguie LJ, Hick JF, Bruen JA, Noller KL, O'Fallon WM, Kurland LT 1985 Congenital malformations among offspring exposed in utero to progestins, Olmstead County, Minnesota, 1936–74. Fertility and Sterility 43: 514–519
41. Check JH, Rankin A, Teichman M 1986 The risk of fetal anomalies as a result of progesterone therapy during pregnancy. Fertility and Sterility 45: 575–577
42. Yovich JL, Turner SR, Pivet RD 1988 Medroxyprogesterone acetate therapy in early pregnancy has no apparent fetal effects. Teratology 38: 135–144
43. Pilarski RT, Pauli RM, Engber WD 1985 Hand reduction malformations: genetic and syndrome analysis. Journal of Pediatric Orthopedics 5: 274–280
44. Hoyme HE, Jones KL, Van Allen MI, Saunders BS, Benirschke K 1982 Vascular pathogenesis of transverse limb reduction defects. Journal of Pediatrics 1: 839–843
45. Hecht JT, Scott CI Jr 1984 Genetic study of an orthopedic referral center. Journal of Pediatric Orthopedics 4: 208–223
46. Janerich DT, Piper JM, Glebatis DM 1974 Oral contraceptives and congenital limb-reduction defects. New England Journal of Medicine 291: 697–700

47. Kricker A, Elliot JW, Forrest JM, McCredie J 1986 Congenital limb reduction deformities and use of oral contraceptives. American Journal of Obstetrics and Gynecology 155: 1072–1078
48. Lammer EJ, Cordero JF 1986 Exogenous sex hormone exposure and the risk for major malformation. Journal of the American Medical Association 255: 3128–3132
49. Gal I, Kirman B, Stern J 1967 Hormonal pregnancy tests and neural tube defects. Nature 216: 83
50. Laurence M, Miller M, Vowles M, Evans K, Carter C 1971 Hormonal pregnancy tests and neural tube defects. Nature 233: 495–496
51. Bauer SB, Retik AB, Colodny AH 1981 Genetic aspects of hypospadias. Urological Clinics of America 8: 559–564
52. Aarskog D 1979 Maternal progestins a possible cause of hypospadias. New England Journal of Medicine 300: 75–80
53. Monteleone RN, Castilla EE, Paz JE 1981 Hypospadias: an epidemiologic study in Latin America. American Journal of Medical Genetics 10: 5–19
54. Czeizel A, Troth J, Eordi E 1979 Aetiological studies of hypospadias in Hungary. Hum Hered 29: 166–171
55. Sweet RA, Schroot HG, Kurland R, Culp OS 1974 Study of the incidence of hypospadias in Rochester, Minnesota, 1940–1970, and a case-control comparison of possible etiologic factors. Mayo Clinic Proceedings 49: 52–58
56. Avellan L 1977 On aetiological factors in hypospadias. Scandinavian Journal of Plastic and Reconstructive Surgery 11: 115
57. David TJ, O'Callaghan SE 1974 Birth defects and oral hormonal preparations. Lancet 1: 1236
58. Wilson JG, Brent RL 1981 Are female sex hormones teratogenic? American Journal of Obstetrics and Gynecology 141: 567–580
59. World Health Organization (WHO) 1981 The effect of female sex hormones on fetal development and infant health. Technical Report Series 657
60. Herbst AL, Ulfelder H, Poskanzer DC 1971 Adenocarcinoma of the vagina: association of maternal stilbestrol therapy with tumor appearance in young women. New England Journal of Medicine 284: 878–881
61. Walker BE, Kurth LA 1995 Multi-generational carcinogenesis from diethylstilbestrol investigated by blastocyst transfers in mice. International Journal of Cancer 61: 249–252
62. Hajek RA, Liang JC, Kaufman RH, Zhao L, Edward CL, Jones LA 1995 Does detection of chromosomal aberrations by FISK in cervicovaginal biopsies from women exposed to DES in utero precede clinically evident disease? Proceedings of American Cancer Research 36: 633 [Abstract]
63. O'Brien PC, Knoller KL, Robboy SJ 1979 Vaginal epithelial changes in young women enrolled in the National Cooperative Diethylstilbestrol Adenosis (DESAD) Project. Obstetrics and Gynecology 53: 300–308
64. Noller KL, Townsend DE, Kaufman RH, Barnes AB et al 1983 Maturation of vaginal and cervical epithelium in women exposed in utero to diethylstilbestrol (DESAD Project). American Journal of Obstetrics and Gynecology 146: 279–285
65. Welch WR, Pratt J, Robboy SJ, Herbst AL 1978 Pathology of prenatal diethylstilbestrol exposure. Pathology Annual 1: 201–216 [Review]
66. Robboy SJ, Young RH, Welch WR, Truslow GY, Prat J, Herbst AL, Scully RE 1984 Atypical vaginal adenosis and cervical ectropion. Association with clear cell adenocarcinoma in diethylstilbestrol-exposed offspring. Cancer 54: 869–875
67. Melnick S, Cole P, Anderson D, Herbst A 1987 Rates and risks of diethylstilbestrol-related clear cell adenocarcinoma of the vagina and cervix. New England Journal of Medicine 316: 514–516
68. Demars LR, Van Lee L, Huang I, Fowler WC 1995 Primary non-clear-cell adenocarcinomas of the vagina in older DES-exposed women. Gynecological Oncology 58: 389–392
69. Herbst AL, Anderson S, Hubby MM, Haenszel WM, Kaufman RH, Noller KL 1986 Risk factors for the development of diethylstilbestrol-associated clear cell adenocarcinoma: a case-control study. American Journal of Obstetrics and Gynecology 154: 814–822
70. Waggoner SE, Anderson SM, Luce MC et al 1996 P53 protein expression and gene analysis and clear cell adenocarcinoma of the vagina and cervix. Gynecological Oncology 6: 339–341
71. Robboy SJ, Noller KL, O'Brien P, Kaufman RH et al 1984 Increased incidence of cervical and vaginal dysplasia in 3980 diethylstilbestrol-exposed young women. Experience of the National Collaborative Diethylstilbestrol Adenosis Project. Journal of the American Medical Association 252: 2979–2983
72. Barnes AB, Colton T, Gundersen J, Noller KL et al 1980 Fertility and outcome of pregnancy in women exposed in utero to diethylstilbestrol. New England Journal of Medicine 302: 609–613
73. Kaufman RH, Adam E, Binder GL, Gerthoffer E 1980 Upper genital tract changes and pregnancy outcome in offspring exposed in utero to diethylstilbestrol. American Journal of Obstetrics and Gynecology 137: 299–308
74. Kaufman RH, Noller K, Adam E, Irwin J et al 1984 Upper genital tract abnormalities and pregnancy outcome in diethylstilbestrol-exposed progeny. American Journal of Obstetrics and Gynecology 148: 973–984
75. Robboy SJ, Toguchi O, Cunha GR 1982 Normal development of the human female reproductive tract and alterations resulting from experimental exposure to diethylstilbestrol. Human Pathology 13: 190–198
76. Herbst AL, Hubby MM, Blough RR, Azizi F 1980 A comparison of pregnancy experience in DES-exposed and DES-unexposed daughters. Journal of Reproductive Medicine 24: 62–69
77. Kaufman RH, Adam E, Noller K, Irwin JF, Gray M 1986 Upper genital tract changes and infertility in diethylstilbestrol-exposed women. American Journal of Obstetrics and Gynecology 154: 1312–1318
78. Noller K, Melton JL, O'Brien PC et al 1990 Medical and surgical diseases associated with in utero exposure to DES. Clinical Practice in Gynecology 2: 1–4
79. Gufstavson C, Gufstavson J, Noller KL, O'Brien PC et al 1991 Increased risk of profound weight loss among women exposed to diethylstilbestrol in utero. Behavioral and Neural Biology 55: 307–312

80. Newbold RR 1993 Gender-related behavior in women exposed prenatally to diethylstilbestrol. Environmental Health Perspectives 101: 208–213
81. Meyer-Bahlburg HFL, Ehrhardt AA, Rosen LR et al 1995 Prenatal estrogens and the development of homosexual orientation. Developmental Psychology 31: 12–15
82. Pillard RC, Rosen LR, Meyer-Bahlburg H et al 1993 Psychopathology and social functioning in men prenatally exposed to diethylstilbestrol. Psychosomatic Medicine 55: 485–491
83. Hileman B 1994 Environmental estrogens linked to reproductive abnormalities. Cancer Chemotherapy and Engemia News 2: 19
84. Greenberg ER, Barnes AB, Resseguie L, Barrett JA et al 1984 Breast cancer in mothers given diethylstilbestrol in pregnancy. New England Journal of Medicine 311: 1393–1398
85. Colton T, Greenberg ER, Noller K, Resseguie L, Van Bennekom C, Heeren T, Zhang Y 1993 Breast cancer in mothers prescribed diethylstilbestrol in pregnancy. Further follow-up. Journal of the American Medical Association 269: 2096–2100 [Review]
86. Wilcox AJ, Baird DD, Weinberg CR, Hornsby PP, Herbst AL 1995 Fertility in men exposed prenatally to diethylstilbestrol. New England Journal of Medicine 332: 1411–1416

44. Clinical aspects of oral contraception

Elizabeth B. Connell

Introduction and historical overview

Despite conventional wisdom to the contrary, contraception and family planning are not the creations of recent generations. Many ancient medical documents have shown that people have always had a strong desire to plan the number and the timing of their children.[1] At some unknown point in time, they apparently correctly concluded that there was a relationship between the male ejaculate and the subsequent development and birth of an infant. Ancient peoples did not know what the factor was that caused this; this was not clear until the Dutch microscopist, Leeuwenhoek, reported seeing sperm in human seminal fluid thousands of years later, in 1677. However, their basic assumption was correct and medical history records an amazing series of contraceptive techniques that our ancestors developed over the centuries.[2]

Folklore from many parts of the world is replete with fascinating and creative approaches that women used to try to avoid unwanted pregnancies. This includes such things as sneezing and jumping backwards after sexual intercourse, burning moxa-balls on their navels and wearing tubes around their waists containing the testicles of a cat or part of the uterus of a lioness. Ancient societies also recognized the necessity of keeping the ejaculate out of the vagina and, therefore, created a number of extremely interesting and exotic barrier techniques. Primary among these were numerous types of pessaries, the first being noted in the Petri Papyrus from Ancient Egypt in 1850 BC. The pessaries were frequently concocted from the dung of strong and powerful animals, such as the elephant and crocodile, to which was added honey, pomegranate pulp, gallnut, whitewash, cedarwood oil, sulfur, tar, alum, quinine and a wide variety of other plant and animal products. The right testicle of a wolf, sponges, balls of oiled silk paper, linen and feathers were also used. Casanova had gold balls made, 18 mm in diameter; he placed these in the vaginas of his many sexual partners prior to intercourse. Each one was said to last for 15 years, although their actual effectiveness remains unknown.

It is particularly interesting, in reviewing the various methods that were devised, to see how many actually made biologic sense and have their modern counterparts in methods we use today. One such example was the placement of half of a lemon in the upper vagina to cover the cervix. Not only was this a barrier but we now recognize that the juice of the lemon, being highly acidic, was undoubtedly spermicidal. Similarly, vaginal fumigation with the smoke of neem wood wax and charcoal, using a special kettle with a long spout, and postcoital douches of wine, garlic, fennel and vinegar administered through tubes of wood and ivory, were undoubtedly also spermicidal. Condoms actually date back to prehistoric times, and pictures of them can be seen drawn on the walls of ancient cave dwellers. The earliest condoms were made from plant materials which were shaped like a pea pod, and from silk and linen. In addition, the bladders of various animals and the caecum of a sheep were commonly employed.

The lengths to which people would go to avoid unwanted pregnancies were also remarkable. Some of the methods that they tried were extremely dangerous and a few were actually lethal. In the Middle Ages many fatalities resulted from the use of agents such as arsenic, lead, copper, iodine and strychnine that women swallowed in their attempts to prevent pregnancy or to induce abortion. Numerous devices, made from a wide variety of materials, were also employed in desperate attempts to interrupt established pregnancies. These were inserted blindly through the vagina and, as would be expected, often resulted in hemorrhage, infection and death. One particularly hazardous technique reported in the ancient medical literature was the jumping up and down on the abdomens of women in an attempt to destroy whatever organs within were essential to the production of pregnancy or to try to produce an abortion.

In more modern times, certain events in the development of new materials and the expansion of medical knowledge have both impacted very heavily on the advances made in contraceptive methods. The vulcanization of rubber made possible today's condoms, diaphragms and cervical caps. The ability to give memory to plastic led to the development of our modern intrauterine devices. The major advances made in our knowledge about the functions of both the male and female reproductive tracts have also contributed greatly to improved methods of fertility regulation. Finally, new information about the roles of the various endocrine organs has permitted the evolution of not only the hormonal methods that we have today but also a number that are currently being developed for use in the future.

CLINICAL CONSIDERATIONS

Medical history

At the time of the first visit of a woman who is seeking advice on contraception, it is essential to obtain a very thorough history.[3] This history has two key components: the first part is medical, the second is personal. The most important medical facts include her age, obstetrical, gynecologic and contraceptive history, and specific diseases, both past and present, that she either has or has had that might impact on the proper choice of a birth control method. These conditions include such things as sexually transmitted diseases (STDs), cardiovascular, liver, renal and breast disease, hypertension, biliary tract disorders and problems related to hemoglobinopathies. In addition to her own medical history, it is also important to elicit any major medical problems that run in her family, particularly those related to cardiovascular diseases and malignancies.

The ascertainment of her personal history is of equal or perhaps even greater importance. Factors of key significance in this instance include the patient's plans regarding future pregnancy, her attitude toward her own sexuality, her general levels of motivation and her reliability in her previous use of medications. Above all, information about certain behavioral patterns with regards to smoking, drinking and substance abuse, and particularly her sexual behavior, including the number of her sexual partners, must be elicited in an empathetic and nonjudgmental fashion.

Examinations

Following this, a complete physical examination should be performed, placing particular emphasis on her breasts (including breast self-exam) and pelvic organs. Laboratory testing should also be carried out whenever possible, including a complete blood count, hematocrit, Papanicolaou smear, smear for gonorrhea, and tests for chlamydia and HIV/AIDS. Depending on the patient's history and the results of her examinations, additional laboratory tests or other studies should be ordered if indicated.

Counseling

Prior to the selection of a specific method of contraception, it is important that a woman be made aware of all of the currently available options. She must be informed about certain key factors regarding each method — its effectiveness, advantages and disadvantages, safety in terms of anticipated side effects, and whether or not it has additional health benefits such as prevention of the transmission of STDs.

Having made a selection, it is essential that extensive counseling in the use of this particular technique be carried out. There is growing evidence that compliance and continuation rates are very strongly influenced not only by the method per se, but also by the accuracy and empathy of the counseling given to an individual prior to her beginning the use of her method.[4] She must be able to distinguish between side effects that are annoying but not significant in terms of being a risk to her health and those that are highly significant and mandate an immediate call for medical attention. In addition, she must be told how to cope with minor side effects and how long she may expect to experience them. Finally, a return schedule should be outlined and the patient encouraged to return at periodic intervals for evaluation and additional information. Continued counseling is of major importance in obtaining proper compliance, particularly in the case of adolescents.[5]

Effectiveness

Contraceptive effectiveness data are traditionally reported using a three classification system. It is essential to recognize that when the various contraceptive methods are being compared, the type of classification for the data for each must be the same if one is to obtain valid comparisons.[3] It must also be recognized that the effectiveness of certain methods, most notably the barrier techniques, may be considerably enhanced by the concurrent use of more than one agent.

The first type of classification — method or theoretical effectiveness — is the rate achieved with correct and consistent use. The second — use effectiveness — is the rate achieved with average use, including both correct and incorrect use. The third — extended use effectiveness — applies to those rates that are achieved once the product is in a postmarketing situation, i.e. extensively used, both correctly and incorrectly, by a wide variety of individuals.[3]

ORAL CONTRACEPTIVES

Background

Hormonal methods of contraception have been and continue to be among our most effective means of preventing unwanted pregnancies. It is fortuitous that when the female sex steroids were being studied as potential fertility-enhancers, it was noted that exactly the opposite was the case — they produced infertility by blocking ovulation. This observation has led to the introduction of a number of hormonal fertility-regulation techniques over the past 30 years and more. Originally approved as oral agents, several other forms of administration have since been developed.[6]

Types of formulations

At the present time there are two major categories of oral contraceptives (OC): the combined pills (COC) and the progestogen-only pills. The original oral contraceptives were the combined monophasic pills, using an estrogen and a progestogen in a number of different formulations. The dosages of both hormones were much higher than those in use today and remained constant throughout the 21 day pill cycle. Next, in order of development, were the sequential pills — estrogen alone followed by estrogen plus a progestogen — ostensibly to simulate the normal menstrual cycle. They were relatively short-lived, being removed from the market based on data from the now-discredited beagle dog and on limited clinical information on the possible induction of endometrial carcinoma. The progestogen-only pill, also known as the mini-pill, is a progestogen given continuously in a low dose with no added estrogen.

The multiphasic COC, both biphasic and triphasic, were developed most recently. These have variable doses of an estrogen and a progestogen, in either two or three different phases. The biphasic COC regimes contain 35 μg of estrogen and a progestogen for 10 days, the progestogen dose being increased for the last 11 days. The triphasic COC have both an estrogen and a progestogen, the dosages varying in the three different phases of the pill cycle. The combined pills are available in 21 or 28 day cycles, the former having 21 days of active therapy followed by a one week pill-free interval and the latter having 21 days of hormone usage followed by seven days with no hormones, during which either iron or a placebo is given.[3]

The oral contraceptives currently available in the United States are listed in Table 44.1.

Mechanism(s) of action

The combination pills work primarily by inhibiting the hypothalamic gonadotropin releasing hormone (GnRH), thus blocking the activity of the pituitary gonadotropins, follicle stimulating hormone (FSH) and luteinizing hormone (LH). This action occurs through a feedback mechanism that suppresses ovulation. The COC also produce thickening of the cervical mucus that helps to inhibit sperm penetration. Finally, the hormonal alterations induced by the COC produce changes in the endometrium that are not conducive to implantation.[3,6]

The progestogen-only pills produce a very inconsistent blockage of ovulation. However, as is the case with all progestogens, they thicken cervical mucus, blocking the penetration of sperm and produce biochemical and physiological changes in the endometrium.[3,6]

Hormonal agents used in COC

The two estrogens that have been used up to the present time in the COC have been ethinyl estradiol (EE) and mestranol.[3,6] In the current pills, EE is far more commonly employed. A number of different progestogens have been used, most of them one of the 19-nortestosterone derivatives. They include norethindrone, ethynodiol diacetate, levonorgestrel, norethindrone acetate and norgestrel. In addition, three new compounds, all derivatives of levonorgestrel, have been studied and marketed in Europe since about 1988; these are desogestrel, gestodene and norgestimate. While these new agents appear to have some advantages in terms of fewer androgenic effects, favorable lipid effects and cycle control, they

Table 44.1 Name and composition of oral contraceptives (USA).

Name	Estrogen	µg	Progestogen	mg	Manufacturer
Brevicon	Ethinyl estradiol	35	Norethindrone	0.5	Syntex
Demulen	Ethinyl estradiol	50	Ethynodiol diacetate	1.0	Searle
Demulen	Ethinyl estradiol	35	Ethynodiol diacetate	1.0	Searle
Genora 1/35	Ethinyl estradiol	35	Norethindrone	1.0	Rugby
Genora 1/50	Mestranol	50	Norethindrone	1.0	Rugby
Jenest-28*	Ethinyl estradiol	35 (21)	Norethindrone	0.5 (7)	Organon
	Ethinyl estradiol	35 (21)	Norethindrone	1.0 (14)	
Levlen	Ethinyl estradiol	30	Levonorgestrel	0.15	Berlex
Loestrin 1.5/30	Ethinyl estradiol	30	Norethindrone acetate	1.5	Parke-Davis
Loestrin 1/20	Ethinyl estradiol	20	Norethindrone acetate	1.0	Parke-Davis
Lo-Ovral	Ethinyl estradiol	30	Norgestrel	0.3	Wyeth
Micronor	None	–	Norethindrone	0.35	Ortho
Modicon	Ethinyl estradiol	35	Norethindrone	0.5	Ortho
NEE 1/35	Ethinyl estradiol	35	Norethindrone	1.0	Lexis
NEE 1/50	Mestranol	50	Norethindrone	1.0	Lexis
Nordette	Ethinyl estradiol	50	Levonorgestrel	0.15	Wyeth
Norinyl 1/35	Ethinyl estradiol	35	Norethindrone	1.0	Syntex
Norinyl 1/50	Mestranol	50	Norethindrone	1.0	Syntex
Norlestrin 1/50	Ethinyl estradiol	50	Norethindrone acetate	1.0	Parke-Davis
Norlestrin 2.5	Ethinyl estradiol	50	Norethindrone acetate	2.5	Parke-Davis
Ortho-Novum 7/7/7*	Ethinyl estradiol	35 (7)	Norethindrone	0.5 (7)	Ortho
	Ethinyl estradiol	35 (7)	Norethindrone	0.75 (7)	
	Ethinyl estradiol	35 (7)	Norethindrone	1.0 (7)	
Ortho-Novum 1/35	Ethinyl estradiol	35	Norethindrone	1.0	Ortho
Ortho-Novum 1/50	Ethinyl estradiol	50	Norethindrone	1.0	Ortho
Ortho-Novum 10/11*	Ethinyl estradiol	35 (10)	Norethindrone	0.5 (10)	Ortho
	Ethinyl estradiol	35 (11)	Norethindrone	1.0 (11)	
Ovcon 35	Ethinyl estradiol	35	Norethindrone	0.4	Mead-Johnson
Ovcon 50	Ethinyl estradiol	50	Norethindrone	1.0	Mead-Johnson
Ovral	Ethinyl estradiol	50	Norgestrel	0.5	Wyeth
Tri-Levlen*	Ethinyl estradiol		Levonorgestrel	0.05 (6)	Berlex
	Ethinyl estradiol		Levonorgestrel	0.075 (5)	
	Ethinyl estradiol		Levonorgestrel	0.125 (10)	
Tri-Norinyl*	Ethinyl estradiol	35 (7)	Norethindrone	0.5 (7)	Syntex
	Ethinyl estradiol	35 (9)	Norethindrone	1.0 (9)	
	Ethinyl estradiol	35 (5)	Norethindrone	0.5 (5)	
Triphasil*	Ethinyl estradiol	30 (6)	Levonorgestrel	0.05 (6)	Wyeth
	Ethinyl estradiol	40 (5)	Levonorgestrel	0.075 (5)	
	Ethinyl estradiol	30 (10)	Levonorgestrel	0.125 (10)	

*Multiphasic product. The number in parenthesis indicates the number of days pills are taken in days each phase of the cycle.

apparently do not represent quantum differences from those currently available.[3,6]

Effectiveness

The method effectiveness rates of the combined pills approach 99%, use-effectiveness rates ranging from the upper 80s to 96%. The mini-pill has a method effectiveness rate of 97% with use-effectiveness rates from the lower 80 s to 92%.[3]

Potency

There has been considerable debate in recent years about the issue of drug potency.[6] Originally, EE was felt to be almost twice as potent as mestranol. However, it now appears that there is no major difference between the two when dosage adjustments are made.

The potency of the various progestogens has been measured in both animals and humans, individual studies showing considerable variation. However, there are major problems in the original concepts about progestogen potency and the subject has fallen somewhat into confusion and disrepute. The potency of a progestogen depends not only on the particular compound being studied but also on the dose, rate and route of administration, and the target organ being evaluated. It is still not generally recognized that the measurement of the potency of a progestogen in one target organ does not necessarily mean that it will have the same degree of impact on all other body tissues. Moreover, when studying a combined medication, one must assess simultaneously the effects of both of the hormonal components in order to determine accurately the overall impact of the drug on the various body organs. It is therefore impossible to measure the potencies of the two components separately and then combine the results, since synergism or antagonism may occur.[3]

Although animal data have been used extensively in the evaluation of progestogen potency, these pose serious problems because of the proven lack of ability to transfer animal data directly to the human. There are major variations from one species to another and even within a single species when such tests as pregnancy maintenance and histology of the reproductive tract are performed. Also, many animal studies have been carried out, particularly ones looking for adverse affects, in dosages considerably higher than those used in studies in the human female.[3]

Noncontraceptive health benefits

Background

Discussions of the oral contraceptives have often started with an elaboration of their potential adverse effects. Given the current state of our knowledge regarding these preparations, this approach no longer seems to be appropriate. Probably the most important information regarding COC that has been accumulated in recent years is that related to the progressive enumeration of their multiple noncontraceptive health benefits.[7–10] These include benefits related to both the improved quality of life and also to the prevention of certain major life-threatening diseases. In fact, for healthy, nonsmoking women, the health benefits clearly outweigh the very minimal health risks associated with the use of low dose COC.

Quality of life benefits

Cycle control. A number of the problems that women experience that are related to their menstrual cycles are helped by the use of the pill. For example, COC have been shown to decrease the amount of uterine bleeding, both intermenstrual bleeding and excessive menses. Often pre-existing menorrhagia will improve and as a result, oral contraceptives help to prevent or ameliorate iron deficiency anemia. Moreover, oral contraceptives frequently convert irregular to regular cycles. Unfortunately, there are new data on cycle control in COC users who smoke that show just the opposite — unfortunate given the increasing rates of smoking today by women, particularly younger women. In addition to the growing incidence of malignancies, deaths from lung cancer now exceeding those from breast cancer, there is well documented cardiovascular, pulmonary and reproductive damage. To this lengthening list must now be added adverse effects on cycle control. Current research suggests that smoking has antiestrogen effects, possibly caused by excessive estrogen catabolism, which are responsible for menstrual problems as well as infertility and early menopause.[11]

Dysmenorrhea. Primary dysmenorrhea also tends to be improved, a matter of great importance, especially to teenage girls. Studies have shown that close to 60% of adolescent girls suffer from dysmenorrhea, 10–15% of whom miss school as a consequence. It is believed that the mechanism of action in this instance is the blocking of ovulation by the use of COC.[3]

Premenstrual tension syndrome. In addition, COC have been noted to reduce premenstrual tension syndrome in some instances. The reason for this decrease in some women and not others remains unclear.

Ovarian cysts/benign breast disease. The risks of developing two other conditions, not life-threatening but quite common and often requiring hospitalization — functional ovarian cysts and benign breast disease — are now well documented to be reduced by the use of COC. In both instances, the prevention appears to be due to the suppression of activity, in the first instance of the ovary and in the second, of the proliferation of breast tissue that is found in the first part of an ovulatory cycle.

The lowered risk of functional ovarian cysts has been demonstrated in several epidemiologic studies.[9] It was estimated in 1983 that 3500 hospitalizations for this condition were averted by COC use.[7] However, in 1987 an anecdotal paper, a case series report on seven patients, described the development of these cysts in patients on phasic pills.[12] In response, a study was carried out in 1989 looking at hospitalizations for this diagnosis and use of phasic pills; no such association was found.[13] In 1992, a case control study was reported, also showing no increased risk.[14]

There is also a lowered incidence of both fibroadenomas and fibrocystic disease of the breast in all age groups.[3] The effect is noted after the first year of pill-taking and lasts at least one year after discontinuation. The lowering of risk appears to be greater with increasing doses of the progestogen and with increasing duration of use. It has been estimated that 23 490 hospitalizations for benign breast disease are prevented annually by COC use.[7] As will be discussed later, the ultimate impact of pill use on the development of breast malignancy remains unknown.

Other possible health benefits

There is also preliminary evidence that the use of the COC may help to reduce the risks of toxic shock syndrome (TSS), endometriosis, uterine fibroids and rheumatoid arthritis. Finally, COC may also protect against the bone loss that occurs in women in their 30s and 40s. The effects are related to the dose of estrogen and the duration of use.[15] If future studies confirm this finding, it could be highly significant since 20 million women in the United States alone have this disease, resulting in more than a million fractures per year and many deaths from hip fractures.[15]

Life-threatening disease benefits

Pelvic inflammatory disease

Despite fears to the contrary, the use of COC by young women may have a positive impact on their future fertility, inasmuch as the incidence of endometriosis, pelvic inflammatory diseases (PID) and ectopic pregnancy are decreased.[3] Since all of these conditions are increasing in incidence in the 15–24 year age group, a lowered risk is highly significant. It has been reported that 15 595 hospitalizations for PID are averted annually by COC use — a 50% reduction. For women using the pill for at least one year, the decrease was 70%.[7] COC have also been shown to decrease the risk of gonorrhea and/or chlamydial salpingitis.[8,16]

This protection against PID is believed to be due to the thickening of cervical mucus induced by the progestogen and also by atrophic changes in the endometrium. In addition, the decreased amount of menstrual blood available to support the growth of pathogenic organisms is probably another key factor since, as has been noted, the pill decreases total blood flow and the duration of flow.[3] However, it is important to counsel women that COC offer no protection against the transmission of the viral sexually transmitted diseases (STDs), including HIV/AIDS. Therefore it is essential that those at high risk for STDs be told to use condoms in addition to their oral contraceptives.

Ectopic pregnancy

Since ovulation does not occur, there is a lowered risk of ectopic pregnancy in pill-takers, the current risk now being assumed to be virtually nonexistent.[9] It has been estimated that 11 695 hospitalizations for ectopic pregnancy are averted each year with pill use.[7] The incidence of this condition continues to rise in the United States, in part due to growing epidemics of PID. Thus, the lowered risk with COC use of both PID and ectopic pregnancy could make a major contribution to lowering the rates of both morbidity and mortality.

Ovarian cancer (see also chapter 67)

The most lethal gynecologic malignancy in women is ovarian cancer, 26 700 new cases and 14 800 deaths being estimated for 1996.[17] Ovarian cancer is now the fourth leading cause of cancer deaths in American women. This cancer is notoriously difficult to diagnose and treat, 60–80% of women only becoming symptomatic because of metastatic spread of the disease. Because of this, death rates are virtually the same as they were in 1930, five-year survivals being only 40%. Thus, it is highly important to note that it has been estimated that 1700 cases of ovarian cancer are averted each year by the use of COC, possibly because of the suppression of 'incessant ovulation'.[7]

The amount of protection increases with increasing duration of use and is greater for nulliparous than parous women.[8] As regards duration of use, the protection goes from three to 11 months, a 30% reduction; from one to two years, 20%; from three to four years, 50%; and at five years, 60%. The amount of protection also varies with the number of pregnancies, i.e. no full term pregnancies, 70%; one to two full term pregnancies, 20%; and more than three, 30%. Data from the Cancer and Steroid Hormone (CASH) study at the Centers for Disease Control (CDC) indicate that this protection continues for at least 15 years after stopping COC use, the end of their current data set with an overall reduction of 40% in 'ever users'.[18]

All four major ovarian epithelial tumors are reduced similarly in risk — mucinous, serous, clear cell and endometroid.[19] In addition, low-dose pills appear to offer the same level of protection as high-dose COC. Given the insidious nature of this disease and its high mortality, this particular health benefit is probably the most important discovered to date.

Endometrial cancer (see also chapter 67)

The most common gynecologic malignancy in women is carcinoma of the endometrium, 34 000 new cases and 6000 deaths being estimated for 1996.[17] It is important to note, parenthetically, that equivalent rates for lung cancer are estimated to be 78 100 new cases and 64 300 deaths in 1996.[17] Two thousand hospitalizations for endometrial cancer are averted each year with COC use.[7] The risk with use of the pill decreases 50% after a year of use and goes up to 66% after five years of use; the protection is greatest in the nulliparous women. The effect lasts, as in the case of ovarian cancer, for at least 15 years after stopping the COC.[20]

All three major types of endometrial cancer are equally reduced in risk — adenocarcinoma, adenoacanthoma and adenosquamous cancer. The reduction is probably mediated by the progestogen in the pill, and is 50% in 'ever users'.[21] All of the current COC formulations appear to produce equal degrees of protection.[19]

Adverse side effects

Background

Side effects of the oral contraceptives have traditionally been divided into minor (nonserious, annoying) and major (serious, life-threatening) categories.[3] However, it has become clear over the years that the so-called minor side effects actually have major effects on compliance and continuation rates.[4] Therefore, it is essential, as was previously pointed out, that initial counseling on pill use be very explicit about what symptoms a woman might expect to experience, how long they might last and what to do about them.

Minor side effects

Skin changes. Use of the oral contraceptives has been shown to produce changes in a number of body organs including the skin. Some patients find that pre-existing acne is improved because estrogens reduce sebin production. On the other hand, the progestogen in the pill may make acne worse in others. To date, the Food and Drug Administration (FDA) has not approved use of the COC for the treatment of acne, although it is sometimes very effective.

Chloasma, or the mask of pregnancy, may occur in some women, particularly those who have had this problem during pregnancy. It is important to recognize that this particular complication often does not disappear entirely, even after stopping the pill.[3,6]

Gastrointestinal changes. Nausea with occasional vomiting may occur with the use of COC. These symptoms are more commonly seen in the early months of pill-taking and usually do not continue to occur in subsequent cycles. It has often been found to be helpful for individuals with this problem to take their COC with food about the time that they go to bed, so that their symptoms will occur primarily during sleep.

Breast changes. There are a number of changes women may notice in their breasts, particularly early in the use of the pill. Some will experience tenderness, even pain, and cyclic enlargement of their breasts. Again, these symptoms are more common in the first few months and tend to disappear with time.

Galactorrhea has been noted on occasion during the administration of COC. This, however, should not be considered to be normal and mandates medical evaluation for other potentially serious causes such as a local breast lesion or a pituitary microadenoma.

Reproductive tract changes

Uterus. As previously noted, the amount of bleeding with the use of COC tends to decrease, as does the incidence of intermenstrual spotting. On occasion this may progress to amenorrhea due to the lack of hormonal stimulation to develop the blood vessels and stroma of the endometrium. Amenorrhea is not an immediate cause for concern if the patient is known, with assurity, to have taken her pills properly. However, after two missed withdrawal bleeding episodes, she should be evaluated for accidental pregnancy. If this is found not to be the case, it is usually recommended that the same preparation be used for several more cycles. It has also been suggested that supplemental estrogen can be tried during this time. When consistent failure to withdraw continues, it is sometimes necessary to move to a pill with a higher estrogen content.[3]

As a result of the impact of the COC on the endometrium, it is also possible that abnormal bleeding may occur, the most common types being excessive withdrawal bleeding and breakthrough bleeding (BTB) and/or spotting during the taking of the active hormone part of the pill cycle.[3] These problems are believed to be due to inadequate hormonal support to the endometrial tissues. If the bleeding is mild, it is usually advisable to continue with the same COC for several more cycles. If it is persistent and/or severe, however, it may be necessary to increase the estrogen dose or to try temporary supplemental estrogen if the bleeding occurs in the early part of the cycle. If it occurs toward the end of the cycle, it may be necessary to increase the amount of progestogen in the pill being administered. If these measures prove to be unsuccessful, local pathology must be ruled out. On occasion, failure to have withdrawal bleeding may occur in conjunction with BTB.[6]

The growth and carneous degeneration of pre-existing leiomyomata, similar to that seen with pregnancy, were not uncommon with use of the earlier high-dose COC. However, this situation is uncommon with the current low dose pills, and is not now a serious cause for concern.[3] As noted previously, there may actually be a reduced risk of developing fibroids during COC use.

Cervix. Changes are also frequently noted in the cervix of a woman using COC. The development of polyploid hyperplasia and hypertrophy are commonly observed, resulting from the hormonal stimulus of the pill. Cervical mucus becomes much thicker, gray and more tenacious, very similar to that seen during the luteal phase of the cycle due to the presence of progesterone. These alterations are believed to help to block the penetration of sperm, a major mechanism of action of the mini-pill. They may well also be responsible for the blockage of certain pathogenic organisms, leading to the lower risk of certain STDs, mentioned as one of the noncontraceptive benefits of COC use.[3,6,16]

Vagina. COC also produce changes in the vagina. Some women notice an increase in vaginal secretions, occasionally quite marked, due to the administered estrogen. This complaint was particularly common when sequential pills were being used, as estrogen was unopposed during the first part of the pill cycle. However, the addition of a progestogen tends to decrease this effect.[3]

Ovary. With continued use of the combined pill, the ovaries become smaller and more atrophic. In the early years of pill use, concern was expressed that the ovarian follicles would be rendered quiescent, beginning their development only after stopping the COC, resulting in midlife pregnancies. However, it is now clear that there is continued maturation of follicles but this is not usually accompanied, except for the mini-pill, by ovulation and the subsequent formation of corpora lutea. As previously noted, there is an overall decrease in functional ovarian cysts. Even though some follicles do undergo development, they rarely reach a size that is clinically significant, most of them becoming atretic.

The current combination COC are highly effective in blocking ovulation, resulting in very few intrauterine gestations and a decreased risk of ectopic pregnancy. On the other hand, the mini-pill has consistently shown a higher intrauterine pregnancy rate and a somewhat higher rate of ectopic pregnancy, possibly due to changes in tubal tissues and/or transport along with the inconsistent suppression of ovulation.

Biliary tract changes

Biliary tract changes have been noted for many years in women taking COC. Estrogens are known to decrease the amount of bile salts that act to keep lipids in solution.[6] Although it was originally felt that cholelithiasis was an adverse effect of the pill and that it came on only after several years of use, it is currently believed that this complication occurs almost entirely in susceptible individuals and usually during the first year of use. Longer use does not appear to produce a net increase in incidence.[3]

Many studies have been conducted on the various oral contraceptives, evaluating their potential impact on liver function. Alterations appear to be minimal with the currently used COC if no liver disease is present. Those individuals with a history of benign cholestatic jaundice of pregnancy are subject to a recurrence with oral contraceptive use. If this complication is going to occur, it usually does so in the first six cycles of use as the result of plugging of bile canaliculi.[6] The jaundice disappears after discontinuation of COC use and leaves no sequelae.[3] The use of the mini-pill may be tried in such patients.[6]

Although uncommon, hepatic artery thrombosis has been observed with pill use, leading to hepatic infarction. In addition, thrombosis of the portal vein and hepatic vein (Budd-Chiari syndrome) have been reported in the medical literature.[6]

The potential for the development of both benign and malignant liver tumors has also been looked at in great detail. The production of a benign tumor, the hepatocellular adenoma (HCA), has been documented. It is uncommon, occurring at a rate of 3.4/100 000 users.[3] Although pathologically benign, this tumor is very vascular and, on occasion, its rupture has produced serious intraperitoneal hemorrhage, requiring emergency surgery, and in a few cases massive bleeding from the tumor has been fatal. HCAs tend to occur after five or more years of use and are more common in women over the age of 30. These tumors are frequently palpable on routine physical examination. They regress when oral contraceptive use is stopped.[3]

There has been considerable debate over the years as to whether or not use of the COC would lead to liver cancer. International data have been difficult to evaluate because of the known association between hepatocellular carcinoma (HCC) and infections with the hepatitis B virus and exposure to aflatoxin.[6] HCC is extremely rare in the United States. Moreover, a large case-control WHO study published in 1989 found no association between the use of combined COC and liver cancer.[22]

Metabolic changes

Carbohydrates. When the earlier high-dose pills were first studied, it was apparent that they had an impact on carbohydrate metabolism, the amount of the impact being related primarily to the dose and potency of the progestogen. In many patients abnormal glucose tolerance tests and elevated serum insulin levels were found as well as changes in the binding affinity of insulin receptors. Estrogens appeared to have little effect on carbohydrate metabolism, even in high doses. Progestogens, on the other hand, decreased insulin receptors and insulin binding and increased insulin resistance.[3]

These alterations generated considerable concern as to whether or not they would lead to premature atherosclerosis and cardiovascular disease (CVD) and to changes in the islet cells of the pancreas, resulting in diabetes mellitus. A number of studies evaluated these hypotheses. Even with high-dose pills, no long-term damage was sustained in normal women who had had an abnormal one hour glucose screening test.[6] One study, based on 317 000 women-years of observation in Great Britain, found no differences in the occurrence of diabetes mellitus when comparing current and past COC users and those who had never taken the pill.[23] Patients with insulin-dependent diabetes similarly showed no adverse effects, some even improving.

Evaluations with low-dose combination and multiphasic COC also showed few or no changes, none at the level of clinical significance.[24] Minor changes were seen with the mini-pill, again, none of which would be a cause for concern.[6]

Lipids. Lipid values were also changed by the use of the high-dose pills. Estrogens were found to increase triglycerides and high density lipoproteins (HDL). Progestogens, on the other hand, decreased HDL, increased very low density lipoproteins (VLDL) and low density lipoproteins (LDL), and decreased the HDL/LDL ratio. The degree of change was found to be directly related to the dosage and potency of the progestogen.[25,26] In general, changes in lipid values varied during the hormonal pill dates, but within normal limits, going back to pretreatment levels during the pill-free week. The mini-pill, being a progestogen-only product, produced very similar but minimal changes.[3,25]

Considerable research has been carried out attempting to evaluate the potential impact of these changes, in particular lipoproteins. It is recognized that HDL is, in general, protective against atherogenesis because it removes cholesterol from cells. VLDL and LDL, on the contrary, take cholesterol to the cells and therefore have an adverse effect, leading to the development of degenerative changes. However, inasmuch as most of the studies on the new lower-dose COC have demonstrated very little, if any, impact on lipids, it is reasonable to conclude that these alterations need not continue to be major concerns for the average healthy woman using COC.[3,6]

Endocrine changes

Background. It has been found that the use of COC produces changes in a number of tests of endocrine function. However, it is important to recognize that most of these are minor, transient and of no clinical significance.[3] Previously, it was feared that these alterations might signal significant impacts on the various target organs, but this was not the case.

Thyroid. Estrogens have been shown to increase thyroid binding globulin (TBG), protein bound iodine (PBI), butanol-extractable iodine (BEI), and bound thyroxin (T4) uptake. They also induce a decrease in triiodothyronine (T3) uptake. These thyroid tests are essentially back to normal one to two months after stopping oral contraceptive usage. No changes have been noted in basal metabolic rate (BMR), T^{131} uptake and unbound thyroxin (T4).

Despite these changes in thyroid tests, believed to be due to the increased hepatic synthesis stimulated by estrogen, there is no evidence that COC use produces clinical thyroid dysfunction. Blood levels, like the thyroid tests, usually return to normal two to three months after discontinuing therapy.[3,6]

Adrenal cortex. As in the case of the thyroid, estrogens increase the synthesis of certain proteins by the liver. Corticosteroid-binding globulin and transcortin levels are increased. This, in turn, produces an increase in serum protein-bound cortisol and free cortisol. On the other hand, COC decrease clearance of urinary metabolites, cortisol metabolite excretion and the response to metyrapone tests.[3] These tests also revert to normal one to two months after stopping use of the COC. No changes have been observed in the adrenal corticotropic hormone (ACTH) stimulation test or in clinical adrenal function. The mini-pill and combined pills containing 20 g of estrogen have not been shown to induce changes in tests of adrenal function.[6]

Anterior pituitary. As previously noted, the major mechanism of action of COC is the blocking of ovulation by the hormonal feedback suppression of the gonadotrophic releasing factors. This suppression appears to be dose-related and to impact LH secretion more than FSH secretion.[6] Pituitary function returns to normal within days after stopping the administration of COC. However, the return of ovulation may be somewhat slower, and appears to be dose-related. There was considerable debate several years ago about whether or not COC increased the risk of developing pituitary microadenomas. It is currently believed that pills do not initiate the development of these lesions. However, a pre-existing tumor may be stimulated to grow by administration of COC.

Weight changes. Women using COC usually undergo no major changes in body weight, despite the fact that it is a common misconception, especially among teenagers, that the pill will make them fat. Investigators have shown that a small percentage of women gain weight and an equally small number lose weight. In general, large amounts of weight gain are almost always traceable to greatly increased food intake.[3]

Depression. It has been shown in a number of studies that depression is rare with COC use by emotionally stable women. However, there are certain groups of individuals who have been found to be at increased risk of developing significant depressive episodes. These are patients with a prior history of severe depression, psychiatric disorders or postpartum depression.[3]

Libido. Many studies have looked at this very complicated subject, attempting to ascertain whether or not COC usage has any impact on libido. It appears that some women experience an increase in libido; this is suggested by the documented increased frequency of sexual intercourse once pill use is begun. However, it has also been recognized that this effect may be due not to the pill, but to the release of anxiety because of the decreased risk of unplanned/unwanted pregnancy. Libido may actually be decreased in some patients, but in these instances it is very often found to be associated with depression and/or the psychosexual conflicts of that particular woman.[3]

MAJOR SIDE EFFECTS

Cardiovascular disease

Hypertension

Hypertension has been found to be associated, on occasion, with the use of COC. It is currently defined as a blood pressure of more than 160 mmHg systolic and 90–100 mmHg diastolic. Hypertension in pill users may occur in one of two forms, the first being the acute form. This particular complication is rare; it usually occurs early in use, often is quite severe and is usually symptomatic. Chronic low grade hypertension is far more common. It tends to occur after several months of administration; it is usually not symptomatic. The elevations in blood pressure in this case are usually mild, in the order of 1–10 mmHg, the values still remaining within normal limits for both systolic and diastolic pressures.[3]

In looking at the etiology of hypertension it needs to be recognized that blood pressure is regulated by two systems that are opposing. First, the liver, stimulated by estrogen, produces angiotensinogen. This is converted to angiotensin which, in turn, constricts blood vessels and raises blood pressure. Second, blood vessels produce prostacycline, particularly under the stimulus of the progestogen component. This opposes angiotensin and produces vasodilation.[3]

In normal women, these two opposing systems remain in balance and, as a result, they do not become hypertensive. In women with abnormal vasculature, however, several events occur. These individuals cannot increase their prostacycline production, therefore, the opposing systems go out of balance and hypertension is the result. This effect is due to both the estrogen and the progestogen, but the progestogen is probably the more important.[3]

The risk of developing hypertension is low in normal women, particularly since the transition to the use of low-dose pills. The likelihood of developing this complication is increased by increasing duration of use and by increasing age. Although it was previously felt that the risk of COC-induced hypertension was greater in women who had had pre-eclampsia, this is no longer believed to be the case.[3]

As far as COC use is concerned, hypertension of 160/100 is usually considered to be an absolute contraindication; milder levels of hypertension are a relative contraindication. Women who are normotensive only because they are taking antihypertensive agents must also be considered to be at somewhat greater risk. If pills are used in this situation and a patient's blood pressure increases, the pills should be stopped.[3]

The long-term clinical significance of a mild but sustained hypertension remains unknown, but its presence does not necessitate discontinuation. Once COC use is stopped, the blood pressure virtually always returns to normal levels within one to three months, demonstrating a cause-and-effect relationship. When severe hypertension develops, this indicates an idiosyncratic reaction and mandates immediate cessation of COC use. Prior oral contraceptive users show no increased incidence of hypertension when followed over a period of time after stopping use of the pill.[3,6]

Thromboembolic disease

Both venous thrombosis and pulmonary embolism have been shown to be associated with pill use. These adverse effects are due primarily to the estrogen component. Estrogens act on the liver and induce changes in the proteins controlling coagulation, resulting in increased levels of factor VII and fibrinogen, and in increased platelet adhesiveness and blood viscosity. In addition, antithrombin III activity and red cell filterability are decreased. The impact of these multiple changes produces an increased tendency for clotting and a decreased ability to dissolve clots.[3]

The risk of a normal woman developing thromboembolic complications using the current low-dose preparations is low. It is increased by major surgery and prolonged immobilization. These complications are more common in women who have a personal or family history of thromboembolic disease. The risk does not appear to increase with increasing age or duration of use. It has now been convincingly demonstrated that many of the earlier reports of higher rates of arterial thromboembolic disease in pill-users were actually related primarily to smoking, not to COC use per se.[10,27,28]

Up until the present time there has been no way to screen and select out specific women who might be at risk for thromboembolic complications other than by history. A new possible etiologic factor for certain cases of venous thrombosis has recently been identified, i.e. poor anticoagulant response to activated protein C (APC).[29-31] It begins to appear that abnormalities in the anticoagulant protein C pathway may explain the high prevalence of venous thrombosis in the majority of thrombophilic patients.[29] It has been documented to occur in certain families; the resistance appears to be transmitted as an autosomal dominant trait.[30] It was concluded in the Leiden Thrombophilia Study that poor response to the APC is the single most important hereditary etiology in cases of venous thrombosis, and it was recommended that it should be tested for in all thrombosis patients.[31]

Women must be made aware of the symptoms that may be related to the development of thromboembolic conditions. These include visual disturbances, sudden severe headaches, chest pain, cough, hemoptysis, abdominal pain, and pain and swelling of the legs. If one of these symptoms should occur, it is important for them to stop the pills immediately and seek medical care.[6]

When individuals taking COC are going to be immobilized or have major elective surgery, it is wise to stop the pill a month in advance and use another form of contraception, only returning to COC use a month after surgery or immobilization, or when the patient has become fully ambulatory. When emergency surgery must be carried out on women using the pill, the best current advice is to stop the pill, institute microheparinization and restart the pill one month after surgery or when the patient is fully ambulatory.[3]

Recent developments regarding venous thromboembolism

Since the end of 1994, there has been a steady stream of publications exploring different aspects of the phenomenon of venous thromboembolism (VTE) in women using different oral contraceptives. An association between COC and VTE has been recognized since the early 1960s,[32] but more recent epidemological research has demonstrated that the relative risk of VTE is only slightly increased over the normal population in women using modern very low-dose COC.[33,34] A recent surge of interest in this rare hazard of COC use has been stimulated by the publication of four papers[35-38] all demonstrating a small but significant increase in relative risk of VTE (RR = 1.4 to 2.2) in users of the third generation COC (containing the progestogens desogestrel, gestodene and norgestimate) compared with second generation users. This finding was sensationalized by the Committee for the Safety of Medicines in the United Kingdom when it made an unequivocal statement that COC containing the third generation progestogens should no longer be routinely prescribed. This statement was issued prior to publication of the data, when the committee was also aware that two of the studies had not been completed. The great majority of other drug regulatory bodies were much more circumspect and urged caution in the interpretation of these preliminary findings.

Since these publications and the storm of subsequent critical correspondence in the columns of the medical journals, especially *The Lancet*, it has become clear that a number of additional factors need to be taken into account in determining the accuracy and the importance of these reports. First, there are several reports which point to selective prescribing (because they were perceived to be safer) of the third generation COC to women who may have higher pre-existing risks for VTE (e.g. first time users, women in the older reproductive years and women with pre-existing medical conditions) which might interact with any COC. Very recent data suggest that VTE risks are no different for first time users of different pills.[39] Secondly, users of the third generation COC may have a significantly reduced risk of myocardial infarction (both fatal and nonfatal).[40] Interestingly, one of the main reasons for introduction of the more expensive third generation COC was the expectation that their 'beneficial' effects on parameters of lipid and carbohydrate metabolism would result in a lower long-term risk of myocardial infarction and stroke.

The third aspect is the recently described interaction between COC and hereditary disturbances of the coagulation cascade in increasing the risk of VTE. It has recently become clear that a mutation of coagulation factor V (Factor V Leiden) results in resistance to activated protein C (APC resistance) in the anticoagulant pathway, leading to increased risk of spontaneous venous thrombosis, usually when the individual is also exposed to other risk factors simultaneously. The presence of the mutation leads to a 7–8 fold increase in relative risk of VTE (from 0.8 to 5.7 per 10 000 per year).[41] This increase in risk is seen in both heterozygotes and homozygotes for the mutation. Controversy has continued following the publication of data purporting to show an even greater increase in risk of VTE in factor V Leiden carriers who were users of third generation COC.[42] Other possible abnormalities of the protein C/protein S pathway and antithrombin III should not be overlooked. Controversy continues to revolve around the extent of possible risk of VTE with third generation COC users compared to second generation users, the increasingly likely reduction in myocardial infarction risk for third generation users, and the role of bias in observational research of this type.[43]

The main message to women, as indicated above, is that both VTE and myocardial infarction are relatively rare in COC users, and that both second and third generation COC are remarkably safe in long-term use. Nevertheless, those women who have a family or personal history of VTE should take appropriate precautions when placed in a situation which may increase VTE risk (elective major surgery, prolonged immobilization or long journeys).

Cerebrovascular disease

There are two main types of stroke: thrombotic and hemorrhagic. Thrombotic strokes are the result of venous clotting; they constitute 85–90% of all strokes.[3] Hemorrhagic strokes, on the other hand, are due to arterial rupture and comprise 10–15% of all strokes. The latter have a higher morbidity and mortality than the thrombotic variety and include subarachnoid hemorrhage, the most common type of stroke in young women. Thrombotic strokes are believed to be related primarily to the estrogen component, whereas hemorrhagic strokes can probably be linked to the progestogen.[6]

As in the case of thromboembolism, reanalyses of the earlier data now reveal that smoking, not the pill, was probably responsible for much of the reported morbidity and mortality attributed to COC.[10,27,28,44] The risk of stroke is very low in normal women who are using low-dose pills. The overall risks are increased by higher doses of estrogen, by hypertension, and above all, by smoking.[3]

If an individual develops a severe headache, hemiparesis or other symptoms suggesting an impending stroke, it is imperative to stop the COC immediately and evaluate the patient. With these symptoms, the decision is clinically easy to make. Much more difficult is the evaluation of the patient complaining of other, more vague, types of headaches. One of the major diagnostic and therapeutic dilemmas in dealing with COC users is the development of a change in the headache pattern experienced by a woman during the use of an oral contraceptive. It is often very difficult to determine precisely why an individual is having headaches. For example, headaches may be part of a symptom complex resulting from systemic diseases, hypertension or allergic conditions.

Certain diagnostic characteristics may be applied to try to distinguish those headaches that are significant from those that are not.[3] The most common type of headache is the one related to tension. It typically is band-like, bilateral, located posteriorly or in the frontal/temporal area, and is associated with tenseness of the neck and shoulder muscles. The pain is usually continuous and nonthrobbing; it ranges from mild to severe and can be relieved by aspirin or acetaminophen. These headaches are often due to some identifiable psychological factor such as stress, anxiety or depression. Of great importance is the fact that there are no associated neurological symptoms.

There has been continuous debate for many years as to whether or not there is any type of association between COC use and migraine headaches.[3] Clinically, these headaches can be distinguished from tension headaches because they present with different symptom-complexes. Vascular in origin, they typically are unilateral, throbbing and severe. The 'classical' migraine headache is preceded by visual aura such as scotomata and is often accompanied by nausea, vomiting and anorexia. Neurological symptoms such as photophobia, phonophobia, dizziness and unilateral numbness and/or weakness may occur. These symptoms disappear when the headache subsides, often during sleep. Migraine headaches are often familial and seem, in some instances, to be triggered by certain foods, alcohol, menses and climatic changes.

As studies were continued on this issue, there was less and less of an apparent relationship between COC and migraine headaches, and as a result, less and less reason to consider them a contraindication to COC use.[45] The one possible exception to this rule was the patient who had classical migraine headaches with visual prodromal aura. In one paper, it was reported that some women with menstrual migraine headaches got worse, some got better, and some had no further headaches.[46] Finally, in the Walnut Creek Contraceptive Drug Study, no relationship could be found between COC use and either tension or migraine headaches.[47] Despite these reassurances, headaches continue to be a source of concern to health care workers and patients alike, particularly among adolescents.[5]

The characteristics of headaches that suggest the possibility of an impending stroke are a family history of migraine and/or cardiovascular disease, sudden onset in a previously asymptomatic woman, and unilateral throbbing severe pain of prolonged duration unresponsive to nonprescription analgesics.[3] Additional reasons for particular concern include neurological symptoms such as dizziness, weakness and numbness of the extremities, and visual symptoms such as blurring and/or temporary loss of vision and scintillating scotomata and/or fortification spectra.[3]

Myocardial infarction

This is the most recently described cardiovascular complication that was believed to be associated with COC use. Myocardial infarction (MI) is rare in young women. It is also rare in young women using COC, no deaths having been reported under the age of 25. There are a number of risk factors for myocardial infarction. These are increasing age, marked obesity, diabetes, hypertension, Type II hyperlipoproteinemia and, above all, smoking.[3,6,48,49]

As in the case of numerous other diseases, cigarette smoking continues to emerge as a key contributor to myocardial infarction, both alone and in association with pill use.[10] In fact, there is growing evidence about the major impact smoking has, not only on women, but also on their infants.[50] With regard specifically to MI, smoking alone poses an increased risk greater than that of COC use alone. Moreover, patients using the pill are more apt to be smokers.[3] Finally, the synergistic risk of heavy smoking (>15 cigarettes/day), increasing age (35 years and older) and COC use is now firmly established.[51]

As estrogen doses in the pill continued to decline, there was a corresponding decrease in cardiovascular disease.[52] Moreover, multiple reanalyses of older epidemiologic data have been carried out, some of them now casting the risks of CVD in a more realistic light.[10,53,54] In addition, long-term follow-up (20 years) failed to show a higher CVD mortality in pill users than in women using an IUD or a diaphragm.[55] Finally, and of great clinical importance, meta-analysis of the Nurses' Health Study data showed no increased rise of CVD after stopping the pill, even with prolonged use of the high-dose COC.[56]

It is now becoming clear that it is necessary to re-evaluate the long-held lipid hypothesis, particularly in light of recent work carried out in the cynomolgus macaque monkey. In this model, the abnormal lipid patterns classically associated with an increased risk of atherosclerosis did not produce the anticipated changes with the administration of COC.[57–59] In fact, the risk appeared to be decreased, possibly due to a direct effect of estrogen on arterial estrogen receptors.

Fetal anomalies (see also chapter 43)

Several years ago a number of reports were published expressing concern about the possible development of fetal anomalies in previous COC users and in women who were taking the pill at the time of ovulation or early in pregnancy. This issue was initially stimulated by a report of an increased incidence of triploidy and spontaneous abortion in such instances.[60] However, these abnormal pregnancies have since been shown not to be related to COC use.[3] There were also a number of studies suggesting an increased risk of genital and nongenital anomalies, such as VACTERL.[61] Cardiovascular birth defects were also ascribed to pill use.[62] Somewhat later, as the result of better studies and careful re-evaluations of the older data, no association has been found between the use of COC and nongenital malformations or Down's syndrome.[51,63–65]

Cervical cancer (see also chapter 67)

The possible stimulation of premalignant and malignant changes in the cervix is another issue that has produced considerable consternation over the years. It was originally felt, from earlier studies, that use of the pill was associated with an increased risk of these conditions. However, it was subsequently noted that in some of these studies, the control groups were composed of women using barrier contraceptives and condoms — a most inappropriate comparison group.[3] Although it was not recognized at that time, measurements were actually being made of the beneficial effects on the cervix of blocking STD organisms by the use of barrier methods of contraception.[51,66]

Many reports have been written attempting to clarify this issue. A number of these have dealt with problems of selection bias. Smoking is now believed to be a previously unrecognized risk factor;[67] the same is true of parity.[68] Other studies have examined various types of potential bias and confounding factors.[69–71] It is currently not universally believed that a clear cause-and-effect relationship has yet been established between the use of COC and the development of cervical dysplasia, carcinoma *in situ* or invasive cervical cancer.[6] Thus, women using COC should have the usual indicated Pap smears, but do not require increased surveillance.[3]

Breast cancer (see also chapter 68)

Breast cancer is one of the most common lesions in women, the overall lifetime risk now being 1 in 8. It has been estimated that in 1996 there will be 184 300 new cases with 44 300 deaths.[17] The possible relationship between COC use and this disease continues to be the most baffling and controversial issue confronting us today. While there is no statistically valid evidence that hormonal stimulation will cause breast cancer *de nouveau*, questions still remain regarding the possible promotional effects of COC on premalignant breast tissue.

Because this is such a critical and volatile matter, a large number of studies have been carried out, often with conflicting results. One study, with considerable methodologic flaws, suggested a relationship with age and high potency progestogens.[72] This finding was not confirmed by later analyses. Further, it was suggested that the risk might be usage specific, i.e. higher in young women having an early menarche (< 13 years) and using the pill for more than eight years and lower for women aged 45–54.[73–75] Two papers from the CDC's Cancer and Steroid Hormone Study (CASH) reached the same conclusion.[76,77]

Another area of concern that was raised was the possibility of an increased risk for women with benign breast disease or with a family history of breast cancer. Two reviews of this issue have failed to establish this correlation.[78,79] When investigators at WHO looked at their data on the pill and breast cancer, a relative risk appeared to be present, but it was not statistically significant.[80] Three reviews, one a meta-analysis, also failed to find an increased risk, even with long-term use.[81–83]

The issue of progestogens and their association with breast cancer continues to be raised.[84] Moreover, there is continuing debate about the statistical validity of the studies on COC published to date.[85–87]

There appears to be a growing consensus that there is no overall increase in the risk of breast cancer in COC users over the age of 45, even in those who have taken the pill for many years.[88] The remaining area of controversy, one which continues to be studied, is whether or not there may be an increased risk in long-term users under the age of 45. There is no evidence of a latency period and no effect noted in recent or current users.[79,88] Finally, no differences have been observed when comparing estrogen doses and types of COC formulations.[88]

Most of the studies on this most important topic have been faulted for different reasons — the potential for various types of bias and the failure to look at a number of confounding effects. Unfortunately, the most negative aspect of this whole debate is the fear and loss of confidence in the pill, often leading to discontinuation of its use, and an unplanned/unwanted pregnancy.[4,5,89]

Malignant melanoma

In 1977, an article was published which raised concern as to whether or not the risk of developing a malignant melanoma might not be increased by the use of COC.[90] However, it was ultimately recognized that the study reporting this association, carried out in California, failed to take into consideration the amount of exposure to sunlight that the patients developing this tumor had received as compared to controls. Other studies since that time have shown no cause-and-effect relationship.[91] Thus, the development of a melanoma is no longer believed to be a matter for concern in COC users.

Special considerations

Pill administration

The current recommendations as to when to start the use of COC, depending on a woman's particular situation, are shown in Table 44.2.[3] There has been considerable confusion about certain aspects of proper pill-taking. It has been variously advised to start the first pack of pills on day 1, day 5 or Sunday. The disadvantage of the Sunday start is that use of a back-up method is usually recommended for the first seven days, in case ovulation has not been prevented by a late start.

Even greater confusion has arisen over the issue of how to handle the 'missed pill' situation. It has long been recognized that missed pills are a major reason for method failures.[92] A number of different regimens have been suggested, none of which has been entirely satisfactory. When one pill is missed, it should be taken as soon as this is recognized and no back-up is required. Missing more than one pill causes greater problems as to how best to deal with this situation. When two are missed in a row in the first two weeks, it is generally advised to take two pills on the day that this is realized, two the next day, and then one a day until the pack is finished along with a back-up barrier method for one week. If three pills in a row are missed, it is usually recommended that the remainder of the pack be discarded and a new one started along with seven days of a back-up method. Recognizing the complexity of the situation, the FDA, after meeting with a group of experts, recommended changes in the COC package inserts, attempting to simplify directions to consumers.[93] These directions apply to 21 and 28 pill packs. The most important thing to stress to women using the mini-pill is that they absolutely must take it at the same time every day.

Table 44.2 Starting dates for COC.

Situation	Start date
Pregnancy termination <12 weeks	Immediately
Pregnancy termination 12–28 weeks	1 week
Pregnancy termination >28 weeks	2 weeks
Term pregnancy/premature births, nonlactating	3–4 weeks
Term pregnancy/premature birth, lactating	Mini-pill while lactating, then combined COC

Contraindications

The contraindications to COC administration have changed over the years, as more data have been gathered on their safety.

Oral contraceptives should not be used in women who currently have the following conditions:

- Thrombophlebitis or thromboembolic disorders
- A past history of deep vein thrombophlebitis or thromboembolic disorders
- Cerebrovascular or coronary artery disease
- Known or suspected carcinoma of the breast
- Carcinoma of the endometrium or other known or suspected estrogen-dependent neoplasia
- Undiagnosed abnormal genital bleeding
- Cholestatic jaundice of pregnancy or jaundice with prior pill use
- Hepatic adenomas or carcinomas
- Known or suspected pregnancy.

Adolescents

The pill has been the contraceptive method of choice selected by most teenagers, since it is safe, effective and readily reversible. Several concerns about COC use in this age group have been raised in the past. The first deals with the issue of the stunting of growth. This does not make any biologic sense, since the major growth spurt is usually over prior to menarche. The second relates to future fertility. As has already been pointed out, COC use actually enhances the possibility of future pregnancy by reducing the risks of ectopic pregnancy, PID and endometriosis as well as avoiding the need for abortions. Third, the potential induction of malignancies, also already addressed, remains a major source of concern for many teenagers, despite evidence that their overall risk of developing a malignancy is actually decreased.[10]

This age group needs especially good counseling. They have repeatedly been shown to have poorer levels of compliance and continuation rates and are far more sensitive to and intolerant of minor side effects than older women.[4,5] Whereas average failure rates for COC are 1–3%, being about 6% during the first year of use, rates as high as 15–20% have been reported for teenagers. Teenagers are particularly concerned that pill use will cause them to gain weight, although it has been shown that COC users do not gain weight any more frequently than those using IUDs or barrier methods.[94] Finally, since many adolescents have multiple sexual partners, it is imperative that they be instructed to use barrier methods in addition to the pill when this is found to be the case.

Older women

For many years, it was recommended that pill use be discontinued at age 35 for smokers and 40 for nonsmokers, based on safety data on high-dose COC.[7] As more information became available on the safety of the low-dose pills, this recommendation was reconsidered. First, the American College of Obstetricians and Gynecologists (ACOG) extended the recommended use by healthy, nonsmoking women to age 44.[95] Then the FDA, on the advice of its Fertility and Maternal Health Drugs Advisory Committee, raised the age limits to the time of the menopause for this group.[96]

There are a number of good reasons to extend the use of the pill.[97–99] Even though ovulation becomes gradually less consistent, the possibility of unplanned and unwanted pregnancy continues to be a major concern. In fact, the rate of unplanned pregnancy in this age group is surpassed only by that of very young teenagers. The risks of significant fetal and maternal morbidity and mortality increase with increasing age, and rates of abortion go up. In addition, the noncontraceptive health benefits are a key factor as well as the prevention of hormonal deficiencies. Risks associated with pregnancy and alternative surgical procedures are greater than those related to use of the low-dose COC and, most importantly, it has been shown that many women who discontinue the pill fail to begin the use of another contraceptive method.[100]

There are two other areas being evaluated for older COC users. Whether or not it is necessary/cost-effective to screen carbohydrate and lipid levels in low risk women over the age of 40 continues to be a matter of debate. The second, when to start hormone replacement therapy (HRT), is now commonly asked, as women continue COC into their late 40s and early 50s. While menopause could be the time chosen, women often become symptomatic earlier. If FSH levels are found to be consistently elevated, it is safe to switch to HRT.

High risk patients

For many years, women with medical problems including such conditions as diabetes mellitus, lipid and coagulation disorders, cardiovascular disease and endocrine problems, have been told not to use COC. With the advent of the very safe low-dose pills and the recognition of their numerous health benefits, these situations are being revisited. In a number of cases, the benefit:risk ratio is gradually moving toward the benefit side of the use of the oral contraceptives.

It is now clear what an important role contraception plays in the management of diabetic women.[101] Both maternal and fetal complications can be minimized by establishing good diabetic control prior to pregnancy. COC can be very useful in this regard, allowing selection of the best time for conception to occur.

Similarly, patients with dyslipidemia were not considered to be appropriate candidates for the use of COC. Today, however, the low-dose pills can be used under carefully controlled conditions, particularly since there is no evidence that COC use will promote atherogenesis.[102]

As noted earlier, many asymptomatic women with a family history of thromboembolism (excluding those with a resistance to APC and older women who continue to smoke) can now be offered COC as a contraceptive option.[29–31,103] In fact, they may be a particularly good choice for women taking oral anticoagulants since they would avoid the risk of intraperitoneal hemorrhage resulting from ovulation, and also because of the known teratogenic effects of the anticoagulants.[103]

Some women with hypertension, angina pectoris and mitral valve prolapse are now being considered, under certain circumstances, to be potential candidates for use of the newer low-dose COC.[104] If the hypertension is well controlled, the patient has no history of coronary artery disease and is a nonsmoker, COC are a possibility.

The animal and human data indicating the possible role of COC in preventing atherosclerosis, already cited, suggest that they may be a reasonable choice for women with angina. However, this would be true only in nonsmokers and those with no additional risk factors.[104] Patients with asymptomatic mitral valve prolapse are now also being evaluated for COC use.

Most women with endocrine disorders are now generally considered to be good candidates for oral contraception. In fact, COC are probably the method of choice for those with polycystic ovary disease, since they inhibit pituitary gonadotropin secretion.[105]

Clearly, women with a variety of medical conditions present their own special problems. Data on COC use in a number of these diseases are often limited. The biggest challenge is to look at our current contraceptive options and the impact of unplanned pregnancy on these women, and decide whether the use of COC is appropriate in any particular situation.

Drug interactions

Little consideration was given until quite recently to the possibility of drug interaction when two or more preparations were being used simultaneously. It is now recognized that, in these instances, there may be changes in the patterns of absorption, or in the therapeutic action of either or both drugs. In the case of the oral contraceptives, griseofulvin, anticonvulsants, sedatives, analgesics, anticoagulants, antidepressants, tranquilizers, bronchodilators, rifampicin, and antihypertensives have been found to exhibit probable drug interactions.[6,51] Numerous other agents have been mentioned as possibly posing a problem but clear interactions have not been specifically proven. The reported interaction with tetracycline has since been disproved, no significant changes being found in the serum concentrations of either drug. The evidence on ampicillin is still contradictory.[6] Where an interaction is possible, that may reduce the effectiveness of the COC, such as griseofulvin, rifampin, anticonvulsants and sedatives, it is wise to use an oral contraceptive with 50 μg of estrogen as opposed to the pill of choice for the average individual, which is an estrogen content between 30–35 μg. In the case of all of the other listed drugs, it is the impact of the COC on their activity that is the significant consideration, changes in dosage, either up or down, possibly being required.[6]

Post-pill fertility

Earlier, concern was expressed about post-pill amenorrhea and a delay in the return of fertility in COC users. It is now clear that short delays of two to three months are not uncommon; longer ones, more than a year, are quite uncommon. In these latter cases, it is frequently found that these individuals had menstrual irregularities before starting COC, due to some gynecologic problem. Such women are not improved or made worse by the administration of COC.[51]

The risk of delayed return of fertility is not increased by increasing duration of use. Moreover, the practice of instituting 'rest periods' should be mentioned only to be condemned; it is of no proven value and has produced a considerable number of unwanted pregnancies.[51]

It is not generally considered necessary to do an infertility evaluation until at least six months have passed in women who were previously apparently normal. Seventy-five percent of patients will resume menses in three months, 50% in six months, and 35% in 12 months.[51]

Perceptions of the pill

Despite mounting evidence regarding the safety of low-dose pills and their health benefits, there continues to be considerable anxiety about their use. This has been shown to be true for both men and women in the United States in a Gallup poll performed for the American College of Obstetricians and Gynecologists.[106] It is quite disheartening to observe very similar data coming from eight developing countries.[107] Even more disheartening is the fact that a repeat poll done in 1994 showed very similiar results; there was less concern about adverse side effects, but the same basic lack of understanding about effectiveness and health benefits.

Numerous myths still exist about the dangers of COC, propagated primarily by inaccurate (but highly saleable) reports in the media. A prime example is the fear generated by reports on the link between COC and breast cancer.[109] Equally concerning are reports on how women, especially adolescents, develop their perceptions about the side effects of the pill.[110] Perhaps the most devastating is a recent report on the risk perceptions drawn from a self-administered survey done at Yale University, again showing a greatly exaggerated perception of risks and virtually no understanding of health benefits.[111]

On a somewhat different note, minor differences between the various COC have often been given more attention than is scientifically warranted. The FDA, recognizing this fact, now demands proof for the use of such claims of superiority.[112]

Compliance

It has been clear for a number of years that compliance in proper pill taking has a major impact on both contraceptive failure rates and the frequency of side effects.[113,114] A major attempt to improve COC compliance is the change in labeling previously mentioned.[93] In addition, numerous attempts have been made to improve pill packaging, going from a 21 to a 28 day system.[3]

Comprehensive counseling, both prior to and during pill use, are also key to good compliance. Equally important is the support given to patients in the event of adverse side effects such as breakthrough bleeding.[114]

'Postcoital pills' (emergency contraception)

It was established a number of years ago that if estrogens are given in adequate amounts to a woman within 72 hours of unprotected sexual intercourse around the time of ovulation, she will be protected in almost all instances against pregnancy.[115] A number of different estrogens have been used over the years. One of the first of the agents used as a 'morning after' pill was diethylstilbestrol (DES). However, the adverse information regarding cervicovaginal carcinomas and genital tract anomalies in the daughters of DES users has made this unacceptable as a form of postcoital contraception.[51] Both synthetic and natural estrogens have been used for this purpose. The preparation used most often today is one of the combined OC, ethinyl estradiol 0.05 mg and norgestrel 0.5 mg.[116] If this preparation is given within 72 hours of exposure, two pills being taken immediately and another two pills 12 hours later, the failure rate is less than 1%. The postcoital pill presumably acts directly on the endometrial glands, putting the endometrial stroma out of phase and thus interfering with implantation. There is a delay of the normal LH surge for seven or more days when the preparation is given just prior to the expected time of the LH surge. It may also exert an effect on tubal motility or the developing corpus luteum.[3]

Some women using this regimen will experience nausea and vomiting.[117] If vomiting is excessive, an inadequate dosage may result. An antiemetic can be given to the patient in case nausea should occur. Other patients may experience mastalgia or menorrhagia.

This form of treatment has not yet been approved by the FDA, although it is widely used, but hopefully this may change in the not too distant future. It is important to tell the individuals being given postcoital contraceptives that this is a technique for emergency use only and should not be relied upon as a continuing form of birth control. They should be urged to select and use another form of family planning in order to avoid another such episode.[51]

FUTURE CONTRACEPTIVE METHODS

For many years, there has been a definition of the ideal contraceptive. It should be safe, reliable, inexpensive, quickly reversible, easy to use, have no significant side effects, prevent STD transmission as well as pregnancy, and be acceptable to both men and women throughout the entire reproductive era. Needless to say no such method exists. Indeed, there is grave doubt that such a method is apt to be found anytime in the foreseeable future. In fact, given the current crisis in contraceptive development, fueled by steadily decreasing interest and support, the entire field is suffering.[118–121]

Despite this unfortunate situation, there are new methods under study that may become available, particularly in the hormonal area, most notably the vaginal contraceptive ring.[122,123] In addition, RU 486, currently under attack and unavailable in the US as an abortifacient, holds some promise for the future. This product is an antiprogesterone that blocks the action of progesterone at the receptor level. It has been studied at a number of different points in the menstrual cycle and during pregnancy. Given at midcycle, it can delay or inhibit the normal LH surge. In the luteal phase, it will induce menses. It is being studied for use as an emergency contraceptive and as a luteolytic agent.[124–126] It can induce labor in women at term and those with a fetal death *in utero*. It is being used at present primarily as an early abortifacient. Thus far, intense opposition to the introduction of this drug into the United States has prevented its availability to American women.

The future of contraception

Some investigators, while conceding major problems in contraceptive development, are more sanguine about the future.[127] However, beyond the purely scientific aspects, problems in the approach taken by both medical and lay publications continue to make contraceptives more of a source of concern and thus less used.[128–131]

Multiple attempts have been made to evaluate factors critical to the successful use of birth control methods.[132–136] Specific groups with special problems have been studied, such as adolescents and lactating women.[134–139] Efforts have also been made to pinpoint failure rates more accurately.[140]

Another area of concern, critical to the future of contraceptive development and use, particularly in the US, is the problem posed by the many social, political and legal deterrents.[118,121] Primary among these are the current crises in medical malpractice and insurance availability and affordability.[141,142]

Aside from the personal, medical and economic aspects of contraception, it is important to note one of our major global problems — overpopulation. A decade or two ago considerable attention was being given to the issues of rapid population growth. It has been estimated that in the 1990s, the equivalent of the total population of East and West Europe will be added. This amounts to two United Kingdoms every 14 months, a Sweden or New Zealand every month or a school class every 10 seconds. It has been estimated that in the first quarter of the next century, depending on what happens in terms of improved contraceptives and contraceptive services, that there will be an addition of 92 million people annually.[143,144]

Conclusion

The oral contraceptives are now over 40 years old; the first one was approved in the United States in 1960. Many review articles have been written, looking back over what we have learned about these agents — the best studied medications in medical history.[3,6,117,145] A number of the older fears about the use of COC have been put to rest. Equally important, numerous health benefits have now been identified. Thus, the oral contraceptives have been and continue to be a major option in our current armamentarium.

REFERENCES

1. Himes N 1970 Medical history of contraception. Schocken Books, New York
2. Finch B, Green H 1964 Contraception through the ages. Charles C. Thomas, Springfield
3. Connell EB, Tatum HJ 1992 Women's reproductive health care. EMIS — Canada, London, Ontario
4. Hillary PJA 1989 The patient's reaction to side effects of oral contraceptives. American Journal of Obstetrics and Gynecology 161: 1412–1415
5. Emans SJ, Grace E, Wood SER, Smith DE, Klein K, Merola J 1987 Adolescents' compliance with the use of oral contraceptives. Journal of the American Medical Association 257: 3377–3381
6. Goldzieher JW 1989 Hormonal contraception: pills, injections and implants. EMIS — Canada, London, Ontario, pp 1–269
7. Ory HW, Forrest JD, Lincoln R 1983 Making choices: evaluating the health risks and benefits of birth control methods. The Alan Guttmacher Institute, New York
8. Ory HW 1982 The noncontraceptive health benefits from oral contraceptive use. Family Planning Perspectives
9. Peterson HB, Lee NC 1989 The health effects of oral contraceptives: misperceptions, controversies, and continuing good news. Clinical Obstetrics and Gynecology 32: 339–355
10. Harlap S, Kost K, Forrest JD 1991 Preventing pregnancy, protecting health: a new look at birth control choices in the United States. The Alan Guttmacher Institute, New York, pp 1–128
11. Rosenberg MJ, Waugh MS, Stevens CM 1996 Smoking and cycle control among oral contraceptive users. American Journal of Obstetrics and Gynecology 174: 628–632
12. Caillouette JC, Koehler AL 1987 Phasic contraceptive pills and functional ovarian cysts. American Journal of Obstetrics and Gynecology 158: 1538–1542
13. Grimes DA, Hughes JM 1989 Use of multiphasic oral contraceptives and hospitalizations of women with functional ovarian cysts in the United States. Obstetrics and Gynecology 73: 1037–1039
14. Holt VL, Daling JR, McKnight B, Moore D, Stergachis A, Weiss NS 1992 Functional ovarian cysts in relation to the use of monophasic and triphasic oral contraceptives. Obstetrics and Gynecology 79(4): 529–533
15. DeCherney A 1996 Bone-sparing properties of oral contraceptives. American Journal of Obstetrics and Gynecology 174: 15–20
16. Louv WC, Austin H, Perlman J, Alexander WJ 1989 Oral contraceptive use and the risk of chlamydial and gonococcal infections. American Journal of Obstetrics and Gynecology 160: 396–402
17. Parker SL, Tong T, Bolden S, Wingo PA 1996 Cancer statistics, 1996. CA-A Cancer J Clin 65: 5–27
18. The Cancer and Steroid Hormone Study of the Centers for Disease Control and the National Institute of Child Health and Human Development 1987 The reduction in risk of ovarian cancer associated with oral contraceptive use. New England Journal of Medicine 316: 650–655
19. Schlesselman JJ 1989 Cancer of the breast and reproductive tract in relation to use of oral contraceptives. Contraception 40: 1–38
20. The Cancer and Steroid Hormone Study of the Centers for Disease Control and the National Institute of Child Health and Human Development 1987 Combination oral contraceptive use and the risk of endometrial cancer. Journal of the American Medical Association 257(6): 796–800
21. World Health Organization 1988 Collaborative Study of Neoplasia and Steroid Contraceptives. Endometrial cancer and combined oral contraceptives. International Journal of Epidemiology 17: 263–269
22. World Health Organization 1989 Collaborative Study of Neoplasia and Steroid Contraceptives. Combined OCs and liver cancer. International Journal of Cancer 43: 254–259
23. Wingrave SJ, Kay CR, Vessey MP 1979 Oral contraceptives and diabetes mellitus. British Medical Journal 1: 23–29
24. Van der Vange N, Klossterboer HJ, Haspels AA 1987 Effect of seven low-dose combined oral contraceptive preparations on carbohydrate metabolism. American Journal of Obstetrics and Gynecology 156: 918–922
25. Godsland IF, Crook D, Simpson R, Proudler T, Felton C, Lees B et al 1990 The effects of different formulations of oral contraceptive agents on lipid and carbohydrate metabolism. New England Journal of Medicine 323(20): 1375–1381
26. Burkman RT, Robinson JC, Kruszon-Moran D, Kimball AW, Kwiterovick P, Burford RG 1988 Lipid and lipoprotein changes associated with oral contraceptive use: a randomized clinical trial. Obstetrics and Gynecology 71: 33–38
27. Mileikowsky GN, Nadler JL, Huey F, Francis R, Roy S 1988 Evidence that smoking alters prostacyclin formation and platelet aggregation in women who use oral contraceptives. American Journal of Obstetrics and Gynecology 158: 1547–1552
28. Goldbaum GM, Kendrick JS, Hogelin GC, Gentry EM 1987 The relative impact of smoking and oral contraceptive use on women in the United States. Journal of the American Medical Association 258: 1339–1342
29. Griffin JH, Evatt B, Wideman C, Fernandez JA 1993 Anticoagulant protein C pathway defective in majority of thrombophilic patients. Blood 82: 1989–1993

30. Svensson PJ, Dahlback B 1994 Resistance to activated protein C as a basis for venous thrombosis. New England Journal of Medicine 330: 517–522
31. Koster T, Rosendaal FR, deRonde H, Briet E, Vandenbroucke JP, Bertina RM 1993 Venous thrombosis due to poor anticoagulant response to activated protein C: Leiden thrombophilia study. Lancet 342: 1503–1506
32. Inman WHW, Vessey MP, Westerholm B, Engelund A 1970 Thromboembolic disease and the steroidal content of oral contraceptives: a report to the Committee on Safety of Drugs. British Medical Journal 2: 203–209
33. Vessey M, Mant D, Smith A, Yeates D 1986 Oral contraceptives and venous thromboembolism: findings in a large prospective study. British Medical Journal 292: 526–529
34. Gerstman BB, Piper JM, Frieman JP et al 1990 Oral contraceptive oestrogen and progestin potencies and the incidence of deep venous thromboembolism. International Journal of Epidemiology 19: 931–936
35. World Health Organization 1995 Collaborative Study of Cardiovascular Disease and Steroid Hormone Contraception. Venous thromboembolic disease and combined oral contraceptives; results of an international multicentre case-controlled study. Lancet 346: 1575–1582
36. World Health Organization 1995 Collaborative Study of Cardiovascular Disease and Steroid Hormone Contraception. Effect of different progestogens in low oestrogen oral contraceptives on venous thromboembolic disease. Lancet 1582–1588
37. Jick H, Jick SS, Gurewich V, Myers MW, Vasilakis C 1995 Risk of idiopathic cardiovascular death and non fatal venous thromboembolism in women using oral contraceptives with differing progestogen components. Lancet 346: 1589–1593
38. Spitzer WO, Lewis MA, Heinemann LAJ, Thorogood M, MacRae KD 1996 Third generation oral contraceptives and risk of venous thromboembolic disorders; an international case-controlled study. British Medical Journal 312: 83–88
39. Suissa S, Blois I, Spitzer WO, Cusson J, Lewis M, Heinemann L 1997 First time use of newer oral contraceptives and the risk of venous thromboembolism. Contraception 56: 141–146
40. Schwingl PJ, Shelton J 1997 Modelled estimates of myocardial infarction and venous thromboembolic disease in users of second and third generation oral contraceptives. Contraception 55: 125–129
41. Vandenbroucke JP, Koster T, Briët E, Reitsma PH, Bertina RM, Rosendaal FR 1994 Increased risk of venous thrombosis in oral contraceptive users who are carriers of factor V Leiden mutation. Lancet 344: 1453–1457
42. Rosing J, Tens G, Nicolaes GAF et al 1997 Oral contraceptives and venous thrombosis: different sensitivities to activated protein C in women using second and third generation oral contraceptives. British Journal of Haematology 97: 233–238
43. Lewis MA, Heinemann LJ, MacRae KD, Bruppacher R, Spitzer WO 1996 The increased risk of venous thromboembolism and the use of third generation progestogens: role of bias in observational research. Contraception 54: 5–13
44. Castelli WP 1996 Reducing risk in OC users who smoke. Contemporary Obstetrics and Gynecology (March): 116–126
45. Benson MD, Rebar RW 1986 Relationship of migraine headache and stroke to oral contraceptive use. Journal of Reproductive Medicine 31: 1082–1088
46. Karsay K 1990 The relationship between vascular headaches and low-dose oral contraceptives. Therapia Hungarica 38: 181–185
47. Ramcharan S, Pellegrin FA, Ray RM, Hsu J 1980 The Walnut Creek contraceptive drug study. A prospective study of the side effects of oral contraceptives. Journal of Reproductive Medicine 25(6): 346–372 (Suppl)
48. Croft P, Hannaford PC 1989 Risk factors for acute myocardial infarction in women: evidence from the Royal College of General Practitioners' oral contraception study. British Medical Journal 298: 165–168
49. Rosenberg L, Palmer JR, Lesko SM, Shapiro S 1990 Oral contraceptive use and the risk of myocardial infarction. American Journal of Epidemiology 131(6): 1009–1016
50. Hoff C, Wertelecki W, Blackburn WR, Mendenhall H, Wiseman H, Stump A 1986 Trend associations of smoking with maternal, fetal, and neonatal morbidity. Obstetrics and Gynecology 68: 317–321
51. Connell EB 1990 Hormonal contraception. In: Kase NK, Weingold AB, Gershenson DM (eds) Principles and practice of gynecology, 2nd edn. Churchill Livingston, New York, pp 993–1020
52. Meade TW, Greenberg G, Thompson GS 1980 Progestogens and cardiovascular reactions associated with oral contraceptives and a comparison of the safety of 50 and 30 μg oestrogen preparations. British Medical Journal 280: 1157–1161
53. Realini JP, Goldzieher JW 1985 Oral contraceptives and cardiovascular disease: a critique of the epidemiologic studies. American Journal of Obstetrics and Gynecology 151: 729–798
54. Thorogood M, Vessey M 1990 An epidemiological survey of cardiovascular disease in women taking oral contraceptives. American Journal of Obstetrics and Gynecology 163: 274–281
55. Vessey MP, Villard-Mackintosh L, McPherson K, Yeates D 1989 Mortality among oral contraceptive users: 20-year follow-up of women in a cohort study. British Medical Journal 299: 1487–1491
56. Stampfer MJ, Willett WC, Colditz GA, Speizer FE, Hennekens CH 1990 Past use of oral contraceptives and cardiovascular disease: a meta-analysis in the context of the Nurses' Health Study. American Journal of Obstetrics and Gynecology 163: 285–291
57. Adams MR, Clarkson TB, Koritnik DR, Nash HA 1987 Contraceptive steroids and coronary artery atherosclerosis in cynomolgus macaques. Fertility and Sterility 47: 1010–1018
58. Clarkson TB, Adams MR, Kaplan JR, Shively CA, Koritnik DR 1989 From menarche to menopause: coronary artery atherosclerosis and protection in cynomolgus monkeys. American Journal of Obstetrics and Gynecology 160: 1280–1285
59. Clarkson TB, Shively CA, Morgan TM, Koritnik DR, Adams MR, Kaplan JR 1990 Oral contraceptives and coronary artery atherosclerosis of cynomolgus monkeys. Obstetrics and Gynecology 75: 217–222

60. Carr DH 1970 Chromosome studies in selected spontaneous abortions. Conception after oral contraception. Canadian Medical Association Journal 103: 343–348
61. Nora AH, Nora JJ 1975 A syndrome of multiple congenital anomalies associated with teratogenic exposure. Archives of Environmental Health 30: 17–21
62. Heinonen OP, Slone D, Monson RR, Hook EB, Shapiro S 1977 Cardiovascular birth defects and antenatal exposure to female sex hormones. New England Journal of Medicine 296: 67–71
63. Wilson JG, Brent RL 1981 Are female sex hormones teratogenic? American Journal of Obstetrics and Gynecology 141: 567–580
64. Linn S, Schonenbaum S, Monson R et al 1983 Lack of association between contraceptive usage and congenital malformations in offspring. American Journal of Obstetrics and Gynecology 147: 923–928
65. Bracken MB 1990 Oral contraception and congenital malformations in offspring: a review and meta-analysis of the prospective studies. Obstetrics and Gynecology 76: 552–557
66. Slattery ML, Overall JC Jr, Abbott TM, French TK, Robison LM, Gardner J 1989 Sexual activity, contraception, genital infections, and cervical cancer: support for a sexually transmitted disease hypothesis. American Journal of Epidemiology 130: 248–258
67. Winklestein W Jr 1991 Smoking and cervical cancer — current status: a review. American Journal of Epidemiology 131: 945–957
68. Parazzini F, La Vecchia C, Negri E et al 1989 Reproductive factors and the risk of invasive and intraepithelial cervical neoplasia. British Journal of Cancer 59: 805–809
69. Swan SH, Petitti DB 1982 A review of problems of bias and confounding in epidemiologic studies of cervical neoplasia and oral contraceptive use. American Journal of Epidemiology 115: 10–18
70. World Health Organization 1985 Collaborative Study of Neoplasia and Steroid Contraceptives. Invasive cervical cancer and combined oral contraceptives. British Medical Journal 290: 961–965
71. Irwin KI, Rosero-Bixby L, Oberle MW, Lee NC, Whatley AS, Fortney JA et al 1988 Oral contraceptives and cervical cancer risk in Costa Rica: detection bias or causal association? Journal of the American Medical Association 259: 59–64
72. Pike MC, Henderson BE, Krailo MD, Duke A, Roy S 1988 Breast cancer in young women and use of oral contraceptives: possible modifying effect of formulation and age at use. Lancet ii: 926–930
73. Stadel BV, Lai S, Schlesselman JJ, Murray P 1988 Oral contraceptives and premenopausal breast cancer in nulliparous women. Contraception 38: 287–299
74. Stadel BV, Schlesselman JJ, Murray PA 1989 Oral contraceptives and breast cancer. Lancet i: 1257–1258
75. Paul C, Skegg DCG, Spears GFS 1990 Oral contraceptives and the risk of breast cancer. International Journal of Cancer 46: 366–373
76. Wingo PA, Escobedo LG, Lee NC et al 1991 Age specific differences in the relationship between oral contraceptive use and breast cancer. Obstetrics and Gynecology 78: 161–170
77. Peterson HB, Wingo PA 1992 Oral contraceptives and breast cancer: any relationship? Contemporary Obstetrics and Gynecology, Breast Health 31–40
78. Murray PP, Stadel BV, Schlesselman JJ 1989 Oral contraceptive use in women with a family history of breast cancer. Obstetrics and Gynecology 73: 977–983
79. Schlesselman JJ 1990 Oral contraceptives and breast cancer. American Journal of Obstetrics and Gynecology 163: 1379–1387
80. World Health Organization 1990 Collaborative Study of Neoplasia and Steroid Contraceptives. Breast cancer and combined oral contraceptives: results from a multinational study. British Journal of Cancer 61: 110–119
81. Romieu I, Berlin JA, Colditz G 1990 Oral contraceptives and breast cancer: review and meta-analysis. Cancer 66: 2253–2263
82. Thomas DB 1991 Oral contraceptives and breast cancer: review of the epidemiological literature. In: Oral Contraceptives and Breast Cancer. Committee on the Relationship between Oral Contraceptives and Breast Cancer. Institute of Medicine, Division of Health Promotion and Disease Prevention. National Academy Press, Washington, DC
83. McGonigle KF 1992 How OCs affect breast disease. Contemporary Obstetrics and Gynecology (May): 156–182
84. Staffa JA, Newschaffer CJ, Jones JK, Miller V 1992 Progestins and breast cancer: an epidemiologic review. Fertility and Sterility 57: 473–491
85. Skegg DCG 1988 Potential for bias in case-control studies of oral contraceptives and breast cancer. American Journal of Epidemiology 127: 205–212
86. Peto J 1989 Oral contraceptives and breast study: is the CASH study really negative. Lancet 1: 552
87. Grimes DA 1992 Progestins, breast cancer, and the limitations of epidemiology. Fertility and Sterility 57(3): 492–494
88. Harlap S 1991 Oral contraceptives and breast cancer. Cause and effect? Journal of Reproductive Medicine 36: 374–395
89. Grimes DA 1995 Breast cancer, the pill and the press. In: Mann RD (ed) Oral contraceptives and breast cancer. Parthenon Publishing, Carnforth, pp 309–322
90. Beral V, Ramcharan S, Faris R 1977 Malignant melanoma and OC use among women in California. British Journal of Cancer 36: 804–809
91. Helmrich SP, Rosenberg L, Kaufman DW, Miller DR, Schottenfeld D, Stolley PD et al 1984 Lack of an elevated risk of malignant melanoma in relation to oral contraceptive use. Journal of the National Cancer Institute 72: 617–620
92. Letterie GS, Chow GE 1991 Effect of 'missed' pills on oral contraceptive effectiveness. Obstetrics and Gynecology 79: 979–982
93. Williams-Deane M 1993 Standardizing the instructions for oral contraceptive use. The Female Patient 18: 77–84
94. Carpenter S, Neinstein LS 1986 Weight gain in adolescent and young oral contraceptive users. Journal of Adolescent Health Care 7: 342–344
95. American College of Obstetricians and Gynecologists 1985 Contraception for women in their later reproductive years. ACOG Committee Opinion Number 41, December
96. F-D-C Reports 1990 February 5, T&G-8

97. Speroff L 1991 A clinician's approach to therapy during a woman's transition years. Contemporary Obstetrics and Gynecology (August): 65–68
98. Connell EB 1992 Oral contraception in the woman over 35. The Female Patient 17: 45–50
99. Mishell DR 1988 Use of oral contraceptives in women of older reproductive age. American Journal of Obstetrics and Gynecology 158: 1657
100. Pratt WF, Bachrach CA 1987 What do women use when they stop using the pill? Family Planning Perspectives 19: 257–266
101. Mestman JH, Schmidt-Sarosi C 1993 Diabetes mellitus and fertility control: contraception management issues. American Journal of Obstetrics and Gynecology 168: 2012–2020
102. Knopp RH, LaRosa JC, Burkman RT 1993 Contraception and dyslipidemia. American Journal of Obstetrics and Gynecology 168: 1994–2005
103. Comp PC, Zacur HA 1993 Contraceptive choices in women with coagulation disorders. American Journal of Obstetrics and Gynecology 168: 1990–1993
104. Sullivan JM, Lobo RA 1993 Considerations for contraception in women with cardiovascular disorders. American Journal of Obstetrics and Gynecology 168: 2006–2012
105. Loriaux DL, Wild RA 1993 Contraceptive choices for women with endocrine complications. American Journal of Obstetrics and Gynecology 168: 2021–2026
106. The Gallup Organization 1985 Attitudes toward contraception. Princeton, NJ
107. Grubb GS 1987 Women's perceptions of the safety of the pill: a survey in eight developing countries. Family Health International. Research Triangle Park, North Carolina
108. The American College of Obstetricians and Gynecologists 1994 Poll shows women still skeptical of contraceptive safety. News release, January 20
109. Grimes DA 1989 Breast cancer, the pill and the press. In: Mann RD (ed) Oral contraceptives and breast cancer. Parthenon, Park Ridge, New Jersey, 309–318
110. Herold ES, Goodwin MS 1980 Perceived side effects of oral contraceptives among adolescent girls. Canadian Medical Association Journal 123: 1022–1026
111. Peipert JF, Gutmann J 1993 Oral contraceptive risk assessment: a survey of 247 educated women. Obstetrics and Gynecology 82: 112–117
112. F-D-C Reports 1991 Oral contraceptive makers must end unproven superiority claims. F-D-C Reports Inc., June 24. 53: T&G-1
113. Chowdhury V, Joshi UM, Gopalkrishna K et al 1980 'Escape' ovulation in women due to the missing of low dose combination oral contraceptive pills. Contraception 22: 241–247
114. Hillard PJA 1989 The patient's reaction to side effects of oral contraceptives. American Journal of Obstetrics and Gynecology 161: 1412–1415
115. Mishell DR 1991 Long-acting contraceptive steroids, postcoital contraceptives and antiprogestins. In: Mishell DR Jr, Davajan V, Lobo RA (eds) Infertility, contraception and reproductive endocrinology, 3rd edn. Blackwell Scientific Publications, Boston, pp 872–894
116. Yuzpe AA, Smith RP, Rademaker AW 1982 A multicenter critical investigation employing ethinyl estradiol combined with dinorgestrel as a postcoital contraceptive agent. Fertility and Sterility 37: 508–513
117. Baird DT, Glasier AF 1993 Hormonal contraception. New England Journal of Medicine 328: 1543–1549
118. Connell EB 1987 The crisis in contraception. Technology review. Massachusetts Institute of Technology, Boston, May/June 477–555
119. Djerassi C 1989 The bitter pill. Science 245: 356–361
120. Tyrer LB, Salas JE 1989 Contraceptive problems unique to the United States. Clinical Obstetrics and Gynecology 32: 307–315
121. Mastroianni L Jr, Donaldson PJ, Kane TT (eds) 1990 Developing new contraceptives: obstacles and opportunities. National Academy Press, Washington, DC
122. Potts DM, Smith JB 1991 The future of hormonal contraception. International Journal of Fertility 36(3): 57–63
123. Issue topic 1981 Comprehensive review of the vaginal contraceptive ring. Contraception 24: 323 (Entire issue on this topic)
124. Baulieu EE 1989 RU-486 as an antiprogesterone steroid: from receptor to contragestion and beyond. Journal of the American Medical Association 262: 1808–1814
125. Stuenkel C, Garzo V, Morris S, Liu JH, Yen SSC 1990 Effects of the antiprogesterone RU 486 in the early follicular phase of the menstrual cycle. Fertility and Sterility 53: 642–646
126. Kekkonen R, Alfthan H, Haukkamaa M, Heikinheimo O, Luukkainen T, Lahteenmaki P 1990 Interference with ovulation by sequential treatment with the antiprogesterone RU 486 and synthetic progestin. Fertility and Sterility 53: 747–750
127. Mishell DR Jr 1992 New and better methods of contraception. Contemporary Obstetrics and Gynecology (September) 15–22
128. Phillips DP, Kanter EJ, Bednarczyk BA, Tastad PL 1991 Importance of the lay press in the transmission of medical knowledge to the scientific community. New England Journal of Medicine 325: 1180–1183
129. Easterbrook PJ, Berlin JA, Gopalan R, Matthews DR 1991 Publication bias in clinical research. Lancet 337: 867–872
130. Koren G, Klein N 1991 Bias against negative studies in newspaper reports of medical research. Journal of the American Medical Association 266: 1824–1826
131. Herold ES, Goodwin MS 1980 Perceived side effects of oral contraceptives among adolescent girls. Canadian Medical Association Journal 123: 1022–1026
132. Forrest JD, Singh S 1990 The sexual and reproductive behavior of American women, 1982–1988. Family Planning Perspectives 22: 206–214
133. Forrest JD 1988 Contraceptive needs through stages of women's reproductive lives. Contemporary Obstetrics and Gynecology (Special Issue) 32: 12–14, 16, 21–22
134. Tanfer K, Cubbins LA, Brewster KL 1992 Determinants of contraceptive choice among women in the United States. Family Planning Perspectives 24: 155–173
135. Forrest JD, Fordyce RR 1988 US women's contraceptive attitudes and practice: how have they changed in the 1980s? Family Planning Perspectives 20: 112–118

136. Mosher WD 1990 Contraceptive practice in the United States, 1982–1988. Family Planning Perspectives 22: 198–205
137. Brown RT, Cromer BA, Fischer R 1992 Adolescent sexuality and issues in contraception. Pediatric and Adolescent Gynecology 19(1): 177–191
138. Wermer MJ, Biro FM 1990 Contraception and sexually transmitted diseases in adolescent females. Adolescent and Pediatric Gynecology 3: 127–136
139. Zacur HA, Gray RH 1992 Contraception during lactation. Contemporary Obstetrics and Gynecology (July): 13–28
140. Trussell J, Kost K 1987 Contraceptive failure in the United States: a critical review of the literature. Studies in Family Planning 18: 237–283
141. Kelly P, Beyler K 1986 Large damage awards and the insurance crisis: causes, effects and cures. Illinois Bar Journal 75: 140
142. US Department of Justice 1986 Report of the policy working group on the causes, extent and policy implications of the current crisis in insurance availability and affordability. US Government Printing Office, Washington, DC
143. Office of Technology Assessment 1981 World population and fertility planning technologies: the next 20 years. Office of Technology Assessment, Washington, DC
144. Green CP 1992 The environment and population growth. Population Report (M). No. 10. Johns Hopkins University Population Information Program, Baltimore, 1–31
145. Goldzieher JW 1991 Thirty years of hormonal contraception: an historical perspective. International Journal of Fertility 36: 10–15

45 Clinical aspects of the use of long-acting hormonal contraception

Edith Weisberg Ian S. Fraser

Introduction

Unintended pregnancy is still a major worldwide problem. It has been estimated by the United Nations Fund for Population Activities (UNFPA) that approximately 910 000 conceptions occur every day worldwide, of which 50% are unplanned and 25% are unwanted. One half of these unintended pregnancies result from contraceptive failures, which are mainly due to user failure to comply with either regular intake of a pill or with application of a contraceptive barrier prior to intercourse. Long-acting contraceptive steroid delivery systems, which reduce the requirement for regular action on the part of the user yet provide safe, effective and reversible contraception totally independent of coitus, are an important development in a world where the need and desire for birth spacing and reduction of family size is immense and where illegal abortion is estimated to result in 500 maternal deaths daily. To be acceptable to a majority of women, these long-acting methods should cause minimal menstrual disruption and have relatively few side effects. Since the appeal of different routes of administration and tolerance of side effects varies greatly from one woman to another, there is a need for a variety of delivery systems releasing differing steroids, especially as experience indicates that the availability of a wide choice of contraceptive methods encourages acceptance and sustained use.[1]

LONG-ACTING DELIVERY SYSTEM

Long-acting hormonal methods of contraception have been under development since the early 1960s. The first systems were all injectable preparations, mainly of 1–3 months duration, but more recently developed systems have become much more sophisticated and provide greatly extended durations of action.[2] Depot medroxyprogesterone acetate (DMPA; Depo-Provera, Upjohn) was first used in the early 1960s in high dosage for the treatment of threatened and recurrent miscarriage and premature labour. It proved ineffective for this purpose, but its contraceptive properties were noted when treated women failed to conceive for prolonged periods after use. Thereupon a number of successful clinical contraceptive trials were instituted.[3]

The addition of estrogen esters to long-acting progestogens to overcome irregular endometrial bleeding problems resulted in the development of combined monthly injectables between 1961 and 1964. In 1964, Folkman and Long[4] reported that small molecules such as steroids diffuse slowly at a constant rate through the membrane of a silicone rubber capsule. Segal and Croxatto, in 1967, demonstrated that silicone rubber capsules filled with a progestogen and placed subcutaneously could be used for long-term contraception.[5] Subsequently the Population Council developed and patented Norplant®, a subdermal implant system consisting of six capsules made of polydimethylsiloxane (Silastic® containing levonorgestrel. Clinical trials of this highly effective, long-acting, reversible method of contraception commenced in 1975. More recently, improved implant systems have been trialed using different progestogens and only one or two silastic rods, which simplify the insertion and removal procedures.

Vaginal contraceptive rings (CVRs), which provide a very effective means of delivering steroids for absorption through the vaginal wall, have been under development since the late 1960s. The initial CVRs containing progestogens alone were of two types: rings releasing relatively high doses of medroxyprogesterone acetate (MPA), norethindrone (NET) or norgestrel which suppressed ovulation and were left *in situ* for three weeks out of four,[6] and rings worn continuously, which released much lower doses of the same progestogens with effects similar to the progestogen-only pill.[7] The first multicentre clinical trials of CVRs took place during 1974–79. A CVR developed by the

World Health Organization (WHO) which released 20 μg levonorgestrel (LNG) over 24 h had a satisfactory clinical profile. More recently, CVRs containing a combination of estrogen plus progestogen, whose actions are similar to that of combined oral contraceptives, have been developed by several groups.

In 1973 clinical trials were started of an intra-uterine system (IUS) based on IUD technology but releasing different doses of natural progesterone. These trials resulted in the marketing of the Progestasert (Alza Corporation) in the United States in 1976, releasing on average 65 μg progesterone/24 hours with a lifespan of 12 months. By increasing the total amount of progesterone contained in the device, the lifespan was increased to three years,[8] however the Progestasert Intra-uterine Progesterone-releasing Contraceptive System (IPCS) has not reached widespread use because of irregular bleeding. The levonorgestrel releasing intra-uterine system has gained much more acceptability. Originally, daily release rates varying from 2–75 μg were studied. The higher release rates could not be sustained for prolonged periods of time, whilst the lowest doses did not provide reliable contraceptive cover. Ultimately an IUS releasing on average 20 μg/24 hours with a lifespan of more than 5–7 years has proved to be not only a very effective contraceptive but, on account of its reduction of menstrual blood loss, an excellent treatment for menorrhagia due to dysfunctional uterine bleeding.[9]

Ethical issues

Long-acting contraceptives have a long association with controversy, starting with the introduction of DMPA in the 1960s. Ironically, the very advantages provided by these methods are among the reasons for the controversy over their use. As a consequence of their high efficacy, ease of administration, long-acting effects and requirement for physician removal, methods such as DMPA and Norplant are more vulnerable to potential abuse. There is concern about their use in women who might not be able to give fully informed consent, such as women with an intellectual disability, a psychiatric disorder or who are substance abusers. There is also concern over the potential 'coercive use' of long-acting methods to control the fertility of low-income, disadvantaged or minority groups.

The concerns of women's health advocates about the need for informed choice, thorough counseling and follow-up are reasonable, but equally applicable to all methods of contraception. To some extent DMPA and other long-acting methods have become a lightning rod for a broad band of political, feminist and social positions about the rights of women and minority groups.[3] There is a need for women to feel that they have control over their decisions, particularly with regard to new contraceptive technology. On the other hand, it is presumptuous for some feminist and consumer groups to think that women are incapable of choosing for themselves when given detailed and balanced information. It is incumbent on health professionals to provide clients and the community with accurate information in a readily understood format and to discuss the concerns of individual women realistically, so that they are well aware of the benefits, risks, advantages and disadvantages of any method of fertility control they are considering. Only if this is done can women make truly informed choices.

Legal issues

Many individuals in modern societies appear to expect that contraceptives can be 'perfect', that is 100% effective and with no adverse or side effects. It is highly unlikely that such an ideal contraceptive will ever exist. Current methods can never be proven to be absolutely safe. Rare but potentially serious side effects might only be demonstrated after very large groups of women have used a method for very long periods of time under careful surveillance. Such post-marketing surveillance is difficult and expensive. Some of the newer 'high-tech' long-acting delivery systems such as Norplant are much more complex in clinical deployment than conventional contraceptives are. Therefore, it is becoming more critical that health personnel are thoroughly trained in their use, including advantages, disadvantages and potential problems. In particular, with implant systems certificated training should be required in insertion and removal techniques. These techniques are not always as simple as they appear at first sight! Experiences in the United States and to a lesser extent in the United Kingdom have shown that western society is becoming increasingly litigious, with the expectation that if an adverse event (even a well recognized one) occurs as a result of contraceptive use someone must be at fault and monetary compensation must be obtained, usually by resorting to the courts. A not inconsiderable number of legal suits are pending in both countries in association with Norplant use, either as a result of technical problems relating to insertion or removal or of perceived failure to fully inform women of possible side effects, such as poor cycle control. Expensive lawsuits are already discouraging pharmaceutical companies from developing and marketing new systems and will ultimately disadvantage women by reducing their contraceptive choices.

Current usage

Marketing approval for DMPA, the first popular long-acting injectable, was first sought in the USA in 1967. It is now approved for use in more than 100 countries and is used by more than nine million women around the world,[10] especially in some developing countries where injections are viewed as beneficial to health. However, it is now also widely regarded as a first choice method in many developed countries.

Early combined estrogen-progestogen injectable formulations had an extremely high rate of effectiveness. However concerns about the possible toxicity of high doses of estrogen delayed their further development. Recent work by the World Health Organization has led to the development, testing and marketing of two very successful and effective once-a-month injectables (Cyclofem and Mesigyna), which are gaining popularity in Mexico and other Latin American countries and in the People's Republic of China.[11]

Clinical trials of Norplant began in 1975 in seven countries and further clinical trials have continued both in developed and developing countries. Norplant was first registered for contraceptive use in Finland in 1983 and since then more than 50 countries, including the USA, have approved the method for distribution. To date 55 000 women have participated in closely supervised trials in 50 countries and well over four million women have used Norplant in countries where it has been approved.[12]

The levonorgestrel IUS (Levonova, Mirena; Leiras & Schering) was initially marketed in Finland in the late 1980s, and has gained steady popularity in Scandinavia and other European countries. More widespread marketing of this innovative and potentially popular system is expected over the next few years.

Different delivery systems

Injectables

DMPA is an aqueous suspension of microcrystals of medroxyprogesterone acetate, a progestogen with a structure very close to that of natural progesterone. Due to the low solubility of this synthetic steroid in the aqueous medium, when given as microcrystals by deep intramuscular injection DMPA has a prolonged release rate from the depot site.[13] The peak serum level of MPA is 10–25 ng/ml at 5–20 days after injection, decreasing to 5–10 ng/ml by 30 days after injection. Detectable levels can still be found in serum 185 days after injection.[14] The duration of its progestational effect is largely dependent on formulation characteristics, particularly crystal size. Some generic formulations have failed to control particle size distribution adequately with significant adverse effects on clinical performance. DMPA is given in a dosage of 150 mg every 12 weeks.

The other widely used long-acting progestogen-only intramuscular injection contains norethisterone (norethindrone) enanthate (NET-EN), the 7-carbon ester derivative of the synthetic progestogen norethindrone in an oily suspension (benzyl benzoate:castor oil, 4:6). Given in a dose of 200 mg, peak serum levels of 8 ng/ml are reached about 10 days after injection and by 98–112 days levels are undetectable.[15] After more than seven injections the rate of decline of serum levels appears to slow in some women. NET-EN is usually given as a 2–3 monthly injection of 200 mg.

Two once-a-month injectables developed by the WHO Special Programme of Research in Human Reproduction contain estradiol valerate 5 mg combined with NET-EN 50 mg (Mesigyna) or estradiol cypionate 5 mg combined with DMPA 25 mg (Cyclofem). These estrogen esters were selected because they exhibited slower hydrolysis rates following intramuscular injections than other formulations. With these preparations progestogen levels reach a peak 3–5 days after administration, slowly decreasing until the next injection, whereas the estrogen serum concentrations decline to reach baseline values by days 10–15 and 7–12 after estradiol cypionate and estradiol-valerate injections, respectively.[16]

Implants

Several biodegradable implants have been developed to provide controlled release of steroids, using bioerodable polymers as carriers. One such system, Capronor, based on poly (ε-caprolactone) and releasing levonorgestrel has been developed by the World Health Organization, National Institutes of Health and the CONRAD program in the United States and has so far been tested in limited phase I and II clinical trials.[17] Serum levels of levonorgestrel showed considerable inter and intrapersonal variation, and the system now seems unlikely to be developed further even though the concept of a biodegradeable implant was an appealing one.

Norplant is a subdermal implant system, consisting of six soft, flexible capsules of Silastic rubber, each containing levonorgestrel 36 mg for a total dose of 216 mg. The dimension of each capsule is 3.6 cm × 2.4 mm. The capsules are inserted under local anesthetic by means of a trocar in a superficial plane in a fan shape under the skin of the inside of the upper arm. Following insertion, the dose of levonorgestrel provided by Norplant is about 85 µg per 24 hours, declining to about 50 µg by 9 months, 35 µg by 18 months and to about 30 µg per 24 hours for the remainder of its recommended use period of five years. Beyond five years of use the release rate becomes less predictable, with pregnancy rates reported to increase significantly except in slim women.[12] Within 24–96 hours of removal of the capsules levonorgestrel levels become undetectable in serum, allowing a rapid return of fertility.[18]

A second generation of Norplant (Jadelle; Schering-Leiras) also developed by the Population Council, and consisting of only two rods that release approximately 30 µg per day of levonorgestrel over three years, has recently received marketing approval in the USA.[19] Each implant is composed of a drug-releasing core, which is a mixture of 50% levonorgestrel and 50% elastomer by weight surrounded by a thin-walled silicone rubber tubing. The rods are 2.5 mm in diameter and 4.3 cm in length with each containing 75 mg levonorgestrel for a total drug load of 150 mg per set.

A single Silastic capsule (Implanon; Organon), 30 mm in length with an outer diameter of 2.4 mm filled with crystalline 3-keto-desogestrel (3-KDG) with an average release rate of 10–15 µg per 24 hours is also close to marketing. It has a probable lifespan of 2–3 years.[20] A single capsule implant, Uniplant (South to South Program), releasing nomogestrol will probably only have an effective lifespan of one year. The Uniplant device consists of a silastic tube 2.4 mm in diameter and 39 mm in length, containing 55 mg nomegestrol acetate, a 19-nor-progesterone derivative.[21] New progestogens such as Nestorone® are also undergoing development as a single rod implant system (Population Council). The reduction in the number of rods increases the ease of insertion and reduces problems with removal but will also reduce the lifespan of each device compared to Norplant.

Contraceptive vaginal rings (CVRs)

CVRs are made of nontoxic dimethylpolysiloxane or similar nonbiodegradable polymer and release steroids in proportion to their surface area and the core loading and inversely in proportion to the thickness of the outer wall. The duration of action of the device is determined by the amount of steroid contained within the reservoir. They are positioned in the upper vagina but do not need to fit around the cervix.

Some original CVRs had the steroid homogeneously impregnated throughout the silastic ring. This resulted in decreasing serum levels of steroid with increasing use due to successive depletion of the drug from the outer layers of the ring. The increasing distance the drug had to travel to the surface of the ring resulted in nonuniform release rates.[22] Core CVRs which have a central core containing the steroid surrounded by a layer of inert silastic through which the drug must travel before reaching the vagina produce a much more constant release rate. The shell ring, in which the steroid-containing portion is centered between a nonmedicated central core and outer band, also provides effective constant steady release of steroid. The thickness of the outer layer, the overall surface area of the ring and the core loading regulate the steroid release rate. The Population Council has developed combined CVRs in which the two contraceptive steroids, norethindrone acetate and ethinyl estradiol, are distributed within two cores made of a mixture of steroid and Dow Corning Medical Adhesive A incorporated into a flexible Silastic ring 58 mm in diameter and 7.6 mm in cross-sectional diameter. These show promise of providing a ring with an effective lifespan of 6–12 months.[23] Organon International (Oss, Netherlands) is working with a combination two-compartment Silastic ring system where the steroids are contained in two ethylene vinyl acetate fiber cores. The mean daily release rate for this ring is 120 µg 3-KDG and 15 µg ethinyl estradiol.[24]

Studies of CVRs indicate a rapid absorption of steroids through the vaginal mucosa into the systemic circulation, but the exact mechanism is uncertain. It might be passive, without a rate-limiting mechanism other than the concentration gradient set up by the accumulation of steroid in the vaginal secretions.[22] There may also be some local absorption into the pelvic tissues with preferential effect on cervical and endometrial cells.

CVRs can release progestogens alone or as a combination of estrogen and progestogen. Rings containing high doses of a variety of progestogens produced variable suppression of ovulation but had unacceptably high incidences of breakthrough bleeding. The most successful early high dose progestogen-only ring was a CVR releasing 100 mg MPA daily.[6]

WHO has developed a continuous use ring that releases levonorgestrel at a low dose of 20 µg/24 hours, with almost constant release rates for three months.[25]

Two dosage levels of 3-keto-desogestrel (15 and 30 µg/24 hrs) have also been studied in progestogen-only CVRs. Both doses produced significant bleeding disturbances and resulted in formation of some persistent follicles but completely prevented ovulation.[24]

Combined CVRs releasing variable doses of ethinyl estradiol have been tested combined with a variety of progestogens, of which the most successful appear to be combinations of ethinyl estradiol 15–20 µg combined with norethindrone acetate (NET-Ac; 1 mg),[23] nestorone (150 µg) or 3-keto-desogestrel (120 µg).[6] The rings are initially inserted on the fifth day of the menstrual cycle, left *in situ* for 21 days, removed for 4–7 days and then reinserted for a further 21 days, providing fairly constant steroid levels.

Steroid releasing intra-uterine systems (IUS)

There are two marketed hormone-releasing intra-uterine systems, one releasing progesterone (Progestasert; Alza Corporation) and the other releasing LNG (Levo-Nova, Mirena; Leiras–Schering). The Progestasert is a T-shaped device with a length of 36 mm and a width of 32 mm. Progesterone from a silicone oil base is released at an expected rate of 65 µg/day through the wall of the ethylene vinyl acetate copolymer stem, which contains the reservoir of progesterone (52 mg).[8]

Levonorgestrel is well absorbed from the uterine cavity, resulting in measurable amounts in serum. By using a Silastic polymer impregnated with LNG and covering it with Silastic tubing, a steady release rate is possible. The incorporation of this system into the Nova-T IUD framework has resulted in the LNG IUS. The effective dose has proved to be 20 µg/24 hours with a lifespan of five years.[9]

Animal toxicology

To meet the requirements of American and other international regulatory agencies, a series of acute and chronic toxicology studies are required in rodents and other laboratory animals utilizing doses which approximate one, three and ten times the proposed human dose. For example, repeated-dose studies indicated that DMPA, administered orally or parentally, at doses up to 10 times the human therapeutic contraceptive dose is nontoxic when administered to dogs and rats over a six month period, to rabbits over a one year period and to monkeys over a 28 month period. As expected, the only changes which were noted were hormonal in nature and included reduced semen volume and a dose-related decrease in adrenal function. Toxicology issues are discussed in further detail in chapter 3. However, controversy has surrounded the use of DMPA as a result of toxicology studies in rhesus monkeys and beagle dogs, which indicated a possible increase in endometrial cancer in monkeys given doses greatly in excess of those used for contraception in women.[27] Beagle bitches responded to injections of DMPA with an increase in breast lumps, some of which became cancerous. In response to these concerns the WHO has reviewed all available data from clinical and basic research and has conducted a number of multinational case control studies. Results from these studies indicate that there is no overall increase in risk of breast, endometrial, ovarian or liver cancer in users of DMPA. The WHO and United States Food and Drug Administration (FDA) as a result have concurred that the beagle dog is not a good species for predicting human risk and therefore no longer require beagle dog studies for marketing approval.[26,27,28]

A first generation combined injectable known as Deladroxate has been widely used in Latin America. It contains dihydroxyprogesterone acetophenide 150 mg and estradiol enanthate 10 mg. There were initial controversies regarding the use of Deladroxate. Animal studies indicated that in some susceptible mammalian species, pituitary and mammary tumours were induced by this drug combination, probably because of high dosage.[29] Evidence of the accumulation of metabolites of the drug in users long after its intended biological action should have disappeared were also reported.

Mechanism of action

The effect of the long-acting methods on pituitary, ovarian, endometrial and cervical function are dependent on the dose and type of steroid delivered by the system. Methods delivering a combination of estrogens and progestogens or high doses of progestogen usually suppress follicular development and ovulation by suppressing the hypothalamic-pituitary axis.[30] Methods releasing lower doses of progestogen alone have a variable effect on hypothalamic-pituitary ovarian function dependent on serum levels of the drug. With higher levels, such as those achieved in the first year of Norplant use, ovulation is usually suppressed. With lower levels, gonadotropin levels are not completely suppressed and follicular activity results in periodic estradiol peaks. However ovulation only occurs infrequently as the circulating progestogen level is usually sufficient to inhibit the positive feedback effect of estradiol on LH release.[31] There is also a direct effect on luteal function resulting in defective progesterone secretion.[12] Landgren and Diczfaluzy summarized four characteristic and distinctly different types of ovarian reaction to low dose progestogens: Group A: no sign of follicular or luteal activity evidenced by low estradiol and progesterone levels; group B: marked cyclical follicular activity but no luteal function; group C: normal follicular activity but inadequate luteal function; and group D: who had estradiol and progesterone levels indistinguishable from their pretreatment ovulatory cycle.[32]

In women using long-acting progestogen-only methods, the endometrium is initially secretory, then suppressed, and eventually atrophic. Progestogens induce significant changes in endometrial infrastructure, including a reduction in the number and diameter of endometrial glands[33] and an increase in microvascular density with more fragile superficial thin-walled vessels due to a disturbance in angiogenesis.[34,35] These changes appear to be accompanied by changes at a cellular level in a variety of parameters, including steroid receptors, prostaglandins, cytokines and growth factors whose significance is poorly understood. They also affect the expression of cell surface receptor molecules such as integrins, which may be very important for implantation (see ch. 36).

Progestogens given alone or combined with estrogens have effects on various properties of cervical mucus and decrease or inhibit sperm transport depending on dose, potency and individual responsiveness. There is a disappearance of ferning and spinnbarkeit and an increase in viscosity and cellularity as well as biochemical changes.[35] Progestogens have been demonstrated *in vitro* to affect both the motility and oxidative metabolism of spermatozoa as well as increasing the permeability of the sperm plasma membrane, compromising the longevity of sperm.[36]

Clinical effects

Efficacy

Contraceptive efficacy of all long-acting methods is high since user failure is reduced. Failure rates for DMPA, demonstrated in large-scale studies in a variety of communities, are below 0.5 per hundred woman-years (HWY).[37] Failure rates with NET-EN are slightly higher but are still usually less than 1/HWY(45).[38] Modern once-a-month injectables also have low failure rates less than 0.5/HWY.[39]

Contraceptive implant systems have remarkably high efficacy levels. The cumulative pregnancy rate for the standard version of Norplant (soft silastic tubing) at the end of five years of use is only 1.1.[40] Studies of an earlier version of Norplant (with hard silastic tubing which reduced the LNG release rate slightly) had indicated a somewhat lower efficacy rate for women weighing more than 70 kg. Serum levels of levonorgestrel with the standard soft silastic tubing are slightly higher in years 4 and 5, producing annual pregnancy rates of around 0.2 per 100 women with no difference in women weighing more than 70 kg.

Pregnancy rates for Jadelle (Norplant II) are not statistically different from those of Norplant. A Chinese study of Jadelle found a gross cumulative pregnancy rate of 0.65 per 100 women at the end of five years.[41] By contrast, the one-year implant, Uniplant, has a 12 month net cumulative pregnancy rate of 0.9%.[42]

CVRs also provide effective contraception. A large multicenter phase III study of the 20 μg levonorgestrel-releasing vaginal ring reported a one year pregnancy rate of 3.7/HWY.[43] There have been no large scale efficacy studies of combined CVRs but smaller studies suggest the one year pregnancy rate is likely to be less than 1.5/HWY. Large scale studies of the LNG-releasing IUS suggest it may be even more effective than Norplant with a pregnancy rate of 0.1 per HWY after five years of use.[44]

Indications for use

Long-acting progestogen-only methods provide a particularly useful choice:

- for most women requiring highly effective long-term reversible contraception
- for women in whom estrogens are contraindicated or not tolerated
- for women older than 35 years who are cigarette smokers
- during lactation
- women with diabetes mellitus, mild hypertension, homozygous sickle cell disease, migraine including focal migraine
- women who are unreliable or unwilling pill takérs.

The combined injectables or CVRs are suitable for women who dislike or are erratic pill takers but desire regular menstrual cycles with highly effective contraception coitally-independent, requiring minimal action on the user's part.

Contraindications: progestogen-only methods

Absolute

- Known or suspected pregnancy

- Undiagnosed abnormal vaginal bleeding
- Injectable methods should be avoided in women with coagulation disorders and those on long-term anticoagulation therapy because of the risk of hematoma at the injection site
- DMPA is unsuitable for women who wish to conceive within the next year
- Women who find irregular bleeding and spotting or amenorrhea unacceptable, especially for cultural reasons

Relative

Women with the following conditions require careful consideration because the potential risks of using a progestogen-only method may outweigh the benefits. Careful medical supervision is required in women with:

- breast cancer as the influence of progestogens on progression is unclear
- diabetes with vascular disease as progestogens may lower HDL-cholesterol and elevate LDL-cholesterol, thus exacerbating the risk of arteriosclerosis
- cerebrovascular or coronary heart disease because of possible lipid changes
- severe hypertension (BP > 180/110) or hypertension with vascular disease
- acute liver disease as progestogens are metabolized by the liver
- chronic liver disease, e.g. cirrhosis with evidence of failure
- history of or current benign or malignant liver tumor
- use of enzyme-inducing drugs as these may lower the efficacy of low-dose progestogen methods
- history of recurrent functional ovarian cysts as these may be more prevalent with low-dose progestogen methods
- immediately postpartum in lactating women (preferably started at six weeks postpartum).

Contraindications: combined estrogen-progestogen long-acting methods

Contraindications are similar to the combined oral contraceptive pill (see Ch. 44).

Contraindications: combined estrogen-progestogen long-acting methods as recommended by the Central Medical Advisory Committee of the International Planned Parenthood Federation.

Absolute

- Confirmed or suspected pregnancy
- Confirmed past or present evidence of thromboembolic disorders
- Cerebrovascular or coronary artery disease
- Focal migraine
- Malignancy of the breast
- Diabetes with vascular complications
- Undiagnosed vaginal bleeding
- Prolonged immobilization
- Four weeks prior to elective surgery if prolonged immobilization is likely (unless prophylactic anticoagulants are given)
- Homozygous sickle cell disease.

Relative

- Heavy smoking (> 20 cigarettes per day) in women over 35
- Severe hypertension (BP > 180/110)
- Hypertension with vascular disease
- Severe cirrhosis or acute liver disease
- Liver tumor, benign or malignant
- Use of hepatic enzyme-inducing drugs.

Effects on lactation

Combined oral contraceptives have been shown in most studies to adversely affect the quantity and quality of breast milk and reduce the duration of lactation, particularly when initiated in the first few months postpartum.[45] There are no data on the effects of combined injectables or CVRs on lactation and infant growth and development. Until these data are available it is advisable that these methods should be avoided during lactation.

Nearly all studies of progestogen-only methods have found either a beneficial or no effect on milk quantity, quality and duration of breast-feeding.[46,47] Small amounts of steroids appear in breast milk, are consumed by the infant, and can be detected in the infant's blood but it has been calculated that the total amount of steroid consumed by the fully breast-fed infant is one hundredth of the maternal dose. The concentration of hormone in breast milk may be influenced by its affinity for steroid-binding proteins in maternal blood as only the unbound steroid can pass into milk.[48] No adverse effects of the ingestion of steroid-containing milk by infants have been reported either on infant growth or development. A long-term study of children exposed to DMPA during breast-feeding followed up to the age of 10–11 years found no differences in physical and mental growth compared to a control group.[49] For the few children who had reached puberty there was also no significant difference in sexual development. However, for most long-acting progestogen contraceptives there are no data on long-term effects of ingestion during breast feeding. This has prompted the development of both implants and vaginal rings releasing Nestorone®, a progestogen poorly absorbed from the gastrointestinal tract and therefore less likely to be absorbed by the breast-fed neonate.

Fetal exposure

Data on teratogenicity of long-acting steroidal methods are sparse as pregnancy during use is rare and if it occurs the pregnancy is often terminated soon after recognition. In humans the only probable teratogenic effect of progestogens is virilization of a female fetus by androgenic progestogens (see ch. 43), but this would occur only with doses well in excess of those being received by women using injectable or implanted progestogen contraceptives.[50] Other anomalies that have been sporadically recorded in association with the use of contraceptive steroids during early pregnancy are cardiac and limb reduction deformities, neural tube defects, vertebral, anal, tracheo-oesophageal and renal defects. To date, there are no good data to support the existence of any link between the contraceptive usage and these anomalies, nor is there any evidence that these methods influence the likelihood of mutagenic abnormalities (ch. 43).

Hormone dependent cancers

Much concern has been generated over the possibility that the use of steroids for contraception could result in an increase in hormone-dependent tumors. Whilst there are extensive data on combined oral contraceptive exposure and various cancers, there are relatively few data on long-acting and progestogen-only contraceptive exposure. These data are discussed thoroughly in chapters 67 and 68. Carefully designed epidemiological studies will also be required to clarify the possible effects of new methods, as it is not advisable to extrapolate from studies of one method to another.

Breast cancer

A recent analysis of breast cancer risk associated with contraceptive steroid use assessed data from 54 studies out of 25 countries which compared 53 297 women with breast cancer and 100 239 controls. Included amongst this sample were 0.8% who had used progestogen-only pills and 1.5% who had used DMPA. The study found that current users of combined oral contraceptives are at a slightly increased risk of detection of breast cancer (RR 1.24) during oral contraceptive use, reducing back to 1.00 by 10 years following cessation.[51] However, because the incidence of breast cancer in young women is low the excess cancers associated with steroid use are very few in number. The data seem to indicate that the risks are similar for DMPA and POP but the numbers of users of these methods are too low to be conclusive. It is not possible to extrapolate from this or other studies as to what the effect of long-acting methods may be on breast cancer risk (ch. 68).

Cervical cancer

The relationship of cervical cancer to steroidal contraceptive use remains unclear due to numerous methodological problems. DMPA has been associated with an increased risk of cervical cancer but this risk becomes nonsignificant when allowance is made for confounding variables such as smoking, sexual activity and sexually transmitted diseases.[52] There are no reliable data on the effect of low-dose progestogens on the development of cervical cancer.[53] Only one published study has looked at the risk of cervical cancer in relationship to combined injectable use, with inconclusive results.[54]

Ovarian cancer

Combined oral contraceptives (COC) have a strong protective effect against ovarian cancer: this persists for 10–15 years after cessation of use.[55] However, although it is thought that the protective effect is due to a reduction in ovulation, a mechanism of action of all combined and long-acting methods, close analogies cannot necessarily be drawn. There are no good data on the effect of low-dose progestogens on ovarian cancer risk. Presumably methods such as Norplant, which do not consistently prevent ovulation, will have a lesser protective effect than COC.

Endometrial cancer

Both the combined pill and DMPA have been shown to reduce the risk of endometrial cancer by 40–60%, a protective effect that lasts for 15 years after cessation of use.[56] There are no data on low-dose progestogen methods, either oral or long-acting, but, based on evidence that the protective effect of COC and DMPA is related to progestogen dose and its antiproliferative effect on the endometrium, it seems likely that other long-acting methods containing progestogen will also have some protective effect on the endometrium.

Noncontraceptive benefits

Whilst a number of substantial noncontraceptive health benefits have been found to result from use of COC, the evidence for progestogen-only and long-acting combined methods is limited. It is likely that similar benefits will accrue but the dosage and route of administration may vary the effect. Data from DMPA users indicate that the total volume of menstrual blood loss is greatly reduced and consequently iron-deficiency anemia is decreased.[37] This is less likely to be the case with progestogen-only implants and CVRs as amenorrhea is less common and irregular bleeding, and spotting are more common. However, preliminary evidence indicates that most women using these methods experience a small decrease in measured blood loss; few will experience an increase. Other menstrual benefits related to DMPA are due to suppression of ovulation and include a decrease in dysmenorrhea, premenstrual symptoms[37] and symptomatic relief in endometriosis.[57] Since ovulation suppression is variable with low-dose long-acting progestogen-only methods, these benefits will occur for some women but will not be consistent. In women with a hemoglobinopathy, DMPA may improve anemia and in sickle cell disease it can decrease the number and severity of sickling crises.[58]

In a small study DMPA has been associated with a reduced incidence of acute pelvic inflammatory disease (PID) in women infected with *Neisseria gonorrhea*.[59] Similar effects have been ascribed to COC use.

The LNG-releasing IUS has a lower discontinuation rate for PID than a copper-bearing device and the incidence of pelvic inflammatory disease amongst users appears to be lower than in the noncontraceptive user population.[60] As this is thought to be due to the effect of progestogen on the tenacity of cervical mucus producing a barrier to bacterial penetration, the endometrium where atrophy decreases the medium for bacterial growth, and possibly decreased tubal contractility, which could reduce upward propulsion of bacteria.[61] It is likely that all long-acting methods will have some protective effect against PID. However, these methods do not provide adequate individual protection against sexually transmissible diseases: women likely to be at risk should be advised to use a condom in addition to their hormonal method.

Although DMPA has been shown to significantly reduce the recurrence rate for vaginal candidiasis there are no data on the effects of other methods.[62]

Side effects

The most consistent and troublesome side effect of long-acting progestogen-only methods is disruption of the menstrual cycle, which is the commonest reason for discontinuation. The experience of bleeding disturbances and assessment of blood loss is a subjective experience that may be perceived differently by the individual. In an attempt at standardization, the Population Council and the WHO have developed a protocol for the reporting of menstrual disturbances.[63] Dividing the menstrual diary recording period into 90 day reference periods from the start of use of the method is a particularly useful concept for all long-acting and particularly progestogen-only methods where cycle length is highly variable. The WHO has developed a computer program which defines bleeding/spotting episodes as one or more consecutive days during which blood loss has been entered in the menstrual diary, with each episode being bounded by intervals of bleeding/spotting-free days. More recent studies of hormonal contraceptive use have tended to use the WHO definitions in order to allow comparison of bleeding patterns between individual methods.

With DMPA the majority of women experience substantial alteration of the menstrual cycle, with 50% developing amenorrhea after 12 months of use.[64] Bleeding appears to be related to the body mass index (BMI). In a Swedish study women with a BMI>25 had a clear tendency towards early amenorrhea and less bleeding disturbances while the opposite was true of women with a BMI <25.[89] Counseling and reassurance are often all that is required to manage bleeding problems but sometimes when bleeding is prolonged, once other medical causes have been eliminated, administration of estrogens is useful. However, the bleeding disturbances often recur after cessation of estrogen therapy.

Bleeding disturbances can also occur after cessation of use, as the effect of DMPA on ovarian suppression is reduced and intermittent follicular development occurs prior to the re-establishment of ovulation.[104] NET-EN users have similar levels of menstrual disruption but only about 30% experience amenorrhea.[64]

In Norplant users, about 60% experience significant menstrual disturbance in the first year of use. The bleeding patterns vary amongst individual women and with duration of use, being more prolonged and irregular during the first year.[65] A detailed analysis of menstrual diaries of women using Norplant showed that 34% had 97 or more days of bleeding in the first year of use and 15% had at least one episode lasting longer than 15 days. In the third year of use these figures were 19% and 7% respectively. Amenorrhea, defined as no bleeding for 90 days or more, was reported by 26% in year 1 and 15% in year 3.[66] The bleeding patterns appear to be partially influenced by the production of endogenous estradiol. As LNG release rates gradually drop with progressive use, and more ovulatory cycles occur, bleeding patterns improve.[67]

Uniplant, the nomogestrol acetate-releasing implant, appears to produce fewer bleeding disturbances, with approximately 56% of women having bleeding patterns similar to normal menstruation.[42]

Progestogen-releasing IUSs have been shown to substantially reduce menstrual blood loss. Progestasert users experience a 40% reduction in volume of blood loss,[68] whilst women using the LNG IUS reported a decrease in both the number of bleeding days and the amount,[69] although during the first one to three months of use of the LNG IUS the number of bleeding/spotting days was greater. Women usually experience a 60% decrease in menstrual blood loss by three months and more than 75% by the end of 12 months use. Amenorrhea has been commonly reported with the LNG-IUS, accounting in initial trials for between 1.6–5.4% of discontinuations in the first year of use. By the end of the five year lifespan of the device, 26% of women are amenorrheic, 71% have regular scanty bleeds and 6% irregular scanty bleeds. Among women who continue use of Mirena with the insertion of a second device, the percentage experiencing amenorrhea increases with increased duration of use. However, with a modification of the counseling given prior to use, amenorrhea or 'no-bleeding contraception', has become a desirable side effect. The bleeding disturbances occurring during LNG IUS use are the result of a local effect of LNG on the endometrium that is characterized by a total loss of cyclical changes; proliferation is strongly suppressed and the endometrium gradually becomes atrophic, with few short, straight glands and a thin decidualized stroma.[34]

The WHO LNG-releasing CVR produced amenorrhea in only 1% of users, normal patterns in 50% and in the remainder the most commonly observed pattern was irregular bleeding.[25] As with implants, the bleeding patterns appear to be influenced by the variable effect of LNG on ovarian function and consequently endogenous estradiol production as well as the direct progestogenic effect on the endometrium.[70] In a comparison of nine methods of contraception and a control group of noncontracepting women,[71] Belsey et al found that women using the WHO CVR had slightly more and longer bleeding/spotting episodes per 90 day period than users of other methods but fewer and shorter episodes than noncontracepting women. Combined estrogen/progestogen CVRs used in a cyclic manner provide good cycle control comparable to COC.[72] Rings containing NET and EE produce slightly more regular bleeding patterns than combinations of estradiol and LNG.

Bleeding patterns with combined injectables are much more regular than long-acting progestogen-only methods but there are still significant deviations from normal. Amongst women using modern once-a-month injectables, 23–25% experienced some irregular bleeding compared with 4.8% of untreated women and 11–13% experienced prolonged bleeding compared with 2.3% of untreated women with 3–6 months of use.[73] During the first 90 days of use there were significantly more bleeding/spotting days and more episodes, presumably reflecting the pharmacokinetics of the drugs, the first bleed occurring 15 days after the first injection as an estradiol withdrawal bleed. Amenorrhea is uncommon, occurring in around 1% of users.

If bleeding during use of progestogen-only long-acting methods is persistently excessively heavy nonsteroidal anti-inflammatory drugs or tranexamic acid can be tried. Estrogens on their own appear to have no effect on heavy bleeding[74] but a low-dose combined pill can be tried, although no data exist on effectiveness. Recently it has been reported that the use of mifepristone can improve bleeding patterns but again no good data are available. If heavy bleeding is likely to affect the health of the woman or if the woman requests it implants should be removed.

Bone density

In 1991 a New Zealand study raised concerns about the effect of long-term DMPA use on bone mineral density (BMD). This small cross-sectional study indicated that women who had used DMPA for five years or more had a reduced bone density of the lumbar spine and femoral neck compared to controls matched for age, race and BMI, but a greater bone density in the lumbar spine when compared to postmenopausal controls.[75] There were a number of methodological problems, as there were double the number of smokers in the DMPA group, baseline

BMDs were unavailable and the study was not controlled for risk factors such as exercise history, family history of osteoporosis and alcohol use. Two subsequent cross-sectional studies from the UK which were reported at the 4th Congress of the European Society for Contraception indicated that the majority of amenorrheic long-term DMPA users had slightly lower BMDs of lumbar spine and hip (96%) compared to age and weight matched controls, with 83% of amenorrheic women in both studies having serum estradiol levels below 100–150 pmol/L. However, both studies found no correlation between duration of DMPA use, period of amenorrhea or estradiol levels and BMD.[76,77] The only randomized study reported to date followed a small group of women allocated to Norplant or DMPA for six months but looked only at forearm BMD. Users of Norplant showed an increase in forearm BMD (2.9%) compared to unchanged values in DMPA users.[78] The changes in bone density were consistent with the changes in biochemical indices for bone metabolism; DMPA users showed signs of increased bone turnover and users of the LNG implant showed increased bone formation, with increased levels of both alkaline phosphatase and osteocalcin.

As women may use progestogen-only methods for many years, an adverse effect on the skeleton may affect the peak bone mass reached in adults as well as the premenopausal bone loss rate, both of which are important for future fracture risk. It appears that there could be a difference in these factors related to either the type, dose or ovarian function effects of different progestogens but further research is required both during prospective use and on cessation.

These concerns about hypoestrogenicity during longterm DMPA use and its possible effect on bone density have raised fears that its use in young women under 16 years could affect the postmenarcheal increase of bone mineral density. The concerns need to be balanced with the obvious benefits of use of a long-acting method when counselling adolescents.

Metabolic changes

Metabolic changes during long-acting contraceptive use depends on the steroid content, delivery method and dose. Progestogen-only methods have been reported to decrease triglyceride and cholesterol levels, to increase LDL-cholesterol and to produce a transient increase in HDL-cholesterol (or a slight decrease); but generally changes remain well within the normal range,[79] suggesting that these methods would not influence the development of cardio-vascular disease. With the combined once-a-month injectables minor changes in lipid levels occurred, reflecting the circulating levels of the two components, but none of the changes were clinically significant and all reverted to baseline after discontinuation of treatment.[80]

None of the progestogen-only long-acting methods appear to have clinically significant effects on blood coagulation or carbohydrate metabolism.[70,79]

Side effects

Side effects reported for long-acting methods are similar to those reported for oral contraceptives and show great individual differences. These include variable effects on weight, with women using DMPA most likely to experience a weight increase averaging about 2 kg at the end of 12 months use. Headache, abdominal bloating, mood change and depression have also been reported.[3] Acne occurs occasionally in women using Norplant. Functional ovarian cysts sometimes occur in users of progestogen-only methods. These are generally asymptomatic but palpable by clinicians, disappear spontaneously and do not require surgical intervention unless a rare complication such as torsion occurs.

The report of erythematous vaginal lesions in 48 out of 139 women using the LNG releasing CVR, which appeared to be related to chronic inflammation, has resulted in redesign of this ring, although the etiology is uncertain.[81] A higher dose ring releasing 300 μg/day, used cyclically for periods varying from 3–6 months, elicited some degree of atrophy of the vaginal rugae at the end of treatment but no ulcerations. A trial of a placebo ring by WHO found no lesions attributable to ring use when the vagina was inspected with a colposcope, suggesting that changes could be related to the effects of some progestogens on the vaginal mucosa. There is also a theoretical concern about a possible adverse effect of high local progesterone concentration on viral transcription and mucosal transfer (e.g. HPV and HIV) in the cervix and vagina.

Following reports of vaginal lesions in women using levonorgestrel-only CVRs, women using combined rings have undergone careful vaginal inspection with a colposcope.[82] Results to date suggest that significant lesions found in combined CVR users are no more common than in a control group of women who did not use CVRs, and that short to medium-term use does not produce serious adverse effects on the vaginal mucosa. However, further long-term studies are required to confirm that use for more than one year does not result in more serious lesions.

Return of fertility

DMPA produces the greatest delay in the return of fertility on cessation of use, but this is relatively short-term with no permanent effect on fertility in nulliparous or parous women.[83] The median conception time is 8–10 months after the last injection is given, i.e. 5–7 months after the drug could have been expected to wear off. Seventy-five percent of women conceive within 15 months of their last injection and 95% within two years. Persistent anovulation, due to very slow metabolism and hence persistence of the drug, produces the delay in return of fertility. This is reversed as soon as the drug is cleared from the system. Prolonged duration of use does not increase the delay in return of fertility.

With other progestogen-only and combined long-acting methods return of fertility is rapid. Pregnancy rates are 50% at three months and 86% at one year in women after removal of Norplant.[84] Similarly, the return of fertility following removal of Jadelle (Norplant II) was within normal limits.[85] With the removal of the LNG IUS, return of fertility is immediate.[44] Data on return of fertility following cessation of combined injectables are sparse but reassuring. In a small group of women given Cyclofem, 52% ovulated during the first posttreatment month and 71% in the second month, whilst on ceasing Mesigyna use 19% women ovulated in the first post-use month and 67% during the second month.[80]

Acceptability and continuation rates

Studies specifically designed to determine acceptability of different contraceptive methods in large representative groups of women are rare. Acceptability rates have largely been extrapolated from discontinuation rates and reasons given by users for stopping the method. Reasons for discontinuation vary with cultural, religious and social factors and are influenced by attitudes of the local media, pressure groups and both the accuracy of information and the level of counseling provided prior to use. Contraceptive acceptability studies can contribute to increased method acceptance and continuation by identifying issues and concerns that can be used to direct the development of informational material which can dispel rumors and correct misinformation. These studies might also be useful in identifying obstacles that stop a woman from using a method even though she finds it acceptable.

Injectables

Continuation rates for DMPA calculated by actuarial life-table methods from WHO multicenter trials ranged from 49–71% at one year,[86] and were similar to those for the COC. Studies in Thailand found that DMPA continuation rates were 50% higher in women who did not desire more children compared to those who did.[87] A Chinese study comparing continuation rates amongst a group of women receiving detailed structured pretreatment and ongoing counseling on the hormonal and probable side effects of DMPA and those receiving standard counseling found continuation rates at 12 months were considerably higher in the former group (89% compared to 58%).[88] A quality of life study of DMPA users in Sweden found 85% to be very satisfied or satisfied with the method after a mean time of 3–4 years of use.[89] Menstrual disturbances are the main reason given for discontinuation. Continuation rates for NET-EN are similar to those for DMPA.[86]

Continuation rates for the once-a-month combined injectables at 12 months are considerably higher than those of DMPA and NET-EN, ranging from 55.9–81.2%.[80] Again, menstrual disturbances were the commonest reason for discontinuation, but this showed variation from country to country, with some indicating amenorrhea as the major concern whilst others cited cycle irregularities, reflecting differences in cultural attitudes and the level of pretreatment and ongoing counseling.

During a large Egyptian trial, overall continuation and satisfaction rates were high.[90] However, those most likely to discontinue were young women with large families who wanted more children, women who were first-time contraceptive users or had menstrual disturbances with previous methods, and those whose neighbors, relatives or husbands had negative views about contraceptive use. Although side effects were given as the major reason for discontinuation, the extent of these did not differ from those experienced by women continuing use. Important factors in discontinuation were a lack of counseling, disatisfaction with clinic services and husbands' attitude to bleeding irregularities (especially in Moslem countries, where menstrual bleeding excludes women from religious and sexual practices).

Implants

Norplant. In large scale pre-introductory trials of Norplant in 17 countries in Latin America, Asia and Africa, total cumulative continuation rates at five years were 40–64.2 per 100 women.[91] Younger women desiring further pregnancies were most likely to discontinue. Cumulative discontinuation rates for menstrual reasons more than doubled between the end of the first and second year of use in 13 of the 17 countries. Continuation rates at 12 months varied from 97.0 per 100 women in Singapore and Ghana to 71.1 in Brazil, with a mean of 91.6 per 100 women. In the UK a survey of 2129 Norplant users reported continuation rates of 85.2% at 12 months.[92] In the USA continuation rates at one year were 85.4% and similar amongst adolescent, clinic patients and those attending private physicians.[93] However, amongst poor Hispanic women in New York the continuation rate at 12 months was only 69.2%.[94] In all the studies, menstrual problems were cited as the most common reason for removal (but the actual disturbances were no different amongst those women who continued with Norplant). Obviously, there are differences in acceptance level of menstrual disturbances, but other factors may also influence the decisions to discontinue use.

A pilot study in Bangladesh found that in a group of women whose husbands were counseled either prior to insertion of Norplant or shortly afterwards, continuation rates at the end of 36 months of use were 10% higher than in the group whose husbands did not receive counseling.[95] In those countries where husbands play an important role in contraceptive decision-making, providing them with information could be expected to increase continuation rates.

Attributes that enhance Norplant acceptability are long duration of use, ease of use, and effectiveness with few side effects, in that order.[96] The attribute most mitigating against Norplant acceptability is the menstrual cycle disruption, which is cited by over 50% of women as the feature most disliked.[96] Other factors which are sometimes disliked, but not to the same extent, are other side effects, the insertion procedure and the appearance and feel of the device after insertion (i.e. palpable under the skin).

Other implants

Cumulative continuation rates for Jadelle do not appear to be substantially different to that of the Norplant capsule system.[41] Both users and providers rated it an acceptable and reliable long-term, contraceptive method. Continuation rates are high; above 71 per 100 at the end of the three year period, but slightly lower (at 61 per 100) for women who stated on entering the study that they wanted more children. For those who had completed their families, the continuation rate was 78 per 100.

There seems to be no good reason to deny a woman the possibility of using an implant if she desires more children; as suggested by some health workers who are concerned about the cost and early discontinuation in these women. The use of implants should probably be discouraged in women who plan to have a pregnancy within the year, but for other women desiring planning a pregnancy within three to five years, implants provide a highly effective method for achieving desired pregnancy spacing.

A multicentre study of Uniplant involving nine countries reported continuation rates of 84.3% at 12 months, the lifespan of the device.[42] A questionnaire completed on removal of the device showed high user satisfaction when compared to their previously used method.[97] The most liked feature for over 50% of women was ease of use with no need to remember anything, while 26% cited high effectiveness. Thirteen per cent reported fewer side effects than with their previous method. When asked about the 'least liked attribute' of Uniplant, almost 50% stated that they disliked nothing, whilst for a third the change in menstrual pattern was the most disliked feature. Two thirds of the women required contraception for longer than 12 months and hence repeated implants, with one third disliking the concept of a new implant annually, mainly because of fear of discomfort at insertion. More than half (56.4%) would have preferred a five year implant. Whilst half the women in the study felt a single implant was ideal, the remaining respondents had no objection to using a two or six implant system.

Contraceptive vaginal rings

There are no reported large studies on combined CVRs, so reliable continuation rates are not available. From the phase 2 studies it appears that CVRs have high levels of acceptability, but women who enter clinical trials might have different characteristics and needs to a general population. In a multicenter study of two different LNG/estradiol releasing CVRs, continuation rates were similar to that of a LNG containing combined oral contraceptive.[72] Discontinuation rates for menstrual problems were similar in pill and CVR users, but vaginal problems were greater in CVR users; discontinuation for other medical reasons was higher amongst COC users. Expulsion of rings from the vagina can be troublesome. A WHO study of a LNG-releasing ring looked at discontinuation rates relating to expulsions and found that 7% of women discontinued as a result of experiencing expulsion of the ring.[98] However, menstrual problems relating to the use of a progestogen alone was the major reason for discontinuation of this ring, not the delivery mode.

Acceptability of a vaginal ring was first demonstrated in a study of different prototypes of non-medicated rings.[99] Convenience and effectiveness were the main attributes of CVRs, leading to high acceptability levels amongst women in Los Angeles and Sydney participating in a study of a combined CVR.[100] Eighty-six per cent rated the ring as very good or good. Other features that contributed to satisfaction were the freedom from daily pill taking, with little to remember apart from removal and reinsertion of the ring to allow withdrawal bleeds, and the feeling of being in control of their method. In earlier studies in Brazil and the Dominican Republic with a different population group, 56% of women rated ease of use as the most liked characteristic of ring use.[101] In a preliminary analysis of a multicentre European study of a combined ethinylestradiol/3-ketodesogestrel-releasing CVR, only 8% of women failed to complete the nine month study for ring-related problems — most frequently expulsions, irregular bleeding and 'foreign body' feeling.[102]

Intrauterine systems

Acceptability of the LNG-releasing IUS is high amongst women who have been well counseled about the menstrual changes induced by the device, including the possibility of erratic bleeding and spotting in the first few months of use and oligo-amenorrhea with increasing duration of use. An independent study of acceptability of the LNG IUS was carried out by Shain et al[103] in which women were interviewed before insertion, three months after insertion and 12 months postinsertion and their satisfaction rates compared to women using the copper-bearing Nova-T IUD and an experimental intracervical LNG-releasing device. Almost all the women using the LNG-IUS found it preferable to their previous IUD; only 3.3% of LNG IUS users were 'less satisfied' or 'much less satisfied' compared to 15.9% of Nova-T users, a highly significant difference.

Characteristics of users

Long-acting contraceptive methods are attractive to some women of all socio-economic groups and all levels of education, including poor, rural indigenous women in many different countries.[93,96,97] Acceptability of these methods is related to effectiveness, ease of use and desire for long-term reliable yet reversible contraception, characteristics that are particularly attractive to the very young and to older women who have completed their families. Age, race and marital status do not seem to influence use of long-acting methods. With progestogen-only methods, attitudes towards bleeding irregularities are particularly important as bleeding disturbances are the most common reason for discontinuation. However, even in groups such as Islamic women, who are excluded from a number of activities when they experience vaginal beeding, attitudes to irregular bleeding vary. In a study of acceptability of monthly injectables in Egypt, some women found bleeding irregularities beneficial, as it exempted them from having intercourse, whereas others discontinued because irregular bleeding excluded them from religious and sexual practices.

Amenorrhea induced by these methods is attractive to many western women, but causes concern in some groups who fear it may indicate pregnancy.

Overall assessment of safety

To date it appears that long-acting methods of contraception are safe for the majority of women, with benefits outweighing risks. All methods cause side effects, most of which are regarded by workers in the field as 'nuisance' or minimal effects, but which can influence an individual woman's quality of life to a major extent. However, apart from menstrual disturbances, the frequency of these side effects appears to be lower than for users of oral contraceptives. Metabolic changes of minor degree (mainly with lipids, carbohydrates and the immune system) have been reported with some methods, but the metabolic changes are usually less than those seen with combined oral contraceptives.[17] Concerns have been expressed about possible risks to infants exposed to long-acting steroidal contraceptives *in utero* or through breast milk, but there is no substantive evidence to support these concerns.

Rare but potentially serious side effects of such low-dose and progestogen-only methods are unlikely to be demonstrated by limited clinical trials prior to marketing. It has been estimated that to detect a possible two-fold increase in risk of venous thrombosis in Norplant users would require a cohort study of 23 000 Norplant users and 23 000 controls followed for five years. To demonstrate a similar possible increased risk for myocardial infarction, breast, ovarian and endometrial cancer would require cohorts of 17 800, 6600, 25 400 and 44 500 respectively. To determine the possible risks of long-acting contraceptive methods with certainly will require considerable time, effort and funding.

Post-marketing surveillance appears to be the only feasible mechanism to establish data on common side effects. However, such studies are unlikely to provide information on cardiovascular and carcinoma risks for many years. An imaginative post-marketing surveillance study of Norplant users has been set up jointly by the WHO, the Population Council and

Family Health International. The study enrolled a cohort of 25 000 women in eight countries of whom half were Norplant users and half IUD users or women who had undergone sterilization.

There are health benefits related to use of some of these long-acting methods, which include a reduction of menstrual blood loss, especially in LNG IUS and DMPA users, with concomittant improvement in hemoglobin levels. These methods do not appear to adversely influence blood pressure or blood clotting making them useful methods for women with related problems. Preliminary evidence suggests that some progestogen-only methods may have a protective effect against endometrial and ovarian carcinoma and reduce the incidence of pelvic inflammatory disease in a similar way to combined oral contraceptives.

Training and counseling

Evidence from studies in a variety of countries indicates that counseling and training are important factors in the successful introduction of long-acting contraceptive methods.[88,93,94] The better a woman and her sexual partner understand the method before accepting its use the more likely they are to find it satisfactory. Women who were adequately informed about the menstrual changes they were likely to experience with DMPA, Norplant or LNG IUS prior to use were more likely to tolerate these side effects and continue use of the method.

The newer long-acting delivery systems are more complex in clinical use than conventional contraceptives, which makes it important that, prior to introduction of the method, health personnel are adequately trained not only in insertion and removal techniques but also in other aspects of use, including advantages, disadvantages and potential problems. The introduction of Norplant has required the establishment of extensive training programs for medical and paramedical staff to ensure safe and effective use of the method. Many of the legal problems facing Norplant in the USA and UK relate to faulty insertion techniques, resulting in difficult removals or failure of women to be adequately informed about possible side effects prior to use.

Introducing these new technologies requires careful planning to ensure that appropriately worded literature is available for potential users and their partners, taking into account ethnic and religious views and traditions. Clinic personnel need to be well informed and trained to provide accurate information and to assist the woman in making an informed choice by answering all her questions and assessing her suitability for the method. Only carefully trained staff who have been adequately assessed should insert or remove devices. Adequate infrastructure must be set up to ensure that suitable protocols, clinical equipment and a supply of devices are in place, as well as an effective follow-up system for acceptors. It is also necessary to develop appropriate advance publicity both for the media and the public.

Characteristics of individual methods

Characteristics of individual methods are summarized in Tables 45.1 and 45.2.

Provision of services

The individual characteristics of long-acting contraceptive methods require consideration when setting up a service for their provision. To ensure continuity of use of combined injectable methods, providers of contraceptive services need to make access easy so that women can come at times that are suitable to them in order to maximize regular administration of injections. Well trained staff should be available to counsel 'clients' and administer the injections.

Provision of Norplant

The provision of Norplant as part of a contraceptive service requires careful planning and training of staff in counseling, insertion and removal techniques prior to commencement. As mentioned above, the medico-legal problems that have arisen with Norplant were associated with women being inadequately informed about possible side effects and problems encountered at insertion and removal of the rods. A detailed review of all Norplant issues has recently been published.[105]

Insertion

Insertions ideally should be carried out during the first seven days of the menstrual cycle to minimize the risk of insertion in the presence of an undiagnosed pregnancy. The rods can also be inserted immediately postabortion or postpartum in nonlactating women and six weeks postpartum in lactating women.

Insertions should only be performed by appropriately trained health care professionals, as difficulties with removal are related to poor insertion techniques. Norplant insertion is a minor surgical procedure carried out under local anesthesia. Using a trocar, the clinician places the Norplant rods through a small incision (approximately 3 mm) under the skin

Table 45.1 Pharmacological and clinical differences of various contraceptive steroid delivery systems.

	Oral		Injectable			Vaginal rings	
	Combined	Minipill	Monthly	Two-monthly	Three-monthly	Progestogen-only	Combined
Estrogen	Ethinyl estradiol	None	Estradiol valerate Estradiol cypionate	None	None	None	Ethinyl estradiol
Estrogen dose	Low	n/a	Medium	n/a	n/a	n/a	Low
Progestogen	LNG, NET, DES, GEST	LNG, NET	DMPA, NET-enanthanate	NET-enanthanate	DMPA	LNG, NES	NET-Ac, NES, 3-KDES
Progestogen dose	Medium	Low	High	High	High	Low	Medium
Frequency of administration	Daily	Daily	30±3 days	60±14 days	84±14 days	3-monthly	3–12 monthly
Blood levels of drug	Fluctuating	Fluctuating	Fluctuating	Fluctuating	Fluctuating	Constant	Constant
First pass through liver	Yes	Yes	No	No	No	No	No
Enzyme induction/ drug interactions	Yes	Yes	*Unlikely	*Unlikely	*Unlikely	*Likely	*Likely
Ovulation inhibition	Yes	Sometimes	Yes	Yes	Yes	Sometimes	Yes
Method efficacy, life-table/100WY	0.5/yr	1–3/yr	<1/yr	<1/yr	<0.5/yr	*Unknown	*<0.5/yr
User efficacy, life-table/100WY	2–6/yr	1–10/yr	<2/yr	<2/yr	<1/yr	*Unknown	*<0.5/yr
Return of fertility	Rapid	Immediate	Short delay	Short delay	Long delay	Immediate	Immediate
Termination of use	User whenever desired	User whenever desired	End of lifespan of injection	End of lifespan of injection	End of lifespan of injection	Immediate by user	Immediate by user
Efficacy margin if delay in next dose	Minimal	Minimal	Moderate	Moderate	Long	Moderate	Moderate
Menstrual pattern	Regular	Some irregularity	Regular	Irregular	Irregular	Irregular	Regular
Amenorrhea	Rare	Occasional	Uncommon	Sometimes	Common	Uncommon	Uncommon
Irregular bleeding	Uncommon	Common	Sometimes	Common	Common	Common	Uncommon
Use in lactation	No	Yes	No	Yes	Yes	Yes	No
Method specific problems	Daily pill routine increases user failure	Efficacy dependent on regular ingestion	Need for monthly injection; similar side effects to COC	Need for more frequent injections than DMPA	Not readily reversible if side effects occur; sometimes long delay in return of fertility	Possible development of erythematous vaginal lesions; ?high P doses in vagina may increase HIV transmission	Nausea on first cycle use of some new ring; same side effects as COC
Method specific benefits	High efficacy; a number of noncontraceptive benefits including menstrual regulation	Suitable for women in whom estrogens are contraindicated	Better cycle control than DMPA; no need for daily pill use improves efficacy	Somewhat better cycle control than DMPA	Amenorrhea welcomed by many women	No daily action required by user but still under user control to terminate use	Good cycle control; no daily action by user but under user control to terminate
Availability	Marketed	Marketed	Marketed	Marketed	Marketed	Phase III	Phase III

LNG: levonorgestrel; NET: norethindrone; DES: desogestrel; GEST: gestodene; DMPA: depot medroxyprogesterone autate; NES: nestorone; 3-KDES: 3 ketodesogestrel; NET-AC: norethindrone acetate; COC: combined oral contraceptive; *inssuficient data

on the inside of a woman's upper arm in a fan-shaped configuration using a template. It is important that the capsules are inserted subcutaneously as deeper insertion makes removal difficult and too superficial insertion, i.e. intradermal, makes the rods more visible and associated with transient discomfort. Use of a strict aseptic technique and keeping the area dry for three days after insertion will minimize the risk of infection at the implant site. Applying a firm but not too tight dressing will minimize the size of the hematoma which sometimes results from the procedure.[106]

Table 45.2 Pharmacological and clinical differences of various contraceptive steroid delivery systems.

	Subcutaneous implants						Intra-uterine system
	Norplant	Jadelle	Implanon	Uniplant	Nestorone	Annuelle	Mirena
Estrogen	None	None	None	None	None	None	None
Progestogen	LNG	LNG	3-ketodesogestrel	Nomogestrol	Nestorone	NET-chol	LNG
Progestogen dose	Low	Low	Low	Low	Low	Low	Low
Frequency of administration	5 years	3–5 years	3 years	1 year	1–2 years	2 years	5 years plus
No. of rods	6	2	1	1	1–2	4–5	n/a
Blood levels of drug	Constant	Constant	Constant	Constant	Constant	Reducing	Constant
First pass through liver	No	No	No	No	No	No	No
Enzyme induction/drug interactions	Yes	*Likely	*Likely	*Likely	*Likely	*Likely	No
Ovulation inhibition	Frequent	Frequent	Frequent	Infrequent	Frequent	Depends on dose	Sometimes
Method efficacy, life-table/100WY	0.2	0.2	*No data	0.94	*No data	*No data	<0.2
User efficacy, life-table/100WY	0.2/yr	0.2/yr	*No data	0.94	*No data		<0.2/yr
Return of fertility	Immediate	Immediate	Immediate	Immediate	Immediate	Gradual	Immediate
Termination of use	Medical intervention	Medical intervention	Medical intervention	Medical intervention	Medical intervention	Depends on erosion rate	Requires medical removal
Efficacy margin if delay in replacement	Long	Long	Data n/a	Data n/a	Data n/a	Data n/a	Long
Menstrual pattern	Irregular	Irregular	Irregular	Some irregularity	Irregular	Irregular	Irregular
Amenorrhea	Moderate	Moderate	Infrequent	Infrequent	Moderate	Moderate	Moderate
Irregular bleeding	Common	Common	Common	Common	Common	Common	Common
Use in lactation	Yes	Yes	Yes	Yes	Yes	Yes	Yes
Method specific problems	Careful training required; removal occasionally difficult; medicolegal problems			Short lifespan of 1 year		Further studies required on optimal number of pellets and lifespan	Training in insertion technique
Method specific benefits	High efficacy, long lifespan	Fewer rods make insertion easier	Injectable insertion system	Easier insertion and removal of single rod	No absorption from GIT of breast-fed infants	Biodegradable; medical removal if early termination desired	Control of menorrhagia, protection of endometrium in ERT and contraceptive cover
Availability	Marketed	Marketed	Marketed	Phase III	Phase II	Phase II	Marketed

LNG: levonorgestrel; NET-chol: norethindrone; GIT: gastrointestinal tract; ERT: estrogen replacement therapy; * insufficient data; n/a: not available

Removal of Norplant capsules

Careful palpation to identify location of all the capsules is important prior to attempting removal. Ultrasonography, plain film x-rays, computerized tomography and fluoroscopy have all been used in an attempt to locate impalpable capsules that are misaligned or inserted too deeply. When Norplant capsules bend, cross, touch one another or are widely spaced, removal will take longer and can be associated with hematoma; large or multiple incisions can be required.[106]

Following difficulties with removal, a number of new techniques have been developed. The standard method requires a small transverse incision (4 mm) at the base of the fan of capsules. Removal of each capsule with mosquito forceps is carried out through this skin incision, after breaking down the fibrous tissue surrounding the implant.[107] The Emory technique is a variation of the standard method with a larger transverse incision (8–10 mm) followed by vigorous breakdown of the fibrous tissue prior to removal.[108] The 'U' technique uses a small longitudinal incision (approximately 4 mm) between the third and fourth capsules to allow lateral grasp of the implants. This technique is quicker and less complicated than the standard technique and results in fewer broken capsules.[109] The 'Pop-out' method uses a small (2–3 mm) incision over the lower end of the most centrally located capsule. The clinician's fingers guide the implants to the incision. A scalpel is used to free the fibrous tissue surrounding the capsule, which is then extracted by hand.

Several needle elevation techniques have been described, whereby local anesthetic is injected deep and perpendicular to the Norplant capsules; the needle is left in place, stabilizing all six capsules and making them easily palpable.[110]

Complications during removal are minimized by careful training. A large multinational study of removals showed that only 4.8% were complicated but the complication rate for untrained clinicians was 2.5 times greater.[111]

Silastic capsules can fracture from grasping with a forceps or excessive tugging to free the capsule from surrounding fibrous tissue. Removal of a broken capsule requires the same careful localization as for an intact capsule, but women should not be subjected to traumatic procedures to remove small pieces of silastic as the remaining drug contents will dissipate rapidly.[106]

Barriers, either financial or persuasive, should not be placed in the way if a woman requests removal of Norplant. Such practices have led to charges of coercion and brought the method into disrepute.

Mirena/Levonova (levonorgestrel releasing intrauterine system)

Insertion of Mirena can be difficult when performed by inexperienced operators. Although most women do not find the initial bleeding problems with Mirena a reason for discontinuation, a small minority who experience irregular or prolonged bleeding or spotting over many months do find this difficult to tolerate. Detailed counseling prior to insertion is important and can especially help many women to accept amenorrhea as a desirable rather than a worrying effect of the device.

Providers need to be aware that as well as providing highly effective contraception, Mirena has been used successfully in the management of menorrhagia. Another medical indication for the use of Mirena is to provide protection of the endometrium in peri and postmenopausal women on estrogen therapy. In perimenopausal women with climacteric symptoms, Mirena provides contraceptive cover that is not provided by usual HRT regimens. It also reduces menstrual bleeding, which is often a problem in this age group.

New methods under development

New implants

Implants releasing different and possibly improved progestogens (e.g. Nestorone®) are at present undergoing phase II trials. These will provide a range of different implants with fewer rods and will lead to improved choices for women seeking contraception.

Annuelle® (Biodegradeable NET:cholesterol implants)

A phase II-A study of a biodegradable subdermal implant containing a combination of norethindrone (NET) and cholesterol has recently been reported. A five pellet and four pellet group containing 266.5 mg and 174 mg NET respectively have been compared.[112] After an initial burst effect within 24 hours of implantation, NET levels reduced gradually in both groups for the first 18 months and remained at a stable level for a further 15 months until they were undetectable at 36 months in the four pellet group, indicating complete biodegradability.

Ovulation occurred in 22% of cycles in the four pellet group and 1% in the five pellet group. As with other progestogen only methods, the main side effect was disturbances of the menstrual cycle, with 65% of cycles normal, 11% amenorrheic and 24% exhibiting intermenstrual bleeding in the four pellet group. In the five pellet group only 43% of cycles were normal, 30% had prolonged irregular bleeding and 23% were amenorrheic. There were no pregnancies up to 24 months. Annuelle points the way for the development of biodegradable implants that provide safe, longterm contraception with the benefit of removability if required. For most women, surgical removal will not be needed.

Contraceptive gels

A pilot study of a gel formulation delivering 0.8 mg of the progestogen Nestorone in 0.4 ml of gel produced favourable therapeutic blood levels when rubbed into the skin on a daily basis. At present, a dose-finding study is being undertaken by the Population Council to determine the optimal contraceptive dose for this progestogen-only gel.

Male steroidal contraception

A WHO multicenter study of weekly injections of 200 mg testosterone enanthate showed that androgens can suppress spermatogenesis to provide reasonably effective contraceptive cover in men with minimal short-term side effects and without affecting sexual function. Ninety-eight percent of men participating in the study achieved azoospermia or oligospermia ($<3 \times 10^6$/ml) within 2–3 months of starting the weekly injections.[113] Complete suppression of spermatogenesis was more likely to occur in Asian men, who also took longer to return to their pretreatment sperm counts. Pregnancy rates were related to sperm concentration, with no pregnancies occurring in the azoospermic group. Amongst oligospermic men, the pregnancy rate was 8.1/100 person years. Side effects were minimal, resulting in only 9.4/100 men discontinuing at 12 months, and included mood swings, aggression, changes in libido and acne. Increases in weight, hemoglobin, creatinine, testosterone and estrogen and decreases in testicular size and urea returned to normal on cessation of therapy.

Weekly intramuscular injections of testosterone produce widely fluctuating and supraphysiological testosterone levels. An attempt to overcome this problem has been the use of subdermal testosterone implants. The insertion of six 200 mg testosterone implants resulted in a more rapid initial fall in sperm concentrations but produced the same percentage of males with oligospermia as the injections. Plasma testosterone and estradiol remained within normal levels with fewer men developing acne or other androgenic side effects.[114] When a progestogen such as DMPA is used in conjunction with testosterone pellets, the dose of testosterone required is lowered further, reducing metabolic and other side effects whilst maintaining the same contraceptive efficacy.[115] Testosterone implants combined with progestogen appear to be an acceptable and reasonably effective method of male contraception but do not overcome the problem of a 2–3 month time-lag from start of therapy to maximal sperm suppression. Additional prospective studies are required to determine whether this approach will have any deleterious cardiovascular or prostatic effects.

Conclusion

The variety of long-acting hormonal contraceptive methods available or in the process of development will provide additional options that will free individuals from daily contraceptive routines, thereby improving efficacy. Implants and intra-uterine releasing systems are particularly useful for people requiring long-term contraception but who are not ready to make the decision to undergo sterilization. The shorter-acting implants and rings will be particularly useful for those requiring effective contraception for the spacing of pregnancies. The provision of progestogen-only methods provides options for women for whom estrogens are contraindicated or unsuitable, whilst combined methods cater for women who find menstrual changes unacceptable. The provision of a larger range of safe effective hormonal contraceptive options utilizing different methods of delivery will make it more likely that individuals or couples can find a suitable method, so that they can achieve their desired family size.

The future holds promise of even better delivery methods, with the development of biodegradable implant systems that could be used for both male and female contraceptive delivery. CVRs with longer lifespans, delivering lower steroid levels whilst maintaining efficacy, are likely and novel methods of drug delivery, such as gels, will have enhanced appeal to prospective users.

REFERENCES

1. Shain RN, Potts M 1984 Need for and acceptability of long acting steroidal contraception. In: Zatuchni GI, Goldsmith A, Shelton JD, Sciarra JJ (eds) Long acting contraceptive delivery systems. Harper & Row, Philadelphia, pp 1–19
2. Fraser IS, Odlind V 1992 Long acting delivery systems. The answer for fertility control. In: Sitruk-Ware R, Bardin CW (eds) Contraception. Newer pharmacological agents, devices and delivery systems. Marcel Dekker, New York, pp 1–22
3. Hickey M, Fraser I 1995 The contraceptive use of depot medroxyprogestrone acetate. Clinics in Obstetrics and Gynecology 38: 849–858
4. Folkman J, Long DM 1964 The use of silicone rubber as a carrier for prolonged drug therapy. Journal of Surgical Research 4: 139–142
5. Segal SJ, Croxatto HB 1967 Single administration of hormones for long-term control of reproductive function. Presentation at the XXIII Meeting of American Fertility Society, Washington DC; November 1967 November
6. Shoupe D, Mishell DR Jr 1992 Contraceptive vaginal rings: efficacy and acceptability. In: Sitruk-Ware R, Bardin CW (eds) Contraception. Newer pharmacological agents, devices and delivery systems. Marcel Dekker, New York, pp 71–89

7. Jackanicz TM 1984 Vaginal ring steroid releasing system. In: Zatuchni GI, Goldsmith A, Shelton JD, Sciarra JJ (eds) Long acting contraceptive delivery systems. Harper & Row, Philadelphia, pp 201–212
8. Edelman DA, Cole LD, Appelo R, Lavin P 1984 Long acting progestasert IUD systems. In: Zatuchni GL, Goldsmith A, Shelton JD, Sciarra JJ (eds) Long-acting contraceptive delivery systems. Harper & Row, Philadelphia, pp 621–627
9. Luukkainen T, Nilsson CG, Allonen H, Haukkamaa M, Toivonen J 1984 Intrauterine release of levonorgestrel. In: Zatuchni GI, Goldsmith A, Shelton JD, Sciarra JJ (eds) Long-acting contraceptive delivery systems. Harper & Row, Philadelphia, pp 601–612
10. Kaunitz A 1992 Injectable contraception: the USA perspective. IPPF Medical Bulletin 26(6): 1–3
11. WHO 1987 Task force on long acting systemic agents for fertility regulation. A pharmacodynamic study of once-a-month injectable contractraceptives 1. Different doses of HRP 112 and of Devo-Provera. Contraception 36: 441–457
12. Bardin CW, Sivin I 1992 Norplant: the first implantable contraceptive. In: Sitruk-Ware R, Barden CW (eds) Contraception. Newer pharmacological agents, devices and delivery systems. Marcel Dekker, New York, pp 23–39
13. Garza-Flores J, Cravioto M, Perez-Palacios G 1992 Steroid injectable contraception: current concepts and perspectives. In: Sitruk-Ware R, Bardin CW (eds) Contraception. Newer pharmacological agents, devices, and delivery systems. Marcel Dekker, New York, pp 41–70
14. Ortiz A, Hiroi M, Stanczyk FZ, Goebelsmann U, Mishell DR Jr 1977 Serum MPA concentrations and ovarian function following intramuscular injection of Depo-Provera. Journal of Clinical Endocrinology and Metabolism 44: 32–38
15. Fotherby K, Howard G, Shrimanker K, Elder MG, Bye PGT 1978 Occurrence of ovulation in women receiving the injectable contraceptive norethisterone enanthate. Contraception 18: 535–542
16. Fraser IS 1989 Systemic hormonal contraception by non-oral routes. In: Filshie M, Guillebaud J (eds). Contraception: science and practice. Butterworths, London, pp 109–125
17. Lewis DH, Tice TR, Myers WE, Cowsar DR, Beck LR 1982 Biodegradable microcapsules for contraceptive steroids. In: Contraceptive delivery systems, 3: Abstract 55. MTP Press, Lancaster, England, p 40
18. Sivin I 1988 International experience with Norplant and Norplant-2 contraceptives. Studies in Family Planning 19: 81–94
19. Olsson SE, Odlind V, Johansson EDB, Nordström ML 1987 Plasma levels of levonorgestrel and free levonorgestrel index in women using Norplant implants or two covered rods (Norplant-2). Contraception 35: 215–228
20. Olsson SE, Odlind V, Johansson EDB 1990 Clinical results with subcutaneous implants containing 3-keto desogestrel. Contraception 42: 1–11
21. Barbosa I, Coutinho E, Athayde C, Ladipo O, Olsson SE, Ulmsten U 1995 The effects of nomogestrol acetate subdermal implant (Uniplant) on carbohydrate metabolism, serum lipoproteins and on hepatic function in women. Contraception 52: 111–114
22. Victor A 1984 Vaginal absorption of contraceptive steroids. In: Zatuchni GI, Goldsmith A, Shelton JD, Sciarra JJ (eds). Long-acting contraceptive delivery systems. Harper & Row, Philadelphia, pp 241–245
23. Ballagh SA, Mishell DR Jr, Lacarra M, Shoupe D, Jackanicz TM, Eggena P 1994 A contraceptive vaginal ring releasing norethindrone acetate and ethinyl estradiol. Contraception 50: 517–533
24. Olsson SE, Odlind V 1990 Contraception with a vaginal ring releasing 3-keto desogestrel and ethinylestradiol. Contraception 42: 563–568
25. Koetsawang S, Gao J, Krishna U, Cuadro A, Dhall GI, Wyss R, Rodriguez J, Andrade ATL, Khan T, Kononova ES 1990 Microdose intravaginal levonorgestrel contraception: a multicentre clinical trial. Contraception 41: 105–110
26. Chilvers C 1994 Breast cancer and depot medroxyprogesterone acetate. A review. Contraception 49: 211–222
27. WHO 1991 Collaborative study of neoplasia and steroid contraceptives. Breast cancer and depot medroxyprogesterone acetate. A multinational study. Lancet 338: 833–838
28. Jordan A 1992 FDA requirements for nonclinical testing of contraceptive steroids. Contraception 46: 499–509
29. Toppozada M 1997 The clinical use of monthly injectable preparations. Obstetrics and Gynecology Survey 32: 335–347
30. Scott JA, Brenner PF, Kletski OA, Mishell DR Jr 1978 Factors affecting pituitary gonadotropin function in users of oral contraceptive steroids. American Journal of Obstetrics and Gynecology 130: 817–821
31. Diczfalusy E, Johannisson E 1984 Endometrial effects of progestogens: their elusive relationship to ovarian function and intermenstrual bleeding. In: Zatuchni GI, Goldsmith A, Shelton JD, Sciarra JJ (eds) Proceedings of an international workshop on long-acting contraceptive delivery systems. Harper & Row, Philadelphia, pp 316–331
32. Landgren BM, Diczfalusy E 1980 Hormonal effects of the 300 μg norethisterone (NET) minipill 1. Daily steroid levels in 43 subjects during a pretreatment cycle and during the second month of NET administration. Contraception 21: 87–113
33. Hickey M, Fraser IS, Dwart ET, Graham S 1996 Endometrial vascular fragility during Norplant use: preliminary results from a hysteroscopic study. Human Reproduction 11(2): 101–110
34. Rogers PAW, Au CL, Affandi B 1993 Endometrial microvascular density during the normal menstrual cycle and following exposure to long-term levonorgestrel. Human Reproduction 8: 1396–1404
35. Moghissi KS 1984 Effects of progestogens on cervical secretion and sperm-cervical mucus interaction. In: Zatuchni GI, Goldsmith A, Shelton JD, Sciarra JJ (eds) Proceedings of an international workshop on long-acting contraceptive delivery systems. Harper & Row, Philadelphia, pp 265–277
36. Trifunac NP, Bernstein GS 1981 Effect of steroid hormones on the metabolism of human spermatozoa. Contraception 24: 523–527

37. Fraser IS, Weisberg E 1981 A comprehensive review of injectable contraception with special emphasis on depot medroxyprogesterone acetate. The Medical Journal of Australia 1 (Suppl 1): 1–19
38. World Health Organization 1983 Task force on long-acting systemic agents for fertility regulation. A multinational comparative clinical trial of long-acting injectable contraceptive norethisterone enantate given in two dosage regimens and depot-medroxyprogesterone acetate. Final report. Contraception 28: 1–20
39. World Health Organization 1988 Task force on long-acting systemic agents for fertility regulation. A multicentred phase 3 comparative study of two hormone contraceptive preparations given once-a-month by intramuscular injection 1. Contraceptive efficacy and side effects. Contraception 37: 1–20
40. Darney PD, Klaisle CM, Tanner S et al 1990 Sustained-release contraceptives. Current Problems in Obstetrics, Gynecology and Fertility 13: 87
41. Gu S, Zhang L, Liu Y, Wang S, Sivin I 1994 A five year evaluation of Norplant® II implants in China. Contraception 50: 27–34
42. Coutinho EM, de Souza JC, Athayde C, Barbosa IC, Alvarez F, Brache V 1996 Multicentre clinical trial on the efficacy and acceptability of a single contraceptive implant of nomogestrol acetate, Uniplant. Contraception 53: 121–125
43. World Health Organization 1990 Special program of research development and research training in human reproduction. Task force on long-acting systemic agents for fertility regulation. Microdose intravaginal levonorgestrel contraception: a multicentre clinical trial 1. Contraceptive efficacy and side-effects. Contraception 41: 105–124
44. Luukkainen T, Allonen H, Haukkamaa M, Lähteenmaki P, Nilsson CG, Toivonen J 1986 Five years experience with levonorgestrel releasing IUDs. Contraception 33: 139–148
45. Croxatto HB, Diaz S, Peralta O, Juez G, Herreros C, Casado ME, Salvatierra AM, Miranda P, Durán E 1983 Fertility regulation in nursing women IV. Long-term influence of a low-dose combined oral contraceptive initiated at day 30 postpartum upon lactation and infant growth. Contraception 27: 13–25
46. Croxatto H, Diaz S, Peralta O, Juez G, Casado ME, Salvatierra AM, Durán E 1982 Fertility regulation in nursing women II. Comparative performance of progesterone implants versus placebo and copper-T. American Journal of Obstetrics and Gynecology 144: 201–208
47. Badraoui M, Askalani H, Mahrous I, Serour G, Hefnawi F 1982 Lactation pattern in Egyptian women using the Progestasert system. Contraceptive Delivery System 3: 53–60
48. Nilsson S, Nygren K-G, Johansson EDB 1978 Ethinyl estradiol in human milk and plasma after oral administration. Contraception 17: 131–139
49. Koetsawang S, Suvanichati S, Paipeekul S 1984 Long-term study of growth and development of children breast-fed by mothers receiving Depo-Provera (medroxyprogesterone acetate) during lactation. In: Zatuchni GI, Goldsmith A, Shelton JD, Sciarra JJ (eds) Long-acting contraceptive delivery systems. Harper & Row, Philadelphia, pp 378–387
50. Simpson JL 1984 Mutagenicity and teratogenicity of injectable and implantable progestins: probable lack of effect. In: Zatuchni GI, Goldsmith A, Shelton JD, Sciarra JJ (eds) Long-acting contraceptive delivery systems. Harper & Row, Philadelphia, pp 334–361
51. Collaborative Group on Hormonal Factors in Breast Cancer 1996 Breast cancer and hormonal contraceptives: further results. Contraception 54: IS–106S
52. World Health Organization 1992 Collaborative study of neoplasia and steroid contraceptives. Depot medroxyprogesterone acetate (DMPA) and risk of invasive squamous cell cervical cancer. Contraception 45: 299–312
53. McCann MF, Potter LS 1994 Progestin-only oral contraception: a comprehensive review. Contraception 50(6): S79 (Suppl 1)
54. Thomas DB 1989 Monthly injectable steroid contraceptives and cervical cancer. American Journal of Epidemiology 130: 237–247
55. World Health Organization 1989 Collaborative study of neoplasia and steroid contraceptives. Epithelial ovarian cancer and combined oral contraceptives. International Journal of Epidemiology 18: 538–545
56. World Health Organization 1991 Collaborative study of neoplasia and steroid contraceptives. Depot medroxyprogesterone acetate (DMPA) and risk of endometrial cancer. International Journal of Cancer. 49: 186–190
57. Fraser IS, Holck S 1983 Depot medroxyprogesterone acetate. In: Mishell DR Jr (ed) Long acting steroid contraception. Raven Press, New York, pp 1–30
58. DeCeulaer K, Gruber C, Hayes R, Serjeant GR 1982 Medroxyprogesterone acetate and homozygous sickle cell disease. Lancet 1: 229–231
59. Ryden G, Fahraeus L, Molin L, Ahman K 1979 Do contraceptives influence the incidence of acute pelvic inflammatory disease in women with gonococcus? Contraception 20: 149–158
60. Sivin I, Stern J, Diaz J, Diaz MM, Faundes A, El Mahgoub S et al 1987 Two years of intrauterine contraception with levonorgestrel and with copper: a randomized comparison of the TCu 380 Ag and levonorgestrel 20 µg/d devices. Contraception 35: 245–255
61. National Institutes of Health Expert Committee on Pelvic Inflammatory Disease 1991 Pelvic inflammatory disease: research directions in the 1990s. Sexually Transmitted Diseases 18: 46–64
62. Dennerstein GJ 1986 Depo-Provera in the treatment of recurrent vulvovaginal candidiasis. Journal of Reproductive Medicine 31: 801–803
63. Belsey EM, Machin D, d'Arcangues C 1986 The analysis of vaginal bleeding patterns induced by fertility regulating methods. Contraception 34: 253–260
64. World Health Organization 1983 Task force on long-acting systemic agents for fertility regulation. Multinational comparative clinical trial of long-acting injectable contraceptives: norethisterone enanthate given in two dosage regimens and depot-medroxyprogesterone acetate. Final report. Contraception 28: 1–20

65. Sivin I, Alvarez-Sanchez F, Diaz S 1983 Three-year experience with Norplant® subdermal contraception. Fertility and Sterility 39: 799
66. Sivin I 1984 Findings in phase III studies of Norplant implants. In: Zatuchni GI, Goldsmith A, Shelton JD, Sciarra JJ (eds) Long-acting contraceptive delivery systems. Harper and Row, Philadelphia, pp 488–500
67. Faundes A, Alvarez-Sanchez F, Brache V, Jimenez E, Tejada AS 1991 Hormonal changes associated with bleeding during low dose progestogen contraception delivered by Norplant subdermal implants. Advances in Contraception 7: 85–94
68. Andrade ATL, Pizarro E 1987 Quantitative studies on menstrual blood loss in IUD users. Contraception 36: 129–144
69. Luukkainen T, Toivonen J 1995 Effect of levonorgestrel-releasing intrauterine device on hormonal profile and menstrual pattern after longterm use. Contraception 52(5): 269–276
70. Landgren BM, Johannisson E, Masironi B, Diczfalusy E 1982 Pharmacokinetic and pharmacodynamic investigations with vaginal devices releasing levonorgestrel at a constant, near zero order rate. Contraception 26: 567–585
71. Belsey EM 1988 Task force on long-acting systemic agents for fertility regulation. Vaginal bleeding patterns among women using one natural and eight hormonal methods of contraception. Contraception 38: 181–206
72. Sivin I, Mishell DR, Victor A 1981 A multicentre study of levonorgestrel-estradiol contraceptive vaginal rings III. Menstrual patterns. An international comparative trial. Contraception 24: 377–392
73. Fraser IS 1994 Vaginal bleeding patterns in women using once-a-month injectable contraceptives. Contraception 49: 399–419
74. Landgren BM, Aedo AR, Johannisson E, Cekan SZ 1994 Studies on a vaginal ring releasing levonorgestel at an initial rate of 27 μg/24 h when used alone or in combination with transdermal systems releasing estradiol. Contraception 50: 87–100
75. Cundy T, Evans M, Roberts H, Wattie D, Ames R, Reid IR 1991 Bone density in women receiving depot medroxyprogesterone acetate for contraception. British Medical Journal 303: 13–16 (Correction in British Medical Journal 1991; 303: 220)
76. Kirkman RJE, Gbolade BA, Murby B 1996 Cross sectional study of bone mineral density in long term users of depot medroxyprogesterone acetate (DMPA). The European Journal of Contraception and Reproductive Health Care (June) 1: 144
77. Ellis S, Randall S 1996 Bone density and depot medroxyprogesterone acetate. The European Journal of Contraception and Reproductive Health Care 1: 135
78. Naessen T, Olsson S, Gudmundson J 1995 Differential effects on bone density of progestogen-only methods for contraception in premenopausal women. Contraception 52: 35–39
79. Johansson E, Odlind V 1983 Norplant: biochemical effects. Long-acting steroid contraception. In: Mishell D (ed) Advances in human fertility and reproductive endocrinology, vol 2. Raven Press, New York, pp 117–125
80. World Health Organization 1993 Facts about once-a-month injectable contraceptives; memorandum from a WHO meeting. Bulletin of the World Health Organization (71)6: 677–689
81. Bounds W, Szarewski A, Lowe D, Guillebaud J 1993 Preliminary report of unexpected local reactions to a progestogen-releasing contraceptive vaginal ring. European Journal of Gynecology and Reproductive Biology 48: 123–125
82. Fraser IS, Lacarra M, Mishell DR Jr, Alvarez F, Brache V, Lähteenmäki P, Weisberg E, Nash HA 1998 Vaginal mucosal appearances in women using vaginal rings for contraception. Contraception (in press)
83. Pardthiasong T, Gray RH, McDaniel EB 1980 Return of fertility after discontinuation of depot medroxyprogesterone acetate and intrauterine devices in Northern Thailand. Lancet 1: 509–511
84. Diaz S, Pavez M, Cadenas H, Croxatto HB 1987 Recovery of fertility and outcome of planned pregnancy after the removal of Norplant subdermal implants or copper T IUDs. Contraception 35: 569–579
85. ICMR Taskforce on Hormonal Contraception 1995 Return of fertility following discontinuation of Norplant® II subdermal implants. Contraception 51: 237–242
86. World Health Organization 1983 Task force on long-acting systemic agents for fertility regulation. Multinational comparative clinical trial of long-acting injectable contraceptives: norethisterone enanthate given in two dosage regimens and depot-medroxyprogesterone acetate. A final report. Contraception 28: 1–20
87. Narkovonnakit T, Bennett T, Balakrishan TR 1982 Continuation of injectable contraceptives in Thailand. Studies in Family Planning 13: 99–105
88. Zhen-Wu L, Chun Wu S, Garceau RJ, Son JS, Qiao-Zhi Y, Wei-Lun W, Vander Meulen TC 1996 Effects of pretreatment counseling on discontinuation rates in Chinese women given depo-medroxyprogesterone acetate for contraception. Contraception 53: 357–361
89. Solheim F 1972 An assessment of quality of life in women treated with Depo-Provera in Sweden. New Zealand Journal of Obstetrics and Gynaecology 5: 80–85
90. Hassan EO, El-Nahal N, El-Hussein M 1994 Acceptability of the once-a-month injectable contraceptives Cyclofem and Mesigyna in Egypt. Contraception 49: 469–488
91. Pre-Introductory Clinical Trials of Norplant® Implants 1995 A comparison of seventeen countries' experience. Contraception 52: 287–296
92. Peers T, Stevens JE, Graham Jo, Davey A 1996 Norplant® implants in the UK: first year continuation and removals. Contraception 53: 345–351
93. Dugoff L, Jones OW III, Allen-Davis J, Hurst BS, Schiaff WD 1995 Accessing the acceptability of Norplant® contraceptive in four patient populations. Contraception 52: 45–49
94. Gerber S, Westhoff C, Lopez M, Gordon L 1994 Use of Norplant® implants in a New York City clinic population. Contraception 49: 557–564
95. Amatya R, Akhter H, McMahan J, Williamson N, Gates D, Ahmed Y 1994 The effect of husband counselling on norplant contraceptive acceptability in Bangladesh. Contraception 50: 263–268

96. Krueger L, Dunson TR, Amatya RN 1994 Norplant® contraceptive acceptability among women in five Asian countries. Contraception 50: 349–361
97. Coutinho EM, Athayde C, Barbosa I, Alvarez F, Brache V, Zhi-Ping GU et al 1996 Results of a user satisfaction study carried out in women using Uniplant contraceptive implant. Contraception 54: 313–317
98. Koetsawang S, Gao J, Krishna U 1990 Microdose intravaginal levonorgestrel contraception: a multicentre clinical trial II. Expulsions and removals. WHO task force on long acting systemic agents for fertility regulation. Contraception 41: 125–141
99. Roumen F, Dieben T, Assendorp R, Bouckaert P 1990 The clinical acceptability of a non medicated vaginal ring. Contraception 43: 201–207
100. Weisberg E, Fraser IS, Mishell DR Jr, Lacarra M, Bardin CW 1995 The acceptability of a combined oestrogen/progestogen contraceptive vaginal ring. Contraception 51: 39–44
101. Faundes A, Hardy E 1981 Acceptability of the contraceptive vaginal ring by rural and urban populations in two Latin American countries. Contraception 24: 393–414
102. Bennink HJT, Assendorp R, Dieben ThOM 1990 First results of a multicentre pilot efficacy study with a contraceptive vaginal ring releasing ethinyloestradiol and 3-ketodesogestrel. Advances in Contraception 6: 293–299
103. Shain R, Ratsula K, Toivonen J, Lähteenmäki P, Luukkainen T, Holden AEC, Rosenthal M 1989 Acceptability of an experimental intracervical device: results of a study controlling for selection bias. Contraception 39: 73–84
104. Schwallie PC, Assenzo JR 1977 The effect of depot medroxyprogestone acetate on pituitary and ovarian function, and the return of fertility following its discontinuation: a review. Contraception 10: 181–202
105. Fraser IS, Tiitinen A, Affandi B, Brache V et al 1998 Norplant® Consensus statement and background review. Contraception 57: 1–9
106. Bromham DR, Oloto EJ 1995 Removal of norplant: a short review. IPPF Medical Bulletin 29(5): 3–4
107. Hatasaka H 1995 Implantable levonorgestrel contraception: 4 years of experience with Norplant®. Clinics in Obstetrics and Gynecology 38: 859–871
108. Sarma SP, Hatcher R 1994 The Emory method: a modified approach to Norplant® implants removal. Contraception 49: 551–556
109. Proptohardjo U, Wibowo S 1993 The 'U'-technique: a new method for Norplant® implants removal. Contraception 48: 526–536
110. Taneepanichskul S, Intaraprasert S, Chaturachinda K 1996 Modified needle elevation technique for misplaced Norplant® implants removal. Contraception 54(2): 87–89
111. Sivin I, Stern J, Diaz S, Pavez M, Alvarez F, Brache V et al 1992 Rates and outcomes of planned pregnancy after use of Norplant capsules, Norplant® rods or levonorgestrel-releasing or copper Tcu 380Ag intrauterine contraceptive devices. American Journal of Obstetrics and Gynecology 166(4): 1208–1213
112. Sing M, Saxena DB, Raghubanshi RS, Ledger WJ, Harmond SM, Leonard RJ 1997 Biodegradeable norethindrone (NET: cholesterol) contraceptive implants phase II — A: a clinical study in women. Contraception 55: 23–34
113. World Health Organisation 1996 Task force on methods for the regulation of male fertility. Contraceptive efficacy of testosterone-induced azoospermia and oligozoospermia in normal men. Fertility and Sterility 65: 821–829
114. Handelsman DJ, Conway AJ, Boylan LM 1992 Suppression of human spermatogenesis by testosterone implants. Journal of Clinical Endocrinology and Metabolism 73: 1326–1332
115. Handelsman DJ, Conway AJ, Howe CJ, Turner HL, Mackey M 1996 Establishing the minimum effective dose and additive effects of depo progestogen in suppression of human spermatogenesis by a testosterone depot. Journal of Clinical Endocrinology and Metabolism 31: 4113–4121

46. Antiprogestogens for contraception, interception and medical termination of pregnancy

Jane E. Norman   Iain T. Cameron

Introduction

Despite our best efforts, the world's population is continuing to rise at an alarming rate. This reflects defects not only in the provision of contraceptive and abortion services, but also in the efficacy of available contraceptive methods. One of the most significant advances in fertility control over the last 20 years has been the development, testing and marketing of effective antiprogestogens, of which mifepristone (RU 486) is the most prominent agent. Antiprogestogens are highly effective medical abortifacients when given in conjunction with prostaglandins, and mifepristone now has a product licence for this indication in four countries. However, antiprogestogens are also effective contraceptives, administered either as a single dose postcoitally, or given in continuous or intermittent fashion to inhibit ovulation or render the endometrium unsuitable for implantation. This chapter aims to review the current and potential future use of antiprogestogens for contraception, interception and medical termination of pregnancy.

PHYSIOLOGY

Action at the pituitary and hypothalamus in nonpregnant women

The complex interplay within the hypothalamo-pituitary-ovarian axis has made it difficult to determine individual sites of action when mifepristone is given during the menstrual cycle. *In vitro* studies and studies in postmenopausal women circumvent this problem. *In vitro*, mifepristone (10^{-12}–10^{-7} M) had no significant effect on basal or GnRH induced LH or FSH secretion from isolated rat pituitary cells.[1] However, in postmenopausal women pretreated with estradiol benzoate (0.625 mg/day), mifepristone (100 or 200 mg per day) suppressed gonadotropin concentrations to premenopausal levels.[2] These effects of mifepristone were mimicked by those of progesterone (25 mg/day), suggesting that mifepristone acted as a progesterone agonist at the pituitary in this situation.

Whilst mifepristone administered to normally cycling women caused a significant reduction in serum LH and FSH concentrations,[3–6] it is not clear whether these effects are primary, or secondary to changes in ovarian steroids. Normal fertile women given mifepristone (5–200 mg as a single dose) in the luteal phase of the cycle showed changes in hypothalamic function (such as temperature drop, thirst and mood change) occurring independently of luteolysis,[7] suggesting that mifepristone had a direct hypothalamic effect. In the late follicular phase, mifepristone antagonized the involvement of progesterone in the midcycle gonadotropin surge.[4] This effect occurred despite preovulatory levels of estradiol, again suggesting that mifepristone had a direct effect on the hypothalamo-pituitary axis.

Therefore, several pituitary actions of mifepristone can be demonstrated, from a progesterone-like effect, through no effect, to progesterone antagonism. During long term administration of mifepristone (100 mg/day for three months to normally cycling women with endometriosis), an increase in mean LH concentrations and pulse amplitude was observed.[8] These effects of LH are difficult to explain, and may represent mifepristone acting as a noncompetitive anti-estrogen.

As an antiglucocorticoid, mifepristone also stimulates ACTH production. It disrupts the negative feedback effect of both the endogenous morning cortisol rise and exogenously administered dexamethasone.[9] Long-term administration of mifepristone causes a rise in ACTH and serum cortisol consistent with antagonism of endogenous cortisol at the pituitary.[8]

Action at the ovary

Though mifepristone-induced changes in the hypothalamo-pituitary axis may influence ovarian steroid production, *in vitro* studies suggest that mifepristone has a direct effect on ovarian steroid production. Mifepristone induces a dose-dependent decrease in the activity of 3β hydroxysteroid dehydrogenase activity in human granulosa cells *in vitro* resulting in suppression of progesterone production.[10] *In vivo* during the follicular phase, mifepristone causes disordered development of the ovarian follicle which can be observed using ultrasound, however these effects may be mediated via the hypothalamo-pituitary ovarian axis.

Action at the endometrium

The action of mifepristone at the endometrium or decidua may be mediated either by changes in ovarian steroids or by a direct action at the endometrial progesterone receptor. An increase in both progesterone and estrogen receptor concentrations was observed in the decidua (largely in stromal cells) following mifepristone.[11,12] In nonpregnant women results of studies on the effect of mifepristone on progesterone receptor numbers were conflicting with an increase[13] and a transient decrease both reported.[14]

Endometrial ultrastructure

Nonpregnant women. Mifepristone induces histological changes in the endometrium in the absence of any change in ovarian steroids. Recent work has extended the classic work on endometrial morphology[15,16] and suggested parameters by which endometrium can be precisely dated throughout the menstrual cycle. Continuous low dose administration of mifepristone (1 mg daily) delayed endometrial maturation without affecting ovarian steroid production.[17] Mifepristone (10 mg) given five and eight days after the LH surge resulted in stromal edema and delayed glandular development.[18] Similar effects were seen when mifepristone, given two days after the LH surge, resulted in delayed endometrial maturation.[14] In other studies, the presence of degenerative changes in capillary endothelial cells was a striking feature.[19] Although mifepristone might be considered to act as an antiprogestogen at the endometrium, it is clear that the effects are not simply those of progesterone withdrawal, as the leucocytic infiltration, local necrosis and hemorrhage seen in the endometrium 2–3 days before the onset of spontaneous menstruation were not features of mifepristone-induced bleeding.[5]

The antiprogestogen induced secretory changes in the endometrium in postmenopausal women given estradiol benzoate 0.625 mg daily for 15 days followed by mifepristone 100 mg or 200 mg on the last six days of treatment.[2] These effects were in contrast to the above studies, but were similar to those observed in women in whom progesterone (25 mg daily) was substituted for mifepristone, again suggesting that mifepristone may act as a progesterone agonist when endogenous concentrations of this steroid are low.

Pregnancy. There are less data on the effect of mifepristone on decidual morphology. One study has shown that the endoplasmic reticulum of decidual capillaries was hyperplastic in women treated with mifepristone compared to that in a control group.[20] No changes were observed by conventional histology.

Endometrial biochemistry

Much of the work on the actions of mifepristone in the endometrium or decidua has focused on its effects on prostaglandin production. Mifepristone and another antiprogesterone, ZK 98734, stimulated prostaglandin production in isolated endometrial cells[21] and decidual cells[22] in culture. Decidua removed from pregnant women pretreated with mifepristone had a greater ability to generate prostaglandins in culture than control decidua.[23,24] Further work indicated that mifepristone inhibited prostaglandin dehydrogenase[25,26] which breaks down prostaglandins. The net effect of mifepristone is therefore to increase local prostaglandin concentrations. This is likely to stimulate uterine contractions and contribute to the abortion process.

Recent work has suggested potential mechanisms by which mifepristone may cause endometrial hemorrhage and extracellular matrix degradation. Mifepristone blocked and reversed progesterone-inhibited plasminogen activator expression.[27] Furthermore, treatment with mifepristone caused a marked increase in prostaglandin E and decrease in prostaglandin E metabolites (identified by immunocytochemistry) particularly around blood vessels.[25] *In vitro*, mifepristone reversed progesterone-induced stromal cell tissue factor protein.[28] This is potentially important as tissue factor is a primary initiator of hemostasis.

As already discussed, mifepristone may also act as a progesterone agonist at the endometrium. In the absence of progesterone (e.g. in postmenopausal women pretreated with estrogens) mifepristone had effects similar to those of progesterone, including a decrease in DNA polymerase alpha and increase in estradiol dehydrogenase activity.[2]

Action at the myometrium

Mifepristone stimulated myometrial contractility both during pregnancy[23] and in the nonpregnant situation.[29] Although an increase in prostaglandin production was not necessary for the mifepristone-induced stimulation of uterine contractions,[23] an increase in decidual prostaglandin synthesis and a decrease in decidual prostaglandin metabolism probably contributed to the uterotonic effects. Alternatively, mifepristone may have stimulated myometrial contractility directly, by inhibition of the relaxant effects of progesterone on the myometrium. These relaxant effects of progesterone include hyperpolarization of smooth muscle cells,[30] decreased intracellular calcium[31] and an increase in the junctional resistance in conditions of progesterone dominance[32,33] presumably by inhibition of gap junction formation. There is clear evidence that mifepristone stimulated gap junction formation in rats[34] and it seems likely that similar mechanisms will operate in the human myometrium.

Action at the cervix

In addition to effects on the endometrium and myometrium, mifepristone induced cervical softening and dilatation, both during pregnancy[35] and in nonpregnant women.[36] The mechanism of this action is unclear. Although it is tempting to speculate that prostaglandins mediate the effects of mifepristone on the cervix there is no evidence to support this. Indeed, a study measuring the bioconversion of arachidonic acid in cervical biopsies of women pretreated with mifepristone showed no change compared with placebo.[37] In another study there was no correlation between ripeness of the cervix and the ability of cervical biopsies to produce lipoxygenase products following treatment with mifepristone *in vivo*.[38] Although a single study using electron microscopy has shown evidence of collagenolysis after mifepristone (100 mg given orally 24 and 12 hours before vacuum aspiration),[39] other authors using histochemical staining of collagen/glycosaminoglycans,[40] or measuring hydroxyproline[41] failed to show any change in collagen content or type. Mifepristone-induced cervical ripening may be mediated by interleukin (IL)-8.[42] This cytokine exhibits a chemotactic effect for neutrophils, synergistic with the actions of prostaglandin E_2. Since the enzymes which ripen the cervix are neutrophil-derived, this is potentially important in the mechanism of cervical ripening.

CONTRACEPTION

Two antiprogestogen actions have been exploited for their contraceptive effect. First, mifepristone inhibits ovulation. Secondly, its administration leads to the development of an endometrium which is unsuitable for implantation. A variety of treatment schedules have been proposed.

Continuous administration

Several studies have shown that continuous daily administration of onapristone (15–50 mg)[43] or mifepristone[43–48] inhibited ovulation. The minimum effective dose is unknown. Croxatto et al found that 5 mg or 10 mg mifepristone, but not 1 mg, was sufficient to inhibit ovulation consistently.[47] Ledger et al gave mifepristone 2 mg or 5 mg to eleven women for 30 days, beginning immediately after an ovulatory placebo cycle.[46] Ovarian activity was monitored by measuring urinary estrone glucuronide or pregnanediol. Despite a rise in estrone glucuronide, suggesting ovarian follicular development, all the treatment cycles were anovulatory, with no significant increase in urinary pregnanediol concentrations. Though the posttreatment cycle showed an inadequate luteal phase in most subjects, one woman conceived. In a further study, six women were given 2 mg mifepristone daily for 30 days, and follicular activity was monitored using ultrasound.[48] Although luteal phase progesterone concentrations suggested ovulation in two cases, the onset of the LH surge was delayed.

These data suggest that daily doses of mifepristone greater than 2 mg are required to inhibit ovulation. However, such doses (or possibly even lower doses) of mifepristone may have rendered the endometrium unsuitable for implantation.[49] In a study where mifepristone (1 mg daily) or placebo was given to 11 normally fertile women, a midluteal phase endometrial biopsy was similar to one obtained from infertile women with luteal phase defects.[17] Similar endometrial findings were confirmed in a further study,[47] suggesting that given in these doses, mifepristone may affect endometrial receptivity. However, whether daily administration of mifepristone will prove to be an acceptable and efficacious contraceptive agent remains to be fully investigated in clinical trials.

Intermittent administration

Animal studies have suggested that intermittent administration of mifepristone may be sufficient to induce the contraceptive effects described above. Ideally, intermittent use of mifepristone would intercept developing follicles before ovulation.[50] However, human studies have been disappointing. When mifepristone, 10 mg or 50 mg was administered weekly for five weeks, elevated progesterone levels consistent with ovulation occurred in two of six women.[51] Another three women were given 50 mg mifepristone for three consecutive days at 10 day intervals and again, one ovulated. Ultrasound examination suggested disordered folliculogenesis/ ovulation in these women, but whether this would prevent conception has yet to be determined. Endometrial biopsies at the end of treatment in the group given 50 mg mifepristone for three consecutive days at 10 day intervals showed either inactive endometrium or disordered development of the endometrium. Further variations on the administration of mifepristone, sometimes with progestogens, continue to show inhibition or disturbance of folliculogenesis and ovulation assessed by a combination of steroid hormone assays and ultrasound.[52] Again, the optimal regimen for intermittent use has yet to be determined, and none of these regimens has been tested for contraceptive effect.

'Once a month' pill

Gestrinone (R2323) is a trienic steroid which binds to the progesterone receptor and exerts a pronounced antiprogestogenic effect. When given to women after ovulation but before implantation, it also results in a decrease in serum progesterone and estradiol concentrations.[53] When given for three days around the time of ovulation, gestrinone can be used as a contraceptive, with a Pearl index of 9.4% including user failures.[54]

When single doses of mifepristone are administered in the luteal phase, disruption of the endometrium and bleeding may be induced.[55–57] As with other regimens, endometrial effects can be observed even in the absence of an ovarian effect. Such endometrial effects have suggested that mifepristone could be administered in the luteal phase as a 'once a month' contraceptive. Although this has advantages in terms of infrequent administration, there are several potential problems with this approach. First, if timing of mifepristone administration is critical, the following menstrual cycle should not be perturbed, otherwise the correct timing of drug administration might become difficult.[58] Secondly, if mifepristone is to be administered in the late luteal phase, it must be able to exert its effects even if fertilization and implantation have occurred. In practice, the contraceptive efficacy of mifepristone given in the late luteal phase is low.[53]

A more successful approach has been to administer mifepristone in the early luteal phase. This has the advantage that the bleeding pattern of both the treatment cycle and the following cycle are less likely to be disturbed.[14] A single dose of 200 mg mifepristone given on the second day after the LH peak retarded the development of the endometrium, thus potentially rendering it unsuitable for implantation.[14] Plasma concentrations of estradiol and progesterone were unaltered, and the lengths of the treatment cycle and subsequent spontaneous cycle were unaffected. Three out of the 24 women had slight vaginal bleeding in association with mifepristone administration. The contraceptive efficacy of this regimen was tested in a clinical trial.[59] Twenty-one sexually active normally cycling women using no other method of contraception were supplied with a rapid urinary LH test. The LH surge was identified in 157 out of 169 treatment cycles. In these 157 cycles, 200 mg mifepristone was taken two days after the LH surge. One pregnancy occurred. Further analysis indicated that for those women at risk of becoming pregnant, the probability was 0.008 after mifepristone, compared with 0.486 after no treatment. As with the preliminary studies above, the main side effect was minimal vaginal bleeding in 35% of cycles. The main disadvantage of the regimen was the necessity to time the LH surge accurately.

Administration of mifepristone in the late luteal phase induced luteolysis and bleeding. However, eleven on-going pregnancies were reported in the three published studies in which mifepristone has been given in this way to 236 women.[60–62] Although the overall failure rate was only 4.7%, measurement of hCG allowed an analysis of the pregnancy rate in women in whom conception had occurred. This was calculated at 14.5%, which was similar to the rate seen when mifepristone was given very early after the missed menses.[63] Not only is this success rate low, but evidence suggests that the interception of early pregnancy, as opposed to contraception, may be less acceptable to the majority of women.

Potential problems using mifepristone as a contraceptive

If mifepristone is to be used as a contraceptive, several issues have to be addressed. The first is efficacy; the contraceptive efficacy of the majority of regimens has yet to be determined in clinical trials. Secondly, there is a theoretical concern that long term administration of an antiprogestogen might lead to unopposed estrogenic activity at the endometrium, with an associated increase in the risk of endometrial carcinoma. In practice, when mifepristone (2 mg/day) or a single postovulatory dose of onapristone (400 mg) was given to premenopausal women, the endometrium was shown histologically to consist of inactive glands and immature stroma despite the demonstration of abundant local estradiol receptors.[49,64] Thirdly, the effects of long-term administration of an antiprogesterone (and in the case of mifepristone, an antiglucocorticoid) are unknown. Studies to date have been reassuring.[8,65] The major adverse effect appeared to be a rise in circulating ACTH concentrations, associated with signs and symptoms compatible with adrenal insufficiency (nausea, vomiting, tiredness). Although these adverse effects were seen following the administration of relatively high doses of mifepristone (100–200 mg), close surveillance will be required to clarify this issue.

Postcoital contraception

Two large randomized studies have evaluated the efficacy of mifepristone as a postcoital contraceptive agent.[66,67] Glasier et al compared 600 mg mifepristone with a regimen using 100 μg ethinyl estradiol and 1 mg norgestrel, both taken twice 12 hours apart. In the study by Webb et al, the two regimens were 600 mg danazol taken twice, 12 hours apart or 100 μg ethinyl estradiol and 500 μg levonorgestrel both taken twice, 12 hours apart. Mifepristone was found to be either as effective[66] or more effective[67] than the alternative treatment. Indeed, none of the 597 women treated with mifepristone became pregnant. Though mifepristone administration was associated with significantly fewer side effects than high dose ethinyl estradiol, a potential disadvantage was a delay in onset of the next menstrual period, seen in around 40% of women.

TERMINATION OF PREGNANCY

Termination of pregnancy can be performed medically or surgically. Prior to the introduction of mifepristone, surgical abortion was the method of choice in the first trimester. Medical abortion using prostaglandins alone is possible but is not widely practised because of side effects, including pain.[68] Surgical abortion involves dilatation of the cervix and evacuation of the uterine contents, usually using a suction curette. The procedure may be performed using either general or local anesthesia. Although surgical abortion is associated with few long-term adverse effects in developed countries, it continues to be a major cause of maternal morbidity and mortality world-wide.

Compounds which reduce endogenous progesterone concentrations have long been sought as medical abortifacients. The synthesis of progesterone was blocked by a variety of synthetic progestogens and indeed by progesterone itself *in vitro*.[69] However, this effect cannot be exploited therapeutically because of the intrinsic progestational activity of these compounds. The group of 3β hydroxysteroid dehydrogenase inhibitors, epostane, trilostane, asastene and cyanoketone inhibit progesterone production but have no agonistic activity themselves. Several studies have examined the efficacy of epostane for menstrual induction. Despite initially promising results[70,71] this work was not continued, partly because of the controversy surrounding medical abortifacients. Gestrinone was used as an agent for menstrual induction, but its effect on progesterone and estradiol concentrations was opposed by hCG from the early embryo.[53]

More recently, the progesterone receptor antagonists mifepristone, ZK 98734 and ZK 98299 have been investigated for their abortifacient activity. Mifepristone was the first of these drugs to undergo clinical trials, and now has a product licence for induction of abortion in China, France, Sweden and the UK.

Antiprogesterones alone

Herrmann et al first published data on the efficacy of mifepristone as an abortifacient.[72] Eleven women requesting legal termination of pregnancy at less than 56 days amenorrhea were given mifepristone 200 mg per day for four days. Eight aborted completely. There was one incomplete abortion and two on-going pregnancies. Although the overall success rate with mifepristone seemed promising, the patient with an incomplete abortion bled heavily and required a blood transfusion. Further trials confirmed similar success rates, with complete abortion occurring in around 60% of women at up to eight weeks gestation.[73–75] Modification of the regimen of administration and of the total dose given does not improve efficacy. However, when treatment was restricted to women within 14 days of the first missed menses, a higher complete abortion rate of 84–85% could be achieved.[63,76] The inverse relationship between gestational age and complete abortion was also illustrated in a study including women of 56–70 days amenorrhea, treated with mifepristone 200 mg daily for a total of four days; only three out of nine women at this later gestation aborted completely.[73] Of the other progesterone receptor antagonists, ZK 98734 (lilopristone) was recently shown to have a similar efficacy to mifepristone for the termination of early pregnancy.

Within each of the above studies, there appear to be few differences between women who abort completely and those in whom treatment is unsuccessful. Differences in plasma concentrations of mifepristone were not demonstrated.[63,76] Factors correlated with treatment success include gestation of less than 49 days, low concentrations of βhCG (< 15000 IU/L) and small gestational sacs (<10 mm diameter).[75]

Mifepristone in combination with prostaglandin

Mifepristone sensitizes the uterus to the contractile action of exogenous prostaglandins.[77] Sequential administration of mifepristone and a prostaglandin is better than either drug given alone. Most early studies used the prostaglandins, sulprostone or gemeprost (Table 46.1). An overall success rate of around 95% was achieved with this combination therapy. Similar outcomes were also seen in a partially randomized comparison of early medical and surgical termination of pregnancy in women with up to 49 days amenorrhea.[78] Mifepristone was licensed for marketing as an abortifacient (in combination with prostaglandin) in 1988 in France and in 1991 in the UK. The administration of mifepristone and prostaglandin for abortion in the UK is dictated by the 1967 Abortion Act which requires treatment to be given in a designated hospital or clinic.

Mifepristone and misoprostol

Recent interest has focused on the orally active prostaglandin misoprostol (Cytotec®, Searle) ([15-S]-15-methyl-PGE_2 methyl ester). This drug is licensed for the treatment of peptic ulcer disease. Its advantage is that it is active orally, and that it has fewer gastrointestinal side effects than other synthetic prostaglandins. The prescription of an oral prostaglandin has several advantages. First, the oral route of administration may be more acceptable than vaginal or intramuscular routes. Secondly, it allows for the possibility of self-administration. Thirdly, the use of mifepristone and misoprostol is significantly cheaper than combination therapy with alternatives such as gemeprost.[79] Although misoprostol alone caused an increase in uterine tone,[80] this was insufficient to

Table 46.1 Efficacy of different combinations of mifepristone and prostaglandin (excluding misoprostol) for medical abortion.

	n	Gestation (days)	Mifepristone (mg)	Prostaglandin (administered vaginally unless otherwise stated)	Complete abortion rate
Cameron et al 1986[86]	39	< 56	600	1 mg gemeprost	95%
Rodger and Baird 1987[110]	100	≤ 56	400–600	0.5–1 mg gemeprost	95%
Dubois et al 1988[61]	106	≤ 49	600	1 mg gemeprost	100%
Silvestre et al 1990[88]	1777	≤ 49	600	0.25–0.5 mg sulprostone	97%
	187		600	1 mg gemeprost	96%
UK Multicentre Trial 1990[87]	588	≤ 63	600	1 mg gemeprost	94%
WHO 1991[83]	181	≤ 49	125	1 mg gemeprost	93%
	187		600	1 mg gemeprost	92%
Wu et al 1992[111]	1572	≤ 59	600	1 mg di-15-methyl $PGF_{2\alpha}$	91%
Somell and Odlund 1993[112]	80	≤ 56	600	1 mg gemeprost	99%
Van Look et al 1993[84]	388	≤ 56	200	1 mg gemeprost	94%
	391		400	1 mg gemeprost	94%
	389		600	1 mg gemeprost	94%
Saxena et al 1994[113]		≤ 56*	200	3 mg 9-methyl PGE_2 (oral) 5 mg 9-methyl PGE_2 (oral)	
Thonneau et al 1994[114]	369	≤ 49	600	0.25 μg sulprostone	93%
Baird et al 1995[82]	391	≤ 63	200	0.5 mg gemeprost	97%
Van Look et al 1995[115]	193	≤ 39**	600	1 mg gemeprost	98%

* = menstrual delay ≤ 7–28 days; ** = menstrual delay ≤ 11 days

Table 46.2 Efficacy of mifepristone combined with misoprostol for medical abortion.

	n	Gestation (days)	Mifepristone (mg)	Misoprostol (μg)	Complete abortion rate
Norman et al 1991[80]	21	≤ 56	200	200–1000 (oral)	86%
Aubeny and Baulieu 1991[116]	100	≤ 49	600	400 (oral)	95%
Thong and Baird 1992[117]	100	≤ 56	200	600 (oral)	93%
Peyron et al 1993[118]	505	≤ 49	600	400 (oral)	97%
	390	≤ 49	600	400–600 (oral)	99%
McKinlay et al 1993[81]	119	≤ 49	200–600	600 (oral)	97%
	101	50–63	200–600	600 (oral)	89%
Sang et al 1994[119]	301	≤ 49	150	600 (oral)	94%
	149	≤ 49	200	600 (oral)	95%
El-Refaey and Templeton 1994[120]	150	≤ 56	200	800 (oral)	93%
El-Refaey et al 1995[121]	130	≤ 63	600	800 (oral)	87%
	133	≤ 63	600	800 (vaginal)	95%
Baird et al 1995[82]	386	< 63	200	600 (oral)	95%
Weeks and Stewart 1995[122]	100	≤ 63	200	?	91%

induce abortion by itself. When misoprostol was given after mifepristone, a further increase in mifepristone-induced contractions was observed, and abortion occurred in the majority of patients.[80] Although mifepristone plus misoprostol was effective in termination of early pregnancy (up to 49 days), the combination had a lower complete abortion rate and a higher ongoing pregnancy rate[81,82] at later gestations than the combination of mifepristone and gemeprost (Table 46.2).

Dose of mifepristone

There is no clear dose response to mifepristone in terms of complete abortion rates using mifepristone alone. This may be because mifepristone circulates bound to an α-1 acid glycoprotein, and unbound drug is rapidly metabolized. Thus serum concentrations of mifepristone increase with increasing doses of drug to doses of 100 mg, thereafter larger doses have little additional effect. Using mifepristone in combination with prostaglandins, lower doses of antiprogestogen appear to be as effective as the recommended 600 mg dose. Two large trials compared the efficacy of a single dose of 600 mg mifepristone with either five doses of 25 mg given at 12 hourly intervals[83] or a single dose of 200 mg or 400 mg.[84] In the first study the overall complete abortion rate was 93%, whilst in the second it was 96%. There were no significant differences between the groups in terms of bleeding pattern, blood loss or side effects. Mifepristone is relatively expensive and a reduction in the dose has considerable advantages, however 600 mg remains the current dose recommended on the data sheet.

Side effects of mifepristone and prostaglandin for termination of pregnancy

Mifepristone alone appeared to cause few side effects other than vaginal bleeding. Following large doses of mifepristone (400 mg per day for four days) headache occurred in up to 30% of women[85] and nausea and vomiting was seen in 80%. However, as these are common pregnancy symptoms, the part played by mifepristone was difficult to quantify.[35,86] Whilst the stimulatory effects of mifepristone on uterine activity may induce abdominal cramps, opiate analgesia was not required. When mifepristone is followed by a prostaglandin, prostaglandin-related gastrointestinal side effects and abdominal pain (presumably due to increased uterine activity) are more common. In a study of over 500 women given mifepristone and gemeprost, 26% and 13% of patients reported vomiting and diarrhea as a new symptom in the four hours following prostaglandin treatment, and 28% required opiate analgesia.[87] In a large French trial of over 2000 women, the reported incidence of vomiting and diarrhea was 15% and 7% respectively, and the overall need for opiate analgesia was 1%.[88] Varying practices in the prescription of antiemetic or antidiarrheal agents should be noted when comparing the results of different studies.

Data on blood loss during mifepristone-induced medical abortion have been conflicting. Initial work suggested that blood loss was similar to surgical abortion at an equivalent gestation,[86,89] i.e. around 80 mL at up to eight weeks gestation. However, further studies showed slightly greater blood loss during medical than during surgical abortion.[90,91] Blood transfusion rates of up to 1% have been quoted.[87]

Women's preferences during abortion

In a UK study, women of up to nine weeks gestation were asked to choose between medical and surgical abortion.[92] Twenty per cent chose medical abortion whilst 26% opted for surgery. Those women who did not express a preference were randomized to either medical or surgical treatment. Each treatment was acceptable to the women who had chosen that particular treatment. In women allocated at random, treatments were equally acceptable to those under 50 days gestation, but between 50–63 days gestation, surgical abortion was found to be more acceptable. In a further study, both medical and surgical abortion led to a similar incidence of psychological benefit.[93]

Second trimester termination of pregnancy

The preferred method of second trimester termination of pregnancy varies in different countries. Surgical dilatation and evacuation (D and E) is the method of choice in the USA. The procedure is usually performed using general anesthesia and has a relatively low morbidity and mortality, comparing well with the intra-amniotic instillation of prostaglandin or hypertonic saline.[94] In the UK, prostaglandin-induced induction of abortion is the preferred treatment option. This involves repeated doses of prostaglandins to induce cervical ripening, uterine contractility and eventual abortion. Oxytocin agonists may be used in addition. Prostaglandin may be administered by the intravenous, intra-amniotic, extra-amniotic or vaginal route. Vaginal gemeprost may offer the best combination of minimal side effects and ease of administration. However, the interval between initiation of prostaglandin treatment and expulsion of the fetus and placenta is over 24 hours in 20% of women.

Compared to either placebo or laminaria, mifepristone was shown to reduce the induction–abortion interval in second trimester abortion, and this reduction in duration of the procedure was associated with lower analgesic requirements.[94–96] Mifepristone may also reduce costs if its use converts second trimester abortion from an in-patient to a day case procedure. More recently, mifepristone has been used in association with misoprostol in second trimester abortion.[97–99] Despite evidence that vaginal administration of misoprostol is superior to oral administration in the first trimester, the use of vaginal misoprostol appears to confer few advantages in the second trimester.[97]

The optimal medical regimen for second trimester termination of pregnancy has yet to be determined. The use of mifepristone has clear advantages, both in terms of shortening the length of the procedure and reducing analgesic requirements. There is no evidence that any one prostaglandin is superior, although misoprostol is cheaper. Formal comparisons between D and E (performed by experienced operators) and medical termination of pregnancy are required, but since adverse outcomes are relatively infrequent with both procedures, large studies will be needed to show any significant difference.

Cervical ripening prior to suction abortion

Surgical approaches to termination of pregnancy require cervical dilatation prior to uterine evacuation. Large forces are necessary to dilate the cervix beyond 9 mm, and this may be associated with cervical damage.[100] There is concern that cervical damage during termination of pregnancy may be associated with cervical incompetence in future pregnancies. In an attempt to avoid this, cervical ripening agents are often given prior to surgical abortion to reduce the force required to dilate the cervix. Many studies have now assessed the efficacy of mifepristone for this purpose.

A large study of the effect of mifepristone on the cervix involved 230 primigravidae of 10–12 weeks amenorrhea given 0–100 mg mifepristone in a double blind randomized fashion 24 and 12 hours prior to surgical termination of pregnancy.[35] Cervical dilation observed at operation was significantly greater in women pretreated with mifepristone (mean 6.5 mm) compared to those treated with placebo (mean 5.4 mm). A similar effect has been observed by others.[36,41,101–104] The WHO study also assessed resistance to further dilatation subjectively at operation. The cervix was significantly easier to dilate in mifepristone-treated women; an effect which was dose-dependent. These results were confirmed by other studies.[37,105,106]

Other benefits of cervical ripening with mifepristone included a reduction in the incidence of excessive operative blood loss (defined as ≥ 400 mL) from 20% in the placebo group to 3%.[107] Mifepristone also decreased operating time and reduced postoperative pain compared with placebo.[105]

FUTURE PROSPECTS

The use of the antiprogestogen mifepristone is likely to continue to expand over the next few years. Although the 'once a month' pill remains elusive, except perhaps for those who are prepared to monitor their menstrual cycle carefully, continuous administration of mifepristone may prove to be an effective contraceptive. Clinical trials are needed to investigate this further. However, for mifepristone to be accepted as a contraceptive agent for widespread use, it will have to compare favorably with currently available preparations of estrogen and progestogen or progestogen alone. Mifepristone-containing preparations could provide an alternative for those women for whom estrogens are contraindicated, where they might be more efficacious than the progestogen-only pill. Long-term studies will be required to evaluate both the adverse and beneficial effects of mifepristone in relation to estrogen and progestogen preparations.

Although mifepristone in combination with a prostaglandin has been shown to be a highly effective abortifacient, the sensitive nature of pregnancy termination, morally, politically and religiously has delayed the introduction of the drug in some countries. Researchers have therefore turned to compounds which are currently available, to determine their efficacy in medical abortion. One such drug is methotrexate. In a recent study of 178 women of up to 63 days gestation, methotrexate followed by 800 μg of misoprostol administered intravaginally 5–7 days later induced complete abortion in 96% of women with no side effects.[108] Methotrexate and misoprostol were less effective in women of 56–63 days amenorrhea.[109] The short and long-term side effects of this combination are not known, and it will be unfortunate if a clinically effective therapy such as mifepristone is dismissed due to political or other pressures.

Mifepristone is also a highly effective postcoital agent, comparing well with the Yuzpe regimen in terms of efficacy and side effects. Some would argue that mifepristone should be the treatment of choice for this indication. Others would go further, suggesting that agents for emergency contraception should be more widely available as 'over the counter' drugs. Those opposed to this view fear that such availability could lead to self-medication for abortion. However a similar argument could be used for misoprostol, which is available over the counter for peptic ulcer disease. Furthermore, with the better provision of accessible and comprehensive family planning services, self-induced abortion should be less necessary.

Conclusion

The last 10–15 years have seen a dramatic expansion in the list of potential applications for antiprogestogens for the medical control of human fertility. In combination with prostaglandins, the drugs are effective abortifacients in the first and second trimesters of pregnancy, and are particularly useful in situations where unwanted pregnancy is a major health issue but large numbers of staff are unavailable to offer surgical procedures. The drugs compare well with estrogen/progestogen preparations for emergency contraception, and might also provide alternatives to the currently available synthetic steroids for long-term hormonal contraception on a daily or monthly basis.

REFERENCES

1. Rojas FJ, O'Conner JL, Asch RH 1985 The antiprogesterone steroid RU-486 does not impair gonadotrophin-stimulated luteal adenylyl cylase activity or gonadotrophin release by pituitary cells. Journal of Steroid Biochemistry 23: 1053–1058
2. Gravanis A, Schaison G, George M et al 1985 Endometrial and pituitary responses to the steroidal antiprogestin RU 486 in post menopausal women. Journal of Clinical Endocrinology and Metabolism 60: 156–163
3. Batista MC, Cartledge TP, Zellmer AW, Nieman LK, Loriaux DL, Merriam GR 1994 The antiprogestin RU486 delays the midcycle gonadotropin surge and ovulation in gonadotropin-releasing hormone-induced cycles. Fertility and Sterility 62: 28–34
4. Batista MC, Cartledge TP, Zellmer AW, Nieman LK, Merriam GR, Loriaux DL 1992 Evidence for a critical role of progesterone in the regulation of the midcycle gonadotropin surge and ovulation. Journal of Clinical Endocrinology and Metabolism 74: 565–570
5. Garzo VG, Liu J, Ulmann A, Baulieu E, Yen SSC 1988 Effects of an antiprogesterone (RU486) on the hypothalamic-hypophyseal-ovarian-endometrial axis during the luteal phase of the menstrual cycle. Journal of Clinical Endocrinology and Metabolism 66: 508–517
6. Shoupe F, Mishell DR, Fossum G, Bopp BL, Spitz IM, Lobo RA 1990 Antiprogestin treatment decreases midluteal luteinizing hormone pulse amplitude and primarily exerts a pituitary inhibition. American Journal of Obstetrics and Gynecology 163: 1982–1985
7. Li TC, Dockery P, Thomas P, Rogers AW, Lenton EA, Cooke ID 1988 The effects of progesterone receptor blockade in the luteal phase of normal fertile women. Fertility and Sterility 50: 732–742

8. Kettel LM, Murphy AA, Mortola JF, Liu JH, Ulmann A, Yen SSC 1991 Endocrine responses to long-term administration of the antiprogesterone RU486 in patients with pelvic endometriosis. Fertility and Sterility 56: 402–407
9. Galliard RC, Riondel A, Muller AF, Herrmann W, Baulieu EE 1984 RU 486: a steroid with antiglucocorticoid activity that only disinhibits the human pituitary-adrenal system at a specific time of day. Proceedings of the National Academy of Sciences 81: 3879–3882
10. DiMattina M, Albertson B, Seyler DE, Loriaux DL, Falk RJ 1986 Effect of the antiprogestin RU 486 on progesterone production by cultured human granulosa cells: inhibition of the ovarian 3β-hydroxysteroid dehydrogenase. Contraception 34: 199–206
11. Wang J-D, Zhu J-B, Shi W-L, Zhu P-D 1994 Immunocytochemical colocalization of progesterone receptor and prolactin in individual stromal cells of human decidua. Journal of Clinical Endocrinology and Metabolism 79: 293–297
12. Perrot-Applanat M, Deng M, Fernandez H, Lelaidier C, Meduri G, Bouchard P 1994 Immunohistochemical localization of estradiol and progesterone receptors in human uterus throughout pregnancy: expression in endometrial blood vessels. Journal of Clinical Endocrinology and Metabolism 78: 216–224
13. Berthois Y, Salat-Baroux J, Cornet D, De Brux J, Kopp F, Martin PM 1991 A multiparametric analysis of endometrial estrogen and progesterone receptors after the postovulatory administration of mifepristone. Fertility and Sterility 55: 547–554
14. Swahn ML, Bygdeman M, Cekan S, Xing S, Masironi B, Johannisson E 1990 The effect of RU 486 administered during the early luteal phase on bleeding pattern, hormonal parameters and endometrium. Human Reproduction 5: 402–408
15. Li TC, Rodgers AW, Dockery P, Lenton EA, Cooke ID 1988 A new method of histological dating of human endometrium in the luteal phase. Fertility and Sterility 50: 52–60
16. Noyes RW, Hertig AT, Rock J 1950 Dating the endometrial biopsy. Fertility and Sterility 1: 3–25
17. Batista MC, Cartledge TP, Zellmer AW, et al 1992 Delayed endometrial maturation induced by daily administration of the antiprogestin RU 486: a potential new contraceptive strategy. American Journal of Obstetrics and Gynecology 167: 60–65
18. Greene KE, Kettel LM, Yen SSC 1992 Interruption of endometrial maturation without hormonal changes by an antiprogesterone during the first half of luteal phase of the menstrual cycle: a contraceptive potential. Fertility and Sterility 58: 338–343
19. Johannisson E, Oberholzer M, Swahn M-L, Bygdeman M 1989 Vascular changes in the human endometrium following the administration of the progesterone antagonist RU 486. Contraception 39: 103–117
20. Schindler AM, Zanon P, Obradovic D, Wyss R, Graff P, Herrmann WL 1985 Early ultrastructural changes in RU 486-exposed decidua. Gynecological and Obstetrical Investigation 20: 62–67
21. Kelly RW, Healy DL, Cameron MJ, Cameron IT, Baird DT 1986 The stimulation of prostaglandin production by two antiprogesterone steroids in human endometrial cells. Journal of Clinical Endocrinology and Metabolism 62: 1116–1123
22. Smith SK, Kelly RW 1987 The effect of the antiprogestins RU 486 and ZK 98 734 on the synthesis and metabolism of prostaglandins $F_{2\alpha}$ and E_2 in separated cells from early human decidua. Journal of Clinical Endocrinology and Metabolism 65: 527–534
23. Norman JE, Kelly RW, Baird DT 1991 Uterine activity and decidual prostaglandin production in women in early pregnancy in response to mifepristone with or without indomethacin *in vivo*. Human Reproduction 6: 740–744
24. Norman JE, Wu WX, Kelly RW, Glasier AF, McNeilly AS, Baird DT 1991 Effects of mifepristone *in vivo* on decidual prostaglandin synthesis and metabolism. Contraception 44: 89–98
25. Cheng L, Kelly RW, Thong KJ, Hume R, Baird DT 1993 The effect of mifepristone (RU 486) on the immunohistochemical distribution of prostaglandin E and its metabolite in decidual and chorionic tissue in early pregnancy. Journal of Clinical Endocrinology and Metabolism 77: 873–877
26. Cheng L, Kelly RW, Thong KJ, Hume R, Baird DT 1993 The effect of mifepristone (RU 486) on prostaglandin dehydrogenase in decidual and chorionic tissue in early pregnancy. Human Reproduction 8: 705–709
27. Lockwood CJ, Krikun G, Papp C, Aigner S, Schatz F 1995 Biological mechanisms underlying the clinical effects of RU 486: modulation of cultured endometrial stromal cell plasminogen activator and plasminogen activator inhibitor expression. Journal of Clinical Endocrinology and Metabolism 80: 1100–1105
28. Lockwood CJ, Krikun G, Papp C, Aigner S, Nemerson Y, Schatz F 1994 Biological mechanisms underlying RU 486 clinical effects: inhibition of endometrial stromal cell tissue factor content. Journal of Clinical Endocrinology and Metabolism 79: 786–790
29. Gemzell K, Swahn ML, Bydgeman M 1990 Regulation of non-pregnant human uterine contractility. Effect of antihormones. Contraception 42: 323–335
30. Marshall JM 1959 Effects of estrogen and progesterone on single uterine muscle fibres in the rat. American Journal of Physiology 197: 935–942
31. Carsten ME 1979 Calcium accumulation by human uterine microsomal preparations: effects of progesterone and oxytocin. American Journal of Obstetrics and Gynecology 133: 598–601
32. Ichikawa S, Bortoff A 1970 Tissue resistance of the progesterone-dominated rabbit myometrium. American Journal of Physiology 219: 1763–1767
33. Bortoff A, Gilloteax J 1980 Specific tissue impedences of estrogen and progesterone-treated rabbit myometrium. American Journal of Physiology 238: C34–C42
34. Garfield RE, Baulieu EE 1987 The antiprogesterone steroid RU 486: a short pharmacological and clinical review, with emphasis on the interruption of pregnancy. Ballière's Clinical Endocrinology and Metabolism 1: 207–221

35. World Health Organization 1990 The use of mifepristone (RU 486) for cervical preparation in first trimester pregnancy termination by vacuum aspiration. British Journal of Obstetrics and Gynaecology 97: 260–266
36. Gupta JK, Johnson N 1990 Effect of mifepristone on dilatation of the pregnant and non-pregnant cervix. Lancet ii: 1238–1240
37. Radestad A, Bygdeman M, Green K 1990 Induced cervical ripening with mifepristone (RU486) and bioconversion of arachidonic acid in human pregnant uterine cervix in the first trimester. Contraception 41: 283–292
38. Heidvall K, Radestad A, Christensen NJ, Lindgren JA 1992 Production of 12-hydroxyeicosatetraenoic acid in pregnant uterine cervix — lack of correlation to mifepristone-induced cervical ripening. Prostaglandins 43: 473–482
39. Radestad A, Thyberg J, Christensen NJ 1993 Cervical ripening with mifepristone (RU 486) in first trimester abortion. An electron microscope study. Human Reproduction 8: 1136–1142
40. Norman JE 1992 Menstrual induction: methods and mechanisms of action. MD thesis, University of Edinburgh
41. Bokstrom H, Norstrom A 1995 Effects of mifepristone and progesterone on collagen synthesis in the human uterine cervix. Contraception 51: 249–254
42. Kelly RW, Leask R, Calder AA 1992 Choriodecidual production of interleukin-8 and mechanism of parturition. Lancet 339: 776–777
43. Croxatto HB, Salvatierra AM, Fuentealba B, Zurth C, Beier S 1994 Effect of the antiprogestin onapristone on follicular growth in women. Human Reproduction 9: 1442–1447
44. Kekkonen R, Heikinheimo O, Alfthan H, Luukkainen T, Haukkamaa M, Lahteenmaki P 1990 Interference with ovulation by sequential treatment with the antiprogesterone RU 486 and synthetic progestin. Fertility and Sterility 53: 747–750
45. Luukkainen T, Heikinheimo O, Haukkamaa M, Lahteenmaki P 1988 Inhibition of folliculogenesis and ovulation by the antiprogesterone RU 486. Fertility and Sterility 49: 961–963
46. Ledger WL, Sweeting VM, Hillier H, Baird DT 1992 Inhibition of ovulation by low-dose mifepristone (RU 486). Human Reproduction 7: 945–950
47. Croxatto HB, Salvatierra AM, Croxatto HD, Fuentealba B 1993 Effects of continuous treatment with low dose mifepristone throughout one menstrual cycle. Human Reproduction 8: 201–207
48. Cameron ST, Thong KJ, Baird DT 1995 Effect of daily low dose mifepristone on the ovarian cycle and on dynamics of follicle growth. Clinical Endocrinology 43: 407–414
49. Cameron ST, Critchley HOD, Thong KJ, Buckley CH,Williams AR, Baird DT 1996 Effects of daily low dose mifepristone on the endometrial maturation and proliferation. Human Reproduction 11: 2518–2526
50. Collins RL, Hodgen GD 1986 Blockade of the spontaneous midcycle gonadotropin surge in monkeys by RU 486: a progesterone antagonist or agonist? Journal of Clinical Endocrinology and Metabolism 63: 1270–1276
51. Spitz IM, Croxatto HB, Salvatierra A-M, Heikinheimo O 1993 Response to intermittent RU 486 in women. Fertility and Sterility 59: 971–975
52. Kekkonen R, Croxatto HB, Lahteenmaki P, Salvatierra AM, Tuominen J 1995 Effects of intermittent antiprogestin RU 486 combined with cyclic medroxyprogesterone acetate on folliculogenesis and ovulation. Human Reproduction 10: 287–292
53. Mora G, Faundes A, Johansson EDB 1975 Lack of clinical contraceptive efficacy of large doses of R2323 given before implantation or after a missed period. Contraception 12: 211–220
54. Sakiz E, Azadian-Boulanger G, Laraque F, Raynaud JP 1974 A new approach to estrogen-free contraception based on progesterone receptor blockage by mid-cycle administration of ethyl norgestrenone (R2323). Contraception 10: 467–474
55. Shoupe D, Mishell DR, Lahteenmaki P et al 1987 Effects of the antiprogesterone RU 486 in normal women. American Journal of Obstetrics and Gynecology 157: 1415–1420
56. Yen S, Garzo G, Liu J 1987 Luteal contraception. Contraception 36(Suppl): 13–25
57. Nieman LK, Choate TM, Chrousos GP et al 1987 The progesterone antagonist RU 486. A potential new contraceptive agent. New England Journal of Medicine 316: 187–191
58. Baird DT, Cameron IT 1985 Menstrual induction: surgery versus prostaglandins. In: CIBA Foundation Symposium 115. Abortion: medical progress and social implications. Pitman, London, pp 179–191
59. Gemzell-Danielsson K, Swahn M-L, Svalander P, Bygdeman M 1993 Early luteal phase treatment with mifepristone (RU 486) for fertility regulation. Human Reproduction 8: 870–873
60. Couzinet B, LeStrat N, Silvestre L, Schaison G 1990 Late luteal phase administration of the antiprogesterone RU 486 in normal women: effects on the menstrual cycle events and fertility control in a long term study. Fertility and Sterility 54: 1039–1043
61. Dubois C, Ulmann A, Baulieu EE 1988 Contragestation with late luteal administration of RU 486 (mifepristone). Fertility and Sterility 50: 593–596
62. van Santen MR, Haspels AA 1987 Interception. IV: Failure of mifepristone (RU 486) as a monthly contragestive, 'lunarette'. Contraception 35: 433–438
63. Couzinet B, LeStrat N, Umann A, Baulieu EE, Schaison G 1986 Termination of early pregnancy by the progesterone antagonist RU 486 (mifepristone). New England Journal of Medicine 315: 1565–1570
64. Cameron ST, Critchley HOD, Buckley CH, Chard T, Kelly RW, Baird DT 1996 The effects of postovulatory administration of onapristone on the development of a secretory endometrium. Human Reproduction 11: 40–49
65. Lamberts SWJ, Koper JW, de Jong FH 1991 The endocrine effects of long-term treatment with mifepristone (RU 486). Journal of Clinical Endocrinology and Metabolism 73: 187–191
66. Glasier A, Thong KJ, Dewar MJ, Mackie M, Baird DT 1992 Mifepristone (RU 486) compared with high-dose estrogen and progestogen for emergency postcoital contraception. New England Journal of Medicine 327: 1041–1044

67. Webb AMC, Russell J, Elstein M 1992 Comparison of Yuzpe regimen, danazol, and mifepristone (RU 486) in oral postcoital contraception. British Medical Journal 305: 927–931
68. Norman JE, Thong KJ, Rodger MW, Baird DT 1992 Medical abortion in women ≤ 56 days amenorrhoea: a comparison between gemeprost (a PGE_1 analogue) alone and mifepristone and gemeprost. British Journal of Obstetrics and Gynaecology 99: 601–606
69. Shinada T, Yokota Y, Igarashi M 1978 Inhibitory effects of various gestagens upon the pregnenolone 3β-ol-dehydrogenase-delta-5-4-isomerase system in human corpora lutea of menstrual cycles. Fertility and Sterility 29: 84–87
70. Birgerson L, Odlund A, Odlind V, Somell C 1987 Termination of early human pregnancy with epostane. Contraception 35: 111–120
71. Crooj MJ, de Nooyer CCA, Rao BR, Berends GT, Gooren LJG, Janssens J 1988 Termination of early pregnancy by the 3β-hydroxysteroid dehyrogenase inhibitor epostane. New England Journal of Medicine 319: 813–817
72. Herrmann W, Wyss R, Riondel A et al 1982 Effet d'un steroide anti-progesterone chez la femme: interruption du cycle menstruel et de la grossesse au debut. Circulation Research Academy of Science, Paris 294: 933–938
73. Vervest HAM, Haspels AA 1985 Preliminary results with the antiprogestational compound RU-486 (mifepristone) for interruption of early pregnancy. Fertility and Sterility 44: 627–632
74. Mishell DR, Shoupe D, Brenner PF et al 1987 Termination of early gestation with the anti-progestin steroid RU 486: medium versus low dose. Contraception 35: 307–321
75. Sitruk-Ware R, Billaud L, Mowszowica I et al 1985 The use of RU 486 as an abortificient in early pregnancy. In: Baulieu E, Segal S (eds) The antiprogestin steroid RU 486 and human fertility control. Plenum Press, New York, pp 243–248
76. Ulmann A 1987 Uses of RU 486 for contragestation: an update. Contraception 36 (Suppl): 27–31
77. Bygdeman M, Swahn M-L 1985 Progesterone receptor blockage. Effect on uterine contractility and early pregnancy. Contraception 32: 45–51
78. Henshaw RC, Naji SA, Russell IT, Templeton AA 1994 A comparison of medical abortion (using mifepristone and gemeprost) with surgical vacuum aspiration: efficacy and early medical sequelae. Human Reproduction 9: 2167–2172
79. Penney GC, McKessock L, Rispin R, El-Refaey H, Templeton A 1995 An effective, low cost regimen for early medical abortion. British Journal of Family Planning 21: 5–6
80. Norman JE, Thong KJ, Baird DT 1991 Uterine contractility and induction of abortion in early pregnancy by misoprostol and mifepristone. Lancet 338: 1233–1236
81. McKinley C, Thong KJ, Baird DT 1993 The effect of dose of mifepristone and gestation on the efficacy of medical abortion with mifepristone and misoprostol. Human Reproduction 8(9): 1502–1505
82. Baird DT, Sukcharoen N, Thong KJ 1995 Randomized trial of misoprostol and cervagem in combination with a reduced dose of mifepristone for induction of abortion. Human Reproduction 10: 1521–1527
83. World Health Organization 1991 Pregnancy termination with mifepristone and gemeprost: a multicenter comparison between repeated doses and a single dose of mifepristone. Fertility and Sterility 56: 32–40
84. Van Look PFA, Henshaw R, Norman J et al 1993 Termination of pregnancy with reduced doses of mifepristone. British Medical Journal 307: 532–537
85. Shoupe D, Mishell DR, Brenner PF, Spitz IM 1986 Pregnancy termination with a high and medium dosage regime of RU 486. Contraception 33: 455–461
86. Cameron IT, Michie AF, Baird DT 1986 Therapeutic abortion in early pregnancy with antiprogestin RU 486 alone or in combination with prostaglandin analogue (Gemeprost). Contraception 34: 459–468
87. UK Multicentre Trial 1990 The efficacy and tolerance of mifepristone and prostaglandin in first trimester termination of pregnancy. British Journal of Obstetrics and Gynaecology 97: 480–486
88. Silvestre L, Dubois C, Renault M, Rezvani Y, Baulieu E-E, Ulmann A 1990 Voluntary interruption of pregnancy with mifepristone (RU 486) and a prostaglandin analogue. A large scale French experience. New England Journal of Medicine 322: 645–648
89. Rodger MW, Baird DT 1989 Blood loss following induction of early abortion using mifepristone (RU 486) and a prostaglandin analogue (gemeprost). Contraception 40: 439–447
90. Chan YF, Ho PC, Ma HK 1993 Blood loss in termination of early pregnancy by vacuum aspiration and by combination of mifepristone and gemeprost. Contraception 47: 85–95
91. Prasad RNV, Choolani M, Roy A, Ratnam SS 1995 Blood loss in termination of early pregnancy with mifepristone and gemeprost. Australian and New Zealand Journal of Obstetrics and Gynaecology 35: 329–331
92. Henshaw RC, Naji SA, Russell IT, Templeton AA 1993 Comparison of medical abortion with surgical vacuum aspiration. British Medical Journal 307: 714–717
93. Henshaw R, Naji S, Russell I, Templeton A 1994 Psychological responses following medical abortion (using mifepristone and gemeprost) and surgical vacuum aspiration: a patient-centered, partially randomised prospective study. Acta Obstetrica and Gynecologica Scandinavica 73: 812–818
94. Urquhart DR, Templeton AA 1990 The use of mifepristone prior to prostaglandin-induced mid-trimester abortion. Human Reproduction 5: 833–886
95. Rodger MW, Baird DT 1990 Pretreatment with mifepristone (RU 486) reduces interval between prostaglandin administration and expulsion in second trimester abortion. British Journal of Obstetrics and Gynaecology 97: 41–45
96. Thong KJ, Baird DT 1992 A study of gemeprost alone, dilapan or mifepristone in combination with gemeprost for the termination of second trimester pregnancy. Contraception 46: 11–17

97. El-Refaey H, Templeton AA 1995 Induction of abortion in the second trimester by a combination of misoprostol and mifepristone: a randomized comparison between two misoprostol regimens. Human Reproduction 10: 475–478
98. El-Refaey H, Hinshaw K, Templeton AA 1993 The abortifacient effect of misoprostol in the second trimester. A randomised comparison with gemeprost in patients pre-treated with mifepristone (RU486). Human Reproduction 8: 1744–1746
99. Weeks AD, Stewart P 1995 The use of mifepristone in combination with misoprostol for second trimester termination of pregnancy. British Journal of Family Planning 21: 43–44
100. Johnstone FD, Beard RJ, Boyd IE et al 1976 Cervical diameter after suction termination of pregnancy. British Medical Journal i: 68–69
101. Radestad A, Christensen NJ, Stromberg L 1988 Induced cervical ripening with mifepristone in first trimester abortion. A double-blind, randomised, biomechanical and biochemical study. Contraception 38: 301–312
102. Durlot F, Dubois C, Brunerie J, Frydman R 1988 Efficacy of progesterone antagonist RU 486 (mifepristone) for pre-operative cervical dilatation during first trimester abortion. Human Reproduction 3: 583–584
103. Lefebrve Y, Proulx L, Elie R, Poulin O, Lanza E 1990 The effect of RU-38486 on cervical ripening. American Journal of Obstetrics and Gynecology 162: 61–65
104. Carbonne B, Brennand JE, Maria B, Cabrol D, Calder AA 1995 Effects of gemeprost and mifepristone on the mechanical properties of the cervix prior to first trimester termination of pregnancy. British Journal of Obstetrics and Gynaecology 102: 553–558
105. Henshaw R, Bjornsson S, Norman J et al 1994 Cervical ripening with mifepristone (RU 486) in late first trimester abortion. Contraception 50: 461–475
106. Cohn M, Stewart P 1991 Pretreatment of the primigravid uterus with mifepristone 30 h prior to termination of pregnancy: a double blind study. British Journal of Obstetrics and Gynaecology 98: 778–782
107. Henshaw RC, Templeton AA 1991 Pre-operative cervical preparation before first trimester vacuum aspiration: a randomised controlled comparison between gemeprost and mifepristone (RU 486). British Journal of Obstetrics and Gynaecology 98: 1025–1030
108. Hausnecht RU 1995 Methotrexate and misoprostol to terminate early pregnancy. New England Journal of Medicine 333: 537–540
109. Creinin MD 1994 Methotrexate and misoprostol for abortion at 57–63 days gestation. Contraception 50: 511–515
110. Rodger MW, Baird DT 1987 Induction of therapeutic abortion in early pregnancy with mifepristone in combination with prostaglandin pessary. Lancet ii: 1415–1418
111. Wu S, Gao J, Wu Y et al 1992 Clinical trial on termination of early pregnancy with RU 486 in combination with prostaglandin. Contraception 46: 203–210
112. Somell C, Odlund A 1993 Induction of abortion in early pregnancy with mifepristone in conjunction with gemeprost. Acta Obstet Gynecol Scand 72: 39–42
113. Saxena BN, Datey S, Gaur LN et al 1994 A multicentre clinical trial with RU 486 followed by 9-methylene-PGE_2 vaginal gel for termination of early pregnancy: a dose finding study. Contraception 49: 87–88
114. Thonneau P, Fougeyrollas B, Spira A 1994 Analysis of 369 abortions conducted by mifepristone (RU 486). Fertility and Sterility 61: 627–631
115. Van Look PFA, Belsey EM, BernersLee N et al 1995 Menstrual regulation by mifepristone plus prostaglandin: results from a multicentre trial. Human Reproduction 10: 308–314
116. Aubeny E, Baulieu E-E 1991 Activite contragestive de l'association au RU 486 d'une prostaglandine active par voie orale. CR Acad Sci 312: 539–545
117. Thong KJ, Baird DT 1992 Induction of abortion with mifepristone and misoprostol in early pregnancy. British Journal of Obstetrics and Gynaecology 99: 1004–1007
118. Peyron R, Aubeny E, Targosz V et al 1993 Early termination of pregnancy with mifepristone (RU 486) and the orally active prostaglandin misoprostol. New England Journal of Medicine 328: 1509–1513
119. Sang GW, Weng LJ, Shao QX, Wu XZ, Lu YL, Cheng LN 1994 Termination of early pregnancy by two regimens of mifepristone with misoprostol and mifepristone with PG05 – A multicentre randomised clinical trial in China. Contraception 50: 501–510
120. El-Refaey H, Templeton AA 1994 Early abortion induction by a combination of mifepristone and oral misoprostol: a comparison between two dose regimens of misoprostol and their effect on blood pressure British Journal of Obstetrics and Gynaecology 101: 792–796
121. El-Refaey H, Rajasekar D, Abdalla M, Calder L, Templeton AA 1995 Induction of abortion with mifepristone (RU 486) and oral or vaginal misoprostol. New England Journal of Medicine 332: 983–987
122. Weeks AD, Stewart P 1995 The use of low dose mifepristone and vaginal misoprostol for first trimester termination of pregnancy, British Journal of Family Planning 21: 85–86

47. Demographic aspects

Sonja McKinlay   Sybil Crawford

Introduction

Menopause is a ubiquitous physiological event in the female of the human species. In all other female animal species, fertility is generally observed until death intervenes, although natural cessation of fertility has been observed in a few long-lived captive primates.

This chapter describes current knowledge concerning the measurement and timing of cessation of fertility as well as the signs and symptoms that accompany this event. It also addresses the relationship between this physiological event and selected diseases or processes as well as the role of declining reproductive hormones in the treatment of these conditions.

AGE AT MENOPAUSE

Some key terms

According to the WHO Scientific Group addressing Research on Menopause[1] the standard definition of menopause is occurrence of a final menstrual period (FMP), either naturally or surgically.

Natural menopause, according to this general definition can only be defined retrospectively after continued amenorrhea in the absence of other causes (such as pregnancy and/or lactation). There is general consensus that amenorrhea for at least 12 months is an acceptable definition in practice.[1,2,3]

Surgical menopause, refers to the surgical cessation of menses through either removal of the uterus or removal of both ovaries. Obviously the immediate hormonal impact of these two surgeries is distinct and women receiving either procedure are usually considered as distinct groups for both research and therapeutic purposes.

Premenopause refers to the time span before FMP and generally includes all fertile years.

Postmenopause refers to the time after FMP.

Perimenopause is a relatively new term that has, to a large extent, replaced the term 'climacteric' to embrace the period of physiological change surrounding FMP. Many researchers use this term more narrowly to describe the period immediately before FMP.

What we know

Our current knowledge concerning the age at FMP focuses almost exclusively on Caucasian populations and can be summarized in the following statements:

- The median age at natural menopause in Caucasian populations is between 51–52 years of age, with an asymmetric range of about 40–55 years.
- There is no evidence that the age at menopause has increased or decreased significantly in the last 2000 years.
- There are no reliable comparative data showing ethnic or racial differences in the age at natural menopause.
- The median age at surgical menopause varies in the range 40–50 years of age, depending on surgical practices of specific health care systems in different countries.
- There is some evidence that African Americans may have an earlier surgical menopause than Caucasian Americans, but the reported difference may be a function of socioeconomic status.
- Current cigarette smoking clearly accelerates FMP by about 1.5 years in Caucasian populations, although the exact physiological mechanism is not clear.
- The impact of other factors on age at natural menopause is relatively very small at best and, in the case of education or income, related strongly to smoking.

The quality of the evidence

In order to assess existing literature and decide what information reliably adds to our knowledge concerning this event that, with few exceptions, effectively terminates fertility, several methodological issues must be identified and included in the evaluation. Each is discussed briefly below.

Median versus mean

Almost all of the data bases from which estimates of the age at natural menopause have been derived have been cross-sectional, requiring varying periods of recall of the date of FMP. Recall of even the year of FMP has been shown to be unreliable, particularly in women who have had more than 12 consecutive months of amenorrhea.[4,5] Moreover, a negative recall bias increases with distance from FMP, causing a consistent underestimate of the mean age and digit clustering at zero.[6,7]

The only reliable method that avoids this negative recall bias and digit clustering is to estimate the median age from a probit or logit analysis of the proportions at each age responding 'No' to the question: 'Have you had a menstrual period or any menstrual bleeding in the last 12 months?'

Interestingly, this unbiased estimation method has been used on more recent surveys, while the negatively-biased mean was used on earlier surveys. As a result, an uncritical review of the literature in the last 50 years or so would seem to support an increase in the age at natural menopause. This apparent increase is entirely due to methodology and is not real.[8]

Retrospective recall versus cross-sectional data

In studies that include *only* postmenopausal women, recall of FMP is entirely retrospective, often over many years, thus further reducing reliability of recall of the year of FMP and increasing the negative bias of mean age estimates. In this study design, the unbiased probit or logit analysis is not usable because all women will answer 'No' to the question, 'Have you had a menstrual period or menstrual bleeding in the last 12 months?'. Thus retrospective data are perhaps the most unreliable, usually collected on women who are 55 years or older. A typical example of this type of design was the early study by the Medical Women's Federation,[9] which demonstrated marked rounding off of reported age at menopause to five or zero.

In cross-sectional studies, data collected on women in the broadest possible age range during which natural menopause is likely to occur are optimal. Age ranges are typically 45–55 or 40–55 or 40–60. Unbiased probit or logit analysis of the question posed above should be reported and the median age corrected for the average recall period (usually 0.5 years).

Truncated data

When women are followed prospectively in order to identify the date of FMP with minimal recall, this is the optimal design for estimating the true average age at FMP. However, in such a cohort study, not all women may be followed until FMP is observed. Such incomplete follow-up results in truncated data (no information on FMP), and, if included in the simple estimation of a mean age, will result in a considerable underestimate. Special analytic techniques are required in order to include truncated data. A recent example is Treloar's study,[3] producing a mean age of 49.5 years.

Competing risk of surgical menopause

Because surgical menopause occurs before natural menopause by definition, and thus prevents observation of the latter, it presents a competing risk for natural menopause that may affect estimation. Two studies[10,11] have demonstrated in cross-sectional and prospective data with varying surgery rates, that this competing risk does not noticeably affect estimation of the age at natural menopause. It is important, however, to verify that any reported age at menopause is not a mixture of natural and surgical events. The average ages for the two types of menopause must be estimated separately.

Impact of smoking

One factor that may profoundly affect the reported age at FMP is the rate of cigarette smoking in a population. Unfortunately, most studies to date have not reported separate estimates for smokers and nonsmokers and/or have not reported the rate of smoking in their data sets. Median ages of over 52 years for natural menopause are likely to have been derived from mostly or only nonsmokers. Conversely, estimates of 51 years or lower (assuming optimal methodology) may reflect a high proportion of smokers.

SIGNS AND SYMPTOMS

The menopausal syndrome — myth or reality?

Since last century, a wide range of symptoms and signs have been associated with menopause, often based on unsystematic clinical observation. The Greenblatt Menopausal Index was a widely referenced early example of an attempt to systematize a syndrome without an adequate data base.[12] Only recently have representative, population-based data sets been analyzed using appropriate multivariate techniques in order to identify consistent signs and symptoms that are associated with the transition to menopause.[13–17]

The following summary represents our current state of knowledge in terms of consistent findings from several studies with well documented, comparable methodologies.

- Hot flashes/flushes, often accompanied by sweats, is the only symptom that is clearly and consistently related to transition to menopause in *Caucasian* populations.
- There is evidence that this symptom may be culturally specific and not universal. For example, the Japanese language does not have a term for this symptom and Japanese women do not appear to identify such a sensation more than 10% of the time.[16,18]
- Depression, sleeplessness, fatigue, irritability have all been variously associated with menopause but no data base has been able to directly link them. Rather, these symptoms may be sequelae of hot flashes and sweats (particularly sleeplessness, fatigue, irritability) or indicators of independently existing conditions.[17]
- There is increasing evidence that depression is not directly related to estrogen decline at menopause[17,19] and that this prevalent condition may be misdiagnosed as 'menopausal' rather than being appropriately treated as clinical depression with other independent causes.[20]
- Weight increase is probably not related to menopause and tends to begin well before menopause.[21,22]
- Changes in menstrual cycles, especially increasing length and irregularity of cycle, length of bleeding episodes, variable blood volume (including flooding or gushing) have all been cited as early indicators of approaching menopause.[23,25] Some change in cycle pattern appears to indicate inception of a transition period.[26,27] However, the best indicators of approaching menopause, in different groups of women (defined by ethnicity or other characteristics) have yet to be determined.
- The use of endocrine markers — specifically elevated serum FSH — has been advocated without good reference data as an early physiological marker indicating transition to menopause. Recent data, however, suggest that FSH is not a good marker, lacking both sensitivity and specificity for predicting (see ch. 49).[28] Currently there is no well-characterized physiological marker that can be used to predict imminent ovarian decline and FMP.
- Recent reports suggest that the years immediately *preceding FMP* are characterized by accelerated physiological change and symptom reporting, not the years *following FMP*.[3,15,29,30] Thus, FMP indicates the near end of the menopausal transition, rather than the beginning.

Preliminary data from one study of Caucasian women indicate that the transition to menopause may last on average about four years, with shorter transitions in smokers and older women.[15] However the marker used for the inception of the transition (perimenopause) was a reported change in cycle regularity, which requires further replication and validation against physiological markers (yet to be identified). There are very sparse data indicating racial or cultural differences in signs and symptoms.

Other complaints including vaginal dryness, incontinence and loss of sexual interest have not been definitively linked to the menopausal decline in ovarian function. Existing literature indicates that sexual activity and interest — at least in couples — declines rapidly in the early 40s — usually well before menopause.[31,32] Vaginal dryness is most likely to be perceived as a problem in a minority of sexually-active women experiencing menopause. One study found that only 3.4% of recently postmenopausal women reported that this symptom was a major problem for them at some time in the prior five years (Massachusetts Women's Health Study, unpublished data).

How should we treat signs and symptoms?

There are several emerging themes in the body of literature relating to menopausal signs and symptoms.

1. The signs and symptoms that have been clearly related to menopause in Caucasian populations (hot flushes/flashes and accompanying sweats, menstrual irregularity and heavy bleeding) send a self-selected minority to the health care system seeking relief — usually close to menopause when these phenomena are most intense or bothersome.[17] Such health care seekers tend to be frequent users,[33] better educated and with increased psychological symptom reporting, including depression.[19,34] The percentage seeking relief has been estimated, reliably, from

population-based studies to range from 25–50% of women in the perimenopause, depending on the definitions used and the symptoms included. From the research available, it is clear that women seeking help for menopause-related symptoms or discomforts are *not representative* of the majority of women making the menopause transition.

2. Menopausal signs and symptoms appear to peak and decline in a relatively narrow perimenopausal window surrounding FMP.[15,35]
3. The extent to which menopause-related symptoms or discomforts are bothersome enough to require medical intervention varies widely across cultures and social systems[16] and is not well understood beyond highly-developed, predominantly Caucasian countries.

The impact of these issues on therapy is multi-faceted. First, therapies developed to alleviate hot flashes may not be appropriate in cultures that do not recognize this symptom. Secondly, therapies should clearly be focused on immediate relief of acute discomforts that will be self-limiting anyway. Thirdly, because the perception of symptoms and degree of discomfort is largely subjective, there is the potential for a considerable placebo effect.

There is a paucity of well-designed randomized trials of candidate therapies for acute menopause-related discomforts. One landmark cross-over trial of hormone therapy[36] demonstrated a considerable (33%) placebo effect. This trial also demonstrated a negative effect of abrupt withdrawal of hormone therapy, causing an intense increase in hot flashes. Figure 47.1, reproduced from that paper, clearly demonstrates these findings. Other suggested treatments have not been subject to the rigorous evaluation of a randomized trial. The need to evaluate, rigorously, alternate therapies is increasingly pressing with recent interest in phytoestrogens and biobehavioral approaches such as self-hypnosis, biofeedback, exercise, etc.

The predominant therapy offered in highly developed countries is some form of exogenous hormones. Recent literature indicates that women experiencing a natural menopause tend to use such therapies for short periods, often adjusting dosages downward and discontinuing treatment as discomforts are alleviated.[37,38,39] The primary indications for such therapy are bothersome hot flashes and/or menstrual irregularity involving heavy, prolonged bleeding. Women experiencing surgical menopause are usually replacing lost ovarian hormones (through bilateral oophorectomy) and tend to continue hormone therapy for longer intervals.

AGING OR MENOPAUSE

What do we know?

Perhaps the least understood aspect of menopause is its relationship to the underlying aging process. Unlike men, women experience a profound physiologic change marked externally by FMP and internally by a

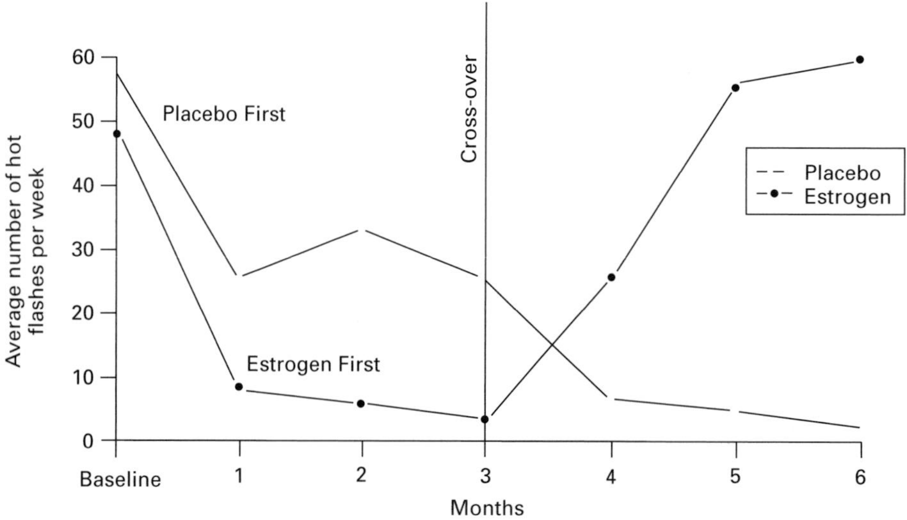

Fig. 47.1 The impact of placebo and of abrupt withdrawal of estrogen on hot flash reporting in a cross-over clinical trial.

decline in ovarian function, inducing infertility. This change occurs, in well-developed societies, about two thirds along the life span and about half-way through adult life. This point is coincident with the emergence of many chronic disease processes and is both preceded and succeeded by decades of aging that may be independent of menopause itself.

There are sparse data that address these relationships and the few reports available tend to focus on a specific disease process. The paragraphs below summarize our knowledge with respect to four key chronic conditions that are known to increase with age in men. Indeed, it is noteworthy that when population data on disease-specific morbidity and mortality are investigated, rates for both men and women tend to show linear relationships with age (possibly requiring a transform for linearity) even though the gender-specific rates may be different.[40]

Bone loss and fracture

Peak bone mass in well-developed Caucasian societies is estimated to occur in the third or fourth decade of life[41,42,43] and subsequently declines. The rate of bone loss, with age, in women has been estimated to be about 1–3% per year.[44,45,46] The hip fracture rate after age 50 for Caucasian women is about two times higher than in men.[47,48]

For the last two decades it has been hypothesized that the higher hip fracture rate in older women (65 years and over) is a direct consequence of a menopause-related acceleration in bone loss.[48,50] However, only recently have prospective studies begun to document such an acceleration.[45,51,52] Moreover these reports indicate that, if this acceleration exists, it begins *before* FMP. Recent reports suggest that chronological age, body mass, smoking, exercise and other life style factors may play a much larger role in bone loss than menopause itself.[45,53]

Reliable estimates of the impact of bone density and prior rates of bone loss on hip fracture have not been produced, primarily because fracture occurs more than 15 years after FMP and prospective follow-up of an adequate cohort of women is expensive. Moreover, the risk of falling appears to contribute considerable predictive information to subsequent fracture, independently of bone density.[54]

Finally, available information on cultural differences in bone density and risk of hip fracture,[55–59] reveals contradictions that underscore first the inability of bone density and rate of loss to reliably predict fracture, and secondly the multiple risk factors likely to predict fracture.

Current knowledge relating bone density to menopause can be summarized as follows:

- Reliable estimates of accelerated bone loss at different bone sites in different populations in the perimenopause are not presently available, although recent reports of data sets in Caucasian women indicate that there may be some accelerated loss associated with menopause.
- Risk factors for accelerated bone loss have not been reliably established from adequate, prospective data bases in different ethnic/racial groups, although several have been proposed.
- The relationship of bone density level and rate of bone loss to subsequent events such as hip fracture has not been well established. Moreover, there is no standard definition of osteoporosis as a disease entity, with a largely retrospective diagnosis based on a combination of diagnosed fractures and bone density levels.
- The role of ovarian decline at menopause in bone loss has been largely inferred through the demonstrated beneficial effect of exogenous hormones in slowing or preventing bone loss in women. It has not been established directly.

Cardiovascular disease

Large prospective databases have established, in Caucasian and African American populations, the primary risk factors for subsequent heart disease. While the relative contributions of risk factors in men and women and in different populations may vary, they include, primarily, cigarette smoking, diabetes, high relative body weight, high and uncontrolled blood pressure and high total cholesterol (and increases in some lipids or lipid fractions). Clearly these and other risk factors such as low level of exercise, and high fat diet, are inter-related.[60,61] Menopause has not been an important risk factor in such data bases.

Recent data indicate that some of these risk factors are established well before menopause, including diabetes, body weight increases and smoking.[22,62] Moreover, there is some evidence that cardiovascular disease is manifest, in terms of myocardial infarcts, in the fourth and fifth decades, before menopause.[63,64] Reported rates of cardiovascular mortality in women, from many countries, indicate smooth exponential trends with age, similar to those in men. Longitudinal data from a population-based study suggest that age-related factors (body mass, exercise) are much more strongly related to cardiovascular risk than is menopause status.[53] Thus the observational, population-based evidence is that cardiovascular disease is age-related and not menopause related.

Most of the controversy regarding heart disease and menopause has arisen through the plethora of observational studies, mostly in the last 15 years, that have compared heart disease risk in women who did or did not use exogenous hormones (predominantly unopposed estrogen). The positive association between hormones and lower rates of heart disease reported by many (but not all) of these studies almost certainly overstates the potential benefit because of selection to hormone use by healthy women and their health care providers (see for example, Matthews et al 1996[65] and the discussion at the end of this chapter).

Decline in sexuality

Menopause is a frequently cited cause of reduced sexual interest and activity in older women. Yet there are no reliable, population-based data that clearly identify a relationship between these two phenomena.

In men, the decline in sexual activity appears to continue with age,[66,67] despite availability of partners. In women, the decline in activity is increasingly a function of not having a viable partner as well as other factors.[31,68] Moreover, sexual drive and interest in women appear not to be related to reproductive hormone levels[69,70] although lower estrogen levels have been associated with vaginal dryness.[71,72] Because hot flashes and vaginal dryness have also been associated with reduced frequency of intercourse,[73,74] it is not clear what the primary relationship is.

Depression

There is no reliable population-based evidence that menopause accelerates this process. Indeed, what reliable evidence exists, indicates that any increase in depressive symptoms associated with menopause is transitory and related more directly to the length of the transition and bothersomeness of accompanying discomforts (including sleep disruption from hot flashes).[17] No direct relationship between depression and decline in reproductive hormones (estradiol, primarily) has been reliably reported. Indeed, Avis and coworkers[78] reported evidence of no direct relationship.

HORMONE THERAPY — THE MAGIC BULLET?

Use of exogenous hormones has been proposed as appropriate therapy to:

- Prevent bone loss
- Prevent heart disease
- Alleviate depression
- Improve elasticity in the vaginal lining and prevent painful intercourse
- prevent Alzheimer's disease and possibly other deterioration in cognitive function.

Only for bone loss is the effectiveness of hormone therapy well-established from the evidence of several well-designed randomized trials producing consistent evidence in women with either natural or surgical menopause and using unopposed estrogens as well as combined therapies.[79]

A first important randomized trial to evaluate the effect of hormone therapies on lipid levels, as well as on blood pressure, in postmenopausal women — the Postmenopausal Estrogen/Progestin Intervention (PEPI) trial — demonstrated statistically significant short-term benefits of active therapy on four lipid measures and none on blood pressure.[75] Of note in the trial results is the placebo effect on total cholesterol and low density lipoprotein levels and the attenuation of initial benefit between six months and three years of therapy. These results do not suggest large and lasting benefits and we still await the results of on-going trials to assess the long-term effect of exogenous hormone therapies on myocardial infarction and other clinical cardiovascular events.

There are no well-designed randomized trials that adequately evaluate the effectiveness of hormone therapies for treating depression, Alzheimer's disease or related conditions. Indeed there is consistent information in recent reports that the risk of suicide is two-fold higher in women taking hormones.[77] This disturbing risk increase is in marked contrast to lower mortality risk of almost all other diseases in women taking hormones (a lower risk consistent with healthy women selecting hormone use). One obvious explanation consistent with this elevated suicide rate is that women with clinical depression are being inappropriately treated with hormones which are ineffective and do not prevent suicide.

How do we know what is effective?

Only a well-designed randomized clinical trial can provide direct, definitive evidence of effectiveness (or the lack thereof) of a therapy although, in rare instances, an accumulation of observational data can provide strong circumstantial evidence. This final section provides guidelines to review and assess the published evidence concerning effectiveness of therapies.

What is a well-designed randomized trial?

There are five key conditions that together result in a well-designed randomized trial. If even one of these criteria are not met, the trial results do not have credibility.

1. Control group. The new experimental therapy must be compared to one or more control groups. These could be: no treatment, usual therapy or standard care, or placebo, depending on the outcome and the type of evidence required. For example, if a new therapy has been developed that is much cheaper to use than an existing standard therapy, then it may be sufficient to demonstrate that the new therapy is as effective as (equivalent to) the standard.

2. Randomization. The patients should be randomly assigned to treatment groups by a well-described, foolproof method that is not administered by the treating physician. Evidence should be provided that the groups are equivalent on a range of key selection characteristics that could affect the outcome.

3. Objective outcome. The primary outcome used to evaluate effectiveness should be either objectively and independently measured or measured in a single or double masked placebo design. For example: all-cause mortality is completely objective while cause-specific mortality is not, as the latter is subject to interpretation. Laboratory assay results are completely objective, provided the laboratory is unaware of treatment assignment and the assay is not affected by the treatment itself. Most trial outcomes are subjectively determined to some extent, requiring placebos and/or masking of outcome assessment.

4. Adequate sample size. Every trial should clearly specify the clinically relevant effect to be observed (usually in the form of a difference between treatment groups). The power to detect this effect should be at least 80%, with a type I error probability (α) of no more than 0.05 (two-sided). If the primary outcome is continuous, the required numbers may be relatively small. However, the vast majority of trials require at least 100 patients in each treatment group and usually substantially more.

5. Appropriate patient population. Every clinical trial to assess efficacy or effectiveness should clearly define the patient population from which trial subjects are selected. Minimally, the inclusion and exclusion criteria should be clearly specified. Preferably, the patients randomized into the trial should be compared to a concurrent registry of potential trial candidates (whether or not they are determined to be eligible or consent to participate).

In order to evaluate the above criteria, the following items should be clear in any report on the results of a randomized trial:

- The treatment groups, patient eligibility and randomized procedure should all be adequately described so that the reader is clear what was actually done.
- The equivalence of treatment groups should be demonstrated for all key selection characteristics likely to affect outcome. If multiple clinical sites are contributing patients, then such equivalence should be described for each clinic site and any differences between sites adequately explained.
- The completeness of follow-up should be clearly documented by treatment group (and by recruitment site, if more than one).
- The primary analysis should include all randomized patients, including dropouts, with appropriate statistical analyses of truncated data. Indeed, analyses should be according to 'intention to treat', regardless of treatment cross-overs or failures.
- The sample size/power justification must be included.

If any of the above items are not clearly discussed in the report, or data presented in the report indicate that any of the five criteria above were not met, then the trial results lack credibility and should certainly not be taken at face value.

And if there is no randomized trial?

In relatively rare circumstances, observational data may meet certain criteria that indicate, from strong circumstantial evidence, that a cause–effect relationship may exist. It is important to note, however, that observational, nonrandomized data have two major limitations that are always present:

- They can only identify *associations* between therapies and possible outcomes, they cannot demonstrate that one causes the other.
- They always include selection biases: subjects selecting themselves for care, providers selecting subjects for therapies.

In order for observational data to have any credibility in providing evidence to support (but not conclusively demonstrate) a cause–effect relationship, the following six conditions must all apply:[77]

1. The reported association between therapy and putative outcome must be strong (usually interpreted as a relative risk of less than 0.5 or greater than 2.0).

2. The reported association must be specific to the outcome(s) under consideration and not observed over a wide range of outcomes.
3. The association must be consistently reported over a number of different studies — the associations must be overwhelmingly in the same direction.
4. There must be a clear temporal sequence, with the hypothesized cause always preceding the supposed effect.
5. There must be a dose–response relationship.
6. There must be a plausible biological mechanism that is consistent with the observed association.

Only if the observational evidence meets all six of these criteria can there be any confidence in the probable existence of a cause–effect relationship. It would be most helpful if literature reviews, in the absence of randomized trials, evaluated the collective evidence against these criteria.

Conclusion

As a final note, it should be clear after reading this section that meta-analysis (the statistical combining of results from similar studies) is only as good as the studies included. If well-designed clinical trials are combined, the meta-analysis may provide an excellent vehicle for identifying important subgroup differences not otherwise detectable in single trials. However, combining observational evidence merely summarizes biased data with misleading precision.

REFERENCES

1. World Health Organization Scientific Group (WHO) 1996 Research on the Menopause in the 1990s. WHO Technical Services Report Series No. 866. Geneva: World Health Organization
2. Kaufert PA, Lock M, McKinlay SM, Bevenne Y, Coope J, Holte A 1986 Menopause research: the Korpilampi Workshop. Social Science and Medicine 22: 1285–1289
3. Treloar AE 1974 Menarche, menopause and intervening fecundability. Human Biology 46: 89–107
4. McKinlay SM, Jefferys M, Thompson B 1972 An investigation of the age at onset of the menopause. Journal of Biosocial Science 4: 161–173
5. McKinlay SM, Bifano NL, McKinlay JB 1985 Smoking and age at menopause. Annals of Internal Medicine 103: 350–356
6. MacMahon B, Worcester J 1966 Age at menopause: United States 1960–1962. Vital and Health Statistics, Series 11, No. 19
7. Benjamin F 1960 The age of the menarche and of the menopause in white South African women and certain factors influencing these times. South African Medical Journal 34: 316–320
8. Flint M 1978 Is there a secular trend in age of menopause? Maturitas 1: 133–139
9. Medical Women's Federation 1933 An investigation of the menopause in one thousand women. Lancet i: 106
10. Krailo MD, Pike MC 1983 Estimation of the distribution of age at natural menopause from prevalence data. American Journal of Epidemiology 117: 356–361
11. Brambilla DJ, McKinlay SM 1989 A prospective study of factors affecting age at menopause. Journal of Clinical Epidemiology 42: 1031–1039
12. Greenblatt RB, Barfield WE, Garner JF et al 1950 Evaluations of an oestrogen, androgen, oestrogen-androgen combination, and a placebo in the treatment of the menopause. Journal of Clinical Endocrinology and Metabolism 10: 1547
13. Greene JG 1976 A factor analytic study of climacteric symptoms. Journal of Psychosomatic Research 20: 425–440
14. Greene JG, Cooke DJ 1980 Lifes stress and symptoms at the climacterium British Journal of Psychology 136: 486–491
15. McKinlay SM, Brambilla DJ, Posner JG 1992 The normal menopause transition. American Journal of Human Biology 4: 37–46
16. Avis NE, Kaufert PA, Lock M, McKinlay SM, Vass K 1993 The evolution of menopausal symptoms. In: Burger H (ed) Baillière's clinical endocrinology and metabolism, pp 17–32
17. Avis NE, Brambilla D, McKinlay SM, Vass K 1994 A longitudinal analysis of the association between menopause and depression: results from the Massachusetts Women's Health Study. Annals of Epidemiology 4: 214–220
18. Lock M 1986 Ambiguities of aging: Japanese experience and perceptions of menopause. Cultural Medical Psychiatry 10: 23–46
19. McKinlay JB, McKinlay SM, Brambilla D 1987 The relative contributions of endocrine changes and social circumstances to depression in mid-aged women. Journal of Health and Social Behavior 28: 345–363
20. Ballinger CB 1977 Psychiatric morbidity and the menopause: survey of a gynecological out-patient clinic. British Journal of Psychiatry 131: 83–89
21. Wing RR, Matthews KA, Kuller LH, Meilhan EN, Plantinga PL 1991 Weight gain at the time of menopause. Annals of Internal Medicine 151: 97–102
22. Casey VA, Crawford SL, Avis NE, McKinlay SM 1996 Weight change during the menopause transition: a longitudinal study. Paper presented at the American Psychological Association Conference on Psychosocial and Behavioral Factors in Women's Health: Research, Prevention, Treatment and Service Delivery in Clinical and Community Settings, Washington, DC
23. Treloar AE, Boynton BG, Behn BG et al 1970 Variation of the human menstrual cycle through reproductive life. International Journal of Fertility 12: 77–126
24. Metcalf MG, Donald RA, Livesey JH 1981 Classification of menstrual cycles in pre- and perimenopausal women. Journal of Endocrinology 91: 1–10

25. Metcalf MG 1988 The approach of menopause: a New Zealand study. New Zealand Medical Journal 101: 103–106
26. Brambilla DJ, McKinlay SM, Johannes CB 1994 Defining the perimenopause for application in epidemiologic investigations. American Journal of Epidemiology 140: 1091–1095
27. Johannes CB, Crawford SL, Longcope C, McKinlay SM 1996 Bleeding patterns and changes in the perimenopause: a longitudinal characterization of menstrual cycles. Clinical Consultations in Obstetrics and Gynecology 8: 9–20
28. Stellato R, Crawford S, McKinlay S, Longcope C 1998 Can follicular-stimulating hormone be used to define menopause status? Endocrine Practice 4: 137–141
29. Whelan EA, Sandler DP, McConnaughey R, Wienberg CR 1990 Menstrual and reproductive characteristics and age at natural menopause. American Journal of Epidemiology 131: 625–632
30. Avis NE, McKinlay SM 1995 The Massachusetts Women's Health Study: an epidemiologic investigation of the menopause. Journal of the American Medical Women's Association 50: 45–63
31. Kinsey AC, Pomeroy WB, Martin CE 1953 Sexual behavior in the human male. WB Saunders, Philadelphia
32. Masters WH, Johnson VE 1966 Human sexual response. Little Brown, Boston
33. Roos NP 1984 Hysterectomies in one Canadian province: a new look at risks and benefits. American Journal of Public Health 75: 39–46
34. Avis NE, McKinlay SM 1989 Health care utilization among mid-aged women. Annals of the New York Academy of Sciences 592: 228–238
35. Dennerstein L, Burrows GD 1978 A review of studies of the psychological symptoms found at the menopause. Maturitas 1: 55–64
36. Coope J, Thomason JM, Poller L 1975 Effects of 'natural oestrogen' replacement therapy on menopausal symptoms and blood clotting. British Medical Journal 4: 139–143
37. Hemminki E, Kennedy DL, Baum C et al 1988 Prescribing of noncontraceptive estrogens and progestins in the United States, 1974–86. American Journal of Public Health 78: 1478–1481
38. Derby CA, Hume AL, Barbour MM et al 1993 Correlates of postmenopausal estrogen use and trends through the 1980s in two southeastern New England communities. American Journal of Epidemiology 137: 1125–1135
39. Johannes CB, Crawford SL, Posner JG, McKinlay SM 1994 Longitudinal patterns and correlates of hormone replacement therapy use in middle-aged women. American Journal of Epidemiology 140: 439–452
40. McKinlay JB, Crawford S, McKinlay SM, Sellers DE 1994 On the reported gender difference in coronary heart disease: an illustration of the social construction of epidemiologic rates. In: Czajkowski NS, Robin-Hill D, Clarkson TP (eds) Women, behavior and cardiovascular disease. US DHHS, Public Health Service, Washington, DC, NIH Pub. No. 94–3309, pp 223–252, 1994
41. Exton-Smith AN, Millard PH, Payne PR et al 1969 Pattern of development and loss of bone with age. Lancet 2: 1154–1157
42. Garn SM 1970 The earlier gain and later loss of cortical bone. Clinics in Orthopedics C. Thomas, Springfield, IL
43. Mazess 1982 On aging bone loss. Clinical Orthopedics 165: 239–252
44. Smith DM, Khairi MR, Norton J, Johnston C Jr 1976 Age and activity effects on rate of bone mineral loss. Journal of Clinical Investigation 58: 716–721
45. Slemenda C, Hui SL, Longcope C, Johnston CC 1987 Sex steroids and bone mass. A study of changes about the time of menopause. Journal of Clinical Investigation 80: 1261–1269
46. Ruegsegger P, Durand EP, Dambacher MA 1991 Differential effects of aging and disease on trabecular and compact bone density of the radius. Bone 12: 99–105
47. Gallagher JC, Melton LJ, Riggs BL et al 1980 Epidemiology of fractures of the proximal femur in Rochester, Minnesota. Clinics in Orthopedics 150: 163–171
48. Farmer ME, White LR, Brody JA et al 1984 Race and sex differences in hip fracture incidence. American Journal of Public Health 74: 1374–1380
49. Newton-John HF, Morgan DB 1970 The loss of bone with age, osteoporosis, and fractures. Clinical Orthopedics 71: 229–252
50. Riggs BL, Wahner HW, Melton LJ et al 1991 Rates of bone loss in the appendicular and axial skeletons of women. Evidence of substantial vertebral bone loss before menopause. Journal of Clinical Investigation 77: 1487–1491
51. Sowers MR, Clark MK, Hollis B et al 1992 Radial bone mineral density in pre- and perimenopausal women: a prospective study of rates and risk factors for bone loss. Journal of Bone Mineral Research 7: 647–657
52. Pouilles JM, Tremollieres F, Ribot C 1993 The effects of menopause on longitudinal bone loss from the spine. Calcified Tissue International 52: 340–343
53. Crawford SL, McKinlay JB, McKinlay SM 1995 Is the midlife increase in coronary heart disease in women attributable to menopause or to normal aging? Paper presented at the Annual Meeting of the American Public Health Association, Epidemiology Section, San Diego
54. Cummings SB 1985 Are patients with hip fractures more osteoporotic? American Journal of Medicine 78: 487–494
55. Yano K, Wasnich RD et al 1984 Bone mineral measurements among middle aged and elderly Japanese residents in Hawaii. American Journal of Epidemiology 119: 751–764
56. Ross PD, Norimatsu H, Davis JW et al 1991 A comparison of hip fracture incidence among native Japanese, Japanese Americans, and American Caucasians. American Journal of Epidemiology 133: 801–809
57. Cummings SR, Cauley JA, Palermo L et al 1994 Racial differences in hip axis lengths might explain racial differences in rates of hip fracture. Osteoporosis International 4: 226–229
58. Villa LM, Marcus R, Delay RR, Kelsy JL 1995 Factors contributing to skeletal health of postmenopausal Mexican-American women. Journal of Bone Mineral Research 10: 1233–1242

59. Perry HM, Horowitz M, Morley JE et al 1996 Aging and bone metabolism in African American and Caucasian women. Journal of Clinical Endocrinology and Metabolism 81: 1108–1117
60. Dyer AR, Stamler J, Paul O et al 1977 Alcohol consumption, cardiovascular risk factors, and mortality in two Chicago epidemiologic studies. Circulation 56: 1067–1074
61. Pooling Project Research Group 1978 Relationship of blood pressure, serum cholesterol, smoking habit, relative weight, and ECG abnormalities to incidence of major coronary events: final report of the Pooling Project. Journal of Chronic Disease 31: 201–306
62. Kuczmarski RJ 1992 Prevalence of overweight and weight gain in the United States. American Journal of Clinical Nutrition 55: 495S–502S
63. Kannel WB, Cupples LA, Gagnon DR 1990 Incidence, precursors and prognosis of unrecognized myocardial infarction. Unpublished manuscript
64. McKinlay JB 1996 Some contributions from the social system to gender inequalities in heart disease. Journal of Health and Social Behavior 37: 1–26
65. Matthews KA, Kuller LH, Wing RR et al 1996 Prior to use of estrogen replacement therapy, are users healthier than non-users? American Journal of Epidemiology 143: 971–978
66. Bungay GT, Vessay MP, McPherson CK 1980 Study of symptoms in middle life with special reference to menopause. British Medical Journal ii: 181–183
67. McKinlay JB, Feldman HA 1993 Changes in sexual activity and interest in the normally aging male. In: Rossi A (ed) Sexuality across the life course (Proceedings of the MacArthur Foundation Research Network on Mid-Life Development), New York
68. Pfeiffer E, Davis G 1972 Determinants of sexual behavior in middle and old age. Journal of the American Geriatrics Society 20: 151–158
69. Ballinger CB, Browning MCK, Smith AHW 1987 Hormone profiles and psychological symptoms in perimenopausal women. Maturitas 9: 235–251
70. Bachman GA, Leiblum SR, Sandler B et al 1985 Correlates of sexual desire in postmenopausal women. Maturitas 7: 211–216
71. Morrel MJ, Dixen JM, Carter CS, Davidson JM 1984 The influence of age and cycling status on sexual arousability in women. American Journal of Obstetrics and Gynecology 148: 66–71
72. Sarrel PM 1987 Sexuality in the middle years. Obstetric and Gynecology Clinics of North America 14: 49–62
73. Cutler WB, McCoy N, Davidson JM 1983 Sexual behavior, steroids, and hot flashes are associated during the perimenopause. Neuroendocrinology 5: 185–189
74. McCoy NL, Cutler W, Davidson JM 1985 Relationships among sexual behavior, hot flashes, and hormone levels in perimenopausal women. Archives of Sexual Behavior 14: 385–394
75. The PEPI Investigators 1995 Effects of estrogen or estrogen/progestin regimens on heart disease risk factors in postmenopausal women: the Postmenopausal Estrogen/Progestin Interventions (PEPI) Trial. Journal of the American Medical Association 273: 199–208
76. Hunt R, Vessey M, McPherson R, Coleman M 1987 Long-term surveillance of mortality and cancer incidence in women receiving hormone replacement therapy. British Journal of Obstetrics and Gynaecology 94: 620–635
77. Lilienfeld D, Stolley PD 1994 Foundations of epidemiology, (3rd edn.) Oxford University Press, Oxford
78. Avis NE, McKinlay SM, Brambilla D, Vass K, Longcope C 1993 Hormone levels, symptoms, and the relationship between menopause and depression. Paper presented at the Seventh International Congress on the Menopause in Stockholm, Sweden
79. Greendale GA, Marcus R, Bush T, Espeland M 1995 Bone mineral density results: the postmenopausal Estrogen/progestins Intervention Study. Paper presented at the Annual Meeting of the North American Menopause Society, San Francisco

48. Pituitary and ovarian changes

Henry G. Burger

Introduction

The menopause has been defined by the World Health Organization as the permanent cessation of menstruation resulting from the loss of ovarian follicular activity. Follicular activity can be assessed in terms both of steroid and of peptide hormone secretion. The major follicular steroid hormone is estradiol (E_2) secreted into the follicular fluid of the Graafian follicle and through the follicular basement membrane into the peripheral circulation. Progesterone is a product of the corpus luteum, the formation of which depends on maturation of the dominant ovarian follicle. Androgens, particularly testosterone and androstenedione, are secretory products of the ovarian stroma, mainly the perifollicular thecal cells. The secretion of the ovarian steroid hormones has been dealt with in chapters 7 and 9.

The other major secretory products of the follicle and its surrounding structures are peptide hormones, the inhibin-related family of proteins. Important advances have been made in this field during the past 10 years. Inhibin (INH) is a dimeric glycoprotein hormone and its major function is the negative feedback regulation of pituitary FSH secretion (ch. 10). INH levels, measured by radio-immunoassay using the 'Monash' assay which is known to cross-react with nonbiologically active α-subunit precursors as well as with biologically active inhibin,[1] have been shown to increase at puberty, to fluctuate during the menstrual cycle and to become undetectable after the menopause.[2] At the time of the cloning of human INH it was recognized that two forms existed, inhibin A and inhibin B, each possessing an identical α-subunit but a different β-subunit, βA or βB. Until recently it had been assumed that both forms were of equal biological potency and significance. However it has become clear that the dominant species of INH present in the plasma of the human male is inhibin B, whilst both inhibin A and inhibin B are present in the human female. Studies using a specific assay for human dimeric inhibin A have shown that its pattern of secretion during the menstrual cycle is similar to that described previously using the less specific 'Monash' assay for INH[3] (Fig. 48.1). Inhibin A levels increase slowly during the follicular phase of the cycle, rise to a midcycle peak coincidentally with the peaks of LH and FSH, fall abruptly and then rise to their highest levels during the midluteal phase, parallel to E_2 and progesterone. Inhibin B levels are maximal in the early follicular phase shortly after the intercycle FSH rise, show no midluteal peak and are low during the luteal

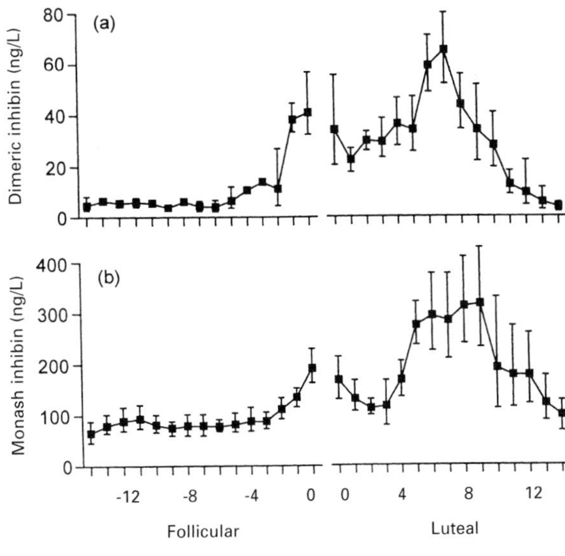

Fig. 48.1 The geometric mean concentrations (± 67% confidence intervals) of (**a**) dimeric inhibin and (**b**) Monash inhibin during the follicular and luteal phases of the female menstrual cycle. Data are aligned round the succeeding LH peak in the follicular phase and the preceding LH peak in the luteal phase.[3]

phase of the cycle. It has been postulated that inhibin B may be important in FSH feedback regulation during the follicular phase of the cycle and that inhibin A may be more important during the luteal phase, although studies of the physiology of inhibin A do demonstrate an inverse relationship between its levels and those of FSH with increasing age in women and during the menopausal transition. Recent data suggest that inhibin B is much less active biologically than inhibin A. These topics have been extensively reviewed recently.[4,5]

REPRODUCTIVE AGING

The morphological basis of hormonal changes

As is discussed in detail below, normal reproductive aging in regularly cycling women is accompanied by increases in serum FSH and slow declines in INH, with little if any change in E_2 production. As the menopause approaches however, estrogen production also declines. This decreasing ovarian hormone production appears to reflect declining ovarian follicle numbers. Richardson and her coworkers[6] extended the earlier studies of Block and Gougeon by estimating follicle numbers in the ovaries of seventeen healthy women, 44–55 years of age, divided into three age matched groups according to their menstrual history over the preceding 12 months. Follicle numbers were counted in sections made from ovaries surgically removed for reasons other than ovarian pathology. Six had had regular menses at 3–5 week intervals and had been asymptomatic, seven had had irregular menses at intervals less than three or greater than five weeks (and were thus in the menopausal transition), and four had not had bleeding for at least 12 months, i.e. were postmenopausal. There was substantial intersubject variability in the first group but overall the ovaries of the regularly cycling subjects contained an average of approximately 1000 primordial follicles. The ovaries of those with irregular menses contained an average of approximately 100 follicles per ovary, whilst in the four postmenopausal women a single follicle was identified in a single ovary of one subject. Block and Gougeon had previously made follicle counts, the former using autopsy specimens from 43 girls and women aged 7–44 years and the latter using ovaries obtained at hysterectomy in 35 women with regular menses aged 19–52 years. Combining the data from the three studies, it is noted that if follicle numbers are plotted semi-logarithmically against age, there is a steady and approximately linear decline from childhood until the age of 40, following which there is a marked acceleration during the last decade before the menopause (Fig. 48.2).

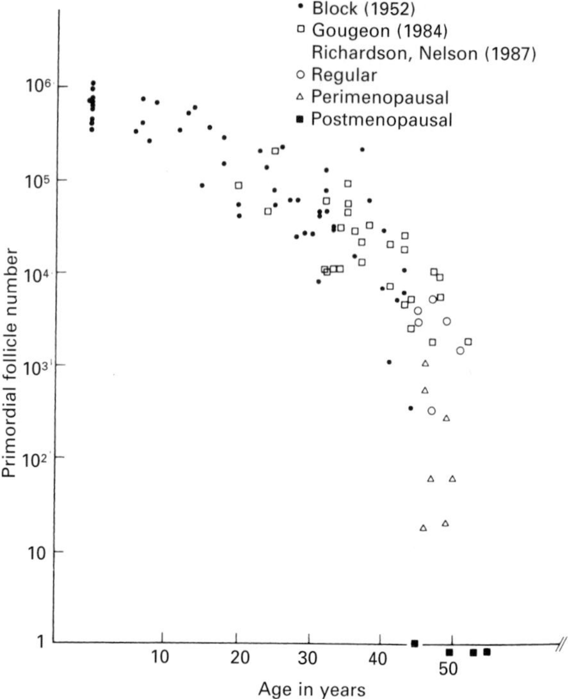

Fig. 48.2 The relationship between age and primordial follicle number is compared using data from the studies of Block (1952, 1953), Gougeon (1984) and Richardson et al (1987).[6]

Faddy and Gosden[7] have developed a mathematical model to describe the rates of growth and death of follicles in human ovaries from women between 19–50 years of age. Their study was based on the numbers of follicles at three successive stages of development, counted in histological sections of ovaries from 52 regularly cycling normal women. Their model predicts that the number of follicles growing from a stage at which there are at least two layers of granulosa cells surrounding an oocyte which has increased in size decreases from 51 per day at age 24–25 to only one per day at age 49–50. They hypothesize that the accelerated decline in follicle number in the last decade before the menopause results from an increase in the rate of atresia of primordial follicles.

Hormonal changes with age in regularly cycling women

This topic has been reviewed extensively in recent publications.[4,5] The major hormonal events which distinguish the regularly cycling woman from her postmenopausal counterpart include marked elevations in the levels of follicle stimulating hormone (FSH) and luteinizing hormone (LH) after the menopause, with a major decline in the level of circulating E_2, a decline in INH and overall little change in androgens. This section describes the hormonal changes observed as a function of age in women who continue to cycle regularly and is followed by a description of changes occurring with reference to the final menstrual period, in particular those occurring during the menopausal transition.

FSH, a dimeric glycoprotein hormone, is stimulated by gonadotropin releasing hormone (GnRH) but has a constitutive component to its secretion in contrast to that of LH which is essentially totally GnRH dependent. The secretion of FSH is under the dual feedback control of ovarian INH and of the steroid hormones, particularly E_2. After the menopause, in the absence of both of these feedback factors, FSH levels rise much more markedly than those of LH but, as women age, particularly over the age of 40, FSH levels rise progressively in the follicular phase and the early postovulatory phase of the menstrual cycle despite the continuance of normal regular cyclic function.

Sherman and Korenman,[8] in a landmark paper describing the hormonal characteristics of the human menstrual cycle throughout reproductive life, compared hormone levels obtained in regularly cycling women aged 18–30 with those in another group aged 46–56. Cycle length in the older group was 24 days compared with 28 in the younger group, due to a shortening of the follicular phase of the cycle. In that study, mean E_2 levels were substantially lower (92 pg/mL≈340 pmol/L) in the older group than in the younger (150 pg/mL≈555 pmol/L) whilst FSH levels were substantially higher. LH and progesterone levels were similar in both groups. Other workers confirmed the elevation of FSH with increasing age. The most extensive study is that of Lee et al[9] which involved 94 regularly cycling women aged 24–50 divided into a young control group aged 24–35 and three comparison groups, aged 36–40, 41–45 and 46–50 years. FSH levels rose during the follicular phase and in the early postovulatory phase as a function of increasing age. They were clearly elevated in the oldest group in whom there was only a very small increase in LH. No changes were noted in the levels of E_2 and progesterone. This study in particular suggested that the rise in FSH required an explanation other than changes in ovarian steroid hormone feedback. The obvious candidate for this was ovarian INH. A subsequent publication from the same group in which samples were obtained from 500 regularly cycling women presenting with infertility showed a progressive increase in FSH levels from age 29–30 onwards. That rise in FSH in inverse to the fall in follicle numbers referred to earlier.

Serum immunoreactive INH levels were measured by two groups in regularly cycling women.[10,11] In one report[10] mean FSH levels in a group of normal cycling women aged 45–49 were more than twice as high as in three younger age groups, while serum INH levels were significantly lower in this oldest age group than in the three younger groups (108 IU/L compared with 239, 235 and 207 IU/L in women aged 20–29, 30–39 and 40–44 respectively). Mean E_2 levels in the oldest group were also significantly lower than in the 30–39 year group but did not differ significantly from those in the other two groups. LH levels did not differ significantly between any of the groups. Both serum INH and E_2 were negatively correlated with FSH. A second study[11] was inconclusive because serum INH levels in a group of six women aged 40–48 were significantly lower than those in one of the two cited control groups (women in nonconception cycles) but not in the other control group (in which samples were obtained from conception cycles). Differences between the INH levels in these younger control groups were unexplained. Serum INH has also been reported to be lower in women presenting to an infertility clinic with presumed incipient ovarian failure although again this observation was not confirmed in another study.[12,13] Thus, in regularly cycling women, several groups have confirmed a selective increase in serum FSH levels as a function of increasing age, while there is persisting controversy regarding whether there are significant declines in E_2 or INH.

The majority of the studies cited above described no change in progesterone levels as a function of age during the luteal phase. However, Reyes et al[14] did observe that luteal progesterone levels were lower in groups of women aged 34–39, 40–44 and 45–50 than they were in a group aged 20–29.

Overall it has been demonstrated unequivocally that serum levels of FSH rise progressively as a function of increasing age in regularly cycling women in a manner inverse to the declining numbers of follicles. The likely explanation of the rise in FSH is a fall in the levels of INH but it may require measurements specifically of inhibin A, inhibin B or of other molecular weight forms of these inhibins to describe comprehensively the changing nature of the ovarian feedback signal which allows levels of FSH to rise.

The author has previously hypothesized that circulating INH concentrations may provide an index of the numbers of follicles which progress in development, a number which declines with increasing age, as do the levels of inhibin. In contrast, provided that a competent follicle is able to develop to dominance, or to a size sufficiently large to maintain steroid production, E_2 levels would be expected to be relatively preserved. It is hypothesized that declining numbers of follicles with declining INH levels lead to reciprocal rises in FSH, which in turn stimulates follicular development and maintains ovarian capacity to develop dominant follicles until late in reproductive life. Preservation of that capacity would result in preservation of circulating E_2 within the normal range and hence allow maintenance of quality of life and bony and vascular health.

HORMONAL CHANGES DURING THE MENOPAUSAL TRANSITION AND IN RELATION TO THE FINAL MENSTRUAL PERIOD

The term 'menopausal transition' is used to describe that period which commences when the first features of approaching menopause begin until one year after the final menstrual period (FMP). In a study of a group of North American women, the transition had a duration of approximately four years.[15] Studies of the hormonal changes occurring during the perimenopause have been based on various experimental designs and definitions. In some investigations, the changes have been recorded as a function of age, with little attention being paid to menstrual cycle status. In the few longitudinal studies reported, the FMP has been used as a reference point, with hormonal changes described in terms of time intervals before and after that point, as reviewed in Burger.[4] Few studies have reported on hormone changes in relation to changes in menstrual cycle characteristics, such as the first self-reported change in menstrual flow or the first change in menstrual frequency or combinations thereof. This approach was adopted in a major study described in more detail below.

FSH, estradiol and progesterone in relation to the final menstrual period

The data of Rannevik[16] are typical of the few published investigations of gonadotropin and steroid levels around the FMP. The authors studied 160 women from the Malmö Perimenopausal Project for a period of 12 years and the data are reproduced in Figure 48.3.[16] A continuous increase was noted in serum FSH and LH from 4.75 years prior to FMP. The increase continued to at least the first sample obtained following FMP, samples being obtained at six monthly intervals. FSH appeared to peak approximately four years after the FMP though the authors noted that a maximum limit of 25 μg/l in their FSH assay 'precluded a systematic statistical analysis of a probable further increase' at that time. They were, however, able to demonstrate a significant decrease in FSH levels from about that time during the last five years of observation. For LH, the peak value observed was the first one following FMP and subsequently there was a statistically significant decrease over the next eight years. Mean LH to FSH ratios decreased continuously during the period of observation.

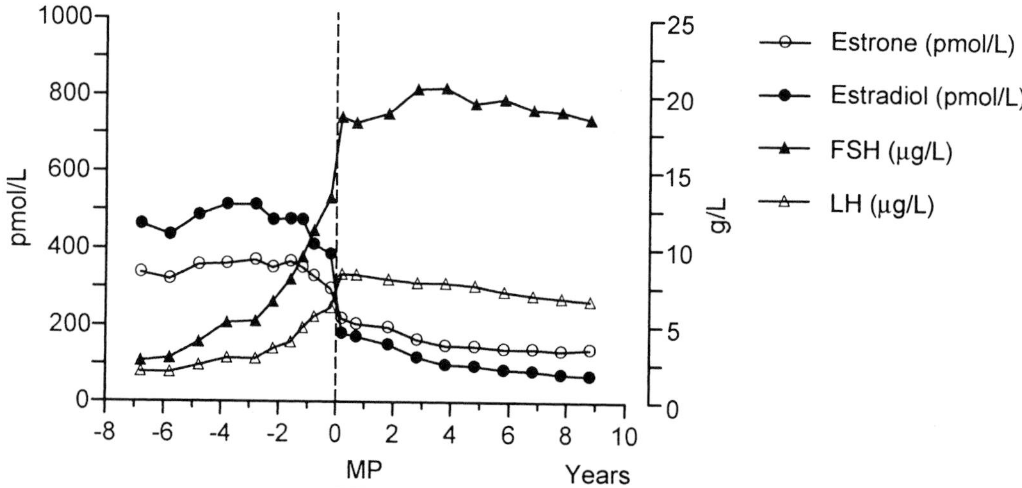

Fig. 48.3 Mean serum levels of FSH, LH estradiol and estrone during the perimenopausal transition.[16]

E_2 levels were also measured for seven years prior to the FMP and remained relatively constant (means of 461–515 pmol/L) until the six month sample prior to the FMP. In 154 observations 1–6 months prior to the FMP, mean E_2 was still 383 pmol/L but had fallen to 182 pmol/L 1–6 months after the FMP, with a further gradual fall to 171 pmol/L by 7–12 months. Ninety seven to 108 months later E_2 levels had reached 72 pmol/L. Levels of estrone were similar in their behavior, with a small fall in the 1–6 months before FMP, a moderate fall 1–6 months afterwards, from 299 to 216 pmol/L, and a gradual fall to 133 pmol/L 97–108 months after the FMP. The data in the postmenopausal period are thus representative of many studies showing a 10–15 fold increase in serum FSH after FMP, a 3–5 fold increase in LH, with *a* >80% drop in E_2 and an approximately 60% drop in estrone during this time. The major circulating estrogen after the menopause is estrone and the majority of this is derived from the extraglandular conversion of adrenal androgen precursors, particularly androstenedione.[17] The major determinant of plasma estrone is the level or rate of production of androstenedione, with the degree of conversion being increased after the menopause. That degree of conversion is a function of excess body fat, with obese women having higher estrone (and E_2) levels than their normal weight counterparts, whilst their gonadotropin levels are lower. Rannevik et al[16] provided no data on geometric mean levels of hormones in their subjects, nor did they report on the relationship between hormonal levels and menstrual cycle status other than FMP. They did, however, note that during the premenopausal period, there was an increase in frequency of inadequate luteal function with low progesterone levels.

Gonadotropin and gonadal steroid levels during the menopausal transition

A large prospective longitudinal study, initiated in 1934, documented patterns of menstrual cyclicity during the reproductive life-span.[18] The median length of the menstrual cycle falls from 28 days at age 20, to 26 days at age 40, resulting primarily from a shortening of the follicular phase. Population studies in which basal body temperature was used to detect possible anovulation indicated that anovulatory cycles become more prevalent e.g. 3–7% of cycles were anovulatory between ages 26–40 years and 12–15% between 41–50 years. The study of luteal phase progesterone levels indicates that the frequency of nondetectable progesterone levels gradually increases as FMP approaches. The lack of a luteal phase rise in progesterone is, of course, a striking feature of the postmenopausal period compared with the reproductive period. Luteal progesterone has been hypothesized to be important in the maintenance of normal bone density.[19] In the large study referred to earlier,[16] the frequency of cycles with progesterone levels indicative of ovulation (taken to be a concentration >10 nmol/L) decreased from 60% to <10% during the six years preceding FMP. Ovulatory progesterone levels were found in 62.2% of women 72–61 months prior to FMP but in only 4.8% who were 6–9 months premenopausal, whilst all progesterone levels were <2 nmol/L postmenopausally.

There are relatively few data which focus specifically on the endocrinology of the menopausal transition, when the most noteworthy characteristic is significant hormonal variability. The study of Sherman and Korenman,[8] referred to earlier, involved 50 complete menstrual cycles in 37 women. They measured hormonal levels daily in two women, one aged 49 and one aged 50, who were clearly in the menopausal transition. Two of those cycles were anovulatory but were characterized by increasing levels of E_2 and initially postmenopausal levels of LH and FSH; these subsequently fell as E_2 rose. It was noteworthy that an anovulatory cycle was followed by a cycle that demonstrated evidence of follicular maturation.

Metcalf and colleagues[20,21] examined the excretion of FSH, LH, estrogens and pregnanediol in weekly urine samples collected for 14–87 weeks from 31 perimenopausal women, aged 36–55 years. The authors stated: 'about the only conclusion that can be made with confidence concerning pituitary-ovarian function in individual perimenopausal women is that it is unsafe to generalise'. In a more recent paper, Metcalf[22] concluded 'in older women, a good menstrual history is probably the single most useful measure of ovarian status'. Hee et al[23] confirmed the variability of perimenopausal gonadotropin and E_2 levels and added data on INH in a small longitudinal study of three volunteer women who had developed irregular cycles at age 45–46. Abrupt decreases in E_2 and INH into the postmenopausal range were followed by levels characteristic of reproductive-age women.

A major recent study has shed further light on the hormonal characteristics of the menopausal transition in relation to self-reported menstrual cycle status. The Melbourne Mid-life Project was based on a cross-sectional survey of a randomly selected population sample of 2001 Australian-born Melbourne women aged between 45–55 years when first interviewed in May 1991.[24] A longitudinal sample of 437 women was studied to examine many aspects of the menopausal transition. The data from the first year of this longitudinal study were subjected to cross-sectional analysis in terms of menstrual cycle history.[25] Twenty seven per cent of the subjects had reported no change in menstrual frequency or flow, 23% reported a change in flow with no change in frequency, 9% a change in frequency without change in flow, 28% a change in both frequency and flow and 13% a lack of flow for at least three months. Mean age increased from 48.5 years in the first group to 51.4 years in the last. The data are illustrated in Figure 48.4. There was a progressive increase in FSH levels across the five groups, the changes being most marked in those experiencing a change in frequency and flow and in those who had not bled for more than three months. E_2 levels were slightly lower in the groups experiencing a change in frequency or a change in frequency and flow. They were statistically significantly lower than those without any change in menstrual function and in those who had had no menses for at least three months, when the geometric mean E_2 concentration was 42% of that observed in the first group. There was a broad spread of E_2 values with some being >1500 pmol/L. Such high levels may reflect hyperstimulation of granulosa cells by elevated FSH levels and could give rise to symptoms of breast fullness and fluid retention. INH levels were significantly lower (71% of group 1) in those experiencing a change in frequency and flow and had fallen to 38% in those with three or more months of amenorrhea. The data were also examined as a function of age and body mass index. FSH levels rose at a rate of 11.8% per year, E_2 fell at 7.8% per year, INH at 9.9% per year and testosterone at 2% per year while there was no change observed in sex hormone-binding globulin or free androgen index.

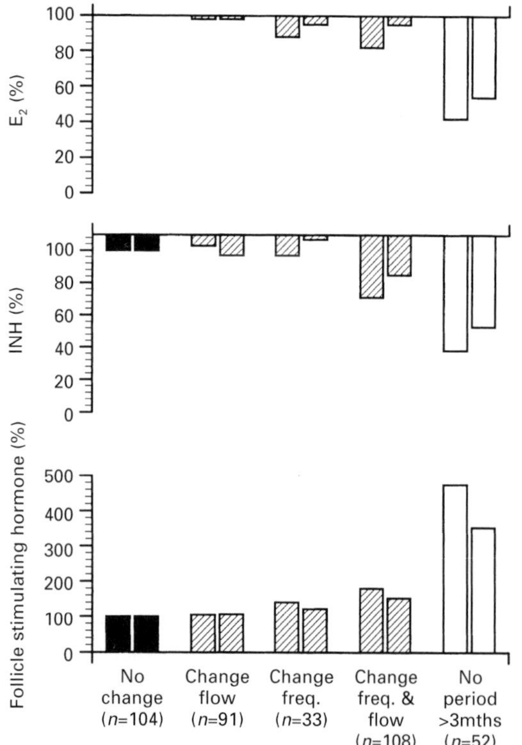

Fig. 48.4 Changes in E_2 (upper), INH (middle) and FSH (lower), as a percentage of levels in Group 1 women from the Melbourne Mid-life Project[25] who had experienced no change in their cycles. The left column is unadjusted, the right is adjusted for age and body mass index.

It was also noteworthy that 43% of the subjects in group 1 had FSH levels above the upper limit seen in young normal subjects during the follicular phase of the cycle, and that figure rose to 94% of those who had not bled for three months or more. Six percent of those without any change in menstrual cycle status had FSH levels in the postmenopausal range, as did 33% of those who had experienced a change in menstrual cycle frequency and 76% of those who had not bled for three months. Conversely, 24% of E_2 levels in the first group were below the lower limit for young women, rising to 60% of those who had not bled for three months. Twenty-two percent of INH levels were low in the first group, 81% in the group with three months amenorrhea or more. A hyperbolic relationship was observed between levels of FSH and both E_2 and INH, both of which were significantly inversely correlated with FSH.

Androgens in relation to the final menstrual period

Variable findings have been reported in regard to the changes in androgens in relation to the FMP. Rannevik et al[16] reported a small but significant decline in testosterone (T), androstenedione (A) and sex hormone-binding globulin (SHBG) during the two years around the menopause. Thus T fell from 1.7 nmol/L 1–6 months before FMP to 1.4 nmol/L 13–24 months afterwards and 1.2 nmol/L 85–96 months afterwards. SHBG fell from 4.0 mg/L 1–6 months before FMP to 3.5 mg/L 85–96 months afterwards, but the T/SHBG ratio was unchanged over that period. The data for A were not listed specifically. Longcope et al[26] did not see any change in T and A over 80 months from the FMP but noted that the mean concentrations of T in all their subjects, including those still having cyclic menses, were significantly less than those of a group of normal young women sampled on days 5–7 of the cycle: they suggested that there is a decrease in the ovarian secretion of T prior to the menopause. It is noteworthy that a recent report[27] found that there was a decline in total serum T concentration with age, such that the levels in a woman aged 40 were approximately 50% of those in a woman aged 21 (0.61 nmol/L compared with 1.3 nmol/L (Fig. 48.5)). Percent free T did not vary significantly with age but free T concentration clearly showed a marked decline. The ratio of dehydroepiandrosterone (DHEA) to T and dehydroepiandrosterone sulfate (DHEAS) to T were age-invariant because of the declines of DHEA and DHEAS with age. Other studies have suggested that total T levels fall by approximately 20% and A by approximately 50% with natural menopause.[28] Vermeulen[29] showed that postmenopausal women aged 51–65 years had lower mean levels of T (1.03 nmol/L), A (3.45 nmol/L) and dihydrotestosterone (DHT) (0.33 nmol/L) in comparison with those in women aged 18–25: T (1.53 nmol/L) A (5.80 nmol/L) and DHT (1.04 nmol/L).

The effects of ovariectomy on androgen profiles were reported by Judd et al[30] and Hughes et al.[31] Before the menopause, removal of the ovaries results in a fall of circulating A and T by about 50%, the fall in the latter being due in large part to the fall in A. Postmenopausally, removal of the ovaries results in a 50% decline in T and a much lesser fall in A. The postmenopausal ovary secretes more T but less A than its premenopausal counterpart.[28]

In the light of the recent report of Zumoff et al[27] and the difficulty in demonstrating a significant decline in T around FMP, it may be that the apparent decline in T at the menopause is related as much to ageing as to decreased ovarian function in those women with intact ovaries. In the Melbourne Mid-life Project, there was no significant change seen in total T or in T/SHBG ratio as a function of changing menopausal status.[25]

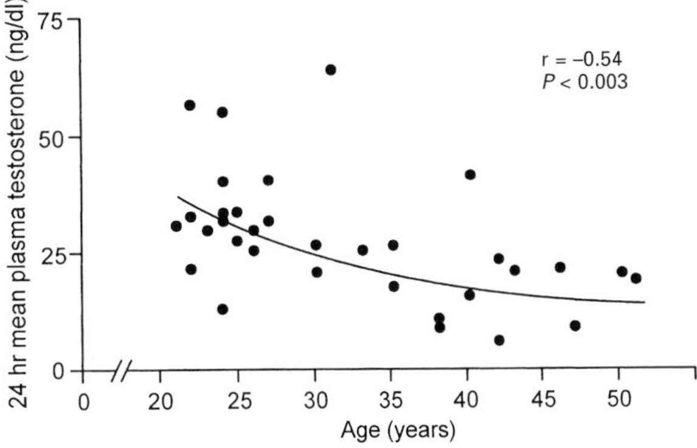

Fig. 48.5 Twenty-four-hour mean plasma total testosterone (T) vs. age in normal females. The regression equation was T (nmol/L) = 37.8 × age (years)$^{-1.12}$. ($r = -0.54$; $P < 0.003$).[27]

Conclusion

The perimenopause is a time of markedly fluctuating hormonal levels. The most striking and most consistently observed hormonal change prior to the FMP is a progressive increase in the levels of FSH. This is seen in women who continue to cycle regularly and becomes much more marked in those experiencing menstrual irregularity. FSH levels probably reach their peak 2–4 years following the FMP and subsequently decline slowly. The levels of E_2 are relatively preserved until close to the FMP. The predictable changes in steroid levels seen during the menstrual cycle are replaced by marked and unpredictable fluctuations once menstrual irregularity becomes established, with E_2 levels varying from low to high. The FMP occurs during a time of falling E_2 levels but it is not possible to describe a specific endocrine status which differentiates the immediately premenopausal woman from the immediately postmenopausal state. The frequency of anovulatory cycles increases as FMP approaches. Substantial changes in androgen concentrations do not appear to occur during the immediate perimenopausal period though postmenopausal androgen levels are lower than those of young regularly cycling women.

Because of the profound and unpredictable fluctuations in hormone levels during the menopausal transition, measurements of such hormones are of little if any diagnostic value and assessment of the average woman's state in relation to the menopause depends on the taking of an adequate history.[32]

REFERENCES

1. Burger HG 1993 Clinical review — clinical utility of inhibin measurements. Journal of Clinical Endocrinology and Metabolism 76: 1391–1396
2. Burger HG 1992 Inhibin. Reproductive Medicine Review. Edward Arnold, 1: 1–20
3. Groome NP, Illingworth PJ, O'Brien M, Cooke I, Ganesan TS, Baird DT et al 1994 Detection of dimeric inhibin throughout the human menstrual cycle by two-site enzyme immunoassay. Clinical Endocrinology 40: 717–723

4. Burger HG 1997 Inhibin and steroid changes in the perimenopause. Serono Symposia (Ed. RA Lobo). The Perimenopause 13: 170–183
5. Burger HG 1996 The endocrinology of the menopause. Maturitas 23(2): 129–136
6. Richardson SJ, Senikas V, Nelson JF 1987 Follicular depletion during the menopausal transition: evidence for accelerated loss and ultimate exhaustion. Journal of Clinical Endocrinology and Metabolism 65: 1231–1237
7. Faddy MJ, Gosden RG 1995 A mathematical model of follicle dynamics in the human ovary. Human Reproduction 10: 770–775
8. Sherman BM, Korenman SG 1975 Hormonal characteristics of the human menstrual cycle throughout reproductive life. Journal of Clinical Investigation 699–706
9. Lee SJ, Lenton EA, Sexton L, Cooke ID 1988 The effect of age on the cyclical patterns of plasma LH, FSH, oestradiol and progesterone in women with regular menstrual cycles. Human Reproduction 851–855
10. MacNaughton J, Bangah M, McCloud P, Hee J, Burger H 1992 Age related changes in follicle stimulating hormone, luteinizing hormone, oestradiol and immunoreactive inhibin in women of reproductive age. Clinical Endocrinology 36: 339–345
11. Lenton EA, de Kretser DM, Woodward AJ, Robertson DM 1991 Inhibin concentrations throughout the menstrual cycles of normal, infertile, and older women compared with those during spontaneous conception cycles. Journal of Clinical Endocrinology and Metabolism 73: 1180–1190
12. Buckler HM, Evans CA, Mamtora H, Burger HG, Anderson DC 1991 Gonadotropin, steroid, and inhibin levels in women with incipient ovarian failure during anovulatory and ovulatory rebound cycles. Journal of Clinical Endocrinology and Metabolism 72: 116–124
13. Cameron IT, O'Shea FC, Rolland JM, Hughes EG, de Kretser DM, Healy DL 1988 Occult ovarian failure: a syndrome of infertility, regular menses, and elevated follicle-stimulating hormone concentrations. Journal of Clinical Endocrinology and Metabolism 67: 1190–1194
14. Reyes Fl, Winter JSD, Faiman C 1977 Pituitary-ovarian relationships preceding the menopause. American Journal of Obstetrics and Gynecology 129: 557–564
15. McKinley SM, Brambilla DJ, Posner JG 1992 The normal menopause transition. Maturitas 14: 102–115
16. Rannevik G, Jeppsson S, Johnell O, Bjerre B, Laurell-Boruli Y, Svanberg L 1995 A longitudinal study of the perimenopausal transition: altered profiles of steroid and pituitary hormones, SHBG and bone mineral density. Maturitas 21: 103–113
17. Sitteri PK, MacDonald PC 1973 Role of extraglandular estrogen in human endocrinology. In: Greep RO, Astwood EB (eds) Handbook of physiology, vol. 2, part 1. Williams & Wilkins, Baltimore, pp 615–629
18. Treloar AE, Boynton RE, Behn BC, Brown BW 1967 Variation of the human menstrual cycle through reproductive life. International Journal of Fertility 12: 77–126
19. Prior JC, Vigna YM, Schechter MT, Burgess AE 1990 Spinal bone loss and ovulatory disturbances. New England Journal of Medicine 323: 1221–1227
20. Metcalf MG, Donald RA, Livesey JH 1981 Pituitary-ovarian function in normal women during the menopause transition. Clincial Endocrinology 14: 245–255
21. Metcalf MG, Donald RA 1979 Fluctuating ovarian function in a perimenopausal woman. New Zealand Medical Journal 89: 45–47
22. Metcalf MG 1988 The approach of menopause: a New Zealand study. New Zealand Medical Journal 101: 103–106
23. Hee J, MacNaughton J, Bangah M, Burger HG 1993 Perimenopausal patterns of gonadotrophins, immunoreactive inhibin, oestradiol and progesterone. Maturitas 18: 9–20
24. Dennerstein L, Smith AM, Morse C, Burger HG, Green A, Hopper J et al 1993 Menopausal symptoms in Australian women. Medical Journal of Australia 259: 232–236
25. Burger HG, Dudley EC, Hopper JL, Shelley JM, Green A, Smith A et al 1995 The endocrinology of the menopausal transition: a cross-sectional study of a population-based sample. Journal of Clinical Endocrinology and Metabolism 80: 3537–3545
26. Longcope C, Franz C, Morello C, Baker R, Conrad-Johnston C Jr 1986 Steroid and gonadatropin levels in women during the peri-menopausal years. Maturitas 8: 189–196
27. Zumoff B, Strain GW, Miller LK, Rosner W 1995 Twenty-four hour mean plasma testosterone concentration declines with age in normal premenopausal women. Journal of Clinical Endocrinology and Metabolism 80: 1429–1430
28. Judd HL 1976 Hormonal dynamics associated with the menopause. Clinical Obstetrics and Gynecology 19: 775–788
29. Vermeulen A 1976 The hormonal activity of the postmenopausal ovary. Journal of Clinical Endocrinology and Metabolism 42: 247–253
30. Judd HL, Lucas WE, Yen SS 1974 Effect of oophorectomy on circulating testosterone and androstenedione levels in patients with endometrial cancer. American Journal of Obstetrics and Gynecology 118: 793–798
31. Hughes CL Jr, Wall LL, Creasman WT 1991 Reproductive hormone levels in gynecologic oncology patients undergoing surgical castration after spontaneous menopause. Gynecological Oncology 40: 42–45
32. Burger HG 1994 Diagnostic role of follicle-stimulating hormone (FSH) measurements during the menopausal transition — an analysis of FSH, oestradiol and inhibin. European Journal of Endocrinology 130: 38–42

49. Hot flashes

Peter R. Brzechffa *Howard L. Judd*

Introduction

The most common and characteristic symptom of the climacteric is an episodic disturbance consisting of sudden flushing and perspiration referred to as a 'hot flush' or 'flash'. These vasomotor events have been documented in up to 85% of women who go through menopause physiologically or secondary to medical intervention, such as ovariectomy, chemotherapy, radiation or medication use.[1–5] Approximately 40% of perimenopausal women also experience hot flashes.[6,7] Unlike other problems encountered at the menopause, hot flashes decrease in frequency and intensity with time. However, they do represent a substantial medical problem with 82% of those suffering from hot flashes experiencing the disturbance more than one year, 25–50% for more than five years and up to 10% for more than 15 years.[2,3,4,8] The aims of this chapter are to review the physiological alterations associated with hot flashes, to describe the hormonal changes associated with these events, and to provide a review of their management.

An excellent description was provided in 1927 of the subjective symptoms associated with hot flashes based on personal interviews with 131 postmenopausal women.[1] Most women indicated that hot flashes begin with a sensation of pressure in the head much like a headache, which increases in intensity until the physiological flash is experienced. The hot flash subsequently produces a feeling of heat or burning in the face, neck and chest followed immediately by an outbreak of perspiration that affects the entire body but is especially prominent over the head, neck, upper chest and back. An increase in pulse rate is also experienced which may be severe enough to produce the sensation of heart palpitations. Less frequently reported signs and symptoms include weakness, fatigue, faintness, vertigo, depression, night sweats and insomnia. Hot flashes typically occur spontaneously without a definitive precipitating event, although women indicate their symptoms are worse in warm humid weather. This is supported by experimental data in which women reported fewer, less intense hot flashes when exposed to a cool ambient temperature.[9] Other often cited triggering factors for hot flashes include stress, alcohol, caffeine and spicy foods.[9–12]

The duration of the subjective discomfort attributed to hot flashes range from 30 seconds to 10 minutes (min); the average length being about 4 minutes (Fig. 49.1). The frequency varies from as often two per hour to as seldom as 1–2 per month. In women with severe flashes the mean frequency is every 54 min.[13] Hot flashes tend to be more prevalent and severe in the first two years following menopause and less commonly occur in women with higher body weight and percent ideal body weights.[14] There is no difference in the temporal pattern of hot flashes between women who have undergone surgical as opposed to natural menopause.[15] However, women in the first year following ovariectomy tend to have an

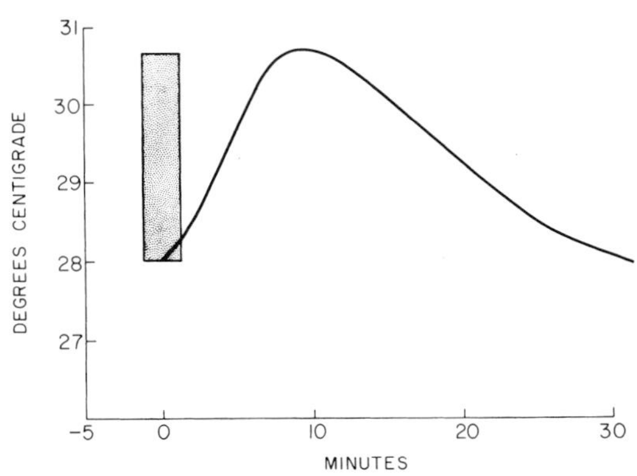

Fig. 49.1 Mean characteristics and typical configuration of finger temperature fluctuations associated with hot flashes. The shaded area delineates the period from the mean beginning to completion of subjective flashing.[13]

increased prevalence and severity of hot flashes as compared to women with naturally occurring menopause.[9] Women with a longer perimenopausal period are more likely to report hot flashes than those with a short perimenopausal period.[16] Other factors thought to predispose women to hot flashes, such as marital or employment status, social class, age at menarche, pregnancy number or other medical ailments have not been positively correlated.[5,17] However, women from western societies do report more commonly the occurrence of hot flashes as compared to those from non-western societies, such as Japan and China.[18,19] It is estimated that up to 20% of women residing in western societies will have hot flash symptoms severe enough that they will seek medical attention.

PHYSIOLOGY

Because of the subjective nature of the complaint, the actual physiologic basis of hot flashes was once questioned. However, several investigators have characterized the physiologic changes associated with these events. These researchers have found that profound changes do occur, indicating that some major disturbance in basic function is responsible for hot flashes.

Initially, limited attempts were made to define changes in physiologic function. One of the earliest studies observed perspiration and alterations of central temperature in a single, symptomatic patient while another study found increases of oxygen consumption and cheek temperature in several women with the disturbance.[20,21] Other observers reported increases in finger vasodilation and face temperature during flashes while demonstrating no change in basal metabolic rate.[22,23]

The first in depth study measured skin temperature of the fingers, toes and forehead, and central temperature at the tympanic membrane and within the rectum, in a woman with frequent hot flashes.[24] Subsequently, several other investigators have conducted similar studies in groups of patients.[13,25–29]

Initially, these reports described a prodromal period between the onset of the subjective feeling and the first recordable change in physiologic function. With development of better methods to assess changes of physiologic function, it was found that the physiologic changes actually precede the onset of the subjective complaint. The first measurable sign of the attack is an increase in cutaneous vasodilation. This has been measured using either a digital plethysmograph or a skin thermosensor to record increases in skin temperature. The vasodilation, as measured by the plethysmograph, begins approximately 1 min before the onset of the subjective flash and continues for approximately 8 min. The skin temperature rise, which reflects cutaneous vasodilation, begins on the average 90 sec after the initiation of the subjective flash, reaches its maximum by 9 min and returns to baseline after about 40 min (Fig. 49.2).[13,24,25,28,29] The magnitude of the skin temperature rise is variable, depending on which area of the body is tested, with the fingers and toes showing the greatest increases.[24] This indicates the cutaneous vasodilation is generalized and not limited to the upper trunk and head. Temperature changes on the forehead, where the symptomatic flash is experienced, are of lesser magnitude probably because of the perspiration and evaporation that occur in this area.[24] For the finger, the average rise in temperature is about 4°C with the maximum being 9°C.[29] The magnitude of the rise shows an indirect correlation with the resting skin temperature (temperature prior to the flash). In other words, the lower the resting skin temperature, the greater the rise will be. During the increase, the skin temperature does not exceed core temperature.

The next measurable sign is a decrease in skin resistance, a measurement of perspiration. This begins on average 45 sec after the onset of the subjective flash, reaches its maximum within 4 min and returns to baseline at about 18 min.

As heat is lost from the body, by cutaneous vasodilation and perspiration, a decline in core temperature occurs. This commences about 4 min after the onset of the subjective symptoms, and returns to baseline in about 30 min.[13,29] The average decrease in core temperature, as measured at the tympanic membrane, is about 0.2°C. Alterations of pulse rate also occur during flashing with increases of 13–20% being reported.[25] Fluctuations of the baseline recording of electrocardiograms are seen, probably reflecting changes in skin resistance.[24,25] Blood pressure and heart rhythm variations have not been observed to occur.[24,25]

These changes in physiologic function do not correspond identically to the subjective symptoms. As mentioned previously, the subjective symptoms begin approximately 1 min after the onset of the first recordable change in cutaneous vasodilation and only last for an average of 4 min.[13] Thus, the physiologic signs continue many minutes after the subjective symptoms have ceased.

The exact mechanism responsible for hot flashes has not been elucidated. Early investigators believed that an imbalance of the autonomic nervous system

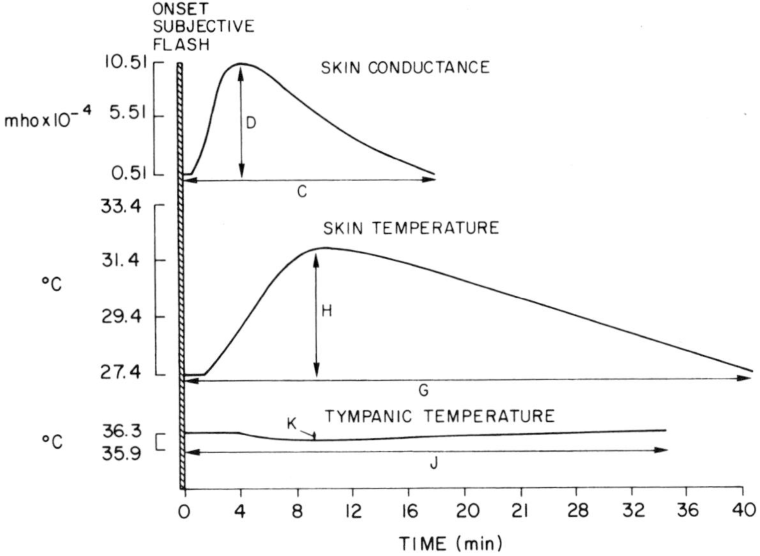

Fig. 49.2 Characteristics of the changes in skin conductance, skin temperature, and tympanic membrane temperature based on observations of 25 hot flashes. All measurements are referenced to the signal by the patient at the onset of the subjective flash.[29]

was somehow responsible, and this could occur because of central or peripheral instability of this system. Based on the physiologic data presented above, it would appear that the climacteric hot flash is the result of a defect in central thermoregulatory function. There are three indications to support this conclusion.

First, the two major physiologic changes associated with hot flashes are the result of different peripheral sympathetic functions. Excitation of sweat glands is by sympathetic cholinergic fibers, while cutaneous vasoconstriction is under the exclusive control of tonic α-adrenergic fibers.[30,31] It is difficult to envision some peripheral event resulting in cholinergic effects on sweat glands and α-adrenergic blockade of cutaneous vessels. However, these are the two basic mechanisms triggered by central thermoregulatory centers to lower core temperature. Thus, a hot flash appears to be a normal thermoregulatory event, occurring at an inappropriate time.

Secondly, during a hot flash, central temperature decreases following cutaneous vasodilation and perspiration. If hot flashes were the result of some peripheral mechanism, the regulatory mechanisms would be expected to prevent the observed decrease in core temperature.

The third indication is the change in behavior associated with the symptom. Women have a conscious desire to try to cool their bodies. They will remove clothing, throw off bedcovers, stand by open windows and doors, etc. All of these actions occur in the face of a normal or decreasing central temperature. An analagous dissociation between perception and central temperature is found at the onset of a fever, when the individual feels cold or a 'chill' prior to any change of central temperature. Because of this 'chill' subjects will modify behavior to conserve heat. This assists in elevating the central temperature, thus the fever.

Most investigators working in the field of temperature regulation consider a fever to be the result of an elevation of the 'set point' of central thermoregulatory centers, particularly those in the rostral hypothalamus.[32,33,34] Pyrogens elevate the central thermoregulatory setpoint and the febrile organism actively raises the central body temperature, using both physiologic (cutaneous vasoconstriction and shivering) and behavioral mechanisms (curling in a ball, putting on more clothes, drinking hot liquids, etc.)[35,36] These activities continue until the core temperature reaches the new set point.

By employing these observations, it is suggested that the menopausal hot flash is triggered by a sudden downward setting of the central, hypothalamic 'thermostats' (Fig. 49.3). Subsequently, heat loss mechanisms are activated to bring the core

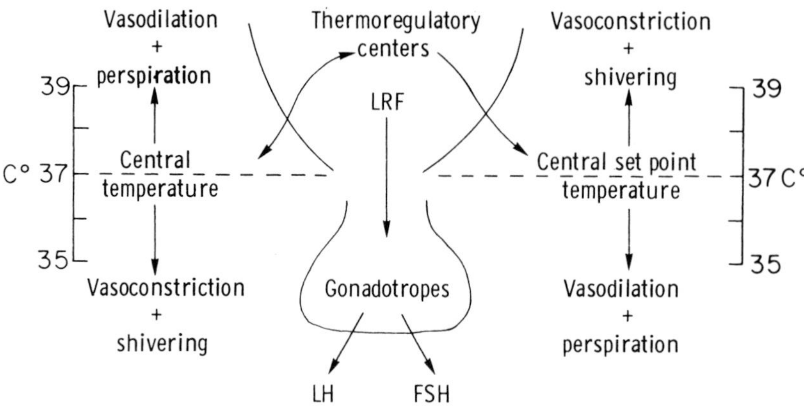

Fig. 49.3 Proposed mechanism of hot flashes is a sudden downward setting of central set point temperature in hypothalamic thermoregulatory centers. Since central temperature would be higher, this would trigger vasodilation and perspiration (hot flash) to dissipate heat.[77]

temperature in line with the new set point, resulting in the fall of core temperature.

HORMONAL STUDIES

The underlying mechanism responsible for initiating the thermoregulatory changes observed during hot flashes has received much investigative study. Because hot flashes occur after the spontaneous cessation of ovarian function or following ovariectomy, it has been presumed that the mechanism is endocrinological, related either to enhancement of pituitary gonadotropin secretion or to reduction of ovarian estrogen secretion. Therefore, numerous investigations have examined the correlation between hot flashes and levels of hormones, particularly gonadotropins and estrogens.

Gonadotropin studies

Several types of studies have been conducted to determine if a direct relationship exists between hot flashes and gonadotropins. Early investigations indicated a correlation of hot flashes with higher levels of plasma luteinizing hormone (LH) while other studies showed no correlation.[37–40] Of particular significance are the reports correlating the occurrence of hot flashes with pulsatile LH release. One study measured hot flashes in six women using continuous finger temperature recordings as well as blood samples which were drawn at 15 minute intervals before and at five minute intervals following the commencement of each episode (Fig. 49.4).[28] During 48 hours of study, 34 hot flashes were recorded along with 31 pulses of LH secretion. Among these, 26 of the 31 LH pulses observed had a close temporal relationship with the occurrence of hot flashes. Independently, other investigators showed the same association.[41] These findings strongly suggested a close temporal relationship between the pulsatile release of LH and the occurrence of hot flashes. Both studies also reported there was no clear association with the occurrence of hot flashes and pulsatile follicle stimulating hormone (FSH) release.

The close temporal relationship between pulsatile LH release and hot flashes suggests LH or the factors that initiate pulsatile LH release are involved with triggering hot flashes. It is doubtful that LH or increased pituitary activity is responsible for hot flashes since these have been described in patients following a surgical hypophysectomy.[42–44] These observations were supported by other investigators who measured hot flashes objectively in two patients with hypoestrogenism secondary to surgically induced pituitary insufficiency (Fig. 49.5).[45] In both of these patients, hot flashes with similar characteristics to those seen in postmenopausal women were observed, despite low plasma LH and no pulsatile release.

Further support that the relationship between these two events is independent of pulsatile LH release is the finding that administration of a potent agonist of

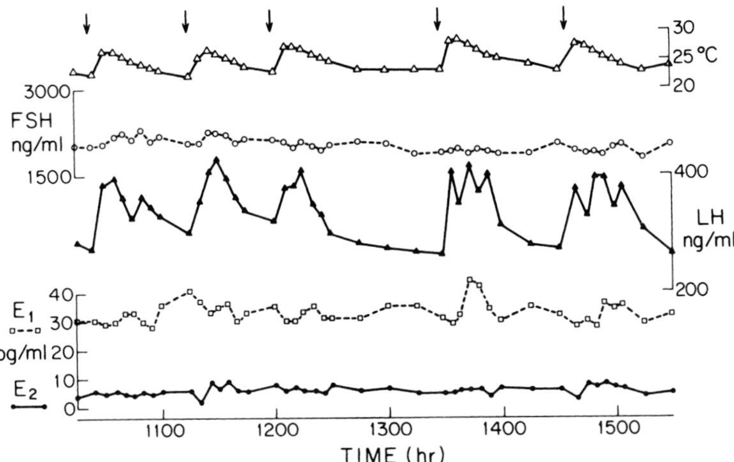

Fig. 49.4 Serial measurements of finger temperature and serum FSH, LH, estrone and estradiol in an individual subject. Arrows mark the onset of the temperature rises.[28]

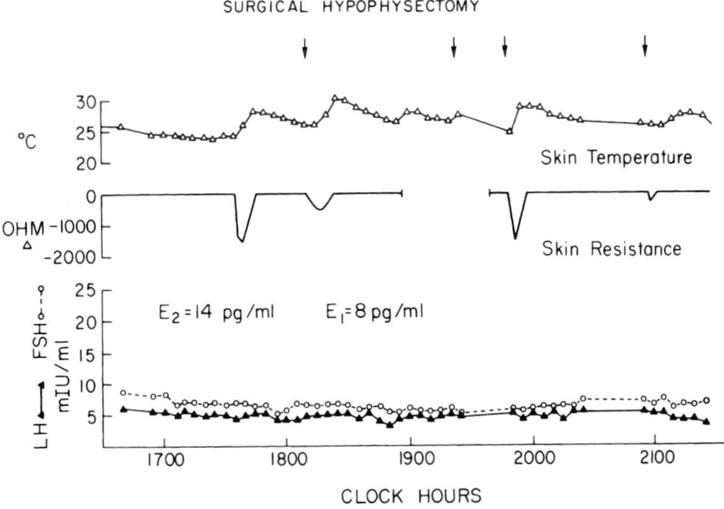

Fig. 49.5 Serial measurements of the skin temperature, skin resistance and serum LH and FSH levels in a woman following partial resection, cryotherapy and irradiation of a chromophobe adenoma of the pituitary. Arrows mark the onsets of subjective flashes.[45]

gonadotropin releasing hormone (GnRH-a) to postmenopausal women obliterates the pulsatile release of LH, but not the occurrence of hot flashes.[46] A similar observation has also been made in premenopausal women given the same class of medication.[47] In subjects with normal menstrual cycles, the daily administration of agonist for one month blocked the pulsatile release of LH from the pituitary presumably through pituitary desensitization. Ovarian function was also obliterated, with estrone and estradiol levels falling to those documented in postmenopausal women. Within three weeks of initiation of agonist administration, hot flashes were induced in three of five subjects. This incidence of occurrence was similar to the 76% incidence observed in 25 premenopausal women who underwent surgical ovariectomy. The characteristics of the hot flashes induced with GnRH-a were also similar to the events observed in the women following surgical ovariectomy.

Based on the physiological and hormonal data presented, it would appear that a suprapituitary mechanism must initiate hot flashes and this is influenced by the hypothalamic factors responsible for pulsatile LH release. Using animal models, several investigators have reported that the hypothalamic hormone, gonadotropin releasing hormone (GnRH), fluctuates in the hypophyseal portal vein blood, and these fluctuations are responsible for pulsatile release of LH from the pituitary.[48,49] One study observed that serum GnRH levels rise prior to the onset of hot flashes, suggesting that GnRH or the factors which influence its secretion from the hypothalamus may trigger these abnormal thermoregulatory events.[50] The hypothalamic site governing the pulsatile release of GnRH is believed to be within the arcuate nucleus and the release of this hypothalamic hormone is modulated by neurotransmitter input to the GnRH neurons. These neurotransmitters, including norepinephrine, dopamine, opioids and prostaglandins, have been shown to influence LH release, presumably via effects on hypothalamic GnRH release. It is conceivable, therefore, that hypothalamic GnRH or the neurotransmitters that influence its release may somehow alter the set point of the hypothalamic thermoregulatory centers to trigger hot flashes under hypo-estrogenic conditions.[30,31] This concept is consistent with the fact that hypoestrogenism enhances norepinephrine turnover rates and augments LH pulses.

Patients with isolated gonadotropin deficiency are believed to have a defect in hypothalamic GnRH secretion.[51,52] Investigators studied five such patients as a model of a spontaneously occurring defect in GnRH synthesis and/or release. These women had received exogenous estrogens for hormone replacement therapy for at least one year.[53] After one month of discontinuation of exogenous estrogens, four of the five subjects showed objectively recorded hot flashes but no pulsatile release of gonadotropins. Since hot flashes occurred in these patients with defects in GnRH synthesis and/or release, it was presumed that hypothalamic GnRH itself is probably not involved in the initiation of these thermoregulatory episodes.

On the other hand, patients with hypothalamic amenorrhea are considered to be models of a defect of neurotransmitter input to GnRH neurons and this abnormal neurotransmitter activity is thought to contribute to the diminished GnRH release from the hypothalamus thereby resulting in hypogonadism and amenorrhea.[54,55] Studies of five patients with hypothalamic amenorrhea were conducted within one year of disease onset and were limited to patients with hypoestrogenism equivalent to that seen following surgical castration.[53] In these subjects no objectively measured hot flashes were recorded. This finding suggests that the same neuroendocrine mechanism responsible for hypothalamic amenorrhea also inhibits the occurrence of hot flashes. Since this disease is probably secondary to abnormal neurotransmitter input to GnRH neurons, these observations suggest that the hypothalamic factors which influence GnRH release, but not GnRH itself, may somehow alter the set point of hypothalamic regulatory centers resulting in the initiation of hot flash episodes. The close proximity of some of the GnRH neurons to the thermoregulatory centers in the preoptic area–anterior hypothalamus is consistent with this concept.[56,57,58]

The observations that brain neurotransmitters, particularly norepinephrine, play roles in both central thermoregulatory function and GnRH release are also consistent with the suggestion that neurotransmitter mechanisms in the hypothalamus are responsible for the simultaneous occurrence of pulsatile LH release and hot flashes.[59,60,61] The findings that the medication clonidine partially blocks the occurrence of objectively measured hot flashes also supports this possibility.[62] The effect of clonidine on hot flashes could be exerted via peripheral or central mechanisms. Clonidine is an α adrenergic receptor agonist that stimulates postsynaptic α adrenergic receptors in the depression site of the vasomotor center of the medulla oblongata.[63] In addition, it may also influence suprabulbar structures such as α adrenergic receptors in the hypothalamus.

Estrogen studies

As a result of the association of hot flashes with the onset of menopause, and of menopause with a drop in circulating levels of estrogen, investigators have sought to determine whether there exists a relationship between estrogen and hot flashes. Several studies demonstrated no correlation between estrogen levels in the blood and the presence or absence of hot flashes in postmenopausal women.[39,64] One investigator measured serum estradiol and estrone levels at 5–15 minute intervals before and after hot flashes and found no association with the occurrence of objectively measured hot flashes.[65] However, postmenopausal women with severe hot flashes were found to have lower levels of circulating estrone and estradiol than asymptomatic women.[66,67] This finding was confirmed in another extensive study where the physical characteristics and serum estrogen levels in postmenopausal women with frequent severe hot flashes were compared with those observed in women who had never experienced the symptom. It was found that women with severe hot flashes had significantly lower mean body weight (% ideal weight) and levels of total estrone and estradiol than the women without the symptom. These findings suggest that body size and its effects on endogenous estrogen metabolism may be a factor in the occurrence of hot flashes in some postmenopausal women.[14]

Hot flashes, however, involve more than just the presence of low plasma estrogen levels. Throughout the postmenopausal period, estrogen levels remain low, yet some women never have hot flashes, while others have severe symptoms. In other circumstances in which estrogen levels are low, such as in prepubertal girls, hot flashes are not reported. What appears to be much more important than absolute levels of estrogen is a drop in estrogen concentration. The abrupt onset of hot flashes following surgical ovariectomy or administration of GnRH analogs, which both cause plasma estrogen levels to fall, strongly support this contention.[39,68,69] This observation was further substantiated by the findings that postmenopausal women with gonadal dysgenesis who never have been exposed to elevated estrogen levels do not experience hot flashes unless they are initially prescribed estrogen and are then withdrawn from it.[41,70] Estrogen replacement therapy has also been shown to ameliorate hot flashes and upon discontinuation of estrogen replacement, hot flashes often resume.

As previously mentioned, hypothalamic dysfunction plays a key role in the genesis of hot flashes. With minor exceptions, the hypothalamus is behind the blood/brain barrier, which can exclude circulating substances which freely diffuse across other capillary beds. Thus, the fraction of circulating estrogens that could influence hypothalamic function should be that portion that is transported across the blood/brain barrier. In the circulation, estradiol can either bind to sex hormone-binding globulin (SHBG) or serum albumin or remain in a free form, and it has been observed that the portion of estradiol not bound to SHBG is the fraction which is transported into the brain across the blood/brain barrier.[71] Interestingly, one study has shown that the mean level of non-SHBG bound estradiol in women who had never experienced a hot flash is twice that observed in symptomatic women, suggesting that this fraction of non-SHBG bound circulating estradiol may be an important determinant for the occurrence of hot flashes.[14]

The specific role of estrogen in the etiology of hot flashes remains to be fully elucidated. In addition to its effect on reproductive tissues, estrogen influences thermoregulatory, neurologic and vascular functioning. The firing rate of thermal sensitive neurons in the preoptic area of the hypothalamus in response to thermal stimuli can be modulated by estrogen as previously described.[72] Estrogen also influences internal body temperature, although the direction of the effect differs extensively between studies.[73,74] The responsiveness of vascular smooth muscle to vasoactive substances such as norepinephrine is affected by estrogen and has been shown to be greater in women with hot flashes than those without hot flashes.[75,76] Thus, estrogen may have peripheral as well as central affects that are important to hot flash physiology.

Androstenedione is the major precursor of circulating estrogens in postmenopausal women and the ovary in the postmenopausal state continues to secrete a small amount of androstenedione and a substantial amount of testosterone.[77,78] However, mean androstenedione and testosterone levels are the same in women with or without hot flashes.[14]

Adrenal studies

In an attempt to define a relationship between hot flashes and adrenal function several investigations have been conducted. Studies examining adrenal medullary function have shown that before, during and after hot flashes there are no changes in peripheral levels of dopamine, norepinephrine or epinephrine.[41,79] Adrenal cortical function, on the other hand, appears to be altered both during and after hot flash episodes with significant increases in plasma cortisol, dehydroepiandrosterone (DHEA) and androstenedione levels being reported.[65] These increases probably represent enhanced adrenal secretions. This increase in adrenal cortical activity may be due to stimulation of the hypothalamic-pituitary-adrenal axis as a manifestation of the stress and discomfort of the hot flash, an increase of adrenocorticotrophic hormone (ACTH) release resulting from a sudden cooling of the hypothalamus or an enhanced steroidogenesis resulting from flash induced increases in adrenal blood flow. Taken together, these observations provide support for the view that hot flashes are triggered by central and not peripheral mechanisms.

Sleep studies

The disruption of the normal sleep pattern of women with hot flashes is a most debilitating ailment for which many seek medical attention. Patients experiencing this symptom frequently complain of night sweats and insomnia and often report frequent awakening episodes and being drenched in sweat, necessitating a change in bedding and clothing. To determine the relationship between sleep disruption and hot flashes, one study recorded sleep stages using polygraphic techniques and the occurrence of hot flashes using objective methods.[80] Women with frequent, severe hot flashes were studied in a sleep laboratory after two nights of conditioning to the laboratory. In nine postmenopausal women, 45 of 47 objectively measured hot flashes, which occurred during sleep, were associated with an awakening episode within 5 minutes before or after the onset of the flash. Although most hot flashes were associated with waking episodes, 40% of waking episodes were not associated with flashes. The onset of the waking episodes usually preceded any measurable change in perspiration or cutaneous vasodilation. These findings suggest that hot flashes can lead to a chronic sleep disturbance and that the onset of waking is due to a central disturbance rather than to the discomfort associated with cutaneous perspiration.

Laboratory investigations confirm that menopausal women take longer to fall asleep, experience more nighttime awakenings and have somewhat less rapid eye movement (REM) sleep than do younger women.[80,81] However, in women with hot flashes sleep efficiency is lower and latency to REM sleep is longer.[82] When these women are treated with estrogen for their hot flashes, they not only report fewer flashes, but also state that they awaken less often during the night and are reported to have a shorter REM latency, and thereby have improved sleep.[80,81,83] Since a chronic sleep disturbance, as seen with hot flashes, can lead to disturbance of psychological function, the above findings provide a plausible explanation for the improvement of both affective and cognitive functions that have been observed with estrogen administration in postmenopausal women experiencing hot flashes.[84] However, this is not the sole explanation for improvement of these brain functions with estrogen, since disturbances of both were also seen in women without hot flashes before estrogen administration.

Management

The important issue of treatment of vasomotor disturbances is considered in detail in chapter 53.

Conclusion

Hot flashes are the most common symptom of the climacteric and represent a substantial medical problem, leading many women to seek medical attention. Hot flashes represent normal thermoregulatory events triggered centrally by altered hypothalamic activity. The hypoestrogenism which follows the loss of ovarian function appears to increase hypothalamic neurotransmitter metabolism, particularly norepinephrine, and augments GnRH output resulting in increased gonadotropin secretion. The enhanced norepinephrine metabolism episodically alters the set point of the thermoregulatory center in the hypothalmus, causing cutaneous vasodilation, perspiration, decrease in core temperature and a subjective feeling of heat and burning (Fig. 49.6). This hypothesis provides new concepts to validate, as well as

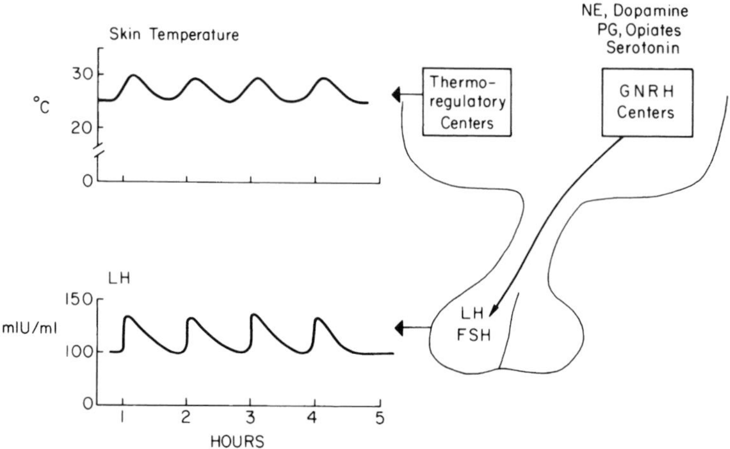

Fig. 49.6 Proposed model of mechanism of menopausal hot flash.

insights into, new treatment methods. Although numerous treatment alternatives have been utilized, estrogen replacement therapy remains the most effective treatment option.

REFERENCES

1. Hannan JH 1927 The flushings of the menopause. Baillière, London
2. Neugarten BL, Kraines RJ 1965 Menopausal symptoms of various ages. Psychosomatic Medicine 27: 266–273
3. Jaszmann L, VanLith ND, Zaat JC 1969 The perimenopausal symptoms. Medical Gynecology and Sociology 4: 268–276
4. Thompson B, Hart SA, Durno D 1973 Menopausal age and symptomatology in general practice. Journal of Biological Science 5: 71–82
5. McKinlay S, Jefferys M 1974 The menopausal syndrome. British Journal of Preventative Social Medicine 28: 108–115
6. Hammar M, Berg G, Fahraeus L 1984 Climacteric symptoms in an unselected sample of Swedish women. Maturitas 6: 345–350
7. Oldenhave A, Jaszmann JB, Haspels AA 1993 Impact of climacteric on well-being. American Journal of Obstetrics and Gynecology 168: 772–780
8. Berg F, Gottvall T, Hammar M 1988 Climacteric symptoms among women aged 60–62 in Linkoping, Sweden in 1986. Maturitas 10: 193–199
9. Kronenberg F 1990 Hot flushes: epidemiology and physiology. Annals of the New York Academy of Science 592: 52–86
10. Voda AM 1981 Climacteric hot flash. Maturitas 3: 73–90
11. Gannon L, Hansel S, Goodwin J 1987 Correlates of menopausal hot flashes. Journal of Behavioural Medicine 10: 277–285
12. Schwingl PJ, Hulka BS, Harlow SD 1994 Risk factors for menopausal hot flashes. Obstetrics and Gynecology 84: 29–34
13. Meldrum DR, Shamonki IM, Frumar AM, Tataryn IV, Chang RJ, Judd HL 1979 Elevations in skin temperature of the finger as an objective index of postmenopausal hot flashes: standardization of the techniques. American Journal of Obstetrics and Gynecology 135: 713–717
14. Erlik Y, Meldrum DR, Judd HL 1982 Estrogen levels in post-menopausal women with hot flashes. Obstetrics and Gynecology 59: 403–407
15. Albright DL, Voda AM, Smolensky MH 1990 Temporal patterns of hot flashes in natural and surgically induced menopause. Chronobiology 4: 731–739
16. McKinley SM, Brambilla DJ, Posner JG 1992 The normal menopause transition. American Journal of Human Biology 4: 37–46
17. Sherman BM, Wallace RB, Bean JA, Chang Y, Schlabaugh L 1981 The relationship of menopausal hot flashes to medical and reproductive experience. Journal of Gerontology 36: 306–309
18. Lock M, Kaufert P, Gilbert P 1988 Cultural construction of the menopausal syndrome: the Japanese case. Maturitas 10: 317–332
19. Lock M 1986 Ambiguities of aging: Japanese experience and perceptions of menopause. Cult Med Psychiat 10: 23–46
20. Albeaux-Fernet M, Deribreux J 1946 La bouffee de chaleur symptome majeur de la menopause. Semaine Hop 22: 1500–1502
21. Collet ME 1949 Basal metabolism of the menopause. Journal of Applied Physiology 1: 629–639
22. Reynolds SR 1941 Dermovascular action of estrogen, the ovarian follicular hormone. Journal of Investigative Dermatology 4: 7–22
23. King JR 1926 Observation on the menopause I. The basal metabolism after the artificial menopause. Bulletin of the Johns Hopkins Hospital 39: 281–303
24. Molnar GW 1975 Body temperature during menopausal hot flashes. Journal of Applied Physiology 38: 499–503
25. Sturdee DW, Wilson RA, Pipili E, Crocker AD 1978 Physiological aspects of menopausal hot flush. British Medical Journal 2: 79–80
26. Molnar GW 1979 Investigation of hot flushes by ambulatory monitoring. American Journal of Physiology 237: R306–310
27. Sturdee DW, Reece BL 1979 Thermography of menopausal hot flushes. Maturitas 1: 201–205
28. Tataryn IV, Meldrum DR, Lu JHK, Frumar AM, Judd HL 1979 LH, FSH and skin temperature during menopausal hot flash. Journal of Clinical Endocrinology and Metabolism 39: 152–154
29. Tataryn IV, Lomax P, Bajorek JG, Chesarek W, Meldrum DR, Judd HL 1980 Postmenopausal hot flushes: a disorder of thermoregulation. Maturitas 2: 101–107
30. Venables R 1967 Methods in psychophysiology. Williams & Wilkins, Baltimore
31. Greenfield AD 1963 The circulation through the skin. Handbook of Physiological Sect 2: 1325–1351
32. Snell ES, Atkins E 1968 The mechanisms of fever, the biological basis of medicine. Academic Press, New York
33. Bligh J 1973 Temperature regulation in mammals and other vertebrates. North-Holland, Amsterdam
34. Kluger MJ 1978 The evolution and adaptive value of fever. Annals of Science 66: 38–43
35. Cooper KE, Cranston WI, Snell ES 1964 Temperature regulation during fever in man. Clinical Science 27: 345–356
36. Reynolds WW, Casterlin ME, Covert JB 1974 Behavioral fever in teleost fishes. Nature 259: 41–42
37. Abe T, Fuguhashi N, Yamaya Y, Wada Y, Hoshiai A, Suzuki M 1977 Correlation between climacteric symptoms and serum levels of estradiol, progesterone, follicle-stimulating hormone, and luteinizing hormone. American Journal of Obstetrics and Gynecology 123: 65–67
38. Hunter DJ, Julier D, Franklin M, Green E 1977 Plasma levels of estrogen, luteinizing hormone, and follicle-stimulating hormone following castration and estradiol implant. Obstetrics and Gynecology 49: 180–185
39. Aksel S, Schomberg DW, Tyrey L, Hammond CB 1976 Vasomotor symptoms, serum estrogens and gonadotropin-levels in surgical menopause. American Journal of Obstetrics and Gynecology 126: 165–169

40. Aitken JM, Davidson A, England P, Govan AD, Hart DM, Kelly A, Lindsay R, Moffatt A 1974 The relationship between menopausal vasomotor symptoms and gonadotropin excretion in urine after oophorectomy. Journal of Obstetrics and Gynecology of the British Commonwealth 81: 150–154
41. Casper RF, Yen SSC, Wilkes MM 1979 Menopausal flushes: a neuroendocrine link with pulsatile luteinizing hormone secretion. Science 205: 823–825
42. Mulley G, Mithell JR 1976 Menopausal flushing: does oestrogen therapy make sense. Lancet 1: 1397–1399
43. Mulley G, Mithell JR, Tattersall RB 1977 Hot flushes after hypophysectomy. British Medical Journal 2: 1062
44. Larsen IF 1977 Hot flashes after hypophysectomy. British Medical Journal 2: 1356
45. Meldrum DR, Erlik Y, Lu JHK, Judd HL 1981 Objectively recorded hot flushes in patients with pituitary insufficiency. Journal of Clinical and Endocrinology Metabolism 52: 684–687
46. Casper RF, Yen SSC 1981 Menopausal flushes: effect of pituitary gonadotropin desensitization by a potent luteinizing hormone-releasing factor agonist. Journal of Clinical Endocrinology and Metabolism 53: 1056–1058
47. DeFazio J, Meldrum DR, Laufer L, Vale W, Rivier J, Lu JHK, Judd HL 1982 Induction of hot flashes in premenopausal women treated with a long acting GnRH agonist. Proceedings of the 29th Annual Meeting of the Society for Gynecological Investigation, Abstract 142
48. Carmel PW, Araki S, Ferrin M 1976 Pituitary stalk portal blood collection in rhesus monkeys: evidence for pulsatile release of gonadotropin-releasing hormone. Endocrinology 99: 243–248
49. Eskay RL, Mical RS, Porter JC 1977 Relationship between luteinizing hormone releasing hormone concentration in hypophyseal blood and luteinizing hormone release in intact, castrated and electrochemically stimulated rats. Endocrinology 100: 263–270
50. Elkind-Hirsch KE, Ravnikar V, Schiff I, Tulchinsky D, Ryan KJ 1981 Determinations of endogenous immunoreactive LHRH levels in the plasma of post-menopausal women. Proceedings of the 28th Annual Meeting of the Society for Gynecological Investigation, Abstract 20
51. DeMorsier G, Gauthier G 1963 La dyplasie olfacto-genitale. Pathological Biology 11: 1267–1272
52. Crowley WF, McArthur JW 1980 Simulation of the normal menstrual cycle in Kallman's syndrome by pulsatile administration of luteinizing hormone releasing hormone. Journal of Clinical Endocrinology and Metabolism 51: 173–175
53. Gambone J, Meldrum DR, Laufer L, Chang J, Lu LHK, Judd HL 1982 Proceedings of the 29th Annual Meeting of the Society for Gynecological Investigation, Abstract 60
54. Yen SSC, Rebar R, Vandenberg G, Judd H 1973 Hypothalamic amenorrhea and hypogonadotropinism: responses to synthetic LRF. Journal of Clinical Endocrinology and Metabolism 36: 811–816
55. Quigley ME, Sheehan KL, Casper RF, Yen SSC 1980 Evidence for increased dopaminergic and opioid activity in patients with hypothalamic hypogonadotropic amenorrhea. Journal of Clinical Endocrinology and Metabolism 50: 949–954
56. Lomax P, Knox GV 1973 The sites and mechanisms of drugs affecting thermoregulation. In: The pharmacology of thermoregulation. Karger, Basel
57. Krey LC, Butler WR, Knobil E 1975 Surgical disconnection of the medial basal hypothalamus and pituitary function in the rhesus monkey. Endocrinology 96: 1073–1087
58. Kobayashi RM, Lu JHK, Moore RY, Yen SSC 1978 Regional distribution of hypothalamic luteinizing hormone releasing hormone in proestrous rats: effects of ovariectomy and estrogen replacement. Endocrinology 102: 98–105
59. Cox B, Lomax P 1977 Pharmacologic control of temperature regulation. Annual Review of Pharmacological Toxicology 17: 341–353
60. Crowley WR, O'Donohue TL, Wachslicht H, Jacobowitz DM 1978 Effects of estrogen and progesterone on plasma gonadotropins and on catecholamine levels and turnover in discrete brain regions of ovariectomized rats. Brain Research 154: 345–357
61. Simpkins JW, Kalra SP 1979 Central site of norepinephrine and LHRH interaction. Federal Proceedings 39: 1107
62. Laufer LR, Erlik Y, Meldrum DR, Judd HL 1982 Effect of clonidine on hot flashes in postmenopausal women. Obstetrics and Gynecology 60: 583–586
63. Houston M 1981 Clonidine hypochloride: review of pharmacologic and clinical aspects. Progress in Cardiovascular Diseases 23: 337–350
64. Stone SC, Mickal A, Rye PH 1975 Postmenopausal symptomatology, maturation index, and plasma estrogen levels. Obstetrics and Gynecology 45: 625–627
65. Meldrum DR, Tataryn IV, Frumar AM, Erlik Y, Lu JHK, Judd HL 1980 Gonadotropins, estrogens, and adrenal steroids during menopausal hot flush. Journal of Clinical Endocrinology and Metabolism 50: 685–689
66. Hagen C, Christiansen C, Christiansen MS, Transbol I 1982 Climacteric symptoms, fat mass and plasma concentrations of LH, FSH, PRL, oestradiol, and androstenedione in the early post-menopausal period. Acta Endocrinologica 101: 87–92
67. Mango D, Scirpa P, Battaglia F, Bini E 1984 Plasma androstenedione and oestrone levels in the climacteric syndrome. Maturitas 5: 245–250
68. DeFazio J, Meldrum DR, Laufer L, Vale W, River J, Lu JHK, Judd HL 1983 Induction of hot flashes in premenopausal women treated with a long acting GnRH-a agonist. Journal of Clinical Endocrinology and Metabolism 56: 445–448
69. Utian WH 1972 The true features of postmenopause and oophorectomy and their response to oestrogen therapy. South African Medical Journal 46: 732–737
70. Yen SSC 1977 The biology of menopause. Journal of Reproductive Medicine 18: 287–296
71. Pardridge WM, Mietus LJ 1979 Transport of steroid hormones through the rat blood-brain barrier: primary role of albumin-bound hormone. Journal of Clinical Investigation 64: 145–154
72. Silva NL, Boulant JA 1986 Effects of testosterone, estradiol, and temperature on neurons in preoptic tissue slices. American Journal of Physiology 250: 625–632
73. Israel SL, Schneller O 1950 The thermogenic property of progesterone. Fertility and Sterility 1: 53–64

74. Marrone BL, Gentry RT, Wade GN 1976 Gonadal hormones and body temperature in rats: effects of estrous cycles, castration, and steroid replacement. Physiology and Behavior 17: 419–425
75. Altura BM 1972 Sex as a factor influencing the responsiveness of arterioles to catecholamines. European Journal of Pharmacology 20: 261–265
76. Ginsburg J, Hardiman P, O'Reilley B 1989 Peripheral blood flow in menopausal women who have hot flushes and in those who do not. British Medical Journal 298: 1488–1490
77. Judd HL 1976 Hormonal dynamics associated with the menopause. Clinics in Obstetrics and Gynecology 19: 775–778
78. Judd HL, Shamonki IM, Frumar AM, Lagasse LD 1982 Origin of serum estradiol in postmenopausal women. Obstetrics and Gynecology 59: 680–686
79. Mashchak CA, Kletzky OA, Artal R, Mishell DR 1984 The relation of physiological changes to subjective symptoms in postmenopausal women with and without hot flushes. Maturitas 6: 301–308
80. Erlik Y, Tataryn IV, Meldrum DR, Lomax P, Bajorek JG, Judd HL 1981 The association of waking episodes with menopausal hot flushes. Journal of the American Medical Association 59: 403–407
81. Schiff I, Regenstein Q, Tulchinsky D, Ryan KJ 1979 Effects of estrogens on sleep and psychological state of hypogonadal women. Journal of the American Medical Association 242: 2405–2407
82. Shaver J, Giblin E, Lentz M, Lee K 1988 Sleep patterns and stability in perimenopausal women. Sleep 11: 556–561
83. Thomson J, Oswald I 1977 Effect of oestrogen on the sleep, mood and anxiety of menopausal women. British Medical Journal 2: 1317–1319
84. Campbell S, Whitehead M 1977 Estrogen therapy and the postmenopausal syndrome. Clinics in Obstetrics and Gynecology 4: 31–47

50. Psychological effects of menopause

Lih-Mei Liao Myra Hunter

Introduction

There is ongoing debate about the psychological sequelae of the normal menopause transition and this is the focus of this chapter. In both the lay and expert literature, menopause is typically linked with a range of psychological problems. For instance, specific symptoms listed in gynecological texts include low energy and drive, cognitive difficulties, irritability, aggressiveness, nervous exhaustion, anxiety, depression, introversion, marital and sexual problems, headache and insomnia. There are inherent difficulties in giving a substantiated account of the psychological effects of menopause; and it may be helpful to understand from where some of these ideas originate, before proceeding to examine the evidence for them.

The word 'uterus' has its root in the Greek word 'hystera'. Its ancient link with emotional instability gave rise to the concept of hysteria in psychodynamic writing. In modern usage, the adjective 'hysterical' means uncontrollably emotional; it is also used colloquially to mean mad, wild or funny. Thus the association between psychopathology and menstruation in women is deeply rooted in the Western mind, bound and sealed by history, culture and myth. Women's emotional experience is at times deemed pathological and attributed to their bodily functioning. The context of that experience is sometimes ignored, though it is often an important determinant. Cross-cultural studies provide some evidence for the importance of context. However, even within the same culture, changes in the social context can alter the women's reporting of their experience of menopause. In his uniquely thorough examination of the historical developments, Wilbush[1] illustrates how social perceptions of menopause and women's own reporting of their experience can shift dramatically, against a background of social change throughout history. Nevertheless, the cultural construction of emotional instability during menopause is often given scientific status and it would be difficult for the most objective investigator to remain uninfluenced.

In the reproductive years, there tends to be more reported negative affect in women than in men.[2] Interpretations of this difference are polarized. Biological explanations emphasize female reproductive physiology as causal factors. Social scientists and feminists view this alleged association as a construction based on the power relationships between the sexes; and they redefine women's higher level of morbidity as a consequence of social and economic factors.[3] For example, emotional distress at menopause has been attributed to women's reaction to being menopausal, which can bring a loss of socially desirable characteristics in the Western world.[4] In the context of such polarized views, it is particularly important to carefully examine the available information.

Studies have tried to gain more accurate accounts from women experiencing menopause but findings from earlier research were inconsistent due to the differing methodologies. Menopausal status was often self-defined[5] or defined by chronological age.[6] Women were often pre-empted into symptom reporting by being given symptom checklists[7] and asked which ones did they experience 'during menopause'. Such retrospective reports could have been biased by stereotyped beliefs about menopause, and by other problems of recall accuracy. Another problem concerns the classification of symptoms which sometimes differed from study to study. For instance, palpitations were classified as psychological by Greene,[8] psychosomatic by Neugarten and Kraines[5] and vasomotor by van Keep.[9] Perhaps the most important drawback of earlier psychological research in relation to menopause is that subjects tended to be clinic attenders and included women with atypical (premature or surgical) menopause. Hence it is difficult to generalize findings to the female population as a whole. Finally, causal interpretations have also been made difficult by the cross-sectional designs used in earlier studies.

More recent studies attempted to rectify some of these problems. The general population samples, prospective designs, clearer definition of menopausal status and use of standardized measures, have helped to provide more consistent information on the normal menopause transition.[10–13]

DEPRESSION

The psychological symptoms listed among the 26 symptoms of estrogen deficiency in the now classic publication by Wilson[14] include 'absent-mindedness', 'irritability' and 'depression'. Among these, depression is perhaps the most commonly reported. In modern medical practice, estrogen treatment is routinely prescribed to alleviate mood problems of mid-aged women. Though widely assumed, the link between hormonal changes at menopause and emotional disturbance remains equivocal; and it is still not clear as to whether or not estrogen is a useful treatment for depression.

The emotional disturbance described in the literature and said to be caused by hormonal changes, can be conceptualized as having three levels. The first is a diagnosable mental illness, i.e. involutional melancholia.[15] This was later retracted. The second proposal is that menopause is a syndrome with a cluster of somatic and psychological symptoms. This concept is now also deemed to have little validity but has not disappeared from medical texts altogether. The third position is a vague version of the second — it does not label menopause as a pathological condition but nevertheless adheres loosely to the idea that psychological problems, especially depression and irritability, are common at menopause due to estrogen deficiency, and that hormonal treatments can solve these problems.

Psycho-endocrinological studies

Using single hormone assessments, Coope[16] found that neither estrogen nor FSH levels correlated with postmenopausal women's scores on the Beck Depression Inventory.[17] In a more detailed study, Ballinger et al[18] took four weekly measures of estradiol, progesterone, FSH, LH and testosterone levels in pre, peri and postmenopausal women. The General Health Questionnaire (GHQ)[19] and standardized interviews were also administered. No significant associations between GHQ scores and hormone levels were observed. If anything, higher GHQ scores (i.e. more depressed) were associated with higher estradiol levels in postmenopausal women. A more recent correlational study was carried out by Avis et al[20] with a random subsample of the Massachesetts cohort. Depression, as assessed by the Centre for Epidemiological Studies — Depression Scale (CES-D)[21] did not correlate with menopausal status as defined by estrogen levels.

There are considerable problems in this type of study due to cyclical and diurnal fluctuations in hormone levels. To obtain an accurate assessment of changes throughout the menstrual cycle in pre and perimenopausal women at least daily samples taken at the same time of the day would be needed.

The association between depression and hormonal changes has also been examined by treatment studies. A randomized controlled study has been carried out to evaluate the efficacy of estrogen in alleviating depression in postmenopausal women.[22] While superphysiological doses of HRT were found to be superior to placebo in its immediate effect on mood, there were no significant differences after four months. Despite this disappointing result, the authors concluded that 'HRT is a useful treatment for depression at menopause'.

Although the evidence between depression and the normal menopause transition is weak, it does not rule out the possibility that there may be an association between depression and sudden estrogen withdrawal — as in the case of oophorectomized or postpartum women. Although the psychological impact of these events cannot be separated from the endocrine factors as causal agents, it would be foolish to dismiss the idea that atypical fluctuations of any systemic steroids might have emotional or behavioral manifestations. However, even if these associations are established, effects of abrupt endocrine changes cannot be assumed to be generalizable to the gradual changes spanning many years in normal menopause.

Psychiatric studies

Dennerstein[23] concluded in her review that there is so far no evidence of a distinct 'major' psychiatric disorder but suggested a prevalence of 'minor' psychological symptoms. This dichotomy between major and minor, psychiatric and nonpsychiatric, is essentially an arbitrary one. Whether or not problems attract professional psychiatric help is often related to extrinsic factors such as those relating to healthcare processes and socio-economics, rather than intrinsic factors, such as symptom severity.

Psychiatric studies have used case registers, field surveys and interviews to estimate the prevalence and incidence of psychiatric problems in women across different age bands. The results, not surprisingly, vary from study to study.[24] In her review of the psychiatric literature, Ballinger[25] concluded that the physiological menopause had little impact on 'mental health' and that studies point to a fall in the prevalence of 'minor psychiatric disorders' in the five years following menopause. Events such as changes in family structure, problems with ageing parents, involvement in outside work and reappraisal of future role seemed to have more impact on well-being at this time than physiological factors. Ballinger[25] attributed the different viewpoints of psychiatrists and gynecologists to the fact that the former see many women with negative affect, of whom only a few are menopausal; while the latter see many menopausal women, of whom a large number report negative affect. Ballinger's frustration at the persistent claims of 'climacteric depression' is keenly felt when she ended her review with: 'It is a tribute to the power of culturally-determined attitudes, media pressure and the promotion of estrogen sales that this menopause myth persists, despite all the evidence to the contrary'.

General population studies

Recent normative studies of women's experience of menopause have yielded clearer evidence. A review by Avis et al[20] demonstrated some of the difficulties in upholding the assumed relationship between estrogen and mood. The studies in Massachusetts, Manitoba and Japan had shared similar data collection techniques developed earlier by Kaufert and Syrotuik.[26] The list of 16 core symptoms for all three studies included diarrhea and constipation, persistent cough, upset stomach, shortness of breath, sore throat, backaches, aches/stiffness in joints, dizzy spells, lack of energy, irritability, feeling blue/depressed, trouble sleeping, loss of appetite, hot flushes and cold/night sweats. To minimize the impact of stereotyping on symptom reporting, the word menopause was not included in the titles of the studies nor in the questions on current symptom experience. Furthermore, the checklist was included in a section dealing with general health rather than menstrual change.

The rates of 'feeling blue' or depressed were generally low, with the highest reported in Massachusetts and lowest in Japan. The highest rates of depressed mood were reported by premenopausal women in the Japanese study and by perimenopausal women in the Massachusetts sample. In the Manitoba sample, there were essentially no differences in mood across the stages. These different patterns argue against a direct or simple link between estrogen and depression.

Hunter[13] did find increased reporting of depressed mood by women as they became peri and postmenopausal. The sample of 36 subjects in the prospective phase of the study was small and results should be interpreted with caution. Hunter's analyses of the cross-sectional and prospective data showed that depressed mood at premenopause accounted for 34% of the variance of depressed mood in the peri and postmenopause. This factor, together with low socioeconomic status and previously held negative beliefs of menopause, accounted for 51% of the variance in peri and postmenopausal depressed mood. In contrast, stage of menopause explained only 2% of the variance in the cross-sectional study. Lifestyle factors, such as stress and lack of regular exercise, were also significant factors in depressed mood.

Holte and coworkers[10] did not find menopause to be accompanied by mood swings or by a deeper feeling of depression among their healthy Norwegian sample. However, they found a reduction in subjective well-being (a sense of happiness and life satisfaction). It is easy to confuse the absence of a sense of well-being with the presence of depression, but the two constructs are not equivalent.[27]

Summary

Earlier studies of clinic populations were not generalizable to general samples. However, the exclusion criteria of some of the recent general population studies may mean that the women studied were healthier cohorts than a truly random general population sample. For instance, Holte[10] did not include hysterectomized women and those receiving HRT; and Matthews et al[28] recruited women who held drivers licenses and excluded women with hypertension, diabetes and those on a number of medications, including psychotropics; Hunter's prospective sample[13] was rather small.

At present, the evidence suggests that, for the majority of women, the experience of menopause may be rather less remarkable than hitherto imagined. Menopausal status alone appears to predict few changes. A large proportion of women experience some vasomotor changes though, for most, these are not unduly debilitating or distressing. Vaginal dryness is reported by just under half of menopausal women, and this symptom can but does not necessarily have a significant impact on sexual behavior, which is also influenced by many other complex factors. These were the only areas of change consistently predicted by menopausal status.

So far there is no clear evidence to support a direct relationship between depressed mood and menopausal status. Psychophysiological studies have not found a relationship between endocrine profile and mood states. HRT has not been shown to directly improve mood over and above the confounding effects of the alleviation of vasomotor symptoms and improved sleep. Certain psychosocial factors have emerged as stronger predictors of depressed mood. Currently large scale prospective studies are in progress in Australia and Sweden and these may further clarify the relationship between hormonal changes and psychological well-being.

PSYCHOLOGICAL DIMENSIONS OF HOT FLASHES

Hot flashes are the most common symptom associated with menopause and there are wide variations in experience. Physiological and psychological hypotheses have been put forward to account for the individual variations. Although there is no apparent difference in the estrogen levels of flashing and nonflashing women, Campbell et al[29] did identify a greater diurnal variation of plasma estradiol levels in the former. Sturdee and Brincat[30] suggested two possibilities: perhaps the rate of change of the plasma estrogen levels trigger flashing; or perhaps there are individual differences in the range of estrogen levels within which flashes will occur but above and below which they will not.

Certain psychological and behavioral factors have also been found to be associated with the subjective experience of hot flashes. Holte[10] found that women who smoked cigarettes were more likely to experience hot flashes. Hunter[13] found that two variables, assessed at premenopause, explained 37% of the variance in hot flash reporting during menopause. These were: a history of premenstrual tension, and having had vasomotor symptoms in the premenopause.

The role of stress has also been examined. Gannon and coworkers[31] asked women to record their hot flashes and the occurrence of stressors daily. They found a significant association between hot flashes and stressors for half of the sample. Women who lead stressful lives may be more prone to symptom reporting at pre, peri or postmenopause, including other symptoms, e.g. PMT. Oldenhave[32] found that vasomotor symptoms were related to the severity of nearly all nonvasomotor symptoms. Alternatively, Ballinger et al[33] suggested that the impact of life stresses might lead to catecholamine and estrogen changes and hence vasomotor changes. Women under stress may be more sensitive to minor fluctuation of hormone levels, or they may have a lower threshold of hot flash occurrence.[28] These explanations are compatible with the observation that some premenopausal women also experience hot flashes.

The impact of hot flashes on quality of life varies between women. Hunter[13] did not find an association between hot flashes and emotional distress but a small proportion of those with the symptom said that it was distressing and interfered with their lives. Some found it embarrassing while other found night sweats more distressing as they can cause, compound or prolong sleep problems.[34]

In a recent psychological study of hot flashes, two separate dimensions were identified.[34] Symptom frequency was unrelated to the extent to which the hot flashes were perceived as a problem (problem factor). The latter was based on the combined ratings of the extent to which hot flashes and/or night sweats were seen as a problem, how distressing the symptoms were and the extent to which they interfered with daily life. The problem factor was positively associated with depressed mood and anxiety, and negatively associated with self-esteem.

Several recent studies evaluated the efficacy of nonmedical interventions for hot flashes. These interventions, which incorporated stress reduction techniques, have been shown to reduce hot flash frequency[35,36,37] and the impact of residual flashes.[37] It is unclear as to why hot flashes can be reduced by modifying central responses. A recent study found that hot flashes can be preceded by anxiety and not by absolute or changes in room temperature.[38] It is possible that techniques such as relaxation counter anxiety thereby removing an important antecedent.

Suffice to say that hot flashes, like most other somatic symptoms, can be influenced by psychological factors and can in turn impact upon psychological well-being. Moreover, they appear to be amenable to psychological interventions and probably self-help strategies.

KNOWLEDGE AND BELIEFS ABOUT MENOPAUSE

When asked, women have often expressed neutral and even positive attitudes about menopause, such as relief about the cessation of menstruation. However, negative stereotypes are nevertheless commonly expressed.[39] Women who have had a surgical menopause, who report current psychological and physical complaints, who are more highly educated, are more likely to express negative attitudes about menopause.[13,40] Standing and Glazer[41] found that white middle class women were more likely to express negative attitudes than a low income multi-ethnic group, and younger women more so than older women. In addition, physicians have been found to hold more negative beliefs about menopause than their female patients[42,43] and female physicians more so than their male counterparts, due perhaps to greater exposure to complaints.[43]

Many women believe in a causal link between menopause and emotional difficulties, especially depressed mood and irritability.[13,34,40] As already discussed, there is no clear evidence from epidemiological research to support this assumption[11] or from correlational studies of hormonal and psychological variables.[25,44] Furthermore, psychosocial factors have often emerged as stronger predictors of mood problems during menopause.[12,45] Even so, the belief that menopause causes psychological problems remains pervasive. This may be a corollary to the more global social construction locating distress within the female body, as discussed at the beginning of this chapter. For instance, Koeske and Koeske[47] found that some women attributed their negatively perceived behaviors to menstrual symptoms, even when situational factors would have provided adequate explanations.

Negative stereotyped beliefs have been found to predict depressed mood during menopause.[13] Previously held negative attitudes also predict higher levels of vasomotor symptoms upon reaching menopause[40] and more psychological complaints in general.[47] In addition, Hunter[13] found certain negative beliefs to be among variables that discriminated between women who sought medical help and those who did not. Negative beliefs about menopause have been found to be associated with lesser perceived personal control of health outcome,[48] which may in turn lead to greater likelihood of seeking professional help. Thus beliefs about menopause and health can be important factors in perceptions and help-seeking during menopause and, as such, they warrant further research and intervention.

In general, personal expectations tend to be more positive than generalized beliefs of menopause. Attitudes can become more positive upon first-hand experience, though not always. Certain stereotyped responses about menopause appear to be routinely expressed, and these are not necessarily modified by personal experience. For instance, when asked, the majority of postmenopausal women considered that their personal experience of menopause had been better than that of most other women.[10] Thus there seems to be a irrefutable myth about menopause, which is perceived to be a problem no matter what actually happens.

Attitudes expressed in relation to menopause seem extremely complex and at times apparently contradictory. For instance, in Leiblum and Swartzman's study,[49] women agreed that menopause should be 'viewed as a medical condition and treated as such'; yet they attributed any psychological problems to stressful life changes rather than hormonal factors and expressed a preference for natural treatment options to hormone replacement therapy. It is possible that women use different constructions about menopause in different contexts. This warrants further investigation using different methodologies.

Studies of attitude to menopause tended not to distinguish between knowledge and beliefs. When assessed, knowledge of menopause has generally been found to be low and many women have often expressed a need for more information.[39,50] Surprisingly, postmenopausal women are no more knowledgeable about menopause than premenopausal women. While published information about menopause has been on the increase, it does not always give a balanced view of menopause. In promoting the efficacy of hormonal treatments on the physical and psychological functioning of mid-aged women, menopause is inadvertently pathologized and the information may not be reassuring. Studies have found that when offered, many women respond to the opportunity for personalized preventative health education interventions relating to menopause.[39,51] This suggests a need for more innovative services. Unfortunately, these services are far and few between at present. Currently the majority of services focus only on the provision of HRT, with little opportunity for women to exercise their choice in the management of health complaints during menopause.

HELP-SEEKING BEHAVIOR

In general, women are more likely to seek medical help than men.[52] Peri and postmenopausal women have not been found to be more likely to seek medical help than premenopausal women.[11,13,27] The seeking of medical help across patient groups is generally predicted by negative health perceptions and health concerns, as well as emotional distress and somatic symptoms.[54] Hunter[13] found that these variables also discriminated between menopause clinic attenders and nonattenders.

In addition, clinic attenders reported greater difficulties in coping and expressed more negative attitude about menopause.

In the same study, HRT use was associated with having seen a doctor for menopausal complaints. Thus treatment uptake may be a consequence of healthcare processes as much as any medical factors. A more recent study by Hay et al[54] yielded similar results. Menopause clinic attenders (nearly all receiving HRT) tend to be characterized by a greater likelihood of having had a surgical menopause, vasomotor symptoms, emotional distress and negative beliefs about menopause.

Since a proportion of menopausal women present both psychological distress and vasomotor symptoms, services need to address psychological as well as medical needs. Women may differ on their choice of treatments, although a recent study of treatment choice in relation to hot flushes found surprisingly few differences between women who chose HRT and those who chose a brief cognitive behavioral intervention.[55] Practical constraints were sometimes presented by women as the deciding factor in treatment choice. For instance, among women who wanted help with reducing their hot flashes, some who did not want HRT nevertheless chose it, because taking a pill was easier than regular attendance at the sessions required by the psychological intervention.

In general, certain psychological approaches have been established as effective interventions for depression and these ought to be considered alongside medical treatments. A proportion of women may require both. A recent pilot study found that problem-solving groups in the primary care context can help menopausal women to alleviate some of their psychological distress.[56] This may be a cost-effective way of dealing with emotional distress and of empowering some of the women who experience menopause adversely.

Conclusion

The current evidence suggests that for the majority of women in the general population, menopause is relatively 'uneventful' and that menopausal status mainly predicts menstrual changes and two symptoms: hot flashes and vaginal dryness. Endocrine factors are significant in these two symptoms but the large individual differences suggest that nonendocrine factors are also involved and that these may interact to effect differential experience. Emotional difficulties reported by some women cannot be explained by menopausal status alone but are associated with a number of psychosocial factors. There appears to be no increase in help-seeking behavior, which is not determined by symptomatology alone but is also related to psychosocial and healthcare factors. Nonendocrine factors that affect women's experience of and behavior at menopause include socio-economic status, general health, attitudes and lifestyle factors such as smoking, stress and employment. Thus if clinics offer hormonal treatment alone, this out of step with menopause as a multi-faceted process, is influenced by various aspects of women's lives and which in turn can impact upon their lives.

This evidence so far challenges the traditional view of menopause as a psychopathogenic process. They inform us that women do not necessarily experience menopause as an adverse life event and that, for whose who do, the context of the women's lives need to be included, in order to develop an adequate understanding of that adversity. However, these studies are in themselves limited. They have not furthered our understanding of what might be the most salient issues of menopause and midlife.

To date, we do not have a psychology of menopause and midlife, other than that which relates to emotional distress and somatic symptoms. Lack of depression does not equate to well-being. Some interesting research is underway using qualitative methodologies[58] but many gaps have still to be filled. For instance, even the more improved studies in recent times, conducted in multicultural societies, have failed to address the potentially differential menopausal experience of women of different ethnic groups within the same society. Information on men's attitudes to menopause and mid-aged women have also not been systematically gathered. Finally, studies have only begun to focus on work, creativity, relationships and other similarly important issues in relation to mid-aged women. More psychological research is needed in future to address these interesting aspects of menopause and midlife.

REFERENCES

1. Wilbush J 1988 Climacteric disorders — historical perspectives. In: Studd JWW, Whitehead MI (eds) The menopause. Blackwell Scientific Publications
2. Paykel ES 1973 Recent life events in the depressive disorders. In: Depue RA (ed) The psychobiology of depressive disorders. Academic Press, New York
3. Ussher J 1992 Research and theory related to female reproduction: implications for clinical psychology. British Journal of Clinical Psychology 31: 129–151

4. Kaufert P 1982 Anthropology and the menopause: the development of a theoretical framework. Maturitas 4: 181–193
5. Neugarten BL, Kraines RJ 1965 'Menopausal symptoms' in women of various ages. Psychosomatic Medicine 27: 266–273
6. Bungay GT, Vessey MP, McPherson CK 1980 Study of symptoms in middle life with special reference to the menopause. British Medical Journal ii: 181–183
7. Blatt MG, Wiesbader H, Kupperman HS 1953 Vitamin E and the climacteric syndrome. American Medical Association Archives of Internal Medicine 91: 792–799
8. Greene JG 1976 A factor analytic study of climacteric symptoms. Journal of Psychosomatic Research 20: 425–430
9. van Keep P 1970 The menopause, a study of attitudes of women in Belgium, France, Great Britain, Italy and West Germany. International Health Foundation, Geneva
10. Holte A 1992 Influences of natural menopause on health complaints: a prospective study of healthy Norwegian women. Maturitas 14: 127–141
11. McKinlay SMA, Brambilla DJ, Prosner JG 1992 The normal menopause transition. Maturitas 14(2): 103–117
12. Kaufert P, Gilbert P, Tate R 1992 The Manitoba Project: a re-examination of the link between menopause and depression. Maturitas 14: 143–156
13. Hunter MS 1992 The south east England longitudinal study of the climacteric and postmenopause. Maturitas 14: 117–126
14. Wilson RA 1966 Feminine Forever. Evans, New York
15. Kraeplin E 1896 Psychiatric, 5th ed. Barth, Leipzig
16. Coope J 1981 Is oestrogen therapy effective in the treatment of menopausal depression? Journal of the Royal College of General Practitioners 31: 124–140
17. Beck A, Ward CH, Mendelson M, Mock J, Erbaugh J 1961 An inventory for measuring depression. Archives of General Psychiatry 4: 561–571
18. Ballinger CB, Browning MCK, Smith AHW 1987 Hormone profiles and psychological symptoms in peri-menopausal women. Maturitas 7: 313–327
19. Goldberg D 1972 The detection of psychiatric illness by questionnaire. Oxford University Press, London
20. Avis NE, McKinlay SMA, Vass K, Brambilla D, Longscope C 1993 Hormone levels, symptoms, and the relation between menopause and depression. Paper presented at the 7th International Congress on the Menopause, Stockholm
21. Radloff 1977 The CES-D scale: a self-report depression scale for research in the general population. Applied Psychological Measurement 1: 385–401
22. Montgomary JC, Appleby L, Brincat M, Versi E, Tapp A, Fenwick PBC, Studd JWW 1987 The effect of oestrogen and testosterone implants on psychological disorders in the climacteric. The Lancet Feb 7: 297–299
23. Dennerstein L 1988 Psychiatric aspects. In: Studd JWW, Whitehead MI (eds) The menopause. Blackwell Scientific Publications.
24. Goldman N, Ravid R 1980 Community surveys: sex differences in mental illness. In: Guttentag M, Salasin S, Belle D (eds) The mental health of women. Academic Press, London
25. Ballinger CB 1990 Psychiatric aspects of the menopause. British Journal of Psychiatry 156: 773–787
26. Kaufert P, Syrotuik J 1981 Symptom reporting at menopause. Social Science and Medicine 15: 173–184
27. Kaufert PA 1994 Menopause and depression: a sociological perspective. In: Berg & Hammar (eds) Modern management of the menopause, Pathenon
28. Matthews KA, Wing RR, Lewis HK, Meilahn EN, Kelsey SF 1990 Influences of natural menopause on the psychological characteristics and symptoms of middle-aged healthy women. Journal of Consulting and Clinical Psychology 58: 345–351
29. Campbell S, Beeson AJ, Kitchen Y, Fergusson IK, Biswas S 1976 Intensive steroid and protein hormone profiles on post-menopausal women experiencing hot flushes. In: Campbell S (ed) The management of the menopause and the post-menopausal years. MTP Press, Lancaster
30. Sturdee D, Brincat M 1988 The hot flush. In: Studd JWW, Whitehead MI (eds) The menopause. Blackwell Scientific Publications
31. Gannon L 1990 Endocrinology of the menopause. In: Fromanek (ed) Meaning of menopause: historical, medical and clinical perspectives. Analytic Press Inc., Hillsdale, NJ
32. Oldenhave A 1991 Well-being and sexuality in the climacteric. International Health Foundation, Geneva
33. Ballinger S, Cobbin D, Krivanek J, Saunders D 1979 Life stresses and depression in the menopause. Maturitas 1: 191–199
34. Hunter MS, Liao KLM 1995 A psychological analysis of menopausal hot flushes. British Journal of Clinical Psychology 34: 589–599
35. Stevenson DW, Delprato DJ 1985 Multiple component self-control programme for menopausal hot flushes. Journal of Behavioural Therapy and Experimental Psychiatry 14: 137–140
36. Germaine LM, Freedman RR 1984 Behavioral treatment of menopausal hot flashes: evaluation of objective methods. Journal of Consulting and Clinical Psychology 52: 1072–1079
37. Hunter MS, Liao KLM 1996 Evaluation of a four-session cognitive-behavioural therapy for menopausal hot flushes. British Journal of Health Psychology 1: 113–125
38. Slade P, Amee S 1995 The role of anxiety and temperature in the experience of hot flushes. Journal of Reproductive and Infant Psychology 13(2): 127–134
39. Liao KLM 1994 Preparation for menopause: development and evaluation of a health education intervention for mid-aged women. Unpublished PhD thesis, University of London
40. Avis NE, McKinlay SMA 1991 Longitudinal analysis of women's attitudes towards the menopause: results from the Massachusetts Women's Health Study. Maturitas 13: 65–79
41. Standing TS, Glazer G 1992 Attitudes of low-income patients towards menopause. Health Care for Women International 13: 271–280
42. Cowan G, Warren LW, Young JL 1985 Medical perceptions of menopausal symptoms. Psychiatry and Women Quarterly 9: 3–13
43. Liao KLM, Hunter MS, White P 1994 Stereotyped beliefs about menopause of general practitioner and mid-aged women. Family Practice 11: 408–412

44. Alder EM, Bancroft J, Livingstone J 1992 Estradiol implants, hormone levels and reported symptoms. Psychosomatic Obstetrics and Gynaecology 13: 223–235
45. Greene JG, Cooke DJ 1980 Life stress and symptoms at the climacterium. British Journal of Psychiatry 136: 486–491
46. Koeske RK, Koeske GF 1975 An attributional approach to moods and the menstrual cycle. Journal of Personality and Social Psychology 31: 474–478
47. Holte A, Mikkelsen A, Moen MH, Skjoerasen J, Jervell J, Stokke KT, Wergeland R 1994 Psychosocial factors and the menopause: results from the Norwegian Menopause Project. In: Berg G, Hammar M (eds) The modern management of the menopause. Parthenon,
48. Liao KLM, Hunter MS 1995 Knowledge and beliefs about menopause in a general population sample of mid-aged women. Journal of Reproductive and Infant Psychology 13: 101–114
49. Leiblum ST, Swarizman LS 1986 Women's attitudes about the menopause: an update. Maturitas 81: 47–56
50. Roberts PJ 1991 The menopause and hormonal replacement therapy: views of women in general practice receiving HRT. British Journal of General Practice 41: 421–424
51. Coope J, Roberts DA 1990 Clinic for the prevention of osteoporosis in general practice. British Journal of General Practitioners 40: 295–299
52. Verbrugge LM, Wingard DL 1987 Sex differentials in health and mortality. Women and Health 12: 103–145
53. Mechanic D 1983 The experience and expression of distress: the study of illness behaviour and medical utilization. In: Mechanic D (ed) Handbook of health, health care and the health professions. Free Press, New York
54. Hay AG, Bancroft J, Johnstone EC 1994 Affective symptoms in women attending a menopause clinic. British Journal of Psychiatry 164: 513–516
55. Hunter MS, Liao KLM 1995 Determinants of treatment choice for menopausal hot flushes: hormonal versus psychological versus no treatment. Journal of Psychosomatic Obstetrics and Gynaecology 16: 101–108
56. Hunter MS, Liao KLM 1995 Problem-solving groups for mid-aged women in general practice. Journal of Reproductive and Infant Psychology 13: 147–151
57. Apter 1995 Secret paths: women in midlife. WW Norton, NY

51. Pharmacological background of estrogen replacement therapy and continuance

Charles B. Hammond Patrick L. Blohm

Introduction

Estrogen therapy for women has received much attention in both lay and medical literature. Much controversy has surrounded its use as a contraceptive agent and also in replacement therapy. Few single-agent therapies (or those in combination with progestogens and/or androgens) can affect a woman's health in so many different ways and in so many parts of her lifespan.

From the onset, the primary route of administration of estrogen therapy (ET) has been oral. Earliest attempts began in western Europe in 1896 when three individuals, Chrobak, Mainzer and Mond reported, almost simultaneously, treatment of menopausal symptoms with orally administered ovarian tissues.[1–3] From then until the late 1920s various methods were used to administer estrogen from a variety of sources (e.g. ovary, placenta and urine).[4] Success was limited in the treatment of menopausal symptoms, primarily because of low bioavailability of the estrogen. In 1929 Butenandt and Doisy successfully isolated estrone.[5] About this time Geist and Spielman (1932)[6] and Sevringhaus (1935)[7] began to use higher purity estrogen preparations to treat menopausal symptoms. However, it was only with the advent of semisynthetic and synthetic estrogens, with their prolonged duration of action, that potent orally active preparations became available for clinical use. The earliest compounds were synthesized in 1938: these were diethylstilbestrol (DES) by Dodds[8] and ethinyl estradiol by Inhoffen.[9] Since then a variety of estrogenic substances, and new formulations of previously identified substances, have been developed and marketed. Today, oral estrogens are one of the largest selling family of drugs throughout the developed world.

Potency

Throughout this chapter, various relative potencies of estrogenic compounds will be discussed. Care must be taken in relating these as many different assays are available for comparisons. Absolute estrogenic potency can be determined in various different assay systems. What is more difficult to determine is which system is most relevant. Finally, there are important variations in potency caused by dose, route of administration, and whether the assay relies on a biochemical end-point such as change in the active hormone/receptor complex in a target cell nucleus,[10] or whether there is a clinical parameter such as change in the maturation index of a vaginal smear, gonadotropin suppression or induction of hepatic protein synthesis. There are many other examples of different biological assays.[11–13] The clinician needs to look at how potencies are compared, decide which are relevant to the particular clinical situation, and then dose and treat appropriately.[14] Table 51.1 gives one view of potency.

The three most important naturally occurring estrogens found in humans, ranked by potency, are estradiol, estrone and estriol. Considerable interconversion occurs between estradiol and needs to be taken into account when considering the effects of various estrogens in women.

AVAILABLE ORAL ESTROGENS

Estradiol

Estradiol is the most potent naturally occurring estrogen.[15] In addition, many of the other naturally occurring estrogens used in oral ET exert at least some of their biologic effects after conversion to estradiol.[16] Estradiol, or estra-1,3,5(10)-triene-3,17β-diol as it is chemically named, appears as a white powder in its pure form. It is almost insoluble in water and only moderately soluble in alcohol.[17]

Natural estradiol, when given orally, is poorly absorbed, undergoes rapid metabolism to estrone and causes a large 'first-pass' effect.[18,19] Because of this,

Table 51.1 Serum estradiol, nonSHBG-bound estradiol, and estrone concentrations (pg/mL) after treatment with different estrogen preparations (mean ± SE).

Estrogen administered (mg)		Estradiol-17β	NonSHBG-bound estradiol-17β	Estrone
EE	0.3	18.5 ± 2	4.3 ± 1	76 ± 14
EE	0.625	39.4 ± 11	11 ± 4	153 ± 31
Estropipate	0.6	34 ± 7	12.4 ± 2	125 ± 25
Estropipate	1.2	42 ± 7	11.4 ± 2	285 ± 52
Estradiol-17β	1	30 ± 7	9.4 ± 2	266 ± 64

most marketed estradiol products are in esterified, micronized or sulfated formulations.

Estradiol valerate is formed by esterification of estradiol with valeric acid at the carbon 17 (C-17) position of the steroid module. A micronized preparation is one which is comprised of drug containing particles of small enough size (<20 μm) to facilitate absorption whole by the intestinal mucosa.[20] Oral micronized estradiol is readily absorbed through the GI tract.[20] Sulfation of estradiol enhances absorption by rendering it water soluble. Regardless of the estradiol preparation, the majority of the drug is metabolized within the intestinal mucosa[21] and liver into estrone (15%) and estrone sulfate (65%).[22] The results are serum levels of estrone that are 3–6 times higher than those achieved for estradiol.[20] After a single 2 mg oral dose of micronized estradiol, mean peak serum levels of 110 pg/mL estradiol were seen at 5 hours with sustained elevation and a slow return to baseline over the next 19 hours. The mean peak estrone level was 467 pg/mL which was noted at 6 hours and remained elevated over the next 18 hours.[20]

Lobo reported mean levels of 65 pg/mL of estradiol and 300 pg/mL of estrone after an oral dose of 2 mg of micronized estradiol. In addition, 1 mg of micronized estradiol was found to generate mean levels of 40–50 pg/mL estradiol and 200 pg/mL estrone.[22] A high serum estrone to estradiol ratio greater than unity is characteristic after oral administration of estradiol and a hallmark of first-pass metabolism. The interconversion between estradiol, estrone and estrone sulfate is a continuous and dynamic equilibrium involving 17β-estradiol dehydrogenases, sulfotransferases and sulfatases and is reversible. Therefore, the elevated levels of estrone, and estrone sulfate (the latter with its relatively long half-life) may circulate as a large stable reservoir of estrogen and estrogen precursors.[23]

The final metabolism of orally administered estradiol is via definitive metabolism of estrone. This is a two-step process. Step one involves the formation of either catecholestrogens by ring A metabolism or formation of estriol via ring D metabolism. Step two involves the formation of sulfate or glucuronide conjugates from the products of step one metabolism and these are then excreted in the urine and to a lesser extent bile.[23]

The relative potency of estradiol has been evaluated in several different ways. Studies comparing serum estradiol and estrone levels have found that similar plasma profiles were obtained with oral administration of 2 mg estradiol valerate, 1.5 mg piperazine estrone sulfate and 1.25 mg of conjugated equine estrogens (CEE).[24,25] Gonadotropin suppression data suggest that estradiol is slightly more potent than piperazine estrone sulfate, slightly less potent than CEE and much less potent than ethinyl estradiol, as shown in Table 51.1.[26] Finally, Archer and coworkers reported therapeutic equivalence, defined as the ability to relieve vasomotor symptoms, between 1 mg estradiol and 0.625 mg of CEE.[27]

Conjugated equine estrogens

The most widely used preparation for oral estrogen replacement therapy (ERT) in the US today is conjugated equine estrogens (CEE). This preparation is actually a combination of up to 10 different estrogenic compounds. These compounds include the sodium sulfated conjugates of estrone, equilin, 17α-dihydroequilin, 17β-dihydroequilin, 17α-estradiol, 17β-estradiol, equilenin, 17α-dihydroequilin, 17β-dihydroequilenin, and Δ 8,9-dehydroestrone.[28]

As already stated, CEE are a mixture of the sodium salts of the sulfate ester forms of various naturally occurring estrogens. Conjugated equine estrogens are still most commonly obtained from natural sources such as extraction from the urine of pregnant mares; however, the major components can be synthesized. A pregnant mare is a potent source of CEE; she may excrete over 100 mg/day. Regardless of the source,

CEE appears as a white powder, and all component estrogens are water soluble.[29]

Importantly, the various preparations of CEE previously marketed may have contained differing quantities of the various estrogens. However, there are now requirements for the total conjugated estrogen content of the preparation as well as the proportion of the two most abundant estrogens, sodium estrone sulfate and sodium equilin sulfate, to exist.[30] Chromatography peaks confirming the presence of the other estrogenic substances are also required, although exact quantitative specifications of these ingredients are not.[31]

The pharmacokinetics of CEE are complex and remain incompletely understood. Part of the complexity is due to extensive metabolization, interconversions and enterohepatic circulation of all of the constituent estrogens. At the center of this interplay is the liver. After oral administration, CEE are rapidly and extensively, if not completely, absorbed in the GI tract.[32] Some of the constituents are absorbed in their original conjugated sulfate forms whereas others are hydrolyzed to unconjugated parent forms within the GI tract prior to absorption. A majority of these estrogens are reconjugated shortly after uptake by the bowel and the liver. Therefore, once absorbed, the estrogens circulate primarily as the sulfate conjugates.[33] Although there is no information on the tissue distribution of CEE preparations, there is also no evidence to suggest that CEE are distributed differently than endogenous estrogens.

After absorption, an equilibrium is established in the systemic circulation between the conjugated (sulfated) and unconjugated forms of the estrogens. This equilibrium is maintained by the liver which normally heavily favors the conjugated forms. The net result, where the serum concentration of the conjugated forms is significantly greater than the unconjugated forms, is the creation of a large, hormonally inert, steroid reservoir. The maintenance of this reservoir depends mainly on high rates of binding to serum proteins. The conjugated forms of CEE constituent estrogens such as estrone sulfate (88%) and equilin sulfate (74%) circulate largely bound to albumin.[35] These same sulfated estrogens appear to interact very little with sex hormone binding globulin (SHBG).[36,37] Albumin binding significantly prolongs the half-life of the sulfated estrogens. In contrast, the unconjugated forms circulate largely bound to SHBG with some binding to albumin.[35] These differences in protein binding of the sulfate conjugates as compared to the unconjugated estrogens are thought to be the principle factor responsible for the differences in the metabolic clearance rates between these components.[38,39] For example, unconjugated estrone and equilin are cleared approximately 10 times faster than their respective sulfate conjugates.[40]

After oral administration of CEE, peak levels of equilin and estrone occur at three and five hours, respectively.[41] Some data exist on plasma estrogen levels following therapeutic doses of CEE. For example, oral doses of 0.625 mg per day of CEE will raise the serum estradiol levels from postmenopausal levels (<20 pg/mL) to values approximating the very early follicular phase of the menstrual cycle. The source of this estradiol is back conversion from estrone. CEE does not contain estradiol. In contrast, serum concentrations of estrone go from baseline values of <40 pg/mL to values 5–10 times higher.

Alternatively, Powers,[42] measuring plasma levels after three days of 1.25 mg CEE, recorded peak 17β-estradiol and estrone levels of about 40 pg/mL and 200 pg/mL respectively and mean serum levels of 31 pg/mL and 152 pg/mL. The biologic impact of these very large increases in serum estrone and estrone sulfate levels is unclear because target cells in hormonally sensitive tissues are relatively inaccessible to sulfated and/or protein bound estrogens.[15] Only the hepatocyte has a membrane relatively permeable to conjugated estrogens. Therefore, a significant proportion of the observed biologic response to oral CEE is thought to be mediated through estradiol regenerated in the liver from the above-described reservoir pool of circulating sulfated estrogens.[16] The remaining biologic effect of CEE is probably largely due to the equine estrogens equilin and equilenin.

Equilin and equilenin, along with 17α-dihydroequilin, 17α-dihydroequilenin, 17β-dihydroequilin, 17β-dihydroequilenin, make up the family of estrogens frequently referred to as 'B ring unsaturated estrogens'. As the name implies, these estrogens differ from the classical human estrogens, estrone, estradiol, estriol, because of one or two additional double bonds in B ring of the steroid molecule. Although not native to the human, these compounds have innate estrogenic activity with the human. Indeed, B ring unsaturated estrogens are relatively potent. Uterotropic assays[43] showed that estrone sulfate and equilin sulfate have approximately equal potency. Rodent vaginal smear[12] and chick oviduct assays[13] have also been implemented to investigate the relative potencies of B ring unsaturated estrogens. Although the results vary depending on the bioassay, the data repeatedly demonstrate that the biopotency of the 'equine' estrogens is equal to or greater than that of the classical human estrogens. Unfortunately, there are fewer human clinical trials that have compared the potency of B ring saturated and unsaturated estrogens. A gonadotropin suppression study reported the following relative potencies: diethyl stilbestrol (DES), 2.5; equilin sulfate, 2.0; CEE, 1; estrone sulfate, 0.4; 17α-dihydroequilin sulfate, 0.12; 17α-estradiol sulfate, 0.6; 17α-dihydroequilenin sulfate, 0.[43] To some degree, equilin is stored in and subsequently slowly released from adipose tissue. In fact, elevated serum equilin levels have been found in patients for up to three months after discontinuation of CEE.[24] Equilin has also been shown to be a significantly more potent inducer of hepatic protein synthesis relative to estrone sulfate.[44] Nevertheless, despite adipose storage and moderate induction of hepatic protein synthesis, there have been no reports of negative sequelae from the prolonged administration of and exposure to B ring unsaturated estrogens.

Complex, reversible metabolic pathways, in addition to extensive enterohepatic circulation, make measurement of estrogen half-life values difficult. However, estimates of the apparent half-life value for various estrogens have been reported. Examples of these include 12 hours for estrone sulfate,[45] 5.4 hours for estrone, 1.9 hours for 17β-estradiol,[46] 3.2 hours for equilin sulfate and 20 minutes for equilin.[34]

It will be obvious by now that the enterohepatic circulation is thought to play a part in the pharmacokinetic profile of any estrogenic compound. This is true not only of CEE components, but also may extend to other estrogenic substances discussed in this chapter. The enterohepatic circulation of any estrogen begins with hepatic conjugation, usually with glucuronic acid. This conjugated estrogen is then excreted into the bile and enters the small bowel. Because of hydrophilicity, conjugates are usually not reabsorbed intact from the small bowel and are transported to the large bowel through gut motility. Bacterial flora present in the colon, particularly *Clostridia* species,[47] metabolize the conjugated estrogen via hydrolysis to regenerate the parent steroid. The newly unconjugated estrogen is reabsorbed and via the portal system is returned to the liver where the process may begin again.

The metabolism of CEE, like the pharmacokinetics, is complex. Administration of only one of the CEE constituent estrogens can result in the appearance in plasma of one or more of the other constituent estrogens. This compounds the difficulty encountered in this area of study. Usually only after repeated hydrolysis, reconjugation, interconversion and enterohepatic circulation, does final metabolism of CEE components occur, with elimination mainly by urinary excretion. Studies involving urinary recovery indicate that orally ingested CEE component estrogens can be excreted as intact glucuronides, sulfates, free phenols, or glucuronide-sulfate conjugate mixtures.[48] The ultimate metabolic pathway for estrone sulfate follows the definitive two-step metabolism of estrone. Step one involves either the formation of catecholestrogens by A ring metabolism, or the formation of estriol via D ring metabolism. Step two involves the formation of sulfate or glucuronide conjugates with the products of step one metabolism, which, in turn, are then excreted in the urine and to a lesser extent bile.[23] Estradiol, after conversion to estrone, is definitively metabolized by this pathway as well. Therefore, the main urinary metabolites of estrone and 17β-estradiol include the glucuronide and sulfate conjugates of estriol, 2-hydroxyestrone, estrone, 16-hydroxyestrone, and 17β-estradiol. Approximately 20 other minor metabolites representing products of permutations of the major metabolic pathways are excreted in the urine.[49]

A small percentage of estrogens secreted into the bile are not reabsorbed from the GI tract via the enterohepatic circulation. They account for the small amount of estrogenic substances excreted in the faeces.

Thus, the liver has a tremendous influence on the metabolism of any circulating estrogen. The converse is also true. Estrogens, to varying degrees, can influence liver function. Orally administered CEE are no exception. Firstly, CEE, like other orally administered estrogens, increase biliary cholesterol concentration, potentially leading to an increased risk of symptomatic gallstone formation.[50,51] This is not just a theoretical risk but has been clinically realized because oral ERT is associated with an increased risk of cholelithiasis. Secondly, and probably more clinically important, is the ability of estrogens to induce an increased production (overproduction) of hepatic proteins and globulins. A nonexhaustive list of these inducible hepatic proteins and globulins includes renin substrate (angiotensinogen), thyroid-binding globulin (TBG), sex hormone-binding globulin (SHBG), cortisol-binding globulin (CBG), hemostatic coagulation factors, transferrin, ceruloplasmin and pregnancy zone protein (PZP).[52] Of these proteins and globulins, changes in SHBG appear to be the most sensitive marker of estrogenic activity and can be used to compare the relative hepatic effects of various oral estrogen preparations.

Fortunately, most estrogens commonly prescribed as oral ERT, including CEE, are used in doses which do not result in clinically relevant sequelae due to enhanced hepatic protein and globulin induction. Additionally, it must be noted that not all estrogenic modulation of hepatic function results in potentially negative effects. For example, certain orally administered estrogens have been found to produce 'favorable' changes in serum lipid and lipoprotein profiles. These changes are thought to be partially responsible for a reduction in the risk of certain cardiovascular diseases. This topic, a major subject in itself, will is discussed in detail in chapter 55.

The potency of equilin has been stated above; however, the potency of composite CEE, absolute and relative to other oral ERT preparations, has also been determined in several assays. Absolute potency data include gonadotropin suppression of FSH to 55% below baseline values by daily administration of 0.625 mg.[53] A threshold dose of 0.3 mg CEE is required to produce a significant change in the urinary calcium/creatinine ratio from baseline menopausal values.[54] Finally, doses of at least 0.625 mg are required to change the maturation index of a vaginal smear significantly.[53,55] As a general statement, CEE potencies relative to other commonly used estrogens as determined by human biologic endpoints are:

estradiol 5 mg = DES 5 mg = CEE 3.75 mg = mestranol 0.08 mg = ethinyl estradiol 0.05 mg.[56]

Esterified estrogens

Esterified estrogens, like CEE, consist of a mixture of sodium salts of the sulfate esters of the naturally occurring estrogens excreted by pregnant mares. The principal difference between esterified estrogen and CEE preparations is the percentage of their two major components, estrone sulfate and equilin sulfate. These two principal components must occur in a combination which represents at least 90% of the total estrogenic content of the preparations.[57] Thus, no more than 10% of the estrogenic content is comprised of other forms of estrogen. Relative to CEE, esterified estrogens contain a smaller percentage of the B ring unsaturated or 'equine' estrogens. These estrogens can be derived from natural sources (equine urine) or can be synthesized. Esterified estrogens are a white amorphous powder and are water soluble.[57]

After oral administration, near complete GI absorption occurs. Esterified estrogens share very similar pharmacokinetics to those described previously for CEE. Metabolism occurs primarily in the liver where sulfate and glucuronide conjugates are produced. A significant proportion of these substances is excreted in the urine. A smaller percentage is secreted into the bile from where enterohepatic recycling takes place. An even smaller percentage of the estrogens pass through the lower GI tract to be excreted in the stool. For relative potencies, please refer to the previous discussion on estrone sulfate and equilin sulfate.

Estropipate has also been called piperazine estrone sulfate. In this preparation, the estrone is rendered soluble by the addition of a sulfate group: the further addition of a piperazine molecule increases stability.

Estrone is a naturally occurring estrogen which differs from estradiol only in the substitution of a keto group for a hydroxyl group at the carbon 17 (C-17) position. The sulfate group conjugated to the 3OH (hydroxy) position on the A ring imparts water solubility to the otherwise water insoluble estrone. The piperazine molecule is pharmacologically inert but aids in buffering and stabilizing the sulfated estrogen. Estropipate has a molecular weight of 436.56 and the chemical name is Estra-1,3,5,(10)-triene-17-one,3-(sulfooxy)-, compound with piperazine (1:1). Estropipate 0.75 mg is equal molar to 0.625 mg estrone sulfate.[58]

GI absorption of estropipate is good after oral administration. Extensive hepatic metabolism takes place as already discussed for the estrone sulfate component of CEE. Estropipate 2.5 mg levels of 16 ng/mL estrone sulfate and 300 pg/mL estradiol sulfate produces 4 hours later. Peak levels of 300 pg/mL estrone and 60 pg/mL estradiol are seen at 6 and 12 hours respectively.[59] The serum estrogen profile after administration of 2.5 mg estropipate is shown in Figure 51.1.

Mean serum estrogen profiles after administration of lower doses of oral estropipate are shown in Table 51.2. As with conjugated equine estrogens, administration of estropipate results in high circulating levels of estrone sulfate which is largely bound to albumin. This results in the formation of a large, hormonally inert reservoir of an estradiol precursor. From this precursor pool, the liver, through estrone/estradiol interconversion, has the ability to maintain steady, sustained plasma levels of estradiol. Much of the biologic effect of estropipate is thought to be mediated through this estradiol. Ultimate metabolism of estropipate is similar to that previously described in detail for the estrone sulfate component of CEE, with excretion of sulfated and glucuronidated metabolites in the urine and, to a lesser extent, the stool.

The potency of estropipate, relative to other estrogens, is best depicted in Table 51.1, where serum

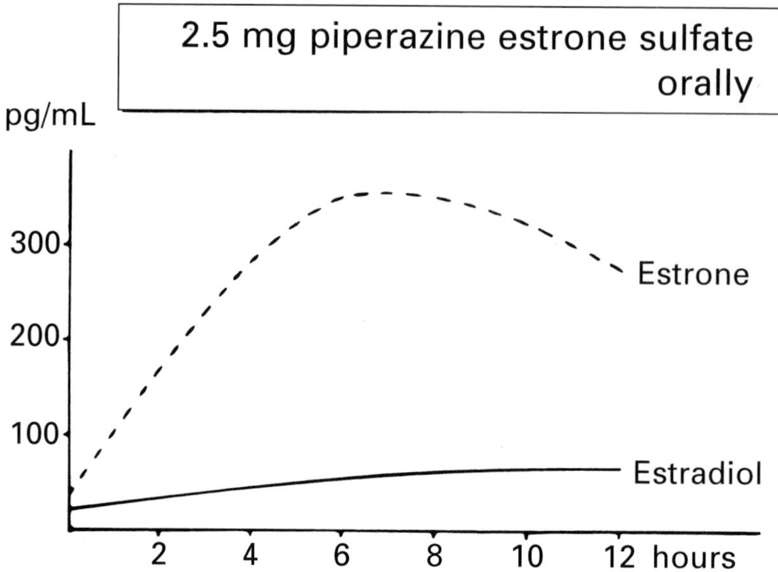

Fig. 51.1 Serum concentrations of estrone and estradiol after oral administration of estrone sulfate.

Table 51.2 Relative potency estimated according to four specific parameters of estrogenicity.

Estrogen Preparation	Serum FSH	Serum CBG-BC	Serum SHBG-BC	Serum angiotensinogen
Estropipate	1.1	1.0	1.0	1.0
Micronized estradiol	1.3	1.9	1.0	0.7
Conjugated estrogens	1.4	2.5	3.2	3.5
DES	3.8	70	28	13
Ethinyl estradiol	(80–200)[a]	(1000)[a]	614	232

[a]Estimated in the absence of parallelism. From Lobo RA et al 1983 Obstetrics and Gynecology 62: 94–98

FSH suppression studies indicate relative potencies of estropipate, estradiol, CEE, DES and ethinyl estradiol to be 1.1, 1.3, 1.4, 3.8 and 80–200, respectively. In general, the hepatic protein induction potency of estropipate is similar to estradiol, less than CEE and significantly less than DES and ethinyl estradiol.[60]

Estriol

Estriol is a naturally occurring estrogenic steroid hormone. Unlike estrone, estriol cannot be converted to estradiol, the usual mediator of estrogenic activity for the naturally-occurring estrogens used in ERT. Therefore, estriol must exert estrogenic activity in its own native form. The relative lack of potency of estriol is due both to rapid metabolism and the short duration of binding to the estrogen receptor.[52]

Orally ingested estriol is rapidly metabolized in the GI tract. Eighty to ninety percent is conjugated to glucuronides which are rapidly excreted. The remaining 10–20% undergoes conjugation to sulfates, which can circulate for longer periods. Of the total estriol dose administered, only 1–2% enters the peripheral circulation unchanged.[23] The half-life of estriol is 9–10 hours, much of which may be due to enterohepatic circulation.[23] Coadministration of food tends to enhance the potency of estriol so there may be some prudence to taking the dose at night to avoid any per dose enhancement of therapeutic effect.[61] Oral administration of estriol does not change the plasma profiles of the other major estrogens seen in postmenopausal women. For example, oral administration of 10 mg estriol daily produced no detectable increase over baseline in the serum values of estrone, estrone sulfate, estradiol, estradiol sulfate or estriol. Only increases in serum estriol sulfate, which is not biologically active, were seen.[62]

Estriol, when given in low and undivided daily doses, does not appear to induce hepatic protein synthesis[63] or endometrial proliferation.[64,65] Although estriol has been used with some success for the treatment of vasomotor symptoms,[66] it may not prevent hypoestrogenic bone loss.[67] As stated earlier, estriol exhibits the shortest binding time to the estrogen receptor of any of the naturally occurring estrogens.[68] That does not mean, however, that estriol is without estrogenic activity. When given orally, suppression of postmenopausal gonadotropin levels was significantly less with estriol than with either piperazine estrone sulfate or estradiol valerate — but suppression still occurred and persisted for seven days after treatment was discontinued.[69] Therefore, although less potent than other naturally occurring estrogens, if given in high and divided daily doses over time, the estrogenic effect of estriol can be substantial.[70]

Ethinyl estradiol

Ethinyl estradiol is a synthetic estrogenic steroid. It has 18 carbon atoms and differs from naturally occurring estradiol by the addition of an acetylene group at carbon 17 (C-17).

Ethinyl estradiol is water insoluble, but is soluble in alcohol and vegetable oils.[17] The C-17 acetylene group conveys extremely potent oral estrogenic activity to the compound. This same group also imparts significant pituitary inhibiting activity, which partially explains why ethinyl estradiol is so popular in combination oral contraceptive preparations.[71]

Ethinyl estradiol has at least 15–20 times the potency of orally administered estradiol,[16] and in some assay systems can be much more potent. To understand the relative potency of ethinyl estradiol better (whereby potency is reduced), reference to the basic metabolism of estradiol is needed. Estradiol metabolism involves a reversible oxidation/reduction reaction occurring at C-17, which permits interconversion of estradiol and estrone. The enzyme responsible is 17β-estradiol dehydrogenase. Further metabolism at the C-3 position leads to sulfation or glucuronidation, which prepares the steroid for excretion. The addition of the acetylene group at C-17 means that ethinyl estradiol is not a good substrate for 17β-estradiol dehydrogenase and so it is resistant to rapid D ring metabolism. Therefore its relative potency is enhanced. Essentially the same estrogenic activity is seen whether ethinyl estradiol is administered orally or parenterally.[17]

After oral administration, ethinyl estradiol absorption in the GI tract is nearly complete. Despite the relative resistance to D ring metabolism imparted by the addition of the acetylene group at C-17, significant hepatic and intestinal metabolism still occurs at other sites in the molecule. In fact, greater than 50% of absorbed ethinyl estradiol may be partially metabolized even before the systemic circulation is reached. Bioavailability of ethinyl estradiol in the peripheral circulation is about 40–50%[71] in one series and almost 60% in another.[72]

Peak serum levels of ethinyl estradiol occur within 1–2 hours of ingestion.[71] A single oral dose of 70 μg ethinyl estradiol was observed to reach an average peak serum level of 174 ng/dL in a study by one investigator.[71] Coadministration of drugs such as ascorbic acid that compete with ethinyl estradiol for intestinal sulfation tend to raise serum levels of circulating free ethinyl estradiol.[73] The drug circulates bound largely (95%) to albumin and minimally to SHBG.[74] Primary storage reservoirs of ethinyl estradiol include the myometrium and fat tissues.[22] The principal product of first-pass hepatic metabolism is ethinyl estradiol-3-sulfate. The ethinyl estradiol to ethinyl estradiol-3-sulfate ratio is usually between 6:1 and 18:1.[73] These ratios are suggestive of significant first-pass metabolism.

It was initially hypothesized that ethinyl estradiol sulfate, like other estrogen sulfates, represented a circulating reservoir of an ethinyl estradiol precursor. This theory, however, is not supported by experimental evidence. Only 13.7% of i.v. administered ethinyl estradiol-3-sulfate and 3.4% of i.v. administered ethinyl estradiol-17-sulfate are converted to ethinyl estradiol. In addition, the observed half-life of ethinyl estradiol sulfates is not significantly different to that of ethinyl estradiol. Together, these data do not suggest a significant 'reservoir' role for ethinyl estradiol sulfates.[75]

The elimination half-life of ethinyl estradiol is 13–27 hours.[71] Ultimately, a majority of the ingested drug, or its intermediate metabolites, undergoes hepatic glucuronide or sulfate conjugation and is excreted in the urine or secreted into the bile. The portion not resorbed by enterohepatic recycling is excreted in the feces.

Seventy per cent of all urinary metabolites of ethinyl estradiol are excreted as glucuronides and 18% are excreted as sulfoconjugates.[76] Drugs which have been shown to enhance or inhibit the activity of the hepatic enzyme cytochrome P-450 IIIA4 will increase or

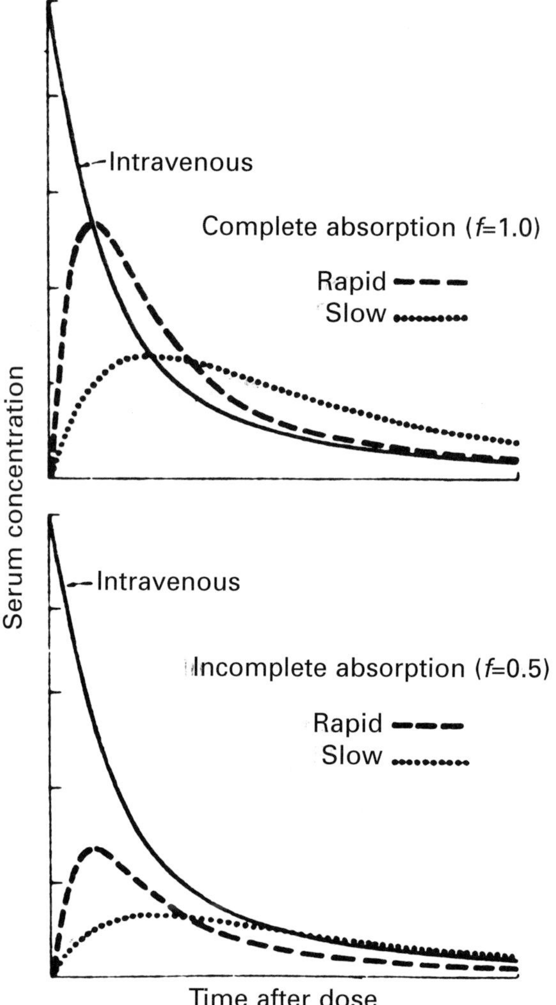

Fig. 51.2 Serum concentrations of drugs after i.v. and oral administration.

decrease ethinyl estradiol metabolism respectively.[77] Although the basic metabolic pathways remain constant, data from pharmacokinetic studies suggest that there is a marked inter- and intraindividual variation in the metabolism of ethinyl estradiol. This may partially explain the seemingly large discrepancies in the literature reporting various pharmacokinetic parameters.

Ethinyl estradiol is a very potent inducer of hepatic protein synthesis and the minimum dose is 5 μg/day.[78] Not all of this effect is due to the classic first-pass metabolism because vaginal administration of ethinyl estradiol also produces significant hepatic induction.[79]

Although approved indications include treatment of vasomotor symptoms and hypogonadism, concerns about the potent hepatic effects of ethinyl estradiol have made its use in postmenopausal oral estrogen replacement therapy uncommon.

Mestranol

Mestranol is the 3-methyl ether derivative of ethinyl estradiol. *In vivo* studies have demonstrated that mestranol does not have any inherent estrogenic activity as it does not bind to the estrogen receptor.[80] Rather, mestranol is a prodrug which is metabolized to, and exerts its estrogenic effects as, ethinyl estradiol. After oral administration, mestranol is well absorbed through the GI tract. Conversion of mestranol to ethinyl estradiol occurs via O-demethylation in the bowel wall and liver prior to entry into the systemic circulation.[81] Peak serum levels of ethinyl estradiol from an oral mestranol dose have been shown to occur 1.7–2.0 hours after ingestion. Similar peak serum ethinyl estradiol levels averaging 175 pg/mL are seen after either 100 μg mestranol or 70 μg ethinyl estradiol. Thus pharmacokinetically, mestranol is 70% as bioavailable as ethinyl estradiol.[71] Doses considered pharmacokinetically equivalent, however, do not automatically imply pharmacodynamic equivalence. In addition, the bioactivity of mestranol relative to ethinyl estradiol varies depending on the endpoint of the assay chosen. For example, Goldzieher and coworkers,[82–86] evaluating endpoints such as endometrial response, gonadotropin suppression, changes in plasma cortisol and testosterone, CBG, and effects on carbohydrate and lipid metabolism, found essentially bioequivalence between mestranol and ethinyl estradiol. In contrast, hepatic protein synthesis assays suggest a more modest mestranol potency of 50% that of ethinyl estradiol.[87] Well described but significant inter- and intraindividual variations in responses to doses of mestranol, like those seen with ethinyl estradiol, may partially explain the seemingly large discrepancies in potency parameters.[88]

After conversion to ethinyl estradiol, mestranol metabolism follows pathways similar to those of ethinyl estradiol. Also, it is to be expected that mestranol exhibits the same potent hepatic induction of protein synthesis as is seen with ethinyl estradiol. For this reason, mestranol, like its active metabolite ethinyl estradiol, is not widely used for postmenopausal estrogen replacement therapy.

Other estrogens

There are other oral estrogens which are used infrequently. These include quinestrol,[17] which has lipophilic storage and only requires up to once a week dosing; diethylstilbestrol,[8,17] a nonsteroidal estrogen which is rarely used today; and chlorotrianisene,[16] another synthetic nonsteroidal estrogen chemically akin to diethylstilbestrol.

ATTRIBUTES OF ORAL ESTROGEN THERAPY

Orally administered estrogenic preparations have been, and for the near future will probably continue to be, the mainstay of treatment for hypoestrogenism associated with the menopause and also for contraceptive purposes. Moreover, there are numerous and varied oral preparations from which the clinician may choose. Other routes of administration for estrogens and these include the transdermal, and the transvaginal using rings, creams and suppositories are available.

The advantages of oral estrogen therapy may be summarized as including:

- Many available agents which have a 'time proven' safety and efficacy
- Oral estrogens have been shown to reduce the risk of cardiovascular disease and to retard hypoestrogenic osteoporosis
- These agents are highly effective in the treatment of vasomotor and vulvovaginal symptoms associated with the menopause
- The cost of oral estrogen therapy is usually equal to or less than alternative modes/routes of therapy.

Disadvantages of oral estrogens include:

- A daily dosing requirement which potentially may reduce compliance or continuance
- Oral administration of naturally occurring estrogens (estriol excepted) yields a nonphysiologic elevation of the E_1 to E_2 ratio
- Oral estrogens, to greater or less degrees, all influence hepatic protein synthesis
- Therapy can result in an increased risk of symptomatic gallbladder disease.

Finally, despite the complex and rapidly changing economics of health care systems, in some countries, exemplified by the USA, one thing remains certain: ultimately, health care goods and services must be paid for. Therefore, the cost of prescription medication is as important to the patient fully covered by a 'prescription plan' as it is to the patient who pays 'out of pocket'. As a group, orally administered estrogen preparations compare favorably in cost to parenterally administered forms of therapy. After inquiry of local retail pharmacies, the clinician should discover that even conservative estimates place the cost of oral estrogen at 30% below the cost of transdermal administration. Given year-round for the remainder of a postmenopausal patient's life, the cost differential between these two forms of hormone replacement therapy may be considerable.

CONTINUANCE

The issues of physician education for patients and prescription and patient continuance with hormonal therapy also need to be addressed. To achieve optimal therapy, as with any drug regimen, both the physician and the patient must accept the therapy. Both need accurate information to make an informed decision and, where possible, these data need to be individualized to optimize each patient's benefits and unique risks and side effects with that particular preparation.

Women are not generally as well informed about menopause as we may think. A recent Harris Survey indicated that only half of working women of menopausal age were able to name any long-term health concerns associated with menopause. Of those who could, 27% named osteoporosis, and only 6% mentioned heart disease.[89] Similar data come from a recently published survey by the American College of Obstetricians and Gynecologists. These showed that a slim majority did know about osteoporosis, but only 1 in 40 knew of an increased risk of heart disease. Importantly, less than one out of three were satisfied with the information provided by their physicians.[89] A recent study by the North American Menopause Society demonstrated that only 44% of women aged 45–60 were satisfied with the information they received about menopause.[90] Physicians were also much more likely to discuss short-term effects of hormonal therapy, such as hot flushes, rather than to provide information regarding long-term health risks such as osteoporosis and heart disease. In addressing treatment, 84% of physicians focused only on hormonal treatment, while only 3% discussed exercise and 2% proper nutrition. Other lifestyle issues were mentioned even less frequently.[90]

Other data from the USA suggest that even when further education is provided, fewer than 20% of postmenopausal women have ever had hormonal therapy prescribed, only 40% or less of those for whom it is prescribed will continue it for more than a year and that overall less than 70% for whom it is prescribed take it according to instructions. Fully 30% for whom prescriptions are written never fill them.[91]

On the other hand, there are data to suggest that not all physicians are fully aware of the role of hormonal therapy for such patients. In one US study, only 13.7% of a group of over 9000 older US women were prescribed estrogen, and those were women who tended to be better educated, of higher socioeconomic class and to have undergone hysterectomy.[92] Physician awareness of the benefits of HRT for osteoporosis and heart disease is particularly lacking among generalists. Although recent evidence indicates that some HRT preparations increase the occurrence of venous thromboembolism, many physicians are unaware of the continued cardiovascular benefits in smokers, hypertensive and diabetic women and patients with coronary artery disease. All of these previously accepted contraindications are now regarded as *indications*.

Patients seem misinformed regarding the occurrence of breast tenderness and the risks of breast cancer and very clearly do not desire to have uterine bleeding. Some even believe such treatment has restored their fertility.[93]

Coope and Marsh have recently published data to show that patient compliance can be markedly improved by educational programs that point out the benefits of estrogen and explain the concerns noted above. I believe it is the responsibility of all physicians who care for women to discuss the potential benefits and risks of such therapies fully, and also to try to individualize the risks and benefits. Additionally, information regarding other concerns of this important era in a woman's life should be presented.[94]

Oral estrogen use for replacement of hypoestrogenism or as part of an oral contraceptive pill has become an accepted and widely used therapeutic modality during the past 50 years. Pros and cons exist, but such therapies have endured the test of time, although many pharmacokinetic mechanisms still remain poorly determined. Continuance remains a major factor in their efficacy, but it is my belief that until other routes of administration have been shown to have the same or better efficacy and continuance, oral routes will remain the mainstay of treatment.

REFERENCES

1. Chrobak R 1896 Uber Einverleibung von Eirstockgewebe. Cbl Gyn 20: 521–524
2. Mainzer F 1896 Behandlung amenorrhoischer und kilmakterischer Frauen mit Ovarialsubstanz. Dtsch Med Wochenschr 25: 393–396
3. Mond R 1896 Kurze Mittheilung uber die Behandlung der Beschwerden bei naturlicher oder durch Operation veranlabter Amenorrhoe mit Eierstocksconserven (Ovarin Merck). Munich Med Wechenschr 14: 314–316
4. Kopera H, van Keep PA 1991 Development and present state of hormone replacement therapy. International Journal of Clinical Pharmacology, Therapeutics and Toxicology 29: 412–417
5. Butenandt A 1929 Progynon: a crystalline female sex hormone. Naturwissenschaften 17: 879
6. Geist SH, Spielman F 1932 The therapeutic value of amniotin in the menopause. American Journal of Obstetrics and Gynecology 23: 697
7. Sevringhaus EL 1935 The relief of menopause symptoms by estrogenic preparations. Journal of the American Medical Association 104: 264
8. Dodds EC, Goldberg L, Lawson W, Robinson R 1938 Oestrogenic activity of alkylated stilboestrols. Nature 142: 34
9. Inhoffen HH, Logemann W, Hohlweg W, Serini A 1938 Untersuchungen in der Sexualhormone-Reihe. Ber 71B: 1024–1032
10. Hammond CB, Maxson WS 1986 Estrogen replacement therapy. Clinics in Obstetrics and Gynecology 29: 407
11. Branham WS, Zehr DR, Sheehan DM 1993 Differential sensitivity of rat uterine growth and epithelium hypertrophy to estrogens and antiestrogens. Proceedings of the Society for Experimental Biology and Medicine 203: 297
12. Grant GA, Beall D 1950 Studies on estrogen conjugates. Recent Progress in Hormone Research 5: 307
13. Dorfman RI, Dorfman AS 1953 The assay of estrogens in the chick by oral administration. Endocrinology 53: 301
14. Blohm P, Hammond CB 1996 Oral estrogen replacement. In: Adashi EY, Rock JA, Rosenwaks Z (eds) Reproductive endocrinology, surgery and technology. Lippincott-Raven, Philadelphia, p 1797
15. Stumpf PG 1990 Pharmacokinetics of estrogen. Obstetrics and Gynecology 75: 9S–17S
16. Barnes RB, Lobo RA 1987 Pharmacology of estrogens. In: Mishell DR (ed) Menopause: physiology and pharmacology. Year Book, Chicago, pp 301–315
17. McEvoy GK et al (eds) 1991 American hospital formulary service. American Society of Hospital Pharmacists, Bethesda
18. Krantz JC, Carr CJ 1958 The pharmacologic principles of medical practice. Williams and Wilkins, Baltimore, p 1049
19. Botella-Llusia J 1973 Endocrinology of Woman. WB Saunders, Philadelphia, p 30
20. Yen SSC, Martin PL, Burnier AM et al 1975 Circulating estradiol, estrone and gonadotropin levels following administration of orally active 17β-estradiol in postmenopausal women. Journal of Clinical Endocrinology and Metabolism 40: 518–521
21. Ryan KJ, Engel LL 1953 Endocrinology 52: 287
22. Lobo RA, Cassidenti DL 1992 Pharmacokinetics of oral 17β-estradiol. Journal of Reproductive Medicine 37: 77–84
23. Kuhl H 1990 Pharmacokinetics of oestrogens and progestogens. Maturitas 12: 171–197
24. Whitaker PG et al 1980 Serum equilin, oestrone and oestradiol levels in postmenopausal women receiving conjugated oestrogens (Premarin). Lancet 1: 14

25. Anderson ABM, Sklovskye A, Sayers L, Steele P, Turnbull A 1978 Comparison of serum oestrogen concentrations in postmenopausal women taking oestrone sulphate and oestradiol. British Medical Journal 1: 140
26. Mashchak CA, Lobo RA, Dozono-Takano R et al 1982 Comparison of pharmacodynamic properties of various estrogen formulations. American Journal of Obstetrics and Gynecology 144: 511–518
27. Archer DF, Fischer LA, Rich D 1992 Estrace versus Premarin for treatment of menopausal symptoms: dosage comparison study. Advances in Therapy 9: 21–31
28. Lyman GW, Johnson RN 1982 Assay for conjugated estrogens in tablets using fused-silica capillary gas chromatography. Journal of Chromatography 234: 234–239
29. Murad F, Kuret JA 1990 Estrogens and progestins. In: Gilman AG, Rall TW, Nies AS, Taylor P (eds) The pharmacological basis of therapeutics. McGraw-Hill, New York, pp 1384–1412
30. The United States Pharmacopeia 1975 19th revision. Mack Publishing, Easton, PA, pp 181–182
31. Fourth Supplement to the USP XIX and NF XIV 1978 (January 31). Mack Publishing, Easton, PA, pp 74–75
32. Adams WP, Hasegawa J, Johnson RN, Haring RC 1979 Conjugated estrogens bioinequivalence: comparison of four products in postmenopausal women. Journal of Pharmaceutical Sciences 68: 986–991
33. Bhavnai BR, Woolever CA, Wallace D, Pan CC 1989 Absorption and metabolism of [^{3}H]equilin-[^{35}S]sulfate and [^{3}H]equilin sulfate following oral and intravenous administration in normal postmenopausal women and men. Journal of Clinical Endocrinology and Metabolism 68: 757–765
34. Bhavani BR, Woolever CA, Benoit H, Wong T 1983 Pharmacokinetics of equilin and equilin sulfate in normal postmenopausal women and men. Journal of Clinical Endocrinology and Metabolism 56: 1048
35. Pan CC, Woolever CA, Bhavnai BR 1985 Transport of equine estrogens: binding of conjugated and unconjugated equine estrogens with human serum proteins. Journal of Clinical Endocrinology and Metabolism 61: 499
36. Rosenthal HE, Pietrzak E, Slaunwhite WR, Sandberg AA 1972 Binding of estrone sulfate in human plasma. Journal of Clinical Endocrinology and Metabolism 34: 806
37. Rosenthal HE, Ludwig GA, Pietrzak E, Sandberg AA 1975 Binding of the sulfate of estradiol-17β to human serum albumin and plasma. Journal of Clinical Endocrinology and Metabolism 41: 1144
38. Longcope C 1972 The metabolism of estrone sulfate in normal males. Journal of Clinical Endocrinology and Metabolism 34: 113
39. Wang DY, Bulbrook RD, Sneeden A, Hamilton T 1967 The metabolic clearance rates of dehydroepiandrosterone, testosterone and their sulfate esters in man, rat and rabbit. Journal of Endocrinology 38: 307
40. Bhavnani BR 1988 The saga of the ring B unsaturated equine estrogens. Endocrine Reviews 9: 396–416
41. Bhavnani BR, Sarda R, Woolever CA 1981 Radioimmunoassay of plasma equilin and estrone in post-menopausal women after administration of Premarin. Journal of Clinical Endocrinology and Metabolism 52: 741
42. Powers MS, Schenkel L, Darley PE, Good WR, Balestra JC, Place VA 1985 Pharmacokinetics and pharmacodynamics of transdermal dosage forms of 17β-estradiol: comparison with conventional oral estrogens used for hormone replacement. American Journal of Obstetrics and Gynecology 152: 1099–1106
43. Dorfman RI, Dorfman AS 1954 Estrogen assays using the rat uterus. Endocrinology 55: 65
44. Lobo RL, Nguyen HN, Eggena P, Brenner PF 1988 Biologic effects of equilin sulfate in postmenopausal women. Fertility and Sterility 49: 234
45. Lobo RA 1987 Absorption and metabolic effects of different types of estrogens and progestogens. The menopause. Obstetric and Gynecology Clinics of North America 14: 143–167
46. Longcope C, Williams KIH 1974 The metabolism of estrogens in normal women after pulse injections of [^{3}H]-estradiol and [^{3}H]-estrone. Journal of Clinical Endocrinology and Metabolism 38: 602–607
47. Chapman CR 1981 Absorption and metabolism of steroid prodrugs. PhD thesis, University of Liverpool
48. Johnson RN, Maasserano RP, Kho BT, Adams WP 1978 Steady-state urinary excretion method for determining bioequivalence of conjugated estrogen products. Journal of Pharmaceutical Sciences 67: 1218–1224
49. Bolt H 1979 Metabolism of estrogens — natural and synthetic. Pharmacological Therapeutics 4: 155–181
50. Boston Collaborative Drug Project, Boston University Medical Center 1974 Surgically confirmed gallbladder disease, venous thromboembolism, and breast tumors in relation to postmenopausal estrogen therapy. New England Journal of Medicine 290: 15
51. Petitti DB, Sydney S, Perlman JA 1988 Increased risk of cholecystectomy in users of supplemental estrogen. Gastroenterology 94: 91–95
52. L'Hermite M 1990 Risks of estrogen and progestogens. Maturitas 12: 215–246
53. Schiff I 1980 Effects of conjugated estrogens on gonadotropins. Fertility and Sterility 33: 333
54. Fishman J, Martucci C 1978 Differential biological activity of estradiol metabolites. Pediatrics 62: 1128
55. Geola FL, Frumar AM, Tataryn IV et al 1980 Biological effects of various doses of conjugated equine estrogens in postmenopausal women. Journal of Clinical Endocrinology and Metabolism 51: 620–625
56. Martinez-Manatou J, Rudel HW 1969 Antiovulatory activity of several synthetic and natural estrogens. In: Greenblatt RB (ed) Ovulation 243
57. Solvay data on file, 1993
58. Ogen packet insert, Abbott Laboratories
59. Aedo AR, Landgren BM, Diczfalusy E 1990 Pharmacokinetics and biotransformation of orally administered oestrone sulphate and oestradiol valerate in postmenopausal women. Maturitas 12(4): 333–343
60. Luotola H, Pyorala T, Loikkanen M 1986 Effects of natural oestrogen/progestogen substitution therapy on carbohydrate and lipid metabolism in postmenopausal women. Maturitus 8: 245–253
61. Englund D, Heimer G, Johansson EDB 1984 Influence of food on oestriol blood levels. Maturitas 6: 71–75

62. Aedo AR, Sunden M, Landgren BM, Diczfalusy E 1989 Effect of orally administered oestrogens on circulating oestrogen profiles in postmenopausal women. Maturitas 11: 159–168
63. Bergink EW, Crona N, Dahlgran E, Samsioe G 1981 Effect of oestriol, oestradiol valerate and ethinyloestradiol on serum proteins in oestrogen-deficient women. Maturitas 3: 241–247
64. Myhre E 1978 Endometrial response to different estrogens. Frontiers of Hormone Research 126–144
65. Schneider HPG 1982 Oestriol and the menopause: clinical results from a prospective study. In: Fioretti P, Martini L, Melis GB, Yen SSC (eds) The menopause: clinical, endocrinological and pathophysiological aspects. Academic Press, New York, pp 523–533
66. Lauritzen C 1987 Results of a 5-year prospective study of estriol succinate treatment in patients with climacteric complaints. Hormone and Metabolism Research 19: 579–584
67. Lindsay R, Hart DM, MacLean A, Garwood J, Clarck AC, Kraszewski A 1979 Bone loss during oestriol therapy in postmenopausal women. Maturitas 1: 279–285
68. Clark JH, Hardin JW, McCormack SC 1978 Estrogen receptor binding and growth of the reproductive tract. Pediatrics 62
69. Aedo AR, Le Donne M, Landgren BM, Diczfalusy E 1989 Effect of orally administered oestrogens on gonadotropin levels in postmenopausal women. Maturitas 11: 147–157
70. Anderson JN, Peck EJ, Clark JH 1975 Estrogen-induced uterine responses and growth: relationship to receptor estrogen-binding by uterine nuclei. Endocrinology 96: 160
71. Goldzieher JW, Brody SA 1990 Pharmacokinetics of ethinyl estradiol and mestranol. American Journal of Obstetrics and Gynecology 163: 2114–2119
72. Orme M, Back DJ, Ward S, Green S 1991 The pharmacokinetics of ethinyl estradiol in the presence and absence of gestodene and desogestrel. Contraception 43: 305–316
73. Back DJ, Madden S, Orme M 1990 Gastrointestinal metabolism of contraceptive steroids. American Journal of Obstetrics and Gynecology 163: 2138–2145
74. Fotherby K 1990 Interactions with oral contraceptives. American Journal of Obstetrics and Gynecology 163: 2153–2159
75. Goldzieher JW, Mileikowsky G, Newburger J et al 1988 Human pharmacokinetics of ethynyl estradiol 3-sulfate and 17-sulfate. Steroids 51: 63–79
76. Williams MC, Goldzieher JW 1980 Chromatographic patterns of urinary ethynyl estrogen metabolites in various populations. Steroids 36: 255–282
77. Guengerich FP 1990 Inhibition of oral contraceptive steroid-metabolizing enzymes by steroids and drugs. American Journal of Obstetrics and Gynecology 163: 2159–2163
78. Mandel FP, Geoia FL, Lu KH et al 1982 Biologic effects of various doses of ethinyl estradiol in postmenopausal women. Obstetrics and Gynecology 59: 673–679
79. Goebelsmann U, Mashchak CA, Mishell DR 1985 Comparison of hepatic impact of oral and vaginal administration of ethinyl estradiol. American Journal of Obstetrics and Gynecology 151: 868–877
80. Kappus H, Bolt HM, Remmer H 1973 Affinity of ethynylestradiol and mestranol for the uterine estrogen receptor and for the microsomal mixed function oxidase of the liver. Journal of Steroid Biochemistry 4: 121–128
81. Bolt HM, Bolt WH 1974 Pharmacokinetics of mestranol in man in relation to its oestrogenic activity. European Journal of Clinical Pharmacology 17: 295–305
82. Goldzieher JW, de la Pena A, Chenault CB, Cervantes A 1975 Comparative studies of the ethynyl estrogens used in oral contraceptives III. Effect on plasma gonadotropins. American Journal of Obstetrics and Gynecology 122: 625–636
83. Goldzieher JW, Chenault CB, de la Pena A, Dozier TS, Kraemer DC 1977 Comparative studies of the ethynyl estrogens used in oral contraceptives: effects with and without progestational agents on plasma cortisol and cortisol binding in humans, baboons and beagles. Fertility and Sterility 28: 1182–1190
84. Goldzieher JW, Chenault CB, de la Pena A, Dozier TS, Kraemer DC 1978 Comparative studies of the ethynyl estrogens used in oral contraceptives: effects with and without progestational agents on plasma androstenedione, testosterone and testosterone binding in humans, baboons and beagles. Fertility and Sterility 29: 388–396
85. Goldzieher JW, Chenault CB, de la Pena A, Dozier TS, Kraemer DC 1978 Comparative studies of the ethynyl estrogens used in oral contraceptives VI. Effects with and without progestational agents on carbohydrate metabolism in humans, baboons and beagles. Fertility and Sterility 30: 146–153
86. Goldzieher JW, Chenault CB, de la Pena A, Dozier TS, Kraemer DC 1978 Comparative studies of the ethynyl estrogens used in oral contraceptives VII. Effects with and without progestational agents on ultracentrifugally fractionated plasma lipoproteins in humans, baboons and beagles. Fertility and Sterility 30: 522–533
87. Teter J, Stupnicki R 1971 A comparative study of the estrogenic potential of two synthetic estrogens (mestranol and ethinylestradiol). Acta Cytologica 15: 167–170
88. Back DJ, Breckenridge AM, Crawford FE, Maciver M, Orme ML'E, Rowe PH 1981 Interindividual variation and drug interactions with hormonal steroid contraceptives. Drugs 21: 46–61
89. Andrews WC 1995 The transitional years and beyond. Obstetrics and Gynecology 85: 1–5
90. Utian WH, Schiff I 1994 North American menopause society — Gallup survey on women's knowledge, information sources and attitudes to menopause and hormone replacement therapy. Menopause, Journal of the North American Menopause Society 1: 39–48
91. Ravmiker VA 1992 Compliance with hormone replacement therapy. Are women receiving the full impact of hormone replacement therapy's preventive health benefits? Women's Health Issues 2: 75–82
92. Cavley JA, Cummings SR, Black DM et al 1990 Prevalence and determinants of estrogen replacement therapy in elderly women. American Journal of Obstetrics and Gynecology 163: 1438–1444
93. Hammond CB 1994 Women's concerns with hormone replacement therapy — compliance issues. Fertility and Sterility 62(S2): 157S–160S
94. Coope J, Marsh J 1992 Can we improve compliance with longterm ERT? Maturitas 15: 141–154

52. General principles of administration of hormone replacement therapy: indications and contraindications, routes of administration, treatment schedules

M.I. Whitehead

Introduction

Terminology

The term 'hormone replacement therapy' (HRT) is widely used throughout Europe, Asia and Australasia to describe the administration of estrogens, with or without a progestogen, to peri and postmenopausal women. In North America, estrogens are still widely prescribed without a progestogen, most probably because of the high numbers of hysterectomies which are performed. Administration of estrogen by itself is termed ERT (estrogen replacement therapy).

The use of the word 'replacement' implies that the recipient will be estrogen deficient. A diagnosis of hypo-estrogenism can usually be made clinically, without recourse to endocrine investigations, in postmenopausal women and those with primary amenorrhea or prolonged secondary amenorrhea. However, the perimenopausal woman experiencing intermittent ovarian activity which results in an irregular cycle length, month by month, presents diagnostic difficulties and therapeutic challenges which are considered further below.

TO PRESCRIBE OR NOT TO PRESCRIBE?

Before considering this question, it is important to remember that no previous generation has been forced to address this issue. This is because, until relatively recently, most women at death were either still premenopausal or had survived but few years into the postmenopausal state. In the United Kingdom, mean female life expectancy was 48 years in 1900 and had risen to 60 years by 1933. The demographic changes which face us over the next decades are considered elsewhere in this book (see ch. 47). Additionally, the first estrogens were not isolated until the late 1920s and synthetic forms were developed shortly thereafter (see ch. 51). Oral HRT, as we know it today, has been available for 45–50 years whereas percutaneous (gel) and transdermal (patch) delivery systems have been developed and introduced into clinical practice only within the last 20 years. Importantly, epidemiological data on common diseases, and how their morbidity and mortality might be influenced by estrogen lack and by use of HRT, have become available only over the last 10–15 years. Even now, our knowledge of the precise nature of many of these relationships remains incomplete.

Attitudes to the use of HRT range from those who regard the menopause as a God-given event to be endured stoically, to those who regard it as an endocrine deficiency state which affects all women and which should be treated by long-term and almost universal use of estrogens.[1] In this author's opinion these extremes are fuelled largely by the lay press. HRT is extolled one week because of benefit and then decried the subsequent week because of risk. Because 25–50% of women use the lay press as their principal source of information about menopause and HRT, it is hardly surprising that so many women are confused by the conflicting evidence, especially when research results are inaccurately quoted by these publications. The recent debacle over the publication of the results of the Collaborative Group on Hormonal Factors in Breast Cancer[2] is an excellent example. To scoop the competition, the *Sunday Times* published a story (October 5th, 1997) from a 'leaked' manuscript before the results were published by the *Lancet*. Unfortunately, the *Sunday Times* got the risk of breast cancer with use of HRT wrong — by a factor of 100-fold! The story in the *Sunday Times* appeared on the front page: the subsequent apology, many weeks later, occupied one inch of newsprint in one of the supplements. Further details of this episode have appeared in an editorial in the *Lancet*[3] which commented 'the *Sunday Times* has a huge circulation. The damage to women's confidence in HRT is likely to be severe'. Unfortunately, a recent postal survey[4]

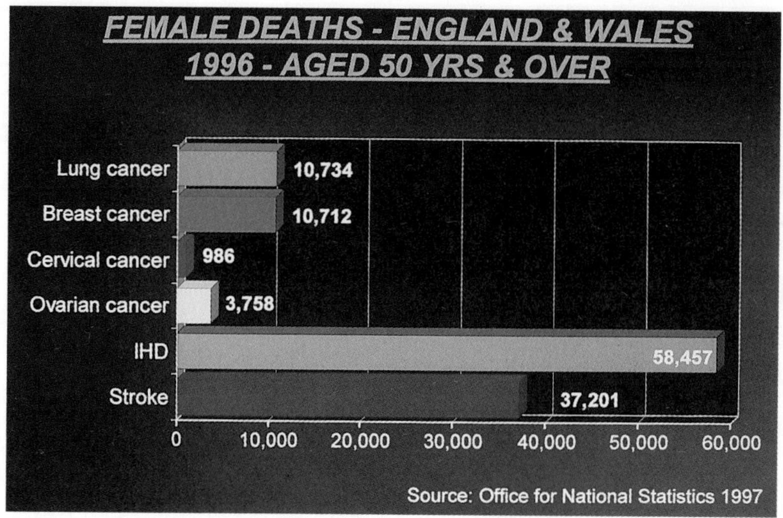

Fig. 52.1 Commonest causes of death in England and Wales in women aged over 50 years. (Source: Office for National Statistics, 1997)

reported that about 50% of women thought that the media provided accurate information on HRT.

Before considering how estrogen lack and estrogen replacement may influence disease morbidity and mortality, it is extremely important that the risk of death from various diseases is put into clear perspective. The commonest causes of death in women aged 50 years and over in England and Wales in 1996 are shown in Figure 52.1. The following should be noted: there were approximately 95 000 deaths from myocardial infarction and cerebrovascular accident, combined. These arterial diseases caused nine times more deaths than breast cancer (10 712 deaths). Additionally, for the first time in England and Wales, more women died from lung cancer (10 734 deaths) than from breast cancer in this age group.

The approach by the editors of this book to the question of whether or not to use HRT has been pragmatic and, hopefully, comprehensive. Each of the next 16 chapters concentrates on a particular target tissue and considers the effects of estrogen withdrawal and of estrogen or progestogen replacement, or both. Generally speaking, estrogens are prescribed either to relieve typical estrogen-deficiency symptoms such as hot flashes, night sweats and/or the symptoms of lower genital tract atrophy; to prevent and treat osteoporosis to reduce the risk of fracture; and to reduce the risk of arterial diseases, especially myocardial infarction, particularly in 'high-risk' groups such as the obese, the hypertensive and those with hypercholesterolemia. Preliminary data also suggest that HRT may reduce the risk of Alzheimer's disease and very preliminary short-term studies suggest a beneficial effect of HRT in women with this diagnosis.

This chapter will provide a detailed review of the administration of HRT to include the benefits and disadvantages of the different delivery systems, and a summary of the different treatment schedules. It will also provide a short resumé of the background to the contraindications and risks covered elsewhere in this book, a discussion of those contraindications and risks not covered elsewhere in this book, and a summary overview of indications for and contraindications and risks of HRT.

ESTROGENS

Philosophy behind the use of estrogens

There are two principal considerations. The first relates to 'replacement' of the estrogen no longer produced by an ovary exhausted of primordial follicles. This is largely scientific and simply requires that a therapeutic serum estrogen concentration be reached with a particular preparation and route of administration. The serum estradiol profile achieved during the reproductive era is *not* mimicked by HRT. Estradiol can be regarded as a by-product of oocyte maturation and reproduction of the peri-ovulatory surge is not required either for symptom relief or for the long-term benefits (skeletal preservation, maintenance of arterial health) in postmenopausal women. Thus, the term hormone *replacement* therapy is, strictly speaking, a misnomer if the premenopausal pattern of estradiol production is used as a comparator.

The second consideration is highly personal and relates to the belief held by the individual patient that the benefits of estrogen outweigh the risks *in her situation*. Numerous factors must be taken into account in this analysis. Many are self-evident and include severity of symptoms and how they impact on the quality of life — bone density and risk of fracture, and risk of arterial disease if HRT is not used — and how these factors change if HRT is taken. Because estrogens are potent sex hormones, use of HRT can never be without risk but, such risks, in an ideal situation, should be clearly understood by the patient and must be less than the benefits of treatment in that individual.

There can be no doubt that, at present, women are poorly informed as to the commonest causes of death (Fig. 52.1). In a recent national survey in the UK, less than 3% of women knew that heart disease was the commonest cause of death in women aged over 50 years. Various surveys have also reported that not only do women greatly underestimate their risk of death from heart disease, but they also greatly overestimate the risk of death from breast cancer — and this applies equally to those of lower and higher educational attainments. Perceived risks from breast cancer and heart disease are illustrated in Figure 52.2 (the subjects providing information on these risks were alumni from Standford University, California, USA).

Women should be aware that the estimate of cumulative absolute risk of cause-specific death in white women aged 50–94 years from coronary heart disease is 31%; from breast cancer: 2.8%; from hip fracture: also 2.8%; and from endometrial cancer: 0.7%.

Finally, the presence of risk factors for use of HRT and how they might impact upon the benefit-risk analysis should be explored with each individual patient. Women are often reluctant to use HRT because of complete misconceptions. Why the myth that HRT causes weight gain is perpetuated by the lay press when so many placebo-controlled studies have disproved this is a mystery.[5] Overweight and obese women are particularly prone to this belief.[6]

Other diseases, often familial, which frighten women away from HRT are cervical cancer, breast cancer and venous thrombosis. The foremost appears unrelated to use of HRT. Data on the association between risk of breast cancer and use of HRT in a woman with a relevant family history are contradictory and the recent report from the Collaborative Group on Hormonal Factors in Breast Cancer found no clear relationship in women with a relevant family history.[2] Too few data are available on the risk of venous thrombosis with use of HRT in women with inherited thrombophilias for a risk to be quoted, although

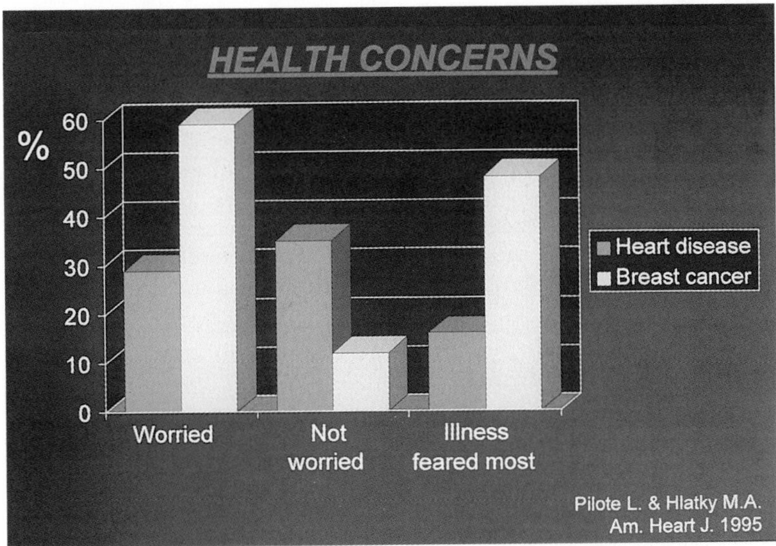

Fig. 52.2 Health concerns of women regarding breast cancer and heart disease. (Adapted from: Pilote L, Hlatky MA 1995 Attitudes of women towards hormone therapy and prevention of heart disease. American Heart Journal 129: 1237–1238)

overall, women on HRT have a significant but small (2–3 fold) increase in risk of venous thrombosis compared with postmenopausal women not on HRT.

As stated at the beginning of this section, no previous generation of middle-aged and more elderly women has been given the opportunity to use HRT sensibly and thereby, perhaps, influence the likelihood of dying from one disease as compared to another. Changing the risk of death will only be widely achieved when women are much better informed, when there is more accurate reporting in the lay media and when medical/nursing attendants provide unbiased and accurate information either by consultation or through other communication devices (videos, leaflets, etc).

Different delivery systems

Before commenting upon the different delivery systems in detail, it should be remembered that the factors influencing absorption, metabolism and excretion of estrogens remain incompletely understood. Furthermore, there is a wide inter-patient variation in the serum levels achieved with the same preparation and route of administration. Most pharmacokinetic data are presented either as means or medians. Scattergrams are seldom used and, thus, the very wide range of values achieved with any estrogen preparation may not be fully appreciated. In clinical practice, failure to relieve typical estrogen deficiency symptoms should lead to an appraisal of the serum estrogen levels achieved with treatment.

Estrogens can be administered through many different routes. These include oral, percutaneous (as gels), transdermal (from patches), parenterally (as implants) and intravaginally as creams, vaginal tablets or from rings. In certain parts of the world (e.g. mainland Europe) injectable forms of estradiol are also available.

Each route of administration has benefits and disadvantages. For oral estrogens, these are summarized in Table 52.1; for gels, in Table 52.2; for patches, in Table 52.3; for implants, in Table 52.4, and for vaginal preparations, in Table 52.5. Logically, the major benefit of the many different routes of administration is that more women will be able to find a form of treatment which is acceptable. However, evidence to support this from prospective studies is lacking (most probably due to the difficulty in designing an appropriate study), but it is well recognized that the introduction of the newer routes of administration, particularly estradiol patches, did not result in large numbers of women on oral therapy changing the route of administration. Quite simply, the numbers of women using HRT increased because many women who had not used HRT started to apply transdermal estradiol. This suggests that women who find oral therapy unacceptable will use an alternative route of administration.

Oral administration (Table 52.1)

Estrogens have been available as tablets for use as HRT for approximately 50 years. Thus, there is a greater clinical and epidemiological experience with this route of administration as compared to the nonoral forms of therapy. This applies particularly to the observational studies of the major benefits (reduction in risk of fracture and arterial disease) and risks (breast cancer and venous thrombosis) of HRT. The majority of these observational data from the USA apply to conjugated equine estrogens (Premarin: Wyeth-Ayerst, Philadelphia, USA), usually given without a progestogen. The majority of European data from long-term observational studies apply to oral estradiol, usually with a progestogen.

As discussed below, there is a surge in serum estrogen values after tablet ingestion. The serum half-life of estradiol and estrone is approximately 4–6 hours and, therefore, to achieve serum values within the therapeutic range (essential for relief of daytime flashes and also nocturnal sweating) a high estrogen dose is required with once daily administration.

Table 52.1 Oral therapy: advantages and disadvantages

Advantages	Disadvantages
• Easy to take • Cheap • Wide choice • Oral progestogen can be co-administered • Elevates HDL and HDL-2 cholesterol	• Daily dosing • High dose required • Variation in absorption • Poor absorption with gastrointestinal dysfunction/post surgery • Alters hepatic protein synthesis • All tablets contain lactose • Elevates or is neutral to triglycerides

Although all estrogen preparations are influenced by enterohepatic recycling, it is probable that the oral route is most influenced by gastrointestinal dysfunction (e.g. malabsorption syndrome; coeliac disease) and by surgery resulting in bowel resection (e.g. Crohn's disease). It is often stated that only oral administration causes nausea: this is untrue. Nausea on initiation of estrogen therapy can occur with any route of administration and is most likely due to a central effect of the rising serum estradiol concentration. Nausea is a common feature of early pregnancy but the estrogen is not administered orally then! Oral progestogens can be co-administered. When combined in the same tablet, progestogen compliance is guaranteed.

Finally, all estrogen tablets contain lactose and cannot be given to lactose-intolerant women.

Percutaneous (gel) administration (Table 52.2)

Percutaneous gels have been available in France for more than 20 years and have been introduced elsewhere more recently. They appear to be favoured, understandably, by women who apply a skin cream on a daily basis.

Until recently, only Oestrogel (Laboratoires Besins-Iscovesco, Paris, France) was available in the United Kingdom but Sandrena (Organon, Oss, Holland) has recently been introduced. The latter is more concentrated. Both appear associated with a low incidence of skin reactions. Both deliver pure estradiol which achieves a more physiological estradiol:estrone ratio than oral therapy. Both provide an almost infinite dosing system because the mass of estrogen which is delivered will depend upon the amount of gel which is applied.

At present, only estradiol can be delivered percutaneously. No progestogen is currently available as a gel but development programmes for progestogen gels are well advanced.

Transdermal (patch) administration (Table 52.3)

The original transdermal therapeutic system (TTS) was membrane-based. The alcohol reservoir, whilst essential for estradiol delivery in this system, also caused skin reactions. The newer matrix dispersal systems deliver estradiol as effectively as the membrane-based systems but do not possess alcohol and therefore are associated with a much lower incidence of skin reactions. Furthermore, reaction to a membrane-based system may not recur with a matrix patch.[7] Because of skin occlusion, it is probable that matrix patches will, like the earlier membrane-based systems[8] cause more skin irritation in hot and humid climates.

Several transdermal matrix patch systems for estradiol are now marketed, the major difference being in the adhesive. As yet, there are no rigorous 'head-to-head' studies comparing the effectiveness of

Table 52.2 Percutaneous gel therapy: advantages and disadvantages

Advantages	Disadvantages
• Low dose pure estradiol	• Daily dosing
• Easy to apply	• More expensive than oral
• Avoids intestinal and liver metabolism	• Variation in absorption
• Physiological E_2:E_1 ratio	• Progestogen cannot be co-administered in gel
• Reduces triglycerides	• Less effect than oral on HDL and HDL-2 cholesterol
• Few skin problems	
• Invariable dosing system	

Table 52.3 Transdermal patch therapy: advantages and disadvantages

Advantages	Disadvantages
• Low dose pure estradiol	• More expensive than oral
• Avoids intestinal and liver metabolism	• Variation in absorption
• Physiological estradiol:estrone ratio	• Not tolerated so well in warm climates because of skin reactions
• Reduces triglycerides	• Less effect than oral on HDL and HDL-2 cholesterol
• Progestogen can be co-administered either sequentially or continuously	• Serum estradiol values decline over time
• Variable dosing system	

estradiol delivery or the incidence of skin irritation between different matrix systems. Such data are needed but may never be readily available because of the manner in which the pharmaceutical industry funds research. All membrane and matrix systems achieve a more physiological estradiol:estrone ratio than oral therapy. The matrix systems also provide an almost infinitely variable dosing system because the mass of estradiol which is delivered depends upon the surface area of the matrix patch. Thus, any dose can be achieved by trimming a patch with skilful use of the kitchen scissors. This practice is not recommended by the manufacturers but such fine tuning is frequently used to good advantage by patients.

Unlike gels, matrix patches are available as sequential therapies with a transdermal progestogen added for 14 days each month (Nuvelle-TS: Schering Health Care, Berlin, Germany; Evorel-Sequi: Janssen-Cilag, New Brunswick, USA) or as continuous/combined estrogen/progestogen regimens (Evorel-Conti: Janssen-Cilag, New Brunswick, USA).

Most recently, patches delivering estradiol over a seven day period have been introduced (Climara: Schering Health Care, Berlin, Germany; Femseven: E. Merck, West Drayton, UK). Published pharmacokinetic data are few. Some indicate fairly constant levels while others suggest an appreciable drop in serum estradiol, from around 70 pg/mL (200 pmol/L) to 40 pg/mL (110 pmol/L) between the second and seventh day. If symptoms return in consequence of such a drop, then it would seem sensible to return to a 3/4 day matrix patch system.

Subcutaneous (implant) administration (Table 52.4)

This is probably the most controversial route of administration. However, because implants contain the natural hormones, estradiol and testosterone, to which female tissues are exposed from puberty, problems with this route of administration result not from the implants per se but from the manner in which they are used. Presently available implants are manufactured from fused crystalline steroid and hence are biodegradable, but at variable rates. Non biodegradable implants producing near zero-order (constant) steroid release are being developed.

Subcutaneous implantation is the only route of administration which guarantees compliance. Additional advantages are the co-administration of testosterone, which appears particularly advantageous in some women following castration. The postmenopausal ovary is a well-recognized source of androgens (see ch. 48). A physiological estradiol:estrone ratio is achieved.

The disadvantages of subcutaneous implantation relate in part to the need for a surgical procedure and, perhaps more importantly, to too frequent re-implantation. As with any surgical procedure, there is a small risk of hemorrhage and bruising but both of these appear uncommon. There are no data on the incidence of infection at the insertion site but this too appears uncommon, although well-recognized. To gain longevity of benefit in terms of symptom relief, there is an initial surge in serum estradiol following implantation and in a small number of women some atypical symptoms begin to return as the serum estradiol values start to fall, not when the pretreatment estradiol value has been reached. Based solely on symptom recurrence, repeated implantation may then be undertaken when serum estradiol is still high. This results in the dichotomy of patients experiencing 'estradiol-deficiency' symptoms, albeit atypical, particularly mood fluctuations, headaches and vague flashing feelings, in the presence of supraphysiological serum estradiol values.

This phenomenon has been called 'tachyphylaxis'.[9] The usual clinical presentation is of a patient requiring, indeed almost demanding, further implants at ever decreasing intervals. Eventually, the implants 'stop working', and the patient often accuses the doctor of 'not putting in a proper implant'. The highest serum

Table 52.4 Implant therapy: advantages and disadvantages

Advantages	Disadvantages
• Low dose pure estradiol	• More expensive than oral
• Pure estradiol	• Surgical procedure
• Six monthly or less frequent insertion	• Unable to control absorption
• High blood levels	• Risk supraphysiological blood levels — tachyphylaxis
• Avoids intestinal and liver metabolism	• Difficult to remove
• Physiological estradiol:estrone ratio	• Very prolonged duration of release in minority of women
• Testosterone implants can be co-administered	
• Compliance is guaranteed	
• Enhanced effect on bone mass	

estradiol value which I have seen in such a patient was of 9300 pmol/L – and the highest I have heard of was 10 400 pmol/L. The average daily serum estradiol value achieved during the ovulatory cycle in women of reproductive age is around 500–520 pmol/L in our laboratory. Management to prevent this problem is much simpler than treatment of the established problem. Prevention can be achieved by routine measurement of serum estradiol (and serum testosterone if co-administered) when the patient requests further implantation, and the delaying of further implants if the serum estradiol or testosterone values 'are elevated'. There is no agreement, at this time, as to what constitutes an 'elevated' value. I try to dissuade patients from further implants if the serum estradiol value exceeds approximately 450 pmol/L and the testosterone value exceeds 1.0 nmol/L. Introduction of this simple measure has eliminated tachyphylaxis in the menopause clinics which I direct.

The management of the miserable, symptomatic woman with tachyphylaxis is much more difficult. I try to dissuade patients from further implantation on the basis that the cycle has to be broken at some time, and that very high serum estradiol values may increase the risk of undesirable side effects such as breast cancer and perhaps venous thrombosis. It is stressed that these are theoretical rather than proven concerns. On the one hand, patients with tachyphylaxis often experience symptoms of estrogen excess. These include breast tenderness, nipple sensitivity, nausea and bloating. On the other hand, they are often tearful, irritable and prone to headaches and severe mood swings. Flashes, in my experience, are not pronounced or are atypical. Treatment involves explanation, sympathy and judicious use of further estrogen therapy by other routes to try to allay symptoms. Occasionally, this means further implantation but with a lower dose of estradiol. More usually, I suggest that patients apply estradiol from either a patch or a gel. Conventional HRT patch and gel dosing will result in a serum increment of estradiol of around 140–200 pmol/L. This will do no more than take the edge off symptoms if the background serum estradiol is 2000–2500 pmol/L — as it often is in a woman with tachyphylaxis.

There are no data on rates of decay of serum estradiol in women with tachyphylaxis. Elevations in serum estradiol sufficient to stimulate the endometrium have been reported 3½ years after the last implant was inserted.[10] In patients with an intact uterus, it is essential that progestogen administration continues, despite no further implant insertion, until the withdrawal bleeding has ceased completely for three months.

One benefit of estradiol alone and of simultaneous estradiol and testosterone implants is the more pronounced effect of the higher serum values on bone mass. As compared to oral, percutaneous and transdermal administration, subcutaneous use of implants has been reported to increase bone mass more in placebo-controlled trials.[11]

Serum products

The different routes of administration can influence the type of estrogen which appears in serum, the so-called 'serum product'. All transdermal (patch), percutaneous (gel) and subcutaneous (implant) estrogen preparations currently available contain only estradiol and give rise, principally, to this estrogen in serum. Oral formulations contain preparations based on estradiol, estrone or equine estrogens. The latter are considered further below. All oral estradiol or estrone-based formulations give rise in serum principally to estrone. Serum profiles for estradiol and estrone, measured at three hourly intervals over 24 hours, are shown in Figures 52.3 and 52.4, respectively. Three groups of postmenopausal women were

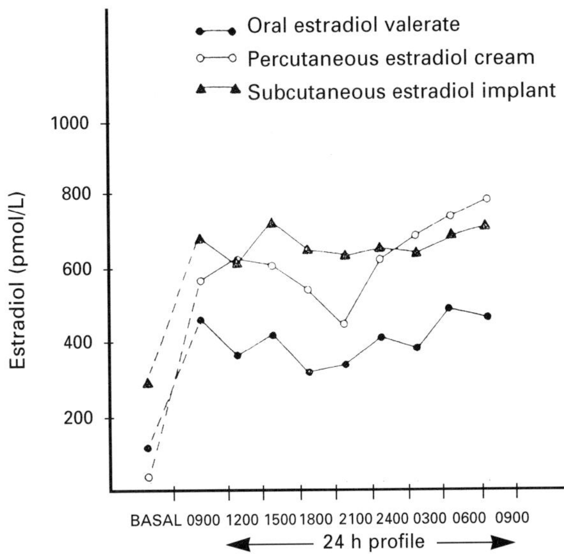

Fig. 52.3 Mean serum estradiol levels in postmenopausal women before and then during therapy with orally, percutaneously or subcutaneously administered estradiol preparations. (From: Campbell S, Whitehead MI 1982 Potency and hepato-cellular effects of oestrogens after oral, percutaneous and subcutaneous administration. In: van Keep PA, Utian W, Vermeulen A (eds) The controversial climacteric. MTP Press, Lancaster, pp 103–125)

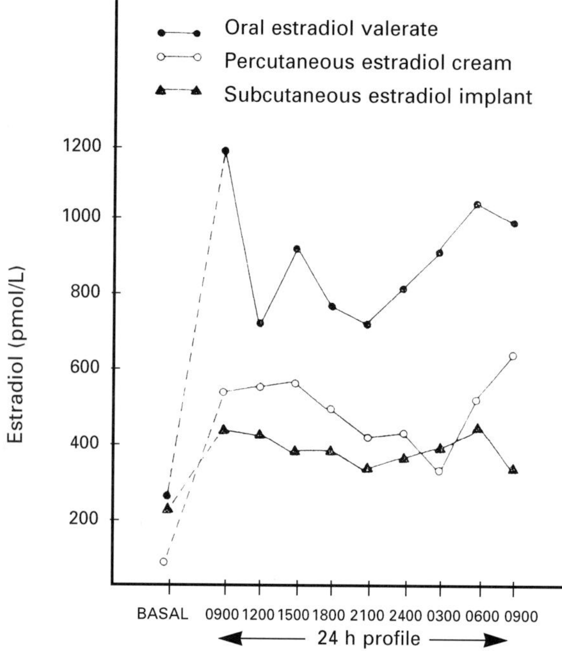

Fig. 52.4 Mean plasma estrone levels in postmenopausal women before and then during therapy with orally, percutaneously or subcutaneously administered estradiol preparations. (From: Campbell S, Whitehead MI 1982 Potency and hepato-cellular effects of estrogens after oral, percutaneous and subcutaneous administration. In: van Keep PA, Utian W, Vermeulen A (eds) The controversial climacteric. MTP Press, Lancaster, pp 103–125)

compared in these studies and all had received treatment for six weeks. One group received oral estradiol (2 mg/day), a second group applied percutaneous estradiol as a gel (2.5 g/day), and a third group had undergone implantation with an estradiol implant (50 mg).

The implant provided the most constant serum estradiol and estrone values over 24 hours. The estrogen tablet was swallowed and the gel was applied at 9.00 pm at night (21.00 hours). Both of these routes were followed by a surge in estrogen values, oral therapy producing a much more marked rise in serum estrone. It is easy to understand why oral estrogens absorbed in a bolus dose directly into the portal system and liver have a greater hepatic effect than the nonoral routes of estrogen administration. In lipid terms, oral estrogens can be expected to increase high density lipoprotein (HDL) and HDL-2 cholesterol more than the parenteral routes and this effect is desirable. However, the oral route, and in particular administration of conjugated equine estrogens, elevates serum triglyceride whereas nonoral administration has either no effect on triglyceride or lowers levels. Triglycerides are a well recognized independent risk factor for death from myocardial infarction in postmenopausal women.[12]

These data also illustrate the more physiological estradiol:estrone ratios achieved with the nonoral as compared to the oral route of administration. However, it is emphasized that the less physiological ratio associated with oral therapy has not been linked to an adverse clinical outcome.

Conjugated equine estrogens are a complex mixture of different estrogens of which 65% is estrone sulphate, the principal serum product. The remaining 35% are equine estrogens such as equilin and equilenin. Conjugated equine estrogens contain almost no estradiol, and the rise in serum estradiol seen with oral administration represents conversion from estrone.

Vaginally administered estrogens (Table 52.5)

Conjugated equine estrogens are also available as a vaginal cream. Other vaginal preparations include an estradiol tablet (Vagifem: Novo Nordisk, Copenhagen, Denmark), and vaginal creams containing dienoestrol (Ortho-dienoestrol: Ortho-Cilag, New Brunswick, USA). For technical reasons it is not possible to measure the level of dienoestrol in serum. More recently developed vaginal preparations include an ultra low-dose vaginal ring (Estring: Upjohn-Pharmacia, Windsor, UK) which delivers sufficient estradiol only for local benefit. This can be highly desirable in a patient with troublesome symptoms due to lower genital tract atrophy who possesses a risk factor for use of systemic estrogens, such as breast cancer. Rings delivering higher doses of estradiol which will significantly increase serum concentrations and result in systemic benefits are on the point of being introduced.

Other vaginal preparations contain the weaker estrogen, estriol. Unlike estradiol and estrone, estriol is not protein-bound but circulates in a 'free' form. It is the only major estrogen excreted by the kidney and the plasma half-life is only a few hours. Thus, once daily vaginal administration of low doses of estriol (1 mg) may help with lower genital tract symptoms, but such low doses will not impart systemic effects such as conservation of bone or endometrial stimulation. When administered at much higher doses (12 mg/day) and also in divided doses, estriol has been linked to endometrial hyperplasia.

The advantages and disadvantages of vaginal administration of estrogens are shown in Table 52.5.

Table 52.5 Vaginal preparations: advantages and disadvantages

Advantages	Disadvantages
• Main action is local if manufacturer's recommendations are followed • Can be used to relieve vaginal symptoms in presence of relative contraindications to use of HRT	• Creams are 'messy' • Risk of creams being used as lubricant — systemic effect in patient and risk of effect in partner • Vaginal tablets and rings are relatively expensive

Many patients find that the creams are 'messy', and the vaginal tablets and rings appear to be more acceptable in this respect. A further potential problem with the vaginal estrogen creams is their misuse not as creams but as lubricants. This often results in overdosage in the patient and many epidemiological studies of the association between HRT and endometrial cancer report an increase in risk in users of vaginal estrogen creams. With excessive use of the cream as a vaginal lubricant there is the additional problem of absorption by the male partner resulting in gynaecomastia, an uncommon but well-recognized side-effect.

PROGESTOGENS

Although prospective data are sparse, clinical experience is that the majority of problems arising with combined estrogen/progestogen HRT are due to the progestogen component. As with estrogens, the effects of progestogens (and particularly the metabolic effects of these) appear related not only to the type or class of drug but also to the route of administration.

Type of progestogen

There are six major classes of progestogen but only two or three are involved in HRT. These are the parent compound, natural progesterone; the C-21 derivatives of progesterone such as medroxyprogesterone acetate (Upjohn: Kalamazoo, Michigan, USA) and dydrogesterone (Duphaston: Solvay Duphar, Southampton, England), and the C-19 nortestosterone derivatives such as norethindrone and levonorgestrel.

In terms of psychological side-effects, much of what is written and believed about the effects of different progestogens appears to be based on opinion and anecdotal comment. A recent, comprehensive literature search through Medline failed to identify a body of robust studies of impeccable methodology showing clear differences in effect between the different types of agents. There are however data clearly showing that lower doses of norethindrone cause fewer psychological and physical side-effects as compared to higher doses[13] and dosage reductions of the other drugs would most probably also minimize potential side-effects.

Traditional teaching has been that the C-21 derivatives of progesterone are less likely than the C-19 nortestosterone derivatives to cause metabolic derangement when added to estrogen in HRT. Certain evidence supports this argument but other research data do not. For example, in one large epidemiological investigation, the addition of a relatively high dose of oral levonorgestrel, 500 μg/day, sequentially to an oral estrogen did not negate estrogen benefits on the risk of coronary artery disease in women under 60 years of age.[14] At present, there are no epidemiologic data which show that, when added to an estrogen, C-21 derivatives are associated with a lower risk of ischemic heart disease (IHD) when compared with the C-19 derivatives. Quite simply, the required epidemiological studies have not been performed and great caution must be exercised in interpreting data which use surrogate markers as endpoints for clinical arterial disease. Thus, the rationale for recommending either a C-21 derivative or one of the new generation of less androgenic C-19 derivatives comes from laboratory-based investigations in which lipid, lipoprotein, carbohydrate, thrombophilia and coagulation changes are used as such surrogates for clinical disease risk. These data are considered in specific chapters elsewhere in this book.

Derivatives of levonorgestrel have been developed which, it is claimed, are less androgenic than the parent compound. These are norgestimate, gestodene and desogestrel. When added to ethinyl estradiol in oral contraceptive formulations, these progestogens cause minimal, if any, potentially adverse lipid and lipoprotein effects. However, natural estrogens, used in HRT, are less potent than synthetic ethinyl estradiol, used in the combined, oral contraceptive pill. When desogestrel was added continuously (every day) to oral estradiol in continuous/combined HRT, potentially undesirable androgenic changes in lipid and lipoprotein metabolism were observed.[15] Many metabolic advantages are anticipated with the introduction of the newer, less androgenic C-19 progestogens: whether these benefits will actually be realized remains to be seen.

Routes of administration

As stated above, one of the major problems with combined estrogen/progestogen HRT is progestogen-induced 'premenstrual tension' (PMT). Because this problem appears dose-related, strategies that are aimed at reducing the daily dose appear logical.

The most obvious approach is to avoid oral administration and to develop a system whereby the progestogen is administered nonorally but systemically. It is argued that by avoiding significant 'first-pass' hepatic metabolism, the total administered dose of the progestogen can be reduced and this should reduce the frequency and severity of unwanted side-effects. The first totally transdermal estrogen/progestogen HRT was Estracombi (Ciba-Geigy, Basle, Switzerland). The transdermal progestogen was norethindrone acetate and the patch was membrane-based, and contained an alcohol reservoir. For reasons stated above, such technology is looking increasingly obsolete with the introduction of matrix patch systems giving less skin irritation.[7] Totally transdermal delivery systems for estradiol and norethindrone acetate (Evorel-Sequi and Evorel-Conti) and also for estradiol and levonorgestrel (Nuvelle-TS) are now available.

The second approach to the problem of progestogen-induced PMT, which also avoids oral administration, is the development of a system which releases the progestogen either within or adjacent to the endometrium and uterine cavity. Leiras has developed a levonorgestrel-releasing intra-uterine system (LNG-IUS). This has already been approved for use in the UK, Scandinavia and elsewhere as a contraceptive, and is marketed as Mirena. It is now being evaluated for use as the progestogen component of combined estrogen/progestogen HRT. This is a logical approach to the problem since the major reason for progestogen use in HRT is for endometrial protection. Regrettably, levonorgestrel has a low 'first-pass' hepatic clearance and, therefore, although the risk of progestogen-induced physical and psychological side-effects is reduced because of the low 20 μg daily dose (serum levonorgestrel values are approximately 200 pg/mL), lipid, lipoprotein and metabolic changes may still occur. When combined with transdermal estradiol 50 μg/day, the LNG-IUS was associated with a decrease in HDL cholesterol of 12.5% and in HDL-2 cholesterol of 27% at one year.[16] Lower dose systems with less systemic absorption are being tested.

Yet another strategy has been to develop a sustained release preparation containing natural progesterone which is delivered into the upper part of the vagina. This has now been approved for use in both the USA and UK and is marketed as Crinone (Wyeth-Ayerst, Philadelphia, USA). The progesterone is dissolved into a bioadhesive gel which adheres to the vaginal skin and which is inserted every 48 hours. Data show that when 90 mg of progesterone is inserted every other day (six insertions over 12 days), sequentially, in combination with oral conjugated equine estrogens, uniform secretory transformation is achieved within the endometrium (Fig. 52.5).[17] Interestingly, the serum progesterone levels can be very variable: some were well within the midluteal phase range (approximately 30 nmol/L) but others were not (much less than 10 nmol/L), yet all endometrial tissue showed evidence of good progestational activity. These data with low serum progesterone levels suggest the existence of a 'pelvic sink' with local distribution to pelvic tissues. Whether this is mediated via the lymphatic system is not known but, clearly, effective doses of progesterone are being delivered to the endometrium yet, because of the low serum values, the risk of PMT is likely to be minimized.

TREATMENT SCHEDULES FOR ESTROGEN AND ESTROGEN/PROGESTOGEN HRT

Worldwide, various schedules of estrogen and progestogen are available. It is most convenient to summarize them as cyclic, sequential, long-cycle, continuous combined or gonadomimetic (Fig. 52.6).

The first regimens to be prescribed were cyclic. The estrogen is administered alone, unopposed by a progestogen, for three weeks out of every four. During the middle 1970s, cyclic estrogen-only regimens began to be associated with an increase in risk of endometrial cancer and, in women with an intact uterus, have largely been replaced by estrogen/progestogen therapy. However, estrogens continue to be prescribed unopposed by a progestogen following hysterectomy, and in premenopausal women who experience typical estrogen-deficiency symptoms premenstrually (see below). With sequential therapies, the older combined regimens administered the estrogen in 21 day cycles with the progestogen being added for 7–10 days each cycle. In modern sequential regimens the estrogen is administered in continuous 28 day cycles and the progestogen is added for either 10, 12 or 14 days each cycle. With sequential therapies the aim is to achieve good cycle control and the majority of users (approximately 85%) have a regular, withdrawal bleed which should resemble menstruation.

The perimenopausal woman often presents a difficult treatment challenge. Typical estrogen-deficiency symptoms such as flashes and sweats may be

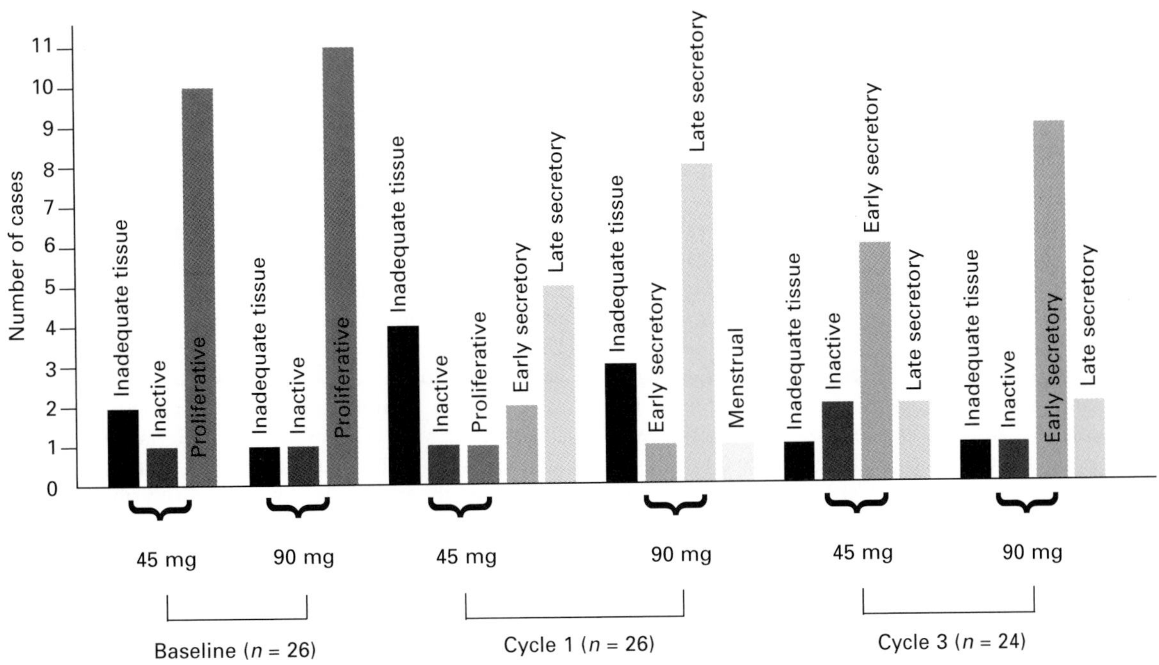

Fig. 52.5 Endometrial histology according to dose of vaginal natural progesterone and cycle of treatment. (From: Ross D, Cooper AJ, Pryse-Davies J, Bergeron C, Collins WP, Whitehead MI 1997 Randomised double-blind, dose-ranging study of the endometrial effects of a vaginal progesterone gel in estrogen-treated postmenopausal women. American Journal of Obstetrics and Gynecology 177: 937–941)

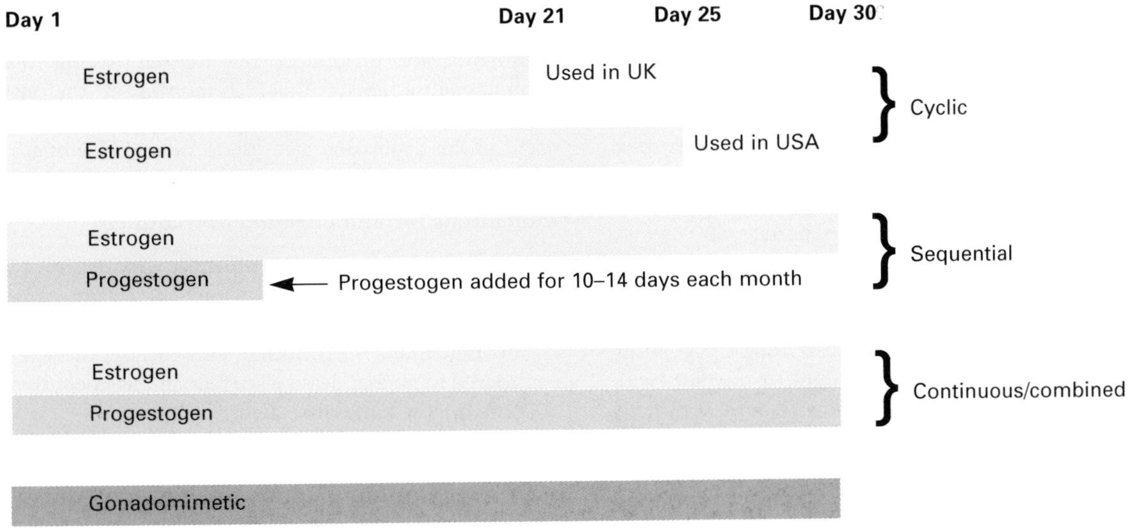

Fig. 52.6 Various schedules for administration of estrogen either alone or in combination with a progestogen.

experienced continuously or just premenstrually. With the latter, and provided that an appropriately timed progesterone level indicates good luteal function, then it seems sensible to prescribe an estrogen unopposed by a progestogen for 7–10 days premenstrually when the symptoms are most severe. The ovarian-derived progesterone should protect the endometrium.

Management of patients with continuous or erratic symptoms or with an irregular cycle is often much more difficult. Use of sequential regimens often results in breakthrough bleeding — one bleed being due to ovarian function and the other to the withdrawal of the progestogen in the HRT. Synchronization of endogenous and exogenous hormonal activity may be impossible if ovarian steroidogenesis is intermittent and unpredictable. In such patients, use of a low dose, monophasic combined estrogen/progestogen contraceptive pill is often ideal because estrogen deficiency symptoms are relieved, spontaneous but intermittent ovarian activity is suppressed, and a regular withdrawal bleed occurs. If symptoms recur during the treatment-free week then this interval can be reduced to 3–4 days or eliminated altogether with the packets of the pill being administered 'back-to-back'.

Women attending menopause clinics (who, presumably, are more likely to be committed to HRT) worry more about breast cancer than withdrawal bleeding. Studies in less selected groups report that the re-establishment of bleeding is regarded as a negative feature. Thus, schedules have been developed for postmenopausal women which aim to minimize or avoid bleeding altogether. These are long-cycle HRT, continuous/combined estrogen/progestogen HRT, and gonadomimetic therapy.

In long-cycle HRT, the frequency of bleeding is reduced because, whilst the estrogen is administered continuously, the progestogen is added only every third month. Data on the safety of such treatments are contradictory. A combination of oral estradiol, 2 mg/day, with medroxyprogesterone acetate, 20 mg/day added for 14 days every three months (Tridestra: Sanofi-Winthrop, Guildford, UK) has not been associated with an increase in incidence of endometrial disease. However, the Scandinavian Long Cycle Study group reported that oral estradiol, 2 mg/day, with norethindrone, 1 mg/day, added for 10 days every third month was associated with a significant increase in the incidence of simple and complex endometrial hyperplasia, and carcinoma.[18] Further data are urgently required to determine whether these observed differences could be due to the different type and dose of progestogen and duration of administration.

Continuous combined HRT aims to cause amenorrhea by inducing endometrial atrophy through the antiproliferative effect of the continuously administered low dose of progestogen. Such treatments have been called 'bleed free' but, for many patients, this is a misnomer. Unfortunately, the continuous progestogen can result in hypertrophy of the endometrial stroma which is highly vascular. As might be predicted, the major problem with continuous combined HRT is that approximately 30–40% of women experience erratic light bleeding especially during the first three to six months, and many women discontinue treatment during this time.[19] However, after this initial phase of erratic bleeding the goal of amenorrhea is usually achieved.

The only currently available gonadomimetic, tibolone (Livial: Organon, Oss, Holland) has an identical aim. Preliminary data from a randomized trial comparing the incidence of bleeding with tibolone and a conventional, continuous combined HRT (Kliofem: Novo Nordisk, Copenhagen, Denmark) have reported, in abstract form, less bleeding with the gonadomimetic than the continuous combined HRT. Further data are required to confirm or refute this difference.

One of the major problems with continuous/combined HRT is the recurrence of vaginal bleeding, albeit light, after a prolonged period of amenorrhea. This might result from poor compliance or concurrent use of antibiotics. However, it might also result from the development of endometrial disease. Thus, the problem is two-fold: when is further investigation warranted and what type of investigation is to be preferred? These issues have recently been extensively reviewed,[20] to which the interested reader is referred. Both continuous combined and gonadomimetic treatments are unsuitable for women during the perimenopause and within 12 months of the last menstrual period. Intermittent ovarian function may occur in this group and give rise to vaginal bleeding.

Indications for and duration of treatment

One of the questions asked most frequently by physicians and patients is 'How long will treatment be prescribed?' The answer, I believe, will depend mainly on the indications for treatment and because these are considered in greater detail elsewhere in this book, they are only briefly considered here.

At present, relief of physical and psychological symptoms remains the major indication for use of HRT. Whilst flashes and sweats resolve spontaneously in the majority of women within five years, a minority, perhaps 5%, experience them for many years. It is often unclear from the history whether psychological symptoms are due to estrogen deficiency or concurrent but coincidental environmental stress. A 'trial of therapy' of HRT of perhaps three months duration is often helpful. Symptoms which respond are clearly due to estrogen lack; the converse also applies.

Rarely, typical estrogen deficiency symptoms do not respond to HRT because the estrogen is not being absorbed. This appears to occur most commonly with oral therapy and can be confirmed by measurement of the appropriate serum product. If oral estrogens, and particularly oral conjugated equine estrogens, are being administered, it is more sensible to measure serum estrone than estradiol. Measurement of serum estradiol, where this assay is available, is indicated to detect the degree of systemic absorption with the non-oral forms of natural estrogen administration. Ethinyl estradiol, dienoestrol and tibolone are not detected by measurements of serum estrone and estradiol.

The durations of treatment required to confer other benefits, such as those on the skeleton and arterial tree, are considered elsewhere in this book.

The use of HRT to relieve vaginal dryness which is so severe as to make intercourse impossible should usually be continued for as long as that woman wishes to remain sexually active. In my experience severe vaginal dryness is *the* symptom which results in very long-term use of HRT. I have many patients on treatment for this indication for over 20 years.

CONTRAINDICATIONS AND RISKS

For the purposes of this chapter, a contraindication is defined as a pre-existing condition which may be adversely affected by the administration of HRT. A risk is the development of a potentially adverse condition in a previously healthy woman. The majority of contraindications and risks are considered in other chapters in this book. This chapter will provide a short resumé of their background and a discussion of those not covered comprehensively elsewhere.

Risks

These are discussed comprehensively in other chapters but are summarized here in Table 52.6. Whilst one or two small placebo-controlled studies have reported on risks, the majority of the data on risks such as breast cancer, endometrial cancer and venous thrombosis have not been derived from prospective, randomized trials. They have been developed, for the most part, from observational epidemiological studies — however methodological flaws and weaknesses are present in this type of investigation. The presence of these biases, to a greater or lesser extent in the various observational studies performed, almost certainly explains, at least in part, the differences in the results obtained by them.

Malignant melanoma

Results from published studies are contradictory, however, it is clear that if postmenopausal estrogen use increases the risk then the impact must be very small. One case-controlled study reported a small increase in risk with long-term use of oestrogen but another case-controlled study did not.[21,22] Three other studies reported slight increases in risk, but none of these achieved statistical significance.[23–25]

An identical problem arose when the relationship between the combined estrogen/progestogen contraceptive pill and risk of malignant melanoma was first investigated. Various small studies reported contrasting results. The prospective cohorts of the Royal College of General Practitioners and Oxford Family Planning Association included adequate patient numbers and also took into account exposure to sunlight; no association between use of the contraceptive pill and risk of malignant melanoma was found.[26,27]

Contraindications (Table 52.7)

Traditionally, contraindications are classified as 'absolute' and 'relative'. This convention is followed here but it is emphasized that such a distinction is largely empiric.

Acute intermittent porphyria is exacerbated during puberty and the reproductive era. In my opinion, this is the only chronic disease which should be considered an absolute contraindication. Breast and endometrial

Table 52.6 Risks of hormone replacement therapy

Breast cancer	Current data suggest a 2.3% increase in incident disease per year of use of HRT; increase in mortality.
Endometrial cancer	Dose and duration-dependent increase in risk with unopposed oestrogens;? reduction in risk to below that in untreated women with continuous combined preparations.
Venous thrombosis	Current data suggest a 2–3 fold increase in risk with use of HRT; risk appears greatest during first 12 months of use; no effect of added progestogen.

Table 52.7 Absolute and relative contraindications to hormone replacement therapy

Absolute	Relative
Acute intermittent porphyria	Endometriosis
?Breast cancer	Fibroids
?Endometrial cancer	?Otosclerosis
?Venous thrombosis with hematological abnormality	?Focal migraine
Undiagnosed abnormal bleeding	?SLE
Pregnancy	?Venous thrombosis without hematological abnormality

cancer are usually included in the list of absolute contraindications but there are no data from well conducted, randomized trials to show whether use of HRT influences the risk of recurrence of either of these cancers. Quite simply, the required studies have not been performed.

Detailed discussions of the relationships between estrogens and progestogens and myomata (fibroids) and these sex hormones and endometriosis are covered in other chapters in this book. Because both myomata and endometriotic tissue can retain some responsiveness to low doses of estrogen and progestogen in postmenopausal women, the potential effects of HRT on these conditions must always be considered.

Regrettably, there are no large-scale, prospective, randomized, studies which have provided clear answers as to whether HRT does or does not cause clinical sequelae in pre-existing myomata and/or endometriosis. Thus, the risk of prolonging/reactivating these diseases is unknown. It is well recognized that the number and size of uterine myomata can occasionally increase with use of HRT.[28] Several case reports have linked the use of HRT with the development of ovarian endometrioma, endometriotic colon obstruction and obstructive uropathy. However, and very importantly, the latter problems can arise in postmenopausal women not exposed to exogenous estrogens.[29] Only one large study investigated whether HRT increased the risk of reactivating pelvic endometriosis. Only one of 85 women who had undergone total abdominal hysterectomy and bilateral salpingo-oophorectomy required further laparotomy within the first five years of administration of estradiol and testosterone implants.[30]

In the absence of randomized controlled trials, practical guidelines with respect to the management of patients with myomata and endometriosis who subsequently receive HRT are based largely on a 'common sense' approach. Myoma size can be monitored clinically and the numbers can be determined by ultrasound examination. It would seem prudent to advise women known to have small myomata, who are about to start HRT, to return for further examination if symptoms occur which may arise from enlarging fibroids (lower abdominal or pelvic pain, increasing urinary frequency, increasingly heavy vaginal bleeding). Identical comments can be applied to the monitoring of patients with mild endometriosis, although the type of symptom may well be different (pelvic pain and deep dyspareunia). More severe endometriotic disease may require surgery before HRT is prescribed. Current thinking is that HRT is not contraindicated in young women who have had to undergo total abdominal hysterectomy and bilateral salpingo-oophorectomy because of severe endometriosis. However, it is not clear whether treatment in this group of women should consist of estrogen alone or estrogen and progestogen. Individualization is probably important. Testosterone can be added to either treatment, as indicated. It should be remembered that the estrogen exposure of pelvic tissues to natural ovarian estrogen secretion is very much higher than from systemic HRT.

The inclusion of otosclerosis in the list of relative contraindications can be challenged. Whilst pregnancy may be associated with episodes of progressive deafness, there is little evidence that normal ovarian function causes deterioration in hearing. The serum estrogen values achieved with HRT are within the lower part of the normal physiological range.

Focal migraine is considered a contraindication to use of the combined, oral contraceptive pill and for this reason is included in this list. However, the estrogenic potency of ethinyl estradiol which is used in the 'pill' is much greater in some tissues than that of the natural estrogens which are prescribed in HRT.

Evidence for considering systemic lupus erythematous (SLE) a relative contraindication is not convincing although individual case reports indicate exacerbations with HRT in some susceptible women. A recent publication[31] reported no adverse effect of estrogens on the progression of SLE.

Recommendations relating to the use of HRT in the presence of a personal or family history of venous thrombosis, with or without hematological abnormality, must be considered anecdotal because, once again, the required prospective studies to determine the risk of further thrombosis with HRT have not been performed. Also, disagreement exists between hematologists with respect to how best to advise women at increased risk of venous thrombosis. Clearly, management will be influenced by legal as well as by medical considerations. In some parts of the world a disclaimer, signed by a fully informed patient and independently witnessed, removes the threat of an allegation of negligence if the subsequent prescription of HRT causes significant morbidity. However, this practice is not universal and is not followed in some countries, such as the USA. In consequence, the use of HRT in an 'at risk' woman is likely to be reduced. In women with a previous history of DVT who need HRT it may be wise to recommend transdermal estradiol rather than oral estrogens since the action on hepatic coagulation factors should be less.

ALTERNATIVES TO HRT

Not all women wish to take HRT and alternative treatments should be developed. Three such treatments will be considered here: phytoestrogens, selective estrogen receptor modulators (SERMs) and natural progesterone cream.

Phytoestrogens

Background

Phytoestrogens are compounds which are derived from plants yet which have an affinity for the estradiol receptor. However, this affinity is much lower than that of estradiol and ranges from about one five-hundredth to about one thousandth of that of estradiol.[32,33] In animal models and in *in vitro* experimental systems, phytoestrogens, like tamoxifen and other selective estradiol receptor modulators, compete with estradiol for the estrogen receptor[34] and appear capable of acting as both estrogen agonists and antagonists.

There are numerous classes of phytoestrogens. The two which have received most attention in relation to human health are the lignans and the isoflavones. Lignans are present in measurable levels in many fiber-rich foods while the isoflavones are confined to legumes, particularly soya beans. Although they possess only a weak affinity for the estradiol receptor, relatively high levels of phytoestrogens can be present in food. For example, an average portion of a soya protein meal provides approximately 45 mg of isoflavones. If this is ingested daily, the urinary levels of isoflavones rise approximately 1000-fold, to up to 8000 mg/day.

When compared with Caucasians in Western-style societies, Japanese women have a lower risk of coronary heart disease, breast cancer and endometrial cancer. It has been suggested that these lower risks are due, at least in part, to differences in diet. Typical plasma isoflavone values of around 100 ng/mL are found in Japanese subjects who consume, on average, 50–100 mg of isoflavones each day from soya products. The average plasma estradiol values of postmenopausal women in Western societies range from around 15–30 pg/mL.[35,36] Thus, phytoestrogen levels in Japanese women may exceed those of endogenous estradiol by one thousandth-fold.

Activity of phytoestrogens in women

In women of reproductive age, controlled studies have shown that phytoestrogen-rich diets (45 mg/day) modify the hormonal status and exert significant physiological effects on the regulation of the menstrual cycle.[37,38] In postmenopausal women, gonadotropin levels are reduced and estrogen-like changes in vaginal cytology occur following administration of phytoestrogens.[39]

Activity of phytoestrogens in animal models

To date, most work in this area has been carried out by the group at Bowman Gray School of Medicine, North Carolina, USA. The animal model is the cynomolgus macaque monkey fed a high cholesterol diet. Various studies have been undertaken and published.[40–43] These have involved feeding young macaque monkeys either casein (to act as a control), or soy with the phytoestrogen component intact (soy+), or soy with the phytoestrogen component extracted by ethanol (soy–).

Soy+ was associated with an approximate 30% reduction in total plasma cholesterol, a 30% increase in high density lipoprotein (HDL) and a 30% reduction in low density lipoprotein (LDL) and very low density lipoprotein (VLDL) cholesterol. Soy+ exerted a significantly greater effect than conjugated equine estrogens in the elevation of HDL cholesterol. Additionally, soy+ decreased iliac artery atherosclerosis by about 80% compared with soy– and casein. Finally, unlike conjugated equine estrogens, soy+ enhanced the dilator responses of atherosclerotic coronary arteries to acetylcholine.

No increase in uterine weight was observed during treatment with soy+.

Selective estrogen receptor modulators (SERMs)

Background

SERMs were previously known as 'anti-estrogens'. They include tamoxifen (Zeneca Pharma, Wilmslow, Cheshire, UK), draloxifene (Pfizer, Sandwich, Kent, UK) and raloxifene (Eli Lilly, Indianapolis, USA). Some classifications also include certain other agents which have been developed by Imperial Chemical Industries (ICI, Wilmslow, Cheshire, UK) and which are known only by number, for example ICI 182,780 and ICI 164,384. The latter are extremely potent anti-estrogens and have little estrogen agonist activity. Almost certainly, their clinical use will be in patients with estrogen dependent cancers. Thus, they will not be considered further in this chapter.

Tamoxifen

The principal reason for the change in name from 'anti-estrogen' to SERM is because the former term is inappropriate. The most well-recognized action of tamoxifen is in the treatment of breast cancer. The definitive meta-analysis published in 1992 by the Early Breast Cancer Trialists' Collaborative Group[44] demonstrated modest but significant benefits associated with its use as an adjuvant therapy in stage 1 and stage 2 disease.

Although the majority of women in this meta-analysis had taken tamoxifen for two years or less, there was a significant trend towards greater delay of recurrence with longer-term use. Additionally, risk of death was also reduced. Furthermore, significant benefits were seen in patients with both estrogen receptor (ER) positive and ER negative tumors, although the benefits were greater in the ER positive group.

In very simple terms, tamoxifen competitively blocks estrogen binding at the ER. The tamoxifen-ER complex will also bind to DNA, but transcription is prevented. Thus, tamoxifen is a partial agonist and, as will be seen, exhibits estrogenic activity in certain tissues.

It was the observation that some women with ER negative tumors benefited from adjuvant tamoxifen which led to a more thorough investigation of its actions. In a carefully designed series of *in vitro* experiments, it was shown that tamoxifen increases the secretion of transforming growth factor-β (TGF-β) in estrogen-responsive breast cancer cell lines.[45] TGF-β can inhibit the growth of ER negative breast cancer cells. It was later shown that tamoxifen induces TGF-β secretion by stromal cells from both ER positive and ER negative tumors, *in vivo*, confirming that this is a truly ER independent process.[46]

In contrast to the effects on breast cancer, tamoxifen exerts conventional estrogenic effects on bone mineral density and a controlled study has demonstrated spinal bone conservation in postmenopausal women with breast cancer.[47] Additionally, in one study, tamoxifen has also been shown to reduce the risk of death from fatal myocardial infarction. The Scottish Adjuvant Trial was established to determine the effects on breast cancer survival but beneficial arterial actions were also observed.[48] A nonsignificant reduction in cardiac mortality was also observed in the Stockholm study.[49]

These effects on bone and the arterial status are clearly compatible with estrogenic activity. Hence, the term SERM is more appropriate than the term anti-estrogen for these actions. Other estrogenic activity of tamoxifen includes a stimulatory effect upon the endometrium. The first of the large randomized studies of adjuvant tamoxifen to report on the risk of endometrial cancer was from Stockholm. This study showed a relative risk of endometrial cancer of 6.4 (95% CI 1.4–28, $p<0.01$) in the treated patients who received tamoxifen 40 mg/day.[50] Prospective studies monitoring endometrial change from the initiation of therapy, using ultrasound and histology, have confirmed that tamoxifen induces some form of endometrial disease in up to 40% of patients.[51] Regrettably, this uterotropic effect of tamoxifen excludes this agent from widespread use amongst primary care physicians for prevention/treatment of osteoporosis and coronary heart disease in postmenopausal women.

Draloxifene and raloxifene

At this time, there are far fewer data on draloxifene as compared to raloxifene. Draloxifene has been shown to be active against advanced breast cancer.[52] The raloxifene database includes results from *in vitro* and animal studies, including large scale, prospective, randomized trials in postmenopausal women. The animal studies demonstrated that raloxifene inhibits estrogen-stimulated MCF-7 breast cancer cell proliferation *in vitro*. Indeed, raloxifene was shown to be more potent than tamoxifen in this system. In mammary carcinoma cell lines which are not estrogen dependent (the androgen sensitive Shionogi mouse mammary carcinoma model), raloxifene has no antiproliferative activity.[53] Raloxifene possesses bone conserving activity in animal models. In 75-day-old ovariectomized rats, given either raloxifene or an orally available form of estrogen daily for five weeks, it was clearly shown by both *ex vivo* single photon analysis of the trabecular rich region of the proximal femur and *ex vivo* dual energy X-ray absorptiometry of the proximal tibial metaphysis that raloxifene exerted a significant protective effect on bone which was statistically indistinguishable from an equivalent dose of estrogen.[54] Other studies using different skeletal sites have reported similar beneficial bone effects with raloxifene.[55]

Raloxifene has also been shown to lower serum cholesterol,[54] and this effect can be maintained for at least 12 months in ovariectomized rats.[55]

The first data from large-scale studies in women have recently been published.[56] In a placebo-controlled study, raloxifene, 30, 60 or 150 mg/day, was administered to postmenopausal women for 24 months. Each dose of raloxifene significantly increased bone mineral density in the lumbar spine and hip as compared to pretreatment values. Decreases in bone mineral density at these sites were observed in those receiving placebo. Serum concentrations of total cholesterol and LDL cholesterol decreased in all the raloxifene groups, whereas the serum concentrations of HDL cholesterol and triglycerides did not change. Importantly, endometrial thickness was similar in the raloxifene and placebo groups at all times during the study. There was no evidence that raloxifene stimulated endometrial proliferation.

Unlike HRT, the proportion of women receiving raloxifene who reported hot flashes or vaginal bleeding was not different to that of women receiving placebo. Thus, whilst raloxifene may not benefit menopausal symptoms, it clearly will conserve bone without causing vaginal bleeding, and may have an effect on arterial disease risk. Further data, particularly on the latter aspect, are urgently required.

Natural progesterone cream

Progest (natural progesterone cream: Professional and Technical Services, Portland, Oregon, USA) has attracted scientific and lay interest. It has been claimed that 'transdermal progesterone is far better than estrogen in reversing postmenopausal osteoporosis and that this action is independent of estrogen'.[57]

Progest can be purchased in the UK and other countries through mail order. In my clinical practice, I met women who had substituted Progest for the progestogen component of combined HRT. Measurement of the serum concentration of progesterone in some of these patients during Progest administration yielded values usually less than 3 nmol/L, which suggests little, if any, systemic absorption. Being unable to find any pharmacokinetic data on Progest, a randomized, double-blind, placebo-controlled, cross-over study to obtain information about absorption, metabolism and urinary excretion of the progesterone component by postmenopausal women was conducted.[58]

In summary, administration of 2–4 times the amount of Progest cream recommended by the manufacturer resulted in a significant increase, as compared to placebo, in urinary pregnanediol-3α-glucuronide (the principal urinary metabolite of progesterone), and in serum progesterone and 17-hydroxyprogesterone values. The data are shown in Table 52.8. However, the median serum progesterone value was only 2.9 nmol/L and this is much below the minimum value associated with normal ovarian function: a day 21 serum progesterone level of at least 30–35 nmol/L is usually observed in fertile women.

A value of serum progesterone of 3 nmol/L will not protect the endometrium from excessive stimulation by estrogen. Thus, Progest should not be substituted for the progestogen in conventional estrogen/progestogen HRT. Additionally, it is not easy to understand how such a small increment will conserve bone. The original article by Lee from which he concluded that 'transdermal progesterone is far better than estrogen in reversing postmenopausal osteoporosis' appeared as a hypothesis.[57] Sixty-three women had serial bone density measurements over three years. However, no methodological details (e.g. precision of the method; details of hardware and software for measuring bone density) were provided. Furthermore, there was no placebo-control group and in addition to Progest most patients also received calcium, 800–1000 mg/day, and conjugated estrogens, 0.3–0.625 mg/day. From the study design it is difficult to justify Lee's claims and in this author's opinion Progest should not be relied upon as an effective bone conserver unless properly designed, prospective, placebo-controlled studies can show clear benefit.

Summary

The marked increase in female life expectancy which has occurred this century has resulted in changes to the patterns of disease which are common and important causes of mortality and morbidity.

Table 52.8 Average pregnanediol-3α-glucuronide (P3G) concentrations in daily samples of early morning urine during treatment, and concentrations of plasma progesterone (P) and 17-hydroxyprogesterone (17-OHP) on the last day of treatment.[58]

	P3G (µmol/L)		P (nmol/L)		17-OHP (nmol/L)	
Treatment	Median	Range	Median	Range	Median	Range
None (baseline)		0.7	0.02–1.7	0.4	0.1–1.4	
Placebo (10 days)	1.1	0.3–2.8	0.8	0.3–1.8	0.4	0.2–0.9
Progest (10 days)	4.2	1.6–13.1***	2.9	0.7–15.00**	1.1	0.3–6.4*

*$p<0.05$; **$p<0.005$; ***$p<0.0001$: Progest versus placebo. All analyses Student's paired 't' test.

The commonest cause of death in women, myocardial infarction, and an important cause of morbidity, osteoporotic fracture (particularly hip fracture), are clearly related to estrogen deficiency. The natural history of other diseases, such as stroke and Alzheimer's disease, may also be modified by estrogen deficiency and replacement. More effort should be made to educate women about these diseases so that choice as to whether to use HRT, or not, is based upon appropriate information.

During the last two decades (and particularly during the last 10 years) novel routes of administration for estrogen have been introduced. Similar methodology is now being applied to the delivery of progestogen: various schedules of estrogen and estrogen and progestogen have been developed for pre and perimenopausal women, for early postmenopausal women and for older women. Thus, treatment is increasingly being 'individualized' and it should be possible to find a regimen acceptable to the great majority of women who wish to use HRT for whatever reason.

Steroid sex hormones are potent and have important biological actions. HRT, when used sensibly, will confer greater benefits than risks. In a tiny number of women use of HRT may be unwise, usually because of pre-existing diseases(s).

Alternatives for HRT are being developed: phytoestrogens and SERMs are actively being researched to define benefits and risks. From data already available it is clear that SERMs conserve bone density. The health food industry is also promoting various treatments incorporating sex hormones or their precursors for the treatment of postmenopausal symptoms and diseases. At this time, the marketing of such products seems far in advance of the research. There is no scientific evidence available from rigorous, placebo-controlled trials to justify the use of such health foods.

REFERENCES

1. Wilson RA 1966 Feminine forever. Allen, London
2. The Collaborative Group on Hormonal Factors in Breast Cancer 1997 Lancet 350: 1047–1059
3. Horton R 1997 ICRF: from mayhem to meltdown. Lancet 350: 1043–1044
4. Griffiths F 1995 Women's decisions about whether or not to take hormone replacement therapy: influence of social and medical factors. The British Journal of General Practice 45: 477–480
5. Campbell S, Whitehead MI 1977 Oestrogen therapy and the menopausal syndrome. In: Greenblatt RB, Studd JWW (eds) Clinics in obstetrics and gynecology, vol. 4, no. 1. The menopause. WB Saunders, Philadelphia and London, pp 31–47
6. O'Connor R, McCaffery M, Pitkin J 1900 (Full title to be advised)
7. Ross D, Rees CMR, Godfree VA, Cooper AJ, Hart DM, Kingsland CJ, Whitehead MI 1997 Randomised cross-over comparison of skin irritiation with two transdermal oestradiol patches. British Medical Journal 315: 288
8. McCarthy T, Dramusic V, Ratnam S 1992 Use of two types of estradiol-releasing skin patches for menopausal patients in a tropical climate. American Journal of Obstetrics and Gynecology 166: 2005–2010
9. Gangar KF, Cust MP, Whitehead MI 1989 Oestrogen deficiency symptoms asssociated with supraphysiological plasma oestradiol concentrations in women with oestradiol implants. British Medical Journal 299: 601–602
10. Gangar KF, Fraser D, Whitehead MI, Cust MP 1990 Prolonged endometrial stimulation associated with oestradiol implants. British Medical Journal 300: 436–438
11. Studd JWW, Holland EF, Leather AT, Smith RN 1994 The dose-response of percutaneous oestradiol implants on the skeletons of postmenopausal women. British Journal of Obstetrics and Gynaecology 101: 787–791
12. Bengtsson C, Bjorkelund C, Lapidus L, Lissner L 1993 Associations of serum lipid concentrations and obesity with mortality in women: 20 year follow-up of participants in a prospective population study in Gothenberg, Sweden. British Medical Journal 307: 1385–1388

13. Magos AL, Brewster E, Singh R, O'Dowd T, Brincat M, Studd JWW 1986 The effects of norethisterone in postmenopausal women on oestrogen replacement therapy: a model for the premenstrual syndrome. British Journal of Obstetrics and Gynaecology 93: 1290–1296
14. Falkeborn M, Persson I, Adami HO, Berstrom R, Eaker E, Mohsen HLR et al 1992 The risk of acute myocardial infarction after oestrogen and oestrogen/progestogen replacement therapy. British Journal of Obstetrics and Gynaecology 99: 821–828
15. Marsh MS, Crook D, Whitcroft SIJ, Worthington M, Whitehead MI, Stevenson JC 1994 Effect of continuous combined estrogen and desogestrel hormone replacement therapy on serum lipids and lipoproteins. Obstetrics and Gynecology 83: 19–23
16. Raudaskoski TH, Tomas EL, Paakkari IA, Kauppila AJ, Laatikainen TJ 1995 Serum lipids and lipoproteins in postmenopausal women receiving transdermal oestrogen in combination with a levonorgestrel-releasing intrauterine device. Maturitas 22: 47–53
17. Ross D, Cooper AJ, Pryse-Davies J, Bergeron C, Collins WP, Whitehead MI 1997 Randomised double-blind, dose-ranging study of the endometrial effects of a vaginal progesterone gel in estrogen-treated postmenopausal women. American Journal of Obstetrics and Gynecology 177: 937–941
18. Cerin A, Heldaas K, Moeller B 1996 Adverse endometrial effects of long-cycle estrogen and progestogen replacement therapy. New England Journal of Medicine 334: 668–669
19. Archer DF, Pickar JH, Bottiglioni F 1994 Bleeding patterns in postmenopausal women taking continuous combined or sequential regimens of conjugated estrogens with medroxyprogesterone acetate. American Journal of Obstetrics and Gynecology 83: 686–692
20. Spencer CP, Cooper AJ, Whitehead MI 1997 Management of abnormal bleeding in women receiving hormone replacement therapy. British Medical Journal 315: 37–42
21. Holly EA, Cress RD, Ahn DK 1994 Cutaneous melanoma in women: ovulatory life, menopause and use of exogenous estrogens. Cancer Epidemiology, Biomarkers and Prevention 3: 661–668
22. White E, Kirkpatrick CS, Lee JAH 1994 Case-control study of malignant melanoma in Washington State 1. Constitutional factors and sun exposure. American Journal of Epidemiology 139: 857–868
23. Holman CDJ, Armstrong BK, Heenan PJ 1984 Cutaneous malignant melanoma in women: exogenous sex hormones and reproductive factors. British Journal of Cancer 50: 673–680
24. Osterlind A, Tucker MA, Stone BJ, Jensen OM 1988 The Danish case-control study of cutaneous malignant melanoma III. Hormonal and reproductive factors in women. International Journal of Cancer 42: 821–824
25. Adami H-O, Persson I, Hoover R, Schairer C, Bergkvist L 1989 Risk of cancer in women receiving hormone replacement therapy. International Journal of Cancer 44: 833–839
26. Green A 1991 Oral contraceptives and skin neoplasia. Contraception 43: 653–666
27. Hannaford PC, Villard-Mackintosh L, Vessey MP, Kay CR 1991 Oral contraceptives and malignant melanoma. British Journal of Cancer 63: 430–433
28. Frigo P, Eppel W, Asseryanis E, Sator M, Golaszewski T, Gruber D, Lang C, Huber J 1995 The effects of hormone substitution in depot form on the uterus in a group of 50 peri-menopausal women — a vaginosonographic study. Maturitas 21: 221–225
29. Kempers RD, Dockerty MB, Hunt AB et al 1960 Significant postmenopausal endometriosis. Surgical Gynecology and Obstetrics 111: 348–356
30. Henderson AF, Studd JWW 1991 The role of definitive surgery and hormone replacement therapy in the treatment of endometriosis. In: Thomas EJ, Rock JA (eds) Modern approaches to endometriosis. Kluwer, London, pp 275–290
31. Arden NK, Lloyd ME, Spector TD, Hughes GR 1994 Safety of hormone replacement therapy (HRT) in systemic lupus erythematosis (SLE). Lupus 3: 11–13
32. Shutt DA, Cox RI 1972 Steroid and phytoestrogen binding to sheep uterine receptors in vitro. Journal of Endocrinology 52: 299–310
33. Verdeal K, Brown RR, Richardson T, Ryan DS 1980 Affinity of phytoestrogens for estradiol-binding proteins and effect of coumestrol on growth of 7,12-dimethylbenz alpha anthracene-induced rat mammary tumours. Journal of the National Cancer Institutes 64: 285–290
34. Messina MJ, Persky V, Setchell KDR, Barnes S 1994 Soy intake and cancer risk: a review of the in vitro and in vivo data. Nutrition and Cancer 21: 113
35. Judd HL 1976 Hormonal dynamics associated with the menopause. Clinical Obstetrics and Gynecology 19: 775
36. Laufer LR, DeFazio JL, Lu JKH 1983 Estrogen replacement therapy by transdermal estradiol administration. American Journal of Obstetrics and Gynecology 146: 533
37. Cassidy A, Bingham S, Setchell K 1994 Biological effects of isoflavones present in soy in premenopausal women: implications for the prevention of breast cancer. American Journal of Clinical Nutrition 60: 333–340
38. Cassidy A, Bingham S, Setchell K 1995 Biological effects of isoflavones in young women — importance of the chemical composition of soya products. British Journal of Nutrition 74: 587–601
39. Wilcox G, Wahlqvist ML, Burger HG, Medley G 1990 Oestrogen effects of plant derived foods in postmenopausal women. British Medical Journal 301: 905–906
40. Anthony MS, Clarkson TB, Hughes CL Jr et al 1996 Soybean isoflavones improve cardiovascular risk factors without affecting the reproductive system of peripubertal rhesus monkeys. Journal of Nutrition 126: 43–50
41. Clarkson TB, Anthony MS, Williams JK et al 1998 The potential of soybean phytoestrogens for postmenopausal hormone replacement therapy. Proceedings of the Society of Experimental Biology and Medicine 217: 365–368
42. Honore EK, Williams JK, Anthony MS 1995 Enhancement of coronary vasodilation by soy phytoestrogens and genistein. Circulation 92 (Suppl. II): 349 (Abstract)
43. Honore EK, Williams JK, Anthony MS et al 1900 Dietary soybean isoflavones prevent intimal hyperplasia after arterial injury in atherosclerotic nonhuman primates. Journal of Vascular Surgery. In press.

44. Early Breast Cancer Trialists' Collaborative Group 1992 Systemic treatment of early breast cancer by hormonal, cytotoxic or immune therapy. Lancet 339: 1–15, 71–85
45. Knabbe C, Lippman ME, Wakefield LM, Flanders KC, Kasid A, Derynck R, Dickson RB 1987 Evidence that transforming growth factor-beta is a hormonally regulated negative growth factor in human breast cancer cells. Cell 48: 417–428
46. Butta A, MacLennan K, Flanders KC, Sacks NPM, Smith I, McKinna A, Dowsett M, Wakefield LM, Sporn MB, Baum M, Colletta AA 1992 Induction of transforming growth factor beta-1 in human breast cancer in vivo following tamoxifen treatment. Cancer Research 52: 4261–4264
47. Love RR, Mazess RB, Barden HS, Epstein S, Newcomb PA, Jordan VC, Carbone PP, DeMets DL 1992 Effects of tamoxifen on bone mineral density in postmenopausal women with breast cancer. New England Journal of Medicine 326: 852–856
48. McDonald CC, Stewart HJ 1991 Fatal myocardial infarction in the Scottish adjuvant tamoxifen trial. British Medical Journal 303: 435–437
49. Rutqvist LE, Mattsson A 1993 Cardiac and thromboembolic morbidity among postmenopausal women with early-stage breast cancer in a randomised trial of adjuvant tamoxifen. Journal of the National Cancer Institute 85: 1398–1406
50. Fornander T, Rutqvist LE, Cedermark B, Glas U, Mattsson A, Silfverswärd C, Skoog L, Somell A, Theve T, Wilking N, Askergren J, Hjalmar M-L 1989 Adjuvant tamoxifen in early breast cancer: occurrence of new primary cancers. Lancet i: 117–120
51. Kedar RP, Bourne TH, Powles TJ, Collins WP, Ashley SE, Cosgrove DO, Campbell S 1994 Effects of tamoxifen on uterus and ovaries of postmenopausal women in a randomised breast cancer prevention trial. Lancet 343: 1318–1321
52. Bruning PF 1992 Draloxifene, a new anti-oestrogen in postmenopausal advanced breast cancer: preliminary results of a double-blind, dose-finding phase II trial. European Journal of Cancer 28A (8/9): 1404–1407
53. Thompson EW, Reich R, Shima TB et al 1988 Differential regulation of growth and invasiveness of MCF-7 breast cancer cells by anti-estrogens. Cancer Research 48: 6764–6768
54. Black LJ, Sato M, Rowley ER et al 1994 Raloxifene LY139481 HCI prevents bone loss and reduces serum cholesterol without causing uterine hypertrophy in ovariectomized rats. Journal of Clinical Investigation 93: 63–69
55. Bryant HU, Turner CH, Frolik CA et al 1995 Long term effects of raloxifene — LY139478 HCI — on bone, cholesterol and uterus in ovariectomized rats abstract. Bone 16 (Suppl): 116S
56. Delmas PD, Bjarnason NH, Mitlak BH, Ravoux A-C, Shah AS, Huster WJ, Draper M, Christiansen C 1997 Effects of raloxifene on bone mineral density, serum cholesterol concentrations, and uterine endometrium in post-menopausal women. New England Journal of Medicine 337: 1641–1647
57. Lee JR 1990 Osteoporosis reversal: the role of progesterone. International Clinical Nutrition Review 10: 384–389
58. Cooper AJ, Spencer C, Whitehead MI, Ross D, Barnard GJ, Collins WP 1998 Systemic absorption of progesterone from Progest cream in post-menopausal women. Lancet (In press)

53. Benefits of treatment: local and general menopausal symptoms

Mary Ann Lumsden

Introduction

The menopause is associated with climacteric symptoms which can cause considerable distress to a woman. A majority of women who take hormone replacement therapy (HRT) do so to obtain relief from these symptoms rather than for prevention of cardiovascular disease or osteoporosis. This chapter discusses some of the benefits of HRT with particular reference to vasomotor symptoms, urogenital atrophy and effects of HRT on the skin. There is also some discussion of the possible use of HRT in the prevention and treatment of Alzheimer's disease. Since the purpose of taking HRT is to improve well-being and quality of life, this will also be discussed and whether this is an independent entity or is related solely to the relief of other symptoms, particularly vasomotor.

POPULATIONS

The effectiveness of any treatment is influenced by patient expectation. With HRT this includes factors such as race and social class.[1] The way women perceive their menopause and the incidence of symptoms varies between different populations. In many Western populations the woman's view of the menopause is negative. This contrasts with women from some countries in Asia and the Far East where, although women know that the menopause will occur, they do not perceive a universal set of associated symptoms; some women do not even acknowledge that there are physical symptoms associated with a decrease in estradiol production: there is no word for 'hot flashes' in Japanese. On the other hand, in Pakistani communities there is a very positive view of the menopause since the women's status is elevated at this time. Menstruation is perceived as unclean and cessation has positive benefits. While if questioned some women do report menopausal symptoms, these are not usually considered to be of very much importance. Although there has been recent questioning of whether this 'absence' of symptoms is merely the culturally-expected answer to Western investigators, overall the perception of menopausal symptoms does appear to be less than in Europe or USA. Table 53.1 summarizes HRT uptake in different communities in recent years. Overall it is low, which suggests that a majority of women consider that the menopause is a natural event, that most of the symptoms are of limited duration or that the risks outweigh the benefits.

Women using estrogens have a higher level of education, a higher income and a healthier overall profile than nonusers. However, it is unlikely that these women experience more symptoms. In Great Britain women doctors have a high uptake of HRT and 50% will continue it for more than ten years. This suggests that knowledge of the advantages of HRT (and also less reliance on the advice of medical practitioners) is of importance.[2]

For a majority of women, the initial exposure to HRT is to provide symptom relief on the short-term; a minority only will take it in the long-term for disease prevention. An important issue in compliance is appropriate expectation concerning how much HRT can be expected to improve quality of life.

Table 53.1 Uptake of HRT in different communities in the early 1990s.

USA	40–60 years	45%
	>65	15%
	>80	7%
Sweden	Perimenopausal	21% (20%)
Netherlands	45–65	12%
Italy	Postmenopausal	2%
France	Postmenopausal	17%
UK	40–69 years	7%
Scotland	33–68 years	9%

VASOMOTOR SYMPTOMS

Vasomotor symptoms are the most common and easily recognizable symptoms of the menopause. The following symptoms are possible:

- Hot flashes
- Night sweats
- Insomnia
- Palpitations
- Headaches
- Dizziness.

They are often the first symptom of the menopause and occur in some women while they are still experiencing regular menstruation. Although for a majority they last for less than one year, for 20% this is not the case. However, hot flashing should not be considered trivial as it may cause considerable distress, particularly when occurring at night, since there is sleep disturbance which may be associated with tiredness and depression. Flashes can occur at any time and may be triggered by a variety of situations. Sleep related events are a common trigger although frequency varies between individuals; duration also varies and may be from a few minutes up to an hour.

Physiology of the hot flash

The physiology of the hot flash has been described in detail elsewhere (ch. 50) It is brought about by a decline in estrogen level, but symptoms may be experienced when a woman is not hypoestrogenic, thought to be due to fluctuating estrogen levels.[3] Although hot flashing is a very common problem it presents no inherent health hazard. It is accompanied by a discrete and reliable pattern of physiological changes associated with the LH surge and temperature changes in the skin. It is thought to be a sudden inappropriate excitation of heat release mechanisms. However, it should be appreciated that it is not dependent on, or due directly to, LH release since it will occur in women treated with gonadotropin releasing-hormone agonists, as described below.

Incidence of hot flashing

In a massive review of hot flashes,[4] it was concluded that exact estimates on prevalence are hampered by inconsistencies and differences in methodologies, cultures and definitions. In the longitudinal follow up of a large number of American women, premenopausal hot flashing occurred in 10%, although others have reported a higher incidence of up to 25%. The incidence is also related to socio-economic factors.[5] Unfortunately the hot flash is a relatively common psychosomatic symptom and women are often unnecessarily treated with estrogen.

The effect of estrogen therapy on hot flashes

The correlation between the onset of flashes and some reduction in estrogen levels is clinically supported by the effectiveness of estrogen therapy and the absence of flashes in hypoestrogenic states such as gonadal dysgenesis. Only after estrogen is administered and withdrawn do hypogonadal women experience a hot flash. Although the clinical impression that premenopausal surgical castrates suffer more severe vasomotor reactions is widely held, this is not consistently borne out in objective studies. Estrogen replacement therapy is the treatment of choice for postmenopausally-related hot flashing and symptom relief usually occurs over the first few weeks starting after about ten days. Relatively low doses of estrogen are sufficient to treat hot flashing but for some with persistent flashes an increase in dose may be appropriate. The alleviation of flashing together with headaches and possible insomnia may improve general well-being.[6,7]

The effect of different routes of administration

Oral. Estrogen was first described as an appropriate treatment for hot flashing by Greenblatt in the 1940s and 1950s[8] when it was demonstrated that oral conjugated equine estrogens were effective in relieving hot flashes and other postmenopausal symptoms. Since this time there have been a number of studies looking at the effect of administering estrogen by different routes on the incidence and severity of hot flashing.

Transdermal therapy. With the advent of transdermal therapy systems during the 1970s and 1980s, comparative studies have been carried out to assess whether there is any difference in efficacy when estrogen is administered by the different routes. Should a difference be demonstrated then this would suggest that hepatic first pass metabolism is important in the relief of hot flashing. However, to be effective, orally administered dosages are relatively high and result in metabolic disturbance. Studies using transdermal systems releasing 100 μg estrodiol daily suggest that the efficacy is similar to oral preparations and that the improvement continues progressively over a matter of 4–6 weeks or more.[9–13] There is a linear reduction in hot flashes as the concentration of estradiol rises, a reduction of 91% occurring at 200 μg

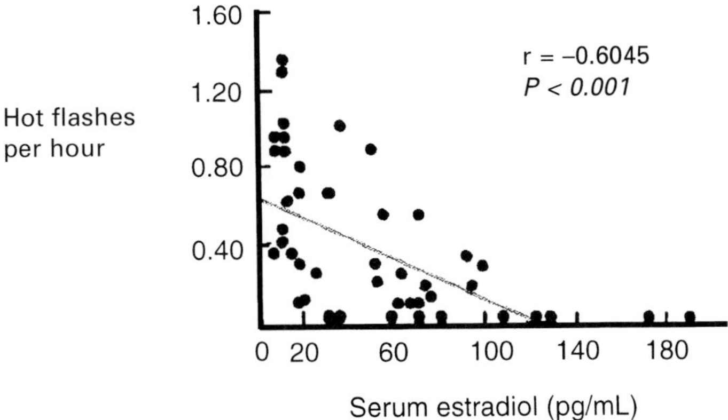

Fig. 53.1 The incidence of hot flashing compared with the circulating concentration of estradiol. Ref 9, with permission.

transdermally. All women using 50 μg or over will experience some relief (Fig. 53.1). Benefit is also obtained when smaller doses of estradiol are administered (50 mg or 25 mg). However, in some instances lower dosages will not be sufficient to prevent flashing. Seven day estradiol transdermal systems have now been developed and comparative studies suggest that the reduction of hot flashes is comparable with that experienced by women using oral estrogens (e.g. Premarin). The effects are dose-related with the 50 μg patch being slightly less effective than Premarin 0.625 mg with 65% as opposed to 75% successfully responding. The onset of efficacy was two weeks after the start of therapy and was fully sustained during the seven day patch period although when there was a 'patch free week', efficacy decreased in line with decreasing estradiol levels.[13] Other studies have failed to demonstrate any recurrence of flashing in the treatment-free week.[15]

Subcutaneous implants. Estradiol implants are also successful in treating vasomotor symptoms.[16,17] This involves insertion under the skin of small crystalline estradiol implants of 25, 50 or 100 mg. The duration of activity is 4–6 months with the 20 mg dose, following which symptoms will start to recur. This is variable from one woman to another. The concept that hot flashing is related to decreases in rather than absolute estradiol levels is further supported by the fact that some women develop tachyphylaxis to estradiol implants. This means that they start to experience symptoms progressively sooner after the implant is inserted, even though circulating estradiol levels are very high. It is thought that this is related to the onset of decreasing levels and it is a problem which is very difficult to treat.

Phytoestrogens. A 'natural' alternative may be the phytoestrogens which occur in soy, wheat flour and a number of other plant sources. Hot flashing is successfully treated in 40% and an improvement in symptoms is noted over the first six weeks of administration.[18]

Combination with progestogens. The efficacy of estrogens in treating vasomotor symptoms is not affected by the addition of a progestogen since progestogens themselves may give benefit from some menopausal symptoms. Studies have compared different oral progestogens as well as the addition of transdermal norethindrone.[19] The effect of combined HRT on hot flashing is largely dependent on the estrogen component. Not all women will experience symptom relief, suggesting that flashing is not always associated with abnormal estrogen levels.

Progestogen therapy

When administration of estrogen is inappropriate then progestogens may be used instead. It is well documented that administration of norethindrone or medroxyprogesterone acetate may give considerable, if not complete, relief of vasomotor systems. Overall their effect on bone is less than with estrogen administration and in some cases there is no protective effect at all. The choice of progestogen may be difficult since norethindrone may offer better protection for the bone than medroxyprogesterone acetate but is frequently associated with more progestational side effects.[20] Trials are underway to look at the effectiveness of megestrol acetate in symptomatic women with breast cancer.

Therapy with other sex steroids

Although testosterone implants are used to improve libido and sexual function, they do not appear to provide benefit for vasomotor symptoms when given alone.[21] However tibolone alone is as successful as the estrogen-containing regimes.[22–24]

Gonadotropin-releasing hormone agonists

Gonadotropin-releasing hormone (GnRH) agonists are frequently used in the treatment of estrogen-dependent gynecological disease, such as endometriosis, for the shrinkage of uterine fibroids and endometrial thinning, as well as in the treatment of hormone-dependent cancers. The mechanism of action is that the drugs produce down regulation of the pituitary gland with a decrease in circulating estradiol levels to the postmenopausal or early follicular phase range. Ovulation is inhibited in all women after the first month of administration. Since the drugs induce a 'pseudomenopause', side effects tend to be identical with those of the natural menopause. Hot flashing occurs in over 80% of women, although its association with cessation of therapy is rare since the drugs tend to be given for a short period only and ovarian function resumes rapidly after administration ceases. However, there is a small group of women in which prolonged administration of GnRH agonists is appropriate. This includes women who are poor operative risks or who have medical problems which render surgical treatment of their condition inappropriate.

GnRH agonists with 'add back' therapy. There are now considerable data on 'add back' therapy. It has been noted that a small amount of estrogen can be replaced in women on GnRH agonist therapy without decreasing the efficacy of the preparation. Combined estrogen/progestogen combinations will relieve symptoms and do not adversely affect the lipid profile. In general, estrogen alone is not prescribed because of its long-term effects on the endometrium. Progestogen regimes have been studied using progestogens at different dosages. Relief of vasomotor symptoms usually occurs with relatively modest doses of progestogen but unfortunately this may not be associated with prevention of osteoporosis (Figs 53.2, 53.3). Tibolone had also been shown to be very effective in this group of women in terms of both symptomatic relief and prevention of bone loss. It is not known if these agents are effective by a mechanism involving estrogen receptor binding, although this would be a possibility since in general moderately large doses of progestogen are necessary to produce therapeutic benefit.

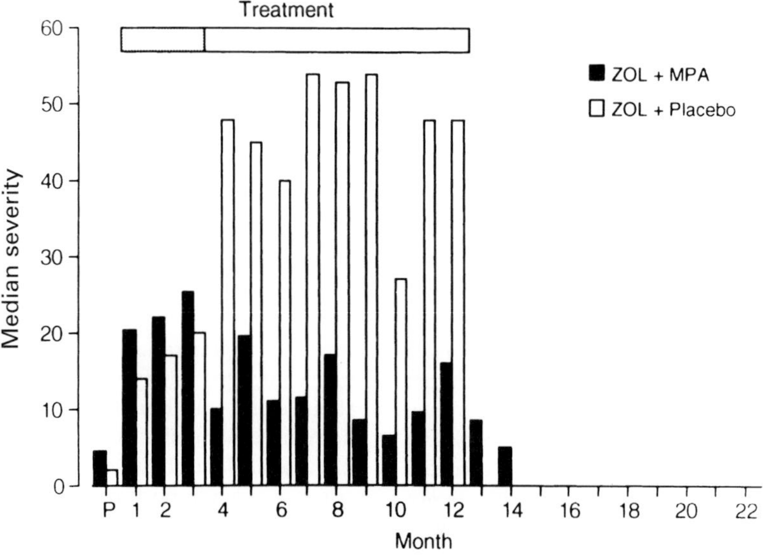

Fig. 53.2 The incidence of hot flashing in women taking goserelin combined with placebo compared with those taking goserelin combined with medroxyprogesterone acetate.[64]

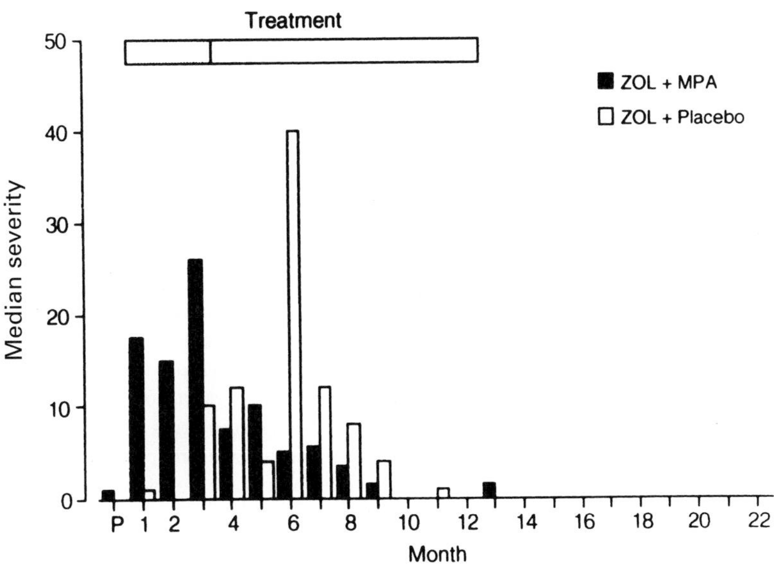

Fig. 53.3 The incidence of night sweats in women taking goserelin combined with placebo compared with those taking goserelin combined with medroxyprogesterone acetate.[64]

Assessment of hot flashes

Objective studies of the effect of hormone replacement therapy on hot flashing are difficult to achieve. Most have involved the statement of the woman regarding her symptoms or the measurement of the elevation in skin temperature which tends to occur after the flash, although this correlates poorly with the woman's actual perception of the event. Studies involving measurement of peripheral blood flow have been performed with some success, however there is no good animal model to explore this further. Although studies have been carried out looking at the effect of acute administration of estradiol on blood flow these have not been performed in the context of looking at change in the incidence of hot flashing.

Estrogen administration decreases forearm blood flow but does not change forearm vascular reactivity, although both factors are increased by tibolone. The dopamine antagonist veralipride, an effective treatment for hot flashing, decreases peripheral vascular responsiveness which might contribute to its beneficial effects.

Other therapies

Behavioral relaxation training can reduce flashing by altering neurotransmitter output since women who flash have an increase in the level of central sympathetic activation.[25] There is also the suggestion that the level of exercise is important.[26]

It is likely that relief of symptoms is due to a receptor-mediated effect of the steroids rather than their effect on transmitter release. Clonidine, which is an alpha agonist, has been used to relieve the vasomotor symptoms of the climactic since it was presumed that the mechanism of action was related to the alpha adrenergic system. However, it has more recently been demonstrated that clonidine is little more effective than placebo and also has no effect on the peripheral blood flow alterations which accompany hot flashing. Dopamine agonists are also being investigated as mentioned above.[27]

ALZHEIMER'S DISEASE

Alzheimer's disease is a leading cause of dementia. There is an inexorable increase in prevalence which doubles every 4.5 years after the age of 65 (i.e. 50% of those aged 85 or over are affected). It is commoner in women, and risk factors include age, family history and a history of head trauma. Of particular importance is a deficit in episodic memory. This is the ability to learn new information that can be recalled minutes, hours or days later. Semantic memory, which includes word names, common facts and memory for over learned general information is less affected.

The pathology of Alzheimer's disease is covered elsewhere. The underlying disorder consists of pathological changes within the brain and a decrease in acetylcholine concentration. Depression is also a very common symptom of Alzheimer's disease.

Dementia is more likely in those who have had a myocardial infarction and in a large prospective study of 9000 women in a leisure world retirement community, Paganini-Hill was able to demonstrate that the risk of developing Alzheimer's was less in estrogen users.[28]

The effect of steroid hormones on the brain

Evidence suggests that sex hormones have an important role in the neuro-organization of cerebral cortex (see ch. 17). There are estrogen and androgen receptors within the brain, although estrogen may also have nonreceptor mediated effects. Some of its effects which may be relevant in a discussion of Alzheimer's disease are as follows:

- Antioxidant properties
- Potentiates neuronal responses
- Augments glucose utilization
- Aids healing of neurological tissue after injury
- Influences neurotransmitter systems
- Increases hippocampal cholinergic markers
- Regulates cytokines.

There have been studies in both the prevention and treatment of Alzheimer's disease.

Memory and cognitive function in the elderly and the effects of HRT

There is a decrease in cognitive efficiency in postmenopausal women, although this is partly age-related. Cognitive function is the process related to acquisition of knowledge and it determines a person's ability to function in day-to-day activities. Estrogens are known to increase the cerebral circulation in postmenopausal women[29] which is also associated with improved cognitive function.[30] Human studies have shown that estrogens improve depression. HRT also reduces the incidence of stroke and thus prevents post-stroke dementia.

The effect of HRT on cognitive function has been investigated by a number of small studies using different preparations and study populations and thus results tend to be variable.[31,34] However, estrogen appears to be superior to placebo in relieving insomnia, irritability, headache, anxiety and memory loss, benefits which are independent of the relief of hot flushing. It has also been demonstrated that there is a positive correlation between cognitive function and estrogen and/or androgen levels.

The prevention of Alzheimer's disease

The place of estrogen in prevention and treatment of Alzheimer's disease is discussed in a recent review.[33] Estrone sulfate levels are lower in those with Alzheimer's disease than those without and estrogen replacement therapy may lower a woman's risk of Alzheimer's disease development. Early ageing females exhibit abnormal neurological function. This is restored by estradiol administration which may be involved in the reparative neuronal response to injury. Also, in a large prospective study, it was demonstrated that the risk of developing Alzheimer's disease among estrogen users was less than among those who had never used estrogen.[28]

Improvement of symptoms of Alzheimer's disease

Estradiol administration influences cholinergic function which may benefit memory and cognitive function. In women a positive effect has been noted on attention span, concentration and also libido. Estrogen replacement therapy improves cognitive function and regional cerebral blood flow in female patients with Alzheimer's disease in short term studies.[32] There have been several small studies involving the study of semantic memory. Improvement has been noted after only one month's administration of hormone replacement therapy. Other studies have found an improvement in attention, orientation and mood as well as less depression. There seems to be a benefit for verbal skills whereas there is disagreement as to whether there is improvement in memory.

In summary it would appear that estradiol deficiency may be one of the factors that contributes to a woman's risk of developing this disorder. However, prospective randomized trials are necessary to determine whether widespread administration of estrogen replacement therapy will alter the onset or progression of Alzheimer's disease.

THE EFFECTS OF HORMONE REPLACEMENT THERAPY ON SKIN

Many women believe that hormone replacement therapy will help prevent the aging changes which occur in the skin, particularly of the face.[35] There have been few placebo-controlled studies in this area. However, it has been suggested that administration of either estriol or estradiol will improve skin thickness. This may be as a result of systemic absorption or local effects. It appears the estrogens influence epidermal and dermal thickness, the structure of elastic fibers, skin vessels and dermal mucopolysaccharide content.[36]

The effect of estrogen on the epidermis

Ovarian failure leads to thinning of the epidermis, which is prevented by HRT, although other hormones and growth factors such as IGF-1 may be involved. Epidermal atrophy corresponds with vascular atrophy, with estradiol treatment then leading to an increase in capillary number as well as dilatation of arterioles and venules which improves the nutrition of the epidermis. Microscopic inspection of the nail fold capillaries of the female demonstrates dependence on menopausal status and hormone replacement therapy.[37] Blood flow through the peripheral microcirculation decreases at the menopause and is increased again after administration of hormone replacement therapy, although morphological changes in vessels are inconsistent.

Progesterone stimulates cell proliferation with a decrease in the cornification rate of epidermal cells and an increase in epidermal thickness.

The effect of HRT on the dermis

A diagram of the constituents of skin is shown in Figure 53.4. The constituents of the dermis are as follows:

- Collagen and elastin fibers
- Fibroblasts
- Ground substance
- Protein (noncollagen)
- Water.

HRT has an effect on a number of these factors which may contribute to the beneficial effects on skin.[36]

The effect of estrogen on skin water content

Much of skin appearance is related to the water-holding capacity of the skin, and pilot studies have been carried out to see if hormone replacement therapy will influence this.[38] Electrical capacitance through the stratum corneum can be measured, which gives an indication of the water flux and transepidermal water loss. Studies are as yet inconclusive but suggest that hormone replacement therapy may increase skin thickness by promoting water retention within the skin. This may result from changes in the elastic fibers in the skin and hyaluronic acid content.

The effect of estrogen on collagen

Estrogen deprivation is classically associated with thin, transparent skin. Skin elasticity and thickness decline in the years after the menopause as estrogen decreases. Collagen accounts for 50% of the total protein of the skin and hormone replacement therapy prevents loss in

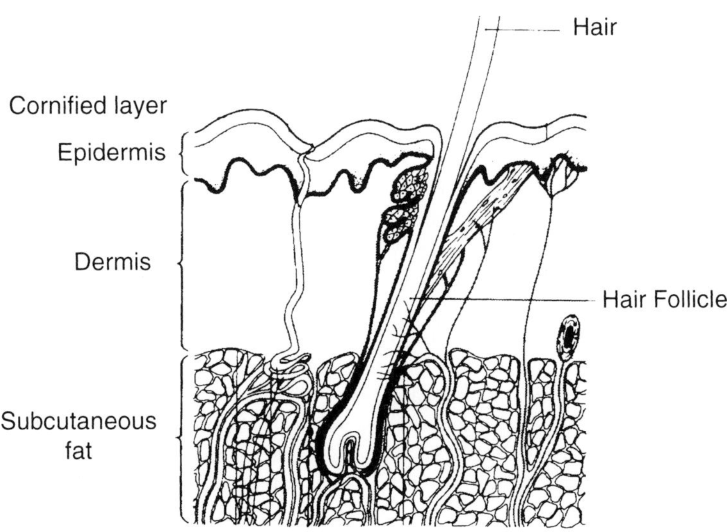

Fig. 53.4 The structure of human skin.

skin as it does in bone, with a consequent increase in skin thickness.[39,40] However, age itself leads to a decrease in skin collagen independent of hormonal status.

It has been suggested that up to 30% of the collagen content will be lost in the first five years after the menopause.[41] Estradiol causes an increase in the production rate of type III collagen which is not affected by the administration of progestogen. Androgen administration has a greater effect: there is enhanced polymerization of soluble collagen to the insoluble form. Degradation is retarded and the half-life of collagen is increased by over 100%.

Other factors

Many women believe that estradiol will prevent age-related skin changes, but objective evaluation suggests that this is probably not the case. Hair follicles contain estrogen and androgen receptors, the content of the former decreasing at the menopause. This may account for postmenopausal thinning of the hair in some women.

Recent studies of the thickness of the wall of the carotid artery suggest that estrogen may have an influence on collagen content of structures other than the skin and bone. Doppler ultrasound studies indicate that the walls are thicker in those treated with hormone replacement therapy than those without. The significance of these studies has as yet to be determined.

UROGENITAL ATROPHY

Menopausal changes in urogenital tissues

The integrity of the tissues of the female reproductive tract is dependent on estrogen. When levels of estrogen decrease after the menopause degenerative changes in these structures occur.[42,43] The vaginal epithelium of postmenopausal women who do not receive estrogen therapy appears pale due to a decrease in vascularity. There is also thinning of the blood vessel walls. They are less well supported and also the blood flow through the vessels themselves is decreased. The net result of all these changes is that the vaginal epithelium is thin, friable and prone to bleeding and infection. The epithelial thinning may mean that there is an increase in transudate, which may lead to increase in discharge. A decrease in elasticity is noted. These effects lead to dyspareunia and vaginal bleeding. Inflammation and ulceration can lead to atrophic vaginitis.

Similar changes occur in the tissues of the urethra and lower parts of the urinary tract. Again, inflammation is a common sequel and patients may complain of dysuria and frequency together with local vaginal discomfort.[44] Urinary symptoms are usually irritative in nature and incontinence as a consequence of estrogen deprivation is uncommon. However, it appears that there is a small increase in incidence of urinary tract infections.

Symptoms of genital atrophy are a later manifestation of the menopause, usually not appearing for 5–10 years. In a study of Swedish women aged over 60 years, Iosif and Bekawsy reported one or more vaginal symptoms in over 50% of subjects and the prevalence of these symptoms increased with age.[45] It is important to recognize that optimal response to treatment will often take a long time (1–2 years).

Methods of administration

Vaginal physiology and function are improved by estrogen, regardless of the route of administration.[43,46] Benefit will usually be obtained when estrogen is administered by the systemic routes. Although a low dose of estrogen such as ethinyl estradiol 10 μg daily will usually be sufficient to relieve vaginal atrophy, supplementation with vaginal estrogen may be beneficial.[47]

Vaginal estrogens

These are useful in the very old since they have few systemic side effects. They can be administered in a variety of ways such as creams, pessaries, tablets or nonbiodegradable long-acting rings.

Most preparations contain either estradiol or estriol and are highly effective at treating local symptoms.[48] In a placebo-controlled study of over 100 women 78.8% of those receiving local estradiol and 81.9% of the placebo group had moderate to severe vaginal atrophy prior to treatment. After eight weeks of therapy only 10.7% of the vaginal estradiol group but 21.9% of the placebo group had the same degree of atrophy.[49] Creams are cheap and effective but tend to be messy to use and compliance is poor. Vaginal tablets are easy for the patient to insert satisfactorily but are expensive. Pessaries are also effective and reasonably acceptable to patients. Vaginal rings under investigation are soft, easily inserted and appear to cause no discomfort for the patient. Recently, a silicon vaginal ring releasing 5–10 μg of estradiol per 24 hours for a minimum of 90 days has been marketed in a few countries. Maturation of the vaginal epithelium improved greatly during treatment as well as symptoms of vaginal dryness, dyspareunia and urinary urgency. Improvement in atrophic vaginitis was noted in over 90% of those using the ring and many found that sexual intercourse became possible.[50,51]

An advantage of low-dose vaginal estrogen administration is that systemic absorption is small and progestogen need not be given with it. It may also be given in addition to systemic treatment in those where atrophic vaginitis continues to be a problem in spite of oral or transdermal HRT.

Alternative local treatment

A preparation is available which absorbs fluid from the surrounding tissues due to its hydrophylic nature. This is also effective in relieving some symptoms of vaginal atrophy.[52]

Urinary symptoms

As stated above, local administration of estrogen may be effective in relieving some urinary symptoms. However, it will only relieve the urinary problems due to atrophy. Estrogens have no affect on the detrusor muscle and so an objective improvement in urgency or urge incontinence is unlikely. There is also no convincing evidence that estrogens improve stress incontinence. Estrogens may be given prior to pelvic floor surgery in those where tissues are thin and of poor quality, otherwise they have little role in the management of stress incontinence.

Aspects of sexuality

Apart from local factors described above, there are other reasons why postmenopausal women may experience a lack of libido. When ovarian function declines, and particularly when the ovaries are removed at hysterectomy, there is a decrease in androgen production which may often be accompanied by a decrease in libido. Libido also tends to decrease with age and for many with very long-standing relationships it is a gradual natural progression. Hormone replacement therapy will improve local factors which may include touch sensation in vaginal tissues.[53] It may also improve the feeling of well-being as described earlier in this chapter, and all of these may contribute to improved libido. Some studies have demonstrated that androgen administration, usually in the form of an implant, may be useful although other studies have been unable to confirm this.

Quality of life

For most women, reaching the age of the menopause is not viewed with regret or resentment. A majority have positive or neutral feelings concerning cessation of menses. However, many do feel that the quality of life is compromised by the presence of menopausal symptoms.[54,55] This would suggest that the use of HRT to relieve symptoms may result in a substantial improvement in quality of life for many. Although motivation for the use of HRT varies significantly between countries, the perceived benefits are generally consistent, including an increase in physical and mental energy levels and an improvement in the psychological condition.[56,57] Uptake and benefits of treatment are associated with the ease with which HRT can be obtained.[26] The improvement in well-being with estradiol is significantly greater than with placebo.[58] There may also be a benefit in treating symptoms such as headache, which may have a psychosomatic component, and which influence well-being.[59]

Women's anticipations reflect the beliefs and values of their cultural world.[60] In the Western world there is frequently a desire to delay the effects of ageing as well as to alleviate symptoms and prevent disease. There is also a desire for HRT to 'fix' damage done by the menopause. There is a hope that youth will be restored and old age postponed. An expectation of HRT is to restore women to their previous level of function irrespective of any natural decline. Inevitably, HRT is unlikely to fulfil these expectations.

The assessment of well-being and quality of life have been largely neglected, emphasis tending to be on the negative. Quality of life is difficult to measure, which explains some of the variation in results documented by the various studies. However, overall the health benefits of postmenopausal estrogen replacement exceed any health risk incurred.[61,62]

Improvement in quality of life is most likely to be dependent on symptom relief. Relief of symptoms such as flashing or sweating will allow better sleep and an improved ability to cope with any problems which may arise. However, some studies have demonstrated that there is an improvement in well-being which is independent of the effects of estradiol on hot flashing and suggest a central effect of the hormones.[63]

Well-being is often assessed merely by a global question asking whether a woman 'feels better than before commencing treatment'. Most estrogen-containing regimes are associated with an improvement in the global assessment independent of the route of administration. Drugs such as tibolone have also been shown to be beneficial.[22]

Conclusion

There is little doubt that HRT is effective in treating vasomotor symptoms. All routes of administration give satisfactory relief and often at low doses. For those in whom estradiol is not appropriate, progestogen alone can be used. In general, HRT is taken for a limited duration only when the principal aim is symptom relief.

Urogenital atrophy is also effectively treated. Benefits may be achieved with oral or other systemic administration although in elderly women local treatment may be the most appropriate since systemic absorption and side effects can be avoided. Atrophic urethritis may be effectively treated but HRT has little effect on detrusor instability or stress incontinence.

Hormone replacement therapy has effects on the skin which may lead to thickening and increased retention of water which can improve the appearance and feel of the skin. However, the effects of age itself cannot be avoided.

The beneficial effects of HRT on prevention and treatment of Alzheimer's disease are less clear. Most studies are too small to be conclusive, but if a beneficial effect were to be confirmed then the implications could be considerable. HRT may also have some influence on the symptoms of depression although this is a complicated field and many of the studies show discrepant results. Psychological and mood symptoms are discussed in more detail in chapter 64.

REFERENCES

1. Abraham S, Perz J, Clarkson R, Llewellyn-Jones D 1995 Australian womens' perceptions of hormone replacement therapy over ten years. Maturitas 21: 91–95
2. Isaacs AJ, Britton AR, McPherson K 1995 Utilisation of hormone replacement therapy by women doctors. British Medical Journal 311: 1399–1401
3. Rannevik G, Jeppsson S, Johnell O, Bjerre B, Laurell-Borulf Y, Svanberg L 1995 A longitudinal study of the perimenopausal transition, sex hormone binding globulin and bone mineral density. Maturitas 21: 103–113
4. Kronnenberg F 1990 Hot flashes: epidemiology and physiology. Annals of the New York Academy of Science 59: 52
5. Schwingl PJ, Hulka BS, Harlow SD 1994 Risk factors for menopausal hot flashes. Obstetrics and Gynecology 84: 29–34
6. Groeneveld FP, Bareman FP, Barentsen R, Dokter HJ, Drogendijk AC, Hoes AW 1996 Vasomotor symptoms and wellbeing in the climacteric years. Maturitas 23: 293–299
7. Studd JW, McCarthy K, Zamblera D, Burger H, Silderberg S, Wren B, Dain MP, Le Lann L, Vandepol C 1995 Efficacy and tolerance of Menorest compared to Premarin in the treatment of postmenopausal women. A randomised, multicentre, double-blind, double-dummy study. Maturitas 22: 105–114
8. Greenblatt RB, Dutran RR 1949 Indications for hormone pellets in the therapy of endocrine and gynaecological disorders. Journal of Obstetrics and Gynaecology of the British Empire 57: 291–301
9. Steingold KA, Laufer L, Ryszard J, Chetkowski J et al 1985 Treatment of hot flashes with transdermal estradiol administration. Journal of Clinical Endocrinology and Metabolism 61: 627–631
10. Padwick ML, Endacott J, Whitehead MI 1985 Efficacy acceptability and metabolic effects of transdermal estradiol in the management of postmenopausal women. American Journal of Obstetrics and Gynecology 152: 1085–1091
11. Place DA, Powers M, Darley PE, Schenkel L, Good WR 1985 A double-blind comparative study of Estraderm and Premarin in the amelioration of postmenopausal symptoms. American Journal of Obstetrics and Gynecology 152: 1092–1099
12. Pornel B, Genazzani AR, Costes D, Dain MP, Lelann L, Vandepol C 1995 Efficacy and tolerability of Menorest 50 compared with Estroderm TTS 50 in the treatment of postmenopausal symptoms. A randomized, multicentre, parallel group study. Maturitas 22: 217–218
13. Gordon SF 1995 Clinical experience with a seven day estradiol transdermal system for estrogen replacement therapy. American Journal of Obstetrics and Gynecology 173: 998–1004
14. Nachtigall LE 1995 Emerging delivery systems for estrogen replacement: aspects of transdermal and oral delivery. American Journal of Obstetrics and Gynecology 173: 993–997
15. McCarthy T, Dramusic V, Carter R, Costales A, Ratnam SS 1995 Randomised crossover study of a 21-day versus a 28-day hormone replacement therapy. Maturitas 22: 13–23
16. Brincat M, Studd JW, O'Dowd T, Magos A, Cardozo LD, Wardle PJ 1984 Subcutaneous hormone implants for the control of climacteric symptoms. A prospective study. Lancet 1: 16–18
17. Cardozo L, Gibb DMF, Tuck SM, Thom MH, Studd JW, Cooper DJ 1984 The effects of subcutaneous hormone implants during the climacteric. Maturitas 5: 177–184
18. Murkies AL, Lombard C, Strauss BJ, Wilcox G, Burger HG, Morton MS 1995 Dietary flour supplementation decreases postmenopausal hot flushes: effect of soy and wheat. Maturitas 21: 189–195
19. Stadberg E, Mattsson LA, Uvebrant M 1996 17β-estradiol and norethisterone acetate in low doses as continuous combined hormone replacement therapy. Maturitas 23: 31–39
20. Pansini F, Albertazzi P, Bonaccorsi G 1994 Hormone replacement therapy and lipids: is transdermal norethisterone acetate better than oral progestogen acetate? Menopause: Journal of North American Menopause Society 1: 119–123
21. Sherwin B, Gelfand MM 1984 Effects of parenteral administration of estrogen and androgen on plasma hormone levels and hot flushes in the surgical menopause. American Journal of Obstetrics and Gynecology 148: 552–557
22. Egarter CH, Huber J, Leikermoser R, Haidbauer R et al 1996 Tibolone versus conjugated estrogens and sequential progestogen in the treatment of cimacteric complaints. Maturitas 23: 55–62

23. Ginsburg J, Prelevic G, Butler D, Okolo S 1995 Clinical experience with tibolone (livial) over eight years. Maturitas 21: 71–76
24. Hardiman P, Nihoyannopoulos P, Kicovic P, Ginsburg J 1991 Cardiovascular effects of Org-OD 14 – a new steroidal therapy for climacteric symptoms. Maturitas 13: 235–242
25. Freedman RR, Woodward S, Brown B et al 1995 Biochemical and thermoregulatory effects of behavioural treatment for menopausal hot flashes. Menopause 2: 211–218
26. Nedstrand E, Ekseth U, Lindgren R, Hammer M 1995 The climacteric among South American women who immigrated to Sweden and age matched Swedish women. Maturitas 21: 3–6
27. Hardiman P, Ginsburg J 1995 Vascular effects of Veralipride, in non-hormonal treatment for climacteric flushing. Menopause 2: 219–223
28. Paganini-Hill A, Henderson VW 1994 Estrogen deficiency and risk of Alzheimers disease in women. American Journal of Epidemiology 140: 256–261
29. Gangar KF, Vyas S, Whitehead M, Crook D, Meire H, Campbell S 1991 Pulsatility index in internal carotid artery in relation to transdermal oestradiol and time since menopause. Lancet 338: 839–842
30. Barrett-Connor E, Kritz-Silverstein D 1993 Estrogen replacement therapy and cognitive function in older women. Journal of the American Medical Association 269: 2637–2641
31. Erkkola R 1994 Effect of ageing and HRT on memory performance and cognitive processes in the female. European Menopause Journal 1: 9–11
32. Ohkura T, Isse K, Akazawa K, Hamamoto M, Yaoi Y, Hagino N 1994 ERT for dementia of the Alzheimer type in women. In: Berg G Hammar M (eds) The modern management of the menopause. Proceedings of the VII International Congress on the Menopause, Stockholm, Sweden, 1993. Parthenon Publishing Group, London, New York, pp 315–333
33. Henderson VW, Paganini-Hill. Estrogen and Alzheimer's disease. In: Progress in Reproductive Medicine (Eds Asch R and Studd J) Parthenon Publishing, UK, pp 185–193
34. Ohkura T, Isse K, Akazawa K et al 1994 Low dose estrogen replacement therapy for Alzheimer disease in women. Menopause 1: 125–130
35. Bauer DC, Grady D, Pressman A et al 1994 Skin thickness, estrogen use and bone mass in older women. Menopause 1: 131–136
36. Schmidt JB, Binder M, Macheiner W, Kainz CL, Gitsch G, Bigglmayer CL 1994 Treatment of skin ageing symptoms in perimenopausal females with estrogen compounds. A pilot study. Maturitas 20: 25–30
37. Haenegi W, Linder HR, Birkhaeuser MH, Schneider H 1995 Microscopic findings of the nail-fold capillaries – dependence on menopausal status and hormone replacement therapy. Maturitas 22: 37–46
38. Piérard-Franchimont C, Latawe C, Goffin V, Piérard GE 1995 Skin water holding capacity and transdermal estrogen therapy for menopause: a pilot study. Maturitas 22: 151–154
39. Meschia M, Bruschi F, Amicarelli F, Barbacini P, Monza GC, Crosignani PG 1994 Transdermal hormone replacement therapy and skin in postmenopausal women: a placebo controlled study. Menopause 1: 79–82
40. Maheux R, Naud F, Rioux M, Grenier R, Lemay A, Guy J, Langevin M 1994 A randomized, double-blind, placebo controlled study on the effect of conjugated estrogens on skin thickness. American Journal of Obstetrics and Gynecology 170: 642–648
41. Castelo-Branco C, Duran M, Gonzalez-Merlo J 1992 Skin collagen changes related to age and hormone replacement therapy. Maturitas 15: 113–119
42. Bergman A, Brenner PF 1987 Alterations in the urogenital system. In: Mishell DR (ed) Menopause: physiology and pharmacology. Yearbook Medical Publishers Inc, Chicago, pp 67–75
43. Semmens JP, Wagner G 1982 Estrogen deprivation and vaginal function in postmenopausal women. Journal of the American Medical Association 248: 445–448
44. Hilton P, Stanton SL 1983 The use of intra-vaginal oestrogen cream in genuine stress incontinence. British Journal of Obstetrics and Gynaecology 90: 940–944
45. Iosif CS, Bekawsy Z 1984 Prevalence of genito-urinary symptoms in the later menopause. Acta Obstetrica Gynecologica Scandinavica 63: 257–260
46. Semmens JP, Tsai CC, Semmens EC, Loadholt CB 1985 Effects of estrogen therapy on vaginal physiology during the menopause. Obstetrics and Gynecology 66: 15–18
47. Mandel FP, Geola FL, Lu JK, Eggena P, Sambhi MP, Hershman JM, Judd HL 1982 Biologic effects of various doses of ethinyl estradiol in postmenopausal women. Obstetrics and Gynecology 59: 673–679
48. Raz R, Stamm WE 1993 A controlled trial of intra-vaginal estriol in postmenopausal women with recurrent urinary tract infection. New England Journal of Medicine 329: 753–756
49. Eriksen PS, Rasmussen H 1992 Low dose 17β oestradiol vaginal tablets in the treatment of atrophic vaginitis: a double-blind placebo controlled study. European Journal of Obstetrics, Gynecology and Reproductive Biology 44: 137–144
50. Smith P, Heimer G, Lindskog M, Ulsten U 1993 Oestradiol-releasing vaginal ring for treatment of postmenopausal urogenital atrophy. Maturitas 16: 145–154
51. Ayton RA, Darling GM, Murkies AL, Forrell EA et al 1996 A comparative study of safety and efficacy of continuous low dose oestradiol release from a vaginal ring compared with conjugated equine oestrogen vaginal cream in the treatment of post menopausal urogenital atrophy. British Journal of Obstetrics and Gynaecology 103: 351–358
52. Bygdeman M, Swahn ML 1996 Replens versus dienoestrol cream in the symptomatic treatment of vaginal atrophy in postmenopausal women. Maturitas 23: 259–263
53. Pearce J, Hawton K, Blake F 1995 Psychological and sexual symptoms associated with the menopause and the effects of hormone replacement therapy. British Journal of Psychiatry 167: 163–173
54. Ledéseert B, Rinea V, Bréart G 1995 Menopause and perceived health status among the women of the French GAZEL cohort. Maturitas 20: 113–120
55. Oldenhave A, Jaszmann LJ, Haspells AA, Everaerd WTh 1993 Impact of climacteric on well-being. American Journal of Obstetrics and Gynecology 168: 772–780

56. Daly E, Gray A, Barlow D, McPherson K, Roche M, Vessey M 1993 Measuring the impact of menopausal symptoms on quality of life. British Medical Journal 307: 836–840
57. Schiff I, Regestein Q, Tulchinsky D, Ryan KJ 1979 Effects of estrogens on sleep and psychological state of hypogonadal women. Journal of the American Medical Association 242: 2405–2407
58. Wiklund L, Karlberg J, Mattsson LA 1993 Quality of life of postmenopausal women on a regimen of transdermal estradiol therapy: a double-blind placebo controlled study. American Journal of Obstetrics and Gynecology 168: 824–830
59. Marcus DA 1995 Inter-relationships of neuro-chemicals, estrogen and recurring headache. Pain 62: 129–139
60. Wardell DW, Engebretson JC 1995 Women's anticipations of hormonal replacement therapy. Maturitas 22: 177–183
61. Gorsky RD, Koplan JP, Peterson JB, Thacker SB 1994 Relative risks and benefits of longterm estrogen replacement therapy: a decision analysis. Obstetrics and Gynecology 83: 161–166
62. Lobo RA 1995 Benefits and risk of estrogen replacement therapy. American Journal of Obstetrics and Gynecology 173: 982–989
63. Swartzman LC, Edelberg R, Kemmann E 1990 The menopausal hot flush: symptom reports and concomitant physiological changes. Journal of Behavioural Medicine 13: 15–30
64. Caird L, West CP, Lumsden MA, Hannan WJ, Gaw SM 1997 Medroxyprogesterone acetate with Zoladex™ for long-term treatment of fibroids: effects on bone density and patient acceptability. Human Reproduction 12: 436–440

54. Benefits of treatment: osteoporosis

L. Joseph Melton III   Sundeep Khosla

Introduction

Osteoporosis is a disease characterized by abnormalities in the amount and architectural arrangement of bone tissue, which lead to impaired skeletal strength and an increased susceptibility to fractures.[1] Except for tooth loss, these fractures are the sole clinical manifestation of the condition. Unfortunately, such fractures are increasingly common in almost every country and exact a devastating social toll.[2] In the United States, for example, at least 1.3 million fractures annually have been attributed to osteoporosis. Because of the resulting disability and cost, this large number of fractures makes osteoporosis an enormous public health problem. It has been estimated that 10% of women with a hip fracture become dependent in the activities of daily living, along with 4% of women with a vertebral fracture and 2% of those with a distal forearm fracture.[3] While fractures of the hip, spine and distal forearm are traditionally linked with osteoporosis, bone is lost throughout the skeleton and most fractures among the elderly are due in part to low bone mass.[4] Direct medical expenditures for these diverse osteoporotic fractures were estimated at $13.8 billion in the United States in 1995[5] and can only rise in the future because fracture rates increase with age and the elderly population is growing rapidly. Thus, the number of hip fractures in the United States could double or triple in the next 50 years.[2] Corresponding increases are anticipated elsewhere in the world as the annual number of hip fractures is expected to rise from 1.7 million in 1990 to 6.3 million by the year 2050.[6]

While it is obvious that the impact of osteoporosis is sufficiently great to justify efforts at prevention, it has been difficult to define a suitable control program because fracture pathogenesis is quite complex. Nonetheless, it is clear that skeletal fragility is strongly correlated with bone mineral density (Fig. 54.1), and population-based studies show that hip fracture incidence is associated with bone density in the proximal femur,[7,8] forearm fracture incidence with bone density in the radius[9–12] and vertebral fracture incidence with bone density in the lumbar spine.[13,14] These data support the notion that any intervention that maintains or improves bone density (e.g. estrogen replacement therapy) is likely to reduce the risk of fractures. On the other hand, fractures result when skeletal loads from trauma (or the activities of daily living in the case of some spine fractures) exceed the breaking strength of bone.[15] Trauma mostly results from falls which are very common,[16] but only about 5% of falls lead to fracture[17] because other factors are important as well. Thus, the likelihood of hip fracture among fallers is influenced by the orientation of the fall, the potential energy of the faller and the amount of soft tissue padding over the hip, as well as by the bone density of the proximal femur.[18] There is also

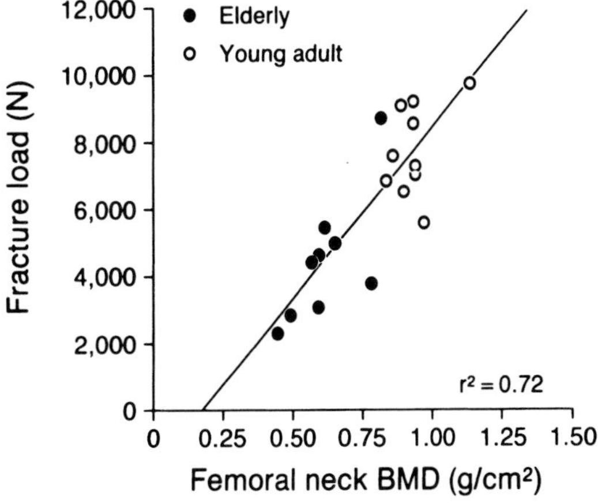

Fig. 54.1 Correlation between fracture load on the proximal femur and bone mineral density (BMD) of the femoral neck. (From Courtney AC, Wachtel EF, Myers ER, Hayes WC 1994 Effects of loading rate on strength of the proximal femur. Calcified Tissue International 55: 53–58)

evidence that various aspects of femoral neck geometry are associated with the risk of hip fractures.[19,20] While prospective studies show that bone density is an important determinant of fracture risk even after adjusting for these other risk factors,[21] the clinical implication is that some fractures will occur even if bone loss can be prevented.

The purpose of this chapter is to review the evidence that estrogen replacement therapy (ERT), with or without the addition of progestogens to protect the endometrium, can reduce the risk of fractures and, thus, prevent osteoporosis-related disability and cost. Consequently, it is necessary to consider the influence of estrogen deficiency on bone loss as well as the efficacy of estrogen replacement in preventing this loss. Due to the existence of nonskeletal risk factors for fractures, it is even more essential to show that estrogen replacement therapy can prevent fractures. Because estrogen treatment has other significant benefits and risks, it is also important to consider whether or not estrogen replacement therapy should be targeted at women who are at increased risk of osteoporosis. Finally, the role of estrogen treatment of women who have already developed osteoporosis must be considered. These different aspects of the problem are covered in the following sections.

PREVENTION OF BONE LOSS

The importance of estrogen in the maintenance of bone mass was described earlier (ch. 18), and randomized controlled trials have consistently shown that estrogen replacement in normal women can halt or at least slow the bone loss that follows natural or surgical menopause.[22–48] Even more numerous observational studies have generally found similar results but are not listed here since the randomized trials provide stronger evidence for this effect. Some studies reveal modest increases in bone mass, which have been explained by reduced bone resorption and increased bone mineralization as bone turnover slows (see Ch. 18). However, positive results are mostly in comparison with placebo-treated patients who are losing bone more rapidly. These trials were formally reviewed by the Office of Technology Assessment, which concluded that almost all of them indicate that estrogens are effective in preventing postmenopausal bone loss soon after the menopause.[49] The wide variety of different estrogen regimens utilized in these trials was judged to have broadly comparable efficacy, with the proviso that doses of 0.625 mg per day of conjugated estrogen or its equivalent were needed to protect the skeleton fully.[50] This is in accord with the recommendations in chapter 52. At this dose, most women seem to respond to treatment.[51] There is also some evidence that progestogens alone can have a similar protective effect.[23,38,52]

However, these trials have been of short duration and there are concerns about long-term compliance with therapy (see ch. 51). Only about 10–20% of postmenopausal women in the United States are on long-term (10 or more years) estrogen treatment.[53–55] Even so, most estrogen use is for reasons unrelated to osteoporosis;[54,56,57] women who had undergone surgical menopause accounted for about 80% of all users in one survey.[55] The prevalence of estrogen replacement therapy among women with a natural menopause is reported to be only 3–8%.[55,58,59] Partly as a result, a substantial proportion of postmenopausal women have osteoporosis by World Health Organization definitions.[60] Based on extrapolations of population-based data, an estimated 30% of postmenopausal white women in the United States might have osteoporosis of the hip, spine or distal forearm;[61] in the proximal femur alone, the prevalence was 16%. This compares with more extensive data from the National Health and Nutrition Examination Survey where an estimated 21% of postmenopausal white women had bone density of the hip that was more than 2.5 standard deviations below the young normal mean.[62] An additional 54% of postmenopausal white women were estimated to have low bone density in the hip, spine or distal forearm.[61] Thus, it is apparent that there is ample room for improvement in the skeletal status of the population.

The controlled clinical trials mentioned above have also focused on perimenopausal women. However, it is increasingly clear that a large proportion of elderly women have high bone turnover similar to that seen following the menopause[63,64] and that many of them are rapidly losing bone.[65] Estrogen, as an antiresorptive agent,[66] should also be effective in this group of women. It was recently estimated, for example, that a quarter of all postmenopausal women have high bone turnover as judged by elevated (> 1 SD above the premenopausal mean) levels of urinary cross-linked N-telopeptides of type I collagen, a marker of bone resorption.[67] Half of the women aged 80 years and over had elevated levels by this definition. Correspondingly, a number of studies indicate that ERT is effective in slowing bone loss when initiated a long time after the menopause, even among women who have already developed osteoporosis.[68–83] In the only randomized controlled trial of ERT in normal elderly women, 27 women on estrogen (Trisequens) and calcium (0.5g/day) gained 3.6% and 8.3% in bone

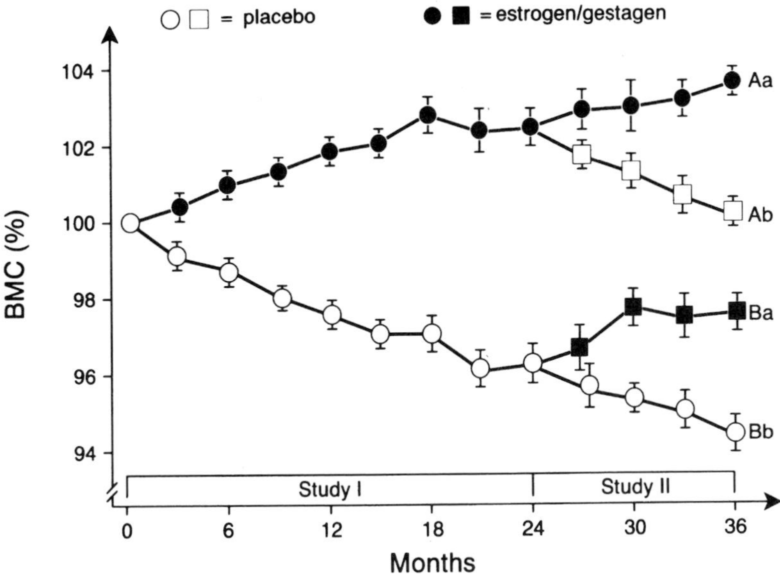

Fig. 54.2 Bone mineral content (BMC) as a function of time and treatment in a cross-over trial of hormone replacement therapy.[27]

mineral content of the distal and ultradistal radius, respectively, compared to 29 women on calcium alone who experienced no change in bone mass over the course of a year.[71] Less than 10% of elderly women are currently on estrogen replacement therapy, however.[56,84–86]

With two exceptions, the randomized clinical trials in this area have assessed the positive influence of estrogen replacement therapy on bone mass rather than fracture risk. Nevertheless, preservation of bone mass should translate directly into fracture reduction unless the protective effect dissipates upon cessation of treatment. Unfortunately, there is some evidence that this is the case. Most studies that have addressed this issue prospectively have shown a resumption of the postmenopausal pattern of rapid bone loss when estrogen treatment is stopped.[27,82,87] This was convincingly illustrated in the cross-over trial of Christiansen and colleagues (Fig. 54.2). Observational studies generally indicate that elderly women on long-term ERT have greater bone density than those never treated. However, a history of short-term use may have little residual protective effect.[88–91] For example, Felson and colleagues showed that bone density at various sites was only 0.1–8.5% (average, 3.2%) greater among women 75 years of age and older who had taken estrogen for seven years or more.[85] However, just 12% of these women were currently on ERT; the rest had stopped therapy many years before.

Prevention of fractures

Since the effects of ERT may wane with time, it is essential to assess its potential for reducing fractures directly for this is the clinical outcome of interest. Only two randomized controlled trials have addressed the efficacy of estrogen replacement therapy in preventing fractures among women without pre-existing osteoporosis. One showed that 4% of 58 oophorectomized women on mestranol (23 mg/day) lost height over nine years compared to 38% of 42 women not on treatment.[25] Almost 90% of the latter group, with height loss, had evidence of vertebral fractures. Moreover, five women in the placebo group developed vertebral crush fractures, compared to only one in the treatment group. The other trial of 84 pairs of women followed for 10 years found only one fracture in the treated group (conjugated estrogen, 2.5 mg/day and medroxyprogesterone, 10 mg/day for seven days each month) compared to seven in the placebo group.[92] A number of epidemiologic studies have also found empirical evidence for a protective effect of ERT on fractures[84,93–109] despite potential confounding by the fact that some estrogen prescribing may have been for treatment of osteoporosis. A report from the American College of Physicians estimated that hip fracture risk was reduced 25% in ever users of estrogen compared to never users[110] based on the evidence shown in Table 54.1. Since most estrogen use is short-term, this may

Table 54.1 Influence of postmenopausal estrogen replacement therapy on hip fracture risk.[108]

	Unopposed estrogen		
	Ever use	*Duration of use*	
Reference	Relative risk	Years of use	Relative risk
Case control studies			
Hutchinson 1979[93]	0.2[a]	>5	0.2[b]
Weiss 1980[94]	0.4[a,b,c]	≥10	0.5[a]
Johnson 1981[95]	0.7		
Paganini-Hill 1981[96]	0.7	>5	0.4[a]
Kreiger 1982[97]	0.4[a]		
Williams 1982[98]	0.4[a]		
Cohort studies			
Hammond, 1979[100]	0.5[a]		
Ettinger, 1985[101]	0.4[a]		
Kiel 1987[102]	0.6[a]		
Naessén 1990[103]	0.8[a]		
Paganini-Hill 1991[104]	1.0	≥15	0.9

[a]$P \leq 0.05$; [b]Risk estimate for hip and distal radius fractures combined; [c]Current estrogen use.

(Modified from Grady D, Cummings SR, Petitti D, Rubin SM, Audet A-M for American College of Physicians 1992. Guidelines for counseling postmenopausal women about preventive hormone therapy. Annals of Internal Medicine 117: 1038–1041.)

underestimate the protective effect of long-term estrogen replacement therapy, which is about 50% in most studies.

However, Cauley and colleagues also found that the protective effect was greatest among those current users of ERT who initiated therapy within five years of the menopause.[108] Compared to current users who started estrogen therapy more than five years after menopause, hip fracture risk was reduced 71% versus 30%, while the risk of all nonspine fractures was reduced 50% versus 25%. Others have reported similar results.[103] This is in accordance with the notion that, once bone mass has decreased substantially, therapeutic options are limited because currently available treatments including estrogen cannot restore osteoporotic bone to biomechanical normalcy. Consequently, it is necessary to predict the likelihood of fracture in an individual (fracture risk) so that intervention can be undertaken before bone loss (and impaired biomechanics) become irreversible. Fortunately, a variety of techniques permit accurate and precise measurement of bone density at different skeletal sites,[60] and studies done in diverse populations consistently show that these measurements can predict fractures.[111]

It has been less easy to show that use of bone densitometry could increase the efficiency of treatment by targeting estrogen replacement therapy only to women at high risk of fracture. Clinical trials to address this issue are impractical given the 30 year delay between the average age of menopause in the population and the average age at hip fracture. The alternative approach has been to rely on simulations that are necessarily based on a variety of assumptions. One study evaluated the cost-effectiveness of screening 50-year-old white women with dual photon absorptiometry of the hip and initiating 15 years of hormone replacement therapy at different bone density thresholds.[112] Under this model, 15 years of treatment was estimated to reduce the lifetime risk of hip fracture from 17% to 9%. Screening appeared to be reasonably cost-effective under a wide range of assumptions, but the analysis was sensitive to the influence of therapy on heart disease and breast cancer. If breast cancer risk with long-term hormone replacement therapy were increased by as much as 25%, then the more selective screening strategies would be preferred but if hormone replacement therapy decreased the risk of death from coronary heart disease by 25% then universal treatment of perimenopausal women might be more cost-effective. The American College of Physicians has recommended the latter approach, with bone density screening reserved for women uncertain about ERT who would take it if they were shown to be at high risk of osteoporotic fracture.[113]

The most comprehensive analysis was recently carried out by the Office of Technology Assessment.[114] A strategy that screened 50-year-old white women with dual energy x-ray absorptiometry measurements of the proximal femur and placed women whose bone density was more than one standard deviation below the mean (about 16% of the population) on ERT for 20 years had an estimated cost-effectiveness of $53 610 per life year saved. More hip fractures were prevented as estrogen use became more widespread, and the Office of Technology Assessment estimated that lifetime hip fracture risk would be reduced from about 17% to 7% by treating all perimenopausal women. Costs would be correspondingly higher, but the cost per life-year saved would improve. Cost-effectiveness also improved with longer duration of estrogen replacement since most of the adverse events prevented by estrogen occur late in life (Table 54.2). This model was dominated by the extraskeletal effects of estrogen replacement therapy, however. For example, the cost per year of life saved might increase from $23 334 for universal treatment for 40 years to $43 765 if a decade of estrogen replacement doubled the risk of breast cancer rather than raising it by 35%, as assumed in the base case analysis. Conversely, the cost per life year saved might be reduced to $7153 if the risk of myocardial infarction while on estrogen replacement were reduced by 80% instead of the presumed 50%.

Cummings et al[115] calculated a 25% reduction in hip fractures in white women by the year 2020 if 50% of them accepted long-term estrogen treatment beginning at age 50 years. In a similar analysis, 25 years of estrogen replacement therapy was estimated to reduce hip fractures by 67% among 50-year-old women at 'average' risk, i.e. without bone density measurements.[116] Another analysis suggested that hip fractures in the population might be reduced by 25% if a quarter of the eligible women undertook long-term estrogen replacement therapy.[117] These benefits are sensitive to assumptions made about the level of compliance with therapy, which may be problematic (see ch. 26). However, the majority of women are uncertain about the benefits of estrogen replacement therapy, and recent studies indicate that knowledge of low bone density increases compliance with ERT.[118] Among women attending an osteoporosis screening clinic, for example, 96% indicated a willingness to consider ERT if bone densitometry showed that they were at an increased risk of fracture.[57] In a population-based screening program in Scotland, nearly half of the postmenopausal women with low bone density were still on hormone replacement therapy after one year compared to only 19% of the women at lower risk.[119] Nevertheless, it is increasingly evident that the protective effects of ERT begin to wane once therapy is halted.[84,94,102,104,108] There was, for example, no reduction in the risk of hip, wrist or all nonspine fractures among elderly women who had taken estrogen for ten or more years (mean 14.6 years) but were not currently on ERT compared to women who had never been treated at all.[108]

Table 54.2 Lifetime hip fracture risk (%) and cost per life-year saved under different strategies for screening 50-year-old women for bone mineral density (BMD) and using estrogen replacement therapy (ERT).[49]

	Screen, BMD threshold			
Duration of ERT	No screening, no ERT	Screen, ERT for BMD < – 1 SD	Screen, ERT for BMD < mean	No screening, all on ERT
No ERT				
Fracture risk	17.0	–	–	–
Cost	Baseline	–	–	–
10 years				
Fracture risk	–	16.0	14.4	12.9
Cost	–	$151 392	$134 644	$126 876
20 years				
Fracture risk	–	15.3	12.4	9.8
Cost	–	$53 610	$42 724	$45 761
30 years				
Fracture risk	–	14.8	11.2	7.8
Cost	–	$28 257	$29 357	$31 059
40 years				
Fracture risk	–	14.7	10.9	7.2
Cost	–	$27 486	$22 431	$23 334

TREATMENT OF ESTABLISHED OSTEOPOROSIS

The majority of women with an osteoporotic fracture have already lost a substantial amount of bone and, because estrogen replacement therapy cannot restore the lost bone, the rationale for ERT among those with established osteoporosis might be questioned. Even in these individuals, however, bone density is a determinant of fracture risk. For example, women with a single vertebral crush fracture had a 5.3 fold increase in the risk of a subsequent vertebral fracture but, among those with a prevalent fracture, the risk of a new vertebral fracture was over twice as high in those with low as compared to high bone mass.[14] Similarly, 94% of elderly individuals who experienced a fall in one study had bone density values of the proximal femur that were below the fracture threshold (2 SD below the young normal mean), yet the likelihood of experiencing a hip fracture in this group still increased almost three fold with each standard deviation decline in bone density of the femoral neck.[18] Thus, by preserving the bone mass that remains, ERT may be expected to reduce the risk of additional fractures. The results of the only randomized controlled trial support this (see below), as do nonrandomized trials.[120]

Indeed, estrogen replacement therapy is more efficacious in this situation than might be expected from its positive influence on bone density. Thus, in a recently reported trial of 75 osteoporotic women with vertebral fractures, those randomized to the estrogen group (17β-estradiol by dermal patches to provide 100 μg/day for days 1–21 and medroxyprogesterone acetate orally at 10 mg/day for days 11–21 of a 28 day cycle) had an average 6.2% increase in lumbar spine bone density during the year of treatment compared with 1.2% for those randomized to the placebo group.[79] However, the vertebral fracture rate was decreased by 61% in the estrogen-treated women compared with controls. When these data were analyzed in more detail,[121] it was clear that the fracture rate in the placebo group was also related to bone turnover, increasing about four fold between low and high levels of turnover (Fig. 54.3A). At all levels of bone turnover, but particularly at lower levels, the risk of vertebral fracture was also inversely related to bone density. However, estrogen treatment eliminated the high levels of bone turnover that were present in the placebo group (Fig. 54.3B). In the presence of normal bone turnover, the inverse relationship between the vertebral fracture rate and spinal bone density was even more evident: a decrease in bone density of the lumbar spine from 0.90 g/cm^2 the fracture threshold, to 0.60 g/cm^2 was associated with a four fold increase in the incidence of new vertebral fractures. These observations suggest that pharmacologic agents could be effective in reducing fracture risk both by slowing bone loss and by eliminating the damaging effect of high bone turnover on the microarchitectural integrity of cancellous bone.[121] This also helps explain the recent epidemiologic observation that current use of ERT has a protective effect on fracture risk that is independent of bone density.[108]

Conclusion

Osteoporosis is a complex, multifactorial chronic disease that may progress silently for decades until characteristic fractures result late in life. Because there are no symptoms until fractures occur, relatively few people are diagnosed in time for effective therapy to be

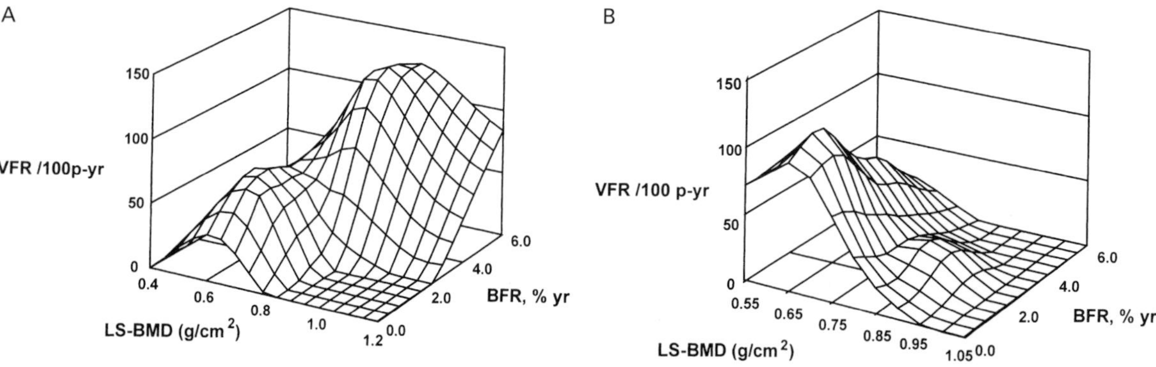

Fig. 54.3 Three-dimensional surface plot of data showing vertebral fracture rate (VFR) as a function of lumbar spine bone mineral density (LS-BMD) and of bone formation rate (BFR) assessed by histomorphometry. **A**: Placebo limb (untreated postmenopausal osteoporosis); **B**: estrogen treatment.[121]

administered during this preclinical phase. Consequently, a large number of individuals experience the pain, expense, disability and decreased quality of life caused by these fractures. Indeed, the lifetime risk of hip, spine and forearm fractures alone has been estimated at 40% for white women and 13% for white men.[122] This important public health problem will worsen in the future as the population ages and, if the enormous costs associated with osteoporotic fractures are to be reduced, increased attention must be given to the design and implementation of effective control programs. It has been estimated from epidemiologic data that an increase in average femoral neck bone density in the community of about 14% should lead to a reduction in femoral neck fractures by roughly one half.[66] Because generally accepted therapies for osteoporosis like ERT cannot restore an osteoporotic skeleton to biomechanical normalcy, this can best be accomplished by using these agents to prevent bone loss rather than to correct bone loss which has already occurred. However, even when bone loss has progressed to the point of fracture, estrogen replacement therapy can still have a positive effect by reducing the very substantial risk of additional fractures among these women.

Acknowledgment The authors wish to thank Mrs Mary Roberts for help in preparing the manuscript. This work was supported in part by research grants AR-27065 and AG-04875 from the National Institutes of Health, United States Public Health Service.

REFERENCES

1. Anonymous 1993 Consensus development conference: diagnosis, prophylaxis, and treatment of osteoporosis. American Journal of Medicine 94: 646–650
2. Melton LJ III 1995 Epidemiology of fractures. In: Riggs BL, Melton LJ III (eds) Osteoporosis: etiology, diagnosis and management, 2nd edn. Lippincott-Raven Publishers, Philadelphia, p 225–247
3. Chrischilles EA, Butler CD, Davis CS, Wallace RB 1991 A model of lifetime osteoporosis impact. Archives of Internal Medicine 151: 2026–2032
4. Seeley DG, Browner WS, Nevitt MC, Genant HK, Scott JC, Cummings SR 1991 Which fractures are associated with low appendicular bone mass in elderly women? The Study of Osteoporotic Fractures Research Group. Annals of Internal Medicine 115: 837–842
5. Ray NF, Chan JK, Thamer M, Melton LJ III 1997 Medical expenditures for the treatment of osteoporotic fractures in the United States in 1995. Journal of Bone and Mineral Research 12: 24–35
6. Cooper C, Campion G, Melton LJ III 1992 Hip fractures in the elderly: a world-wide projection. Osteoporosis International 2: 285–289
7. Melton LJ III, Wahner HW, Richelson LS, O'Fallon WM, Riggs BL 1986 Osteoporosis and the risk of hip fracture. American Journal of Epidemiology 124: 254–261
8. Cummings SR, Black DM, Nevitt MC et al 1993 Bone density at various sites for prediction of hip fractures. The Study of Osteoporotic Fractures Research Group. Lancet 341: 72–75
9. Hui SL, Slemenda CW, Johnston CC Jr 1988 Age and bone mass as predictors of fracture in a prospective study. Journal of Clinical Investigation 81: 1804–1809
10. Eastell R, Riggs BL, Wahner HW, O'Fallon WM, Amadio PC, Melton LJ III 1989 Colles' fracture and bone density of the ultradistal radius. Journal of Bone and Mineral Research 4: 607–613
11. Kelsey JL, Browner WS, Seeley DG, Nevitt MC, Cummings SR 1992 Risk factors for fractures of the distal forearm and proximal humerus. The Study of Osteoporotic Fractures Research Group. American Journal of Epidemiology 135: 477–489
12. Gärdsell P, Johnell O, Nilsson BE, Gullberg B 1993 Predicting various fragility fractures in women by forearm bone densitometry: a follow-up study. Calcified Tissue International 52: 348–353
13. Melton LJ III, Atkinson EJ, O'Fallon WM, Wahner HW, Riggs BL 1993 Long-term fracture prediction by bone mineral assessed at different skeletal sites. Journal of Bone and Mineral Research 8: 1227–1233
14. Ross PD, Davis JW, Epstein RS, Wasnich RD 1991 Pre-existing fractures and bone mass predict vertebral fracture incidence in women. Annals of Internal Medicine 114: 919–923
15. Melton LJ III, Chao EYS, Lane J 1988 Biomechanical aspects of fractures. In: Riggs BL, Melton LJ III (eds) Osteoporosis: etiology, diagnosis, and management. Raven Press, New York, pp 111–131
16. Winner SJ, Morgan CA, Evans JG 1989 Perimenopausal risk of falling and incidence of distal forearm fracture. British Medical Journal 298: 1486–1488
17. Gibson MJ 1987 The prevention of falls in later life. Danish Medical Bulletin 34 (Suppl 4): 1–24
18. Greenspan SL, Myers ER, Maitland LA, Resnick NM, Hayes WC 1994 Fall severity and bone mineral density as risk factors for hip fracture in ambulatory elderly. Journal of the American Medical Association 271: 128–133
19. Faulkner KG, Cummings SR, Black D, Palermo L, Glüer C-C, Genant HK 1993 Simple measurement of femoral geometry predicts hip fracture: the study of osteoporotic fractures. Journal of Bone and Mineral Research 8: 1211–1217
20. Glüer C-C, Cummings SR, Pressman A et al 1994 Prediction of hip fractures from pelvic radiographs: the study of osteoporotic fractures. The Study of Osteoporotic Fractures Research Group. Journal of Bone and Mineral Research 9: 671–677
21. Cummings SR, Nevitt MC, Browner WS et al 1995 Risk factors for hip fracture in white women. The study of Osteoporotic Fractures Research Group. New England Journal of Medicine 332: 767–773
22. Aitken J, Hart DM, Lindsay R 1973 Oestrogen replacement therapy for prevention of osteoporosis after oophorectomy. British Medical Journal 3: 515–518

23. Lindsay R, Hart DM, Purdie D, Ferguson MM, Clark AS, Kraszewski A 1978 Comparative effects of oestrogen and a progestogen on bone loss in postmenopausal women. Clinical Science and Molecular Medicine 54: 193–195
24. Christiansen C, Christensen MS, McNair P, Hagen C, Stocklund KE, Transbøl I 1980 Prevention of early postmenopausal bone loss: controlled two-year study in 315 normal females. European Journal of Clinical Investigation 10: 273–279
25. Lindsay R, Hart DM, Forrest C, Baird C 1980 Prevention of spinal osteoporosis in oophorectomised women. Lancet 2: 1151–1154
26. Christiansen C, Christensen MS, Rodbrø P, Hagen C, Transbøl I 1981 Effect of 1,25-dihydroxy-vitamin D_3 in itself or combined with hormone treatment in preventing postmenopausal osteoporosis. European Journal of Clinical Investigation 11: 305–309
27. Christiansen C, Christensen MS, Transbøl I 1981 Bone mass in postmenopausal women after withdrawal of oestrogen/gestagen replacement therapy. Lancet 1: 459–461
28. Lindsay R, Hart DM, Clark DM 1984 The minimum effective dose of estrogen for prevention of postmenopausal bone loss. Obstetrics and Gynecology 63: 759–763
29. Christiansen C, Rodbrø P 1984 Does oestriol add to the beneficial effect of combined hormonal prophylaxis against early postmenopausal osteoporosis? British Journal of Obstetrics and Gynaecology 91: 489–493
30. Gotfredsen A, Nilas L, Riis BJ, Thomsen K, Christiansen C 1986 Bone changes occurring spontaneously and caused by oestrogen in early postmenopausal women: a local or generalised phenomenon? British Medical Journal 292: 1098–1100
31. Riis B, Thomsen K, Christiansen C 1987 Does calcium supplementation prevent postmenopausal bone loss? A double-blind, controlled clinical study. New England Journal of Medicine 316: 173–177
32. Riis B, Thomsen K, Strom V, Christiansen C 1987 The effect of percutaneous estradiol and natural progesterone on postmenopausal bone loss. American Journal of Obstetrics and Gynecology 156: 61–65
33. Civitelli R, Agnusdei D, Nardi P, Zacchei F, Avioli LV, Gennari C 1988 Effects of one-year treatment with estrogens on bone mass, intestinal calcium absorption, and 25-hydroxyvitamin D-1 alpha-hydroxylase reserve in postmenopausal osteoporosis. Calcified Tissue International 42: 77–86
34. Munk-Jensen N, Pors Nielsen S, Obel EB, Bonne Eriksen P 1988 Reversal of postmenopausal vertebral bone loss by oestrogen and progestogen: a double blind placebo controlled study. British Medical Journal (Clinical Research Edition) 296: 1150–1152
35. Riis BJ, Johansen J, Christiansen C 1988 Continuous oestrogen-progestogen treatment and bone metabolism in post-menopausal women. Maturitas 10: 51–58
36. Genant HK, Baylink DJ, Gallagher J, Harris ST, Steiger P, Herber M 1990 Effect of estrone sulfate on postmenopausal bone loss. Obstetrics and Gynecology 76: 579–584
37. Williams SR, Frenchek B, Speroff T, Speroff L 1990 A study of combined continuous ethinyl estradiol and norethindrone acetate for postmenopausal hormone replacement. American Journal of Obstetrics and Gynecology 162: 438–446
38. Gallagher JC, Kable WT, Goldgar D 1991 Effect of progestin therapy on cortical and trabecular bone: comparison with estrogen. American Journal of Medicine 90: 171–178
39. Harris ST, Genant HK, Baylink DJ et al 1991 The effects of estrone (Ogen) on spinal bone density of postmenopausal women. Archives of Internal Medicine 151: 1980–1984
40. Prince RL, Smith M, Dick IM, Price RI, Webb PG, Henderson NK, Harris MM 1991 Prevention of postmenopausal osteoporosis: a comparative study of exercise, calcium supplementation, and hormone-replacement therapy. New England Journal of Medicine 325: 1189–1195
41. Castelo-Branco C, Martínez de Osaba M, Pons F, González-Merlo J 1992 The effect of hormone replacement therapy on postmenopausal bone loss. European Journal of Obstetrics, Gynecology and Reproductive Biology 44: 131–136
42. Svendsen OL, Hassager C, Marslew U, Christiansen C 1992 Changes in calcanean bone mineral occurring spontaneously and during hormone replacement therapy in early post-menopausal women. Scandinavian Journal of Clinical and Laboratory Investigation 52: 831–836
43. Marslew U, Overgaard K, Riis BJ, Christiansen C 1992 Two new combinations of estrogen and progestogen for prevention of postmenopausal bone loss: long-term effects on bone, calcium and lipid metabolism, climacteric symptoms, and bleeding. Obstetrics and Gynecology 79: 202–210
44. Field CS, Ory SJ, Wahner HW, Herrmann RR, Judd HL, Riggs BL 1993 Preventive effects of transdermal 17β-estradiol on osteoporotic changes after surgical menopause: a two-year placebo-controlled trial. American Journal of Obstetrics and Gynecology 168: 114–121
45. Castelo-Branco C, Pons F, González-Merlo J 1993 Bone mineral density in surgically postmenopausal women receiving hormonal replacement therapy as assessed by dual photon absorptiometry. Maturitas 16: 133–137
46. Aloia JF, Vaswani A, Yeh JK, Ross PL, Flaster E, Dilmanian A 1994 Calcium supplementation with and without hormone replacement therapy to prevent postmenopausal bone loss. Annals of Internal Medicine 120: 97–103
47. Haines CJ, Chung TKH, Leung PC, Hsu SYC, Leung DHY 1995 Calcium supplementation and bone mineral density in postmenopausal women using estrogen replacement therapy. Bone 16: 529–531
48. Wimalawansa SJ 1995 Combined therapy with estrogen and etidronate has an additive effect on bone mineral density in the hip and vertebrae: four-year randomized study. American Journal of Medicine 99: 36–42
49. US Congress, Office of Technology Assessment 1995 Appendix C: Evidence on HRT and bone loss. In: Effectiveness and costs of osteoporosis screening and hormone replacement therapy, vol. II. Evidence on benefits, risks, and costs OTA-BP-H-144. US Government Printing Office, Washington, DC, pp 19–33

50. US Congress, Office of Technology Assessment 1995 Appendix E: Hormonal replacement therapy regimens. In: Effectiveness and costs of osteoporosis screening and hormone replacement therapy, vol. II. Evidence on benefits, risks, and costs, OTA-BP-O-H-144. US Government Printing Office, Washington, DC, pp 49–63
51. Hassager C, Jensen SB, Christiansen C 1994 Non-responders to hormone replacement therapy for the prevention of postmenopausal bone loss: do they exist? Osteoporosis International 4: 36–41
52. Trémollières F, Pouilles JM, Ribot C 1993 Effect of long-term administration of progestogen on post-menopausal bone loss: result of a two-year, controlled randomized study. Clinical Endocrinology 38: 627–631
53. Avis NE, McKinlay SM 1990 Health-care utilization among mid-aged women. Annals of the New York Academy of Sciences 592: 228–238
54. Scalley EK, Henrich JB 1993 An overview of estrogen replacement therapy in postmenopausal women. Journal of Women's Health 2: 289–294
55. Derby CA, Hume AL, Barbour MM, McPhillips JB, Lasater TM, Carleton RA 1993 Correlates of postmenopausal estrogen use and trends through the 1980s in two southeastern New England communities. American Journal of Epidemiology 137: 1125–1135
56. Cauley JA, Cummings SR, Black DM, Mascioli SR, Seeley DG 1990 Prevalence and determinants of estrogen replacement therapy in elderly women. American Journal of Obstetrics and Gynecology 163: 1438–1444
57. Garton M, Reid D, Rennie E 1995 The climacteric, osteoporosis and hormone replacement; views of women aged 45–49. Maturitas 21: 7–15
58. Standeven M, Criqui MH, Klauber MR, Gabriel S, Barrett-Connor E 1986 Correlates of change in postmenopausal estrogen use in a population-based study. American Journal of Epidemiology 124: 268–274
59. Johannes CB, Crawford SL, Posner JG, McKinlay SM 1994 Longitudinal patterns and correlates of hormone replacement therapy use in middle-aged women. American Journal of Epidemiology 140: 439–452
60. Report of a WHO Study Group 1994 Assessment of fracture risk and its application to screening for postmenopausal osteoporosis. WHO Technical Report Series 843. World Health Organization, Geneva
61. Melton LJ III 1995 Perspectives: how many women have osteoporosis now? Journal of Bone and Mineral Research 10: 175–177
62. Looker AC, Johnston CC Jr, Wahner HW et al 1995 Prevalence of low femoral bone density in older US women from NHANES III. Journal of Bone and Mineral Research 10: 796–802
63. Garnero P, Sornay-Rendu E, Chapuy M-C, Delmas PD 1996 Increased bone turnover in late postmenopausal women is a major determinant of osteoporosis. Journal of Bone and Mineral Research 11: 337–349
64. Melton LJ III, Khosla S, Atkinson EJ, O'Fallon WM, Riggs BL 1997 Relationship of bone turnover to bone density and fractures. Journal of Bone and Mineral Research 12: 1083–1091
65. Kanis JA, Adami S 1994 Bone loss in the elderly. Osteoporosis International 4 (Suppl 1): S59–S65
66. Riggs BL, Melton LJ III 1992 The prevention and treatment of osteoporosis. New England Journal of Medicine 327: 620–627
67. Melton LJ III, Khosla S, Atkinson EJ, O'Fallon WM, Riggs BL 1995 Impact of high bone turnover on bone loss and fractures in the elderly. Journal of Bone and Mineral Research 10(Suppl 1): S263
68. Lindsay R, Hart DM, Aitken JM, MacDonald EB, Anderson JB, Clarke AC 1976 Long-term prevention of postmenopausal osteoporosis by oestrogen: evidence for an increased bone mass after delayed onset of oestrogen treatment. Lancet i: 1038–1041
69. Recker RR, Saville PD, Heaney RP 1977 Effect of estrogens and calcium carbonate on bone loss in postmenopausal women. Annals of Internal Medicine 87: 649–655
70. Nordin BEC, Horsman A, Crilly R, Marshall DH, Simpson M 1980 Treatment of spinal osteoporosis in postmenopausal women. British Medical Journal 280: 451–455
71. Jensen GF, Christiansen C, Transbøl I 1982 Treatment of post-menopausal osteoporosis. A controlled therapeutic trial comparing oestrogen/gestagen, 1,25-dihydroxy-vitamin D_3 and calcium. Clinical Endocrinology 16: 515–524
72. Caniggia A, Delling G, Nuti R, Lore F, Vattimo A 1984 Clinical, biochemical and histological results of a double-blind trial with 1,25-dihydroxyvitamin D_3, estradiol, and placebo in postmenopausal osteoporosis. Acta Vitaminologica et Enzymologica 6: 117–128
73. Quigley ME, Martin PL, Burnier AM, Brooks P 1987 Estrogen therapy arrests bone loss in elderly women. American Journal of Obstetrics and Gynecology 156: 1516–1523
74. Christiansen C, Riis BJ 1990 17β-estradiol and continuous norethisterone: a unique treatment for established osteoporosis in elderly women. Journal of Clinical Endocrinology and Metabolism 71: 836–841
75. Lindsay R, Tohme JF 1990 Estrogen treatment of patients with established postmenopausal osteoporosis. Obstetrics and Gynecology 76: 290–295
76. Moore M, Bracker M, Sartoris D, Saltman P, Strause L 1990 Long-term estrogen replacement therapy in postmenopausal women sustains vertebral bone mineral density. Journal of Bone and Mineral Density Research 5: 659–664
77. Resch H, Pietschmann P, Krexner E, Woloszczuk W, Willvonseder R 1990 Effects of one-year hormone replacement therapy on peripheral bone mineral content in patients with osteoporotic spine fractures. Acta Endocrinologica 123: 14–18
78. Garnett T, Studd J, Watson N, Savvas M 1991 A cross-sectional study of the effects of long-term percutaneous hormone replacement therapy on bone density. Obstetrics and Gynecology 78: 1002–1007
79. Lufkin EG, Wahner HW, O'Fallon WM et al 1992 Treatment of postmenopausal osteoporosis with transdermal estrogen. Annals of Internal Medicine 117: 1–9
80. Marx CW, Dailey GE III, Cheney C, Vint VC II, Muchmore DB 1992 Do estrogens improve bone mineral density in osteoporotic women over age 65? Journal of Bone and Mineral Research 7: 1275–1279

81. Hasling C, Charles P, Jensen FT, Mosekilde L 1994 A comparison of the effects of oestrogen/progestogen, high-dose oral calcium, intermittent cyclic etidronate and an ADFR regime on calcium kinetics and bone mass in postmenopausal women with spinal osteoporosis. Osteoporosis International 4: 191–203
82. Davis JW, Ross PD, Johnson NE, Wasnich RD 1995 Estrogen and calcium supplement use among Japanese-American women: effects upon bone loss when used singly and in combination. Bone 17: 369–373
83. Kohrt WM, Birge SJ Jr 1995 Differential effects of estrogen treatment on bone mineral density of the spine, hip, wrist and total body in late postmenopausal women. Osteoporosis International 5: 150–155
84. Kanis JA, Johnell O, Gullberg B et al 1992 Evidence for efficacy of drugs affecting bone metabolism in preventing hip fracture. British Medical Journal 305: 1124–1128
85. Felson DT, Zhang Y, Hannan MT, Kiel DP, Wilson PW, Anderson JJ 1993 The effect of postmenopausal estrogen therapy on bone density in elderly women. New England Journal of Medicine 329: 1141–1146
86. Handa VL, Landerman R, Hanlon JT, Harris T, Cohen HJ 1996 Do older women use estrogen replacement? Data from the Duke established populations for epidemiologic studies of the elderly (EPESE). Journal of the American Geriatric Society 44: 1–6
87. Lindsay R, Hart DM, MacLean A, Clarke AC, Kraszewski A, Garwood J 1978 Bone response to termination of oestrogen treatment. Lancet 1: 1325–1327
88. Wasnich R, Yano K, Vogel J 1983 Postmenopausal bone loss at multiple skeletal sites: relationship to estrogen use. Journal of Chronic Diseases 36: 781–790
89. Sowers MR, Wallace RB, Lemke JH 1985 Correlates of mid-radius bone density among postmenopausal women: a community study. American Journal of Clinical Nutrition 41: 1045–1053
90. Melton LJ III, Bryant SC, Wahner HW et al 1993 Influence of breastfeeding and other reproductive factors on bone mass later in life. Osteoporosis International 3: 76–83
91. Nguyen TV, Jones G, Sambrook PN, White CP, Kelly PJ, Eisman JA 1995 Effects of estrogen exposure and reproductive factors on bone mineral density and osteoporotic fractures. Journal of Clinical Endocrinology and Metabolism 80: 2709–2714
92. Nachtigall LE, Nachtigall RH, Nachtigall RD, Beckman EM 1979 Estrogen replacement therapy I: a 10-year prospective study in the relationship to osteoporosis. Obstetrics and Gynecology 53: 277–281
93. Hutchinson TA, Polansky SM, Feinstein AR 1979 Post-menopausal oestrogens protect against fractures of hip and distal radius: a case-control study. Lancet 2: 705–709
94. Weiss NS, Ure CL, Ballard JH, Williams AR, Daling JR 1980 Decreased risk of fractures of the hip and lower forearm with postmenopausal use of estrogens. New England Journal of Medicine 303: 1195–1198
95. Johnson RE, Specht EE 1981 The risk of hip fracture in postmenopausal females with and without estrogen drug exposure. American Journal of Public Health 71: 138–144
96. Paganini-Hill A, Ross RK, Gerkins VR, Henderson BE, Arthur M, Mack TM 1981 Menopausal estrogen therapy and hip fractures. Annals of Internal Medicine 95: 28–31
97. Kreiger N, Kelsey JL, Holford TR, O'Connor T 1982 An epidemiologic study of hip fracture in postmenopausal women. American Journal of Epidemiology 116: 141–148
98. Williams AR, Weiss NS, Ure CL, Ballard J, Daling JR 1982 Effect of weight, smoking, and estrogen use on the risk of hip and forearm fractures in postmenopausal women. Obstetrics and Gynecology 60: 695–699
99. Wasnich RD, Ross PD, Heilbrun LK, Vogel JM, Yano K, Benfante RJ 1986 Differential effects of thiazide and estrogen upon bone mineral content and fracture prevalence. Obstetrics and Gynecology 67: 457–462
100. Hammond CB, Jelovsek FR, Lee KL, Creasman WT, Parker RT 1979 Effects of long-term estrogen replacement therapy. I. Metabolic effects. American Journal of Obstetrics and Gynecology 133: 525–536
101. Ettinger B, Genant HK, Cann CE 1985 Long-term estrogen replacement therapy prevents bone loss and fractures. Annals of Internal Medicine 102: 319–324
102. Kiel DP, Felson DT, Anderson JJ, Wilson PWF, Moskowitz MA 1987 Hip fracture and the use of estrogens in postmenopausal women: The Framingham Study. New England Journal of Medicine 317: 1169–1174
103. Naessén T, Persson I, Adami H-O, Bergström R, Bergkvist L 1990 Hormone replacement therapy and the risk for first hip fracture: a prospective, population-based cohort study. Annals of Internal Medicine 113: 95–103
104. Paganini-Hill A, Chao A, Ross RK, Henderson BE 1991 Exercise and other factors in the prevention of hip fracture: the Leisure World study. Epidemiology 2: 16–25
105. Spector TD, Brennan P, Harris PA, Studd JW, Silman AJ 1992 Do current regimes of hormone replacement therapy protect against subsequent fractures? Osteoporosis International 2: 219–224
106. Kreiger N, Gross A, Hunter G 1992 Dietary factors and fracture in postmenopausal women: a case-control study. International Journal of Epidemiology 21: 953–958
107. Grisso JA, Kelsey JL, Strom BL et al 1994 Risk factors for hip fracture in black women. The Northeast Hip Fracture Study Group. New England Journal of Medicine 330: 1555–1559
108. Cauley JA, Seeley DG, Ensrud K, Ettinger B, Black D, Cummings SR 1995 Estrogen replacement therapy and fractures in older women. The Study of Osteoporotic Fractures Research Group. Annals of Internal Medicine 122: 9–16
109. Maxim P, Ettinger B, Spitalny GM 1995 Fracture protection provided by long-term estrogen treatment. Osteoporosis International 5: 23–29
110. Grady D, Rubin SM, Petitti DB et al 1992 Hormone therapy to prevent disease and prolong life in postmenopausal women. Annals of Internal Medicine 117: 1016–1037

111. Johnston CC Jr, Melton LJ III 1995 Bone densitometry. In: Riggs BL, Melton LJ III (eds) Osteoporosis: etiology, diagnosis and management, 2nd edn. Lippincott-Raven Publishers, Philadelphia, pp 275–297
112. Tosteson ANA, Rosenthal DI, Melton LJ III, Weinstein MC 1990 Cost effectiveness of screening perimenopausal white women for osteoporosis: bone densitometry and hormone replacement therapy. Annals of Internal Medicine 113: 594–603
113. Anonymous 1992 Guidelines for counseling postmenopausal women about preventive hormone therapy. American College of Physicians. Annals of Internal Medicine 117: 1038–1041
114. US Congress, Office of Technology Assessment 1995 Effectiveness and costs of osteoporosis screening and hormone replacement therapy, vol. I. Cost-Effectiveness Analysis, OTA-BP-H-160. US Government Printing Office, Washington, DC
115. Cummings SR, Rubin SM, Black D 1990 The future of hip fractures in the United States: numbers, costs, and potential effects of postmenopausal estrogen. Clinical Orthopaedics and Related Research 252: 163–166
116. Gorsky RD, Koplan JP, Peterson HB, Thacker SB 1994 Relative risks and benefits of long-term estrogen replacement therapy: a decision analysis. Obstetrics and Gynecology 83: 161–166
117. Johnell O, Stenbeck M, Rosen M, Gullberg B, Kanis JA 1993 Therapeutic strategies in the prevention of hip fracture with drugs affecting bone metabolism. Bone 14 (Suppl 1): S85–S87
118. Rubin SM, Cummings SR 1992 Results of bone densitometry affect women's decisions about taking measures to prevent fractures. Annals of Internal Medicine 116: 990–995
119. Torgerson DJ, Donaldson C, Russell IT, Reid DM 1995 Hormone replacement therapy: compliance and cost after screening for osteoporosis. European Journal of Obstetrics, Gynecology and Reproductive Biology 59: 57–60
120. Riggs BL, Seeman E, Hodgson SF, Taves DR, O'Fallon WM 1982 Effect of the fluoride/calcium regimen on vertebral fracture occurrence in postmenopausal osteoporosis: comparison with conventional therapy. New England Journal of Medicine 306: 446–450
121. Riggs BL, Melton LJ III, O'Fallon WM 1996 Drug therapy of vertebral fractures in osteoporosis: evidence that decreases in bone turnover and increases in bone mass determine antifracture efficacy. Bone 18 (Supplement): 1975–2015
122. Melton LJ III, Chrischilles EA, Cooper C, Lane AW, Riggs BL 1992 How many women have osteoporosis? Journal of Bone and Mineral Research 7: 1005–1010

55. Effects of hormone replacement therapy on the cardiovascular system

Jane A. McCrohon David S. Celermajer

Introduction

This chapter will examine the issue of hormone replacement therapy and its role in modifying the increased cardiovascular risk that occurs in the female population after the menopause. Throughout the premenopausal period, adult women have a lower risk of coronary heart disease than men of similar age. This female advantage declines steadily after the menopause,[1–3] with women having an equivalent cardiovascular risk to the male population by the eighth decade of life. Epidemiologic studies have shown that estrogen replacement therapy might be associated with a reduction of approximately 50% in the incidence of cardiovascular events in postmenopausal women.[2,4–11] In western populations, where cardiovascular disease is the major contributor to total mortality for both sexes, the impact of this potential benefit on public health may be enormous.

The mechanisms by which estrogen might exert this cardiovascular benefit remain largely unresolved. Estrogen has a well documented beneficial effect on the lipid profile,[3,12–14] however this may account for only 25–30% of the observed benefit.[3] Animal studies have shown that estrogen therapy reduces the accumulation of lipids in the arterial wall, even without significant reduction in plasma levels of lipoproteins or total cholesterol.[15–17] In addition, both human and animal studies demonstrate that estrogen may improve arterial function independent of lipid effects,[18–20] suggesting that estrogen may influence the development of atherosclerosis and reduce cardiovascular events by direct action at the arterial wall level.

Many postmenopausal women who have not undergone hysterectomy require progesterone as part of their hormone replacement, to minimize the risk of endometrial cancer and the abnormal uterine bleeding which may occur during unopposed estrogen therapy.[21,22] Although information is beginning to emerge, less is known about the effects of progesterone on the incidence of clinical vascular disease or on atherogenesis and arterial function. Some investigators have suggested that the addition of progesterone might attenuate the estrogen-related cardiovascular benefit,[13,23] and this requires further study.

The effects of estrogens and other sex steroid hormones on coagulation, other blood constituents and carbohydrate metabolism may also provide additional means whereby postmenopausal women who take hormones might derive a cardiovascular benefit. The interest in the mechanism of sex steroid effects has generated a large number of both experimental animal and human studies, with at times conflicting results. To a large extent the answers remain unclear, awaiting the outcome of large prospective clinical trials, such as the Women's Health Initiative, and the results of basic science research into the possible mechanisms. There is no doubt, however, that the field of sex steroid hormones and the cardiovascular system has and will continue to generate much interest over the next few years as this information emerges.

EPIDEMIOLOGIC EVIDENCE

Most studies that have so far examined the potential benefits of hormone replacement therapy have depended on epidemiologic data. Nevertheless, the relatively consistent finding of 40–50% reduction in cardiovascular morbidity and mortality suggested by these data, although not conclusive, remains too important to ignore. These observational studies have prompted interest in prospective clinical trials, such as the Postmenopausal Estrogen/Progestin Interventions (PEPI) trial published in 1995[24] and the Women's Health Initiative, due to be completed by the end of the decade.

In 1985, evidence from the Framingham Study[1] suggested that noncontraceptive estrogen use increased the risk of cardiovascular disease in postmenopausal women, with an estimated increase in risk of 50% ($P<0.01$) in postmenopausal estrogen users. Separate analyses of these data,[2] examining subgroups based on age and time since estrogen therapy was last taken, have suggested that the original analysis possibly underestimated the benefits of postmenopausal estrogen use, especially considering the small number of women on hormone replacement in the study (<15%). Since that time however, multiple clinical, animal and autopsy studies have opposed this view, demonstrating that exogenous estrogens are associated with reduced development of atherosclerotic lesions and a decreased incidence of clinical cardiovascular events. Table 55.1 summarizes eight of the prospective studies reported in the literature.[4–11] The results show a reduction in cardiovascular endpoints with hormone replacement therapy in all studies, varying between 46–84%, with the exception of the Framingham study, which at final analysis, showed an increase in cardiovascular risk of 20% in estrogen users, although this was not statistically significant. Table 55.2 includes 11 published case-control studies of varying size and statistical significance,[25–35] with the majority showing a favorable effect of estrogen replacement on cardiovascular risk. In 1991, Bush,[2] using meta-analysis and weighting factors for study type, population size and currency of estrogen use, concluded that based on the 21 studies available at that time, estrogen use reduced the risk of cardiovascular disease in women by approximately 50%. Of note, there is only one randomized, prospective clinical trial of estrogen use in women in this group.[36] This was a 10 year study and also

Table 55.1 Observational studies; prospective.

Observational studies	*n*	% users of ERT	Mean follow-up (yrs)	Event	Relative risk	
Lafferty (1985)[4]	124	49%	C	8.6	MI	0.16*
Stampfer (1986)[5]	32 317	58%	C	4.0	All CVD	0.30*
Hammond (1979)[6]	610	49%	C	5.0	All CVD	0.33*
Bush (1987)[3]	2270	26%	C	8.5	CVD death	0.34*
Potocki (1971)[7]	198	47%	C	10.0	CHD	0.47
Henderson (1988)[8]	8807	56%	E	4.5	MI	0.54*
Wilson (1985)[10]	1234	24%	E	10.0	All CVD	1.94
Stampfer (1991)[11]	48 470	47%	C	10.0	All CVD All death	0.72* 0.89*

C: current user; E: ever user; CVD: cardiovascular disease; MI: myocardial infarction; *$P<0.05$ for incidence of MI
Reproduced from Bush and Stampfer,[2,11] with permission from the publisher.

Table 55.2 Observational studies; case control.

Case control	*n* (cases/controls)	Current use	Event	Risk estimate
Talbott (1977)[25]	64/64	Yes	Sudden death	0.34
Gruchow (1988)[26]	154/779	Yes	Severe occlusion	0.37*
Sullivan (1988)[27]	1444/744	Yes	>70% occlusion	0.44*
Rosenberg (1976)[28]	336/6730	Yes	MI	0.47
McFarland (1989)[29]	137/208	Yes	>70% occlusion	0.50*
Beard (1989)[30]	86/150	No	MI/sudden death	0.55
Avila (1990)[31]	103/721	Yes	MI	0.70
Adam (1981)[32]	76/151	Yes	MI	0.79
Szklo (1984)[33]	36/39	No	MI	0.83
Rosenberg (1980)[34]	105/160	Yes	MI	1.05
La Vecchia (1987)[35]	116/160	Yes	MI	1.62

MI: myocardial infarction; *$P<0.05$
Reproduced from Bush,[2] with permission from the publisher.

involved progestogen administration. The results showed a 70% reduction in myocardial infarction (MI) and no increase in cancer risk. However, due to the small population size, the results were not statistically significant.

The majority of epidemiologic evidence has compared relative risk in women using unopposed estrogen therapy versus controls. Due to the well-documented increase in endometrial hyperplasia and neoplasia with estrogen use alone,[24] the question arises as to whether combined estrogen/progestogen therapy will yield the same cardiovascular benefit. Several studies have raised the concern that progestogens may attenuate some or all of the beneficial estrogenic effects, particularly on the lipoprotein profile.[13,23] As mentioned previously, the effect of sex steroids on plasma lipid/lipoprotein levels may explain only approximately 30% of the observed clinical benefit.[2] It may be that the more important effect of sex steroids is their influence on the manner in which the arterial wall interacts with and processes lipid (e.g. lipoprotein oxidation, macrophage uptake of cholesterol ester), as well as their effects at many other levels (coagulation factors, receptor interactions, endothelial function and blood flow). In some animal studies, addition of progesterone attenuates the estrogen-related benefit on atherosclerosis (e.g. in cynomolgus monkeys),[37] however in other animal models, progesterone has not affected the estrogen-induced benefit on arterial wall lipid accumulation (e.g. in ovariectomized rabbits).[38] Possible explanations for these apparently contradictory findings will be discussed under the lipid section later in this chapter.

In humans, the data on the effects of added progestogens are also conflicting. Some cross-sectional studies have shown that added progestogen is associated with a significant attenuation of the estrogen-related lipid altering effects,[13,23] notably a lowering of the high-density lipoprotein (HDL) cholesterol and in particular the HDL-2 subfraction (thought to be associated with the most cardiovascular benefit). However, other studies have suggested that added progestogens have no detrimental effect on the lipid profile and that there may even be a greater improvement in cardiovascular risk factors in the estrogen/progestogen group than in women using estrogens alone. Nabulsi et al[12] showed similar levels of HDL cholesterol, LDL cholesterol, apolipoproteins A1 and B, lipoprotein (a) and triglycerides in women taking either combined HRT or unopposed estrogen, compared to controls. In this study, the lipid profile in hormone users showed a reduction in LDL cholesterol levels of 0.40 mmol/L, an increase in HDL cholesterol of 0.23 mmol/L, and a reduction in fibrinogen levels of 0.16 g/L, yielding a total estimated reduction of 42% in the risk of coronary artery disease. This did not include the additional benefits on carbohydrate metabolism and factor VII levels that were also seen in the combined estrogen/progestogen group. The preservation of cardiovascular benefit with added progestogen has been further supported by the recent prospective and randomized PEPI trial results,[24] demonstrating improved lipoprotein levels and reduced fibrinogen levels in all hormone users compared with controls, with the greatest benefit in the unopposed estrogen users and those women in the combined group using micronized progesterone.

In many areas, there is currently still more contradiction than clarity. Much of this apparent contradiction arises from the fact that work in this field has involved many different hormone regimes, different populations of women and largely observational studies. In this research area it is often difficult to control certain variables, such as the definition of the onset of menopause, the fluctuation in hormone levels in relation to study times and levels of patient compliance. It is hoped that large prospective trials, such as the Women's Health Initiative (WHI), which commenced in 1991, will provide clearer recommendations for practitioners and their patients and ease some of the anxiety that the issue of hormone replacement therapy has engendered in the community, media and the medical profession in recent years. Several randomized prospective trials, such as the HERS, ERA and European secondary prevention trials and the North American primary prevention trials, the largest being the Women's Health Initiative, are examining the effects of a variety of different HRT regimens on a number of cardiovascular and/or noncardiac end-points. Despite this, it is possible that these studies may still leave unanswered important questions relating to the prescription of combination therapy, including the best choice of preparation, dosage and method of administration. Furthermore, results of the large WHI trial may not be available for several years. Until this time, it will remain the responsibility of the individual doctor to appraise the currently available evidence for and against hormone replacement therapy, for each individual patient.

THE PHYSIOLOGIC EFFECTS AND MECHANISMS OF ACTION OF HORMONE REPLACEMENT THERAPY

The commonest single cause of mortality in postmenopausal women in industrialized countries is coronary artery disease.[39] A wealth of epidemiologic work has now shown that postmenopausal hormone replacement may alter a woman's risk of developing coronary disease, by both an effect on lipids and, probably more importantly, by beneficial direct effects on the artery wall.

Animal and human studies have documented improvements in cardiac function and arterial wall physiology (both structural and functional) with the use of estrogen therapy. Less information has been obtained using the clinically relevant combination of estrogen/progestogen therapy. The studies that have used combined therapy have varied in their results — some showing an augmentation of estrogen's beneficial effect, no change or an attenuation of the estrogen effect, without destroying the benefit completely.

Cardiac effects

The major sex steroids certainly influence cardiac contractility, however this may be largely due to systemic arterial vasodilatation rather than to an intrinsic myocardial inotropic effect. Estrogen and progestogen receptor sites do exist at the atrial and ventricular fiber level of the heart,[40] however their presence is scanty and possible function unclear. Animal studies have consistently shown that estradiol increases the cardiac output, mostly by a significant effect on systemic vasodilatation.[41,42]

Estrogens have been shown to stimulate muscarinic and β-adrenergic cardiac receptors in rats and in humans.[43,44] In addition, estradiol reduces arterial impedance in the carotid and uterine arteries of postmenopausal women as measured by the pulsatility index.[45] In the uterine studies, the reduction in pulsatility index with estrogen use was moderately attenuated by the addition of C-19 progestogens. Work published by Prelevic et al,[46] demonstrated that left ventricular systolic flow parameters increased on both estrogen and combined therapy. The increase in flow velocity integral reflected both an increase in stroke volume and preserved myocardial contractility. There may be hormone-related improvement in left ventricular diastolic function as well. Manolio et al,[47] have found that past or present estrogen users have a lower incidence of subclinical cardiac disease, with reduced LV mass on ECG and better E/A ratios on doppler assessment of mitral inflow (a measure of cardiac diastolic function). A protective benefit of estrogens on diastolic function is significant since this age-related change in most hearts accounts for a large proportion of cardiac morbidity (e.g. cardiac failure, decreased exercise tolerance and predisposition to atrial arrhythmias) in older age groups. These findings, suggesting improved left ventricular systolic and diastolic function in women taking hormone replacement, may be another factor contributing to an observed survival benefit.

Arterial effects

Lipids

Both surgical and natural menopause is associated with a detrimental effect on the lipid profile, with elevation in the atherogenic low-density lipoprotein (LDL) cholesterol and total triglycerides and a decrease in the atheroprotective high-density lipoprotein (HDL) levels and apoproteins A1 and A2.[12,48] Hence the overall LDL/HDL ratio is shifted unfavorably even if the total serum cholesterol is unaltered. In contrast, exogenous estrogen administration leads to an increase in the rate of production of large VLDL (very low density lipoprotein) particles and the clearance of their potentially atherogenic remnants. Plasma LDL levels are reduced due to increased clearance by induction of hepatic LDL receptors, however there is a shift towards smaller, more dense cholesterol-depleted LDL particles, which have been associated with a higher incidence of myocardial infarction.[49] Hence, it is not completely clear whether the reduction in LDL cholesterol with estrogens are equivalent in benefit to the changes obtained by other lipid lowering treatments. Triglyceride levels were marginally raised in women on hormone replacement in the PEPI study,[24] although other trials have shown a variable effect. The increase in triglycerides is due to increased production and is not affected by the addition of progestogens.

The PEPI investigators postulate that this change may not be atherogenic but note that their study excluded women with high baseline triglyceride levels who might have been at greatest risk. Estrogen therapy favorably promotes elevations in HDL cholesterol, notably the important HDL-2 subclass, due to increased rates of production of HDL associated lipoproteins, particularly ApoA1, and suppression of hepatic lipase activity. The addition of progestogens induces hepatic lipase activity, increasing the breakdown of HDL-2 and HDL cholesterol without significant effects on LDL cholesterol levels.[48] Nabulsi et al showed that users of both unopposed estrogen and combined therapy had similar levels of HDL, HDL-2 and HDL-3, total cholesterol, apolipoproteins A-1 and B, LDL cholesterol and the atherogenic lipoprotein (a).[12] The majority of women using combined therapy were taking medroxyprogesterone acetate (MPA), which has lower levels of androgenic activity than progestogens such as levonorgestrel and norethisterone. The recent PEPI trial provides the most accurate results to date and confirms that hormone replacement therapies as a group are associated with improvement in the lipid profile over controls. However it unequivocably demonstrates that unopposed estrogen has a more favorable effect on HDL cholesterol than combined therapy, and of the progestogens used, micronized progesterone attenuates this benefit far less than the commonly prescribed medroxyprogesterone acetate.[24] HDL cholesterol levels are inversely correlated with cardiovascular risk,[12] however no prospective clinical studies have as yet confirmed that increasing HDL reduces the risk of heart disease in the female population.

Of particular interest, lipoprotein (a) levels have been shown to be reduced by sex steroid administration.[12,50,51] Lipoprotein (a) is similar in composition to LDL, with the addition of an extra apoprotein, and is considered particularly atherogenic.[52] Lipoprotein (a) (Lp(a)) levels are significantly correlated with cardiovascular risk and appeared to be influenced only by genetic factors, independent of environmental and lifestyle modifications, until the finding that estrogen tharapy may reduce Lp(a) levels. Lp(a) levels fluctuate in pregnant women, returning to basal levels after delivery, and also vary within stages of the menstrual cycle.[53,54] Testosterone-related steroids such as stanozol have been shown to reduce Lp(a) levels by up to 65% in postmenopausal women, and estrogen used in men with prostate cancer has reduced levels of Lp(a) by up to 50%.[55,56] Studies with both unopposed estrogen and combination estrogen/progestogen therapy have also shown reductions of up to 15% in Lp(a) levels.[51] These studies have observed levels of Lp(a) before and after treatment using the individual as their own controls. Two cross-sectional studies however, the Framingham Offspring Study and the FINRISK Haemostasis Study,[52,57] were unable to show a significant difference in Lp(a) levels associated with hormone replacement therapy. The population size in these studies was large and therefore the discrepancy may best be explained by the cross-sectional nature of these latter two studies, different types of HRT studied or the possibility that different populations may have different responses to hormone replacement for genetic and/or environmental reasons. Assuming a positive effect, it is unclear whether these hormones act through increased catabolism or decreased synthesis of Lp(a).

Structurally, Lp(a) bears homology to plasminogen and may compete with the latter during fibrinolysis. Therefore elevated levels of Lp(a) might be detrimental to the breakdown of thrombotic lesions and predispose the individual to both atherosclerosis and possibly acute coronary syndromes, such as unstable angina and myocardial infarction.

The route of steroid administration may be important in determining the magnitude of the effects of hormones on the lipid profile. Several studies have indicated that transdermal estrogens have a less marked effect on plasma lipid and lipoproteins than the oral estrogens.[14,58] Oral estrogens may reach higher concentrations in the portal circulation compared to transdermally absorbed hormones, and this may account for their greater effect on hepatic lipid metabolism.[14] Based on an analysis of the multiple studies examining the hormone/lipid profile interaction, it has been estimated that plasma lipid effects account for approximately 25–50% of the arterioprotective benefit of estrogen replacement.[2] For this reason, much research attention has focussed on the direct effect of sex steroids on the arterial wall, which may further explain the clinically observed benefit of hormone replacement therapy in postmenopausal women.

Arterial wall structure

The sex steroids estrogen and progesterone have been shown to affect both the extent and the structure of atherosclerotic lesions in both animal and human studies. In animal models of atherosclerosis, estrogens prevent collagen and elastin accumulation in the aortic wall of normotensive rats,[59] and suppress thickening of the aorta in hypertensive rats.[60] Haarbo and colleagues,[15] demonstrated that estrogen therapy reduces accumulation of intra-arterial lipid and therefore the development of athersclerosis in cholesterol-fed rabbits. In this model, the estrogen-related benefit was not attenuated by the use of combined therapy with the 19-nortestosterone progestogens, norethisterone acetate and levonorgestrel. Although the lipid profile was not adversely affected by the use of progestogens in this particular study, other studies have raised the concern that the possible detrimental effects of these agents on the lipid profile might attenuate or even eliminate any long-term arterial wall benefit. Adams et al have recently performed a similar experiment on the atheroprotective effects of hormone replacement in cynomolgus monkeys.[37] In this study they tested one of the most common estrogen/progestogen combinations

— oral conjugated equine estrogen with medroxyprogesterone acetate. With unopposed estrogen therapy, atherosclerosis extent was decreased by 70% compared with controls, however the addition of progesterone eliminated the estrogen-related benefit. In contrast to Haarbo's work, this particular study used medroxyprogesterone acetate and was associated with unfavorable changes in the lipid profile. It is possible that this difference in results is due to different actions of various progestogens, and/or species differences, highlighting the need to determine which combination will yield greatest clinical benefit in humans. Medroxyprogesterone acetate may attenuate estrogen's beneficial vascular effects more than other progestogens in several studies,[23,24] despite the fact that it has less androgenic properties and less effect on lipoprotein lipase than most other progesterones. More work is needed to clarify these differing results.

In humans, autopsy studies dating as far back as the 1930s have documented the increased amount of atherosclerosis in females who undergo a premature menopause compared to the normally low prevalence of coronary disease in premenopausal women or young postmenopausal women.[61,62] Colditz et al,[63] suggested that the women who had received a hysterectomy with *bilateral* oopherectomy were at highest risk of coronary disease (risk ratio of 2.2), and that this risk was reversed with postmenopausal estrogen replacement. They observed no difference in coronary disease in those women undergoing natural menopause or hysterectomy with unilateral or bilateral ovarian preservation as compared to premenopausal controls. The study, however, only included young postmenopausal females.

The search for possible mechanisms for reduced atherosclerotic plaque formation during estrogen therapy has generated much interest. As mentioned previously, the effects of hormone replacement involve more than just an effect on *plasma* lipid levels. This includes the interaction of sex hormones and cholesterol within the arterial wall. The amount of lipid that accumulates in an arterial wall is thought to be determined by several processes: the process of lipid uptake into the artery from the plasma and, probably more importantly, the retention of this lipid in the arterial wall by various means, including interaction of lipid with intercellular matrix components such as proteoglycans.[64] In conditions where lipid retention times in the arterial wall are increased, lipid may be more likely to undergo atherogenic changes such as LDL cholesterol oxidation, increased LDL binding to arterial wall components and increased uptake of cholesterol into macrophages to form foam cells, an important component of early atherosclerotic lesions.

Haarbo has shown that aortic permeability to LDL (i.e. the influx of LDL into the wall from plasma) is not altered significantly by estrogen.[65] Assuming this is correct, the finding by Wagner et al[66] of an inhibitory effect of estrogen on the sum accumulation of LDL in the arterial wall suggests that estrogen may act by stimulating a greater efflux of LDL cholesterol from the arterial wall (i.e. reducing the retention time of potentially atherogenic lipid). This could be due to a reduction in the affinity for and LDL-binding capacity of the intercellular matrix components (via changes in proteoglycans, collagen and/or elastin expression), which in turn may reduce the arterial wall transit time whereby LDL could be made more atherogenic (e.g. by oxidation and incorporation into macrophages for foam cell formation). This area of sex steroid effect on arterial wall structure and lipid interaction remains an active area of research and possibly explains the reason why the effects of estrogens on *plasma* lipid levels alone accounts for only a relatively small proportion of the observed clinical cardiovascular benefit.[2]

Arterial function

Estrogen can improve arterial function as well as structure, with important physiological consequences. Rosano et al[67] demonstrated that acute administration of sublingual estradiol-17β improves exercise tolerance and reduces myocardial ischemia in postmenopausal women with known coronary disease. Several studies have also shown that estrogen is a potent vasodilator, in both coronary and several peripheral vascular beds,[68–70] supporting the hypothesis that estrogen exerts a benefit not only in reducing the amount of atherosclerotic plaque, but also through improved arterial function and flow dynamics. Possible mechanisms for this beneficial effect on arterial physiology include an improvement in endothelial function and/or smooth muscle dilator effects, calcium-channel blocking actions of estrogen and interaction with the sex steroid receptors that have been demonstrated in human vascular smooth muscle cells and endothelium.[71–73]

The endothelium plays a critical role in the regulation of arterial tone and vascular reactivity. Disruption or damage to the integrity of the endothelium is thought to be a key factor in the development of atherosclerosis and the occurrence of acute cardiac syndromes.[74] Endothelial cells release endothelium-derived relaxing factor, or nitric oxide. Nitric oxide (NO) or a related nitrosothiol is a powerful vasodilator released by healthy endothelium, in response to various chemical triggers including acetylcholine, serotonin, thrombin, substance P, and physical stimuli such as increases in blood flow, pulsatile pressure and shear forces.[75] Arterial reactivity is a delicate balance between this vasodilator mechanism, and the vasoconstrictor actions of other hormones (such as endothelin-1), neurotransmitters and platelet-release factors. In atherosclerosis, endothelium-dependent vascular relaxation is abnormal,[76] probably as a consequence of endothelial layer damage and disruption to NO production. Estrogen has been shown in both animal and human studies to benefit endothelium-dependent dilatation, as assessed by acetylcholine-induced or flow-mediated arterial vasodilation.[20,68–70,77–79] This vasodilation is probably mediated by nitric oxide — either an increased production from the endothelium, reduced breakdown of nitric oxide and/or increased sensitivity to its effect. Vascular release of nitric oxide in the uterine artery increases throughout pregnancy,[80] with increased urinary nitrates from nitric oxide catabolism. There is also an increase in serum nitrate levels and an improvement in nitric oxide-related arterial dilation seen during the follicular phase of the menstrual cycle when the estrogen surge occurs.[81,82] Rabbit studies have also shown a higher basal release of NO in females compared to males.[83]

It is likely that a significant part of the cardiovascular benefit of hormone replacement therapy in postmenopausal women is related to an improvement in and preservation of endothelial function. Celermajer et al[84] have demonstrated that ageing is associated with progressive arterial endothelial dysfunction. This decline in endothelial function occurs approximately ten years later in women compared to men, and coincides with the onset of female menopause, suggesting a protective effect of estrogen on the arterial wall.

Animal work has examined the effect of sex steroid hormones in ovariectomized, cholesterol fed rabbits[15] and cynomolgus monkeys.[18] Williams et al showed that both long-term and short-term estrogen treatment prevented impaired acetylcholine-induced dilatation of atherosclerotic coronary arteries in surgically postmenopausal cynomolgus monkeys.[18] This acute effect of estrogen administration has been duplicated in human studies in postmenopausal women,[20,68–70] most notably by Gilligan et al who demonstrated this benefit at physiologic concentrations of plasma estradiol with levels measured before and after intravenous estrogen infusion.[18,77] This is important, because previous experiments showing a positive effect of estrogen on vasomotor function may well have been demonstrating a direct smooth muscle-relaxant effect alone, due to supraphysiologic concentrations of estradiol in the bloodstream.

In addition to invasive techniques, where endothelium-dependent arterial vasodilation is assessed by the direct infusion of acetylcholine into the coronary and peripheral circulations, a significant amount of work has examined endothelium-mediated vasoreactivity by noninvasive ultrasound techniques. This involves studying changes in the diameter of the human brachial artery using changes in arterial flow produced by a forearm sphygmomanometer cuff, as a measure of endothelial function under a variety of conditions.[85] Flow-mediated dilation (FMD) of peripheral arteries is known to be mainly mediated by release of nitric oxide,[86] and therefore provides a marker of endothelial health and integrity. It has been shown to correlate well with changes in the coronary circulation as measured by invasive intra-arterial techniques.[87] In a prospective study, Lieberman et al showed that estrogen replacement therapy administered for nine weeks, improves flow-mediated endothelium-dependent vasodilation in postmenopausal women (13.5% for the 1 mg/day oral estradiol group versus 6.8% in the placebo group).[70] As concerns combined HRT, we recently compared the endothelium-dependent dilatation of the brachial artery in healthy postmenopausal women taking hormone replacement therapy versus controls, and found improved arterial function in the former group, consistent with a protective effect of estrogen only and combined therapy on large arterial function.[88] However, Dorup et al,[89] in a smaller prospective study, were unable to demonstrate any benefit of combined hormone replacement therapy compared to controls.

The effect of long-term hormone replacement therapy, as most frequently used in clinical practice, is hard to assess. The question is, whether the benefits observed with short-term estrogen administration translate into vascular benefit for those women taking hormone replacement every day over many years. Williams et al[77] demonstrated a coronary vasodilator response to acetylcholine in ovariectomized, cholesterol-fed cynomolgus monkeys given long-term estrogen therapy for two years. Histology at autopsy showed that the degree of intimal thickening and atherosclerotic burden was less in the estrogen-supplemented group, compared to hormone deficient controls. Thus it is possible that the observed vasomotor benefit may be the result of reduced atherosclerosis in general, rather than a specific action of long-term estrogen on arterial wall function. Of interest, a recent study by Gilligan et al,[90] has shown that the vasodilator response generated by acute estradiol infused intra-arterially into the human forearm vasculature is not reproducible after three weeks of chronic transdermal estradiol, although the original effect could be reproduced by repeat intra-arterial hormone administration. These results are at odds with the animal experiments of Williams et al using long-term estrogen[77] and Lieberman's study in humans.[70] Possible explanations may relate to species differences, to differences between coronary and peripheral arterial responses, to a tolerance effect (unlikely in view of the return of effect with the same dose intra-arterially as before), or the possible need for the estradiol levels to be high (as in midcycle) in order to demonstrate endothelium protective effect.

The concern that added progestogens may negate positive estrogenic effects at the endothelial level has been investigated in several studies. Williams et al showed an attenuation of the dilator response in the coronary arteries of monkeys treated with estrogen with the addition of the progestogen medroxyprogesterone acetate.[78] Similar studies of sufficient power to detect a negative progestogen effect have not been performed as yet in humans. This is a significant issue, since most postmenopausal women will have an intact uterus, and many will be prescribed the progesterone component of therapy to counteract the risk of endometrial atypia/neoplasia. A recent study[91] has shown that serum nitrite/nitrate levels are significantly higher in postmenopausal women treated with combined hormone replacement therapy compared with untreated postmenopausal controls. These results suggest that part of the cardioprotective effect of HRT may be mediated by an increase in circulating NO. However, a separate analysis of results from serum samples collected on those days when the women were taking estrogen and progestogen did not yield any significant difference in circulating NO levels compared to controls. This study suggests, but does not prove, that added progestogen may oppose estrogen's beneficial effect. We will need to await the results of further prospective clinical studies to adequately assess the effects of combination therapy and which compounds from each steroid group will yield the most benefit.

Estrogen also acts directly at the arterial wall via calcium-dependent mechanisms. Recent work by Weiner at al has shown that sex hormones are capable of inducing calcium-dependent nitric oxide synthases in estrogen-fed or pregnant guinea pigs.[92] Experiments in rabbit coronary arteries measuring tension development showed that 17β estradiol inhibited arterial contraction stimulated by prostaglandin F2α and endothelin-1, probably by inhibiting calcium influx in smooth muscle cells.[93] This arterial vasodilation was maintained after the endothelium had been removed, further confirming an endothelium-independent effect. A recent study in isolated porcine coronary arteries also demonstrated the calcium channel blocker-like action of 17β estradiol.[94] Further data supporting a direct effect of estrogen on the arterial wall has arisen from the examination of vascular smooth muscle cells in culture. Nichols et al[95] demonstrated decreased protein synthesis in rat vascular smooth muscle cells in culture when exposed to estrogen. In humans, research by Karas et al demonstrated that vascular smooth muscle cells express estrogen-receptor mRNA and protein and that estrogen action at this receptor leads to gene activation.[72] Human studies examining the coronary arteries from autopsies of pre and postmenopausal women with and without heart disease have also demonstrated the presence of estrogen receptors on vascular smooth muscle cells.[73] The greater the expression of estrogen receptors, the less the degree of atherosclerosis, particularly in the premenopausal group where the expression of estrogen receptors is highest.

There is also evidence for estrogen receptors on endothelial cells. Colburn[71] demonstrated that cytosol extracted from endothelial cells in culture binds to estradiol with high affinity and specificity. The possible attenuation of the vasomotor benefits of estrogen by progestogens cannot readily be explained by receptor action. A recent study[96] examining 20 transplanted hearts (eight having normal coronary arteries) failed to show any evidence of progestogen receptor expression in either normal or atherosclerotic coronary specimens. It is also possible that there is an interaction of these sex hormones at sites such as the muscarinic receptors on vascular smooth and/or endothelial cells.

Blood pressure

Studies examining the effects of hormone replacement therapy on blood pressure have produced differing results. Due to reports of increased blood pressure with earlier high dose oral estrogen replacements,[97] hypertension was initially considered a relative contraindication to hormone replacement. Possibly supporting this effect, Pallas et al,[98] found that oral conjugated estrogens were associated with an increase in plasma renin substrate and renin activity but no increase in the plasma renin level itself. Soon after, however, a comprehensive review by Maschak and Lobo[97] of epidemiologic, prospective and cross-over trials conducted during the 1970s and 80s clearly indicated that hormone replacement therapy does not increase the incidence of hypertension or aggravate pre-existing hypertension. Surprisingly, there have even been reports of reduced diastolic and systolic blood pressure with combination therapy, not seen in groups treated with estrogen alone.[99] Recent work by Proudler et al,[100] showed that after six months of hormone replacement therapy, serum angiotensin converting enzyme activity was reduced by 20%. The most recent information to date is the results of the prospectively designed PEPI trial,[24] which showed no significant change in either diastolic or systolic blood pressure values during the three years of hormone replacement. All these women were normotensive at the commencement of the trial. Despite these favorable results, the occasional occurrence of estrogen-induced hypertension or instability of blood pressure control cannot be disregarded; therefore careful monitoring of blood pressure changes should be performed after the commencement of hormone replacement therapy, particularly in the subgroup of women with pre-existing hypertension.

Coagulation

The process of thrombosis is recognized to play an important role in the development of clinical cardiovascular events, based on the observation that acute cardiac syndromes (myocardial infarction, unstable angina) are due to coronary artery thrombosis, even in the absence of severe coronary stenosis. The propensity of an individual to acute thrombosis is mediated by the balance between prothrombotic factors, such as fibrinogen, von Willebrand factor, platelets and plasminogen activator inhibitor (PAI-1), and prothrombolytic factors such as plasminogen and tissue plasminogen activator. These and various other mediators of thrombosis have been studied in women and it appears that the risk of developing cardiovascular disease is associated with high levels of coagulation factor VII and von Willebrand factor, fibrinogen and (PAI-1).[101] All of these markers increase with age, however the effect of hormone replacement therapy on these levels varies,[12,57] influencing primarily the level of fibrinogen and the fibrinolytic capacity by modulating PAI-1 levels. Gebara et al[102] demonstrated a beneficial reduction in PAI-1 levels in postmenopausal women taking hormone replacement and that this effect was greater in women taking unopposed estrogen, although numbers were small in the combined hormone therapy group. The mechanism for this reduction in PAI-1 is unclear, and randomized prospective clinical trials are needed to determine whether estrogen consistently reduces PAI-1 levels and if this confers a decrease in cardiovascular morbidity and mortality.

Several observational studies have noted a decrease in fibrinogen levels in postmenopausal women on hormone replacement, as compared to controls. Nabulsi et al[12] showed lower levels of fibrinogen in both estrogen and combined estrogen/progestogen therapy groups and this was further validated in the PEPI trial, where the magnitude of reduction in fibrinogen levels might represent a reduction of 50% in cardiovascular risk, based on estimates from the Framingham women's data.[103] The cross-sectional FINRISK Haemostasis Study[57] also documented a significant reduction in fibrinogen, but as with other studies, the effect on factor VII (and its parallel interplay with triglyceride level), von Willebrand factor and plasminogen levels was less clear. In addition, animal work in rabbits[104] has shown that estrogen reduces the formation of the potent platelet aggregator and vasoconstrictor thromboxane A2, hence altering the thromboxane A2:prostacyclin (PGI2) ratio favorably, the latter acting as a vasodilator and anti-aggregating platelet agent. Therefore, in summary, hormone replacement in currently prescribed dosages possibly decreases the tendency to vascular thrombosis in postmenopausal women.

IN PRACTICE, WHOSE CARDIOVASCULAR SYSTEM NEEDS HORMONE REPLACEMENT THERAPY?

The benefits of hormone replacement therapy in reducing cardiovascular morbidity and mortality in postmenopausal women by as much as 50%[2] is impressive, although based largely on epidemiologic rather than prospective, randomized studies. Cardiovascular disease is the main cause of death in this age group in industrialized countries, and in general women tend to fare less well in the survival stakes once they do present clinically.[105] The reasons for this are probably multifactorial. Often, women present at a later stage of their disease; their disease may be more severe than their symptoms suggest and, historically, the diagnosis and referral for intervention and treatment is deferred in women. At a practical level, women tend to have smaller coronary arteries than males, possibly making an equivalent atherosclerotic load more detrimental. Furthermore, the possibility of interventional procedures such as angioplasty, coronary stenting and coronary artery bypass grafting may be technically more difficult, less beneficial and less attractive as treatment options than in their male counterparts. In addition, many of the recent advances in cardiovascular protection, such as cholesterol-lowering, are based on results that are derived from studies recruiting mostly or exclusively men,[106,107] and may not necessarily be applicable to female patients. For these reasons, the possibility that hormone replacement therapy could provide coronary atheroprotection in postmenopausal females, at a time when the endogenous protective effect of the body's own hormones is declining, has provided much excitement and also considerable intellectual and emotional debate.

The decision to prescribe hormone replacement therapy for each woman, for disease prevention, depends on estimates of that woman's *absolute* risk of dying from each potential cause, and how that risk is altered by prescription of HRT. For the average postmenopausal woman, the risk of dying of heart disease is approximately 40%, whereas the chance of developing breast cancer is at most 5.5%, with approximately a 1% chance of mortality.[108] Hence, breast cancer in postmenopausal women, may have a more indolent course than in younger females, and is not always the cause of death in these patients.[109] In a woman with previous breast cancer, her absolute risk of breast malignancy is higher (approximately three-fold),[108] and the benefit/risk ratio of HRT is consequently lower. On the other hand, a woman who has had a coronary event but no history of breast cancer has a higher benefit/risk ratio for taking HRT than average. These considerations of absolute rather than relative risk must be applied by each physician, when making decisions about HRT for each individual woman.

Therefore, in an ideal world, it might be advisable to prescribe hormone replacement therapy to most women, to relieve perimenopausal symptoms and to provide longer-term benefit to their skeletal[4] and cardiovascular system. In reality, however, the data on cardiovascular benefit is incomplete and occasionally confusing, and the possibility of breast cancer with long-term treatment (although small in comparison to the seeming benefits),[11] still raises concern at a community level. To confirm an absolute risk reduction requires prospective, randomized clinical trials documenting improved total and cardiovascular end-points of morbidity and mortality over at least 5–10 years, and possibly even longer in terms of quantifying the risks of cancer. The risk of endometrial cancer is acceptably small with combination estrogen/progestogen therapy,[110,111] and although not definite, the risk of dying from breast cancer is likely to be small, especially with regular surveillance using mammograms. The data as to whether a doctor should prescribe postmenopausal hormones to females with a family history of breast cancer are unclear and likely to depend on doctor-patient wishes, however a patient with previous breast or endometrial cancer should probably be excluded from HRT, although there are no controlled studies showing that this group fares worse than the general population on combined therapy.

Hormone replacement tharapy has been shown unequivocally to benefit several major cardiovascular risk factors, including HDL cholesterol and plasma fibrinogen levels. In addition, prospective trials will confirm whether the multiple cardiovascular benefits of HRT demonstrated in cross-sectional studies will be validated and translate into clinical benefit.

Ultimately, if these benefits are borne out, the value of HRT in the postmenopausal age group and its public health implications will be undeniable. Hopefully, such results will put an end to the common retort that previous epidemiologic work is selecting a subgroup of postmenopausal females who, by the very nature of their interest in health, place them at a lower cardiovascular risk than age-matched controls in the general population.

Even with the results of large prospective trials such as the Women's Health Initiative, the questions concerning which hormone preparations yield the best clinical benefit will probably still remain unclear. It appears from the PEPI study[24] (a large placebo-controlled, randomized clinical trial over a three year period) that micronized progesterone provides more benefit than the more commonly used medroxy-progesterone acetate. In this study, oral conjugated equine estrogen was used. Although the unopposed estrogen arm showed the most beneficial elevation of HDL cholesterol, the high rates of endometrial hyperplasia observed make this therapy potentially unacceptable in all women with an intact uterus. In PEPI, cyclic administration of micronized progesterone yielded the most favorable elevation in HDL from the combined therapy group. Possible differences between the routes of administration of hormone replacement is also an important issue and not yet adequately studied. A Canadian study compared treatment with cyclic oral micronized progesterone and either oral conjugated equine estrogens or percutaneous 17β estradiol.[112] This demonstrated a greater attenuation by progesterone of the elevation in HDL levels in the percutaneous group whereas the combined oral preparation tended to increase HDL cholesterol and apo A1 levels. In contrast, Stevenson et al,[113] showed no difference in HDL levels but a lowering in triglycerides and improved glucose tolerance in the transdermal estrogen group. Hence more information is needed to confirm whether the reduced hepatic metabolism of estrogen in the transdermal group, which produces less metabolic change and certainly a more physiological method of administration, translates into a significant difference in terms of clinical effect. Unfortunately, many of the current prospective trials are not designed to answer this question. At present the choice of route of administration probably rests with patient preference.

Therefore, based on currently available evidence, we recommend that postmenopausal women should take the following steps to reduce their lifetime risk of heart disease. Low fat diets, regular exercise, smoking cessation and control of hypertension remain the cornerstones of primary cardiovascular prevention. Women with two or more risk factors for atherosclerosis, or who have established vascular disease, should be considered for HRT, if there is no contraindication. In those with no uterus, unopposed estrogen therapy should be prescribed. In those with a uterus, unopposed estrogen can be prescribed, but causes excessive uterine bleeding in many women, and necessitates regular endometrial sampling. We prefer the prescription of estrogen with progesterone. Which route, dose and drug is optimal is not known, and the evidence comparing these aspects of HRT is confusing and inconclusive. Currently, it is reasonable for each physician and patient to decide together about their favored combination of HRT. Women with a past history of breast cancer should not receive long-term HRT, even if they have cardiovascular disease. Finally, the majority of postmenopausal women will be healthy, without known disease of heart, breast or bone. In such women, prescription of HRT is justifiable based on current evidence, but this decision should be individualized for each woman, and made by each woman after appropriate information has been given by her treating physician.

Conclusion

The evidence supporting a reduction in cardiovascular morbidity and mortality with the use of long-term hormone replacement in postmenopausal women is thus far quite convincing, but not conclusive. In combination with menopausal symptom relief and prevention of osteoporosis, a reduction of cardiovascular risk makes hormone replacement therapy a potentially attractive health option to offer the ageing female population. From a cardiac viewpoint, epidemiologic and some prospective work has shown that unopposed and combined estrogen/progestogen therapy favorably influences a number of cardiac risk factors, including plasma lipid levels, several hemostatic factors, arterial vasoreactivity and probably the development of atherosclerosis. However the lack of results from long term, randomized, prospective clinical trials, particularly for combined estrogen/progestogen therapy in regards to the main end-points of cardiac and total morbidity and mortality, make it difficult to give a general recommendation for the use of hormone replacement in all members of the female postmenopausal population. It is hoped that prospective trials that are currently in progress, such as the Women's Health Initiative, will clarify some of these issues. In the meantime, the information thus far seems in favor of postmenopausal hormone replacement in those women without absolute or relative contraindications, after thorough discussion between the individual patient and physician of the risk to benefit ratio.

REFERENCES

1. Kannel WB, Hjortland MC, Mcnamara P, Gordon T 1976 Menopause and risk of cardiovascular disease. The Framingham Study. Annals of Internal Medicine 85: 447–452
2. Bush TL 1991 Extraskeletal effects of estrogen and the prevention of atherosclerosis. Osteoporosis International 2: 5–11
3. Bush TL, Barett-Connor E, Cowan LD et al 1987 Cardiovascular mortality and non-contraceptive estrogen use in women: results from the Lipid Research Clinics Program follow-up study. Circulation 75: 1102–1109
4. Lafferty FW, Helmuth DO 1985 Post-menopausal estrogen replacement: the prevention of osteoporosis and systemic effects. Maturitas 7: 147–159
5. Stampfer MJ, Willett WC, Colditz GA et al 1986 A prospective study of postmenopausal estrogen therapy and coronary heart disease. New England Journal of Medicine 313: 1044–1049
6. Hammond CB, Jelovsek FR, Lee KL et al 1979 Effects of long-term estrogen replacement therapy I. Metabolic effects. American Journal of Obstetrics and Gynecology 133: 525–536
7. Potocki J 1971 Wplyw leczenia estrogenami na niewydolnose wiencowa u kobiet po menopauzie. J Pol Tyg Lek 216: 1812–1815
8. Henderson BE, Paganini-Hill A, Ross RK 1988 Estrogen replacement therapy and protection from acute myocardial infarction. American Journal of Obstetrics and Gynecology 159: 312–317

9. Wilson PWF, Garrison RJ, Castelli WP 1986 Postmenopausal estrogen use and heart disease (letter). New England Journal of Medicine 315: 135
10. Wilson PWF, Garrison RJ, Castelli WP 1985 Postmenopausal estrogen use, cigarette smoking, and cardiovascular morbidity in women over 50: the Framingham Study. New England Journal of Medicine 313: 1038–1043
11. Stampfer MJ, Colditz GA, Willett WC, Manson JE, Rosner B, Speizer FE, Hennekens CH 1991 Postmenopausal estrogen therapy and cardiovascular disease: ten-year follow-up from the Nurses' Health Study. New England Journal of Medicine 325: 756–762
12. Nabulsi AA, Folsom AR, White A, Patsch W, Heiss G, Wu KK, Szklo M 1993 Association of hormone-replacement therapy with various cardiovascular risk factors in postmenopausal women. New England Journal of Medicine 328: 1069–1075
13. Sacks FM, Walsh BW 1990 The effects of reproductive hormones on serum lipoproteins: unresolved issues in biology and clinical practice. Annals of the New York Academy of Science 592: 272–285
14. Sitruk-Ware R, Ibarra de Palacios P 1989 Oestrogen replacement therapy and cardiovascular disease in post-menopausal women. A review. Maturitas 11: 259–274
15. Haarbo J, Leth-Espensen P, Stender S, Christiansen C 1991 Estrogen monotherapy and combined estrogen-progestogen replacement therapy attenuate aortic accumulation of cholesterol in ovariectomized cholesterol-fed rabbits. Journal of Clinical Investigation 87: 1274–1279
16. Adams MR, Kaplan JR, Manuck SB, Koritnik DR, Parks JS, Wolfe MS, Clarkson TB 1990 Inhibition of coronary artery atherosclerosis by 17-β estradiol in ovariectomized monkeys. Arteriosclerosis 10: 1051–1057
17. Kushwaha RS, Lewis DS, Carey KD, McGill HC 1991 Effects of estrogen and progesterone on plasma lipoproteins and experimental atherosclerosis in the baboon. Arteriosclerosis and Thrombosis 11: 23–31
18. Williams JK, Adams MR, Herrington DM, Clarkson TB 1992 Short-term administration of estrogen and vascular responses of atherosclerotic coronary arteries. Journal of the American College of Cardiology 20: 452–457
19. Jiang C, Sarrel PM, Lindsay DC, Poole-Wilson PA, Collins P 1991 Endothelium-independent relaxation of rabbit coronary artery by 17β-oestradiol in-vitro. British Journal of Pharmacology 104: 1033–1037
20. Reis SE, Gloth ST, Blumenthal RS, Resar JR, Zacur HA, Gerstenblith G, Brinker JA 1994 Ethinyl estradiol acutely attenuates abnormal coronary vasomotor responses to acetylcholine in postmenopausal women. Circulation 89: 52–60
21. Paterson M, Wade-Evans T, Sturdee D, Thom M, Studd JWW 1980 Endometrial disease after treatment with oestrogens and progestogens in the climacteric. British Medical Journal i: 822–824
22. Armstrong BK 1988 Oestrogen therapy after the menopause – boon or bane? Medical Journal of Australia 148: 213–214
23. Tikkanen MJ, Kuusi T, Sipinen S 1986 Post-menopausal hormone replacement therapy: effects of progestogens on serum lipids and lipoproteins: a review. Maturitas 8: 7–17
24. The Writing Group for the PEPI Trial 1995 Effects of estrogen or estrogen/progestin regimens on heart disease risk factors in postmenopausal women. The postmenopausal estrogen/progestin interventions (PEPI) trial. Journal of the American Medical Association 273: 199–208
25. Talbott E, Kuller LH, Detre K et al 1977 Biologic and psychologic risk factors of sudden death from coronary disease in white women. American Journal of Cardiology 39: 858–864
26. Gruchow HW, Anderson AJ, Barboriak JJ et al 1988 Postmenopausal use of estrogen and occlusion of coronary arteries. American Heart Journal 115: 954–963
27. Sullivan JM, Vander Zwaag R, Lemp GF et al 1988 Postmenopausal estrogen use and coronary atherosclerosis. Annals of Internal Medicine 108: 358–363
28. Rosenberg L, Armstrong B, Jick H 1976 Myocardial infarction and estrogen therapy in post-menopausal women. New England Journal of Medicine 294: 1256–1259
29. McFarland KF, Boniface ME, Hornung CA et al 1900 Risk factors and non-contraceptive estrogen use in women with and without coronary disease. American Heart Journal
30. Beard CM, Kottke TE, Annegers JS et al 1989 The Rochester Coronary Heart Disease project: effect of cigarette smoking, hypertension, diabetes and steroidal estrogen use on coronary heart disease among 40 to 59-year-olds, 1960–82. Mayo Clinic Proceedings 64: 1471–1480
31. Avila MH, Walker AM, Jick H 1990 Use of replacement estrogens and the risk of myocardial infarction. Epidemiology 1: 128–133
32. Adam S, Williams V, Vessey MP 1981 Cardiovascular disease and hormone replacement treatment: a pilot case-control study. British Medical Journal 282: 1277–1278
33. Szklo M, Tonascia J, Gordis L et al 1984 Estrogen use and myocardial infarction risk: a case-control study. Preventive Medicine 13: 510–516
34. Rosenberg L, Slone D, Shapiro S et al 1980 Non-contraceptive estrogens and myocardial infarction in young women. Journal of the American Medical Association 244: 339–342
35. La Vecchia C, Francuschi S, Decarli A et al 1987 Risk factors for myocardial infarction in young women. American Journal of Epidemiology 125: 832–843
36. Nachtigall LE, Nachtigall RH, Nachtigall RD et al 1979 Estrogen replacement therapy. A prospective study in the relationship to carcinoma and cardiovascular and metabolic problems. Obstetrics and Gynecology 54: 74–79
37. Adams MR, Golden DL 1900 Atheroprotective effects of estrogen replacement therapy are antagonized by medroxyprogesterone acetate in monkeys. Abstract from the 68th scientific sessions, American Heart Association
38. Haarbo J, Svendsen OL, Christiansen C 1992 Progestogens do not affect aortic accumulation of cholesterol in ovariectomized cholesterol-fed rabbits. Circulation Research 70: 1198–1202

39. Kaplan NM 1985 Estrogen replacement therapy: effect on blood pressure and other cardiovascular risk factors. Journal of Reproductive Medicine 39 (Suppl): 802–803
40. Strumpf WE, Sar M, Aumuloer G 1977 The heart: a target organ for estradiol. Science 1: 319–321
41. Rosenberg CR, Morriss FH, Battaglia FC, Makowski EL, Meschia G 1976 Effects of estrogens on the uterine blood flow to reproductive and non-reproductive tissues in pregnant ewes. American Journal of Obstetrics and Gynecology 124: 618–629
42. Killam AP, Rosenberg CR, Battaglia FC, Makowski EL, Meschia G 1973 Effects of estrogens on blood flow of oopherectomized ewes. American Journal of Obstetrics and Gynecology 115: 1045–1052
43. Maddox YT, Falcon JG, Ridinger M, Cunard CM, Ramwell PW 1980 Endothelium-dependent gender differences in the response of the rat aorta. Journal of Pharmacology and Experimental Therapeutics 40: 452–457
44. Silva de Sá MF, Meirelles RS 1977 Vasodilation effect of estrogen on the human umbilical artery. Gynecological Investigation 8: 307–313
45. Ganger KF, Vyas S, Whitehead M, Crook D, Meire H, Campbell S 1991 Pulsatility index in internal carotid artery in relation to transdermal oestradiol and time since menopause. Lancet 338: 839–842
46. Prelevic GM, Beljic T 1994 The effect of oestrogen and progestogen replacement therapy on systolic flow velocity in healthy postmenopausal women. Maturitas 20: 37–44
47. Manolio TA, Furberg MD, Shemanski L, Psaty BM, O'Leary DH, Tracy RP, Bush TL 1993 Associations of postmenopausal estrogen use with cardiovascular disease and its risk factors in older women. Circulation 88: 2163–2171
48. Hazzard WR 1989 Estrogen replacement and cardiovascular disease: serum lipids and blood pressure effects. American Journal of Obstetrics and Gynecology 161: 1847–1853
49. Campos H, Sacks FM, Walsh BW, Schiff I, O'Hanesian MA, Krauss RM 1993 Differential effects of estrogen on low density lipoprotein subclasses in healthy postmenopausal women. Metabolism 42: 1153–1158
50. Farish E, Rolton HA, Barnes JF, Hart DM 1991 Lipoprotein (a) concentrations in postmenopausal women taking norethisterone. British Medical Journal 303: 694
51. Soma M, Fumagalli R, Paoletti R, Meschia M, Maini HC, Crosignani PG et al 1991 Plasma Lp(a) concentration after oestrogen and progestogen in postmenopausal women. Lancet 337: 612
52. Jenner JL, Ordovas JM, Lamon-Fava S, Schaefer M, Wilson PWF, Castelli WP, Schaefer EJ 1993 Effects of age, sex and menopausal status on plasma lipoprotein (a) levels. Circulation 87: 1135–1141
53. Zechner R, Desoye G, Schweditsch MO, Pfeiffer KP, Kostner GM 1986 Fluctuations of lipoprotein (a) concentrations during pregnancy and post-partum. Metabolism 35: 333–336
54. Saha AL, Armentrout MA, Hassell SM, Vella FA, Kannan K, Silberman SR 1989 Lipoprotein (a) quantitation by enzyme-linked immunoassay: correlations within normal female menstrual cycle. Arteriosclerosis 9: 760a
55. Alber JJ, Taggart HM, Appelbaum-Bowden D, Haffner S, Chestnut CH, Hazzard WR 1984 Reduction of lecithin-cholesterol acyltransferase, apolipoprotein D and the Lp(a) lipoprotein with the anabolic steroid stanozol. Biochim Biophys Acta 795: 293–303
56. Henriksson P, Angelin B, Berglund L 1992 Hormonal regulation of serum Lp(a) levels; opposite effects after estrogen treatment and orchidectomy in males with prostatic carcinoma. Journal of Clinical Investigation 89: 1166–1171
57. Salomaa V, Rasi V, Pekkanen J, Vahtera E, Jauhiainen M, Vartiainen E, Ehnholm C, Tuomilehto T, Myllylä 1995 Association of hormone replacement therapy with hemostatic and other cardiovascular risk factors. The FINRISK hemostasis study. Arteriosclerosis, Thrombosis and Vascular Biology 15: 1549–1555
58. Stanczyk FZ, Shoupe D, Nunez V, Macias-Gonzalez P, Vijod MA, Lobo A 1988 A randomized comparison of non-oral estradiol delivery in postmenopausal women. American Journal of Obstetrics and Gynecology 159: 1540–1546
59. Fischer GM, Swain ML 1977 Effect of sex hormone on blood pressure and vascular connective tissue in castrated and noncastrated male rats. American Journal of Physiology 232: H617–H621
60. Wolinsky H 1972 Effects of estrogen and progestogen treatment on the response of the aorta of male rats to hypertension: morphological and chemical studies. Circulation Research 30: 341–349
61. Levy H, Boas EP 1936 Coronary artery disease in women. Journal of the American Medical Association 107: 97–102
62. Clawson BJ 1941 The incidence of types of heart disease among 30,265 autopsies, with special reference to age and sex. American Heart Journal 22: 607–624
63. Colditz GA, Willett WC, Stampfer MJ, Rosner B, Speizer FE, Hennekens CH 1987 Menopause and the risk of coronary heart disease in women. New England Journal of Medicine 316: 1105–1110
64. Williams KJ, Tabas I 1995 The response to retention hypothesis of early atherogenesis. Arteriosclerosis, Thrombosis and Vascular Biology 15: 551–561
65. Haarbo J, Nielsen LB, Stender S, Christiansen C 1994 Aortic permeability to LDL during estrogen therapy. A study in normocholesterolaemic rabbits. Arteriosclerosis and Thrombosis 14: 243–247
66. Wagner JD, Clarkson TB, St Clair RW, Schwenke DC, Shicely CA, Adams MR 1991 Estrogen and progesterone replacement therapy reduces low-density lipoprotein accumulation in the coronary arteries of surgically postmenopausal cynomolgus monkeys. Journal of Clinical Investigation 88: 1995–2002
67. Rosano GMC, Sarrel PM, Poole-Wilson PA, Collins P 1993 Beneficial effect of oestrogen on exercise-induced myocardial ischaemia in women with coronary artery disease. Lancet 342: 133–136
68. Gilligan DM, Badar DM, Panza JA, Quyyumi AA, Cannon RO 1994 Acute vascular effects of estrogen in postmenopausal women. Circulation 90: 786–791
69. Gilligan DM, Quyyumi AA, Cannon RO 1994 Effects of physiological levels of estrogen on coronary vasomotor function in postmenopausal women. Circulation 89: 2545–2551

70. Lieberman EH, Gerhard MD, Uehata A, Walsh BW, Selwyn AP, Ganz P, Yeung AC, Creager MA 1994 Estrogen improves endothelium-dependent, flow-mediated dilation in postmenopausal women. Annals of Internal Medicine 121: 936–941
71. Colburn P, Buonassisi V 1978 Estrogen-binding sites in endothelial cell cultures. Science 201: 817–819
72. Karas RH, Patterson BL, Mendelsohn ME 1994 Human vascular smooth muscle cells contain functional estrogen receptor. Circulation 89: 1943–1950
73. Losordo DW, Kearney M, Kim EA, Jekanowski J, Isner JM 1994 Variable expression of the estrogen receptor in normal and atherosclerotic coronary arteries of premenopausal women. Circulation 89: 1501–1510
74. Ross R, Glomset JA 1976 The pathogenesis of atherosclerosis. New England Journal of Medicine 295: 369–377
75. Vanhoutte PM, Houston DS 1985 Platelets, endothelium, and vasospasm. Circulation 72: 728–734
76. Ludmer PL, Selwyn AP, Shook TL, Wayne RR, Mudge GH, Alexander RW, Ganz P 1986 Paradoxical vasoconstriction induced by acetylcholine in atherosclerotic coronary arteries. New England Journal of Medicine 315: 1046–1051
77. Koudy Williams J, Honoré EK, Washburm SA, Clarkson TB 1994 Effects of hormone replacement therapy on reactivity of atherosclerotic coronary arteries in cynomolgus monkeys. Journal of the American College of Cardiology 24: 1757–1761
78. Williams JK, Shively CA, Clarkson TB 1994 Determinants of coronary artery reactivity in premenopausal female cynomolgus monkeys with diet-induced atherosclerosis. Circulation 90: 983–987
79. Keaney JF, Shwaery GT, Xu A, Nicolosi RJ, Loscalzo J, Foxall TL, Vita JA 1994 17β-estradiol preserves endothelial vasodilator function and limits low-density lipoprotein oxidation in hypercholesterolemic swine. Circulation 89: 2251–2259
80. Magness RR, Rosenfeld CR 1989 Local and systemic estradiol-17 beta: effects on uterine and systemic vasodilation. American Journal of Physiology 256: E536–542
81. Roselli M, Imthurm B, Macas E, Keller PJ, Dubey RK 1994 Circulating nitrite/nitrate levels increase with follicular development; indirect evidence for estradiol-mediated NO release. Biochemical and Biophysical Research Communications 202: 1543–1552
82. Hashimoto M, Akishita M, Eto M, Ishikawa M, Kozaki K, Toba K et al 1995 Modulation of endothelium-dependent flow-mediated dilatation of the brachial artery by sex and menstrual cycle. Circulation 92: 3431–3435
83. Hyashi T, Fukoto JM, Ignarro LJ, Chaudhuri G 1992 Basal release of nitric oxide from aortic rings is greater in female rabbits than male rabbits: implications for atherosclerosis. Proceedings of the National Academy of Science, USA 89: 11259–11263
84. Celermajer DS, Sorensen KE, Spiegelhalter DJ, Georgakopoulos D, Robinson J, Deanfield JE 1994 Aging is associated with endothelial dysfunction in healthy men years before the age-related decline in women. Journal of the American College of Cardiology 24: 471–476
85. Celermajer DS, Sorensen KE, Gooch VM, Spiegelhalter DJ, Miller OI, Sullivan ID, Lloyd JK, Deanfield JE 1992 Non-invasive detection of endothelial dysfunction in children and adults at risk of atherosclerosis. Lancet 340: 1111–1115
86. Joannides R, Haefeli WE, Linder L, Richard V, Bakkali EL, Thuillez C, Lüscher TF 1995 Nitric oxide is responsible for flow-dependent dilatation of human peripheral conduit arteries in vivo. Circulation 91: 1314–1319
87. Anderson TJ, Uehata A, Gerhard MD, Meredith IT, Knab S, Delagrange D et al 1995 Close relationship of endothelial function in the human coronary and peripheral circulations. Journal of the American College of Cardiology 26(12): 35–41
88. McCrohon JA, Adams MR, McCredie R, Robinson J, Pike A, Keech A, Celermajer DS 1995 Hormone replacement therapy is associated with improved endothelial function in post-menopausal women (abstract). Australian and New Zealand Journal of Medicine 25(5): 616
89. Dorup I, Hermann AP, Sorensen KE 1996 Hormone replacement therapy does not protect women against the age-related decline in endothelial function. Abstract from the American College of Cardiology meeting.
90. Gilligan DM, Badar DM, Panza JA, Quyyumi AA, Cannon RO 1995 Effects of estrogen replacement therapy on peripheral vasomotor function in postmenopausal woman. American Journal of Cardiology 75: 264–268
91. Roselli M, Imthurn B, Keller PJ, Jackson EK, Dubey RK 1995 Circulating nitric oxide levels in postmenopausal women substituted with 17-beta estradiol and norethisterone acetate. A two-year follow-up study. Hypertension 25: 848–853
92. Weiner CP, Lizasoain I, Baylis SA, Knowles RG, Charles IG, Moncada S 1994 Induction of calcium-dependent NO synthases by sex hormones. Proceedings of the National Academy of Science, USA 91: 5212
93. Jiang C, Sarrel PM, Lindsay DC, Poole-Wilson PA, Collins P 1991 Endothelium-independent relaxation of rabbit coronary artery by 17β-oestradiol in vitro. British Journal of Pharmacology 104: 1033–1037
94. Han SZ, Karaki H, Ouchi Y, Akishita M, Orimo H 1995 17β-estradiol inhibits calcium influx and calcium release induced by thromboxane A2 in porcine coronary artery. Circulation 91: 2619–2626
95. Nichols NR, Olsson CA, Funder JW 1987 Steroid effects on protein synthesis on cultured smooth muscle cells from rat aorta. Journal of Pharmacology and Experimental Therapeutics 240: 392–395
96. Rivali S, Vidali A, Cannon PJ, Kelly A 1995 Progesterone receptors are not expressed in normal and atherosclerotic coronary arteries. Abstract from the American Heart Association 68th scientific session.
97. Maschak CA, Lobo RA 1985 Estrogen replacement therapy and hypertension. Journal of Reproductive Medicine 30: 805–810
98. Pallas KG, Holzwarth GJ, Stern MP et al 1977 The effect of conjugated estrogens on the renin-angiotensin system. Journal of Clinical Endocrinology and Metabolism 44: 1061–1068

99. Barrett-Connor EL, Wingard DL, Criqui MH 1989 Postmenopausal estrogen use and heart disease risk factors in the 1980s: Rancho Bernardo Calif., revisited. Journal of the American Medical Association 261: 2095–2100
100. Proudler AJ, Ahmed AI, Crook D, Fogelman I, Rymer JM, Stevenson JC 1995 Hormone replacement therapy and serum angiotensin-converting-enzyme activity in postmenopausal women. Lancet 346: 89–90
101. Meade TW, Mellows S, Brozovic M et al 1986 Haemostatic function and ischaemic heart disease: principal results of the Northwick Park Heart study. Lancet 2: 533–537
102. Gebara OCR, Mityelman MA, Sutherland P, Lipinska I, Matheney T, Xu P et al 1995 Association between increased estrogen status and increased fibrinolytic potential in the Framingham Offspring Study. Circulation 91: 1952–1958
103. Kannel WB, Wolf PA, Castelli WP, D'Agostino RB 1987 Fibrinogen and the risk of cardiovascular disease: the Framingham Study. Journal of the American Medical Association 258: 1183–1186
104. Fogelberg M, Vesterqvist O, Diczfalusy U, Henriksson P 1990 Experimental atherosclerosis: effects of oestrogen and atherosclerosis on thromboxane and prostacyclin formation. European Journal of Clinical Investigation 20: 105–110
105. Newman KP, Sullivan JM 1996 Coronary heart disease in women: epidemiology, clinical syndromes, and management. Menopause 1: 51–59
106. Shepherd J, Cobbe SM, Ford I, Isles CG, Lorimer AR, Macfarlane PW et al 1995 Prevention of coronary heart disease with pravastatin in men with hypercholesterolaemia. New England Journal of Medicine 333: 1301–1307
107. The Scandinavian Simvastatin Survival Study Group 1994 Randomized trial of cholesterol lowering in 4444 patients with coronary heart disease (4S). Lancet 344: 1383–1389
108. Henderson C 1991 Breast cancer. Harrison's principles of internal medicine, 12th edn. ch 303, p 1613
109. Bergkvist L, Adami HO, Persson I et al 1989 Prognosis after breast cancer diagnosis in women exposed to estrogen and estrogen-progesterone replacement therapy. American Journal of Epidemiology 130: 221–228
110. Breckwoldt M, Keck C, Karck U 1995 Benefits and risks of hormone replacement therapy. Journal of Steroid Biochemistry and Molecular Biology 53(1–6): 205–208
111. Palacios S 1994 Cancer surveillance during HRT. International Journal of Fertility and Menopausal Studies 39 (Suppl 2): 93–98
112. Moorjani S, Dupont A, Labrie F, De Lignieres B, Cusan L, Dupont P, Mailloux J, Lupien PJ 1991 Changes in plasma lipoprotein and apolipoprotein composition in relation to oral versus percutaneous administration of estrogen alone or in cyclic association with utrogestan in menopausal women. Journal of Clinical Endocrinology and Metabolism 73(2): 373–379
113. Stevenson JC, Crook D, Godsland IF, Lees B, Whitehead MI 1993 Oral versus transdermal hormone replacement therapy. International Journal of Fertility and Menopausal-Studies 38 (Suppl 1): 30–35

56. Progestogen therapy in malignant tumors of the uterus and ovary

Juan C. Felix Robert J. Kurman

Introduction

Progestogen therapy has been an integral part of the therapeutic armamentarium for hormonally related tumors of the uterus and ovary for nearly four decades. Efforts at hormonal intervention were reported as early as 1959 by Kistner[1] who reported efficacious treatment of six patients with endometrial hyperplasia and one patient with early endometrial carcinoma with Enovid and hydroxyprogesterone caproate. In 1961, Kelly and Baker[2] reported a 29% response rate in the treatment of advanced endometrial carcinoma with progesterone or hydroxyprogesterone caproate. Since those first reports, many other investigators have confirmed the therapeutic efficacy of progestational agents in endometrial and ovarian carcinoma, albeit with a large disparity in reported efficacy. Factors favoring the use of progestogens in the therapy of advanced carcinomas of the endometrium and ovary include achievable responses following failure of prior radiation therapy and chemotherapy, the extremely low morbidity and mortality, and the benefits of increase in appetite and an improved feeling of well-being experienced by most patients so treated.

ENDOMETRIAL CARCINOMA

A large body of literature has been accrued in the last three decades examining the efficacy of progestational agents in the treatment of advanced or recurrent endometrial carcinoma. Initial reports noted a response rate of advanced endometrial carcinoma of approximately one third of patients treated. Kauppila reviewed 17 different trials using either medroxyprogesterone acetate (MPA), megestrol acetate, or hydroxyprogesterone caproate.[3] He found a response rate of 34% in 1068 evaluable patients, with a duration of response of 16–28 months and a survival of 18–33 months. In addition, patients who responded to progestational therapy were shown to have an improved survival over patients who failed to respond. Refenstein reported an increase in median survival, with a median of 26 months among responders when compared to a median of 4 months for nonresponders.[4] However, more recent data from the Gynecologic Oncology Group reported only a 14% overall response rate using a 150 mg dose of MPA, with a median survival of just 10 months.[5] Similarly, reports from Piver et al[6] and Podratz et al[7] demonstrated lower response rates of 15.8% and 11.2% respectively. The recent data are summarized in Table 56.1.

Results examining the use of progestogens as adjuvants to primary surgical treatment of endometrial carcinoma have been disappointing. Both Lewis et al[8] and Vergote et al[9] saw no advantage in giving adjuvant progestogens to patients undergoing hysterectomy for early stage endometrial carcinoma. Small series examining the use of hormonal therapy in combination with cytotoxic chemotherapeutic agents are more encouraging. Hoffman et al[10] reported a 33% response rate in advanced endometrial cancer to a combination of cisplatin, doxorubicin, cyclophosphamide and megestrol acetate. Lovechio et al[11] reported a response rate of 60% with a similar combination.

The variation in response rates noted in the literature follow certain understandable variables. Response rates to progestational therapy are higher in patients with low grade endometrial carcinomas when compared to more aggressive tumors.[7,12] Most of the more recent reports, such as Thigpens and Pivers, had a large proportion of cases in which the tumors were of high histologic differentiation. Similarly, patients with tumors rich in progesterone receptors have been shown to have a higher response rate than those tumors with absent or low progesterone receptors. Kaupilla's review of five studies[3] showed that 86% of patients with progesterone receptor-rich tumors responded to progestational therapy compared with only 17% of patients with receptor-poor tumors.

Table 56.1 Response of advanced endometrial carcinoma to progestogen therapy.

Study	Progestogen	Dose	Total cases	CR (%)	PR (%)	Stable (%)
Thigpen et al (1991)[33]	MPA	200 mg/d	138	17	9	—
		1000 mg/d	140	10	8	—
Thigpen et al (1986)[5]	MPA	150 mg/d	331	10	8	50
Podratz et al (1985)[7]	Megestrol	320 mg/d	81			
	DMPA	1–3 g/wk	33			
	Medroxy-progesterone	800 mg/d	26	6*	5*	40*
Piver et al (1980)[6]	HPC	1 g/wk	51	14**		20
	MPA	1 g/wk	37	19**		30

*Combined percentages of the three treatment groups; **Complete plus partial response; MPA: Medroxyprogeoterone acetate; DMPA: depot medroxyprogesterone acetate; HPC: hydroxyprogesterone caproate.

Although low grade and high receptor content are often associated,[13] Chambers reported a five year survival rate of 48% for patients with grade 3, receptor-rich tumors compared to 20% for patients with grade 3, receptor-poor tumors,[14] suggesting that receptor content was an independent predictor of response. Recent reports with poor or no response to progestational therapy examined data of patients following failure with chemotherapeutic regimens that included platinum based agents and/or taxol. These studies show markedly decreased response rates when compared to studies in the era when alkylating agents alone were the standard of therapy. Although data are limited, recurrences or persistence of tumors following platinum based chemotherapy seem to show a decrease of receptor-rich tumors when compared to older, pre-platinum series.[15–18]

In addition to the absolute presence or absence of estrogen and progesterone receptors in tumors, receptor heterogeneity seems to offer an additional explanation for hormonal treatment failure in cases of advanced endometrial carcinoma. Zaino et al[19] noted that within a single tumor mass, various populations of tumor cells differed in either absolute expression or relative quantity of estrogen and progesterone receptors expressed. These and other investigators postulate that a receptor negative subpopulation within a receptor positive tumor will fail to respond to progestational agents and select itself as the new predominant cell line refractory to further attempts at hormonal intervention. This hypothesis could also explain the transitory effect of progestational therapy in patients who do have an initial response.

Since progesterone receptor presence in endometrial carcinomas correlate with therapeutic response, pretreatment of patients with agents that increase or stabilize progesterone receptor content would seemingly increase the efficacy of progestational therapy. Carlson et al[20] reported an increase in progesterone receptor positivity from 52 to 84% following tamoxifen treatment. The same group reported a 25% response rate of advanced endometrial cancer with combined tamoxifen and progestational therapy. Rendina et al[21] saw a 47% response rate in patients who had failed to respond to either tamoxifen or medroxyprogesterone therapy alone when the drugs were used in combination. Subsequent reports, however, have been less enthusiastic, with a response rate of just 5% reported by Kline et al.[22] Similarly, Pandya found no improvement with combination tamoxifen and progestogen therapy over progestogen therapy alone.[23] Despite the variation in reported clinical responses, experimental models show dramatic inhibition of tumor growth using the combination of tamoxifen and progestogens, particularly with progesterone receptor-positive tumors.[24] Such experimental successes support the continued investigation of these therapeutic strategies.

The mechanism of action of progestational agents in endometrial carcinoma is not well established. Both estrogen and progesterone receptors belong to a superfamily of ligand-activated transcription factors.[25,26] The receptor protein acts as a transducer, binding the hormone and transporting the bound complex to the nucleus. Once in the nucleus, a cascade of enzymatic and molecular events trigger the transcription and expression of putatively specific genes. Examples of these specific actions include increased expression of BCL-2 and the upregulation of p53.[27] These interactions with cell cycle specific genes are thought to account in part for the decrease in cell division and reduced proliferation seen in progestogen responsive carcinomas. Better described actions of the progesterone ligand-receptor complex include a decrease in the expression of estrogen receptor.[28] This reduction in estrogen receptor is thought to account for inhibition of the estrogen-dependent proliferation of endometrial cancer cells.[29] The mechanisms of high dose progestogen therapy could involve actions other than local tumor receptor interactions, however, Blossey et al[30] showed that MPA also exerted antitumor activity in a dose-related fashion by interfering with the hypothalamo-pituitary-adrenal axis and suppressing adrenal steroid secretion. The molecular events that give rise to the genetic expression responsible for the secretory differentiation and maturation of endometrial carcinoma seen histologically in some tumors treated with progestogens remain undiscovered. Elucidation of such mechanisms could provide future direction for both hormonal and genetic manipulation of these tumors.

Examination of different progestational agents in various clinical trials has shown very little variability in efficacy between the different progestogens used.[3] Podratz et al found response rates of 11%, 9% and 12% respectively for megestrol acetate, hydroxyprogesterone caproate and medroxyprogesterone acetate.[7] Similarly, little difference is noted in examining the route of administration. Sall et al showed that oral MPA achieved comparable or higher serum levels than an intramuscular route[31] and Kaupilla[7] noted a similar or slightly more favorable response rate with oral versus intramuscular MPA. It is mainly the ease and comfort of oral administration that has made it the preferred route of progestogen administration.

Evaluation of dosage efficacy presents more difficulty, due to conflicting results in the recent literature. An improved dose response effect was shown early by Geisler,[32] who reported response rates of 48% with 160 mg/d of megestrol acetate compared to rates of only 14% for a 40 mg/d dosage. Initial efforts of the Gynecologic Oncology Group to directly compare standard dose progestational therapy (200 mg/d MPA) to higher dose regimen (1000 mg/d MPA) resulted in response rates of 26% and 18% respectively, showing a disturbing trend of poorer response with the higher dosed regimen.[33] However later studies by this group showed a nonstatistically significant increase in activity of high dose progestogen therapy (800 mg/d megestrol acetate) when compared to traditional dosage, with a 24% overall response rate and duration of response of 6.5–27 months (median 8.9).[34] Clearly, the question of optimal dosage is not yet resolved and further investigation in this area is warranted. However, if a higher dose regimen is selected it would seem that megestrol acetate would be the preferred agent since a standard dose of 160 mg/d achieves the effectiveness of 1000 mg/d of medroxyprogesterone acetate[35] and significantly higher dosages such as the 800 mg/d regimen can be achieved with relative ease orally.

Toxicity and complications with hormonal therapy are uncommon. The most widely reported serious toxic effects are vascular. Lentz et al reported that four of 54 patients experienced vascular thrombosis with high-dose (800 mg/d) megestrol acetate use; three patients had pulmonary emboli and one had an arterial thrombosis. He reported that these complications could have contributed to the demise of three patients.[34] The incidence of spontaneous venous thrombosis in women with advanced cancer is significant, and it is unclear how much greater it is with high-dose progestogens. In addition to the vascular complications, weight gain is noted in most patients using progestogens,[36] however grade 3 weight gains (greater than 20% gains) were reported by Lentz in the same series and grade 3 or 4 hyperglycemia observed in three patients.

Due to this relative low toxicity (in a cancer-treatment context), progestational agents have gained wide usage in patients with endometrial cancer, particularly those with advanced disease. However in patients with a history of previous pulmonary emboli, deep venous thrombosis, severe heart disease or severe diabetes, alternative hormonal therapy such as tamoxifen should be considered. Antiestrogen therapy for endometrial cancer was first reported by Swenerton who noted a response to tamoxifen in seven patients who had failed progestogen therapy.[37] Subsequent reports in the literature have confirmed a beneficial effect of tamoxifen in advanced or recurrent endometrial carcinoma, but it appears that it is ineffective in most patients who do not respond to progestogens.[38–40]

Early endometrial carcinoma

Fertility-preserving hormonal therapy for early carcinoma of the endometrium was first reported in 1959, when Kistner[1] reported that progestational therapy was efficacious in six patients with endometrial hyperplasia and one patient with *in situ* endometrial carcinoma. Initial attempts with hormonal therapy in early endometrial carcinomas were no doubt derived from the successful experience in the hormonal therapy of endometrial hyperplasia. While treatment results vary between series depending on the histological criteria used to define the hyperplasia, a response rate of about 70% is generally agreed upon.[41,42] Using strict criteria for the stratification of hyperplasia, Ferenczy and Gelfand[43] reported 80% regression, 20% persistence and 0% progression to carcinoma of patients with endometrial hyperplasia without atypia, in patients treated with medroxyprogesterone acetate (20 mg/d), compared with about 25% regression, 50% persistence and 25% progression to carcinoma in untreated patients. Again, as with advanced carcinoma, failure to respond to progestational therapy in hyperplasia seems to be related at least in part to tissue receptor status. Masuzawa et al noted the absence of estrogen receptor down-regulation in cases of endometrial hyperplasia that failed to respond to progestogen therapy, revealing the potential for continued estrogen-related stimulation.[44]

Three series have recently been published evaluating the efficacy of primary progestational therapy for the treatment of early endometrial carcinoma in which the histologic diagnosis of endometrial adenocarcinoma is clearly defined.[45–47] All three series evaluated patients under the age of 40 who desired to preserve fertility and were willing to accept the risk of disease progression. Kim et al[46] reported seven patients with grade 1 histology who were treated with 160 mg/d megestrol acetate. Of the seven patients, four (57%) showed resolution of their lesion, while the remaining three patients failed and underwent hysterectomy. One initial responder had a recurrence, responded to a second trial of progestational therapy, but subsequently showed carcinoma (confined to the uterus at the time of hysterectomy). All patients in this series were alive and disease-free at last follow-up.

Randall and Kurman[47] reviewed their experience in treating women with atypical hyperplasia and early endometrial carcinoma with primary progestogen therapy (160 mg/d megestrol acetate). Of 12 patients with grade 1 endometrial carcinoma treated, there were nine regressions (75%) and three persistent carcinomas. Two of the patients with persistence were shown at time of hysterectomy to have endometrial carcinoma limited to the endometrium, as well as synchronous ovarian endometrioid carcinomas arising in endometriosis. The third patient with persistence showed only atypical hyperplasia at the time of hysterectomy. In no case did patients progress to higher stage lesions. The median length of treatment required for tumor regression was nine months. In this series, of the 25 women treated with progestational therapy for hyperplasia or carcinoma who desired pregnancy, seven conceived and five (20%) had full term pregnancies. Three women with an initial diagnosis of endometrial carcinoma delivered full term infants and remained disease-free at last follow-up.

Finally, Bohkman[45] reported 15 patients with grade 1 carcinoma treated with primary progestogen therapy (oxyprogesterone caproate 500 mg/d i.m.) and four patients with grade 2 endometrial carcinoma treated with hydroxyprogesterone caproate 500 mg/d i.m. plus cyclophosphamide, methotrexate and vincristine. Fifteen of 19 patients (84%) responded within six months of initiating therapy. Four patients who failed therapy underwent hysterectomy. Of the four failures, two showed carcinoma limited to the corpus and two showed no residual tumor at the time of hysterectomy. These series are summarized in Table 56.2.

In addition to these series, 14 additional patients have been reported in the literature[48–54] in which primary progestational therapy was used to treat early endometrial carcinoma in patients aged 15–35; nine

Table 56.2 Summary of primary progestogen therapy for early endometrial carcinoma.

Study	Progestin	Dose	Cases	Response (%)	Failure (%)
Kim et al (1997)[46]	Megestrol	160 mg/d p.o.	7	4 (57%)	3 (43%)
Randall and Kurman (1997)[47]	Megestrol	160 mg/d p.o.	12	9 (75%)	3 (25%)
Bokhman et al (1985)[45]	Oxyprogesterone caproate	500 mg/d i.m.	19*	15 (79%)	4 (21%)

*Four patients with grade 2 tumors received concurrent cyclophosphamide, methotrexate and vincristine.

(64%) responded to therapy. Of the five failures, four had hysterectomies showing stage I endometrial carcinoma, while one was lost to follow-up. Importantly, one of the initial responders was reported to have serial endometrial biopsies with 'atypical cells'.[51] Breakthrough bleeding in this patient prompted hysterectomy and revealed stage III endometrial carcinoma. This patient went on to develop regional metastases 27 months after surgery and radiation, and progestogens were used for further treatment.

Despite the high rate of success of primary progestational therapy in these reports and the tremendous amount of enthusiasm generated by this fertility-preserving treatment, a great deal of caution should be adhered to when treating patients with endometrial carcinoma using progestational therapy alone. Although failure rates are low and disease is usually contained to the uterus, at least one case, described above, clearly progressed to a higher stage during the period of observation. Therefore, if a patient being treated with primary progestational therapy for endometrial carcinoma has persistence of disease or atypical findings on more than one follow-up biopsy, consideration should be given to terminating medical therapy in favor of hysterectomy. As well as the possibility of progression during therapy, a few patients were lost to follow-up in these series, at least one of whom had persistent disease. For this reason, patient selection is critical in order to insure the greatest likelihood of good patient compliance. Optimal candidates should be 40 years of age or younger and have a strong desire to preserve and pursue fertility. This latter criterion increases the likelihood of continued medical follow-up during and following therapy for their malignancy as they seek fertility and eventual obstetrical care. Patients who are unable or unwilling to participate in long-term medical treatment and surveillance should also be offered hysterectomy after child bearing has been completed or the pursuit of fertility abandoned.

Finally, even though young patients generally have low grade lesions that are usually confined to the endometrium, some young patients will have more advanced disease. Gitsch et al[55] reported findings of patients 45 years and younger with endometrial carcinoma. He found synchronous ovarian malignancies in five of 17 cases (29%) compared to 4.6% in women older than 45, as well as metastatic endometrial carcinoma of the ovary in three patients (17%). Although unlike most of the experience reported in the literature, the data from Gitsch further underscore the need for careful patient selection and pretreatment evaluation.

Endometrial stromal sarcoma

Endometrial stromal sarcoma (ESS), also known as 'endolymphatic stromal myosis' and 'endometrial stromatosis', is a low grade sarcoma that exhibits an insidious growth pattern in both the uterus and in metastatic sites. Due to its rarity, ESS has not been studied in randomized or even collected series. Only sporadic reports of few cases exist in the literature. Despite this lack of objective data, little doubt exists over the value of progestational agents in the treatment of this rare lesion. First reports of this tumor revealed a strong hormonal influence. Both Gloor[56] and Krieger and Gusberg[57] reported less frequent recurrences and longer disease-free periods in patients after bilateral oophorectomy. Gros et al[58] showed control of metastases following surgical or radiation induced castration. These initial data gave way to several reports of control of recurrences or metastases using progestational therapy.[59–63] In all, 13 cases of recurrent or metastatic ESS treated with progestational therapy for periods of 16–62 months were reported to show a response (six patients) or stabilization of disease (seven patients). Responses were often impressive and included radiographic disappearances of pulmonary, bladder and abdominal recurrences. As with endometrial cancer, response of ESS to progestational therapy seems to be correlated to the presence of progesterone receptors. Katz et al[64] reported response to progestational therapy in all progesterone receptor-rich tumors.

Intravenous leiomyomatosis is an extremely rare neoplastic process arising in the vascular spaces of the myometrium. Like ESS, these tumors have been found to be hormonally influenced[65] and have been reported to respond to progestational therapy. Due to their rarity, therapeutic trials in patients with intravenous leiomyomatosis have not been performed. Despite the paucity of data, however, their indolent nature makes them rather well suited for progestational therapy.

OVARIAN CARCINOMA

Progestational therapy for ovarian carcinoma is reserved almost exclusively for the palliative treatment of patients refractory to all forms of cytotoxic chemotherapy. It is therefore not surprising that the reported efficacy of progestational therapy against ovarian carcinoma is significantly lower than for endometrial carcinoma. Although an initial report by Geisler[66] detected a 48% response rate in 23 patients using high-dose megestrol therapy, subsequent series have failed to repeat such favorable results. Careful review of this report shows that, unlike subsequent series, few patients reported by Geisler received previous platinum based therapy. This selection bias could have accounted for the better response rates. Review of the three recent phase II trials evaluating the efficacy of megestrol acetate on advanced or recurrent ovarian carcinoma show very low response rates. Ahlgren et al[67] found no responders among 30 assessable patients treated with megestrol. Veenhof et al[68] saw only one partial response in 54 evaluable patients so treated, with nine others remaining with stable disease. Finally Sikic et al[69] reported one complete remission, three partial responses, three minimal responses and five patients with stable disease. In this last series, survival in responders was statistically significantly improved from 26 months in nonresponders to 57 months in responders. These three studies are summarized in Table 56.3. Major adverse effects to progestogen in therapy in all three studies were comparable to those reported for endometrial carcinoma.

Various explanations have been given for the lower response of ovarian carcinoma to progestational therapy. Perhaps the currently favored theory is that the number of progesterone receptor-rich ovarian carcinomas is lower than that of endometrial carcinomas. The more recent studies place primary tumor progesterone receptor positivity at only 40–50%.[70,71] Interestingly, however, although differences in tumor cell types show variances in progesterone receptor content, efficacy of progestogen therapy has not shown cell type to be a major variable.

However low the response rate of ovarian carcinoma to progestational agents might be, their use for palliative purposes should continue to be considered. Despite discouraging results, occasional patients have true, long lasting responses to progestational therapy with minimal adverse effects. Progestogens continue to provide the oncologist with an active agent to offer patients who are often moribund and could not tolerate further cytotoxic therapy, yet who are asking for more intervention.

A great deal of attention is currently being focused on alternative hormonal therapy for ovarian carcinoma. Of the agents currently available, tamoxifen has been the one most widely utilized. Ahlgren reported five responses among 29 patients (17%) treated with tamoxifen, with two of the responses exceeding five years' duration. A similar experience was reported in a study by the Gynecologic Oncology Group.[72] As with other hormonal agents, inconsistent reports in the literature dampen enthusiasm. Neither Shirley et al[73] nor Slevin et al[74] found any objective responders among, respectively, 23 and 22 evaluable patients. Although some differences in dosage, schedules and patient selection were present between these studies, the differences were not thought to account for the major differences in response rates. There is no doubt that continued interest in the therapeutic effects of tamoxifen, leuprolide acetate (and other GnRH analogs), as well as other forms of hormonal manipulation, will be the target of continued investigation.

Cervical cancer

Although rare studies have suggested that cervical carcinoma cells could be hormonally influenced[75,76] we are not aware of a convincing report of response to hormonal therapy in patients with advanced cervical carcinoma.

Table 56.3 Summary of phase II trials evaluating progestogen therapy in advanced ovarian carcinoma.

Study	Progestogen	Cases	Response (%)	Nonresponders (%)	Stable (%)
Ahlgren et al (1993)[67]	Megestrol 800 mg/d	30	0 (0%)	30 (100%)	—
Veenhof et al (1994)[68]	Megestrol 800 mg/d	54	1 (2%)	53 (98%)	9 (17%)
Sikic et al (1986)[69]	Megestrol 800 mg/d	47	4 (8%)	43 (92%)	8 (17%)*

*Includes three patients with 'minimal responses'.

REFERENCES

1. Kistner RW 1959 Histological effects of progestins on hyperplasia and carcinoma in situ of the endometrium. Cancer 12: 1106–1122
2. Kelly RM, Baker WH 1961 Progestational agents in the treatment of carcinoma of the endometrium. New England Journal of Medicine 264: 216–222
3. Kaupilla A 1984 Progestin therapy of endometrial, breast, and ovarian carcinoma. Acta Obstetrica Gynecologica Scandinavica 63: 441–450
4. Reifenstein EF 1974 Treatment of advanced endometrial cancer with hydroprogesterone correlate. Gynecological Oncology 2: 377–382
5. Thigpen T, Blessing J, DiSaia P et al 1986 Oral medroxyprogesterone acetate in advanced or recurrent endometrial carcinoma: results of therapy and correlation with estrogen and progesterone receptor levels. The Gynecologic Oncology Group experience. In: Baulier EE, Iacobelli S, McGuire WW (eds) Endocrinology and Malignancy. Parthenon Publishers, Pearl River, NY, pp 446–454
6. Piver MS, Barlow JJ, Lurain JR et al 1980 Medroxyprogesterone acetate (Depo-Provera) vs. hydroxyprogesterone caproate (Delalutin) in women with metastatic endometrial adenocarcinoma. Cancer 45: 268–272
7. Podratz KC, O'Brien PC, Malkasian GD et al 1985 Effects of progestational agents in treatment of endometrial carcinoma. Obstetrics and Gynecology 66: 106–110
8. Lewis GC, Slack NH, Mortel R et al 1974 Adjuvant progestogen therapy in the primary definitive treatment of endometrial cancer. Gynecological Oncology 2: 368–376
9. Vergote I, Kjorstad K, Abeler V et al 1989 A randomized trial of adjuvant progestagen in early endometrial cancer. Cancer 64: 1011–1016
10. Hoffman MS, Roberts WS, Cavanaugh D et al 1989 Treatment of recurrent and metastatic endometrial cancer with cisplatin, doxorubicin, cyclophosphamide, and megestrol acetate. Gynecological Oncology 35: 75–77
11. Lovechio JL, Averette HE, Lichtinger M et al 1984 Treatment of advanced or recurrent endometrial adenocarcinoma with cyclophosphamide, doxorubicin, cis-platinum, and megestrol acetate. Obstetrics and Gynecology 63: 557–560
12. Kohorn KI 1976 Gestagens and endometrial carcinoma. Gynecological Oncology 4: 398–411
13. Creasman WT, Soper JT, McCarty KS Jr et al 1985 Influence of cytoplasmic steroid receptor content on prognosis of early stage endometrial carcinoma. American Journal of Obstetrics and Gynecology 151: 922–932
14. Chambers JT, MacLusky N, Eisenfeld A et al 1988 Estrogen and progestin receptor levels as prognosticators for survival in endometrial cancer. Gynecological Oncology 31: 65–71
15. Kaupilla A, Kujansuu E, Vihlo R 1982 Cytosol estrogen and progestin receptors in endometrial carcinoma of patients treated with surgery, radiotherapy, and progestin. Cancer 50: 2157–2165
16. Sutton GP, Senior MB, Strauss JF et al 1986 Estrogen and progesterone receptors in epithelial ovarian malignancies. Gynecological Oncology 23: 176–182
17. Richman CM, Holt JA, Lorincz MA et al 1985 Persistence and distribution of estrogen receptor in advanced epithelial ovarian carcinoma after chemotherapy. Obstetrics and Gynecology 65: 257–263
18. Runowicz CD, Nuchtern LM, Braunstein JD et al 1990 Heterogeneity in hormone receptor status in primary and metastatic endometrial cancer. Gynecological Oncology 38: 437–442
19. Zaino RJ, Clark CL, Mortel R et al 1988 Heterogeneity of progesterone receptor distribution in human endometrial adenocarcinoma. Cancer Research 48: 1889
20. Carlson JA, Allegra JC, Day TG et al 1984 Tamoxifen and endometrial cancer: alterations in estrogen and progesterone receptors in untreated patients and combined hormonal therapy in advanced neoplasia. American Journal of Obstetrics and Gynecology 149: 149–153
21. Rendina GM, Donadio C, Fabri M et al 1984 Tamoxifen and medroxyprogestertone therapy for advanced endometrial carcinoma. European Journal of Obstetrics, Gynecology and Reproductive Biology 17: 285–291
22. Kline RC, Freedman RS, Jones LA et al 1987 Cancer Treatment Reports 71: 327–328
23. Pandya KJ, Yeap BY, Davis TE 1989 Phase II study of megestrol and megestrol + tamoxifen in advanced endometrial carcinoma: an Eastern Cooperative Oncology Group study. Proceedings of the Annual Meeting of the American Association of Cancer Research 30: A1037 (Abstr)
24. Zaino RJ, Mortel R, Satyaswaroop PG 1985 Hormonal therapy of human endometrial carcinoma in a nude mouse model. Cancer Research 45: 539–546
25. Evans R 1998 The steroid and thyroid hormone receptor superfamily. Science 240: 889–891
26. Green S, Chambon P 1988 Nuclear receptors enhance our understanding of transcriptional regulation. Trends in Genetics 4: 309–314
27. Bu SZ, Yin DL, Ren XH et al 1997 Progesterone induces apoptosis and up regulation of p53 expression in human ovarian carcinoma cell lines. Cancer 79: 1944–1950
28. Uchima FD, Edery M, Iguchi T et al 1991 Growth of mouse endometrial luminal cells in vitro: functional integrity of the estrogen receptor system and failure of estrogen to induce proliferation. Journal of Endocrinology 128: 115–120
29. Katsuki Y, Shibutani Y, Aoki D et al 1997 Dienogest, a novel synthetic steroid, overcomes hormone-dependent cancer in a different manner than progestins. Cancer 79: 169–176
30. Blossey HC, Wander HE, Koebberling J et al 1984 Pharmacokinetic and pharmacodynamic basis for treatment of metastatic breast cancer with high dose medroxyprogesterone acetate. Cancer 54: 1208–1215
31. Sall S, DiSaia P Morrow CP et al 1979 A comparison of medroxyprogesterone serum concentrations by the oral or intramuscular route with persistent or recurrent endometrial carcinoma. American Journal of Obstetrics and Gynecology 135: 647–650

32. Geisler HE 1973 The use of megestrol acetate in the treatment of advanced malignant lesions of the endometrium. Gynecological Oncology 1: 340–344
33. Thigpen T, Blessing J, Hatch K et al 1991 A randomized trial of medroxyprogesterone acetate (MPS) 200 mg versus 1000 mg daily in advanced or recurrent endometrial carcinoma: A Gynecologic Oncology Group (GOG) study. Journal of Clinical Oncology 10: 185 (Abstr)
34. Lentz SS, Brady MF, Major FJ et al 1996 High-dose megestrol acetate in advanced or recurrent endometrial carcinoma: a Gynecologic Oncology Group study. Journal of Clinical Oncology 14: 357–361
35. Miller AA, Bechter R, Schmidt CG 1988 Plasma concentrations of medroxyprogesterone acetate and megestrol during long-term follow-up in patients treated for metastatic breast cancer. Journal of Cancer Research and Clinical Oncology 114: 186–190
36. Tchekmedian NS, Tait N, Moody M et al 1986 Appetite stimulation with megestrol acetate in cachectic cancer patients. Seminars in Oncology 13: 37–43
37. Swenerton KD, Shaw D, White GW et al 1979 Treatment of advanced endometrial carcinoma with tamoxifen. New England Journal of Medicine 301: 106–111
38. Slavik M, Petty WM, Blessing JA et al 1984 Phase II clinical study of tamoxifen in advanced endometrial adenocarcinoma: a Gynecologic Oncology Group study. Cancer Treatment Reports 68: 809–813
39. Edmonson JH, Krook JE, Hilton JF et al 1986 Ineffectiveness of tamoxifen in advanced endometrial carcinoma after failure of progestin treatment. Cancer Treatment Reports 70: 1019–1022
40. Quinn MA, Campbell JJ 1989 Tamoxifen therapy in advanced/recurrent endometrial carcinoma. Gynecological Oncology 32: 1–7
41. Wentz WB 1974 Progestin therapy in endometrial hyperplasia. Gynecological Oncology 2: 362–367
42. Eichner E, Abellera M 1971 Endometrial hyperplasia treated by progestins. Obstetrics and Gynecology 38: 739–742
43. Ferenczy A, Gelfand M 1989 The biologic significance of cytologic atypia in progestogen-treated endometrial hyperplasia. American Journal of Obstetrics and Gynecology 160: 126–131
44. Masuzawa H, Badokhon NH, Nakayama K et al 1994 Failure of down-regulation of estrogen receptors and progesterone receptors after medroxyprogesterone acetate administration for endometrial hyperplasias. Cancer 74: 2321–2328
45. Bohkman JV, Chepick OF, Volkova AT et al 1985 Can endometrial carcinoma Stage I be cured without surgery and radiation therapy? Gynecological Oncology 20: 139–155
46. Kim YB, Holshneider CH, Ghosh K et al 1997 Progestin alone as primary treatment of endometrial carcinoma in premenopausal women: a report of seven cases and review of the literature. Cancer 79: 320–327
47. Randall TC, Kurman RJ 1997 Progestin treatment of atypical hyperplasia and well differentiated carcinoma of the endometrium in women under age 40. Obstetrics and Gynecology 90: 434–440
48. Kempson RL, Pokarny GE 1968 Adenocarcinoma of the endometrium in women aged 40 and younger. Cancer 21: 650–662
49. O'Neill RT 1970 Pregnancy following hormonal therapy for adenocarcinoma in Stein-Levinthal syndrome. American Journal of Obstetrics and Gynecology 108: 318–321
50. Fechner RE, Kaufman RH 1974 Endometrial adenocarcinoma in Stein-Levinthal syndrome. Cancer 34: 444–452
51. Greenblatt RB, Gambrell RD, Stoddard LD 1982 The protective role of progesterone in the prevention of endometrial carcinoma. Pathology Research Practice 174: 297–318
52. Farhi DC, Nosanchuk J, Silverberg SG 1986 Endometrial adenocarcinoma in women under 25 years of age. Obstetrics and Gynecology 68: 741–745
53. Lee KR, Scully RE 1989 Complex endometrial hyperplasia and carcinoma in adolescents and young women 15 to 20 years of age: a report of 10 cases. International Journal of Gynecological Pathology 8: 201–213
54. Kimmig R, Strowitzki T, Muller Hocker J et al 1995 Conservative treatment of endometrial cancer permitting subsequent triplet pregnancy. Gynecological Oncology 58: 255–257
55. Gitsch G, Hanzal E, Jensen D et al 1995 Endometrial cancer in premenopausal women 45 years and younger. Obstetrics and Gynecology 85: 504–508
56. Gloor E 1978 La myose endolymphatique, sarcome 'low grade' du stroma endometrial. II: Clinique. Journal of Gynecology, Obstetrics and Biology of Reproduction 7: 447–459
57. Krieger PD, Gusberg SB 1973 Endolymphatic stromal myosis — a grade I endometrial sarcoma. Gynecological Oncology 1: 299–313
58. Gros CM, LeGal Y, Keiling R 1965 De l'endometriose cytogene endolymphatique. Nouv Press Med 73: 2195–2198
59. Baggish MS, Woodruff JD 1972 Uterine stromatosis: clinicopathologic features and hormone dependency. Obstetrics and Gynecology 40: 487–498
60. Pellillo D 1968 Proliferative stromatosis of the uterus with pulmonary metastases. Remission following treatment with a long-acting synthetic progestin: a case report. Obstetrics and Gynecology 31: 33–39
61. Krumholz BA, Lobovsky FY, Halitsky V 1973 Endolymphatic stromal myosis with pulmonary metastases. Remission with progestin therapy: report of a case. Journal of Reproductive Medicine 10: 85–89
62. Jacobsen KB, Haram K 1975 Endolymphatic stromal myosis. Report of a case surgically treated and with hormones. Virchovs Archives (Pathological Anatomy) 369: 173–179
63. Gloor E, Schneider P, Cikes M et al 1982 Endolymphatic stromal myosis. Surgical and hormonal treatment of extensive abdominal recurrence 20 years after hysterectomy. Cancer 50: 1888–1893
64. Katz L, Merino MJ, Sakamato H, Schwartz PE 1987 Endometrial stromal sarcoma: a clinicopathologic study of 11 cases with determination of estrogen and progestin receptor levels in three tumors. Gynecological Oncology 26: 87–97
65. Evans AT, Symmonds RE, Gaffey TA 1981 Recurrent pelvic intravenous leiomyomatosis. Obstetrics and Gynecology 57: 260–264

66. Geisler HE 1985 The use of high-dose megestrol acetate in the treatment of ovarian adenocarcinoma. Seminars in Oncology 12 (Suppl 1): 20–22
67. Ahlgren JD, Ellison NM, Gottlieb RJ et al 1993 Hormonal palliation of chemoresistant ovarian cancer: three consecutive phase II trials of the Mid-Atlantic Oncology Program. Journal of Clinical Oncology 11: 1957–1968
68. Veenhoff CHN, van der Burg MEL, Nooy M et al 1994 Phase II study of high-dose megestrol acetate in patients with advanced ovarian carcinoma. European Journal of Cancer 30A: 697–698
69. Sikic BI, Scudder SA, Ballon SC et al 1986 High-dose megestrol acetate therapy of ovarian carcinoma: a Phase II study by the Northern California Oncology Group. Seminars in Oncology 13 (Suppl 4): 26–32
70. Slotman BJ, Kuhnel R, Rao BR et al 1989 Importance of steroid receptor and aromatase activity in the prognosis of ovarian cancer: high tumor progesterone receptor levels correlate with longer survival. Gynecological Oncology 33: 76–81
71. Harding M, Cowan S, Hole D et al 1990 Estrogen and progesterone receptors in ovarian cancer. Cancer 65: 486–491
72. Hatch KD, Beecham JB, Blessing JA et al 1991 Responsiveness of patients with advanced ovarian carcinoma to tamoxifen: a Gynecologic Oncology Group study of second-line therapy in 103 patients. Cancer 57: 269–271
73. Shirley DR, Kavanaugh JJ Jr, Gershenson DM et al 1985 Tamoxifen therapy of epithelial ovarian cancer. Obstetrics and Gynecology 66: 575–578
74. Slevin ML, Harvey VJ, Osborne RJ et al 1986 A phase II study of tamoxifen in ovarian carcinoma. European Journal of Cancer and Clinical Oncology 22: 309–312
75. Potish RA, Twigs LB, Adcock LL et al 1986 Prognostic importance of progesterone and estrogen receptors in cancer of the uterine cervix. Cancer 58: 1709–1713
76. Bhattacharya D, Redkar A, Mittra I et al 1997 Oestrogen increases S-phase fractions and oestrogen and progesterone receptors in human cervical cancer in vivo. British Journal of Cancer 75: 554–558

57. Use of estrogens and progestogens in women with breast cancer

John A. Eden

Introduction

In most Western countries, breast cancer is now the commonest malignancy affecting nonsmoking women (Table 57.1). It is interesting to examine the changing patterns of death over the last century. In Australia at the turn of the century, infection was the single commonest cause of death, causing 35% of all female deaths (Table 57.1).[1] The common infectious causes included tuberculosis, diphtheria, typhoid and the childhood illnesses such as measles and whooping cough. Pregnancy killed three times as many women as breast cancer. Over the first 50 years of this century there was a dramatic rise in relative mortality from breast cancer. This rise predated the introduction of the oral contraceptive pill and hormone replacement therapy (HRT). This sharp rise in breast cancer mortality was paralleled by similar rises in the mortality from cardiovascular disease and other common cancers, such as bowel cancer. The main reason for this rising mortality from cardiovascular disease and cancer was 'disease substitution'. In other words, as public health measures such as clean water, sewerage and immunization reduced mortality from infectious causes, women began living long enough to die from the diseases of aging, namely cardiovascular disease and cancer. It is interesting to note that for women under the age of 40 years, the death rate from breast cancer has remained at 9 per 100 000 for nearly 100 years (Fig. 57.1). The substantial rise in breast cancer mortality has occurred in older women. Both breast cancer incidence and mortality rise significantly with age (Fig. 57.2). An absolute rise in breast cancer mortality this century comes probably from the changing patterns of reproduction (Fig. 57.1). Age at first full term pregnancy is a particularly potent risk factor for breast cancer. In recent times, women are delaying their first pregnancy for social and economic reasons, and thus inadvertently increasing their risk of developing breast cancer. Table 57.2 summarizes some of the important risk factors for the development of breast cancer.[2] See also chapter 68.

Table 57.1 Causes of death in Australian women 1909 and 1992.[1]

Cause of death	1909	1992
Infection	35.3%	2.5%
Pregnancy	3.1%	0.02%
All cardiovascular disease	16.7%	48.4%
Ischemic heart disease	9.2%	25.5%
Stroke	5.1%	9.7%
All cancer	8.1%	25.3%
Breast cancer	1.1%	4.2%
Bowel cancer	0.9%	3.5%

The use of HRT by a woman who has had breast cancer remains controversial. However, the medical management of the menopausal woman who has had breast cancer presents the clinician with two difficult problems. First, some women will have severe symptoms from estrogen deprivation that will need treatment, or else quality of life will be poor. Secondly, long term complications such as osteoporosis and cardiovascular disease can be more important for these women than their risk of developing a tumor recurrence or a new breast cancer. These important issues will be addressed in this chapter.

PATHOPHYSIOLOGY OF SEX STEROIDS AND BREAST CANCER

Estrogen

Estrogen has long been implicated as the main sex hormone in the initiation and promotion of breast cancer. The case against estrogen is summarized:[2–10]

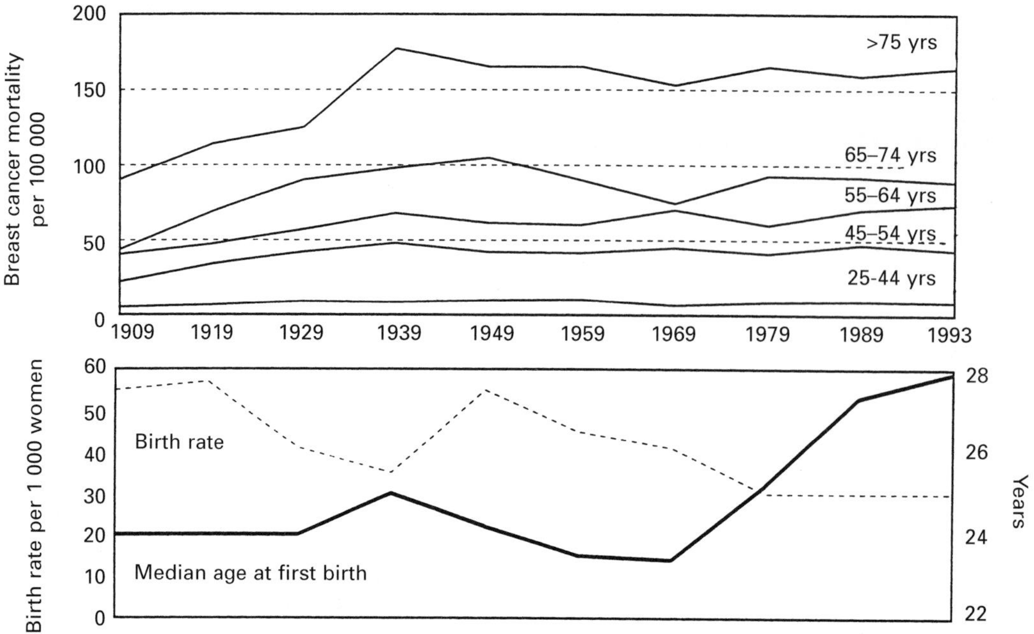

Fig. 57.1 Secular changes in annual breast cancer mortality for Australian women (per 100 000), 1909–93 (upper graph compared with the birth rate and median age at first birth over the same time (lower graph).

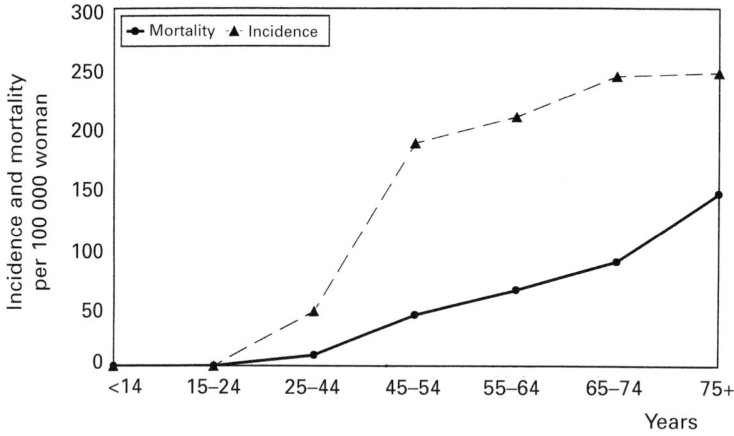

Fig. 57.2 Annual breast cancer incidence and mortality for Australian women (per 100 000) in 1993.

1. Breast cancer is much more common in women than it is in men
2. Estradiol (E_2) stimulates some breast cancer cell lines in culture
3. Estrogen stimulates breast ductal tissue
4. Risk factors for the development of breast cancer relate to reproductive markers such as age at menopause, age at menarche, parity, breast feeding and age at first full term pregnancy
5. Oophorectomy palliates some breast cancers
6. Stopping HRT can induce a remission in women with metastatic breast cancer who had been using HRT
7. Premature menopause reduces the risk of developing breast cancer.

However, many of these epidemiological risk factors can be explained in other ways. For example the reason

Table 57.2 Some risk factors for breast cancer incidence.[2,3]

Factor	Comparison group	Approximate relative risk
Age 70–74 years	Age 25–29 years	56
United States of America	Japan	5
Two or more affected first degree relatives	No affected first degree relative	5
Two alcoholic drinks a day	Non-drinker	1.7
Age at menarche 11 years	Menarche at 16 years	1.3
Age at first birth >30 years or nulliparous	<20 years	1.9
Age at menopause <45 years	Menopause at 45–50 years	0.7
Proliferative disease on breast biopsy	No breast biopsy	2.0
Atypical hyperplasia on breast biopsy	No breast biopsy	3.0
History of cancer in other breast	No history of breast cancer	5.0

why women rather than men develop breast cancer could simply relate to the fact that women have more breast ductal tissue than men. The relationship between breast cancer incidence and reproductive markers can be explained in terms of other hormones, such as androgen and progesterone.[1] Many estrogen-sensitive breast cancer cell lines also have their growth stimulated by insulin and other peptide growth factors.[6,7] Pharmacological doses of estrogen were in fact one of the earliest successful endocrine treatments for advanced breast cancer.[8] Direct comparisons between high dose estrogen therapy and tamoxifen show that both therapies are equivalent in terms of efficacy.[18] Tamoxifen has replaced high dose estrogen therapy principally because of its lower rate of side effects.[18]

Two popular theories have been proposed that implicate estrogen and progesterone as the main determinants of breast cancer risk. The first was proposed by Henderson and colleagues[9] and suggests that it is a woman's total lifetime exposure to estrogen that determines breast cancer risk; thus a woman who has an early menarche and late menopause will have a higher risk of developing breast cancer than a woman who has an average age of menopause and menarche. According to this theory, taking 10–15 years of HRT will also increase the risk of developing breast cancer. This theory was modified by Pike and colleagues[10] who suggested that not only does estrogen increase the risk of breast cancer development but so does progesterone — and the two together have a synergistic adverse effect. However, these theories fail to explain the marked protective effect of early first pregnancy and parity.

Pregnancy is associated with markedly elevated levels of estrogen and progesterone, so a woman who has an early first pregnancy and subsequently has many babies should have a *higher* risk of breast cancer than a nulliparous woman. The converse is the case. It is clear that the effect of sex steroids on the breast is complicated. Most researchers believe that a critical 'window' of carcinogenesis is left open during the teenage years and closed by the first pregnancy. Strategies aimed at substantially reducing the incidence of breast cancer will probably need to focus on the first 25 years of life rather than the postmenopausal years.

Many aspects of the relationship between estrogen and the breast remain unclear. For example it is not clear how much serum-derived E_2 is actually taken up by the breast.[11,12] Breast tissue levels of E_2 are around 20 times higher than in serum and this gradient is maintained both before and after the menopause.[11,12] It is apparent that the breast itself is capable of local synthesis of estrogen.[11,12,13] It has been shown that most of breast cancers are surrounded by fat with higher aromatase activity than fat taken from different quadrants within the same breast.[14] Bullbrook and colleagues reviewed the case that estrogen is the main endocrine promoter of breast cancer.[11] They were unable to show a relationship between serum (total and free), urinary or salivary estrogens and breast cancer risk. The breast is also capable of metabolizing E_2 into weaker or biologically inert estrogens such as estrone sulfate and, especially, catecholestrogens; some of the catecholestrogens have been shown to bind irreversibly to the estrogen receptor (ER), which is thereby permanently activated.[15] Thus it would seem likely that local breast estrogen metabolic pathways are more important than serum derived E_2.

Progesterone and progestogens

The effect of progesterone and progestogens upon the breast is just as complicated: it depends upon the type, dosage and duration of use of the progestogen. During the luteal phase of the menstrual cycle large amounts of progesterone are produced. Going and colleagues examined breast biopsies and correlated them with the menstrual cycle.[16] They showed that both mitosis and apoptosis were maximal in the midluteal phase.[16] However when mitosis is correlated to breast tissue concentrations of E_2 or progesterone, the lowest mitotic index is observed in the tissue samples with the highest concentrations of progesterone; the highest mitotic index was found in those tissues with the greatest E_2 concentrations.[17] At the cellular level, continuous exposure to progestogen reduces breast cell E_2 content and promotes pathways leading to the depletion of intracellular E_2 levels.[6] Continuous large doses of progestogens have been shown to be as effective as tamoxifen when given to women with advanced breast cancer.[18] Clarke and Sutherland[6] and Musgrove and colleagues[7] have performed a series of elegant experiments with progestogens on human breast cancer cell lines *in vitro*. They have shown that progestogens do not directly stimulate resting breast cells to proliferate. Instead, cells that are already entering the S phase are hurried through the cell cycle only to have their growth arrested in early G1 phase. Thus a modest increase in mitotic activity is seen over the first 24 hours, followed by a profound and continued inhibition of breast cell mitotic activity as long as the progestogen is given. Progestogens appear to have no effect on quiescent breast cells.[6] Progestogens have also been shown to inhibit the production of cathepsin-D, a protein that is mitogenic and could play a role in tumor invasion.[6]

THE ENDOCRINE TREATMENT OF BREAST CANCER

A wide variety of endocrine agents have been used to treat metastatic breast cancer. A 30–35% response rate has been found regardless of whether the treatment has been tamoxifen, aminoglutethimide, estrogens, progestogens or androgens.[18]

Tamoxifen

Tamoxifen, the attenuated estrogen, is the most studied endocrine therapy for breast cancer. It has been shown to be safe and effective for advanced cases and, because of beneficial effects other than the treatment of metastases, is being increasingly used to treat most menopausal women who have had breast cancer.[18–22] The annual incidence of new primary breast cancers among breast cancer survivors is 14 per 1000, compared with an incidence of 2 per 1000 in the general population.[19] Tamoxifen reduces the risk of contralateral breast cancers in women with a history of breast cancer.[19] Among eight prospective randomized trials, tamoxifen reduced the risk of new breast cancer by 35%.[19] Tamoxifen has also been shown to reduce the risk of osteoporotic fractures,[21] to improve the lipoprotein profile[19] and to reduce the risk of adverse cardiovascular events. The main clinical side-effects of tamoxifen include an aggravation of hot flushes, a slightly increased risk of thromboembolic disease[22] and a two to threefold increased risk of endometrial cancer.[22–24]

Opinions differ over the best way of monitoring the endometrium of women on tamoxifen. Ross and Whitehead[23] describe the lack of agreement on the best method of screening. Transvaginal ultrasound is a relatively noninvasive investigation, but has a high false positive rate in women on tamoxifen, in whom benign conditions such as endometrial polyps commonly occur.[23] Other possibilities include endometrial biopsy and outpatient hysteroscopy. Some authorities suggest annual screening of women on tamoxifen, whereas others suggest investigation only when there is abnormal bleeding.[23–25] Because of the reduced risk of contralateral breast cancer amongst women with a personal history of breast cancer, clinical trials are under way to see whether tamoxifen can reduce the risk of development of breast cancer among women at high risk.[19,22] Tamoxifen is most efficacious when estrogen receptors (ER) are present but can still be effective when they are absent.[4,5] Tamoxifen has been shown to influence a number of growth regulating factors, including epidermal growth factor and cathepsin-D.[26]

As a treatment for breast cancer, tamoxifen is thus safe and effective. Highly significant reductions in the annual rates of recurrence and death are achieved.[4,5] The reduced risk of recurrence is chiefly seen during the first four years of therapy. Benefit is seen in women with ER positive or ER negative tumors, as well as in women with node positive or node negative disease.[3,4] For women with node positive disease, the absolute improvement in 10 years survival is around 12 deaths avoided per 100 women treated.[3,4] When one takes into account the non-breast-related benefits of tamoxifen, it is difficult to justify denying tamoxifen therapy to any postmenopausal woman who has had breast cancer.[27]

Other endocrine treatments

Rose and Mouridsen[18] have reviewed the endocrine management of advanced breast cancer. They point out that despite the rationale for combined endocrine therapy, most trials have failed to show a benefit. Single agents seem to have the highest response rate when used as first line therapy: estrogens, tamoxifen and progestogens all have a similar response rate — around 35%. Rose and Mouridsen also reviewed trials that compared tamoxifen with other endocrine therapies and which failed to show a significant difference. The majority of these endocrine therapies have concentrated on postmenopausal women. In general, premenopausal women seem less responsive to endocrine therapies — with the one notable exception of bilateral oophorectomy.[4,5] The Early Breast Cancer Trialists Collaborative Group reviewed ovarian ablation trials that included more than 3000 subjects.[4,5] They showed that ovarian ablation in premenopausal women with axillary gland involvement produced a similar improvement in survival to that of chemotherapy. This large review also showed some benefit for using chemotherapy in a selected group of postmenopausal women with breast cancer.

Although tamoxifen has been clearly established as the main endocrine therapy for breast cancer,[27] it is not a pure anti-estrogen, having some estrogenic effects in addition to its anti-estrogenic actions. Wolf and Fuqua[26] have recently reviewed the efforts to produce a pure anti-estrogen and the efforts to understand tamoxifen resistance. Pure anti-estrogens are exemplified by the compounds ICI 164 384 and ICI 182 780.[26] These substances are derived from 17β-estradiol by the addition of a substituted alkyl side chain at the 7α position; they inhibit ER binding to DNA, increase the turnover of ER, and competitively inhibit E_2 binding to the ER.[26] Like tamoxifen, it seems probable that these new agents also exert antiproliferative actions independent of the ER. It remains to be seen whether these newer agents will replace tamoxifen. Pure anti-estrogens might not exert the nonbreast benefits seen with tamoxifen, namely lowering lipids, inhibiting bone loss and reducing the risk of cardiovascular complications.

OTHER CONSIDERATIONS IN BREAST CANCER

Contraception

There are no data examining the safety of combined oral contraceptive pills given to young women who have had breast cancer. It can be argued that modern pills probably deliver similar tissue levels of estrogen and progestogen to those seen in the normal ovarian cycle. However it would seem prudent to avoid estrogen containing contraceptive pills unless all the other options have been exhausted. Other methods of contraception, including intra-uterine devices, barrier methods and sterilization might be better options. It would also seem logical to consider a progestogen only contraceptive pill before an estrogenic combined contraceptive pill.

Managing the menopause

The medical management of the menopausal woman who has had breast cancer can be divided into two main themes: control of menopausal symptoms and long-term management.

Control of menopausal symptoms

For most women, the symptoms for which they seek therapy are hot flushes and vaginal dryness. Hot flushes can disappear with time, but this is not always the case. Stress reduction (e.g. using yoga, meditation, hypnotherapy or relaxation tapes) and avoidance of known aggravators such as overheating, alcohol and spicy foods can all be helpful. Clonidine has been used with variable success.[28-29] Moderate doses of progestogens such as medroxyprogesterone acetate (MPA) 20–100 mg daily or norethindrone (NET) 5–10 mg daily have been shown to be effective in placebo-controlled studies.[30,31] These are probably the least controversial endocrine therapies to consider for these women.

Another common problem is the woman who was well until she started tamoxifen as an endocrine therapy for her breast cancer but then has aggravation of menopausal flushes. After discussion with the oncologist, consideration should be given to temporarily stopping the tamoxifen — a maneuver that may be a better option than adding HRT to the tamoxifen treatment. In many cases the tamoxifen can be restarted 12 months later, commencing with a lower dose (e.g. 5 mg per day) and increasing the dose slowly up to 20 mg.

Vaginal symptoms can usually be managed with nonhormonal vaginal moisturizers such as Replens (Winthrop), weakly absorbed, topical estrogens such as Vagifem (Novo Nordisk), or estriol creams and pessaries. The older topical preparations such as dienestrol and conjugated equine estrogen creams should probably be avoided, because they can be well absorbed across the vaginal mucosa.

In a small group of women, menopausal symptoms will not be controlled by these measures alone and consideration will have to be given to using proper

Table 57.3 Published studies where estrogen replacement therapy has been given to women with a personal history of breast cancer.[45]

Authors	Number	Follow-up (months)	% relapse
Wile et al[41]	25	35	12%
Disaia[42]	77	59	8%
Stoll and Parbhoo[43]	50	24	0%
Powles et al[44]	35	43	6%
Eden et al[32]	90	72	7%

estrogen replacement. Quality of life has to be balanced against the theoretical risk of induction of the tumor. Our group in Sydney now have some experience with using HRT after breast cancer. In our 1995 case-controlled study,[32] we compared 90 women who were mostly using an oral estrogen such as conjugated equine estrogen 0.625 mg daily combined with a moderate dose of continuously administered progestogen (usually MPA 50 mg daily) with a matched control group (n = 180). The risk of tumor recurrence was significantly lower amongst the HRT users compared with the control. A number of other groups have published small series of patients given HRT after breast cancer with apparent safety (Table 57.3). Prospective randomized trials have begun around the world and the results of these studies are eagerly awaited.

LONG-TERM MANAGEMENT OF BREAST CANCER

With the advent of screening mammography, many women are having their breast cancer detected at an early stage. Most of these women will survive over 20 years and, like other women, will be concerned about their risk of osteoporotic fracture and cardiovascular disease complicating treatment. For the reasons already outlined, one strategy being increasingly considered for these women is the use of tamoxifen 20 mg daily as a preventive strategy. Because of the increased risk of endometrial cancer among tamoxifen users, it is prudent to monitor the endometrium of these women. Possible strategies include transvaginal ultrasound, outpatient hysteroscopy, endometrial sampling or using a progestogen challenge test (which precipitates bleeding if there has been significant estrogenic effect). There is also a high rate of benign uterine pathology amongst tamoxifen users.[23,24] Consideration should be given to performing serial bone mineral density measurements on women who have had breast cancer. If significant bone loss is apparent, then nonestrogen strategies can be followed to prevent fractures; the options include the use of calcitriol and the bisphosphonates.[33–35] Cardiovascular risk can be reduced by encouraging these women to adopt a healthy lifestyle, including a diet high in fruit, vegetables, cereals and low in animal fat; to exercise at least four hours a week; to avoid cigarette smoking; to maintain normal blood pressure; and to correct any serum lipid abnormality. It is particularly relevant to note that there are studies that show that women who exercise this way not only reduce their risk of cardiovascular disease but also reduce their risk of developing breast cancer.[3]

Cobleigh and colleagues[36] have proposed that tamoxifen and HRT might be prescribed together (HRT and tamoxifen have been administered simultaneously, apparently without ill-effect).[36] They postulate that the cardiac benefits of tamoxifen and HRT could be synergistic. They further suggest that although tamoxifen slightly increases the risk of vascular thrombosis, premenopausal women receiving tamoxifen do not experience a higher incidence of thrombosis compared with postmenopausal women receiving tamoxifen, so combining natural estrogen with tamoxifen should not have a synergistic adverse effect on thrombosis.[36] Tamoxifen is now offered to virtually all postmenopausal women who have had breast cancer, so they argue that it is reasonable to ask whether tamoxifen and HRT can be administered safely.

Prevention of breast cancer

The tamoxifen breast cancer prevention trial has raised the possibility of using a chemotherapeutic agent that might delay or prevent the appearance of breast cancer. There is still considerable debate over the wisdom of giving tamoxifen to healthy women,[19,22] but this important trial has at least increased discussion of the concept that breast cancer *can* be prevented. The interested reader is directed to several recent reviews.[19,22,36]

Genetics

Overall only around 10% of breast cancer is attributable to familial predisposition; about half of this risk is attributable to dominantly inherited genes. Women who carry the BRCA1 gene have an 85% chance of developing breast cancer by the age of 80.[3] The BRCA 1 gene has been cloned and sequenced.[37] Several mutations have been found in this gene as well as the BRCA2 gene. Unfortunately, the management of such affected individuals remains unclear, but options include screening mammograph, or bilateral mastectomy; tamoxifen prophylaxis remains to be proven.

Hormones

Reproductive factors have already been discussed and, even though age at first pregnancy is a potent risk factor, it is hardly practical to ask women to have their first child before 25 years just to reduce their risk of breast cancer. However there is increasing interest in the concept of designing a contraceptive pill that might reduce the risk. This remains hypothetical.

Diet

A number of studies have focused on dietary fat, but it seems not to be a significant predictor of breast cancer risk.[38] Several other food constituents have been proposed to alter breast cancer risk, including vitamin A and retinoids, the deltanoids (vitamin D analogs) and plant estrogens such as the isoflavones found in soya bean.[3]

Lifestyle factors

Substantial exercise has been shown to reduce the risk of breast cancer in pre- and postmenopausal women.[39] More than moderate alcohol consumption has been shown to increase the risk of breast cancer, so it seems prudent to advise women to minimize their exposure to alcohol.

Environmental exposures

Concern has been raised concerning exposure to pesticides because a number of these agents appear to be weak estrogens. At least one study has failed to show an association between pesticide concentrations and breast cancer risk.[40]

Conclusion

Estrogen and progesterone act on the breast. With regard to estrogen, it remains unclear whether E_2 produced within the breast is more important than E_2 derived from serum. The effect of progesterone and progestogens on the breast depends upon the type, dosage and duration of exposure. Tamoxifen is being increasingly prescribed to postmenopausal women who have had breast cancer. This therapy should reduce their risk of tumor recurrence, new breast cancer, osteoporotic fractures and cardiovascular events. Non-estrogen osteoporosis therapies can be prescribed for women with low bone mass.

For a small group of women after treatment of breast cancer, menopausal symptoms will be so severe that consideration should be given to using some form of hormonal therapy. Progestogens alone in a moderate dose will often be effective treatment for hot flashes. Weakly absorbed topical estrogens or vaginal moisturizers can be used for vaginal symptoms. However for a few women menopausal symptoms will not respond to these treatments and continuous combined estrogen-progestogen replacement therapy can be considered.

REFERENCES

1. Castles I 1992 Causes of death, Australia. Australian Bureau of Statistics (3303.0)
2. Gail MH, Benichou J 1992 Assessing the risk of breast cancer in individuals. Cancer Prevention 1: 1–15
3. Hulka BS, Stark AT 1995 Breast cancer: cause and prevention. Lancet 346: 883–887
4. Early breast cancer trialists collaborative group 1992 Systemic treatment of early breast cancer by hormonal, cytotoxic or immune therapy. Lancet ii: 1–15
5. Early breast cancer trialists collaborative group 1992 Systemic treatment of early breast cancer by hormonal, cytotoxic or immune therapy. Lancet ii: 71–85
6. Clarke CL, Sutherland RL 1990 Progestin regulation of cellular proliferation. Endocrinology Reviews 11(2): 266–301
7. Musgrove EA, Lee CSL, Sutherland RL 1991 Progestins both stimulate and inhibit breast cancer cell cycle progression while increasing expression of transforming growth factor α epidermal growth factor receptor, c-fos c-myc genes. Molecular and Cell Biology 11(10): 5032–5043
8. Haddow A, Watkinson JM, Paterson E 1944 Influence of synthetic estrogens upon advanced malignant disease. British Medical Journal (Sept 23): 4368–4373
9. Henderson BE, Ross R, Berstein L 1988 Estrogens as a cause of human cancer. Cancer Research 48: 246–253

10. Key TJ, Pike MC 1988 The role of estrogens and progestogens in the epidemiology and prevention of breast cancer. European Journal of Cancer 24: 29–43
11. Bulbrook RD, Leake RE, George WD 1989 Estrogens in the initiation and promotion of breast cancer. In: Beck JS (ed) Estrogen and the human breast. Royal Society of Edinburgh, Edinburgh, pp 67–76
12. Blankenstein MA, Szymczakj J, Daroszewski J et al 1992 Estrogens in plasma and fatty tissue from breast cancer patients and women undergoing surgery for non-oncological reasons. Gynecological Endocrinology 6: 13–17
13. Miller WR, Mullen P 1993 Factors influencing aromatase activity in the breast. Journal of Steroid Biochemistry and Molecular Biology 44: 597–604
14. Bulun SE, Price TM, Aitken J, Mahendroo MS, Simpson ER 1992 A link between breast cancer and local estrogen biosynthesis suggested by quantification of breast adipose tissue aromatase cytochrome P450 transcripts using competitive polymerase chain reaction after reverse transcription. Journal of Clinical Endocrinology and Metabolism 77: 1622–1628
15. Fishman J, Schneider J, Herschcopf RJ et al 1994 Increased estrogen 16α hydroxylase activity in women with breast and endometrial cancer. Journal of Steroid Biochemistry 20: 1077–1081
16. Going J, Anderson T, Battersby S 1988 Proliferative and secretory activity in human breast during natural and artifical menstrual cycles. American Journal of Pathology 130: 193–204
17. Barrat J, de Lignieres, B, Marpeau L 1990 Effet in vivo de l'administration locale de progesterone sur l'activité mitotique des galactophores humains. Journal of Gynecology, Obstetrics and the Biology of Reproduction 19: 269–274
18. Rose C, Mauridsen HT 1989 Endocrine management of advanced breast cancer. Hormone Research 32 (Suppl 1): 189–197
19. Vogel VG, Saenz M 1995 Tamoxifen for the prevention of breast cancer: yes. In: De Vita VT, Hellman S, Rosenberg SA (eds) Important advances in oncology. Lippincott, Philadelphia, pp 187–200
20. McDonald CC, Stewart HJ 1991 Fatal myocardial infarction in the Scottish adjuvant Tamoxifen trial. British Medical Journal 303: 435–437
21. Love RR, Mazzess RB, Barden HS et al 1992 Effects of tamoxifen on bone density in postmenopausal women with breast cancer. New England Journal of Medicine 326: 852–856
22. De Gregorio MW, Maenpaa JU, Wiebe VJ 1995 Tamoxifen for the prevention of breast cancer: no. In: De Vita VT, Hellman S, Rosenberg SA (eds) Important advances in oncology. Lippincott, Philadelphia, pp 175–185
23. Ross D, Whitehead W 1995 Hormonal manipulation and gynaecological cancer; the tamoxifen dilemma. Current Opinion in Obstetrics and Gynecology 7: 63–68
24. Van Leeuwen FE, Benraadt J, Coebergh JWW et al 1994 Risk of endometrial cancer after tamoxifen treatment of breast cancer. Lancet 343: 448–452
25. Neven P, Shepherd JH, Lowe DG 1993 Tamoxifen and the gynaecologist. British Journal of Obstetrics and Gynaecology 100: 893–897
26. Wolf DM, Fuqua SAW 1995 Mechanisms of action of anti-estrogens. Cancer Treatment Reviews 21: 247–271
27. Jaiyesimi IA, Buzdadar AU, Decca DA Hortobagyi GN 1995 The use of tamoxifen for breast cancer; 28 years later. Journal of Clinical Oncology 13(2): 513–529
28. Wren BG, Brown LB 1986 A double-blind trial with clonidine and a placebo to treat hot flushes. Medical Journal of Australia 144: 369–370
29. Clayden JR, Bell JW, Pollard P 1974 Menopausal flushing: a double blind trial of a non-hormonal medication. British Medical Journal 1: 409–412
30. Schiff I, Tulchinsky D, Kramer D et al 1980 Oral medroxyprogesterone in the treatment of postmenopausal symptoms. Journal of the American Medical Association 244(13): 1443–1445
31. Paterson MEL 1992 A randomized double blind cross-over trial into the effect of norethisterone on climacteric symptoms and biochemical profiles. British Journal of Obstetrics and Gynaecology 89: 464–472
32. Eden JA, Bush T, Nand S, Wren BG 1995 A case controlled study of combined continuous estrogen-progestin replacement therapy among women with a personal history of breast cancer. Journal of the North American Medical Society 2(2): 67–72
33. Storm T, Thamsborg G, Steiniche T et al 1990 Effect of intermittent cyclical etidronate therapy on bone mass and fracture rate in women with postmenopausal osteoporosis. New England Journal of Medicine 322: 1265–1271
34. Tilyard MW, Spears GFS, Thomson J, Dovey S 1992 Treatment of postmenopausal osteoporosis with calcitriol or calcium. New England Journal of Medicine 326: 357–362
35. Liberman UA, Weiss SR, Broll J et al 1995 Effect of oral alendronate on bone mineral density and the incidence of fractures in postmenopausal osteoporosis. New England Journal of Medicine 333: 1437–1443
36. Cobleigh MA, Berris RF, Bush T et al 1994 Estrogen replacement in breast cancer survivors — a time for change. Journal of the American Medical Association 272: 540–545
37. Miki Y, Swensen J, Shattuck-Eidens D et al 1994 A strong candidate for the breast and ovarian cancer susceptability gene BRCA 1. Science 226: 66–71
38. Hunter DJ, Spiegelman D, Adami H et al 1996 Cohort studies of fat intake and the risk of breast cancer — a pooled analysis. New England Journal of Medicine 334: 356–361
39. Freidenreich CM, Rohan TE 1985 A review of physical activity and breast cancer. Epidemiology 6: 311–317
40. Kreiger N, Wolff MS, Iliat RA, Rivera M, Vogelman J, Orentreich N 1994 Breast cancer and serum organochlorines: a prospective study amongst white, black and Asian women. Journal of the National Cancer Institute 86: 589–599
41. Wile AG, Opfell RW, Margileth DA 1993 Hormone replacement therapy in previously treated breast cancer patients. American Journal of Surgery 165: 372–375
42. Disaia PJ 1993 Hormone replacement therapy in patients with breast cancer. Cancer 71 (Suppl): 1490–1500
43. Stoll BA, Parbhoo S 1988 Treatment of menopausal symptoms in breast cancer patients. Lancet i: 1278–1279
44. Powles TJ, Hickish T, Casey S et al 1993 Hormone replacement therapy after breast cancer. Lancet 342: 60–61
45. Sands R, Boschoff C, Jones A, Studd J 1995 Current opinion: Hormone replacement after a diagnosis of breast cancer. Journal of the North American Menopause Society 2(2): 73–80

58. Sex steroid production from ovarian tumors

Robert P.S. Jansen

Introduction

It is convenient to think of luteinized ovarian stromal cells as producing androgens (especially androstenedione), follicular cells aromatizing such androgens to estradiol, luteinized granulosa cells secreting only progesterone, and hilus cells producing testosterone. In reality, steroid production in the ovaries is not so rigidly compartmentalized: aromatization occurs in luteinized thecal cells too[1,2] and estradiol is produced by both major steroidogenic cell types of the mature corpus luteum.[3] So it should not cause surprise to observe that structure-function relationships among the steroid-producing hyperplasias and neoplasms of the ovary are relatively loose.[4] In addition, nonsteroid products from ovarian tumors can substantially modify secreted or circulating steroids and their clinical effects, making the study of peptide and glycoprotein hormones from ovarian tumors an integral part of the subject under discussion.

FORM AND FUNCTION IN REPRODUCTIVE TUMORS

The cells that proliferate in normal and neoplastic tissues are relatively undifferentiated stem cells. Especially in neoplasms, such stem cells often leak proteins and other substances that have a primitive ontological origin (characteristically we find cell products that we normally associate with early embryonic cells).[4] A small, persistent background production of unglycosylated human chorionic gonadotropin (hCG) in both adult males and females is a good example,[5] hCG having been among the organism's very first gene-products after conception, synthesized within a week of fertilization of the egg by the sperm.[6]

The morphological appearance of a neoplasm is the result of the degree of 'down-the-line' differentiation of the proliferating stem cells. Such differentiation is needed for cellular production of the active polypeptides, biogenic amines and prostaglandins that lie behind the commonest endocrinologically important 'ectopic hormone syndromes'.[7] These hormones are mostly phylogenetically ancient:[8] ACTH is found, for example, in protozoa; hCG is found in bacteria.

Morphological and functional differentiation coincide in neoplasms more often than not.[4] Thus germ cell tumors that differentiate as endodermal sinus tumors (recapitulating the yolk sac, which is the first tissue to manufacture albumin in the embryo) are marked by production of the fetal albumin, alpha fetoprotein (AFP); those which differentiate to contain multinucleated giant cells (recapitulating syncitiotrophoblast), such as choriocarcinoma, some embryomas and occasional dysgerminomas, produce those typical products of normal trophoblast, human placental lactogen and (well-glycosylated) hCG; they also often contain the aromatases needed to convert circulating Δ^5 androgens to estrogens. As well as the steroid hormone products elaborated upon below, granulosa cell tumors, recapitulating cells of the ovarian follicle, secrete inhibin,[9] and ovarian Sertoli cell tumors typically secrete anti-Müllerian hormone.[10] AFP production has been reported in Sertoli cell tumors.[11,12]

Differentiation of neoplastic tissues to the point of secreting steroid hormones has been described only for tumors of tissues steroidogenic in their normal non-neoplastic state. Steroidogenic function follows morphological form only up to a point, however, and departures from apparent parent tissue steroid specialization are frequent. Moreover, the influences of the systemic and intratumoral peptide hormone environment and the opportunities for steroid conversion in both intratumoral and extratumoral tissues usually need to be taken into account.

PATHOPHYSIOLOGY OF CLINICAL PRESENTATIONS

Ovarian hyperplasias

Stromal cell hyperplasia is dependent on high levels of hCG in pregnancy, or even longer-term high levels of LH in the polycystic ovary syndrome or, especially, after the menopause.[13] Focal or nodular *stromal cell hyperplasia* (especially as a *luteoma* of pregnancy), often results in androstenedione secretion.[14] There can be peripheral conversion to testosterone, for masculinization in pregnancy of the mother (and, less often, of a female fetus) or, with hyperplasias outside of pregnancy, to amenorrhea, hirsutism and virilization;[15,16] or there can be conversion to estradiol, causing endometrial hyperplasia and acyclical bleeding. Hilus cell hyperplasia produces large amounts of testosterone — and virilization — classically and typically after the menopause.[17]

Ovarian cystic hyperplasias in pregnancy of luteal origin — such as *hyperreactio luteinalis* (seen with high hCG levels of trophoblastic disease) and *ovarian hyperstimulation syndrome* (after FSH plus hCG treatment for multiple ovulation induction) — are characterized by very high levels of estradiol and progesterone. Attribution of such overproduction to the ovaries is hindered in clinical practice, however, by the fact that these same steroids are secreted also by placental trophoblast. A distinction can be made by noting high levels of the ovarian progestogen 17-α hydroxyprogesterone,[18,19] which is not synthesized in trophoblast, and which, with the normal decline of the corpus luteum of pregnancy, is usually baseline by the end of the first trimester. During such pregnancies serum 17-hydroxyprogesterone levels correlate well with ultrasound appearances of the ovaries.

Steroid production by 'nonfunctioning' ovarian tumors

In high hCG or LH environments, a number of ovarian tumors that do not ordinarily produce sex hormones are able to virilize. This can happen in *pregnancy*[4,20,21] or after the *menopause*.[4,22] The luteinizing action of the hCG or LH is on the stromal cells around the tumor.[23] What the tumors capable of producing this phenomenon at first sight have in common is the presentation of a large, internal, tumor-stromal interface, which somehow induces a theca-like stromal cell differentiation[21,24] and which gives the stroma the capacity to produce large amounts of androstenedione. It is also possible, however, that some of these tumors themselves produce hCG,[25] which then acts on the stroma in a paracrine fashion.

The ovarian tumors that most commonly result in hormonally active stromal activation are the cystadenomas (usually mucinous, sometimes endometrioid, very rarely serous), Brenner tumors and (metastatic) Krukenberg tumors;[17,25,26] granulosa cell tumors (see below) can be virilizing in pregnancy owing to reactive surrounding thecal elements. Depending on other circumstances, such as the amount of body fat to aromatize androgens to estrogens, postmenopausal endocrine manifestations caused by these tumors in high LH environments can also be feminizing.[22]

In the normally highly feminizing circumstance of pregnancy, only androgenizing effects will become clinically apparent. If virilization occurs, a female fetus, although to some extent protected by the aromatizing capacity of the placenta, can be affected as well as its mother. These indirectly sex hormone-producing tumors outnumber directly-secreting sex cord-stromal neoplasms, particularly in pregnancy. Whereas in the nonpregnant state intrinsically nonfunctioning tumors constitute 20% of virilizing tumors, in pregnancy the proportion is 45–50%, and after the menopause the proportion is higher still.[4]

Ovarian stromal and sex cord neoplasms

The sex cord stromal ovarian tumors vary in their admixture of stromal and sex cord elements, with either element predominating, and sometimes present in pure form. The age incidence of the classic varieties, surveyed from the literature, is shown in Figure 58.1.

Pure stromal tumors such as fibromas are usually endocrinologically (and morphologically) inert. The more luteinized the neoplastic stromal cell cytoplasm appears (in the form of a thecoma or lipid cell tumor), the more likely it is that there will be a steroid product. The histological appearance, however, cannot predict what steroid will be produced[4] and hence what, if any, the clinical consequences might be. Thecomas can feminize through the direct production of estradiol or through the peripheral conversion of androstenedione to estrogens.[27] Cortisol production has been revealed in excised tissue *in vitro*, but there are no reported cases of Cushing's syndrome.[28] Hilus cell, or Leydig cell, tumors almost aways secrete testosterone and are particularly virilizing.[29]

Pure sex cord tumors, such as highly differentiated Sertoli cell tumors and granulosa cell tumors, can be endocrinologically inert, except for their protein products anti-Müllerian hormone and inhibin, which can be used as tumor markers.[9,10] More often, the tumors have admixed sex cord and stromal cell components and are hormonally active. There is variably differentiated recapitulation of either a female

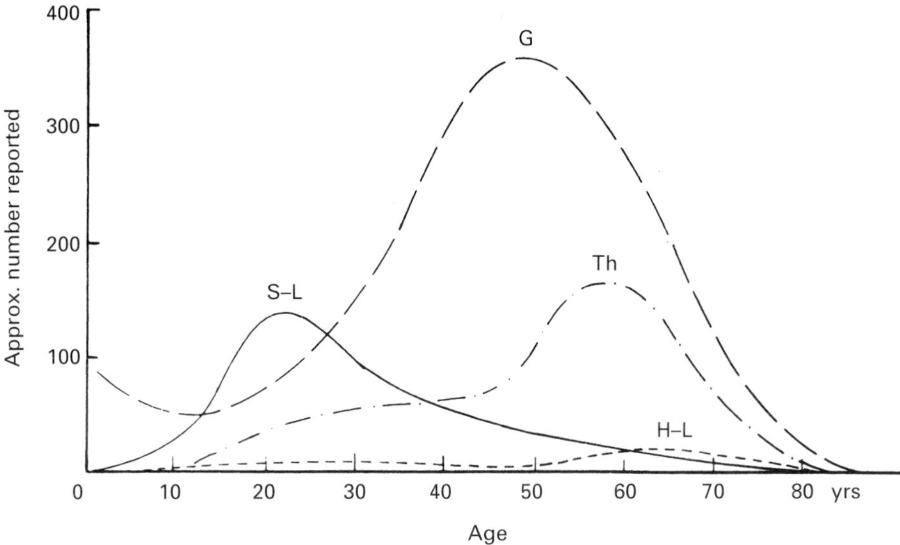

Fig. 58.1 Age-incidence of reported sex cord stromal tumors of the ovary. Tumors include Sertoli-Leydig cell tumors (S-L), granulosa cell tumors (G), thecomas (Th) and hilus or Leydig cell tumors (H-L).[4]

gonadal structure (granulosa-thecal cell tumor) or male gonadal structure (Sertoli-Leydig cell tumor, or 'arrhenoblastoma'). The commonest predominant steroid products are, respectively, estradiol[30] and testosterone,[31] but either morphological form can produce the other hormone (with androgens predominating in some cystic granulosa cell tumors in girls[32] and aromatization of androgens leading to feminization having been reported among Sertoli-Leydig cell tumors even in boys).[33] In some sex cord tumors, production of the weaker product, androstenedione, predominates.[4] The usual clinical endocrine manifestations can thus be feminizing or virilizing. When sex cord-stromal tumors occur before puberty, precocious puberty can manifest.

Three granulosa cell tumors have been reported with luteinized granulosa cell components and the production of large amounts of progesterone.[4,34] There are two reports in the literature of life-threatening production of aldosterone from ovarian Sertoli cell tumors, with hypokalemia and severe hypertension.[35,36]

Ovarian trophoblastic tumors

Germ cell tumors can recapitulate syncitiotrophoblast, manifesting giant cells capable of secreting significant quantities of hCG. In decreasing order of likelihood, hCG-secreting giant cells may be found in primary ovarian choriocarcinomas, embryomas and dysgerminomas. If these tumors occur before puberty, precocious puberty can result.[4,37,38]

It is immediately appealing to suppose that the mechanism of precocious puberty from germ cell tumors is the neoplastic production of effectively glycosylated chorionic gonadotropin leading to stimulation of ovarian stroma, with consequent production of steroid hormones. If this were the case, though, the predominant steroid in girls would be androstenedione, which is relatively weak. The evidence from a reported case of a dysgerminoma in a boy with precocious puberty suggests a different mechanism — but one which equally well demonstrates the association between form and function in the trophoblastic component of these tumors.[39] In addition to evidence of hCG-induced Leydig cell production of testosterone, it was inferred that, as is the case with normal trophoblast, the giant cells in this boy were converting the normally-occurring high prepubertal circulating levels of dehydroepiandrosterone (DHA), a Δ-5,16-hydroxylated steroid and essentially inert, into the potent steroid product, estradiol.

Because childhood ovaries contain few hilus cells and little or no luteinized stromal tissue, placenta-like 16-dehydroxylation and aromatization of circulating DHA might thus be the predominant mechanism for precocious puberty in girls who have germ cell tumors that secrete hCG. It can be noted too that estrogenic effects from giant cell-containing, hCG-producing tumors might not be confined to tumors of germ cell origin: several cases have been reported of particularly aggressive endometrial adenocarcinomas (usually estrogen dependent tumors) in which multinucleated hCG-containing cells were found within the tumor;[40] although peripheral hCG levels were elevated, circulating estradiol levels were unfortunately not reported.

PRINCIPLES OF MANAGING OVARIAN ENDOCRINE TUMORS

Hormonal independence from gonadotropins

Upon investigating a girl or woman who presents with *virilization* (amenorrhea, hirsutism, breast atrophy, frontal alopecia, clitoromegaly, voice deepening), *feminization* (anovulatory dysfunctional uterine bleeding, often with endometrial hyperplasia on ultrasound, hysteroscopy or curettage), or *precocious puberty* (feminizing or virilizing), it can be difficult to distinguish a hyperplastic state from a neoplastic one. The distinction can be important, because hyperplasias might, in principle, be managed with suppressive endocrine therapy, whereas autonomous tumors should be removed.

A major clue, in many contexts, will be the serum levels of the two gonadotropins, FSH and LH. When FSH and LH are suppressed in association with high levels of, for example, testosterone, autonomous production of this steroid can be inferred.[4] Similarly, prolonged elevation of estradiol, particularly with suppression of FSH, should always lead to further investigation. In ambiguous cases, suppression therapy (e.g. the oral contraceptive pill) can be tried — but it should be pointed out that, upon commencement of ovarian suppression with an estrogen in high androgen situations, the first hormonal consequence to expect will be a substantial *rise* in serum testosterone levels owing to induction of sex hormone-binding globulin synthesis in the liver; proper suppression of serum testosterone might not be apparent for six weeks.

Suppression for diagnostic purposes can be achieved more rapidly using a GnRH analog. If an agonist is used there will be a few days of increased FSH and LH, resulting in a flare of increased steroid production that also lasts several days, if the tumor is sensitive to gonadotropins, followed then by a sustained reduction in steroid levels over ensuing weeks.[41] GnRH-antagonists, as they become available for use, should inhibit gonadotropins and dependent steroid production within days.

Steroids in treatment

In principle, gonadotropin-dependent hyperplasia and gonadotropin-independent neoplasia ought to be distinguishable. In practice the situation is often blurred. On the one hand, suppression of long established hyperplastic ovarian states with ovarian steroid therapy can be imperfect. On the other hand, suppression of gonadotropins might still be clinically useful in the treatment of some ovarian cancers.

Ovarian granulosa cell tumors, for example, can display FSH receptors,[42] implying sensitivity to FSH. Although granulosa tumors occur at any age (Fig. 58.1), they are commonest after the menopause,[17,43] when their prognosis is worse than it is in premenopausal women. Consequently, FSH suppression with exogenous estrogen might be useful for reducing the risk of recurrence of granulosa cell tumors.[44]

Detection of the tumor

How to go about localizing a tumor producing sex steroids or sex steroid effects will depend on the size the tumor might be expected to be. Normal tissues are almost always more efficient in producing steroid hormones than abnormal, particularly neoplastic, tissues. For example, if a preovulatory follicle has a diameter of 2 cm, one might suppose that a granulosa cell tumor would need to be several times this size to secrete a comparable amount of estrogen. A stromal tumor with clinical endocrine consequences will need to be bigger than a corpus luteum, for the same reasons. This means that the great majority of ovarian sex hormone (or, for that matter, trophoblastic) tumors cause obvious enlargement of the ovary, detectable on palpation or with vaginal ultrasonography.[4] The exception is the hilus cell tumor, which is composed of differentiated Leydig or Leydig-like cells that produce close to adult male levels of testosterone without the presence of testicular tubules to push the size of the tumor to that typical of a normal testis.

Hilus cell tumors, almost all of which occur after the menopause (Fig. 58.1), can be microscopically sized.[29,45] The differential diagnosis is generally a subcapsular adrenal testosterone-producing adenoma, which can be sensitive to hCG and LH,[43,46] and which likewise can be too small reliably to be detected with ultrasound, computed tomography or magnetic resonance imaging. Almost alone among the steroid producing tumors, preoperative localization of hilus or adrenal Leydig-like tumors can require selective catheterization of adrenal and ovarian veins to detect the place of high testosterone production. Arguably, however, laparoscopy with bilateral ovariectomy is not much more invasive than multiple retrograde venous cannulation, and will lead to treatment as well as diagnosis in most such cases.

REFERENCES

1. Batta SK, Wentz AC, Channing CP 1980 Steroidogenesis by human ovarian cell types in culture: influence of mixing cell types and effect of added testosterone. Journal of Clinical Endocrinology and Metabolism 50: 274–279
2. Dennefors BL, Janson PO, Knutson F, Hamberger L 1980 Steroid production and responsiveness to gonadotropin in isolated stromal tissue of human postmenopausal women. American Journal of Obstetrics and Gynecology 136: 997–1002
3. Ohara A, Mori T, Shunzo T, Chiaki B, Narimoto K 1987 Functional differentiation in steroidogenesis of two types of luteal cells isolated from mature human corpora lutea of menstrual cycle [sic]. Journal of Clinical Endocrinology and Metabolism 65: 1987–1200
4. Jansen RPS 1992 Oncological endocrinology. In: Coppleson M (ed) Gynecologic oncology. Fundamental principles and clinical practice. Churchill Livingstone, Edinburgh, pp 135–171
5. Yoshimoto Y, Wolfsen AR, Hirose F, Odell WD 1979 Human chorionic gonadotropin-like material: presence in normal human tissues. American Journal of Obstetrics and Gynecology 134: 729–733
6. Hearn JP, Webley GE, Gidley-Baird AA 1991 Chorionic gonadotrophin and embryo-maternal recognition during the peri-implantation period in primates. Journal of Reproduction and Fertility 92: 497–509
7. Odell W, Wolfsen A, Yoshimoto Y, Weitzman R, Fisher D, Hirose F 1977 Ectopic peptide synthesis: a universal concomitant of neoplasia. Transcripts of the Association of American Physicians 90: 204–227
8. Roth J, LeRoith D, Shiloach J, Rosenzweig JL, Lesniak MA, Havrankova J 1982 The evolutionary origins of hormones, neurotransmitters, and other extracellular chemical messengers. Implications for mammalian biology. New England Journal of Medicine 306: 523–527
9. Lappöhn RE, Burger HG, Bouma J, Bangah M, Krans M, De Bruijn HWA 1989 Inhibin as a marker for granulosa-cell tumors. New England Journal of Medicine 321: 790–793
10. Gustafson ML, Lee MM, Scully RE, Moncure AC, Hirakawa T, Goodman A, Muntz HG, Donahoe PK, MacLaughlin DT, Fuller AFJ 1992 Müllerian inhibiting substance as a marker for ovarian sex-cord tumor. New England Journal of Medicine 326: 466–471
11. Larsen WG, Felmar EA, Wallace ME, Frieder R 1992 Sertoli-Leydig cell tumor of the ovary: a rare cause of amenorrhea. Obstetrics and Gynecology 79 (Suppl): 831–833
12. Motoyama T, Watanabe H, Gotoh A, Takeuchi S, Tanabe N, Nashimoto I 1989 Ovarian Sertoli-Leydig cell tumor with elevated serum alpha-fetoprotein. Cancer 63: 2047–2053
13. Yin P-H, Sommers SC 1961 Some pathologic correlations of ovarian stromal hyperplasia. Journal of Clinical Endocrinology and Metabolism 21: 472–477
14. Rice BF, Savard K 1966 Steroid hormone formation in the human ovary: IV. Ovarian stromal compartments; formation of radioactive steroids from aurate-1-^{14}C and action of gonadotropins. Journal of Clinical Endocrinology and Metabolism 26: 593–609
15. Braithwaite SE, Erkman-Balis B, Avila TD 1978 Postmenopausal virilization due to stromal hyperthecosis. Journal of Clinical Endocrinology and Metabolism 46: 295–299
16. Garcia-Bunuel R, Berek JS, Woodruff JD 1975 Luteomas of pregnancy. Obstetrics and Gynecology 45: 407–414
17. Taylor HB 1966 Functioning ovarian tumors and related conditions. Pathology Annual 1: 127–147
18. Osathanondh R, Goldstein DR, Tulchinsky D, Finn AE 1977 Serum 17-α hydroxyprogesterone in patients with gestational trophoblastic neoplasms. Obsterics and Gynecology 49: 77–79
19. Forest MG, Orgiazzi J, Tranchant D et al 1978 Approach to the mechanism of androgen overproduction in a case of Krukenberg tumor responsible for virilization during pregnancy. Journal of Clinical Endocrinology and Metabolism 47: 428–434
20. Verhoeven ATM, Mastboom JL, Van Leusden HAIM, Van der Velden WHM 1973 Virilization in pregnancy coexisting with an (ovarian) mucinous cystadenoma. A case report and review of virilizing ovarian tumors in pregnancy. Obstetrics and Gynecology Survey 28: 597–622
21. Quinn MA, Baker HWG, Rome R, Fortune D, Brown JB 1983 Response of a mucinous ovarian tumor of borderline malignancy to human chorionic gonadotropin. Obsterics and Gynecology 61: 121–126
22. MacDonald PC, Grodin JM, Edman CD, Vellios F, Siiteri PK 1976 Origin of estrogen in a postmenopausal woman with a nonendocrine tumor of the ovary and endometrial hyperplasia. Obsterics and Gynecology 47: 644–650
23. Hughesdon PE 1958 Thecal and allied reactions in epithelial ovarian tumors. Journal of Obstetrics and Gynaecology of the British Empire 65: 702–709
24. Scott JS, Lumsden CE, Levell MJ 1967 Ovarian endocrine activity in association with hormonally inactive neoplasia. American Journal of Obstetrics and Gynecology 97: 161–170
25. Matias-Guiu X, Prat J 1990 Ovarian tumors with functioning stroma: an immunohistochemical study of 100 cases with human chorionic gonadotropin monoclonal and polyclonal antibodies. Cancer 65: 2001–2005
26. Ireland K, Woodruff JD 1976 Masculinizing ovarian tumors. Obstetrics and Gynecology Survey 31: 83
27. Sternberg WH, Dhurander HN 1977 Functional ovarian tumors of stromal and sex cord origin. Human Pathology 8: 565
28. Imperato-McGinley J, Peterson RE, Dawood MY, Zullo M, Kramer E, Saxena BB, Arthur A, Huang T 1981 Steroid hormone secretion from a virilizing lipoid cell tumor of the ovary. Obsterics and Gynecology 57: 525–531

29. Dunnihoo DR, Grieme DL, Woolf RB 1966 Hilar-cell tumors of the ovary. Report of 2 new cases and a review of the world literature. Obsterics and Gynecology 27: 703–713
30. Gaffney EF, Majmudar B, Hertzler GL, Zane R, Furlong B, Breding E 1983 Ovarian granulosa cell tumors — immunohistochemical localization of estradiol and ultrastructure, with functional correlations. Obsterics and Gynecology 61: 311–319
31. Savard K, Gut M, Dorfman RI, Gabrilove JL, Soffer LJ 1961 Formation of androgens by human arrhenoblastoma tissue in vitro. Journal of Clinical Endocrinology and Metabolism 21: 165–174
32. Norris HJ, Taylor HB 1969 Virilization associated with cystic granulosa tumors. Obsterics and Gynecology 34: 629–635
33. Coen P, Kulin H, Ballantine T, Zaino R, Frauenhoffer E, Boal D, Inkster S, Brodie A, Santen R 1991 An aromatase-producing sex-cord tumor resulting in prepubertal gynecomastia. New England Journal of Medicine 324: 317–322
34. Li TC, Hill AS, Duncan SLB, Radstone DJ, Parsons MA, Cooke ID 1990 Granulosa cell tumour of the ovary producing both oestrogen and progesterone. Case report. British Journal of Obstetrics and Gynaecology 97: 649–652
35. Todesco S, Terribile V, Borsatti A, Mantero F 1975 Primary aldosteronism due to a malignant ovarian tumor. Journal of Clinical Endocrinology and Metabolism 41: 809–819
36. Ehrlich EN, Dominguez OV, Samuels LT, Lynch D, Oberhelman H, Warner NE 1963 Aldosteronism and precocious puberty due to an ovarian androblastoma. Journal of Clinical Endocrinology and Metabolism 23: 358–367
37. Ueda G, Hamanaka N, Hayakawa K et al 1972 Clinical, histochemical, and biochemical studies of an ovarian dysgerminoma with trophoblasts and Leydig cells. American Journal of Obstetrics and Gynecology 114: 748–754
38. Castleman B, Scully RE, McNeely BU 1972 Case records of the Massachusetts General Hospital. Case 11–1972. New England Journal of Medicine 286: 594–600
39. Kirschner MA, Wider JA, Ross GT 1970 Leydig cell function in men with gonadotrophin-producing testicular tumors. Journal of Clinical Endocrinology and Metabolism 30: 504–511
40. Pesce C, Merino MJ, Chambers JT, Nogales F 1991 Endometrial carcinoma with trophoblastic differentiation: An aggressive form of uterine cancer. Cancer 68: 1799–1802
41. Chico A, García JL, Matias-Guiu X, Webb SM, Rodríguez J, Prat J, Calaf J 1995 A gonadotrophin dependent stromal luteoma: A rare cause of post-menopausal virilization. Clinical Endocrinology 43: 645–649
42. Davy M, Torjesen PA, Aakvaag A 1977 Demonstration of an FSH receptor in a functioning granulosa cell tumor. Acta Endocrinologica 85: 615–623
43. Horvath E, Chalvardjian A, Kovacs K, Singer W 1980 Leydig-like cells in the adrenals of a woman with ectopic ACTH syndrome. Human Pathology 11: 284–287
44. Goldston WR, Johnston WW, Fetter BF, Parker RT, Wilbanks GD 1972 Clinicopathologic studies in feminizing tumors of the ovary I. Some aspects of the pathology and therapy of granulosa cell tumors. American Journal of Obstetrics and Gynecology 112: 422–429
45. Casthely S, Diamandis HP, Pierre-Louis R 1977 Hilar cell tumor of the ovary: diagnostic value of plasma testosterone by selective ovarian vein catheterization. American Journal of Obstetrics and Gynecology 129: 108–110
46. Wong T-W, Warner NE 1971 Ovarian thecal metaplasia in the adrenal gland. Archives of Pathology 92: 319–328

59. An overview of side effects

Philip Darney

Introduction

Synthetic estrogens and progestogens are widely used by both younger and older women. Women who rely solely on hormonal contraceptives during the fertile years and continue hormone replacement therapy (HRT) until death could accumulate 70 years of exposure to exogenous sex steroids. Most of the epidemiologic evidence reviewed in this book shows that prolonged use of sex steroids for contraception premenopausally and replacement afterward confers, on balance, important health benefits. The purpose of this chapter is to examine the so-called 'minor' side effects that occur with the administration of estrogens and progestogens. These side effects are not a direct threat to health, but they often lead to early discontinuation of therapy so that long-term benefits are not achieved. In this way, the 'minor' side effects associated with estrogens and progestogens can not only have adverse consequences for current 'quality of life' but can also become important determinants of future health.

A survey of nearly 10 000 former combined oral contraceptive (COC) users in the USA found moderate differences in the reasons for discontinuation, depending on whether the former user had quit on her own or because of her doctor's advice (Table 59.1).

The effects discussed in this chapter are commonly dose-related, vary with route of administration and type of sex steroid and can be modulated by concomitant use of other drugs. Consideration of these factors helps the clinician plan the treatment of a particular side effect. Many side effects of hormonal contraception or HRT require only explanation and reassurance but some must be ameliorated by some means so that use of hormones can be continued.

CHANGES IN BLEEDING PATTERNS

Irregular uterine bleeding is a major problem for women using hormones for contraception or replacement. Unexpected bleeding (or the unexpected absence of bleeding) gives rise to fears and concerns; it is aggravating and can be embarrassing. Therefore, before starting hormonal therapy of any kind, patients must be fully informed about what menstrual or other bleeding changes are possible, their significance and the possibility of treatment. This knowledge will help candidates for hormonal treatment decide which regimen, if any, might be best for them. And, once they begin treatment, this knowledge will help avoid discouraging surprises that may cause discontinuation before the benefits of long-term treatment are realized.

Bleeding patterns with combined oral contraceptives (COC) (See also ch. 45)

With COC there are two characteristic breakthrough bleeding problems: irregular bleeding in the first few months after starting and unexpected bleeding after many months of use. The bleeding problem should be managed in a way that allows the patient to remain on low dose oral contraception.

Table 59.1 Some reasons for discontinuation of COC use by women in a large USA survey.[1]

Reason	Doctor's advice (%)	Own volition (%)
Headache	12.0	6.4
Bleeding	11.8	6.0
Weight gain	3.4	11.4
Nausea	3.5	10.2
Vascular disease	10.4	3.2
Blood pressure	11.8	1.2

These data and data presented later in this chapter demonstrate that the so-called 'minor' side effects are important determinants of continuation for hormonal contraception as well as hormone replacement therapy.

There is no evidence that the onset of bleeding is associated with decreased efficacy, no matter what oral contraceptive formulation is used, even the lowest dose products. Breakthrough bleeding does not correlate with changes in the blood levels of the contraceptive steroids.[2] An exception to this general statement may be the changes in blood levels which occur with concurrent drug treatment with rifampicin and anti-epileptic drugs.

The most frequently encountered breakthrough bleeding is that which occurs in the first few months of COC use. The incidence is greatest in the first three months, ranging from 10–30% in the first month to less than 10% in the third.

Figure 59.1 shows 'breakthrough bleeding' defined as requiring the use of a pad or tampon (BTB), 'breakthrough spotting' in which no protection is needed (BTS), and all intermenstrual bleeding (IMB) for a large number of women participating in a clinical trial of a desogestrel-ethinyl estradiol (DSG/EE), low dose COC over an 18 month period.[3] This type of bleeding is best managed by encouragement and reassurance. This bleeding usually improves after the third cycle in the majority of women. If necessary, even this early pattern of breakthrough bleeding can be treated as outlined below. It is helpful to explain to the patient that this bleeding represents tissue breakdown as the endometrium adjusts from its usual thick state to the relatively thin state allowed by the hormones in oral contraceptives.

Breakthrough bleeding which occurs after many months of oral contraceptive use is a consequence of progestogen-induced decidualization and suppression. This endometrium is shallow and the vessels tends to be fragile and prone to breakdown with asynchronous bleeding. Management advice tends to be anecdotal, but is often very effective for individual users. If bleeding occurs just before the end of the pill cycle, it can be managed by having the patient stop the pills, wait seven days and start a new cycle. If breakthrough bleeding is prolonged or if it is aggravating for the patient, regardless of the point in the pill cycle, control of the bleeding can usually be achieved with a short course of exogenous estrogen. Conjugated estrogen, 1.25 mg, or estradiol, 2 mg, is administered daily for seven days when the bleeding is present, no matter where the patient is in her pill cycle. The patient continues to adhere to the schedule of pill taking. Usually one course of estrogen solves the problem, and recurrence of bleeding is unusual (but if it does recur, another seven day course of estrogen tends to be effective).

Responding to irregular bleeding by having the patient take two or three pills is not effective. The progestogen component of the pill will always dominate, hence doubling the number of pills will also double the progestational impact and its decidualizing,

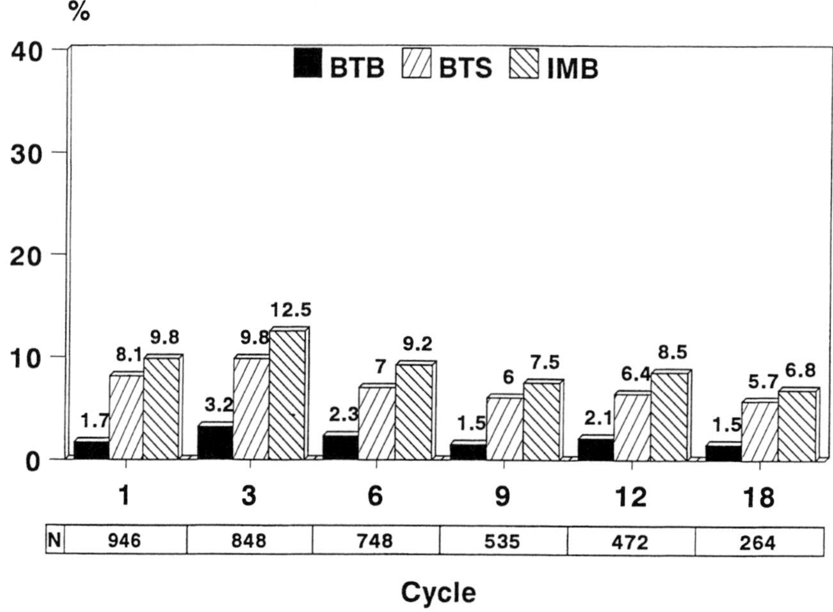

Fig. 59.1 Incidence of cycle control irregularities with triphasic desogestrel-ethinyl estradiol (DSG/EE).

atrophic effect on the endometrium. The addition of extra estrogen while keeping the progestogen dose unchanged is logical and effective. This allows the patient to remain on the low dose formulation with its advantage of greater safety. Breakthrough bleeding is not sufficient reason to expose patients to the marginally increased risks associated with higher dose oral contraceptives. Any bleeding which is not handled by this routine requires investigation for the presence of cervical or endometrial chlamydial infection or neoplasia.

There is no good evidence that any oral contraceptive formulations that are approximately equivalent in estrogen and progestogen dosage are significantly different in the rates of breakthrough bleeding. Clinicians often become impressed that switching to another product effectively stops the breakthrough bleeding. It is more likely that the passage of time is the responsible factor, and bleeding would have stopped regardless of switching and regardless of product.

Amenorrhea

With low dose pills, the estrogen content is not sufficient in some women to stimulate endometrial growth. The progestational effect dominates to such a degree that a shallow atrophic endometrium is produced, lacking sufficient tissue to yield withdrawal bleeding. Permanent atrophy of the endometrium does not occur, and resumption of normal ovarian function will restore endometrial growth and development. Users of COC should be assured that there is no harmful, permanent consequence of amenorrhea while on oral contraception because they may fear that their lack of bleeding signifies current pregnancy, illness or future infecundity.[4,5]

The incidence of amenorrhea in the first year of use with modern, low dose oral contraception is about 2%.[3] This incidence increases with duration, reaching perhaps 5% after several years of use. It is important to alert patients upon starting oral contraception that diminished bleeding and possibly no bleeding may ensue. These effects can then be perceived as benefits preventing unnecessary blood loss and anemia rather than signs of illness.

Amenorrhea is a difficult management problem if the COC user is concerned about risk of pregnancy. A sensitive urine pregnancy test will allow reliable diagnosis even in early gestation. However, routine, repeated use of such testing is expensive and annoying, and may lead to discontinuation of oral contraception. A simple test for pregnancy which the author has found helpful is to assess the basal body temperature during the end of the pill-free week; a basal body temperature less than 98°F is not consistent with pregnancy and oral contraception can be continued.

Many women are reassured with an understanding of why there is no bleeding and are able to continue on the pill despite the amenorrhea. Some women cannot reconcile themselves to a lack of bleeding, and this is an indication for trying other formulations (a practice unsupported by any clinical trials and, therefore, the expectations are uncertain). But the problem does not warrant exposing patients to the slightly greater risks of major side effects associated with estrogen doses of 50 μg or more.

Some clinicians have anecdotally observed that the addition of extra estrogen for one month (1.25 mg conjugated estrogens or 2 mg estradiol daily throughout the 21 days while taking the oral contraceptive) will rejuvenate the endometrium, and withdrawal bleeding will resume, persisting for many months.

Bleeding irregularities with progestogen-only contraception

In view of the unpredictable effect on ovulation, it is not surprising that irregular menstrual bleeding is the major clinical problem with low dose progestogen-only contraceptives like the 'mini pill' and Norplant®. The daily progestational impact on the endometrium contributes to this problem. Patients may experience any menstrual pattern from normal, ovulatory cycles (40%), short, irregular cycles (40%), or a total lack of cycles ranging from irregular bleeding to spotting and amenorrhea (20%). This unpredictability is the major reason why women discontinue progestogen-only methods of contraception.[6] (See also ch. 45.)

Contraceptive implants

Bleeding patterns are more variable among users of Norplant® who use it for the full five years than among users of progestogen-only pills because serum concentrations of the progestogen (levonorgestrel) gradually drop by half from the first to the fifth year of Norplant® use. Some alteration of menstrual patterns will occur during the first year of use in approximately 80% of users.[7,8] The changes include alterations in the interval between bleeding, the duration and volume of menstrual flow and spotting. Oligomenorrhea and amenorrhea also occur, but are less common—fewer than 10% of women after the first year. Irregular and prolonged bleeding are more likely during the first year. Although bleeding problems occur much less frequently after the second year, they can occur at any time (Fig. 59.2).[8,9]

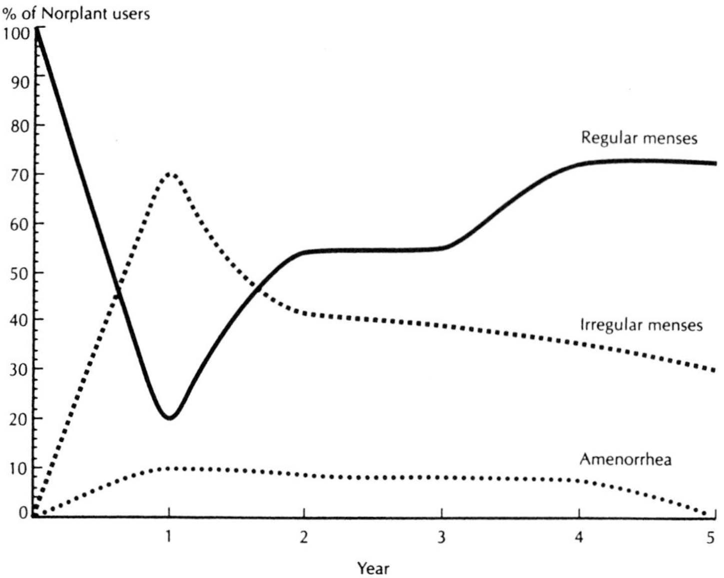

Fig. 59.2 Incidence of different menstrual patterns during long-term use of Norplant®.

Despite an initial increase in the number of spotting and bleeding days over preinsertion menstrual patterns, hemoglobin concentrations rise in Norplant® users because of a decrease in the average volume of menstrual blood loss.[10,11] Although more than 80% of women using Norplant® will experience abnormal bleeding patterns, the majority are not bothered by it if they know what to expect (Table 59.2).[12]

Norplant® users who can no longer tolerate the presence of prolonged bleeding will benefit from a short course of oral estrogen: conjugated estrogens, 1.25 mg, or estradiol, 2 mg, administered daily for seven days. COC (50 µg of ethinyl estradiol and 250 µg of levonorgestrel) taken daily for 20 days were more effective than ethinyl estradiol 50 µg alone in a study by Alvarez and colleagues, but prolonged, high doses of estrogen with or without a progestogen may be contraindicated in women using Norplant® if they are using the progestogen-only method because of risk of thromboembolism.[13] A therapeutic dose of one of the prostaglandin inhibitors given during the bleeding also helps to diminish flow, but estrogen is more effective.[14]

Although the Norplant® system is very effective, pregnancy must be considered in women reporting amenorrhea who have been ovulating previously, as evidenced by regular menses prior to an episode of amenorrhea. A sensitive urine pregnancy test should be obtained. Women who remain amenorrheic throughout their use of Norplant® are most unlikely to become pregnant.[8] It is important to explain to patients the mechanism of the amenorrhea: the local progestational effect causing decidualization and atrophy.

Table 59.2 Changes in menstruation reported by implant users: family planning clinic, San Francisco General Hospital.[3]

Menstrual changes	Total (n=205)	Percent current users (n=140)	Past users* (n=65)
Experienced changes	86	89	82
Very/moderately bothered	31	21	51
Slightly/not bothered	69	79	49

*Discontinuers

Bleeding with injectable progestogens

Depot medroxyprogesterone acetate (DMPA; Depo-Provera; Pharmacia and Upjohn) is the most commonly used injectable progestogen. It finds widest use as a highly effective contraceptive when 150 mg are injected every three months, but is also used in much higher doses to treat endometriosis and endometrial and breast cancers. The relative serum concentrations of progestogen from DMPA injections are much higher than from progestogen (mini) pills or implants (Norplant®). Follicular suppression is more complete and ovarian estradiol secretion is less; with estradiol concentrations in the low-normal range combined with high progestogen exposure the endometrium eventually becomes atrophic.[15] Norethindrone enanthate (NET-EN), 200 mg each two months, is an injectable contraceptive that is slightly less effective than DMPA, but is equally disruptive to the menstrual cycle.

Up to 25% of injectable progestogen users discontinue in the first year because of irregular bleeding.[16] The bleeding is rarely heavy; in fact, hemoglobin values rise in DMPA users. The incidence of irregular bleeding is 70% in the first 6–12 months and 10% thereafter. Bleeding and spotting decrease progressively with each re-injection so that after five years, 80% of users are amenorrheic (compared to 10% of Norplant® users) (Fig. 59.3).[17] NET-EN is less likely to cause amenorrhea, but many women prefer absence of bleeding to unpredictable bleeding.

Once-a-month injectable contraceptives which contain estrogen in addition to progestogen have fewer bleeding problems. They are available in only a few countries. Examples include Mesigyna (norethindrone enanthate, 50 mg, and estradiol valerate, 5 mg) and Cyclofem (DMPA, 25 mg, and estradiol cypionate, 5 mg). Mesigyna is associated with better bleeding patterns. The addition of estrogen is generally accepted as limiting the use of these injectables to women at low risk of thromboembolic diseases.

As with Norplant®, bleeding can be treated with exogenous estrogen, 1.25 mg conjugated estrogens or 2 mg estradiol, given daily for seven days. A non-steroidal anti-inflammatory product given for a week is also helpful. Giving the DMPA injection earlier (more frequently) sometimes improves the bleeding pattern, but this has not been shown in all studies.[18] Most women can wait for amenorrhea or hypomenorrhea without treatment if they know what to expect with time.

About half of the women who discontinue DMPA can expect normal menses to return in six months after the last injection, but 25% will wait a year before resumption of a normal pattern.[17]

Hormone replacement therapy (HRT) and bleeding (See also ch. 52)

As with contraceptive estrogens and progestogens, the most common cause of discontinuation of HRT is

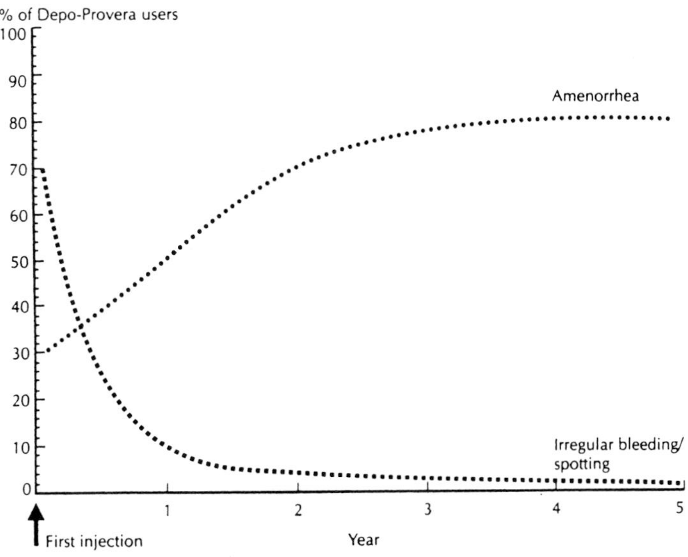

Fig. 59.3 Incidence of different menstrual patterns during long-term use of DMPA.

abnormal bleeding. Since HRT is used at a time in life when women expect not to have vaginal bleeding, any bleeding at all can be a problem. Bleeding may be unacceptable not just to women receiving HRT, but also to the clinicians providing it, who, when bleeding occurs, must worry about endometrial disease and weigh the need for biopsy.[19]

With daily dosage of estrogen (either every day or the first 25 days of each calendar month) and sequential progestogen (usually the first 12–14 days of each calendar month or the last 12–14 days of estrogen use) withdrawal bleeding occurs in 80–90% of patients.[20] A reduction of the progestogen dose from 10 to 5 mg of medroxyprogesterone acetate (MPA) or its equivalent, sometimes reduces side effects such as breast tenderness, fluid retention, depression and bleeding, but the lowest effective dose of progestogen for endometrial protection has not been clearly established, so the standard for sequential therapy remains 10 mg of MPA.

Continuous (combined) administration of estrogen (conjugated, 0.625 mg, or micronized estradiol, 1.0 mg) and progestogen (MPA, 2.5 mg, or norethindrone, 0.35 mg) eliminates withdrawal-type bleeding, but breakthrough bleeding occurs in about half of the patients during the first six months of treatment, decreasing to 20% after the first year. Increasing the progestogen dose yields only a small improvement in this bleeding rate, and may cause other side effects.[21] If significant breakthrough bleeding persists after two years, sequential administration to obtain orderly withdrawal bleeding and reduce anxiety about endometrial cancer may be the better choice. It is not necessary to biopsy the endometrium whenever bleeding occurs unless there are other reasons to suspect endometrial cancer. Since the progestogen effect predominates, a biopsy almost always produces only atrophic endometrial tissue. If bleeding persists after a year of combined therapy, a transvaginal ultrasound scan or hysteroscopic search for endometrial polyps or myomas is worthwhile. Delivery of levonorgestrel with an intra-uterine device has been shown to protect the endometrium while reducing the incidence of bleeding.[22]

WEIGHT GAIN

Increasing body weight is a frequent complaint among users of hormonal contraception and a common reason for discontinuation. The magnitude of weight gain is difficult to document, but seems to vary widely by population studied and by method of contraception. The greatest weight gain occurs in users of DMPA, less in Norplant® users, and least in COC users. Weight gain is less often stated as a problem associated with HRT.

Weight and COC

The complaint of weight gain is frequently cited as a major problem with COC continuation, but studies of the low dose preparations fail to demonstrate a significant mean weight gain with users of oral contraception, and show no major differences among the various products.[23] This may be a problem of perception and may involve confusion with abdominal bloating. The clinician has to carefully reinforce the lack of association between low dose oral contraceptives and weight gain and focus the patient on diet and level of exercise. Most women gain a moderate amount of weight as they age, whether they take oral contraceptives or not. Nevertheless, there is the occasional individual in whom increased weight gain does appear to have been associated with COC use, and the increase ceases with COC discontinuation.

Weight and DMPA

Although clinicians generally accept that DMPA causes more weight gain than other contraceptives, attempts to document a greater weight gain specifically associated with DMPA have not been successful.[24] As with oral contraception, the weight gain may not usually be hormone-induced, but more reflect lifestyle and ageing. Studies of long-term use show a progressive mean gain of about 2 kg per year, but this may be due to the population studied rather than DMPA.[25]

Weight and progestogen implants (Norplant®)

Women using Norplant more frequently complain of weight gain than of weight loss, but findings are variable. In the Dominican Republic, 75% of those who changed weight actually lost, while in San Francisco, two-thirds gained. Assessment of weight change in Norplant® users is confounded by changes in exercise, diet and ageing. Only 36% of women reporting weight gain with Norplant® in San Francisco said that they lost weight after having the implants removed (Table 59.3).[26] It seems unlikely that the low levels of levonorgestrel with Norplant® have significant anabolic effect. Counselling for weight changes should include dietary review and focus on dietary habits. Indeed, a five year follow-up of 75 women with Norplant® implants could document no increase in

Table 59.3 Primary and secondary reasons for discontinuation of Norplant use and resolution of symptoms at follow up among users at San Francisco General Hospital, 1989 (n = 200).*

Reason for discontinuation	Primary(%)	Secondary(%)	Resolution of symptoms Resolved(%)	Unresolved(%)	Unknown(%)
Completed 5 years of use	19	0	–	–	–
Menstrual changes	17	11	61	5	34
Prolonged bleeding	9	2	71	5	24
Irregular menses	4	3	54	0	46
Menorrhagia	3	2	78	0	22
Dysmenorrhea	2	4	40	20	40
Amenorrhea	1	1	33	0	67
Headache	11	4	76	14	10
Weight gain	10	4	36	28	36
Not sexually active	8	4	–	–	–
Moving from area	7	2	–	–	–
Desires pregnancy	6	2	–	–	–
Mood changes	6	5	57	10	33
Weight loss	2	3	63	37	0
Acne	1	5	73	17	10
Other personal and medical	15	7	64	15	21

*Percentages do not add up to 100 due to rounding.

the body mass index (nor was there a correlation between irregular bleeding and body weight).[27]

ANDROGENIC EFFECTS OF CONTRACEPTIVE PROGESTOGENS

When weight gain occurs it is more likely due to the progestogenic effect of appetite stimulation rather than the androgenic effect of anabolism. This idea is supported by evidence that DMPA, which is a very weak binder to androgen receptors, causes more weight gain than does levonorgestrel — a strong binder. Side effects related to the skin are classified as 'androgenic' because they occur more frequently with progestogens which bind avidly to androgen receptors. Acne, hirsutism and alopecia are examples of these effects. They occur more commonly with levonorgestrel implants than with DMPA. COC users can experience them if the androgenic effect of the COC progestogen overcomes the contrary effect of the COC estrogen. Since androgenic progestogens are not commonly used in HRT, complaints related to skin changes are rare.

Acne

Low dose oral contraceptives tend to improve acne regardless of which product is used.[28] The low progestogen doses (including levonorgestrel formulations) currently used are insufficient to stimulate an androgenic response, but acne is more responsive to COC containing the less-androgenic progestogens[29] because these compounds lower free androgen concentrations more.[30] An example of this effect is shown in Figures 59.4 and 59.5 for levonorgestrel as compared to the less androgenic desogestrel. Cyproterone acetate-containing COC may be more effective because of the antiandrogenic effect of the cyproterone.

The levonorgenstrel minipill may occasionally cause acne. The mechanism is similar to that seen with Norplant®. The androgenic activity of levonorgestrel decreases the circulating levels of sex hormone-binding globulin (SHBG). Therefore, free steroid levels (levonorgestrel and testosterone) are increased despite the low dose. This is in contrast to the action of combined oral contraception where the effect of the

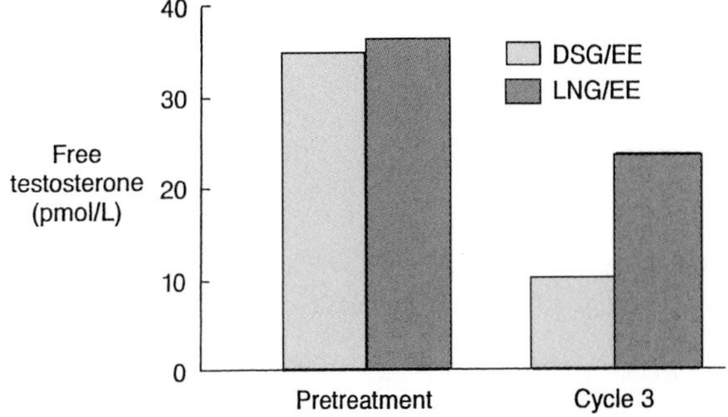

Fig. 59.4 Free testosterone concentrations with two monophasict (COC) combined oral contraceptives.

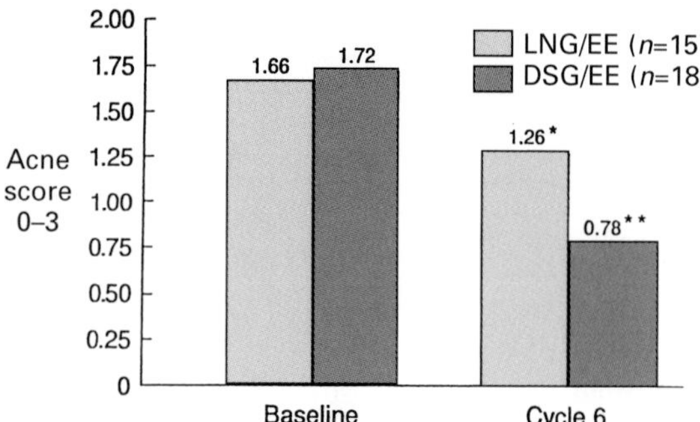

Fig. 59.5 Acne score: comparison trial of levonorgestrel-ethinyl estradiol (LNG/EE) and desogestrel-ethinyl estradiol (DSG/EE). (* = $P < 0.01$; ** = $P < 0.001$)

progestogen is countered by the estrogen-induced increase in SHBG.[31]

Acne is rarely seen with DMPA, even though serum concentrations of the progestogen are relatively much higher than with the minipill or Norplant®. Medroxyprogesterone acetate does not bind readily to androgen receptors and, therefore, does not decrease SHBG concentrations or displace bound testosterone from SHBG.[32] Cyproterone acetate is an example of a progesterone derivative with moderate antiandrogenic activity. In combination with ethinyl estradiol, it is used to treat acne as well as prevent ovulation. It is available widely throughout the world but not in the USA.

Acne, with or without an increase in oil production, is the most common skin complaint among Norplant® users. The acne is caused by the androgenic activity of the levonorgestrel which produces a direct impact and also causes a decrease in sex hormone-binding globulin (SHBG) levels leading to an increase in free steroid levels (both levonorgestrel and testosterone).[33] This is in contrast to combined oral contraceptives which contain levonorgestrel, where the estrogen effect on SHBG (an increase) produces a decrease in unbound (free) androgens. Common therapies for complaints of acne include dietary change, practice of good skin hygiene with the use of soaps or skin cleansers, and oral tetracyclines or application of topical antibiotics (e.g. 1% clindamycin solution or gel, or topical erythromycin). Use of local or oral antibiotics helps most users to continue Norplant® despite acne (see Table 59.3).

Alopecia, hirsutism and acanthosis nigricans are other androgenic side effects that have been reported in users of Norplant® and, less frequently, in COC and DMPA users. These are unusual effects which cannot be demonstrated to occur more commonly in users of contraceptive progestogens than in nonusers. No well controlled trials have specifically examined the incidence of these androgenic side effects. COC are often used to treat hirsutism and alopecia because they lower androgen levels,[34] but some women complain of these conditions after beginning COC. For such patients switching to a COC containing a less androgenic progestogen (desogestrel, norgestimate, gestodene, or cyproterone acetate) may be helpful.[35,36]

NONANDROGENIC CHANGES IN SKIN PIGMENTATION

Melasmic (chloasmic) hyperpigmentation can occur during treatment with sex steroids. Unlike the androgenic changes described above, hyperpigmentation, which commonly affects the areolar and genital skin during pregnancy, is thought to be due to the effects of increased melanocyte-stimulating hormone (MSH) or estrogen and progesterone on epidermal melanocytes.[37] During pregnancy these changes are occasionally diffuse, most commonly involving the face (forehead, cheeks, and nose bridge — the so-called 'mask' of pregnancy), but sometimes other sun-exposed areas. Melasma usually disappears as sex steroid levels decline after delivery.

Similar changes can occur with the use of COC, but much less commonly than during pregnancy. COC-associated melasma is dose-related so that COC containing 50 μg or more of estrogen are more likely to cause skin darkening and postmenopausal hormone replacement therapy is least likely to. Melanotic nevi may rarely be stimulated by estrogens, but there is no evidence that, when sun exposure is taken into account, COC increase the risk of malignant melanoma.[38,39]

Women who experience facial melasma during pregnancy should avoid prolonged sun exposure and use topical sunscreens (sun protection factor 15 or greater) if they take COC. If melasmic changes do not regress after discontinuing COC, topical hydroquinone bleaching creams, tretinoin or chemical peels may help.

Progestogen-only contraceptives (oral, implants or injections) are also occasionally associated with melasma, but much less frequently than COC. The mechanism is unclear: progestogen-only contraceptives decrease endogenous production of estrogen and progesterone to varying degrees. Acanthosis nigricans, an androgenically-stimulated skin darkening that is associated with diabetes, should not be mistaken for benign melasma.

Hyperpigmentation can occur directly over the site of contraceptive implants in about 5% of users, most often those with dark skin. It usually disappears slowly after implant removal and is not usually associated with hyperpigmentation of the face or other areas.

OTHER SIDE EFFECTS

Benign breast changes

Breast changes occur commonly in users of contraceptive steroids and uncommonly with HRT. These are benign and usually self-limited (the possible association of exogenous estrogens and progestogens with breast cancer is reviewed in detail in chapter 68). The most common complaint with COC is breast swelling or tenderness later in the pill cycle in the first three or four months of use. These symptoms are most common with higher-dose COC and uncommon with modern, low-dose preparations. If symptoms persist beyond the first few cycles of COC use, a lower-dose pill should be tried.

Use of COC for more than two years has been associated with a reduced incidence of fibrocystic breast symptoms,[40] but this benefit is not clearly established for progestogen-only contraceptives.

Among progestogen implant (Norplant®) users bilateral mastalgia, often occurring premenstrually, and associated with complaints of fluid retention occurs in less than 1% of women.[26] After pregnancy has been ruled out as a cause of breast pain, reassurance and therapy aimed at symptomatic relief are indicated. This symptom may be due to temporary follicular estradiol production which is greater in those women with lower levels of levonorgestrel. Most Norplant® users improve spontaneously or respond to treatment and do not elect to remove the implants. Breast complaints are uncommon among users of progestogen-only pills, DMPA or HRT.

Careful assessments of the relationship between methylxanthines and mastalgia have failed to demonstrate a link. Nevertheless, avoiding coffee, tea and chocolate seems to help some women. The most effective treatments for breast pain are the following: danazol (200 mg/day), vitamin E (600 units/day), bromocriptine (2.5 mg/day) or tamoxifen (20 mg/day), but there are no studies of these treatments in users of contraceptive steroids.

Galactorrhea

Galactorrhea is more common among women who begin a steroid contraceptive during or upon discontinuation of lactation. Pregnancy and prolactin-secreting tumors should be ruled out by performing a pregnancy test and, if indicated by other symptoms, a prolactin determination. Patients should be reassured that mild galactorrhea is not unusual among implant and oral contraceptive users. Decreasing the amount of breast and nipple stimulation may decrease the symptoms.

Ovarian cysts

Oral contraceptives and DMPA completely suppress ovulation in almost all users; this effect is the source of obvious benefits like reduced incidence of ovarian cancer and cysts and ectopic pregnancy. The magnitude and mechanisms of these protective effects are covered elsewhere in this book, but the ovulatory effects of low-dose progestogen-only contraceptives are included here because they can result in side effects that cause discontinuation.

Unlike oral contraception, the low serum progestogen levels maintained by Norplant® or progestogen-only pills do not suppress FSH which continues to stimulate ovarian follicle growth in most users. The LH peak during the first two years of Norplant® use, on the other hand, is usually abolished so that these follicles do not ovulate.[41] However, some continue to grow and cause pain or be palpated at the time of pelvic examination.[42] Adnexal masses are approximately eight times more frequent in Norplant® users compared to normally cycling women. Because these are simple follicular cysts (and most regress spontaneously within one month of detection), they need not be sonographically or laparoscopically evaluated. Further evaluation is indicated if they became large and painful or fail to regress. Regular ovulators are less likely to form cysts so the situation is likely to improve after two–three years of Norplant® use. Those who continue to be bothered should be switched to contraceptives that suppress ovulation — COC or DMPA.

Headaches

The central nervous system effects of estrogens and progestogens which lead to depression, altered libido and other mood changes are complex and incompletely understood. They are addressed in chapters 17 and 64. The cerebral symptom that is most common and most likely to prompt discontinuation of contraception or HRT is headache.

Among Norplant® users, for example, the most common side effect reported is headache; about 20%

of women who discontinue use do so because of headache.[12,43] As shown in Table 59.3, when women with headaches discontinued Norplant®, 76% reported three months later that the headaches had resolved, but a significant proportion found no relief. In a large international study of DMPA, the most common medical reason for discontinuing was headache, followed by weight gain, dizziness, abdominal pain and anxiety.[44,45] Whether DMPA actually causes these side effects is difficult to know since they are very common complaints in nonusers[46], and they are also frequently reported during placebo use.

As shown in Table 59.1, headache is also a principal cause of COC discontinuation.[1] True migraine headaches are more common in women, while tension headaches occur equally in men and women. There have been no well-executed studies to determine the impact of oral contraception on migraine headaches. Patients may report that their headaches are worse, unchanged or better.

Early observational studies with high-dose pills suggested that focal migraine was linked to a risk of stroke. More recent studies reflecting the use of low-dose formulations yield mixed results. One failed to find a further increase in stroke in patients with migraines who use oral contraception, another concluded that the use of oral contraception by those with migraines was associated with a four fold increase of the already increased risk of ischemic stroke.[47,48] Because of the seriousness of this potential complication, the onset of focal visual or sensory symptoms or severe headaches requires evaluation. If the patient is at a higher dose, a move to a low-dose formulation may relieve the headaches. Switching to a different brand is worthwhile, if only to assess a placebo response. True vascular headaches (classic migraine) may be an indication to avoid or discontinue oral contraception. If a patient insists on using oral contraception, a product containing 20 mg estrogen should be used, if available.

In a small minority of women, a relationship exists between their fluctuating hormone levels during a menstrual cycle and migraine headaches, with the onset of headaches characteristically coinciding with menses. Headaches may be alleviated by eliminating the menstrual cycle, either with the use of continuous daily oral contraceptives or the daily administration of a progestational agent (such as 10 mg medroxyprogesterone acetate). Some women with migraine headaches have extremely gratifying responses. Women who experience an exacerbation of their headaches with oral contraception should consider one of the progestogen-only methods.

Nausea and edema

A final group of side effects occurring with estrogen treatment are nausea, leg edema, and a feeling of 'bloating' or abdominal swelling. These symptoms are more common with higher dose COC; with lower doses they usually disappear after two or three cycles if they are present at all. The low doses of estrogen used in HRT are less commonly associated with these symptoms.

Some women using low-dose progestogen pills or implants report symptoms of edema and 'bloating' like those which previously accompanied their menses. If nausea or swelling persist beyond the first few months of COC use, a different, preferably lower-dose, preparation should be tried. Women who have 'premenstrual' symptoms on progestogen-only contraceptives may feel better on COC. All such symptoms can be more persistent among users of DMPA because it can take several months for the drug to leave the circulation. For heavier women, it takes longer.

Conclusion

Estrogen and progestogen administration for contraception and hormone replacement therapy is associated with side effects which sometimes make continuation of the hormones difficult for women. Some of these side effects, such as bleeding abnormalities and androgenic skin changes, are clearly related to the type and dose of steroid, but others, such as weight change and headache, are not clear and direct results of the hormones. In either case, changes in dose, type of progestogen or route of administration often relieves symptoms, allowing the hormone user to obtain the long-term health benefits of exogenous estrogen and progestogen treatment.

REFERENCES

1. Pratt WF, Bachrach CA 1987 What do women use when they stop using the pill? Family Planning Perspectives 19: 257
2. Jung-Hoffman C, Kuhl H 1990 Intra- and interindividual variations in contraceptive steroid levels during 12 treatment cycles: no relation to irregular bleedings. Contraception 42: 423
3. Darney P 1993 Safety and efficacy of a triphasic oral contraceptive containing desogestrel: results of three multicenter trials. Contraception 48: 328

4. Furuhjelm M, Carlstrom K 1973 Amenorrhea following use of combined oral contraceptives. Acta Obstetrica Gynecologica Scandinavica 52: 373
5. Jacobs HS, Knuth UA, Hull MGR, Franks S 1977 Post 'pill' amenorrhoea — cause or coincidence? British Medical Journal 2: 940
6. Brache V, Faundes A, Johansson E, Alvarez F 1985 Anovulation, inadequate luteal phase, and poor sperm penetration in cervical mucus during prolonged use of Norplant implants. Contraception 31: 261
7. Sivin I, Alvarez-Sanchez F, Diaz S, Holma P, Coutinho E, McDonald O, Robertson DN, Stern J 1983 Three-year experience with Norplant subdermal contraception. Fertility and Sterility 39: 799
8. Shoupe D, Mishell DR Jr, Bopp B, Fiedling M 1991 The significance of bleeding patterns in Norplant implant users. Obstetrics and Gynecology 77: 256
9. Sivin I, Diaz S, Holma P, Alvarez-Sanchez F, Robertson DN 1983 A four-year clinical study of Norplant implants. Studies in Family Planning 14: 184
10. Nilsson C, Holma P 1981 Menstrual blood loss with contraceptive subdermal levonorgestrel implants. Fertility and Sterility 35: 304
11. Fakeye O, Balogh S 1989 Effect of Norplant contraceptive use on hemoglobin, packed cell volume, and menstrual bleeding patterns. Contraception 39: 265
12. Darney PD, Elizabeth A, Tanner S, MacPherson S, Hellerstein S, Alvarado A 1990 Acceptance and perceptions of Norplant among users in San Francisco, USA. Studies in Family Planning 21: 152
13. Alvarez-Sanchez F, Brache V, Thevenin F, Cochon L, Faundes A 1996 Hormonal treatment for bleeding irregularities in Norplant implant users. American Journal of Obstetrics and Gynecology 174: 919
14. Diaz S, Croxatto HB, Pavez M, Belhadj H, Stern J, Sivin I 1990 Clinical assessment of treatments for prolonged bleeding in users of Norplant implants. Contraception 42: 97
15. Mishell DR Jr, Kharma KM, Thorneycroft IH et al 1972 Estrogenic activity in women receiving an injectable progestogen for contraception, American Journal of Obstetrics and Gynecology 113: 372
16. Cromer BA, Smith RD, Blair JM, Dwyer J, Brown R 1994 A prospective study of adolescents who choose among levonorgestrel implant (Norplant), medroxyprogesterone acetate (Depo Provera), or the combined oral contraceptive pill as contraception. Pediatrics 94: 687
17. Gardner JM, Mishell DR Jr 1970 Analysis of bleeding patterns and resumption of fertility following discontinuation of a long-acting injectable contraceptive. Fertility and Sterility 21: 286
18. Harel Z, Biro FM, Kollar LM 1995 Depo-Provera in adolescents: effects of early second injection or prior oral contraception. Journal of Adolescent Health 16: 379
19. Ravnikar VA 1987 Compliance with hormonal therapy. American Journal of Obstetrics and Gynecology 156: 1332
20. Strickland DM, Hammond TL 1988 Postmenopausal estrogen replacement in a large gynecologic practice. American Journal of Gynecological Health 2: 33
21. Archer DF, Pickar JH, Bottiglioni F, for The Menopausal Study Group Bleeding patterns in postmenopausal women taking continuous combined or sequential regimens of conjugated estrogens with medroxyprogesterone acetate. in press.
22. Andersson K, Mattsson L, Rybo G, Stadberg E 1992 Intrauterine release of levonorgestrel—a new way of adding progestogen in hormone replacement therapy. Obstetrics and Gynecology 79: 963
23. Carpenter S, Neinstein LS 1986 Weight gain in adolescent and young adult oral contraceptive users. Journal of Adolescent Health Care 7: 342
24. Moore LL, Valuck R, McDougall C, Fink W 1995 A comparative study of one-year weight gain among users of medroxyprogesterone acetate, levonorgestrel implants, and oral contraceptives. Contraception 52: 215
25. Mainwaring R, Hales HA, Stevenson K, Hatasaka HH, Poulson AM, Jones KP, Peterson CM 1995 Metabolic parameters, bleeding, and weight changes in US women using progestin only contraceptives. Contraception 51: 149
26. Darney PD, Klaisle CM, Tanner ST, Alvarado AM 1990 Sustained release contraceptives. Current Problems in Obstetrics, Gynecology and Fertility 13: 87
27. Pasquale SA, Knuppel RA, Owens AG, Bachmann GA 1994 Irregular bleeding, body mass index and coital frequency in Norplant contraceptive users. Contraception 50: 109
28. van der Vange N, Blankenstein MA, Kloosterboer HJ, Haspels AA, Thijssen JHH 1990 Effects of seven low-dose combined oral contraceptives on sex hormone binding globulin, corticosteroid binding globulin, total and free testosterone. Contraception 41: 345
29. Lemay A, Dewailly SD, Grenier R, Huard J 1990 Attenuation of mild hyperandrogenic activity in postpubertal acne by a triphasic oral contraceptive containing low doses of ethynyl estradiol and d,1-norgestrel. Journal of Clinical Endocrinology and Metabolism 71: 8
30. Palatsi R, Hirvensalo E, Liukko P et al 1984 Serum total and unbound testosterone and sex hormone binding globulin in female acne patients treated with two different oral contraceptives. Acta Derm Venerol (Stockh) 64: 517
31. Hammond G, Langley M, Robinson P et al 1984 Serum steroid binding protein concentrations and bioavailibility of testosterone with oral contraceptives. Fertility and Sterility 42: 44
32. Jeppson S, Gershagen S, Johansson EDB et al 1982 Plasma levels of medroxyprogesterone acetate (MPA), sex-hormone binding globulin, gonadal steroids, gonadotrophins and prolactin in women during long-term use of depo-MPA (Depo Provera) as a contraceptive agent. Acta Endocrinologica 99: 339
33. Affandi B, Cekan SZ, Bookasemsanti, Samil RS, Diczfalusy E 1987 The interaction between sex hormone binding globulin and levonorgestrel released from Norplant, an implantable contraceptive. 35: 135
34. Darney P 1995 The androgenicity of progestins. American Medical Journal 98 (Suppl 1A): 104
35. Cullberg G, Hamburger L, Mattsson L et al 1985 Effects of desogestrel/ethinyl estradiol hirsutism, androgens and SHBG. Acta Obstetrica Gynecologica Scandinavica 64: 195
36. Porcile A, Gallardo E 1991 Oral contraceptives containing desogestrel in hirsutism. Contraception 44: 533

37. Altmeyer P, Bernd A, Holymann M et al 1989 Alpha-MSM and pregnancy. 2 Houtkr 64: 577
38. Hannaford PC, Villard-Mackintosh L, Vessey MP, Kay CR 1991 Oral contraceptives and malignant melanoma. British Journal of Cancer 63: 430
39. Green A 1991 Oral contraceptives and skin neoplasia. Contraception 43: 653
40. World Health Organization 1990 Collaborative study of neoplasia and steroid contraceptives, breast cancer and combined oral contraceptives: results from a multinational study. British Journal of Cancer 61: 110
41. Alvarez F, Brache V, Tejada AS, Faundes A 1986 Abnormal endocrine profile among women with confirmed or presumed ovulation during long-term Norplant use. Contraception 33: 111
42. Faundes A, Brache V, Tejada AS, Cochon L, Alvarez-Sanchez F 1991 Ovulatory dysfunction during continuous administration of low-dose levonorgestrel by subdermal implants. Fertility and Sterility 56: 27
43. Gu S, Du M, Zhang L, Liu YL, Wang SH, Sivin I 1994 A 5-year evaluation of Norplant contraceptive implants in China. Obstetrics and Gynecology 83: 673
44. World Health Organization 1986 A multicentered phase III comparative clinical trial of depot-medroxyprogesterone acetate given three-monthly at doses of 100 mg or 150 mg I. Contraceptive efficacy and side effects. Contraception 34: 223
45. World Health Organization 1983 A multinational comparative clinical evaluation of two long-acting injectable contraceptive steroids: norethisterone enanthate and medroxyprogesterone acetate. Final report. Contraception 28: 1
46. Westhoff C, Weiland D, Tiezzi L 1995 Depression in users of depomedroxyprogesterone acetate. Contraception 51: 351
47. Tzourio C, Tehindrazanarierelo A, IglÇsias S, AlpÇrovitch, Chgedru F, d'Anglejan-Chatillon J, Bousser M-G 1995 Case-control study of migraine and risk of ischaemic stroke in young women. British Medical Journal 310: 830
48. Lidegaard O 1995 Oral contraceptives, pregnancy and the risk of cerebral thromboembolism: the influence of diabetes, hypertension, migraine and previous thrombotic disease. British Journal of Obstetrics and Gynecology 102: 153

60. Non-therapeutic beneficial effects

Gabor T. Kovacs

Introduction

The two broad groups of hormonal therapeutic agents that will be considered in this section are the oral contraceptives and hormones used for replacement therapy during and after the menopause.

ORAL CONTRACEPTIVES

These preparations were revolutionary when first introduced in that they were being administered not for the treatment of an established disease, the accepted role for medication, but as a way of preventing 'disease'. This concept of prophylactic therapeutics was rather revolutionary in the 1960s, especially when we consider that the 'disease' they were to prevent was not life threatening, but life producing, i.e. pregnancy. Nevertheless they soon became widely accepted and used, with over 80 million women taking them worldwide by 1977.[1] It also was accepted that such benefits as oral contraceptives had to offer were not without some risks, and case reports of side effects such as pulmonary embolism,[2] cerebrovascular accidents[3] and coronary thrombosis[4] were reported within a couple of years of initial marketing in the United Kingdom. Subsequently a retrospective study by the Royal College of General Practitioners (RCGP) Birmingham Research Unit was the first to establish a significant association between the use of oral contraceptives and venous thrombosis.[5] These findings led to the establishment of a prospective study by the RCGP which published its first report in 1974.[6] This report examined total morbidity and benefits in pill users, and showed that the benefits outweighed the risks. When this study was expanded[7] and its findings published in 1977, they confirmed that there was increased risk of death from cardiovascular disease in oral contraceptive users, but this particularly applied to women over 35 years of age, women who smoked, and appeared to be related to continuous pill use of over five years. The debate about the rate of cardiovascular complications continues to the present day, with several recent reports suggesting that the third generation progestogen (desogestrel and gestodene) containing oral contraceptives result in an increased incidence of thromboembolic disease compared with second generation formulations. These studies are discussed in detail in chapter 44 and an excellent brief summary of the situation can be found in the Lancet Commentary, December 1995.[8]

This section however will concentrate on the beneficial 'side effects' of oral contraceptives, that is effects that are not the primary function of preventing pregnancy, but other beneficial effects on body systems that are a by-product of their hormonal action. An excellent review of the benefits of oral contraceptives was presented in the 1989 Jephcott Lecture by Vessey.[9]

Menstrual effects

Regularization and control of menstrual cycle

Without doubt, the most significant beneficial side effect of oral contraceptives is on the menstrual cycle. In an Australian survey[10] in 1985 it was found that 20% of 1377 young women on no medications had visited their doctor because of menstrual problems. Of these, 38% attended because of menstrual irregularity. A postal survey carried out in Oxford found that women on oral contraceptives were much less likely to have irregular cycles.[11]

When the first pill Enovid was licensed by the American Food and Drug Administration in 1959, it was marketed as a hormone preparation which was taken for 21 days, with seven day breaks, so as to convert all women into the perfect menstrual pattern of 28 day cycles. This may be a great benefit for women whose cycles were irregular. Many women have been prescribed oral contraceptives to regulate their cycles and produce predictable menstruation.

It has been widely believed that women like to menstruate regularly, and are reassured by the appearance of menses. However an Australian study of 1377 young women in 1985 found that 80% found menstruation inconvenient and embarrassing.[10] The use of the oral contraceptive not only allows irregular cycles to be regulated, but can also allow for menstruation to be less frequent. The concept of less frequent menstruation on oral contraceptives was first reported by Loudon and colleagues,[12] and was recently reactivated[13] when we reviewed our experience through Family Planning Victoria. The main disadvantage of the method is some initial breakthrough bleeding with breast tenderness and headaches as the other reported disadvantages. These studies concluded that the trimonthly regimen is a useful and much appreciated method for many women, and should be more widely offered.

Another advantage of prolonged administration of hormone and less frequent pill-free days, is that there is less chance of inadvertent pregnancy if pills are omitted or malabsorbed.[14]

In summary, one of the most significant beneficial side effects of oral contraceptives is their ability to re-regulate the menstrual cycle. Although conventionally oral contraceptives are prescribed on a 'three weeks on one week off' basis, many women use it to regulate their menstruation, and consideration should be given to recommending to women that they may use it in bimonthly or trimonthly regimens.

Decreasing dysmenorrhea

The 'menstrual cycle problems survey' of Abrahams and colleagues[10] found that dysmenorrhea was second only to cycle irregularity as the reason for consulting the doctor about menstrual problems, accounting for 35% of consultations. Menstrual pain is discussed in detail in chapters 31 and 32, including its mechanisms, etiology and pathogenesis. It suffices here to say that dysmenorrhea is most uncommon in anovulatory cycles, and oral contraceptives significantly improve most (about 70–80%) cases of primary dysmenorrhea. This again is confirmed in the Oxford postal survey.[11] A Tasmanian survey of women using oral contraceptives[15] found that dysmenorrhea improved from a score of 3.1 to 2.3 on an analog score from 1 to 5. If dysmenorrhea is not relieved or significantly improved by anovulants, then a pathological cause such as endometriosis or pelvic inflammatory disease must be excluded.

Decreasing menorrhagia

Menorrhagia is another of the most common presenting symptoms in gynecology clinics, yet in the 'menstrual cycle problems survey' of Abrahams and colleagues[10] surprisingly it accounted for only 4% of general practitioner consultations. One of the first lines of treatment of menorrhagia in young women is to use a monophasic and progestogenic combined oral contraceptive pill. Most women with menorrhagia report decreased menstrual loss with oral contraceptives, and there is a significant decrease in the incidence of anemia for women on the pill.[16] Objective measurement of menstrual bloodloss and hemoglobin levels confirm this. The Tasmanian women taking oral contraceptives[15] reported that the quantity of their menstruation decreased significantly on oral contraceptives from 3.4 to 2.6 on an analog scale of 1 to 5.

Decreasing premenstrual syndrome

The physiology of premenstrual syndrome is poorly understood, and chapter 33 discusses its epidemiology and pathophysiology in detail. There is also a very detailed account of the numerous medical and psychosocial approaches to therapy. Sufficient here to say that many women who suffer from premenstrual syndrome find that the symptoms improve with combined oral contraceptives.[19] The accepted explanation for this is that rather than the physiological fluctuations of estrogen, and more importantly progesterone, during the menstrual cycle, the pharmacological administration of the same dose of estrogen and progestogen continuously throughout the cycle smooths these symptoms. Supportive evidence comes from the finding that monophasic oral contraceptives are associated with less premenstrual syndrome (PMS) than triphasics. Interestingly, in the 'menstrual cycle problems survey' of Abraham and colleagues[10] only 2% of consultations for menstrual problems were premenstrual tension related. It also needs to be pointed out that the Oxford postal survey did not find a decrease in PMS in pill takers.[11]

Functional ovarian cysts

During the normal menstrual cycle an ovarian follicle develops, ruptures at ovulation and then forms into a corpus luteum. Should the follicle not rupture but keep growing, a follicular cyst results. Should the corpus luteum seal over and fill with blood or secretions, a corpus luteum cyst develops. With the follicular and ovulation inhibition activity of monophasic oral contraceptives, follicles do not usually develop, and functional cysts are uncommon.[20] Not only does this prevent unnecessary intervention in many women, but also, should an ovarian cyst be detected in someone on monophasic oral contraceptives, it is more likely to be neoplastic and therefore needs to be investigated. This may not apply to the very low dose and triphasic combined preparations and certainly does not apply to progestogen-only formulations where follicular 'cysts' can be noted from time to time. The actual incidence is uncertain.

Ovarian carcinoma (epithelial tumors)

The influence of steroids on the incidence of gynecological cancers is considered in detail in chapter 67, but the beneficial effect of the combined oral contraceptive pill on prevention of ovarian cancer is so significant that it warrants special mention under beneficial side effects. Several studies, both case control and cohort, have shown a significant decrease in the incidence of epithelial ovarian tumors in oral contraceptive users. The most detailed study was that undertaken by the Cancer and Steroid Hormone Study (CASH) in the United States[21] which found that the effect was observed within six months of use, with a relative risk of 0.2 after 10 years, an effect which lasted for at least 15 years.

Endometrial carcinoma

This is also discussed in chapter 67, but it needs to be highlighted that women who have taken combined oral contraceptives have a significant decrease in the incidence of subsequent endometrial carcinoma. The CASH study[21] showed an effect within 12 months, maximal at two years with a relative risk of 0.4, and persisting for at least 15 years.

Thyroid disease

It was suggested by the RCGP study in 1978[22] that women who use combined oral contraceptives have a decreased incidence of thyroid disease. The mechanism for this is not clear, and the more recent publication from the Oxford FPA study is far less impressive.[23] Whether the combined oral contraceptive decreases the risk of thyroid disease has to be stated as a possible benefit, yet unproven.

Endometriosis

The histological effect of the oral contraceptive is to produce a relatively inactive, suppressed secretory 'pill endometrium'. It may therefore be anticipated that oral contraceptives may have a preventative or even therapeutic role with regards to endometriosis. Unfortunately there are few data available, and there is contradictory evidence from different reports. A protective role for oral contraceptives comes from Buttram[24] who in a series of 172 women studied retrospectively found no relationship between disease severity and the use of oral contraceptives, but reported a trend to mild rather than severe disease with longer use. In another series Sensky and Liu[25] found that in a series of 163 endometriosis patients only 13% had been on oral contraceptives, which was much lower than expected, and consequently postulated that the oral contraceptives may protect. In a large series of women undergoing laparoscopic sterilization Krishon's group[26] found no significant difference between women affected by endometriosis and controls with regards to a past history of oral contraceptive use. In contrast a study by Paparazzini and colleagues[27] found a relative risk of 2.1 (95% CI 1.2–3.6) for the use of oral contraceptives in women with ovarian endometriosis, a trend that increased with duration use.

There is therefore no consensus on the effect of oral contraceptives on endometriosis. Any analysis of findings is compounded by the use of oral contraceptives for the control of symptoms of endometriosis such as pain and premenstrual bleeding. It can probably be concluded that it either has no effect or a small protective effect.[28]

Arthritis (especially rheumatoid)

Another observation that was made from the RCGP study[29] was that combined oral contraceptive users had decreased incidence of rheumatoid arthritis. However other studies have not shown this reduction.[30] There is no consensus, and there are methodological problems, most important of which are the difficulty of diagnosis and incomplete reporting. At most a reduction in rheumatoid arthritis can be claimed as a possible advantage. Furthermore there is no suggestion for a decrease in osteoarthritis.

Benign breast disease

The effect of estrogen and progesterone on the breast is discussed in detail in chapter 16, and its treatment in chapter 39. In summary, there is significant evidence to show that benign breast lumps are less common in women who use oral contraceptives.[31] The protective effect is only in current users, increases with duration and is probably less with modern 'low dose pills'.

Decreased pelvic inflammatory disease (PID)

There is good evidence to show that the risk of acute and subacute PID is decreased in the users of oral contraceptives,[32] thought to be due to the progestogen effect on cervical mucus. This protective effect does not seem to relate to chlamydial cervicitis.[33] It is possible that oral contraceptives increase the chance of development of a large ectropion which may became infected with chlamydia, but decrease the risk of transfer of organisms into the upper tract by an effect on mucus.

Uterine fibroids

There is also conflicting evidence with regard to uterine fibroids and oral contraceptives. The RCGP study found that fibroids were less common in pill users, and the Oxford/FPA study found no effect of the pill on fibroids. However, in occasional women on the pill fibroids have been found to enlarge quite quickly, but this might have occurred anyway. There is no suggestion that combined oral contraceptive (COC) ingestion will decrease the size of fibroids, but it will often diminish the amount of bleeding.

Hirsutism and acne

The etiology of hirsutism is quite complicated and is usually due to increased circulating free androgen levels combined with increased local androgen action through metabolism of receptors in the skin. It is often significantly influenced by hereditary factors.[34] The mechanism that causes hirsutism also seems responsible for acne. Whatever its cause, the aims of hormonal therapy are to decrease blood levels of androgenic hormones, and inhibit their end-organ actions. The main line of therapy is to administer an estrogen-progestogen combination at the same time as an antiandrogen. Androgen production (mainly from the ovary) is usually dependent on the secretion of LH, and this is suppressed with the COC.[35] A medium dose estrogen pill may be preferable, and biphasic preparations with relatively low progestogen effect have been widely used.[36] A novel and useful COC preparation is Diane 35 (Schering, Berlin), containing 2 mg cyproterone acetate and 35 μg ethinyl estradiol which is better than most COCs at suppressing the symptoms of mild hyperandrogenism, such as acne and mild hirsutism.[37] This is because cyproterone acetate is also an effective antiandrogen, although much higher doses are used in a reverse sequential regimen for maximal clinical effect (50–100 mg daily).

Duodenal ulcers

Duodenal ulcers may be less common in women who use COCs. It has been postulated that a possible explanation for this is that anxious women may avoid the pill.[38]

Wax in ears

The RCGP study first reported that there was a decreased incidence of wax in the ears of oral contraceptive users. It is likely that steroid hormones reduce sebaceous gland secretions within the ear canal.

HORMONE REPLACEMENT THERAPY AT AND AFTER THE MENOPAUSE

There are two extreme schools of thought with regard to hormone replacement therapy (HRT) in the menopause/postmenopause. One extreme point of view is that the menopause is natural and therefore no treatment is indicated. The opposite point of view is that humans were not originally 'designed' to live past menopause and have not evolved to cope with the estrogen deficiency syndrome resulting from ovarian failure. In concept, this situation is no different from thyroid deficiency in myxedema, or diabetes with insulin deficiency, and all women should therefore undergo HRT during the postmenopause.[39] Aspects of symptomatic treatment of menopausal symptoms were discussed in chapters 90–53. Some of these areas, however, deserve further highlighting under the heading of nontherapeutic beneficial side effects.

One of the best recent population studies was performed by a detailed telephone survey of 2000 Australian born women between 45–55 years of age.[40] Twenty-two specific symptoms were enquired about and most common were those of joint stiffness or aches, lack of energy, backaches, sleeping difficulties, nervous tension and hot flashes. The administration of estrogen replacement therapy significantly improves most of these symptoms with particular efficiency for vasomotor symptoms.

Musculoskeletal symptoms

Interestingly, in the Australian population study[40] the commonest of 22 symptoms reported by all three groups (premenopausal, perimenopausal and post-menopausal) was aches and stiff joints. There is often a substantial improvement of these symptoms with HRT.

Psychological changes

This area is discussed in detail in chapters 50 and 64, including a discussion of the range of psychological problems reported in the menopause, and a discussion of the correlation between endocrinological and psychological data, as well as a review of studies investigating the frequently beneficial effects of HRT on the emotional wellbeing of women at menopause.

It has been shown that estrogens and progestogens can affect mood, behavior, memory, coordination and learning. Steroid receptors have been localized in amygdala, hippocampus and locus ceruleus, where they may mediate effects on psychological functioning. Other studies suggest that steroids and their metabolites can modulate neurotransmitter receptors for excitory or inhibitory amino acids.[41] In general estrogens have an excitatory and progestogens an inhibitory effect on the central nervous system. Studies in animals and humans have shown that elevated levels of estrogens result in better sensory perception with improved limb coordination and enhanced attention and short term memory. Hormone replacement therapy may result in an improvement of psychological state and mental functioning.

Lower urinary tract changes

The effect of estrogen and progesterone on urinary tract, bladder and pelvic floor was described in detail in chapter 20. There are three major areas of urinary problems in the menopause: incontinence, voiding dysfunction and sensory bladder problems.

Incontinence can be urge (loss of urine with a powerful urge to urinate) or stress (loss of urine on raised intra-abdominal pressure), but often there is a combination of both. Genuine stress incontinence is due to structural change and it rarely improves with HRT, whilst urge is due to detrusor instability and is sometimes improved when HRT or local estrogen administration by vaginal cream, tablet or pessary ring is instituted.[42,43] Urge and stress incontinence increases with age through and beyond menopause.

The problem of voiding dysfunction is far less well documented in women than in men. Inadequate emptying may lead to recurrent infections and HRT appears to be of benefit in preventing recurrences.

Sensory disorders include frequency, urgency and dysuria. In postmenopausal women estrogen deficiency is often the causative factor, and symptoms may dramatically improve with HRT.[44] Recurrent urinary tract infection is not uncommon in postmenopausal women, and its frequency has been shown to be decreased by HRT.[45] In the absence of improvement with HRT other causes such as bladder calculi, bladder tumors, interstitial cystitis, urethral diverticulum or previous radical pelvic surgery or irradiation should be excluded.

The prevention of osteoporosis

The effects of estrogens and progestogens on bone are discussed in chapter 18 whilst osteoporosis including its prevention and treatment are the subject of chapter 54. As the prevention of osteoporosis is one of the most significant side effects of HRT, it warrants a short overview in this chapter.

It has been recently highlighted that osteoporosis is the emerging epidemic of the 1990s, with the estimated annual Australian treatment cost of $779 million per year for osteoporotic fractures.[46] Wark also concludes that systemic estrogen-progestogen therapy remains the first line approach for the prevention of menopausal bone loss and in many women, for the treatment of osteoporosis. Much epidemiological evidence supports the efficacy of long term estrogen use in preventing fractures.[47]

Bone loss after the menopause occurs at 3–6% per year for 5–10 years, with an ongoing loss thereafter of 1%. The administration of estrogen not only prevents this rapid postmenopausal bone loss, but if an adequate dose is used, will initially increase bone density at about 1% per year.[48] It has been hypothesized that about 10–15% of the skeletal mass is estrogen dependent, and it is this proportion which is rapidly lost after the menopause if estrogens are not taken, or when HRT is discontinued.[49]

In order to minimize the risk of osteoporotic fractures clinicians would have to recommend that HRT commence at the time of the menopause, and continue lifelong. This would result in a decrease of bone density at the age of 80 years by about 10% versus a reduction of 30% in a woman who had never taken HRT, and this improvement of bone density would reduce fracture risk by about two-thirds.[50] In order to minimize the duration of exogenous estrogen ingestion an alternate approach has been proposed to commence HRT many years after the menopause, and then to continue for the rest of the woman's life. If started at say, 70 years, bone density would increase by about 10% in the first two years, and then bone loss would slow to 0.5–1% per year, resulting in overall 20% reduction of bone density from premenopausal levels to the age of 80, rather than the 30% in untreated women. This has been estimated to give a reduction of fracture risk by about one third.

Alternatively, HRT could be delayed until after the first osteoporotic fracture, thus treating only those women who are at highest risk of recurrent fracture. The drawback of this policy is that many women who could have had osteoporosis prevented will experience a fracture. All of these strategies consider the therapeutic side effect of bone sparing of estrogens in isolation and do not take into account effect on balance and coordination. In reality, the beneficial effect on bone density is part of the several desirable therapeutic outcomes that the use of estrogens and progestogens produce in the menopause.

The decrease of cardiovascular risk factors

The physiological effects of estrogen and progesterone on blood vessels are discussed in detail in chapter 19, and the effects of therapy on the vascular system in chapter 55.

Cardiovascular disease, including coronary artery disease, stroke and other vascular disease is the commonest cause of death in Western society, accounting for approximately 50% of female deaths. Furthermore, nonfatal myocardial infarction and cerebrovascular disease are far more common than fatal disease, so cardiovascular disease causes major morbidity in women. It has been postulated that as men below 60 years of age develop cardiovascular disease at twice the rate of women, estrogens are cardioprotective, but even in the eighth decade men experience cardiovascular disease at 1.4 times the rate of women. Studies that show higher rates for female cardiovascular disease after the menopause may be confounded by failing to take smoking into account.[51] Nevertheless, there is now overwhelming evidence from epidemiological studies that postmenopausal administration of estrogens generally results in halving of the risk of death from coronary heart disease, and possibly all cardiovascular disease.[52] Green and Bain state that over 30 epidemiological studies on the relationship of estrogen replacement therapy (ERT) and cardiovascular disease (CVD) have been published, most of which were case-control or cohort studies, with only one prospective randomized study. They also highlight the meta-analysis of Stampfer and Colditz[53] which found a relative risk for CVD for women on ERT of 0.56 (95% CI 0.50–0.61). Although these studies suffer to various degrees from the weaknesses of selection bias, observation bias and confounding, it is probably reasonable to conclude that ERT reduces the risk of CVD morbidity and mortality in postmenopausal women by 40%. This is probably the most significant beneficial therapeutic effect of ERT. The mechanism of action appears to be at several levels including favorable effects on lipid levels and direct effects on the arterial wall. However, information on the relative benefits of the type of estrogen preparation, its mode of administration, duration of use, and any confounding effects of progestogen[54] is limited.

Beneficial effects on brain function

The effects of estrogen and progesterone on the central nervous system are discussed in detail in chapter 17, and the effects on psychological mood and central nervous system in chapter 64.

What effect estrogens and progestogens, or rather their decreased levels after the menopause, have on cerebral function and psychogenic conditions is much debated. There is some evidence from longitudinal studies that mental health deteriorates with estrogen deficiency after the menopause.[55,56] There is little consensus on the psychological benefits of HRT in the menopause, and many clinicians believe that any improvement is due to the relief of physical problems such as improved sleep patterns, fewer vasomotor disturbances and relief of atrophic symptoms. However, some studies have reported improvement in psychological symptoms independent of any physical symptomatic improvement after the administration of estrogens.[57,58] The addition of progestogen may result in a dampening of the beneficial effect of estrogen.[59]

There is also increasing evidence that the development of Alzheimer's disease in older women may be due to estrogen deficiency, and that estrogen replacement may be useful in preventing or delaying the onset of this dementia.[60] Paganini-Hill and Henderson investigated 8877 female Leisure World residents, of whom 2529 died between 1981–92. They matched the 138 women with dementia against four controls and compared the use of estrogens. They found that the risk of Alzheimer's disease and related dementia was less in estrogen users than nonusers (odds ratio 0.69, confidence limits 0.46–1.03). The risk decreased significantly with dose and duration of use. However, a similar study from Puget Sound, Seattle, of 107 females with Alzheimer's disease compared to 120 matched controls, found that roughly 50% of both cases and controls had received estrogens, and they concluded that their study provided no evidence that estrogen replacement has an effect on the risk of Alzheimer's disease.[61]

The possible therapeutic effect of estrogens on established Alzheimer's disease comes from a handful of small studies. The first of these[62] reported a significant improvement in attention, mood orientation and social interaction in three out of seven women treated with micronized estradiol 2 mg daily for six weeks. In Japan, Honjo and colleagues reported similar improvement in six out of seven women treated with estrogens, when compared to untreated controls assessed on the Japanese National Institute of Mental Health and Hasegawa scale.[63] Ohkura and colleagues also found that low dose ERT may improve or slow the rate of cognitive decline in patients with mild to moderate Alzheimer's disease when ten women were treated with 0.625 mg/day of conjugated equine estrogen, compared to untreated controls.

One part of the pathophysiological basis of these changes is probably the finding that estrogens exert their effect on brain cells throughout life to maintain maximally dense meshwork of neural fibers. This facilitates sympathic activity maintaining cognitive thought and memory. Toran-Allerand's group has shown that estrogen sensitizes neurons to nerve growth factor, a peptide which is involved with the growth and maintenance of axons and dendrites.[64] It has also been shown in animal experiments that the enzyme choline acetyltransferase is induced by the administration of estrogen, resulting in an increase in the concentration of acetylcholine.[65] In Alzheimer's disease there is a diminution in acetylcholine. Other neurotransmitters (serotonin and dopamine) whose activity is reduced in Alzheimer's disease have been shown to be stimulated by estrogens. Whether estrogens really have significant beneficial effects on the prevention and treatment of dementia will not be definitively proven until larger prospective controlled clinical studies have been carried out.

REFERENCES

1. Kay CK 1980 The happiness pill? The Journal of the Royal College of General Practitioners 30: 8–19
2. Jordan WM 1961 Pulmonary embolism. Lancet 2: 1146
3. Lorentz IT 1962 Parietal lesion and 'Enovid'. Lancet 2: 1191
4. Boyce J, Fawcett JW, Noall EWP 1963 Coronary thrombosis and Conovid. Lancet 1: 111
5. Royal College of General Practitioners 1967 Oral contraception and thrombo-embolic disease. Journal of the Royal College of General Practitioners 13: 267–279
6. Royal College of General Practitioners 1974 Oral contraceptives and health. Pitman Medical, London
7. Royal College of General Practitioners Oral Contraception Study 1977 Mortality among oral-contraceptive users. Lancet ii: 727–731
8. Weiss N 1995 Third-generation oral contraceptives: how risky? Lancet 346: 1570
9. Vessey MP 1990 The Jephcott Lecture, 1989. An overview of the benefits and risks of combined oral contraceptives. In: Mann R D (ed) Oral contraceptives and breast cancer. Parthenon Publishing, New Jersey, 121: 132
10. Abraham S, Fraser I, Gebski V et al 1985 Menstruation, menstrual protection and menstrual cycle problems. Medical Journal of Australia 142: 247–251
11. Brown S, Vessey M, Stratton I 1988 The influence of method of contraception and cigarette smoking on menstrual patterns. British Journal of Obstetrics and Gynaecology 95: 905–910
12. Loudon NB, Foxwell M, Potts DM, Guild AL, Short RV 1977 Acceptability of an oral contraceptive that reduces the frequency of menstruation: the tri-cycle pill regimen. British Medical Journal 2: 487–490
13. Kovacs GT, Rusden J, Evans A 1994 A trimonthly regimen for oral contraceptives. The British Journal of Family Planning 19: 274–275
14. Kakouris H, Kovacs G 1992 Pill failure and non-use of secondary precautions. The British Journal of Family Planning 18: 41–44
15. Riddoch GG, Duncombe P, Kovacs G 1996 Tasmanian survey of pill symptoms. Australian Family Physician 25(Suppl 1): S38–S40
16. Zadeh JA, Karabus CD, Fielding J 1967 Haemoglobin concentration and other values in women using an intrauterine device or taking corticosteroid contraceptive pills. British Medical Journal 4: 708–711
17. Nilsson L, Rybo G 1971 Treatment of menorrhagia. American Journal of Obstetrics and Gynecology 110: 713–720
18. Fraser IS, McCarron G 1991 Randomised trial of 2 hormonal and two prostaglandin inhibiting agents in women with a complaint of menorrhagia. Australian and New Zealand Journal of Obstetrics and Gynaecology 31: 66–70
19. Herzberg B, Coppen A 1970 Changes in psychological symptoms in women taking oral contraceptives. British Journal of Psychiatry 116: 161–164
20. Vessey MP, Metcalfe A, Wells C, McPherson K, Westhoff C, Yeates D 1987 Ovarian neoplasms, functional ovarian cysts and oral contraceptives. British Medical Journal 294: 1518–1520
21. Cancer and Steroid Hormone Study 1987 The reduction in the risk of ovarian cancer associated with oral contraceptive use. New England Journal of Medicine 316: 650–655
22. Frank P, Kay CR 1978 Incidence of thyroid disease associated with oral contraceptives. British Medical Journal 2: 1513
23. Vessey M, Villard-Mackintosh L, McPherson K, Yeates D 1987 Thyroid disorders and oral contraceptives. British Journal of Family Planning 13: 124–127
24. Buttram VC 1979 Cyclic use of combination oral contraceptives and the severity of endometriosis. Fertility and Sterility 31: 347–348
25. Sensky TE, Liu DTY 1980 Endometriosis: associations with menorrhagia, infertility and oral contraceptives. International Journal of Gynaecology and Obstetrics 17: 573–576
26. Krishon B, Poindexter AN 1988 Contraception: a risk factor for endometriosis. Obstetrics and Gynecology 71: 829–831

27. Paparazzini F, LaVecchia C, Franceschi S, Negri E, Cecchetti G 1989 Risk factors for endometrioid, mucinous and serous benign ovarian cysts. International Journal of Epidemiology 18: 108–112
28. Vercellini P, Crosgnani PG 1992 Epidemiology of endometriosis In: Brosens I, Donnez J (eds) The current status of endometriosis. Proceedings of the 3rd World Congress on Endometriosis. Parthenon, Carnforth, pp 111–130
29. Royal College of General Practitioners Oral Contraception Study 1978 Reduction in incidence of rheumatoid arthritis associated with oral contraceptives. Lancet 1: 569–570
30. Vessey MP, Villard-Mackintosh L, Yeates D 1987 Oral contraceptives, cigarette smoking and other factors in relationship to arthritis. Contraception 35: 457–464
31. Brinton LA, Vessey MP, Flavel R, Yeates D 1981 Risk factors for benign breast disease. American Journal of Epidemiology 113: 203–214
32. Rubin G, Ory HW, Layde PE 1982 Oral contraceptives and pelvic inflammatory disease. American Journal of Obstetrics and Gynecology 144: 630–635
33. Washington AE, Gove S, Schachter J, Sweet RL 1985 Oral contraceptives, Chlamydia trachomatis infection, and pelvic inflammatory disease. Journal of the American Medical Association 253: 2246–2250
34. Greenblatt RB 1987 Hirsutism: ancestral curse or endocrinopathy? In: Greenblatt et al (eds) The cause and management of hirsutism. Parthenon, Carnforth, pp 17–29
35. Givens JR 1983 Role of oral contraceptives in the treatment of hyperandrogenism of hirsute women. In: Mahesh VB, Greenblatt RB (eds) Hirsutism and virilism. John Wright PSG Inc, Boston, pp 351–367
36. Kovacs GT, Marks R 1987 Contraception and the skin. Australian Journal of Dermatology 28: 86–92
37. Spona J, Huber J, Schmidt JB 1987 Ovulation inhibitory effect of SH B 209 AE (Diane-35 R) — a new antiandrogen-estrogen combination. In: Schindler AE (ed) Antiandrogen-estrogen therapy for signs of androgenization. Walter de Gruyter, Berlin, pp 51–58
38. Guillebaud J 1993 Contraception, your questions answered. Churchill Livingstone, Edinburgh, p 125
39. Wren BG 1985 Oestrogen replacement therapy. The management of an endocrine deficiency disease. Medical Journal of Australia 142: S3–S15
40. Dennerstein L, Smith AMA, Morse C, Burger G, Green A, Hopper J, Ryan M 1993 Menopausal symptoms in Australian women. Medical Journal of Australia 159: 232–236
41. Smith SS 1994 The modern management of the menopause. Proceedings of the VIIth International Congress on the Menopause, 1993. Parthenon Carnforth, UK, pp 257–268
42. Walter S, Wolf H, Barlebo H, Jensen HK 1978 Urinary incontinence in postmenopausal women treated with oestrogens. Urologia International 33: 135–139
43. Cardozo L 1988 Sex and the bladder. British Medical Journal 296: 587–588
44. VonSchoultz B 1987 Estrogens and urogenital epithelial function. Acta Obstetrica Gynecologica Scandinavica 140: 28–32
45. Brandberg A, Mellstrom D, Samsioe G 1987 Low dose estriol treatment in elderly women with urogenital infections. Acta Obstetrica Gynecologica Scandinavica 140: 33
46. Wark JD 1996 Osteoporosis: the emerging epidemic. Medical Journal of Australia 164: 327–328
47. Maxim P, Ettinger B, Spitalny GM 1995 Fracture protection provided by long-term estrogen treatment. Osteoporosis International 5: 23–29
48. Garnett TJ, Savval M, Studd JW 1991 Osteoporosis prevention with oestrogens and progestogen. Consensus. In: Sitruk-Ware R, Utian WH (eds) The menopause and hormone replacement therapy. Marcel Dekker Inc, New York, pp 247–256
49. Heaney RP 1990 Estrogen-calcium interactions in the postmenopause: a quantitative description. Bone Minerals 11: 67–84
50. Ettinger B, Grady D 1993 The waning effect of postmenopausal oestrogen therapy on osteoporosis. New England Journal of Medicine 329: 1192–1193
51. Burger HG 1992 Menopause; implications for coronary disease. In: Kelly DT (ed) Women and coronary disease. Excerpta Medica, Edgecliffe, pp 15–22
52. Green A, Bain C 1993 Epidemiological overview of oestrogen replacement and cardiovascular disease. Baillière's Clinical Endocrinology and Metabolism 7: 95–112
53. Stampfer MJ, Colditz GA 1991 Estrogen replacement therapy and coronary heart disease: a quantitative assessment of the epidemiological evidence. Preventative Medicine 20: 47–63
54. Lobo RA, Speroff L 1994 International consensus conference on postmenopausal hormone therapy and the cardiovascular system. Fertility and Sterility 61: 592–595
55. Hallstrom T 1973 Mental disorder and sexuality in the climacteric: a study in psychiatric epidemiology. Scandinavian University Books, Gotenburg, Sweden,
56. Bungay GT, Vessey MP, McPherson CK 1980 Study of symptoms in middle life with special reference to the menopause. British Medical Journal 281: 181–183
57. Campbell S, Whitehead M 1977 Oestrogen therapy and the menopausal syndrome. Clinics in Obstetrics and Gyneacology 4: 31–47
58. Dennerstein L, Burrows GD, Hyman GJ, Sharpe K 1979 Hormone therapy and affect. Maturitas 1: 247–259
59. Sherwin BB, Gelfand MM 1989 A prospective one year study of estrogen and progestin in postmenopausal women: effects on clinical symptoms and lipoprotein lipids. Obstetrics and Gynecology 73: 759–766
60. Paganini-Hill A, Henderson VW 1994 Estrogen deficiency and risk of Alzheimer's disease in women. American Journal of Epidemiology 140: 256–261
61. Brenner D, Kukull WA, Stergachis A, van Belle G, Bowen JD, McCormick WC, Teri L, Larson EB 1994 Postmenopausal estrogen replacement therapy and the risk of Alzheimer's disease: a population-based case-control study. American Journal of Epidemiology 140: 262–267
62. Fillit H, Weinreb H, Cholst I, Luine V, McEwen B, Amador R, Zabriskie J 1986 Observations in a preliminary open trial of estradiol therapy for senile dementia-Alzheimer's type. Psychoneuroendocrinology 11: 337–345

63. Honjo H, Ogino Y, Naitoh K, Urabe M, Kitawaki J, Yasuda J, Yamamoto T, Isihara K, Namabara T 1989 In vivo effects by oestrone sulfate on central nervous system-senile dementia (Alzheimer's type). Journal of Steroid Biochemistry 34: 521–525
64. Sohrabji F, Miranda RC, Toran-Allerand D 1994 Estrogen differentially regulates estrogen and nerve growth factor receptor RNA in adult sensory neurons. Journal of Neuroscience 14: 459–471
65. McEwen BS, Biegon A, Fischette CT, Luine VN, Parsons B, Rainbow TC 1984 Toward a neurochemical basis of steroid hormone action. In: Martini L, Ganong WF (eds) Frontiers in neuroendocrinology. Raven Press, New York, ch 8, pp 153–176

61. Effects on carbohydrate metabolism

Ian F. Godsland

Introduction

Concerns have been expressed over changes in carbohydrate metabolism during clinical use of female sex steroids since the observation by Waine in 1963 that the newly-introduced estrogen/progestogen combined oral contraceptive was associated with deterioration in glucose tolerance.[1] Since then, the enormous proliferation of small, safety-oriented studies of the effects of estrogens and progestogens on glucose tolerance has led to considerable confusion over the effects of these steroids on carbohydrate metabolism. Careful review of the literature does, however, allow a rationale to be developed, which, in turn, can provide some insights into the possible clinical implications of sex steroid-induced changes in carbohydrate metabolism.

CLINICAL SIGNIFICANCE OF CHANGES IN CARBOHYDRATE METABOLISM

Metabolism of carbohydrates via glucose to carbon dioxide and water is central to the body's energy economy, and insulin's involvement in promotion of this process is central to its control. Classically, disruption of the normal relationship between glucose and insulin leads to diabetes mellitus, but increasing attention is being given to the risks of cardiovascular disease that may accompany such disruption.[2]

Insulin secretion and diabetes

Type I or insulin-dependent diabetes mellitus almost certainly involves autoimmune destruction of the pancreas, and both genetic and environmental factors are important in this process.[3] Type II or noninsulin-dependent diabetes (NIDDM) develops later in life and carries a two to threefold increase in risk of coronary heart disease (CHD). This is especially marked in women, who, after they develop NIDDM, appear to entirely lose the protection from CHD that they enjoy relative to men.[4]

The pancreatic insulin response to glucose consists of distinct first and second phases, the first phase comprising a large bolus output of insulin from the pancreas, and the second phase a more measured, feedback-controlled response, which more accurately re-establishes basal glucose levels. A deficient first phase response appears to be an early marker of predisposition to NIDDM, but this will also be accompanied by resistance to insulin's various actions.[5] Whatever the predisposing factors, there must be a deficient pancreatic insulin response to glucose for NIDDM to manifest.

Insulin resistance and cardiovascular disease

Stimulation of peripheral uptake of glucose into muscle and adipose tissue, and suppression of hepatic glucose production are amongst the principal actions of insulin, both of which combine to maintain normoglycemia. The sensitivity of these processes to insulin can be affected by a number of factors, including dietary and exercise habits, genetic factors, vascular function and female sex steroid administration. Where there is a normal pancreatic insulin response to glucose, insulin release varies according to the degree of insulin resistance (the inverse of insulin sensitivity) to maintain normal glucose levels.[6] Thus, insulin concentrations rise to overcome insulin resistance. Such elevations in insulin levels have been linked in two large prospective epidemiological studies to the subsequent development of coronary heart disease.[7,8] Moreover, there is experimental evidence that insulin can promote smooth muscle cell proliferation and arterial lipid deposition, both early events in atherogenesis.[9] Hyperinsulinemia is thus considered to be a potential risk factor for cardiovascular disease. This possibility has been strengthened by the observation that insulin can

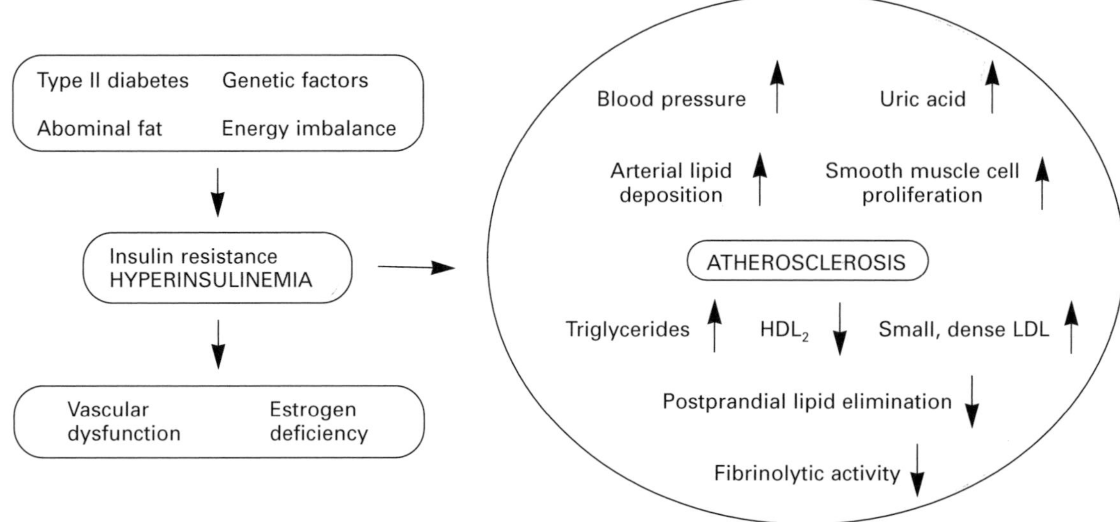

Fig. 61.1 Factors contributing to insulin resistance and hyperinsulinemia, and components of the metabolic syndrome.

increase catecholamine release, stimulate renal sodium reabsorption and enhance vascular smooth muscle cell reactivity (thus potentially increasing blood pressure),[10] that insulin may stimulate hepatic triglyceride release (thus inducing dyslipidemia),[11] and that insulin can stimulate hepatic synthesis of the antifibrinolytic factor, plasminogen activator inhibitor-1 (thus adversely affecting the hemostatic system).[12]

The status of insulin as a cardiovascular risk factor has recently come under criticism: there has been a series of negative or equivocal prospective epidemiological studies[13,14] and increasing uncertainty over some of the supposed adverse biochemical and physiological effects of insulin.[15] The more recent epidemiological studies can be criticized for low power and confounding due to pre-existing morbidity, and the uncertainties over the adverse effects of insulin, at least on blood pressure, may result from experiments having been performed in states of normal insulin sensitivity. Hyperinsulinemia therefore remains a potential risk factor, but attention has shifted towards the wider issue of insulin resistance.

In addition to maintaining normoglycemia, insulin suppresses adipose tissue lipolysis and acts as a potent vasodilator. When there is insulin resistance, impaired suppression of adipose tissue lipolysis results in increased supply of nonesterified fatty acids to the liver, increased production of triglyceride-enriched very-low-density lipoprotein, an increased proportion of small, dense low-density lipoprotein and reduced levels of high-density lipoprotein.[16] This dyslipidemic pattern is associated with increased risk of cardiovascular disease, particularly in women.[17] Insulin-induced vasodilation is impaired in insulin resistant states,[18] and this impairment may be responsible for the associations that have been reported between insulin resistance and hypertension, since, in the absence of insulin-induced vasodilation, the effects of insulin-induced sympathetic activity may come to predominate. If one includes the potential metabolic and physiological effects of the hyperinsulinemia associated with insulin resistance, it will be apparent that insulin resistance can set in train an entire syndrome of adverse changes in risk factors for cardiovascular disease.[19] The concept of a 'metabolic' or 'insulin resistance' syndrome has become increasingly influential in recent years. Although it is difficult to study epidemiologically, the theoretical justification and observational evidence for such a cardiovascular risk syndrome has been sufficiently strong for it to become one of the principal considerations in cardiovascular risk (Fig. 61.1).

SEX STEROIDS AND CELLULAR AND PHYSIOLOGICAL ASPECTS OF CARBOHYDRATE METABOLISM

An accurate picture of the biochemical and physiological effects of estrogens and progestogens comes both from animal studies and clinical studies of glucose tolerance, insulinemia and insulin resistance in users of reproductive steroids, primarily oral contraceptives and hormone replacement therapy.

Effects on insulin secretion

Estrogens

Interest in the effects of estrogens on pancreatic insulin secretion dates back to the 1930s, when the possibility that suppression of pituitary activity might ameliorate the development of diabetes led investigators to explore the influence of estrogens in animal models of diabetes.[20] These experiments culminated in the observation that estrogens could substantially reduce the development of diabetes in the subtotally pancreatectomized rat.[21] The development of procedures for studying insulin secretion from isolated islets and of radioimmunoassay for direct measurement of insulin concentrations enabled further confirmation of the beneficial effects of estrogens on insulin secretion, both in intact[22,23] and ovariectomized animals.[23,24]

Estrogens appear to affect the pancreas directly: there is receptor binding specific for estradiol in the pancreas;[25] estradiol can directly enhance insulin release from the isolated perfused rat pancreas;[26] and protection against development of diabetes in animal models is still seen in adrenalectomized or hypophysectomized animals, thus arguing against secondary effects mediated by other hormones.[27] Nevertheless, there is some evidence for a permissive effect of estrogen-induced increases in corticosteroid activity. Evidence for a beneficial effect of estrogens on insulin secretion in humans comes from the observation that the pancreatic insulin response to glucose declines sharply at the menopause.[28]

Progesterone and progestogens

In studies of isolated islets from animals treated with progesterone, significant increases in insulin output were detected.[22,24] Direct stimulatory effects of progesterone and 17β hydroxyprogesterone-derived progestogens were seen in isolated islet culture.[29] Further support for a direct effect of progesterone on the pancreatic islets comes from the demonstration that progesterone can enter the islet cells, bind to specific cytosolic receptors and subsequently undergo transfer to the cell nucleus.[30,31]

Effects on insulin resistance

Estrogens

An estrogen-induced increase in the sensitivity of insulin-dependent glucose uptake in diaphragm and skeletal muscle has been reported in several studies, using both estradiol-17β and ethinyl estradiol.[32] In accord with these effects, specific binding of estrogens to rat skeletal muscle and adipose tissue has been reported. Improved sensitivity of adipose tissue glucose metabolism to insulin has also been described.[33]

Given this strong evidence for estrogen-induced improvements in insulin sensitivity, it is paradoxical that estrogen is almost certainly responsible for the insulin resistance seen in premenopausal women taking combined oral contraceptives below. A resolution of this paradox is suggested by careful review of the literature on the effects of estrogen deficiency, estrogen replacement and estrogen administration on carbohydrate metabolism in pre and postmenopausal women. Estrogen deficiency following the menopause is associated with a progressive increase in insulin resistance which relates to increasing time since menopause rather than chronological age.[34,35] The weight of evidence then shows that estrogen replacement with estradiol improves carbohydrate metabolism,[36,37] low dose (0.625 mg/day) conjugated equine estrogens are beneficial or neutral,[38–40] the majority of studies of high dose (1.25 mg/day or more) conjugated equine estrogens indicate deterioration in carbohydrate metabolism,[37,41] and, likewise, the potent alkylated estrogens, mestranol and ethinyl estradiol, used in oral contraceptives are associated with deterioration in carbohydrate metabolism.[42–45] This suggests that estrogen replacement improves carbohydrate metabolism whereas excessive estrogen action causes a deterioration. The improvement is consistent with the effects of estrogens at the cellular level. It is then necessary to explain why excessive estrogen action is associated with the opposite effect.

There are several candidate mechanisms, but the weight of evidence favors an increase in corticosteroid activity as the critical factor in estrogen-induced deterioration in glucose tolerance. Estrogen administration increases glucocorticoid concentrations, corticosteroid-binding globulin levels and plasma free cortisol levels, and reduces elimination of exogenously administered corticosteroids.[46] Increases in free cortisol have also been seen in women taking oral contraceptives containing 50 or 30 μg of alkylated estrogen.[47,48] Progestogens appear to have no effect on corticosteroid metabolism.[46] Two further strands of investigation provide compelling evidence for an involvement of increased corticosteroid activity in estrogen-induced deterioration in carbohydrate metabolism. First, raised blood pyruvate levels during an OGTT are a characteristic effect of glucocorticoid administration and were consistently seen in users of high and medium dose oral contraceptives.[49,50] Increased tryptophan metabolism is the other 'metabolic signature' left by increased corticosteroid activity. The enzyme, tryptophan pyrrolase, controls the first, and rate-limiting, step in the catabolism of tryptophan. Activity of this enzyme is increased in pregnancy and by estrogen administration and these effects are mediated by increased glucocorticoids.[51] Increased tryptophan metabolism leads to signs of vitamin B_6 deficiency,[52] which may be aggravated by estrogen conjugates competitively inhibiting binding of pyridoxal phosphate to its enzyme.[53] Tryptophan catabolism is directed towards formation of xanthurenic acid and away from quinolinic acid. Reduced levels of quinolinic acid would be expected to result in a lifting of inhibition of the gluconeogenic enzyme phosphoenolpyruvate carboxykinase by quinolinic acid. Pyridoxal phosphate administration results in a significant improvement in oral glucose tolerance test (OGTT) glucose, insulin and pyruvate responses following pyridoxal phosphate supplementation in those women with measureable vitamin B_6 deficiency.[54] This observation confirms the role of at least one consequence of excessive glucocorticoid activity in estrogen-induced deterioration in glucose tolerance. In concentrations above those seen in premenopausal women, estrogens:

- Increase plasma corticosteroid concentrations
- Increase plasma corticosteroid-binding globulin levels
- Decrease plasma cortisol elimination
- Increase plasma free cortisol concentrations
- Induce metabolic changes typical of increased corticosteroid activity
- Promote corticosteroid-induced increases in tryptophan catabolism.

These observations support the importance of increased corticosteroid activity in the deterioration of carbohydrate metabolism induced by estrogen excess.

Progesterone and progestogens

Insulin-mediated glucose metabolism is impaired in isolated diaphragm and skeletal muscle from progesterone-treated animals.[32,55] This impairment has also been reported in isolated adipocytes with both progesterone and progestogens.[55] As with estrogens, the mechanisms underlying these direct effects at the tissue level remain unknown. In contrast to estrogens, the effects of progestogens *in vivo* are generally in accord with these effects at the tissue level. Effects of progestogens *in vivo* vary according to progestogen type. These effects are described in detail below. The effects of estrogens and progestogens at the tissue levels are summarized as follows:

Estrogens

- Augment the pancreatic insulin response to glucose
- Increase the sensitivity of muscle and adipose tissue glucose metabolism to insulin.

Progesterone

- Augments the pancreatic insulin response to glucose
- Decreases the sensitivity of muscle and adipose tissue glucose metabolism to insulin.

ORAL CONTRACEPTIVE THERAPY

The great majority of oral contraceptive prescribing has involved estrogen/progestogen combined formulations. Nevertheless, progestogen-only contraception continues to constitute an important minority of contraceptive therapies, and the effects of different progestogens on carbohydrate metabolism are also considered here because they provide necessary background for the interpretation of combined formulation effects.

Progestogen-only therapy

Evidence from *in vivo* studies of progesterone and the majority of pregnane progestogens is too limited to draw any general conclusions, but, in general, medroxyprogesterone acetate, administered as an intramuscular depot (150 mg every three months), has been found to cause deterioration of glucose tolerance or hyperinsulinemia or both.[56–58] It is noteworthy that medroxyprogesterone acetate has glucocorticoid actions which are not seen with progesterone.[59,60] The gonane progestogen, levonorgestrel, has been consistently linked with deterioration in carbohydrate metabolism.[61–63] Effects of the other commonly-used gonane progestagens, desogestrel, gestodene and norgestimate, on glucose metabolism and insulin levels do not appear to have been studied. The weight of evidence suggests that the estrane progestogens ethynodiol diacetate and norethisterone are relatively neutral with regard to carbohydrate metabolism.[62,64,65,66] The effects of progestogens and estrogens *in vivo* in humans are summarized as follows:

- Estrogen deficiency induces insulin resistance
- Estrogen replacement restores insulin sensitivity
- Estrogen excess induces insulin resistance
- Medroxyprogesterone acetate and levonorgestrel induce insulin resistance
- Norethindrone has no effect on insulin sensitivity.

Combined oral contraceptive therapy

The development of overt, clinical diabetes mellitus has never been linked with oral contraceptive use in case-control or prospective epidemiological studies. This is, at first sight, surprising, since changes in glucose tolerance diagnostic of diabetes mellitus have been reported in oral contraceptive users, particularly in those taking high estrogen dose combinations.[49,67–69] It is possible that the trophic effect of estrogens on the pancreas, demonstrated in the early animal studies, are ameliorating any potential adverse effect of oral contraceptive therapy on the long-term progression of diabetic changes. In a recent analysis of data gathered as part of a large cross-sectional study, it was noted that the age-related decline in glucose tolerance seen in premenopausal women (aged 18–44) was not present in oral contraceptive users.[70] A similar pattern was seen with regard to the first phase plasma insulin response to intravenous glucose, which declined with age in nonusers, but remained steady in oral contraceptive users (Fig. 61.2). As mentioned previously, a decline in first phase insulin response is one of the principal early indices of developing diabetes, the first phase response being highly dependent on the net mass of functioning islet cell tissue.

Subclinical elevations in post-load plasma glucose levels and increased insulin concentrations have been reported in users of virtually all types of combined oral contraceptive.[71–73] It is almost certain, however, that in the population of oral contraceptive users as a whole there is considerable variation in individual response and there may be significant increases, not only in mean values, but also in the prevalence of individuals with degrees of deterioration in glucose tolerance or hyperinsulinemia at the upper extreme of the frequency distribution, which would be expected to be most clinically important. Using the 95th percentile limit for the OGTT 120 minute plasma glucose concentration in a group of 639 healthy premenopausal women not taking oral contraceptives, it was found that the proportion of outlying values in a group of 229 women taking a combination of 0.03 mg ethinyl estradiol and 0.15 mg levonorgestrel was increased 2.5 times.[74] This increase in prevalence agrees well with the United States National Health and Nutrition Examination Survey (1976–80) figure for the prevalence of impaired glucose tolerance in women using oral contraceptives: 15.4% compared with 6.3% in nonusers.[75]

In a large cross sectional comparative study of users of seven different currently available low estrogen dose (30–40 µg) combinations, the degree of deterioration

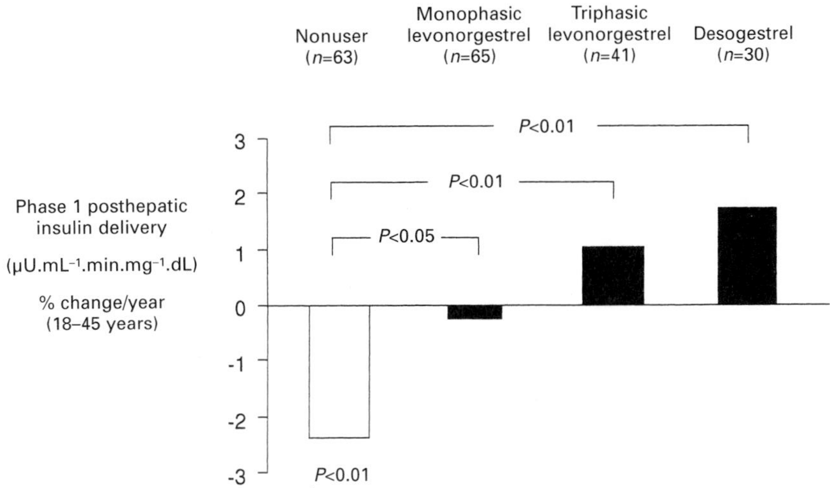

Fig. 61.2 The percentage change in first phase pancreatic insulin delivery per year in premenopausal women not taking combined oral contraceptives, or taking low-estrogen dose formulations containing levonorgestrel (monophasic or triphasic) or desogestrel progestogens.[70]

in glucose tolerance, measured using the oral glucose tolerance test, did not appear to vary appreciably with oral contraceptive formulation.[62] This accords with the estrogen component (ethinyl estradiol) being the component of the combination primarily responsible for oral contraceptive-induced deterioration in glucose tolerance. Further support for this possibility comes from an analysis of oral contraceptive-induced insulin resistance.[66] Intravenous glucose tolerance tests (IVGTT) were carried out in 95 nonuser controls and 296 oral contraceptive users, the formulations studied being two different levonorgestrel-containing combinations, a desogestrel combination, a norethindrone combination and formulations comprising norethisterone or ethynodiol diacetate alone (considered together since the latter is metabolized to norethindrone before becoming metabolically active). All combinations caused a similar decline in glucose elimination rate and a similar degree of insulin resistance, whereas the estrane progestogen-only formulations had no effect (Fig. 61.3). A multivariate analysis indicated that the estrogen component contributed 77% of oral contraceptive-induced variation in insulin sensitivity, and the net progestogenicity (dependent on dose and type of progestogen) of the combination contributed 23%.[76]

Although deterioration in glucose tolerance and insulin resistance were primarily related to the estrogen component of the combined oral contraceptives in the two cross-sectional studies described above, there was marked variation in glucose tolerance test insulin response with oral contraceptive progestogen content. This variation was strikingly similar regardless of whether the oral or intravenous glucose tolerance test was employed (Fig. 61.4),[66] the greatest degree of hyperinsulinemia being seen with levonorgestrel-containing combinations and the least with norethindrone-containing combinations. A similar degree of hyperinsulinemia associated with levonorgestrel-containing combinations was seen in earlier large comparative studies, both cross-sectional and longitudinal.[77]

Using OGTT incremental insulin area as a measure of insulin response it was found that the proportion of values above the 95th percentile limit derived in nonuser controls was increased in users of low estrogen dose oral contraceptives, depending on the progestogen content:[76] levonorgestrel-containing combinations increased the prevalence five to seven-fold whereas low dose norethindrone and desogestrel combinations increased the prevalence about two-fold. In general, significant upward shifts in mean values were accompanied by an equivalent increase in the proportion of outlying values. An interesting exception

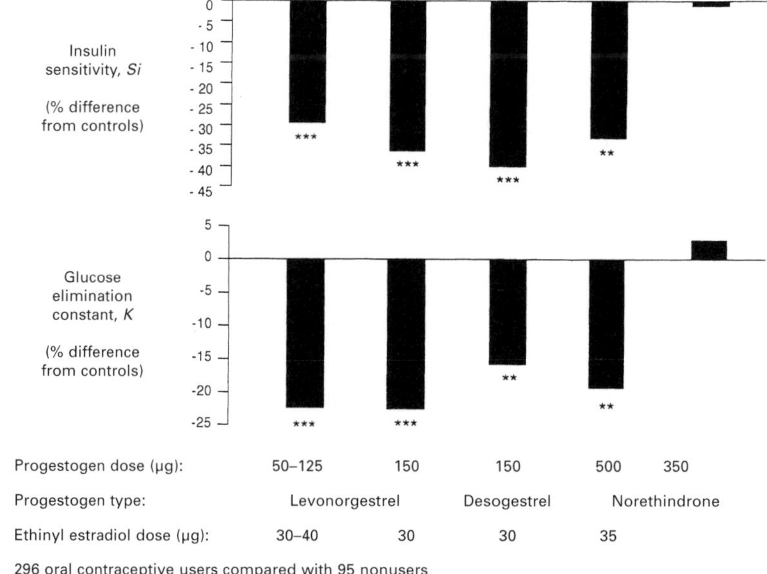

Fig. 61.3 Percentage differences in insulin sensitivity (*Si*) and intravenous glucose tolerance test glucose elimination rate (*k*) between women not taking oral contraceptives and users of four different low-estrogen dose combined oral contraceptives and one progestogen-only oral contraceptive.[66] Significances ***$P<0.001$; **$P<0.01$.

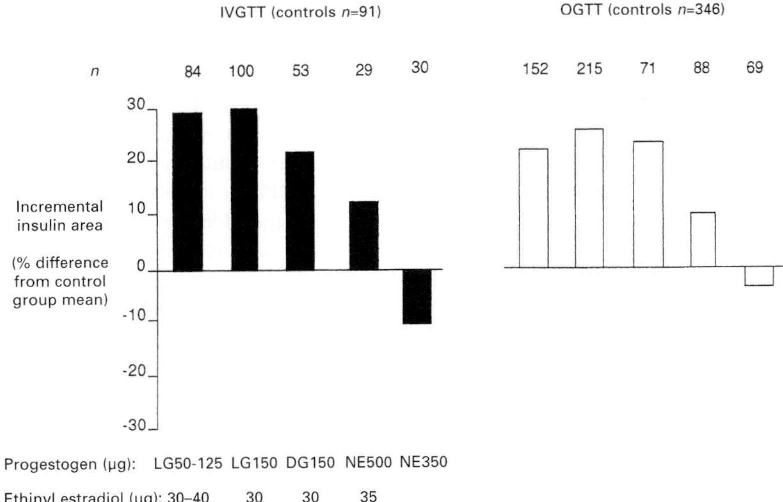

Fig. 61.4 Percentage differences in oral glucose tolerance test (OGTT) and intravenous glucose tolerance test (IVGTT) insulin response between women not taking oral contraceptives and users of four different low-estrogen dose combined oral contraceptives and one progestogen-only oral contraceptive.[66]

to this was found in the combination of 0.03 mg ethinyl estradiol with 0.15 mg desogestrel. In this case an appreciable increase in mean OGTT insulin response was accompanied by relatively little increase in the proportion of outlying values, compared with nonuser controls.[78] An explanation for this variation in hyperinsulinemic response is probably to be found in progestogen-induced variations in plasma insulin half-life.[66,79]

It is important to note that, despite inducing insulin resistance, combined oral contraceptives either have no effect or tend to reduce fasting glucose and insulin levels. This almost certainly results from the specific antagonism that estrogens exert both on the action and secretion of glucagon. This effect has been reported by several groups,[80,81] its net result being a marked increase in the basal hepatic portal insulin:glucagon molar ratio. This reduces the basal activity of the critical gluconeogenic enzyme, phosphoenol pyruvate carboxykinase, thus reducing basal glucose levels.[82]

POSTMENOPAUSAL HORMONE REPLACEMENT THERAPY (HRT)

Alleviation of symptoms of the menopause can be achieved by estrogen replacement. Recognition that estrogens alone, unopposed by a progestogen, can cause endometrial hyperplasia has led to increasing use of estrogen/progestogen combined HRT in postmenopausal women with an intact uterus. There is a distinct difference between combined oral contraceptive and postmenopausal hormone replacement therapies. For effective steroidal contraception there must be sufficient estrogenic activity to completely suppress ovulation. Oral contraceptive therapy is therefore, of necessity, a state of estrogen excess, and is generally associated with insulin resistance. In postmenopausal HRT, only the therapeutic effect of estrogen replacement is required, and a range of effects on carbohydrate metabolism are seen.

Unopposed estrogen replacement

Studies of the effects of unopposed estrogens have been summarized in the previous section on insulin resistence and estrogens. Physiological replacement with transdermal estradiol was, in general, associated with improved carbohydrate metabolism, and one of these studies provided evidence for improved insulin sensitivity, secretion and elimination with estradiol therapy.[36] Higher doses of conjugated equine estrogens (1.25 mg/day) and the potent alkylated estrogens, ethinyl estradiol and mestranol, were generally associated with deterioration in carbohydrate metabolism. The simplest interpretation of these differentials was that estrogen replacement improves insulin sensitivity, whereas excessive estrogen action is associated with insulin resistance as a result of secondary effects on corticosteroid metabolism. The possibility remains that the non-native estrogens have pharmacological effects on corticosteroid metabolism, dependent on their characteristic chemical structures. Resolution of this uncertainty would require detailed elucidation of estrogen-insulin sensitivity dose–response relationships with each type of estrogen, and some standardization to a measure of endogenous estrogen activity. Route of administration is unlikely to be an important consideration in estrogen-induced changes in carbohydrate metabolism: improvements have been seen with both parenteral and oral administration of estradiol and, at least in animal studies, deterioration in *in vivo* carbohydrate metabolism has been seen with parenteral administration of alkylated estrogens.[83]

Estrogen/progestogen combined hormone replacement therapy

Interactions between combined HRT and carbohydrate metabolism are complicated by the predominance of the progestogen effects, since the administration of estrogen is to restore a lack of the hormone rather than impose an excess. This is seen with HRT regimes involving cyclical administration of medroxyprogesterone acetate. During the estrogen plus progestogen phase of the treatment cycle, a significant increase in insulin resistance has been reported (Fig. 61.5).[38,84] This has also been seen with a HRT formulation containing levonorgestrel, but not with one containing norethindrone acetate (Fig. 61.5).[85] These are effects that would be expected from the independent effects of these progestogens on insulin resistance see above.

The most commonly used combination in the USA comprises conjugated equine estrogens and medroxyprogesterone acetate. In the study by Nabulsi et al, fasting glucose and insulin concentrations were lower in postmenopausal women taking a combination of conjugated equine estrogens and medroxyprogesterone acetate,[86] but, as described previously, suppression of glucagon secretion and action by estrogens make such differences in fasting levels difficult to interpret in terms of differences in insulin sensitivity. Other studies also found a similar drop in fasting glucose levels, but these studies also included evaluation of changes during an OGTT; the weight of evidence favored deterioration in glucose tolerance as the predominant effect of the combination.[39,40,41] Interestingly, in the study of Lobo et al, OGTT

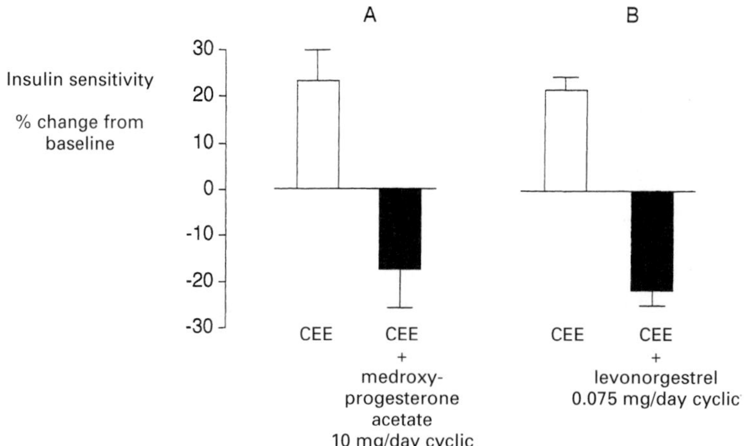

Fig. 61.5 Induction of insulin resistance by inclusion of medroxyprogesterone acetate or levonorgestrel as progestogen in combined postmenopausal hormone replacement therapy. **A**: Percentage change in insulin sensitivity, measured as the glucose elimination constant following insulin injection, in five women given conjugated equine estrogens (CEE: 0.625 mg/day, open bar), and five women given the same dose of estrogens plus cyclical medroxyprogesterone acetate (10 mg/day, closed bar) for two months.[38] **B**: Percentage change in insulin sensitivity, measured by modelling analysis of intravenous glucose tolerance test glucose and insulin concentrations, in 30 women taking conjugated equine estrogens (0.625 mg/day) and cyclical levonorgestrel (0.075 mg/day), tested during the estrogen alone phase (open bar) and the estrogen plus progestogen combined phase (closed bar) of the third treatment cycle.[85]

glucose response was significantly increased during at least one of the three cycles studied (cycles 3, 6 and 13) in the combination users, but not in the users of estrogen alone, and OGTT insulin response was reduced in all groups, primarily during the early part of the OGTT.[39]

Glucose tolerance was similarly affected when conjugated equine estrogens were given with the progestogen levonorgestrel.[85] The impairment in glucose tolerance was associated with some increase in IVGTT insulin response, but there was no overall reduction in insulin sensitivity when compared with baseline levels. Mathematical modeling analysis revealed that the initial plasma insulin response to glucose was markedly reduced, a finding which recalls the reduction in insulin response during the early part of the OGTT in users of conjugated equine estrogen, medroxyprogesterone actetate combinations, reported by Lobo et al.[39] It seems likely that it was this that resulted in the deterioration in glucose tolerance. The increase in insulin concentrations during the latter part of the IVGTT would then be due to feedback on the pancreas by the elevated glucose levels. These changes also recall the pattern seen with high estrogen dose oral contraceptives.[77]

A norethindrone containing HRT combination improved glucose tolerance in women with impaired glucose tolerance, but had no effect on either OGTT glucose or insulin levels in diabetic women or women with normal glucose tolerance.[87] A similar lack of effect on IVGTT glucose and insulin levels was seen when norethisterone acetate was administered transdermally, in a cyclical regime with transdermally administered estradiol.[85] Neither insulin resistance nor any other measure of insulin metabolism was affected. Norethindrone therefore appears to be neutral, but may oppose the favorable effects of estradiol.

Conclusion

Depending on formulation and context of administration, improvement or deterioration in carbohydrate metabolism may be seen with administration of estrogens and progestogens, given alone or in combination. In general, estrogen deficiency is associated with deterioration in carbohydrate metabolism; this is restored by estrogen replacement, but estrogen excess again causes deterioration in carbohydrate metabolism, by secondary effects on corticosteroid metabolism. Progestogens then modify the degree of hyperinsulinemia associated with estrogen-induced insulin resistance, primarily by effects on insulin elimination.

The degree of post-glucose load hyperglycemia seen in users of currently available low estrogen dose combined oral contraceptives generally falls far short of criteria for diabetes. Diabetic hyperglycemia is associated with protein glycosylation and glucose toxicity, but these effects are unlikely to be important with the degrees of hyperglycemia seen in combined oral contraceptive users. The insulin resistance induced by combined oral contraceptives is also problematic, since the underlying mechanism may differ from that associated with cardiovascular disease. Candidates for the mechanism of vascular disease-associated insulin resistance include impaired transendothelial insulin transport, impaired action of insulin-sensitive enzymes of glucose metabolism, impaired intracellular signaling mechanisms and metabolic competition from nonesterified fatty acids. So far, increased corticosteroid activity has not emerged as a prominent candidate. In any case, there appears to be little opportunity for diminishing oral contraceptive-induced insulin resistance except by abandoning the alkylated estrogen component.

Combined oral contraceptive therapy is unusual since modification of insulin elimination by the progestogen component means that there is dissociation between insulin resistance and hyperinsulinemia. Given current knowledge, it would seem prudent to minimize oral contraceptive-induced hyperinsulinemia, and this is indeed possible by appropriate selection of progestogen type and dose. This recommendation is strengthened by a recent analysis of correlations between oral glucose tolerance test insulin response and other risk factors. Adverse associations with blood pressure and HDL cholesterol concentrations were stronger in 633 users of low-estrogen dose combined oral contraceptives than in 346 nonuser controls (Table 61.1). The possible long-term beneficial effects of oral contraceptive therapy on pancreatic insulin secretion are, at present, highly speculative. The only insight that might be gained into this issue would require comparison of long-term diabetes incidence in oral contraceptive users compared with women not taking oral contraceptives, who had similar degrees of deterioration in carbohydrate metabolism to those seen in oral contraceptive users.

Development of non-insulin dependent diabetes mellitus (NIDDM) in women accelerates appreciably in middle age,[88] and is accompanied by loss of protection against coronary heart disease.[4] Whether menopausal estrogen deficiency contributes to these effects is unknown, but, as described above, there are theoretical reasons to suppose that it might. Studies

Table 61.1 Cardiovascular risk factor inter-relationships in combined oral contraceptive (COC) users: univariate correlations between metabolic syndrome risk factors in women not taking COC and COC users. Reproduced with permission from Ref. 89.

	Non users (n=346)	COC (n=674)
OGTT insulin/OGTT glucose	0.19*	0.24***
OGTT insulin/triglycerides	0.15*	0.03
OGTT insulin/HDL cholesterol	–0.03	–0.17**
OGTT insulin/systolic blood pressure	0.06	0.16**
OGTT insulin/diastolic blood pressure	0.07	0.11*
Triglycerides/HDL cholesterol	–0.26**	–0.08

OGTT: oral glucose tolerance test; HDL: high density lipoprotein; *P<0.05; **P<0.01; ***P<0.001

relating development of NIDDM to time of menopause would help resolve this issue. All else being equal, HRT combinations that either improve or do not adversely affect carbohydrate metabolism would seem preferable. These considerations may become more important in diabetics. Clearly HRT need not be contraindicated in diabetics, but it would seem unwise to use combinations that suppress the initial pancreatic insulin response to glucose and cause insulin resistance and deterioration in glucose tolerance. Combinations that improve insulin secretion or insulin sensitivity might even come to be positively indicated in diabetic postmenopausal women, but this area needs considerable further study to determine whether potential improvements in diabetic control and incidence of complications are indeed realized.

REFERENCES

1. Waine H, Fieden E, Caplan H 1963 Metabolic effects of Enovid in rheumatoid patients. Arthritis and Rheumatology 6: 796–797
2. Godsland IF, Stevenson JC 1995 Insulin resistance: syndrome or tendency. Lancet 346: 100–103
3. Eisenbarth GS 1986 Type 1 diabetes mellitus: a chronic autoimmune disease. New England Journal of Medicine 314: 1360–1368
4. Barrett-Connor EL, Cohn BA, Wingard DL, Edelstein SL 1991 Why is diabetes mellitus a stronger risk factor for fatal ischaemic heart disease in women than in men? The Rancho Bernardo Study. Journal of the American Medical Association 265: 627–631
5. Groop LC 1995 Early metabolic abnormalities in NIDDM. Diabetes Review International 4: 9–12
6. Hollenbeck C, Reaven GM 1987 Variations in insulin-stimulated glucose uptake in healthy individuals with normal glucose tolerance. Journal of Clinical Endocrinology and Metabolism 64: 1169–1173
7. Pyörälä K 1979 Relationship of glucose tolerance and plasma insulin to the incidence of coronary heart disease: results from two population studies in Finland. Diabetic Metabolism 13: 345–349
8. Ducimetiere P, Eschwege E, Papoz L, Richard J, Claude J, Rosselin G 1980 Relationship of plasma insulin levels to the incidence of myocardial infarction and coronary heart disease in a middle-aged population. Diabetologia 19: 205–210
9. Stout R 1990 Insulin and atheroma: 20-yr perspective. Diabetes Care 13: 631–654
10. Morris AD, Petrie JR, Connell JMC 1994 Insulin and hypertension. Journal of Hypertension 12: 633–642
11. Reaven G 1988 Banting Lecture 1988: role of insulin resistance in human disease. Diabetes 37: 1595–1607
12. Kooistra T, Bosma P, Töns H, van den Berg A, Meyer P, Princen H 1989 Plasminogen activator inhibitor 1: biosynthesis and mRNA level are increased by insulin in cultured human hepatocytes. Thrombosis and Haemostasis 62: 723–728
13. Hargreaves AD, Logan RL, Elton RA, Buchanan KD, Oliver MF, Riemersma RA 1992 Glucose tolerance, plasma insulin, HDL cholesterol and obesity: 12-year follow-up and development of coronary heart disease in Edinburgh men. Atherosclerosis 94: 61–69
14. Ferrara A, Barrett-Connor EL, Edelstein SL 1994 Hyperinsulinaemia does not increase the risk of fatal cardiovascular disease in elderly men or women without diabetes: the Rancho Bernardo Study, 1984–1991. American Journal of Epidemiology 10: 857–869
15. Haffner SM 1993 Insulin and blood pressure: fact or fantasy? Journal of Clinical Endocrinology and Metabolism 76: 541–542
16. Frayn K 1993 Insulin resistance and lipid metabolism. Current Opinion in Lipidology 4: 197–204
17. Miller Bass K, Newschaffer CJ, Klag MJ, Bush TL 1993 Plasma lipoprotein levels as predictors of cardiovascular death in women. Archives of Internal Medicine 153: 2209–2216
18. Baron AD 1994 Hemodynamic actions of insulin. American Journal of Physiology 267: E187–E202
19. Després J-P, Marette A 1994 Relation of components of insulin resistance syndrome to coronary disease risk. Current Opinion in Lipidology 5: 274–289

20. Barnes B, Regan J, Nelson W 1933 Improvement in experimental diabetes following the administration of amniotin. Journal of the American Medical Association 101: 926–927
21. Houssay BA, Foglia VG, Rodriguez RR 1954 Production and prevention of some types of experimental diabetes by oestrogens or corticosteroids. Acta Endocrinologica 17: 146–164
22. Costrini N, Kalkhoff R 1971 Relative effects of pregnancy, estradiol and progesterone on plasma insulin and pancreatic islet insulin secretion. Journal of Clinical Investigation 50: 992–999
23. Faure A, Haourari M, Sutter B-C-J 1985 Insulin secretion and biosynthesis after oestradiol treatment. Hormone and Metabolism Research 17: 378
24. Bailey C, Ahmed-Sorour H 1980 Role of ovarian hormones in the long-term control of glucose homeostasis. Diabetologia 19: 475–481
25. Tesone M, Chazenbalk G, Ballejos G 1979 Estrogen receptor in rat pancreatic islets. Journal of Steroid Biochemistry 11: 1309–1314
26. Sutter-Dub M-T 1979 Effects of pregnancy, progesterone and/or oestradiol on the insulin secretion and pancreatic insulin content in the perfused rat pancreas. Diabetic Metabolism 5: 47–56
27. Rodriguez R 1965 Influence of oestrogens and androgens on the production and prevention of diabetes. In: Leibel B, Wrenshall G (eds) On the nature and treatment of diabetes. Excerpta Medica, New York, pp 288–307
28. Walton C, Godsland I, Proudler A, Wynn V, Stevenson J 1993 The effects of the menopause on insulin sensitivity, secretion and elimination in nonobese, healthy women. European Journal of Clinical Investigation 23: 466–473
29. Neilsen J 1984 Direct effect of gonadal and contraceptive steroids on insulin release from mouse pancreatic islets in organ culture. Acta Endocrinologica 105: 245–250
30. Green I, Howell S, ElSeifi S, Perrin D 1978 Binding of ^{3}H progesterone by isolated rat islets of Langerhans. Diabetologia 15: 349–355
31. Winborn W, Sheridan P, McGill H Jr 1987 Localization of progestin receptors in the islets of Langerhans. Pancreas 2: 289–294
32. Rushakoff R, Kalkhoff R 1981 Effects of pregnancy and sex steroid administration on skeletal muscle metabolism in the rat. Diabetes 30: 545–550
33. Gilmour K, McKerns K 1966 Insulin and estrogen regulation of lipid synthesis in adipose tissue. Biochem Biophys Acta 116: 220–228
34. Proudler A, Felton C, Stevenson J 1992 Ageing and the response of plasma insulin, glucose and C-peptide concentrations to intravenous glucose in postmenopausal women. Clinical Science 83: 489–494
35. Godsland IF, Crook D, Stevenson JC, Collins P, Rosano GMC, Lees B, Sidhu M, Poole-Wilson PA 1995 The insulin resistance syndrome in postmenopausal women with cardiological syndrome X. British Heart Journal 74: 47–52
36. Cagnacci A, Soldani R, Carriero P, Paoletti A, Fioretti P, Melis G 1992 Effects of low doses of transdermal 17β-estradiol on carbohydrate metabolism in postmenopausal women. Journal of Clinical Endocrinology and Metabolism 74: 1396–1400
37. Lindheim SR, Duffy DM, Kojima T, Vijod MA, Stancxyk FZ, Lobo RA 1994 The route of administration influences the effect of estrogen on insulin sensitivity in postmenopausal women. Fertility and Sterility 62: 1176–1180
38. Lindheim SR, Presser SC, Ditkoff EC, Vijod MA, Stanczyk FZ, Lobo RA 1993 A possible bimodal effect of estrogen on insulin sensitivity in postmenopausal women and the attenuating effect of added progestin. Fertility and Sterility 60: 664–667
39. Lobo RA, Pickar JH, Wild RA, Walsh B, Hirvonen E 1994 Metabolic impact of adding medroxyprogesterone acetate to conjugated estrogen therapy in postmenopausal women. Obstetrics and Gynecology 84: 987–995
40. PEPI; The Writing Group for the PEPI Trial 1995 Effects of estrogen or estrogen/progestin regimens on heart disease risk factors in postmenopausal women: the postmenopausal estrogen/progestin interventions (PEPI) trial. Journal of the American Medical Association 273: 199–208
41. Barrett-Connor E, Laakso M 1990 Ischaemic heart disease risk in postmenopausal women: effects of estrogen use on glucose and insulin levels. Arteriosclerosis 10: 531–534
42. Larsson-Cohn U, Wallentin L 1977 Metabolic and hormonal effects of post-menopausal oestrogen replacement treatment. Acta Endocrinologica 86: 583–596
43. Polderman KH, Gooren LJG, Asscheman H, Bakker A, Heine RJ 1994 Induction of insulin resistance by androgens and estrogens. Journal of Clinical Endocrinology and Metabolism 79: 265–271
44. Gow S, MacGillivray I 1971 Metabolic, hormonal and vascular changes after synthetic oestrogen therapy in oophorectomised women. British Medical Journal 2: 73–77
45. Spellacy W, Buhi W, Birk S 1982 The effects of two years of mestranol treatment on carbohydrate metabolism. Metabolism 31: 1006–1008
46. Burke C 1970 The effects of oral contraceptives on cortisol metabolism. Journal of Clinical Pathology 23 (Suppl 3): 11–18
47. Lindholm J, Schultz-Möller N 1973 Plasma and urinary cortisol in pregnancy and during estrogen-gestagen treatment. Scandinavian Journal of Clinical Laboratory Investigation 31: 119–122
48. Meulenberg P, Hofman J 1990 The effects of oral contraceptive use and pregnancy on the daily rhythm of cortisol and cortisone. Clin Chim Acta 190: 211–222
49. Wynn V, Doar J 1966 Some effects of oral contraceptives on carbohydrate metabolism. Lancet ii: 715–719
50. Wynn V, Doar J 1969 Some effects of oral contraceptives on carbohydrate metabolism. Lancet ii: 761–766
51. Braidman IP, Rose DP 1971 Effects of sex hormones on three glucocorticoid-inducible enzymes concerned with amino acid metabolism in rat liver. Endocrinology 89: 1250–1255
52. Rose DP 1972 Aspects of tryptophan metabolism in health and disease: a review. Journal of Clinical Pathology 25: 17–25
53. Adams PW, Wynn V, Rose DP, Seed M, Folkard J, Strong R 1973 Effect of pyridoxine hydrochloride (vitamin B_6) upon depression associated with oral contraception. Lancet i: 897–904

54. Adams PW, Wynn V, Folkard J, Seed M 1976 Influence of oral contraceptives, pyridoxine (vitamin B_6), and tryptophan on carbohydrate metabolism. Lancet i: 759–764
55. Sutter-Dub M-T, Dazey B 1981 Progesterone antagonises insulin effect: in vivo and in vitro studies. Hormone and Metabolism Research 13: 241–242
56. Gershberg H, Zorrilla E, Hernandez A, Hulse M 1969 Effects of medroxyprogesterone acetate on serum insulin and growth hormone levels in diabetics and potential diabetics. Obstetrics and Gynecology 33: 383–389
57. Spellacy W, McLeod A, Buhi W, Birk S 1972 Depot medroxyprogesterone acetate and carbohydrate metabolism: measurement of glucose, insulin and growth hormone after twelve months' use. Fertility and Sterility 23: 239–244
58. Vermeulen A, Thiery M 1974 Hormonal contraceptives and carbohydrate tolerance. II Influence of medroxyprogesterone acetate and chronic oral contraceptives. Diabetologia 10: 253–259
59. Edgren RA, Hambourger WE, Calhoun DW 1959 Production of adrenal atrophy by 6-methyl-17-acetoxy progesterone with remarks on the adrenal effects of other progestational agents. Endocrinology 65: 505–507
60. Siminoski K, Goss P, Drucker DJ 1989 The Cushing syndrome induced by medroxyprogesterone acetate. Annals of Internal Medicine 111: 758–760
61. Spellacy W, Buhi W, Birk S 1976 The effects of norgestrel on carbohydrate and lipid metabolism over one year. American Journal of Obstetrics and Gynecology 125: 984–986
62. Godsland I, Crook D, Simpson R, Proudler T, Felton C, Lees B, Anyaoku V, Devenport M, Wynn V 1990 The effects of different formulations of oral contraceptive agents on lipid and carbohydrate metabolism. New England Journal of Medicine 323: 1375–1381
63. Singh K, Viegas O, Liew D, Singh P, Ratnam S 1988 The effects of norplant-2 rods on clinical chemistry in Singaporean acceptors after 1 year of use: metabolic changes. Contraception 38: 453–463
64. Goldman JA, Eckerling B 1970 Glucose metabolism during the menstrual cycle. Obstetrics and Gynecology 35: 207–210
65. Goldman J 1975 Effect of ethynodiol diacetate and combination type oral contraceptive compounds on carbohydrate metabolism. I Six months intravenous glucose tolerance study. Diabetologia 11: 45–48
66. Godsland I, Walton C, Felton C, Proudler A, Patel A, Wynn V 1992 Insulin resistance, secretion and metabolism in users of oral contraceptives. Journal of Clinical Endocrinology and Metabolism 74: 64–70
67. Gersgberg H, Javier Z, Hulse M 1964 Glucose tolerance in women receiving an ovulatory suppressant. Diabetes 13: 378–382
68. Peterson WF, Steel Jr MW, Coyne RV 1966 Analysis of the effect of ovulatory suppressants on glucose tolerance. American Journal of Obstetrics and Gynecology 95: 484–488
69. Halling GR, Michals EL, Paulsen CA 1967 Glucose intolerance during ethynodiol diacetate-mestranol therapy. Metabolism 16: 465–468
70. Godsland IF 1996 Interactions of oral contraceptive use with the effects of age, exercise habit and other cardiovascular risk modifiers on metabolic risk markers. Contraception 53: 9–16
71. Kalkhoff R 1975 Effects of oral contraceptive agents on carbohydrate metabolism. Journal of Steroid Biochemistry 6: 949–956
72. Gaspard UJ 1987 Metabolic effects of oral contraceptives. American Journal of Obstetrics and Gynecology 157: 1029–1041
73. Godsland I, Crook D, Wynn V 1990 Low-dose oral contraceptives and carbohydrate metabolism. American Journal of Obstetrics and Gynecology 163: 348–353
74. Godsland IF, Crook D, Stevenson J, Wynn V 1989 Estrogen/progestin combinations and carbohydrate metabolism. International Proceedings Journal 1: 74–80
75. Russell-Briefel R, Ezzati TM, Perlman JA, Murphy RS 1987 Impaired glucose tolerance in women using oral contraceptives: United States, 1976–1980. Journal of Chronic Disease 40: 3–11
76. Godsland IF, Crook D 1994 Update on the metabolic effects of steroidal contraceptives and their relationship to cardiovascular disease risk. American Journal of Obstetrics and Gynecology 170: 1528–1536
77. Wynn V, Adams P, Godsland I, Melrose J, Niththyananthan R, Oakley N, Seed M 1979 Comparison of the effects of different combined oral-contraceptive formulations on carbohydrate and lipid metabolism. Lancet i: 1045–1049
78. Godsland I, Crook D, Wynn V 1991 Coronary heart disease risk markers in users of low-dose oral contraceptives. Journal of Reproductive Medicine 36 (Suppl): 226–237
79. Srivastava M, Oakley N, Tompkins C, Sonksen P, Wynn V 1975 Insulin metabolism, insulin sensitivity and hormonal responses to insulin infusion in patients taking oral contraceptive steroids. European Journal of Clinical Investigation 5: 425–433
80. Thomas J 1963 Modification of glucagon-induced hyperglycaemia by various steroidal agents. Metabolism 12: 207–212
81. Ahmed-Sorour H, Bailey CJ 1980 Role of ovarian hormones in the long-term control of glucose homeostasis: interaction with insulin, glucagon and epinephrine. Hormone Research 13: 396–403
82. Mandour T, Kissebah A, Wynn V 1977 Mechanism of oestrogen and progesterone effects on lipid and carbohydrate metabolism: alteration in the insulin:glucagon molar ratio and hepatic enzyme activity. European Journal of Clinical Investigation 7: 181–187
83. Beck P, Venable R, Hoff D 1975 Mutual modification of glucose-stimulated serum insulin responses in female rhesus monkeys by ethinyl estradiol and nortestosterone derivatives. Journal of Clinical Endocrinology and Metabolism 41: 44–53
84. Elkind-Hirsch K, Sherman L, Malinak R 1993 Hormone replacement therapy alters insulin sensitivity in young women with premature ovarian failure. Journal of Clinical Endocrinology and Metabolism 76: 472–475
85. Godsland I, Gangar K, Walton C, Cust M, Whitehead M, Wynn V, Stevenson J 1993 Insulin resistance, secretion and elimination in postmenopausal women receiving oral or transdermal hormone replacement therapy. Metabolism 42: 846–853

86. Nabulsi AA, Folsom AR, White A, Patsch W, Heiss G, Wu KK, Szklo M 1993 Association of hormone replacement therapy with various cardiovascular risk factors in postmenopausal women. New England Journal of Medicine 328: 1069–1075
87. Luotola H, Pyörälä T, Loikkanen M 1986 Effects of natural oestrogen/progestogen substitution therapy on carbohydrate and lipid metabolism in post-menopausal women. Maturitas 8: 245–253
88. Harris MI, Hadden WC, Knowler WC, Bennett PH 1987 Prevalence of diabetes and impaired glucose tolerance and plasma glucose levels in US population aged 20–74 yr. Diabetes 36: 523–534
89. Godsland IF 1996 Sex steroids and changes in the cardiovascular system: carbohydrate metabolism. Gynecological Endocrinology 10 (Suppl 2): 59–64

62. Effects of estrogens and progestogens on plasma lipids and lipoproteins

David Crook

Introduction

The metabolism of cholesterol and other lipids has been intensively researched over the past 40 years in response to the finding that many myocardial infarction patients have an abnormal plasma lipoprotein profile. Plasma lipid and lipoprotein levels are under some degree of genetic control but are also influenced by factors such as age, diet and obesity. Interest in the influence of sex hormones (estrogens, androgens and progestogens) on plasma lipid and lipoprotein metabolism arose from the observation that the gender difference in the plasma lipoprotein profile matches the gender difference in the incidence of coronary heart disease (CHD) in the young and middle-aged.[1] Subsequently, administration of sex hormones as combined oral contraception (COC) or postmenopausal hormone replacement therapy (HRT) was found to alter the plasma lipoprotein profile, raising the possibility of an effect on CHD events.

This hypothesis has aroused much controversy ever since the introduction of COC and has become an equally contentious issue in the context of HRT. This overview is intended to summarize current concepts of plasma lipoprotein metabolism, to review the influence of sex hormones (both given alone and in therapeutic combinations) and to assess the clinical significance of such changes.

OVERVIEW OF PLASMA LIPOPROTEIN METABOLISM

Lipids such as cholesterol, triglycerides and phospholipids are by definition relatively water-insoluble and so circulate in the plasma by complexing with specific proteins ('apolipoproteins') to form large macromolecules ('lipoproteins'). As hundreds of individual molecules may be combined within a single lipoprotein particle, there is enormous potential for heterogeneity and indeed dozens of different lipoprotein types have been identified. Various nomenclature systems have been proposed, of which the most enduring is based on particle density, in turn the product of the chemical composition (lipid-to-protein ratio) of the particle (Table 62.1). The major advances in lipoprotein biochemistry seen during the last few decades have been reviewed recently.[2–6]

Triglyceride-rich lipoproteins

Triglyceride-rich lipoproteins fall into two broad categories: those which transport lipid mainly of dietary ('exogenous') origin and those which transport lipid mainly derived from hepatic ('endogenous') synthesis. Their structure is rather similar in each case: a globule of triglyceride and other nonpolar lipids stabilized by a thin coat of apolipoproteins and more polar lipids such as free cholesterol and phospholipids.

Triglyceride-rich lipoproteins of exogenous origin

Dietary triglycerides (the major food lipid) are hydrolyzed by pancreatic lipase into a mixture of mono- and diglycerides suitable for absorption by the cells of the intestinal mucosa. These cells re-esterify glycerides into triglycerides and then combine them with other lipids to form large particles ('chylomicrons'), each stabilized by a single molecule of a specific apolipoprotein, apoB$_{48}$. Chylomicrons are secreted into the intestinal lymph, entering the plasma compartment via the thoracic duct. During this process, chylomicrons interact with other lipoproteins, receiving extra apolipoproteins which regulate for their subsequent catabolism. Within the plasma compartment chylomicrons are rapidly attacked by lipoprotein lipase, an endothelial-bound enzyme which cleaves fatty acids from the glycerol backbone of the triglyceride molecule. These fatty acids may be used immediately as a source of energy or may be taken up

Table 62.1 A simplified classification of plasma lipoproteins.

Triglyceride-rich lipoproteins
(Chylomicrons and very low density lipoproteins [VLDL])

Function: Transport of dietary triglycerides and other lipids (in the case of chylomicrons) or endogenously synthesized triglycerides and other lipids (in the case of VLDL) to adipose and other peripheral tissues and to the liver.
Origin: Intestine (chylomicrons) or liver (VLDL).
Atherogenicity: Larger triglyceride-rich particles are involved in coagulation and fibrinolysis. Smaller particles, such as VLDL remnants, can invade the subendothelial space and be taken up by macrophages, leading to the formation of foam cells. Oxidized lipoproteins may be especially atherogenic.

Cholesterol-rich lipoproteins
(Low density lipoproteins [LDL] and lipoprotein(a) [Lp(a)])

Function: Transport of cholesterol (both dietary and newly-synthesized) to peripheral tissues for use in cell membranes and synthesis of steroid hormones (LDL); involvement in coagulation/fibrinolysis (Lp(a)).
Origin: Endproduct of VLDL catabolism (LDL) or hepatic synthesis (Lp(a)).
Atherogenicity: Both LDL and Lp(a) can accumulate within the subendothelial space and participate in the atherogenic process. Oxidized lipoproteins may be especially atherogenic. The combination of high levels of both LDL and Lp(a) may be very damaging.

Protein-rich lipoproteins
(High density lipoproteins [HDL])

Function: Multiple, including transport of cholesterol from cells to the liver for disposal; regulation of triglyceride metabolism; protection of LDL from oxidation; regulation of platelet and endothelial function.
Origin: Hepatic synthesis; minor contribution from intestine. Extensively remodelled within the plasma compartment.
Atherogenicity: Anti-atherogenic (consistent with known functions).

by nearby adipocytes and re-esterified into triglycerides, an efficient way of storing energy. Few other classes of molecule can condense as much energy into a given volume of a relatively inert material.

Thus chylomicron metabolism involves a lipolytic cascade in which triglycerides are systematically stripped from the particle. This process results in smaller lipoproteins, depleted of triglycerides but now rich in cholesteryl esters due to the action of lipid transfer enzymes. Normally, these 'remnant' particles are rapidly taken up by the liver. Delays in their removal from the plasma compartment may be atherogenic as remnants can be taken up by macrophages in the arterial wall, causing these cells to become overloaded with cholesterol.[7] In contrast, newly-synthesized chylomicrons are not considered to be atherogenic, partly because their size restricts their entry into the subendothelial space and partly because of their low cholesterol content.

Triglyceride-rich lipoproteins of endogenous origin

Lipoproteins containing endogenously-synthesized lipid (very low density lipoproteins, VLDL) are smaller than chylomicrons and carry less triglyceride per particle. A further distinction is the presence of the full length version of the apoB molecule, $apoB_{100}$. The discovery[8] of an mRNA editing process by which intestinal cells synthesize $apoB_{48}$, from the same gene that codes for $apoB_{100}$ is one of the major advances in lipoprotein biochemistry in recent years. VLDL undergo a lipolytic cascade analogous to that seen with chylomicrons, complete with transfers and exchanges of lipids and apolipoproteins to and from other lipoproteins. Some VLDL remnants are taken up by the liver but others persist in the circulation, becoming enriched with cholesteryl esters obtained from high density lipoproteins (HDL). Subsequent remodelling of remnants produces the cholesterol-rich lipoprotein, LDL.

The atherogenicity of VLDL is controversial.[6] Most epidemiological studies find that elevated fasting triglyceride levels (mostly due to VLDL) increase CHD risk, especially in women.[9] However, this relationship is confounded by the low HDL levels often seen in such individuals. As with chylomicrons, it is likely that a subset of VLDL may be atherogenic, perhaps those remnants that become susceptible to lipid peroxidation due to their delayed residence time within the plasma compartment.

Cholesterol-rich lipoproteins

The end-product of VLDL catabolism is LDL, the major carrier of plasma cholesterol in human plasma.

LDL contain about 50% of cholesterol by weight, derived both from diet and from endogenous synthesis. The main function of LDL is to transport this lipid to peripheral tissues for use in the synthesis of cell membranes and steroid hormones. Some LDL are taken up by the liver. These processes involve the $apoB_{100}$/E receptor, which recognizes the single $apoB_{100}$ molecule present in each LDL particle. Compared to the catabolism of triglyceride-rich lipoproteins, LDL uptake is a relatively slow process, increasing the possibility of deleterious interactions between LDL and the arterial wall. Peroxidation of LDL may lead to fragmentation of $apoB_{100}$ and thus affect receptor-mediated uptake of this lipoprotein. Recent evidence suggests that oxidatively-modified LDL can damage the endothelium and so interfere with vascular function. Accelerated ingress of LDL into the subendothelial space may lead to further oxidative damage and to an imbalance whereby the ability of macrophages and other cells to scavenge these lipoproteins is saturated. The pathological consequences of such an imbalance may be serious. Aside from leading to a net accumulation of cholesterol, the oxidized lipids trapped within this space may have adverse effects on other components of the arterial wall.

Analytical techniques such as ultracentrifugation and gel electrophoresis reveal that LDL are not a homogenous population of lipoproteins but comprise of an array of different subclasses. 'Small, dense' LDL appear to be more atherogenic than other fractions.[10] One reason may be that small, dense LDL are easily oxidized and so would be expected to accelerate atherogenesis once trapped within the subendothelial space. Individuals with small, dense LDL also tend to have low levels of HDL and high levels of triglycerides, to have prolonged postprandial lipemia and to be insulin-resistant and hypertensive. Not surprisingly, the relative contribution of these metabolic disorders to the increased CHD risk seen in individuals with small, dense LDL is currently the subject of intense research investigation.

Lipoprotein(a) [Lp(a)], an intriguing variant of LDL, carries a unique polypeptide (apo(a)) that is disulphide-linked to the single $apoB_{100}$ molecule present in all LDL. The metabolism of Lp(a) differs from that of LDL in that Lp(a) are not formed by catabolism of VLDL. The catabolism of Lp(a) is not understood at present, although the $apoB_{100}$/E receptor does not appear to be critical. Apo(a) displays an extraordinarily high degree of structural homology with plasminogen, and there is some evidence that Lp(a) can interfere with fibrinolysis. Prospective studies show that individuals with high Lp(a) levels are at increased risk of CHD, especially if their LDL levels are also high.[11]

Protein-rich lipoproteins

A shared feature of both triglyceride- and cholesterol-rich lipoproteins is the presence of the apoB ligand. As an alternative to apoB, HDL contain a complex array of proteins including receptor ligands, enzymes, cofactors and inhibitors, reflecting the central regulatory role of this lipoprotein.

HDL form a strikingly heterogenous population of lipoproteins. Most (>99%) particles contain apoAI, a protein synthesized by the liver and, to a lesser extent, the intestine. Some particles contain additional proteins, such as apoAII, apoAIV and apoE, and some may contain *only* these proteins, to the exclusion of all others. The simplest approach to classifying this heterogeneity has been to recognize two main subfractions, HDL_2 and HDL_3 (HDL_1 being almost undetectable in normal individuals). HDL_2 are larger and more lipid-rich than are HDL_3. Further subfractionation has revealed lipoproteins such as HDL_{2b}, the largest particles in the HDL spectrum. Alternative classifications have been devised which rely on the antigenicity of the apolipoproteins carried by these lipoproteins.

The classic function of HDL is the maintenance of cholesterol homeostasis. Cholesterol in peripheral tissues must be transported back to the liver where it may be excreted through the intestine as bile or recycled to extrahepatic tissues. As no cells can break down the cholesterol nucleus, this phenomenon of 'reverse cholesterol transport' must be critical to the maintenance of normal cell function and the avoidance of cholesterol accumulation within cells, in particular those within arteries.

Four steps of reverse cholesterol transport have been identified:

1. Efflux of free cholesterol from cell membranes to small HDL acceptor particles within interstitial fluid
2. Esterification of this cholesterol within HDL via the lecithin:cholesterol acyltransferase (LCAT) reaction, both in the plasma and the interstitial fluid
3. Transfer of these cholesteryl esters to other plasma lipoproteins via cholesteryl ester transfer protein (CETP)
4. Delivery of these cholesteryl esters to the liver through HDL or other lipoproteins.

Thus a cholesteryl ester molecule which may once have formed part of a cell membrane could be delivered directly to the liver from within an HDL particle (following the action of hepatic lipase and/or through receptor-mediated or receptor-independent mechanisms) or could be delivered as part of an LDL or VLDL particle, again through receptor-mediated or receptor-independent mechanisms. Such a molecule could eventually find itself being delivered to nonhepatic tissues, perhaps even to the cell of origin. The study of cholesterol homeostasis is, not surprisingly, rather problematical. One complication is that the HDL system involves extensive recycling and remodeling, in which large HDL particles transfer some of their lipid load to other lipoproteins, giving rise to smaller HDL particles, which then rejoin the cycle. Lipid-poor or free apoAI may play an important role in these processes.

Individuals with low HDL levels are generally, but not always, at higher risk from CHD than are those with high levels.[12] In women, a low HDL level is a stronger predictor of CHD than is a high LDL or triglyceride level.[13]

In addition to reverse cholesterol transport, HDL regulate the metabolism of triglyceride-rich lipoproteins and prevent the accumulation of remnant lipoproteins. HDL may exert beneficial effects on endothelial function by inhibiting LDL oxidation (and thus uptake by macrophages), by controlling expression of vascular cell adhesion molecule 1 (VCAM-1), and by regulating thromboxane and prostacyclin metabolism. The control of endothelial function by HDL may be relevant to the current debate over sex hormones and arterial disease as the clinical significance of hormonally-induced changes in HDL has often been challenged on the basis that any changes in the incidence of CHD are lost once therapy is discontinued. A role for HDL as a regulator of endothelial function would be consistent with such an observation.

One role of HDL which is assuming an increasing degree of importance is as an inhibitor of LDL oxidation. This may be a critical factor within the subendothelial space, where the number of HDL particles greatly exceeds that of LDL and other particles. This anti-oxidant property involves specific enzymes associated with the HDL particle, such as paraoxonase and platelet-activating factor aryl hydrolase.[14]

One of the more contentious issues in current HDL research is the relative anti-atherogenicity of the different subclasses. HDL_2 (and especially HDL_{2b}) have in the past been considered to be more closely involved in the prevention of atherogenesis than HDL_3, but this distinction is not supported by prospective studies. Small, lipid-poor HDL such as pre-β_1-Lp-AI and γ-LpE may be rate-limiting in reverse cholesterol transport[15] and so may prove to be the more clinically-important players. The limitation here is that the assay of such particles is currently restricted to a few laboratories worldwide and so the demonstration of their clinical validity is proceeding at a slow pace.

THE EFFECTS OF ENDOGENOUS SEX HORMONES ON PLASMA LIPOPROTEINS

Background

Any understanding of the metabolic effects of treating women with estrogens, androgens or progestogens will benefit from an appreciation of the effects of endogenous changes in their plasma levels. Each and every component of the plasma lipoprotein system is under the influence of sex hormones to some degree.[1] Such tight linkage between lipid metabolism and the endocrine system is iilustrated well in the case of pregnancy, in which the ability to increase plasma lipoprotein levels could help satisfy the increased demand for cholesterol to make hormones and cell membranes. The rationale behind other changes, for example the fall in HDL levels induced by testosterone, is less clear. One possibility is that sex hormones determine the pattern of body fat deposition: Wingard[16] had proposed that the gender difference in adiposity (android vs. gynoid) is responsible for the gender difference in plasma lipoprotein levels and ultimately the gender difference in CHD incidence.

Premenopausal women have lower plasma levels of total cholesterol and triglycerides than do men of the same age, due to lower levels of LDL and VLDL, respectively. They also tend to have higher levels of HDL, in particular HDL_2. Apolipoproteins $apoB_{100}$ and apoAI show gender differences consistent with these differences in plasma lipoprotein levels, being lower and higher, respectively, in women of childbearing age. Small, dense LDL are less common in premenopausal women than in age-matched men. Individuals living in nonindustrialized countries tend to have lower plasma lipid and lipoprotein levels with less of a gender difference, suggesting that the genetic determinants of plasma lipoprotein levels are influenced by environmental factors such as diet. Plasma levels of Lp(a) do not appear to be influenced by gender, further evidence for the unusual nature of this lipoprotein.

Puberty

The study of the effects of puberty on plasma lipoprotein levels is substantially confounded by concurrent changes in estradiol and testosterone and by changes in adiposity. The most consistent finding is that HDL levels fall in boys but remain stable in girls. As both sexes are born with similar HDL levels, this finding implies that the sex difference in HDL is due more to a HDL-lowering effect of testosterone than to a HDL-raising effect of estrogen.

The menstrual cycle

Despite numerous studies, there is little consensus as to the effects of the menstrual cycle on plasma lipids and lipoproteins: different studies arrive at different findings. One major problem is that the half-life of lipoproteins such as LDL and HDL is measured in days and weeks, and so an observation of a change in plasma levels of a particular lipoprotein may not reflect the endocrinological milieu at that precise time.

Pregnancy

Pregnancy is associated with substantial (two to three-fold) rises in plasma levels of VLDL, LDL, Lp(a) and HDL. Serial measurement of hormones during gestation indicates that the hyperlipidemia of pregnancy is influenced not only by estradiol and progesterone but by insulin and hPL.

Menopause

The study of such a gradual and poorly-defined condition as the climacteric is confounded by the effects of ageing, but most studies have found an increase in plasma LDL levels of approximately 0.5 mmol/L,[17] with lesser increases in those of VLDL, Lp(a) and small dense LDL. Intriguingly, there is little or no effect of the menopause on HDL levels, consistent with the lack of an increase during female puberty. Plasma lipoprotein levels are not affected by 'chemical' castration with drugs such as gonadotrophin releasing hormone (GnRH) agonists.[18]

THE EFFECTS OF SEX HORMONE THERAPY ON PLASMA LIPOPROTEINS

General considerations

The effects of sex hormones on plasma lipoprotein levels depend on the dose administered, on the route of administration and on factors such as cigarette smoking. Measurement of total cholesterol is of limited use in the context of sex hormone safety evaluation as a fall in plasma total cholesterol levels could be equally due to a fall in LDL levels, which would be perceived as being a beneficial action, or to a fall in those of HDL, which would be perceived as being detrimental.

In general, oral estrogens reduce plasma total cholesterol levels (by reducing those of LDL) and increase those of triglycerides and HDL. Androgens tend to induce the opposite pattern: increases in LDL levels and falls in those of triglycerides and HDL. Androgens share with estrogens the ability to lower plasma levels of Lp(a), further evidence of the atypical nature of this lipoprotein. The changes induced by progestogens such as levonorgestrel, medroxyprogesterone acetate or norethindrone depend very much on the androgenic (or anti-estrogenic) nature of these steroids. Natural progesterone and progesterone derivatives such as dydrogesterone have little or no impact on plasma lipoprotein metabolism, whereas steroids such as levonorgestrel can induce a typically androgenic response in the plasma lipoprotein profile if given at sufficiently high dose. The chemical structure of progestogens provides few clues as to the likely effect of these steroids on plasma lipoprotein levels. For example, desogestrel and gestodene have strikingly less impact on plasma lipoprotein levels than does their parent compound, levonorgestrel.

Detailed information concerning the effects of sex steroids on plasma lipoprotein metabolism can be found in review articles.[19–28] When given in combinations, as in combined oral contraceptives (COC) and combined hormone replacement therapy (HRT), sex hormones influence plasma lipoprotein levels in a simple additive manner. Thus combining an oral estrogen with a progestogen such as levonorgestrel will blunt the increase in HDL seen with estrogen alone. Many studies of combined therapies are limited by their use of a single on-treatment sample, usually taken at the end of the progestogen phase. A further concern is the lack of a control group in many studies. The Postmenopausal Estrogen/Progestogen Interventions (PEPI) Trial[29] found mean plasma levels of some lipids and lipoproteins to drift by 5% in women randomized to placebo; claims that a steroid hormone induces changes of this order need to be treated with caution.

Estrogen therapy: effects on plasma lipoproteins

Triglyceride-rich lipoproteins

Oral estrogens increase fasting plasma triglyceride levels by increasing those of VLDL, leading to a triglyceride-enrichment of LDL and HDL. The effect on VLDL is due to the 'first pass' effect of oral estrogen on the hepatic synthesis of the major VLDL protein, $apoB_{100}$. Oral estrogens differ in their ability to increase fasting triglyceride levels: a rough order (weight-for-weight) would be:

ethinyl estradiol conjugated equine estrogens (CEE) > 17β estradiol > estrone.

At the doses most commonly used for COC and HRT, ethinyl estradiol (30–35μg/d) increases fasting triglyceride levels by about 60%, CEE (0.625–1.25 mg/d) by about 30% and micronized 17β-estradiol (1–2 mg/d) by 0–15%. Transdermal estradiol (50–200 μg/d) does not increase fasting triglyceride levels, consistent with the ability of this route to avoid acutely-high steroid levels in the hepatic portal vein. In some studies, transdermal estradiol reduces fasting triglyceride levels by 10–20%, consistent with the physiological effects of this hormone: premenopausal women tend to have lower fasting triglyceride levels than do age-matched men.

These increased fasting triglyceride levels are not thought to increase CHD risk (see later) although the possibility of triglyceride-induced activation of the hemostatic system is a concern. There is a very rare risk of gross hypertriglyceridemia in genetically-predisposed individuals given COC or HRT, sometimes presenting as severe and life-threatening pancreatitis.[30] Oral estrogens can reduce the extent of postprandial lipemia despite increasing fasting levels.[31] Such as paradox complicates the assignment of clinical significance to estrogenic increases in fasting triglyceride levels. It may be that the increased fasting triglyceride levels, thought by some to be an unwanted side-effect, are eclipsed by the potentially significant improvement in postprandial triglyceride levels.

Cholesterol-rich lipoproteins

All estrogens can reduce plasma total cholesterol levels by reducing those of LDL. In premenopausal women LDL levels are typically low and the doses of ethinyl estradiol used in COC have little effect. Postmenopausal women have higher LDL levels and estrogen therapy with CEE (0.625–1.25 mg/d) or micronized 17β estradiol (1–2 mg/d) causes them to fall by about 10%. More substantial falls may be seen in hypercholesterolemic women. Despite initial reports of a lack of effect on LDL, transdermal estradiol (50–200 μg/d) reduces LDL levels by about 5%.

These falls in LDL levels are achieved by upregulating LDL ($apoB_{100}$/E) receptors in the liver and at other sites. As the major protein component of LDL, $apoB_{100}$ is a ligand for these receptors, LDL particles are rapidly taken up from the plasma compartment, so reducing their plasma levels. Alterations in the synthesis and clearance of LDL precursors such as VLDL may also be important.

Estrogens also reduce LDL levels by reducing the cholesterol content of LDL. This is an unwanted effect, but the atherogenic potential of small dense LDL may be due to their increased susceptibility to lipid peroxidation. As estrogens inhibit lipid peroxidation (although this is controversial), the reduction in LDL particle size seen with estrogens may not be associated with an increase in CHD risk. Estrogens reduce plasma Lp(a) levels by up to 10%, especially in postmenopausal women.

Protein-rich lipoproteins

Estrogens increase HDL levels, but only if given orally. Ethinyl estradiol at doses of 30–35 μg increases HDL levels by 10–15%. Conjugated equine estrogens (0.625–1.25 mg/d) and micronized 17β estradiol (1–2 mg/d) increase HDL levels by about 10%. Higher doses of CEE induce only slightly greater increases, implying that the underlying mechanisms are becoming saturated. The increase is seen in both HDL_2 and HDL_3 subfractions. The major mechanism involves increased hepatic synthesis of the key HDL apolipoprotein, apoAI, resulting in overproduction of HDL. Although estrogens also inhibit the activity of hepatic lipase, an important enzyme in HDL catabolism, this effect may have limited significance *in vivo*.

Transdermal estradiol (50–200 μg/d) has little or no effect on HDL levels, consistent with the avoidance of an acute effect on hepatic protein synthesis.

Androgen and progestogen therapy: effects on plasma lipoproteins

Triglyceride-rich lipoproteins

Androgens and progestogens with androgenic activities lower fasting plasma triglyceride levels by up to 50%, mainly through their ability to activate lipoprotein lipase (LPL), the endothelial-bound enzyme responsible for VLDL catabolism. Nonoral administration of these hormones, for instance as contraceptive implants, may also lower fasting triglyceride levels, confirming the nonhepatic mechanism behind this change. Natural progesterone and progestogens with little or no androgenic activity, such as desogestrel and dydrogesterone, do not affect LPL activity and so do not affect fasting triglyceride levels. Tibolone, a steroid metabolized to hormones displaying both estrogenic and androgenic activities, given at a dose of 2.5 mg/d, reduces fasting triglyceride levels by 20–30%. There are few data on the effects of any of these hormones on postprandial lipemia.

Cholesterol-rich lipoproteins

High doses of testosterone and other androgens can increase plasma cholesterol levels by up to 30% by increasing those of LDL. This is accomplished partly by inhibiting the activity of LDL ($apoB_{100}$/E) receptors, but also by stimulating the LPL-mediated conversion of VLDL to LDL, as described above. Progestogens with androgenic activity such as levonorgestrel increase LDL levels, but not at the doses currently used in COC and HRT. Natural progesterone and progestogens with low androgenic activity do not affect LDL levels. Tibolone (2.5 mg/d) has no effect on LDL levels, a puzzling finding as the effects of this steroid on other lipoproteins are so typically androgenic.

The effects of androgens and progestogens on LDL oxidation and LDL particle size are being evaluated at present. Androgens and progestogens with androgenic activity induce striking falls in Lp(a) levels, for example, tibolone (2.5 mg/d) reduces Lp(a) levels by 50%. The mechanisms behind these changes, unmatched by any other class of drug, are at present unknown.

Protein-rich lipoproteins

Androgens (including the therapeutic steroid danazol), progestogens with androgenic activities and tibolone all reduce HDL levels by 10–50%, according to dose. This reduction is achieved primarily by increasing hepatic lipase (HL) activity and so promoting HDL catabolism; there is little evidence for an effect on apoAI synthesis. Transdermal administration of testosterone reduces HDL by less than 10%; similar falls have been seen with contraceptive implants containing levonorgestrel or medroxyprogesterone acetate (MPA) and with progestogen intra-uterine devices and vaginal rings. Natural progesterone and progestogens with low androgenic activity have little effect on HDL at the doses currently used for COC and HRT.

Oral contraceptives: effects on plasma lipoproteins

Progestogen-only oral contraceptives have little or no effect on plasma lipoprotein metabolism. The net effect of COC on plasma lipoprotein metabolism will depend on the balance between the estrogen (ethinyl estradiol) and the progestogen components. This balance is determined not only by the doses of the two components but by the precise type of progestogen. Relatively androgenic steroids such as levonorgestrel are more effective at opposing estrogen-induced changes in plasma lipoproteins than are steroids such as norethindrone and desogestrel. Surprisingly, when the estrogen dose is reduced to 20 μg with desogestrel-containing COC the lipid profile is only slightly altered from that seen with 30 μg ethinyl estradiol.

Triglyceride-rich lipoproteins

The most striking metabolic effect of the earliest COC was the increase in fasting plasma triglyceride levels.[27] Despite 30 years of reformulation this side-effect remains: the balance of current low-dose formulations is such that none of the progestogens is able to overcome the effect of the ethinyl estradiol component on VLDL synthesis. Even formulations containing high doses (250 μg) of levonorgestrel increase fasting plasma triglyceride levels. Those containing norethindrone, gestodene or desogestrel induce 50% increases; norgestimate formulations may have slightly less effect.

Cholesterol-rich lipoproteins

In contrast, the substantial (30%) increases in LDL levels seen with the early COC formulations are no longer evident.[27] Current low dose formulations have little effect on this lipoprotein. Those containing desogestrel may induce a small (~ 5%) fall in LDL cholesterol levels, but only in older women aged greater than 35 years.[32] COC also reduce LDL particle size and may protect LDL from oxidation. There are some reports of a reduction in Lp(a) levels in women using COC. Levels of apoB are usually raised by current COC, partly due to the contribution of the raised VLDL levels.

Protein-rich lipoproteins

The relatively large doses of progestogens used in the early COC formulations were capable of overcoming the ability of the estrogen component to increase HDL levels, leading to a net reduction of perhaps 20%.[27] Because of the increased risk of CHD seen with these COC, a key feature in the development of current COC formulations has been the desire to avoid such a fall. This has been achieved partly by adjustment of the estrogen-progestogen balance, but even the minimum doses of levonorgestrel needed for clinical efficacy can

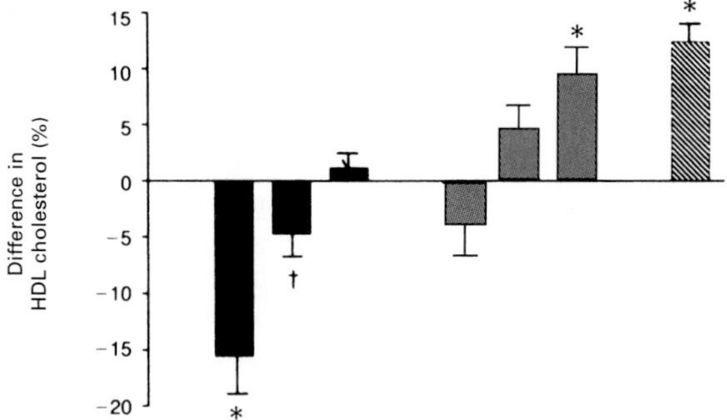

Fig. 62.1 Percent differences in HDL cholesterol levels between women taking one of seven combination oral contraceptives and those not taking contraceptives. Bars 1–3: formulations combining 30–40 μg ethinyl estradiol with 250, 150 or 50–125 (phasic) μg levonorgestrel. Bars 4–6: formulations combining 35 μg ethinyl estradiol with 1000, 500–1000 (phasic) or 500 μg norethisterone. Bar 7: formulation combining 30 μg ethinyl estradiol with 150 μg desogestrel. The T-bars indicate 1 SD. The asterisk ($P < 0.001$) and dagger ($P < 0.01$) indicate significant differences between users and nonusers in the mean values for the principal metabolic variables.[33]

oppose the estrogenic increase in HDL. One potential advantage of progestogens with less androgenic nature, such as desogestrel and gestodene, is that the estrogenic increase in HDL persists (Fig. 62.1).[33]

Hormone replacement therapy: effects on plasma lipoproteins

The plasma lipid profile in users of combined HRT containing micronized natural progesterone or relatively nonandrogenic progestogens, such as dydrogesterone or medrogesterone, is virtually identical to that seen with estrogen monotherapy. In contrast, and in close analogy to the position with COC, progestogens with androgenic properties such as levonorgestrel can oppose and in some cases overcome estrogenic effects on the lipid profile. This is why there has been a move to develop metabolically 'transparent' progestogens which allow the estrogenic effect on plasma lipoproteins to predominate.

The Postmenopausal Estrogen/Progestogen Interventions (PEPI) trial[29] has provided invaluable information on the effect of progestogens on plasma lipoprotein levels. Some of the outstanding features of this clinical trial include a rigorous design (randomized, double-blind, placebo-controlled trial), comparison of four different HRT formulations, a three-year study duration and exemplary lipid and lipoprotein assays.

Triglyceride-rich lipoproteins

The PEPI study[29] shows that low doses of progestogens such as MPA and natural progesterone only weakly oppose the increase in fasting plasma triglyceride levels induced by unopposed oral conjugated equine estrogens (CEE; 0.625 mg/d) (Fig. 62.2). Thus most of the *oral* HRT formulations in current use increase fasting plasma triglyceride levels, regardless of whether they contain a progestogen. Tibolone is a notable exception; as shown above this steroid can lower fasting plasma triglyceride levels. When estrogen is administered nonorally, for instance through a transdermal patch or gel, co-administration of a progestogen lowers fasting plasma triglyceride levels even further. Both combined and estrogen-only HRT reduce postprandial lipemia; the effects of tibolone are not known at present.

Cholesterol-rich lipoproteins

The PEPI study[29] found that the doses and types of progestogen used in current HRT formulations do not oppose estrogenic reductions in LDL levels, and indeed there was a trend towards even lower LDL levels with MPA combinations (Fig. 62.2). A similar — and unexpected — effect has been noted with levonorgestrel-containing therapies. Continuous combined therapies employ lower doses of progestogens but the net progestogen load often approaches that seen with cyclical therapies. A meta-analysis[34] has shown that LDL cholesterol levels are lowered to the same extent as with cyclical therapy.

The impact of combined therapies on plasma Lp(a) levels, LDL particle size and LDL oxidation is currently being evaluated.

Protein-rich lipoproteins

Our understanding of the impact of combined HRT on HDL levels has recently been challenged by evidence that HRT-induced changes in plasma levels of this lipoprotein are transient. This is based on a survey of 292 postmenopausal women, 84 of whom took unopposed estrogen (mostly CEE), 38 of whom took combined therapy (mostly CEE plus MPA) and 170 of whom took no therapy.[35] HDL levels were equally raised in the two HRT groups, compared to the nonusers.

The PEPI study[29] is of particular interest in this respect. In women randomized to CEE monotherapy (0.625 mg/d), HDL cholesterol levels rose by 12% within six months. Addition of medroxyprogesterone acetate (MPA), either cyclically (10 mg/d for 12

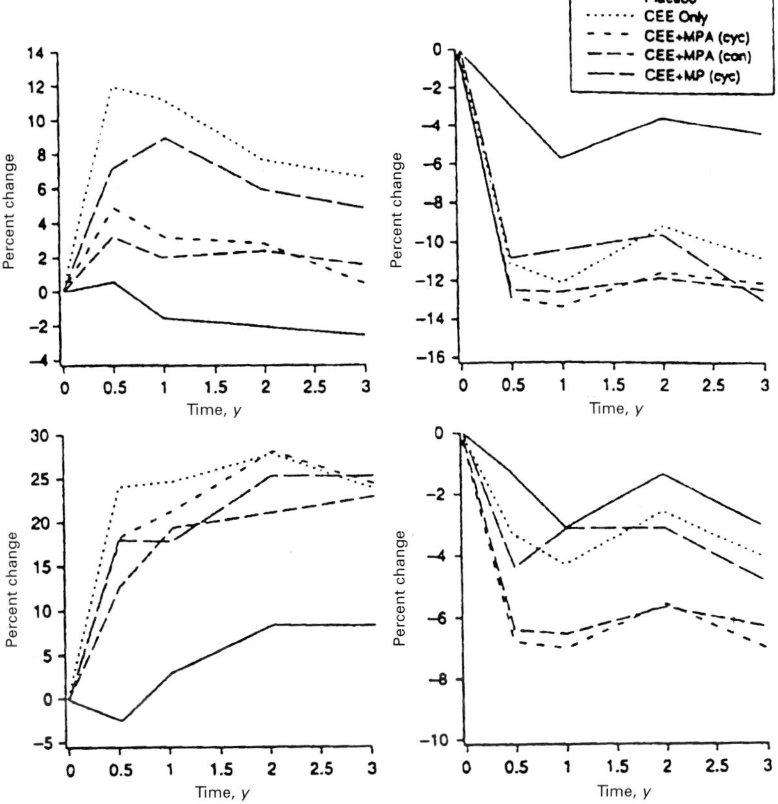

Fig. 62.2 Mean percent change from baseline by treatment arm for HDL cholesterol (top left), LDL cholesterol (top right), triglycerides (bottom left) and total cholesterol (bottom right) in women taking one of four HRT regimens or placebo.[29]

d/month) or continuously (2.5 mg/d), increased HDL cholesterol levels by 3–5%; cyclic micronized progesterone (200 mg/d for 12 d/month) was associated with less opposition to the estrogenic effect and HDL cholesterol levels rose by about 7%. HDL cholesterol levels then fell over the remainder of the duration in all groups, but inspection of these data (Fig. 62.2) shows that the effect of HRT on HDL remained constant relative to women randomized to placebo.

This and other controlled clinical trials show that progestogens such as levonorgestrel, norethindrone and MPA can oppose the estrogenic increase in HDL. This fall is seen with both cyclical and continuous combined therapies.[34] Natural progesterone, dydrogesterone and medrogesterone will not oppose the increase in HDL levels. Tibolone reduces HDL levels by approximately 20%.

The issue of transience of HDL changes needs to be resolved: if the differential effect of various HRT formulations on this potentially important lipoprotein is only expressed for the first five years or so then the attention paid to plasma lipoprotein metabolism may have been excessive. However, there are no known mechanisms for any such 'adaptation' of plasma lipoprotein levels. Long-term randomized trials may be able to resolve this issue.

WHAT IS THE CLINICAL SIGNIFICANCE OF THESE CHANGES IN PLASMA LIPOPROTEINS?

Measurement of the response of the plasma lipoprotein profile to the administration of estrogens, androgens or progestogens has acquired great prominence over the last 30 years, mainly in response to the emerging role of plasma lipoproteins as predictors of CHD. As lipoprotein studies are relatively inexpensive (compared to epidemiological programs) and noninvasive they have become widely used as surrogates for the 'hard' end-points of CHD such as myocardial infarction. This prominence has arisen both from a defensive position (in order to explain the high incidence of CHD seen with older brands of COC) as well as from a more positive way (in order to understand how HRT may reduce this risk). Such lines of enquiry have now merged so that current interest is now firmly directed towards the possibility of improving women's — and, more recently, men's — health by maximizing the beneficial effects of steroid therapies on plasma lipoprotein metabolism. Indeed, the results of plasma lipoprotein studies have contributed to the development of both COC and HRT, the most notable example of this being the introduction of desogestrel as COC progestogen.

Has this emphasis on plasma lipoprotein levels been justified? There is a long and honorable history of studies in fat-fed cynomolgous monkeys and other experimental animals but the findings of such research cannot be directly extrapolated to myocardial infarction events in women. The more appropriate evaluation is to look at the effects of these therapies on the incidence of 'hard' endpoints in women. In terms of COC, the most rigorous comparison would be made between users of formulations containing desogestrel or gestodene versus those containing levonorgestrel, with all women taking similar doses of ethinyl estradiol. At the time of writing (November 1997) this issue is controversial as the apparent protection associated with these newer progestogens, consistent with their effects on HDL, has been suggested to reflect differences in the health care of these women.[36] CHD is an extraordinarily rare event in young women and in the continued absence of any form of randomized controlled trial design perhaps none of the existing studies is capable of resolving this issue.

CHD is more common in older women and there are correspondingly more opportunities in which to evaluate this 'lipid hypothesis'. Here the simplest comparison will be between women using oral estrogen monotherapy and those using oral combined (estrogen-progestogen) therapy. This latter group have traditionally been assumed to lose some of the cardiovascular benefit associated with estrogen monotherapy, mainly due to the blunting of the rise in HDL levels.[37]

There are no randomized controlled trials of the impact of such therapies on CHD. However, observational studies do *not* support the hypothesis that progestogenic/androgenic effects on HDL will translate into a loss of cardiovascular benefit.[38] In the Nurses' Health Study[39] the relative risk of CHD in women using combined therapy compared to nonusers (0.39, 95% confidence interval [CI] 0.19–0.78) was similar to that seen with women using estrogen monotherapy (0.60, 95% CI 0.43–0.83). The number of CHD cases (eight) who used combined therapy was small, but the inability of such studies to demonstrate a progestogen 'problem' in terms of CHD needs to be more widely discussed. This is especially appropriate as the negative image of testosterone and other androgens is itself under question.[40] Thus we are faced with a serious discrepancy between what has been expected (based on changes in the plasma lipoprotein profile) and what has been found (based on clinical events). Perhaps the existing epidemiological database is too weak to be reliable? The debate over bias and confounding in observational studies initiated by the recent studies of COC and venous thromboembolism continues unabated and it is likely that randomized controlled trials — at least in the case of HRT — will be needed to resolve these issues. Such trials are currently in progress in the UK and USA.

Other factors may explain this conflict. Perhaps there has been over-reliance on the power of the plasma lipoprotein profile to predict CHD events, to the exclusion of other aspects of metabolic risk, such as fibrinolysis? Similarly, the direct effects of steroid hormones on endothelial function, vasomotion and plaque stability have only recently been addressed.

One intriguing possibility is that pharmacological changes in plasma lipoprotein levels may not necessarily have the expected effects on atherosclerosis, due to the heterogeneity of the plasma lipoprotein system. The clearest example here is the increased fasting triglyceride levels seen with oral estrogens: this hepatic response involves oversynthesis of large VLDL, not the impaired catabolism of the more atherogenic small VLDL particles. Similarly, the reductions in HDL levels induced by testosterone and related steroids may not impair the anti-atherogenic properties of this lipoprotein. For example, HDL-mediates triglyceride metabolism but triglyceride levels are reduced, not increased, by testosterone and related steroids. The effects of these steroids on other HDL functions, such as reverse cholesterol transport, need to be evaluated.

Conclusion

- All aspects of the plasma lipoprotein system are implicated in CHD.
- Interest in conventional lipid risk factors, such as plasma lipid levels, is moving towards areas such as oxidative damage to lipoproteins, interactions with the endothelium and the postprandial phase.

- Estrogens and androgens affect *all* aspects of the plasma lipoprotein system; progestogens related to natural progesterone have little or no effect whereas those related to testosterone behave as androgens within this system.
- Oral estrogens reduce LDL and Lp(a) levels but increase those of HDL and fasting triglycerides; nonoral estrogens induce smaller falls in LDL and Lp(a) levels and have no effect — or even reduce — those of HDL and fasting triglycerides.
- Androgens and progestogens with androgenic activity, such as levonorgestrel, can increase LDL levels and reduce levels of Lp(a), HDL and fasting triglycerides.
- The traditional view has been that oral estrogens will reduce CHD risk but that progestogens with androgenic properties will oppose any such benefit.
- Recent development of COC and HRT has therefore been driven by the search for 'lipid-friendly' or 'lipid-neutral' progestogens, such as desogestrel and dydrogesterone.
- The epidemiological validation of this approach is still awaited.

REFERENCES

1. Godsland IF, Wynn V, Crook D, Miller NE 1987 Sex, plasma lipoproteins and atherosclerosis: prevailing assumptions and outstanding questions. American Heart Journal 114: 1467–1503
2. Shepherd J 1994 Lipoprotein metabolism — an overview. Drugs 47(Suppl 2): 1–10
3. Packard CJ 1996 Plasma lipid and lipoprotein metabolism in the 1990s — what we know and what we need to know. In: Betteridge J (ed) Lipids: current perspectives. Martin Dunitz, London, pp 1–20
4. Young SG, Parthasarthy S 1994 Why are low-density lipoproteins atherogenic? Western Journal of Medicine 160: 153–164
5. von Eckardstein A, Huang Y, Assmann G 1994 Physiological role and clinical relevance of high-density lipoprotein subclasses. Current Opinion in Lipidology 5: 404–416
6. Hamsten A, Karpe F 1996 Triglycerides and coronary heart disease — has epidemiology given us the right answer? In: Betteridge J (ed) Lipids: current perspectives. Martin Dunitz, London, pp 43–68
7. Zilversmit DB 1995 Atherogenic nature of triglycerides, postprandial lipidemia, and triglyceride-rich remnant lipoproteins. Clinical Chemistry 41: 153–158
8. Scott J, Navaratnam N, Bhattachanya S et al 1994 The apolipoprotein B messenger RNA editing enzymes. Current Opinion in Lipidology 5: 87–93
9. Hokanson JE, Austin MA 1996 Plasma triglyceride level is a risk factor for cardiovascular disease independent of high-density lipoprotein cholesterol level: a meta-analysis of population-based prospective studies. Journal of Cardiovascular Risk 3: 213–220
10. Krauss RM 1991 The tangled web of coronary risk factors. American Journal of Medicine 90(Suppl 2A): 36–41S
11. Maher VMG, Brown BG 1995 Lipoprotein (a) and coronary heart disease. Current Opinion in Lipidology 6: 229–235
12. Jacobs DR, Mebane IL, Bangdiwala SI, Criqui MH, Tyroler HA 1990 High density lipoprotein cholesterol as a predictor of cardiovascular disease mortality in men and women: the follow-up study of the Lipid Research Clinics prevalence study. American Journal of Epidemiology 131: 32–47
13. Bass KM, Newschaffer CJ, Klag MJ, Bush TL 1993 Plasma lipoprotein levels as predictors of cardiovascular death in women. Archives of Internal Medicine 153: 2209–2216
14. Mackness MI, Mackness B, Durrington PN, Connelly PW, Hegele RA 1996 Paraoxonase: biochemistry, genetics and relationship to plasma lipoproteins. Current Opinion in Lipidology 7: 69–81
15. von Eckardstein A, Huang Y, Wu S, Funke H, Noseda G, Assmann G 1995 Reverse cholesterol transport in plasma of patients with different forms of familial HDL deficiency. Arteriosclerosis, Thrombosis and Vascular Biology 15: 691–703
16. Wingard DL 1990 Sex differences and coronary heart disease. Circulation 81: 1710–1711
17. Stevenson JC, Crook D, Godsland IF 1993 Effects of age and menopause on serum lipids and lipoproteins in healthy women. Atherosclerosis 98: 83–90
18. Howell R, Edmonds DK, Dowsett M, Crook D, Lees B, Stevenson JC 1995 Gonadotrophin releasing-hormone analogue (goserelin) plus hormone replacement therapy for the treatment of endometriosis: a randomised controlled trial. Fertility and Sterility 64: 474–481
19. Crook D 1996 Oral contraceptives and vascular disease: role of serum lipids and lipoproteins. Gynecological Endocrinology 10(S2): 65–68
20. Krauss RM 1994 Lipids and lipoproteins and effects of hormone replacement. In: Lobo RA (ed) Treatment of the postmenopausal woman: basic and clinical aspects. Raven Press Ltd, New York, pp 235–242
21. Gevers Leuven JA 1994 Sex steroids and lipoprotein metabolism. Pharmacological Therapeutics 64: 99–126
22. Newnham HH 1993 Oestrogens and atherosclerotic vascular disease — lipid factors. In: Burger HG (ed) Baillière's clinical endocrinology and metabolism, vol 7. The Menopause. Baillière Tindall, London, pp 61–93
23. Bush TL, Miller VT 1987 Effects of pharmacological agents used during the menopause: impact on lipids and lipoproteins. In: Mishell DR (ed) Menopause: physiology and pharmacology. Year Book Medical Publishers, Chicago, pp 187–208
24. Crook D 1996 Postmenopausal hormone replacement therapy, lipoprotein metabolism and coronary heart disease. Journal of Cardiovascular Pathology 28 (Suppl 5): S40–45
25. Crook D, Godsland IF. Safety evaluation of modern oral contraceptives: effects on lipoprotein and carbohydrate metabolism. Contraception (In press)
26. Fotherby K 1985 Oral contraceptives, lipids and cardiovascular disease. Contraception 31: 367–394

27. Burkman RT 1988 Lipid and lipoprotein changes in relation to oral contraception and hormonal replacement therapy. Fertility and Sterility 49: 39S–50S
28. Crook D 1997 The metabolic consequences of treating postmenopausal women with non-oral hormone replacement therapy. British Journal of Obstetrics and Gynaecology 104(16): 4–18
29. The Writing Group for the PEPI Trial 1995 Effects of estrogen or estrogen/progestin regimens on heart disease risk factors in postmenopausal women. Journal of the American Medical Association 273: 199–208
30. Crook D 1998 HRT and hypertriglyceridemias. In: Whitehead MI (ed) The prescriber's guide to hormone replacement therapy. Parthenon (In Press).
31. Westerveld HT, Kock LAW, van Rijn HJM, Erkelens DW, de Bruin TWA 1995 17β-estradiol improves postprandial lipid metabolism in postmenopausal women. Journal of Clinical Endocrinology and Metabolism 80: 249–253
32. Lobo RA, Skinner JB, Lippman JS, Cirillo SJ 1996 Plasma lipids and desogestrel and ethinyl estradiol: a meta-analysis. Fertility and Sterility 65: 1100–1109
33. Godsland IF, Crook D, Simpson R et al 1990 The effects of different formulations of oral contraceptive agents on lipid and carbohydrate metabolism. New England Journal of Medicine 323: 1375–1381
34. Udoff L, Langenberg P, Adashi EY 1995 Combined continuous hormone replacement therapy: a critical review. Obstetrics and Gynecology 86: 306–316
35. Paganini A, Dworsky R, Krauss RM 1996 Hormone replacement therapy, hormone levels, and lipoprotein cholesterol concentrations in elderly women. American Journal of Obstetrics and Gynecology 174: 897–902
36. World Health Organization 1997 Collaborative study of cardiovascular disease and steroid hormone contraception. Acute myocardial infarction and combined oral contraceptives: results of an international case-control study. Lancet 349: 1202–1209
37. Henderson BE, Ross RK, Paganini-Hill A, Mack TM 1986 Estrogen use and cardiovascular disease. American Journal of Obstetrics and Gynecology 154: 1181–1186
38. Psaty BM, Heckbert SR, Atkins D et al 1994 The risk of myocardial infarction associated with the combined use of estrogens and progestins in postmenopausal women. Archives of Internal Medicine 154: 1333–1339
39. Grodstein F, Stampfer MJ, Manson JE et al 1996 Postmenopausal estrogen and progestin use and the risk of cardiovascular disease. New England Journal of Medicine 335: 453–461
40. Crook D 1996 Testosterone, androgens and the risk of myocardial infarction. British Journal of Clinical Practice 60: 180–181

63. Effects on the immunological system

Warren R. Jones

Introduction

Considerations of the effects of exogenous estrogens and progestogens on the immune system cover several related areas. These include the physiological influences of sex steroid hormones on the immune system during the menstrual cycle and pregnancy and the behavior of infections and immunological disorders in relation to these physiological states. The pharmacological effects of exogenous estrogens and progestogens can likewise be considered both in normal individuals and in disease states which directly or indirectly involve the immune system.

Many of the data in these areas are contentious, particularly in animal models, sometimes with directly opposed effects ascribed to the same agent. For this reason, and because the emphasis in this chapter is clinical, reference will be made primarily to human studies supplemented by experimental animal data only where these provide reasonably unequivocal information. It must be stated, however, that the physiological effects of ovarian and placental hormones on the immune system are still relatively poorly understood so that a degree of background 'noise' underlies the assessment of the immunopharmacology of exogenous sex steroids.

Despite these caveats, there is general evidence from several areas of research and clinical practice that gonadal steroids play a significant role in immune function.[1–7] This contention is supported by several fundamental tracts of information:

1. The sexual dimorphism of the immune response
2. Alterations in the immune response during pregnancy
3. The presence of gonadal steroid hormone receptors on cells of the immune system
4. The female preponderance of autoimmune diseases and the increased levels of autoantibodies found in normal women
5. Alterations in immune responses induced by exogenous sex steroids (the primary subject of this chapter).

PHYSIOLOGICAL EFFECTS OF ENDOGENOUS ESTROGENS AND PROGESTOGENS ON THE IMMUNE SYSTEM

Experimental studies in animals and laboratory and clinical evidence in humans demonstrate complex inter-relationships between the endocrine and immune systems. The two physiological circumstances in which these phenomena might become most apparent are during the phases of the menstrual cycle and in pregnancy.

Menstrual cycle

There is clear evidence of an influence of ovarian steroid hormones on the genital tract and that this varies throughout the menstrual cycle. The mucosal immune system has evolved within the female reproductive tract to resist infectious pathogens but not, normally, spermatozoa, thereby allowing successful reproduction to occur. In order to meet these challenges the menstrual endocrine control system regulates genital tract immunity mostly at the level of the uterine cervix. The end result is that sperm are ensured access to the upper tract at midcycle but there is a relative protection against ascending infection at other times in the cycle, particularly in the luteal phase.[8–10] It has been shown, for example, that local immunoglobulin (SIgA, IgG) levels in cervical mucus, and possibly in the Fallopian tube, are relatively low during the estrogen-dominated preovulatory phase and high in the luteal phase in response to escalating progesterone production.[8]

Pregnancy

There has been extensive and continuing interest in

immunoregulatory mechanisms in mammalian pregnancy.[11,12] Whilst estrogens and progesterone clearly participate in the complex immunobiological phenomena which insure successful reproduction in placentate species, their role is probably indirect and marginal. Along with a miriad of other pregnancy-associated molecules they mediate immunological effects in experimental models. Progesterone is broadly immunosuppressive at high dosage levels corresponding to those present in pregnancy. Data for estrogens are somewhat conflicting; at low dosage they stimulate reticuloendothelial activity, but at higher doses they appear to depress cell mediated immune responses in some experimental systems either directly by effects on T lymphocyte subsets, or indirectly by influencing thymic function.[2,13] On balance, in terms of sex steroid activity, the immunosuppressive action of progesterone seems to be the dominant effect in pregnancy.

EFFECTS OF ENDOGENOUS ESTROGENS AND PROGESTERONE ON IMMUNE DISEASES AND INFECTIONS

Once again there is relevant information to be found in this area with regard both to the menstrual cycle and pregnancy.

Menstrual cycle

There are threads of evidence that the activity of autoimmune diseases may fluctuate during the menstrual cycle in a manner that is consonant with the progesterone-dominated immunosuppressive environment of the luteal phase. For obvious reasons, such information is derived from the study of disorders such as the autoimmune connective tissue diseases and arthritides such as rheumatoid arthritis where features such as arthritis/arthralgia and vasculitis are dynamic enough to exhibit discernible changes over the relatively short phasic time-scale involved.[14–17]

There is no clear evidence for altered susceptibility to infection, or lowered responsiveness to vaccination, in relation to the phases of the menstrual cycle.

Pregnancy

The behaviour of most autoimmune diseases is not modified by the potential immunosuppressive influence of pregnancy. The exceptions appear to be systemic lupus erythematosus (SLE) and related diseases, and rheumatoid arthritis (RA). Most studies indicate that SLE tends to exacerbate postpartum,[18,19] perhaps as a rebound manifestation of release from the 'protective' immunosuppressive effect of pregnancy, although it is clear that the behaviour of this complex disease in pregnancy and the puerperium is influenced by many factors including recent advances in therapy. Polyarteritis nodosa behaves similarly.

There has been much interest in the effect of pregnancy on RA. It is now well documented that the disease regularly tends to ameliorate during pregnancy and, variably, to relapse post-partum.[19,20] This phenomenon has an interesting historical background. The first comprehensive observation of the beneficial effect of pregnancy on RA was made by Hench[21] and led to his Nobel prize-winning discovery of the corticosteroids. We now understand that the immunosuppressive role of the increased levels of free cortisol in pregnancy is part of a broader and complex influence mediated by estrogen, progesterone and a variety of pregnancy-associated or pregnancy-specific glycoproteins.[19]

There is no evidence that the prognosis or natural history of autoimmune diseases is altered by pregnancy.[19] The finding of a protective effect for RA of a prior pregnancy that is independent of family history or HLA status[22] is interesting but its implication of some long-term influence on the immune system of exposure to sex steroids is open to question (see below).

The possibility that the hormone-induced systemic immunosuppression of pregnancy may predispose to maternal infection has been widely canvassed but the data are somewhat contentious. Although there is no evidence for a general susceptibility to infection, it appears that there may be depressed resistance to, and increased morbidity in, some infections, particularly those of viral origin.[23]

Skin test reactivity to ubiquitous antigens remains largely unimpaired in pregnancy,[24] as does the ability to respond effectively to immunizations. Therefore, the clinical effects of altered cell mediated immunity (CMI) in pregnancy are marginal and confined mainly to quantitative deficiencies in defence against viral infections.

EFFECTS OF EXOGENOUS ESTROGENS AND PROGESTOGENS ON THE IMMUNE SYSTEM

The 'experiments of nature' associated with the interplay between the endocrine and immune systems in health and disease have provided evidence for immunomodulatory effects of estrogen and progesterone — mostly in the direction of immunosuppression. The effects of exogenous ovarian steroids will now be considered in relation both to various immunological parameters and the (relatively rare) reports of their role in provoking immunopathology.

Most of the data on the effects of exogenous steroid are based on generic groups of agents, i.e. estrogens, progestogens, oral contraceptives (OC), etc.; information on specific steroids, synthetic analogs and components is sorely lacking.

Estrogens

Estrogens in general, and estradiol in particular, have the following effects on the immune system in both physiological and pharmacological dosage:[2,4,5,7,13,25–34]

1. Reversible involution of the thymus; no effect on the spleen
2. Stimulation of antigen-specific primary antibody responses and production of immunoglobulins by lymphocytes after polyclonal activation. This effect is mediated by an inhibitory action of estrogens on T suppressor lymphocytes which allows an increasing activation of maturing B lymphocytes leading to enhanced immunoglobulin production
3. Interaction with specific receptors within the immune system. Receptors are present in the thymus, spleen, and T suppressor (CD8-positive) cells
4. Along with added mitogens *in vitro*, stimulation of CD8 positive cells with a possible simultaneous low level direct activation of effector T helper lymphocytes (CD4-positive cells)
5. Mediation of the production of a variety of immunoregulatory factors in the thymus
6. Depression of *in vivo* CMI responses in experimental systems, including delayed type hypersensitivity skin reactions (e.g. to tuberculin and corneal allografts)
7. Regulation of production of interferon gamma and other lymphokines
8. Stimulation of the general reactivity of the reticuloendothelial system and phagocytosis with enhancement of antigen presenting cells and macrophage activity.

Progestogens

As indicated above, most data on the effects of exogenous progestogens are derived from studies using progesterone in experimental animals. Different classes of progestogens have not been studied individually. 17 OH progestogens might be expected to influence the immune system in a manner similar to the natural hormone. On the other hand the 19-nor compounds might have more complicated effects due to their combined progestogenic and androgenic activity. In this context it can be stated that, in general, androgens have an immunosuppressive effect (and 'protect' against autoimmune disease). They appear to exert a low level inhibition of both T and B lymphocytes.[29,35,36]

Less is described of the effects of progestogens than of estrogens on immune responses and many of the findings overlap. Progestogens, therefore, may cause the following effects:[2,37,38]

1. Suppression of CMI responses
2. Enhancement of T suppressor cell activity
3. Inhibition of mitogen-induced lymphocyte proliferation
4. Activation of macrophages and monocytes.

Despite the overlap of effects of estrogens and progestogens on immunophysiology, there are important differences in their influences on experimental and clinical autoimmune diseases (see below).

Oral contraceptives (OC)

There appear to be no published data on possible specific effects of the various classes of OC (or for that matter of injectable or implantable hormonal contraceptives) on immune responses. Any such effects need to be inferred from the information presented above on estrogens and progestogens, either alone or in combination.

By contrast, there is a respectable literature on the effects of estrogens, progestogens and hormonal contraceptives on autoimmune diseases and, to a lesser extent, on infections (see below).

Estrogens and progestogens causing immunopathology

A syndrome of autoimmune progesterone dermatitis, though rare, is now well documented. Herzberg et al[39] reviewed the condition and were able to cite 42 cases in the English and German literature. To these can be added a further three cases.[40–42] Progesterone sensitivity has also been implicated in a case of recurrent acute anaphylaxis.[43] Stevens et al[41] have described a case of 'estrogen sensitive dermatitis' but the uniqueness of this report suggests that this phenomenon may not be a distinct clinical entity.

Urticaria, erythema multiforme and an eczematous eruption are the most common features of autoimmune progesterone dermatitis; oral and perineal lesions may also occur. The cutaneous eruption appears, or is exacerbated in, the luteal phase of the menstrual cycle and resolves or improves after the menses. The condition abates during periods of amenorrhoea or (variably) in pregnancy. The diagnosis is confirmed by an intradermal progesterone test. Both Type I (immediate) and Type IV (delayed) types of reactions or mixtures can be elicited. Sensitization due to prior exposure to OC or other exogenous ovarian steroids has been proposed as a causative factor, however only 12 of 35 cases reviewed in detail by Herzberg et al[39] fell into this category. In addition Stevens et al[41] were unable to demonstrate cross-sensitivity to estrogen in a study of four cases of autoimmune progesterone dermatitis. Treatment of the condition involves ovulation inhibition with non-progesterone containing compounds. Tamoxifen, Danazol and GnRH agonists have been used with effect.[39,42] Corticosteroids, both topical and systemic, give only temporary relief.

Erythema nodosum is reported as an extremely rare complication of OC use (reviewed in Samter[44]). It remains uncertain whether this disorder is related to estrogen, progestogen or both.

EFFECTS OF EXOGENOUS ESTROGENS AND PROGESTOGENS ON AUTOIMMUNE DISEASES AND INFECTIONS

There is an extensive literature addressing the influence of exogenous estrogens and progestogens on occult and established autoimmune disease. Many of the clinical reports relate to combined oral contraceptives (COC). Comprehensive data on the role of these steroids in the clinical behavior of infections are deficient, perhaps because there is an established tacit assumption that they increase susceptibility to infectious diseases as a consequence of their presumed general 'immunosuppressive' activity. This contention will be examined in detail below.

Autoimmune diseases

Combined oral contraceptives (COC) can initiate SLE and related connective tissue diseases in individuals with an autoimmune diathesis,[45] and can exacerbate established disease and increase the risk of associated complications and manifestations such as vasculitis and pulmonary hypertension.[46,47] The estrogen component of COC appears to be the basis of these deleterious effects.[48,49] This accords with its action in experimental animal models of SLE[50,51] and is mediated by its inhibition of suppressor T cells and antigen-specific T cell reactions, and promotion of B cell hyperreactivity. Some influence on the role of CD5 positive B cells is reported in experimental animals.[52] These cells are increased in number in the blood of patients with some autoimmune diseases including Sjögrens syndrome and RA (but see below). There is also some evidence of altered metabolism of estrogens in SLE whereby increased 16 alpha hydroxylation leads to an accumulation of biologically potent 16 alpha metabolites of estradiol.[53,54]

Progestogens appear to have no deleterious effects on SLE and related disorders.[45,48] The benign (even favorable) effects of different progestogens appear to be unrelated to their progestational properties.[55] In any event, progestogens in general, administered by the oral, depot or implant routes are the hormonal contraceptives of choice in these disorders.

In contrast to their effects in SLE, exogenous ovarian steroids, including OC and agents used for postmenopausal hormone replacement therapy (HRT) have ameliorating effects on established RA.[48,56,57] As is the case with prior pregnancy, the question whether previous or current use of OC or HRT protects against the development of RA is the subject of a contentious literature (for review see Bird[58]).

Once again, estrogen appears to be the major influence in the sex steroid effects on RA.[59] It has been reported that women who have active RA improve on small doses of ethinyl estradiol.[49] These effects are presumably augmented by progestogens in COC. The reasons for the apparently paradoxical effects of estrogens on RA compared with SLE relate to the difference(s) in pathogenesis of the two groups of disorders. RA is a T cell dependent autoimmune disease whereas SLE, in simplistic terms, is B cell dependent.[46] Estradiol suppresses the development, incidence, and severity of Type II collagen-induced arthritris (CIA) in rats and lowers anti-collagen autoantibody levels. Progesterone alone has no effect but when administered together with estradiol the effect is greater than with estradiol alone.[60]

Infections

The possible effects of OC on infection have been a matter of conjecture for many years. Animal and *in vitro* studies have provided little information of value and clinical studies have either been inconclusive or unable to dissect out possible immune influences from the many confounding variables inherent in the epidemiology of OC usage and sexual activity.

Whilst local, nonimmunological effects of OC in the female genital tract (e.g. on cervical mucus) might be expected to protect against sexually transmitted diseases there is no clear evidence that this is so.[61] Equally there is no evidence that the influence of OC on the immune system is manifest in any alteration in the prevalence or behavior of these diseases.

It is a common assumption that the OC usage increases susceptibility to, and severity of, viral diseases such as varicella, herpes simplex and infectious hepatitis. Once again there is no clear and consistent evidence to support this contention. It must therefore be assumed that, on balance, the complicated *in vitro* effects of estrogens and progestogens on immune mechanisms are incapable of abrogating effective defence against infection.

REFERENCES

1. Talal N 1979 Sex factors, steroid hormones and the host response. Arthritis and Rheumatology 22: 1154–1156
2. Grossman CJ 1984 Regulation of the immune system by sex steroids. Endocrine Reviews 5: 435–455
3. Ahmed SA, Penhale WJ, Talal N 1985 Sex hormones, immune responses and autoimmune diseases. Mechanisms of sex hormone action. American Journal of Pathology 121: 531–557
4. Stimson WH 1987 Sex steroids, steroid receptors, and immunity. In: Berczi I, Kovacs K (eds) Hormones and immunity. MTP Press, Lancaster, pp 93–119
5. Pathak SK, Mathur RS 1988 Immune-endocrine interactions. In: Mathur S, Fredericks CM (eds) Perspectives in immunoreproduction — conception and contraceptives. Hemisphere, New York, pp 22–34
6. Lahita RG 1990 Sex hormones and the immune system — part I, human data. Baillière's Clinical Rheumatology 4: 1–12
7. Paavonen T 1994 Hormonal regulation of immune responses. Annals of Medicine 26: 255–258
8. Schumacher GFB 1980 Humoral immune factors in the female reproductive tract and their changes during the cycle. In: Dhindsa G, Schumacher GFB (eds) Immunological aspects of infertility and fertility regulation. Elsevier, Amsterdam, pp 93–141
9. Wira CR, Stern J 1991 Endocrine regulation of the mucosal immune system in the female reproductive tract: control of IgA, IgG and secretory component during the reproductive cycle, at implantation and throughout pregnancy. In: Pasqualini JR, Scholler R (eds) Hormones and foetal pathophysiology. Marcel Decker, New York, pp 343–367
10. Wira CA, Prabhala RH 1993 The female reproductive tract is an inductive site for immune responses: effect of estradiol and antigen on antibody and secretory component levels in uterine and cervico-vaginal secretions following various routes of immunization. In: Griffin PD, Johnson PM (eds) Local immunity in reproductive tract tissues. Oxford University Press, Oxford, pp 271–293
11. Billingham RE, Beer AE 1984 Reproductive immunology: past, present and future. Perspectives in Biology and Medicine 27: 259–275
12. Sargent IL, Redman CWG 1989 Maternal immune responses to the fetus in human pregnancy. In: Stern CMM (ed) Immunology of pregnancy and its disorders. Kluwer Academic, London, pp 115–141
13. Stimson WH 1983 The influence of pregnancy-associated serum proteins and steroids on the maternal immune response. In: Wegmann TG, Gill TJ, Cumming CD (eds) Immunology of reproduction. Oxford University Press, New York, pp 281–301
14. Rose E, Pilsbury DM 1944 Lupus erythematosus (erythematoides) and ovarian function, observations on a possible relationship with a report of 6 cases. Annals of Internal Medicine 21: 1022–1034
15. Rudge SR, Kowanko IC, Drury PL 1983 Menstrual cyclicity of finger joint size and grip strength in patients with rheumatoid arthritis. Annals of Rheumatic Diseases 42: 425–430
16. Steinberg AD, Steinberg BJ 1985 Lupus disease activity associated with the menstrual cycle. Journal of Rheumatology 12: 816–817
17. Bhalla AK 1989 Hormones and the immune response. Annals of Rheumatic Diseases 48: 1–6
18. McHugh NJ, Maddison PJ 1990 Systemic lupus erythematosus: biological effects and management. In: Scott JS, Bird HA (eds) Pregnancy, autoimmunity and connective tissue disorders. Oxford University Press, Oxford, pp 81–113
19. Silver RM, Branch DW 1992 Autoimmune disease in pregnancy. Bailliere's Clinical Obstetrics and Gynaecology 6: 565–600
20. Griffin J 1990 Rheumatoid arthritis: biological effects and management. In: Scott JS, Bird HA (eds) Pregnancy, autoimmunity and connective tissue disorders. Oxford University Press, Oxford, pp 140–162
21. Hench PS 1938 The ameliorating effect of pregnancy on chronic atrophic (infectious rheumatic) arthritis, fibrosis and intermittent hydrarthrosis. Proceedings of Staff Meetings, Mayo Clinic 13: 161–167
22. Hazes JM, Dijkmans BA, van den Broucke JP, de Vries RR, Cats A 1990 Arthritis and Rheumatology 33: 1770–1775
23. Falkoff R 1987 Maternal immunologic changes during pregnancy: a critical appraisal. Clinical Reviews of Allergy 5: 287–300
24. Hawes CS, Kemp AS, Jones WR, Need JA 1981 A longitudinal study of cell-mediated immunity in pregnancy. Journal of Reproductive Immunology 3: 165–173
25. Ahmed SA, Aufdemorte TB, Chen JR, Montoya AI, Olive D, Talal N 1989 Estrogen induces the development of auto antibodies and promotes salivary gland lymphoid infiltrates in normal mice. Journal of Autoimmunity 2: 543–552
26. Kuhn H, Gross M, Schneider M, Weber W, Mehlis W, Stegmuller M, Tanbert H 1983 The effect of sex steroids and hormonal contraceptives upon thymus and spleen in intact rates. Contraception 28: 587–601
27. Holmdahl R, Carlsten H, Jansson L, Larsson P 1989 Oestrogen is a potent immunomodulator of murine experimental rheumatoid disease. British Journal of Rheumatology 28: 54–58

28. Sarvetnick N, Fox HS 1990 Interferon gamma and the sexual dimorphism of auto immunity. Molecular Biology in Medicine 7: 323–331
29. Paavonen T, Andersson LC, Adlercreutz H 1981 Sex hormone regulation of in vitro immune response. Estradiol enhances human B cell maturation via inhibition of suppressor T cells in pokeweed mitogen-stimulated cultures. Journal of Experimental Medicine 154: 1935–1945
30. Sthoeger ZM, Chiorazzi N, Lahita RG 1988 Regulation of the immune response by sex hormones. In vitro effects of estradiol and testosterone on pokeweek mitogen induced human B-cell differentiation. Journal of Immunology 141: 91–98
31. Stimson WH 1988 Estrogen and human T lymphocytes: presence of specific receptors in the T suppressor/cytotoxic subset. Scandinavian Journal of Immunology 28: 345–350
32. Athreya BH, Pletcher J, Zulian F, Weines DB, Williams WV 1993 Subset specific effects of sex hormones and pituitary gonadotrophins on human lymphocyte proliferation in vitro. Clinical Immunology and Immunopathology 66: 201–211
33. Cohen JHM, Davel L, Cordier G, Saez S, Revillard JP 1983 Sex steroid receptors in peripheral T cells: absence of androgen receptors and restriction of estrogen receptors to OKT8 positive cells. Journal of Immunology 131: 2767–2771
34. Hu SK, Mitcho YL, Rath NC 1988 Effect of estradiol on interleukin-1 synthesis by macrophages. International Journal of Immunopharmacology 10: 247–252
35. Lehmann DD 1988 Andogens inhibit proliferation of human peripheral blood lymphocytes in vitro. Clinical Immunology and Immunopathology 46: 122–128
36. Dunkel L, Taino WM, Savilahti E 1985 Effect of endogenous androgens on lymphocyte populations. Lancet ii: 440–441
37. Flynn A 1986 Expression of Ia and the production of interleukin 1 by peritoneal exudate macrophages activated in vivo by steroids. Life Science 38: 2455–2460
38. Holdstock GI, Chastenay BF, Krawitt EL 1982 Effects of testosterone, estradiol and progesterone on immune regulation. Clinical and Experimental Immunology 47: 449–456
39. Herzberg AJ, Strohmeyer CR, Cirillo-Hyland VA 1995 Autoimmune progesterone dermatitis. Journal of the American Academy of Dermatology 32: 333–338
40. Lee CW, Yoon KB, Yi JU, Cho SH 1992 Autoimmune progesterone dermatitis. Journal of Dermatology 19: 629–631
41. Stephens CJ, McFadden JP, Black MM, Rycroft RJ 1994 Autoimmune progesterone dermatitis: absence of contact sensitivity to glucocorticoids, oestrogen and 17 alpha-OH-progesterone. Contact Dermatitis 31: 108–110
42. Yee KC, Cunliffe WJ 1994 Progesterone-induced urticaria: response to buserelin. British Journal of Dermatology 130: 121–123
43. Meggs WJ, Pescovitz OH, Metcalf D, Loreaux DL, Cutler G, Kalmer M 1984 Progesterone sensitivity as a cause of recurrent anaphylaxis. New England Journal of Medicine 311: 1236–1238
44. Samter M (ed) 1988 Immunological diseases, vol. 2. Little, Brown, Boston, p 1248
45. Travers RL, Hughes GR 1978 Oral contraceptive therapy and systemic lupus erythematosus. Journal of Rheumatology 5: 448–451
46. Jungers P, Dougados M, Pelissier C et al 1982 Influence of oral contraceptive therapy on the activity of systemic lupus erythematosus. Arthritis and Rheumatology 25: 618–623
47. Miller MH 1987 Pulmonary hypertension, systemic lupus erythematosus and the contraceptive pill. Annals of Rheumatic Diseases 46: 159–161
48. Barrett C, Neylon N, Snaith ML 1986 Oestrogen induced systemic lupus erythematosus. British Journal of Rheumatology 25: 300–301
49. Schuurs AHWM, Verheul HAM 1989 Sex hormones and autoimmune disease. British Journal of Rheumatology 28: 59–61
50. Talal N 1981 Sex steroid hormones and systemic lupus erythematosus. Arthritis and Rheumatology 24: 1054–1056
51. Holmdahl R 1989 Estrogen exaggerates lupus but suppresses T-cell dependent autoimmune disease. Journal of Autoimmunology 2: 651–656
52. Ahmad SA, Dauphinée MJ, Montoya AI, Talal N 1989 Estrogen induces normal murine CD5+ B cells to produce auto antibodies. Journal of Immunology 142: 2647–2653
53. Lahita RG, Bradlow HL, Kunkel HG, Fishman J 1981 Increased 16 alpha hydroxylation of estradiol in SLE. Journal of Clinical Endocrinology and Metabolism 53: 174–178
54. Bucala R, Lahita RG, Fishman J, Cerami A 1985 Increased levels of 16α-dydroxyestrone modified proteins in pregnancy and systemic lupus erythematosus. Journal of Clinical Endocrinology and Metabolism 60: 841–847
55. Verheul HAM, Schot LPC, Deckers GHJ, Schuurs AHWM 1986 Effects of tibolone, lynestrenol, ethylestrenol and desogestrel on autoimmune disorders in NZB/W mice. Clinical Immunology and Immunopathology 38: 198–208
56. Kay CR, Wingrave SJ 1983 Oral contraceptives and rheumatoid arthritis. Lancet 1: 1437 (letter)
57. Lahita RG 1985 Sex steroids and the rheumatic diseases. Arthritis and Rheumatology 28: 121–126
58. Bird HA 1990 The epidemiology of rheumatic diseases in relation to hormonal factors. In: Scott JS, Bird HA (eds) Pregnancy, autoimmunity and connective tissue disorders. Oxford University Press, Oxford, pp 68–80
59. Bijilsma JW, Huber-Bruning O, Thijssen J-H 1987 Effect of oestrogen treatment on clinical and laboratory manifestations of rheumatoid arthritis. Annals of Rheumatic Diseases 46: 777–779
60. Jansson L, Holmdahl R 1989 Oestrogen-induced suppression of collagen arthritis IV. Progesterone alone does not affect the course of arthritis but enhances the oestrogen-mediated therapeutic effect. Journal of Reproductive Immunology 15: 141–150
61. Burkman RT 1994 Non-contraceptive effects of hormonal contraceptives. American Journal of Obstetrics and Gynecology 170: 1569–1575

64. Psychological, mood and central nervous system effects

Nicholas Panay Robert Sands
John W. W. Studd

Introduction

Reproductive steroids often have profound psychological effects and may be used specifically for the treatment of psychological symptoms. This chapter will consider the data for the effects of reproductive steroids on the central nervous system and through this explain their effects and possible therapeutic benefits on psychological symptoms in the clinical setting.

The effects of reproductive steroids on the CNS are twofold: those affecting neuronal structure and synaptic connectivity (genomic) and those affecting neurotransmission (nongenomic). Genomic effects are permanent and control neural architecture. During fetal life, estrogen exerts organizational effects on brain development that control neural architecture. In adulthood, estrogen has activational effects on brain function via its transitory regulation of brain plasticity and the concentrations of specific neurotransmitters.[1] These effects are described in detail in chapter 17.

Estrogen receptors mediating the genomic effects in the CNS are primarily found in the preoptic area, hypothalamus and amygdala and to a lesser degree in the hippocampus, cerebellum, septal area and inferior colliculus.[2] Progesterone receptors are found in the caudate, cerebellum, cortex, habenula, hippocampus, hypothalamus, olfactory lobe, lamina terminalis and area postrema. Limbic system functions, which subserve emotion and behavior, can therefore be influenced by circulating reproductive steroids. Nongenomic effects alter the chemical/electrical status of the neuron; for example, the progesterone metabolites 3α5α THP and allopregnenolone may bind with the $GABA_A$ receptor to enhance chloride flux. This is one mechanism by which progesterone might have a mood depressant effect on the CNS.

The action of estrogen on CNS neuroreceptors can alter the concentration and availability of neurotransmitter amines, including serotonin and norepinephrine.[3] Estrogen increases the rate of degradation of monoamine oxidase, the enzyme that catabolizes serotonin.[4] Estrogen has been shown to displace tryptophan from its binding sites to plasma albumin[5] allowing more free tryptophan to be available to the brain where it can be metabolized to serotonin. Finally, estrogen enhances the transport of serotonin. The effect of estradiol on neurotransmitter receptors for excitatory amino acids would explain how estrogen may affect mood, particularly as depression is largely due to a serotonin deficit. The decline of estrogen at the menopause may therefore affect mood in some women.

PSYCHOLOGICAL MOOD AND CNS EFFECTS OF ENDOGENOUS REPRODUCTIVE STEROIDS

Depressive illness

Prevalence studies of mental disorders have revealed that males suffer more often from substance abuse and hostility/conduct disorders, whereas women are more prone to develop anxiety disorders and depressive illness. Early experience, social and cultural factors interact with the biological substrate to produce sex differences.[6] It is as yet unclear whether these biological differences are related to the circulating gonadal hormones or due to the action of hormones during sexual differentiation. It is clear that estrogens generally have an excitatory role, activating the central nervous system through neurotransmitter receptor activation in estrogen responsive neurons, leading to elevated mood, increased activity and antidepressant effects. Later on in this chapter we shall consider the evidence for the therapeutic role of estrogen as an antidepressant.

Progesterone is depressant on the central nervous system and in high doses can be anesthetic. It is clear that the times in life when estrogen levels are low, i.e. post-partum and postmenopause, or when progesterone levels are high, i.e. premenstrually, is when the greatest excess of depression occurs on a regular cyclical basis.

Cognitive and sensorimotor functioning

Estrogens play an important role in cognitive functioning in women. Although in humans sexual behavior is not tightly linked to the reproductive cycle it is evident that there are effects of cyclical variation of estradiol on performance of spatial tasks and paired-associate learning. High midcycle estrogen levels have been positively correlated with activation of sensorimotor function, i.e. increased sensory perception such as fine touch, two point discrimination, hearing, olfaction, visual signal detection and increased locomotor activity such as walking, typing, finger tapping.[7] There also appears to be improved limb coordination. The progesterone dominant part of the luteal phase has been linked to increased ability in perceptual restructuring tasks requiring a response delay. These tasks include mental subtraction, time estimation and solving of maze and embedded number problems.[8]

It is thought that the facilitating action of estradiol on cognitive functions such as learning, short term memory and attention may be directly related to genomic estrogenic effects as a growth factor on estrogen responsive dendritic neurons with synapse formation.[9]

Premenstrual syndrome

There are indications it is the high luteal phase progesterone levels which exacerbate PMS symptoms such as depression and mood swings. This is supported by the fact that abolition of ovulation with GnRH analogs or percutaneous estrogens alleviates symptoms.

Dementia

Estrogens may also have a direct effect on the vasculature of the central nervous system leading to smooth muscle relaxation and improved perfusion. This may partly explain the benefits of hormone replacement therapy (HRT) in subjects predisposed to multi-infarct and Alzheimer's dementia.

Other CNS effects of reproductive steroids

Catamenial epilepsy varies according to the menstrual cycle, with the peak frequency of occurrence corresponding to the lowest ratio of progesterone to estradiol during the cycle.[10] In addition to a genetic and/or developmental predisposition to express seizures there may also be at least three types of hormone actions involved in the cyclical occurrence of epilepsy and protection from seizures. First, estrogen may induce excitatory synapses in the hippocampus leading to reduced seizure thresholds. Secondly, progesterone can act via steroid metabolites through the $GABA_A$ receptor to reduce excitability, and thirdly, the reproductive steroids can act on the liver to increase clearance rates of antiseizure medication.[6] Estrogens are also recognized to exacerbate symptoms of Parkinson's disease. This effect supports the anatagonistic action of estradiol on the dopaminergic system which is a postulated mechanism for its antidepressant effects.

PSYCHOLOGICAL, MOOD AND CNS EFFECTS OF HORMONE REPLACEMENT THERAPY

Effect of the menopause on the CNS

There is now much evidence to suggest that changes in brain function with increasing age are mainly as a result of changes in the levels of reproductive steroids. The menopause is associated with a reduction of central content and activity of certain neurotransmitters and neuropeptides which is improved by estrogen administration. Climacteric depression is at its worst 2–3 years before the periods stop and it is the women who are still having regular periods whose depression may respond to estrogens rather than the postmenopausal women.[11] Correction of vasomotor instability, insomnia and painful intercourse will help mood in what is called the 'domino effect', but there is also a mental tonic effect of estrogens that occurs irrespective of other climacteric symptoms. Estrogen replacement appears to enhance mood in a dose-dependent manner and also enhances or maintains aspects of cognitive functioning. See chapter 17 for more detailed discussion on physiological CNS effects.

Effects of HRT on the CNS of menopausal women

Cognition

Reports of estrogen effects on cognition have not been unanimous but the consensus appears to be that some modalities, particularly memory, are improved. Philips and Sherwin,[12] studying 19 bilaterally oophorectomized women given estradiol valerate, found that only immediate recall and associative learning improved whereas delayed recall, visual reproduction and digit span did not improve. In a large study by Barrett-Connor and Kritz-Silverstein,[13] 800 women including current, past and never users of mainly conjugated equine estrogens aged 65–95 years were studied. No improvement was seen in the estrogen user groups in terms of mental status, visual and verbal memory. Finally, in a study by Kampen and Sherwin,[14] 71 healthy postmenopausal women receiving various types of estrogen were found to have an improvement in verbal memory but no difference in spatial ability or attention. From these and other studies we must conclude that HRT improves several but not all cognitive constructs and it is uncertain if it can be targeted for specific cognitive tasks. It is still unknown if estrogen effects are different in different age groups, nor is it known whether its effect is only preventative or might also be restitutional.

Depression

There are few adequate studies that have looked at oral estrogen in adequate doses but climacteric depression has been shown to improve with percutaneous estrogens, either patch or implant. Montgomery et al[11] demonstrated significant elevation of mood in climacteric depression in women treated with estrogen and testosterone implants (Fig. 64.1). The benefits were not transient but were maintained until the end of a 23 month follow up (Fig. 64.2).

Many studies have evaluated whether mood is worsened during the climacteric by studying overall quality of life. For example, Daly et al[15] found that 63 women with complaints of menopausal symptoms, age 45–60, had improved well-being after estrogen therapy. Limouzin-Lamothe et al[16] also showed that general well-being, in 499 women with a mean age of 51, was improved by estrogen therapy. Ditkoff et al[17] studying 36 asymptomatic women aged 45–60 found that they had significantly improved Beck depressive scores following therapy with conjugated estrogens. Finally, Best et al[18] found that 16 healthy hysterectomized postmenopausal women had improved Hamilton Depression scores after estradiol implants.

The effect of hormone replacement therapy on mood has been studied by many workers but few have concentrated on patients with major depressive disorder. One of the earliest and most convincing studies as to the benefits of estrogen in depression is that of Klaiber et al[19] who studied the use of oral equine estrogens in severely depressed inpatients who had been unresponsive to conventional treatments such as electroconvulsive therapy, antidepressants and psychotherapy. According to DSM criteria, these patients all had primary, recurrent unipolar major depressive disorders. Conjugated equine estrogens were commenced on huge doses, starting with a dose of 5 mg and increased weekly in 5 mg increments to a maximum of 25 mg daily, a dose achieved in 50% of those receiving active treatment. The results were impressive in that there were highly significant reductions in depression scores in the estrogen-treated group, as well as clinically significant improvements in mood as observed by trained personnel (Fig. 64.3).

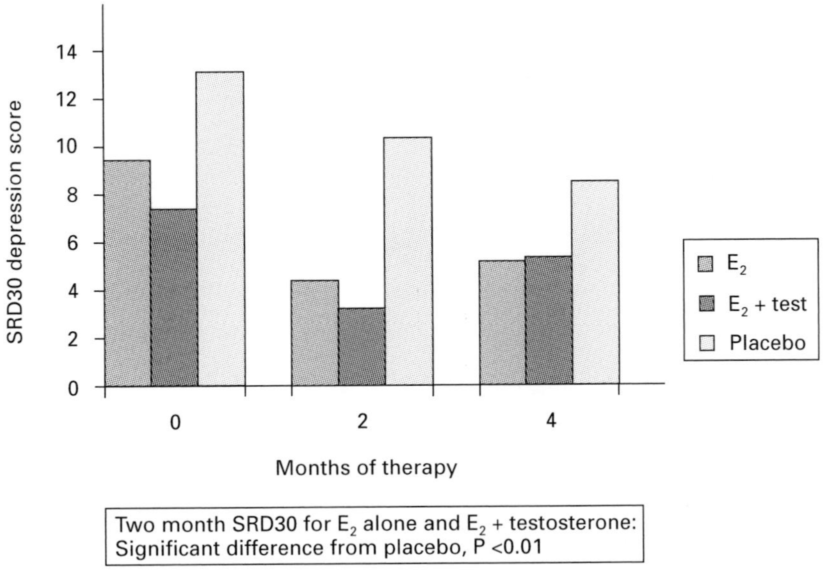

Fig. 64.1 Effect of estradiol/testosterone implants in perimenopausal women.[14]

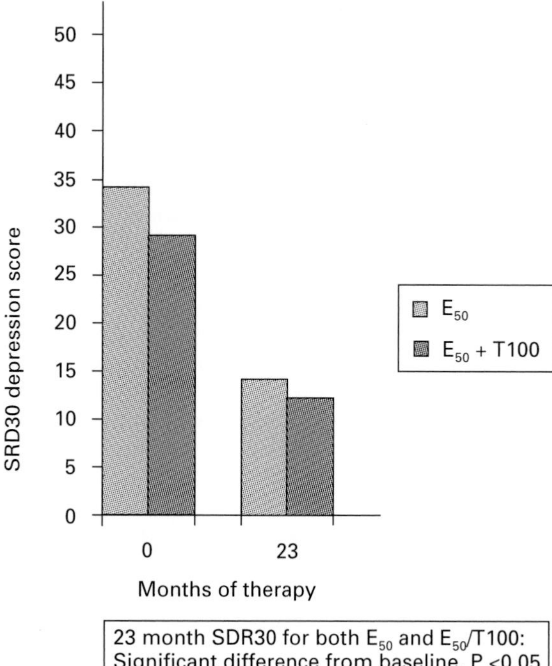

Fig. 64.2 Perimenopausal depression and hormone implants: 23 month results. (From Montgomery J, Studd JWW: unpublished data, used with permission.)

This important study was overlooked because of fears of high dose estrogens and is only recently being corroborated.

Some studies on depressed patients have not found the response to estrogen to be as promising. Coope et al[20] assessed the response of 55 depressed patients, aged 40–60, to piperazine estrone sulfate in a double-blind placebo-controlled cross-over study. There was no significant improvement in the Beck depression scores but a low dose of weak estrogen was used. Shapira et al[21] also found no improvement with estrogen supplementation of eight depressive postmenopausal women on imipramine therapy. It may be that the dosage and hence serum levels of estrogen achieved in these study patients were inadequate to produce an effect. The most acceptable treatment for climacteric depression in our opinion are estradiol patches, 200 μg twice weekly, which will produce estradiol levels of about 600 pmol/L. There are anxieties about overtreatment with estrogens but these levels are still within the normal range of the ovarian cycle.

Dementia

Estrogens may have a direct effect on the vasculature of the central nervous system, increasing blood flow. Studies have demonstrated that estrogen replacement therapy may improve cerebral perfusion and cognition in postmenopausal women with cerebrovascular disease.[22] In the long term this may prevent diseases with a vascular etiology such as vascular dementia[23] and Alzheimer's disease, as the vasculature is clearly involved in this.[24] Two studies of elderly female Alzheimer's patients have revealed improvements in

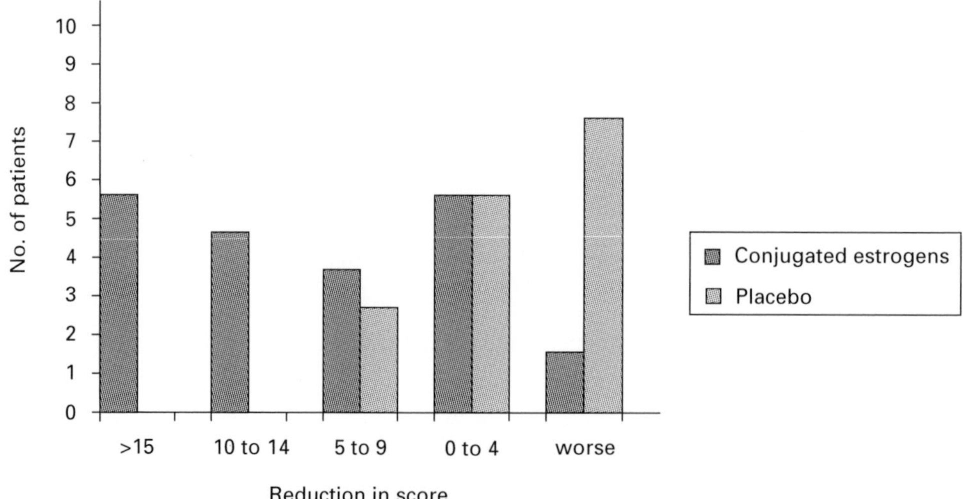

Fig. 64.3 Effect of high dose conjugated equine estrogens on major depression.[19] Improvement in Hamilton depression scores: Conjugated estrogens vs placebo.

tests of mental status over a period of six weeks of estrogen replacement therapy.[25,26]

PSYCHOLOGICAL, MOOD AND CNS EFFECTS OF CONTRACEPTIVE THERAPY

Combined oral contraceptive (COC)

There has been controversy as to the psychological effects of the combined oral contraceptives (COC). Research has suggested that oral contraceptives can cause depression by inducing tryptophan oxygenase, which leads to pyridoxine deficiency in some women.[27] The observation by Forrest of a steady increase in depression scores during the menstrual cycle seemed to support the theory of a metabolic cause for the increase in pill-associated depression.[28] Other workers showed that the alteration in tryptophan metabolism is usually well compensated in nonsusceptible individuals but may accentuate or precipitate the development of depression in susceptible individuals.[29]

There are indications that certain women are sensitive to production of negative mood changes by progestogens. Cullberg[30] showed that only women who had previously suffered from PMS reacted badly when taking COC. This suggests that women with PMS are more sensitive to hormonal provocation than women without. There are also some endocrine indications the hypothalamo-pituitary unit is more sensitive to ovarian hormones in women with PMS than in controls.[31] This is important as it suggests that it would be possible to predict which patients would experience negative mood changes during COC use and HRT. In women taking COC, a triphasic pill is more likely to provoke symptoms than a monophasic pill.[32] Qualitative differences appear to exist between different types of progestogenic compounds. In Cullberg's study, desogestrel was found to be less likely to provoke symptoms than levonorgestrel.[30]

Others have been unable to demonstrate an increased incidence of depression in COC users. Fleming and Seager[33] in a cross sectional study found that the incidence of depression in 335 women taking the pill was no higher than among matched controls not taking such medication. The intensity of depression was related more to age, personality and occupation than to use of the pill. A higher proportion of users than of controls experienced sexual satisfaction. In a more recent study, 4112 women's well being and sexual interest were studied retrospectively by questionnaire.[34] Oral contraceptive users, although found to have broadly similar patterns of well-being, were less likely to show peaks and troughs of well-being and highs and lows of sexual interest. This was more evident in the monophasic than triphasic pill users.

The Royal College of General Practitioners study[35] found no episodes of depression requiring hospitalization and only a slight excess of mild to moderate depression which was mainly in higher dose pill users, i.e. greater than 35 μg of ethinylestradiol. In balance, it appears that with modern low dose pills the incidence of psychological problems is extremely low. In women with depressive symptoms, use of a pill with a different type of progestogen may improve symptoms. A course of pyridoxine may also help, which may have to be taken for two months before benefits are seen.[36]

Progestogen-only pill (POP)

Psychological disturbances and the premenstrual syndrome have been found to be more a problem with the combined oral contraceptive than the POP.[37] In fact there have been no studies where the POP has been implicated as specifically causing clinically significant depression. In those patients where ovulation suppression occurs (approximately 50%) there may even be improvement of depressive symptoms associated with premenstrual syndrome.

Depot progestogens

Little work has been done specifically on the psychological side-effects of depot progestogens such as depot medroxyprogesterone acetate (DMPA — Depo Provera®, Pharmocia and Upjohn) and levonorgestrel implants (Norplant® Hoechst). Theoretically, one would expect these progestogens to produce PMS-type side effects (depression, mood swings, irritability and headaches). This, to a certain extent, is counteracted by the ovulation suppressant effects (especially DMPA), so much so that many users, particularly those who are amenorrheic, appear to have an improvement in their PMS symptoms.[36] Nevertheless, depression and mood change have been reported to occur in some users of DMPA.[38]

One of the few studies that has specifically looked at psychological symptoms in Norplant® users,[39] found that a small but significant number of women suffered from nervousness and depression following implant insertion. More importantly, these psychological problems seemed to be more important than bleeding problems in determining whether removal of the implants was requested by the user. It has been suggested that mental problems related to Norplant® have received too little attention and that satisfaction was highest in carefully selected users among older women. This is supported by Wagner and Berenson's[40] case reports of two women, aged 18 and 29 years, who developed depression and panic disorder one to two months after insertion of Norplant®. The symptoms worsened over the following year and resolved within one month of removal. These authors also stressed the importance of careful case selection for Norplant® usage and that patients should be informed of the risk of psychiatric disorders with this contraceptive method.

The levonorgestrel intra-uterine system (LNG-IUS — Mirena® Schering HC), which releases 20 µg of levonorgestrel every 24 hours, appears to have predominantly a local effect on the endometrium producing very low and constant systemic levels.[41,42] Psychological side-effects such as depression and irritability, are minimal and are usually worst in the first three months.[43,44] It has been proposed as the ideal method of providing progestogenic opposition in women using hormone replacement therapy who are progestogen intolerant and would otherwise not comply with treatment.[45,46]

PSYCHOLOGICAL, MOOD AND CNS EFFECTS OF OTHER GYNECOLOGICAL THERAPEUTIC REGIMENS USING REPRODUCTIVE STEROIDS

The premenstrual syndrome

The complex mood and psychological aspects of premenstrual syndrome are thoughly reviewed in chapter 33.

Although the underlying cause of PMS remains unknown, cyclical ovarian activity appears to be an important factor.[47] A logical treatment for severe PMS, therefore, is to suppress ovulation and thus suppress the cyclical endocrine/biochemical changes which cause the cyclical symptoms.[48] Estrogens and progestogens have been used for this. A treatment of proven efficacy in a placebo-controlled trial which appears suitable for long-term usage is continuous 17β estradiol combined with cyclical progestogen. This was first administered as a 100 mg implant and proved to be highly effective in every Moos cluster of symptoms compared to placebo (Fig. 64.4).[49]

The drawback with this is that the implants last for a long period of time.[50] Fertility is suppressed for 12–24 months and progestogens must be continued for at least 18 months until the stimulatory estrogenic effects on the endometrium have ceased.

Transdermal estradiol patches have also been used with success. In the first study, Estraderm TTS® 200 µg patches were shown to suppress ovulation.[51] This dose was subsequently tested against placebo in a cross-over trial and found to be highly effective in the treatment of PMS (Fig. 64.5).[52]

Another theory about the action of estradiol in PMS is that it may act directly by elevating mood.[11,17,19] The observation in the Smith et al[53] study that estradiol 100 µg was equally as effective as estradiol 200 µg in treating PMS strongly suggests the principal

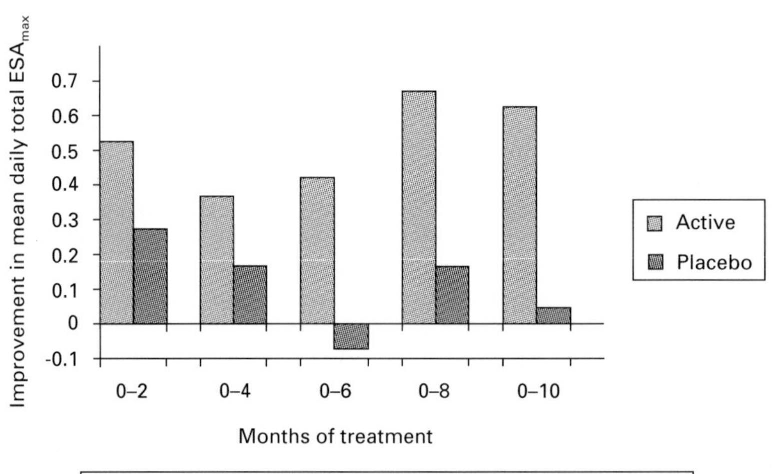

Fig. 64.4 Subcutaneous estradiol and PMS improvement in total Moos MDQ score with time: estradiol versus placebo.[49]

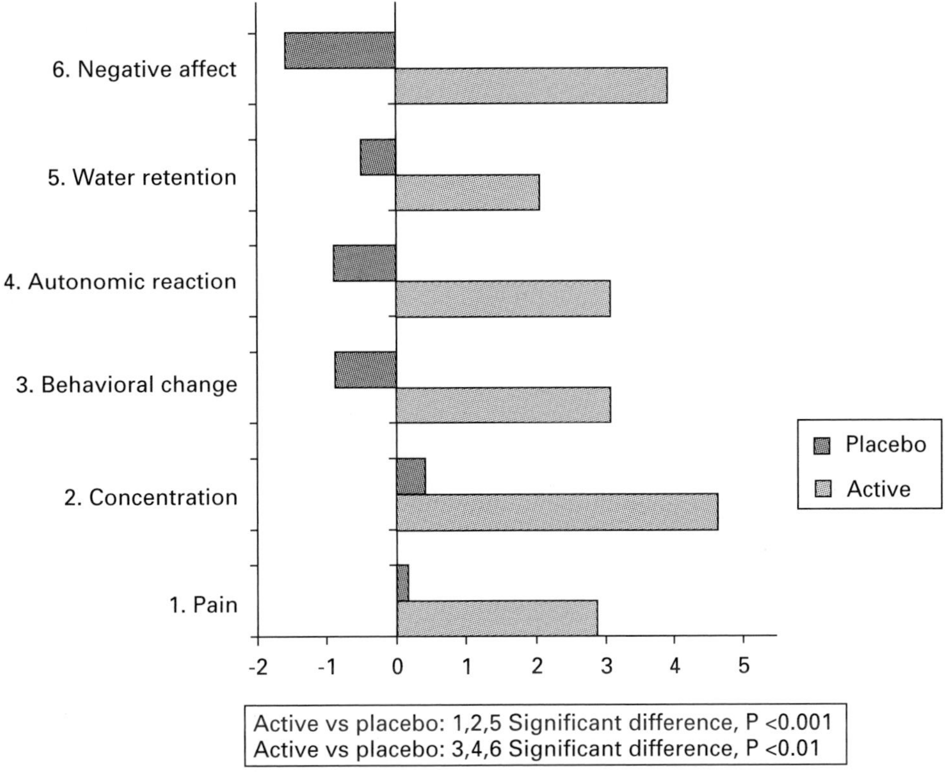

Fig. 64.5 Percutaneous estradiol and PMS improvement in adverse Moos symptom clusters.[52]

mechanism of action is ovarian suppression, although the logical study of luteal phase support by transdermal or oral estrogen has yet to be performed.

Estrogen therapy in women with postnatal depression

Postnatal depression will affect approximately 10–15% of women following childbirth and will persist for longer than a year in approximately 40% of those affected.[54]

The possibility of a biological etiology for postnatal depression has been proposed because of various pieces of evidence. These include: the increasing incidence of mood disorders at times of rapidly fluctuating, mainly falling, hormone levels, e.g. premenstrually, post-partum and perimenopausally; the relatively constant time interval between delivery and the onset of each post-partum disorder; the lack of overall influence of psychosocial and background factors in determining post-partum disorders; the possible association between premenstrual syndrome and post-partum depression; and finally the estrogen responsiveness of both PMS and postnatal depression.[55]

Wagner[56] has postulated that the high circulating estrogen levels of pregnancy protect against depression and the rapid decline of levels at birth removes this effect. Although a clear link has not as yet been established between the reproductive steroids and postnatal depression in studies carried out so far,[57,58] this may be due to methodological problems of such research. Alder,[59] who assessed breastfeeding patterns and contraceptive use post-partum, stressed the importance of taking these factors into account when conducting biological studies into post-partum depressive illness.

We have already seen that a number of studies using estrogens[11,15–19] have produced significant improvements in levels of depression in perimenopausal women using hormone replacement therapy. There are also data to support the hypothesis that therapy with 200 μg transdermal estradiol both significantly reduces depression scores and accelerates recovery in women with postnatal depression.[60] Data recently published from our unit provide further evidence of the benefits of estradiol in this condition (Fig. 64.6).[61]

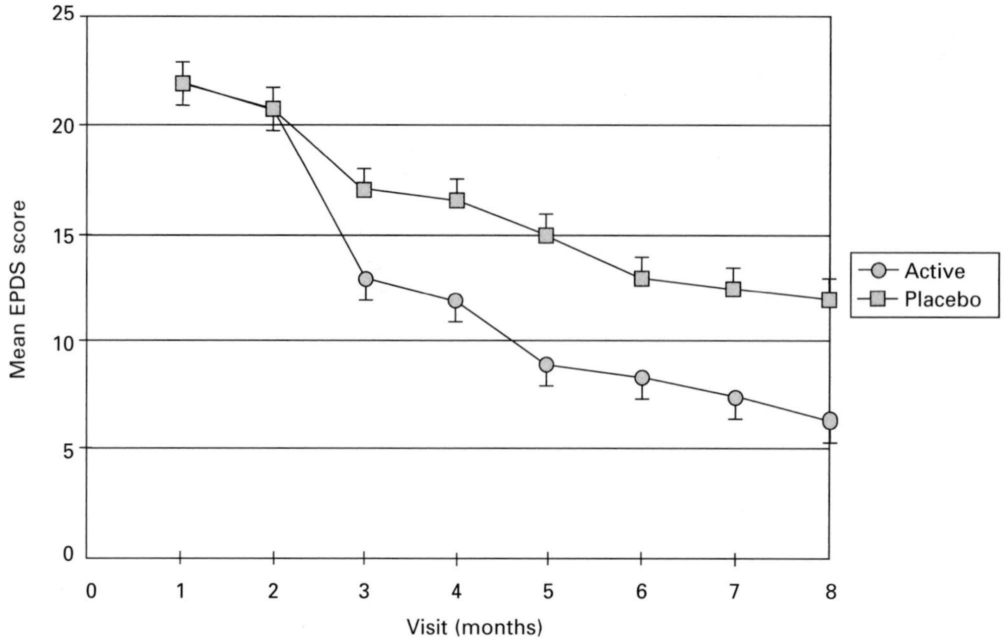

Fig. 64.6 Transdermal estradiol for severe postnatal depression.[61] Subject's Edinburgh postnatal depression scores (EPDS) are shown before (<2 months) and after (>2 months) starting a placebo-controlled trial of transdermal therapy with 17β estradiol, 200 μg per day for postnatal depression. The pretreatment scores of the two groups are very similar. On the third visit, i.e. after 1 month of treatment, there is already a significant difference between active and placebo groups, which is then maintained. Mean scores (+/– SE) are shown for each group.

Noncontraceptive progestogen/progesterone regimens

The following progestogen and progesterone therapeutic regimens will be discussed in the context of possible psychological effects: the cyclical treatment of conditions such as dysfunctional uterine bleeding (DUB) and secondary dysmenorrhea and progestogenic opposition in estrogen therapy; continuous high dose regimens used for the treatment of endometriosis, endometrial hyperplasia and carcinoma; cyclical regimens with progesterone used for the treatment of recurrent miscarriage, PMS and support of early pregnancy; and antiprogestogens used in the induction of abortion and in the treatment of PMS.

Cyclical progestogenic regimens

Most workers studying the psychological effects of cyclical therapeutic progestogens in recent years have concentrated on the effects of progestogens used in sequential opposition to estrogen therapy. One of the most frequently encountered problems with progestogen therapy has been that of negative mood effects, especially depression, anxiety and cognitive impairment.[62] In the study by Smith et al,[53] 44% of PMS patients receiving either dydrogesterone 10 mg for 10 days each month or medroxyprogesterone acetate (MPA) 5 mg for 10 days each month experienced side effects attributable to the progestogen. There was no significant difference in the total incidence of side effects between women taking dydrogesterone and those taking MPA. An even higher incidence of side effects (58%) has been observed in women using the more androgenic progestogen norethindrone in women being treated for PMS with estradiol implants.[63] Problems with progestogenic side effects have also been demonstrated in menopausal patients using hormone replacement therapy.[64] In a study by Magos et al[65] the PMS-type effects of norethindrone were demonstrated in postmenopausal women.

Compliance with cyclical progestogenic treatment has been shown to be poor, particularly when used in sequential HRT regimens.[66] Therapy is often discontinued because of the physical and psychological side effects. Women receiving combined therapy will occasionally resort to hysterectomy and bilateral oophorectomy so that unopposed estrogens can be used.[67]

Clinicians must therefore try to find ways in which to minimize these side effects and thus maximize compliance. This can be achieved by reducing the dose and duration of progestogen in combined regimens. For instance, it is acceptable in PMS patients to give only seven to ten days of progestogen with close monitoring of withdrawal bleeds and a low threshold for endometrial sampling. In combined HRT, small amounts of progestogen, e.g. 2.5 mg medroxyprogesterone acetate, can be given on a daily basis to protect the endometrium and minimize side effects.

Alterative progestogens such as the 17-hydroxyprogesterone-derived pregnanes, medroxyprogesterone acetate and dydrogesterone, should be used as first line therapy, rather than the 19 nortestosterone-derived estranes such as norethindrone which have more psychological as well as other side effects. The third generation gonane progestogens such as desogestrel and gestodene appear to have superior psychological side effect profiles compared to older generation progestogens.[30] It is unfortunate that, in combination with ethinylestradiol, these contraceptive pills have recently been shown to be associated with twice the risk of non-fatal thromboembolism compared to first and second generation progestogen-containing combined pills. It is possible that this association is due predominantly to 'higher risk' women preferentially using these pills. In women who are severely progestogen intolerant and do not have risk factors for thromboembolism these progestogens may be a useful alternative.

Finally, the oral route can be avoided altogether by using the levonorgestrel or progesterone-releasing intra-uterine systems, reducing CNS and systemic side effects even further. These systems are not yet licensed for use as progestogenic opposition for estrogen therapy but trials are currently underway to confirm this benefit.

Continuous progestogen regimens

Continuous progestogens have been given in high doses to women with endometrial hyperplasia, carcinoma and endometriosis. Although there may be a reduction in general well-being and depression of mood, suppression of ovulation in non-oophorectomised women can occasionally improve cyclical depressive symptoms.

Progesterone regimens

Progesterone, like progestogens, has been used in the management of various gynecological disorders including endometrial hyperplasia, menopausal symptoms, dysfunctional uterine bleeding, amenorrhea, luteal phase inadequacy and premenstrual syndrome. Oral micronized progesterone has been developed to overcome absorption problems which meant in the past it had to be given by injection or rectally. Unlike oral progestogens, psychological and other side effects are uncommon with progesterone administration. Dalton,[68] using low dose progesterone as an uncontrolled treatment for PMS, did not detect any adverse effects in 40 women treated over 10 years for PMS. High dose micronized oral progesterone therapy, especially when given with food which increases its absorption, is associated with transient drowsiness.[69]

Progesterone has been advocated as a treatment for premenstrual syndrome but most double-blind studies have failed to show any efficacy of progesterone over placebo.[70] Only Dennerstein et al,[71] in a double-blind placebo-controlled cross-over study using oral micronized progesterone, claimed a slight improvement in mood symptoms such as anxiety, depression and stress, but Magos and Studd[72] in correspondence showed that there was no improvement if the appropriate statistical method was used. These findings of a lack of efficacy for progesterone are not surprising if one considers the CNS depressant effect of endogenous progesterone and that premenstrual symptoms are at their worst during the luteal phase of the cycle when natural progesterone levels are at their highest.

Antiprogestogens

Since most of the mood changes and associated symptoms of PMS occur during the luteal phase of the menstrual cycle when progesterone levels are at their highest, it would seem logical that antiprogesterone treatment may alleviate the symptoms of PMS.[73] Two well conducted studies using mifepristone (RU486) for the treatment of PMS have been published so far.[74,75] Unfortunately, neither of these showed any improvement in either the physical or psychological symptoms of PMS suggesting that antiprogestogens have no significant application in the treatment of PMS.

Conclusions (see Table 64.1)

Endogenous estrogens have been shown to have an excitatory role on central nervous system

Table 64.1 Key points: psychological, mood and CNS effects of therapeutic reproductive steroids.

Estrogens	Progesterone/progestogens
Affect neurotransmitters and their receptors in similar manner to antidepressants	Effect of progesterone on CNS neurotransmitters can cause depressed mood
Improvement in selective cognitive functioning	Progesterone anesthetic in large doses
Physiological doses modulate mood in nondepressed women	Improvement in selective cognitive functioning in luteal phase of cycle
Pharmacological doses treat major depressive illness	PMS-like psychological side effects (depression, mood swings, irritability) with cyclical progestogens and triphasic combined oral contraceptives
Good evidence for preventative and therapeutic effects in Alzheimer's and multi-infarct dementia	Occasional improvement of PMS symptoms with depot medroxyprogesterone, ovulation-suppressing doses of other continuous progestogens and LNG IUS
No evidence for major depressive illness in women using low dose combined oral contraceptive	Evidence for depressive illness in some users of depot levonorgestrel implants
Physiological doses effectively treat premenstrual syndrome	No significant depression with therapeutic doses of progesterone
Physiological doses effectively treat postnatal depression	No significant improvement of PMS with progesterone or antiprogestogens

neurotransmitters. We have seen that therapeutic estrogens can produce significant improvement in the triad of estrogen-responsive psychological disorders: postnatal depression, premenstrual depression and climacteric depression. There is also strong evidence that estrogens can protect against and improve the symptoms of Alzheimer's disease and multi-infarct dementia. There is no good evidence that modern low dose combined oral contraceptives produce clinically significant depression or any improvement in the condition.

Endogenous progesterone has depressant effects on the CNS. Therapeutic progestogens, especially when given cyclically, can have adverse psychological effects producing PMS-like symptoms such as depression, irritability and loss of concentration. These effects can be reduced by giving a smaller amount and duration of less androgenic progestogens or by avoidance of the oral route, specifically directing treatment to the endometrium where it is required, via an intra-uterine system.

Future research should be directed at confirming the role of estrogen as a treatment for the triad of depressive disorders previously mentioned so that inappropriate treatment with antidepressant medication and electroconvulsive therapy can be avoided. We should also concentrate our efforts on finding increasingly sophisticated ways of avoiding the problem of progestogen intolerance which at present reduces treatment effectiveness and compliance in many women.

REFERENCES

1. Sherwin BB 1996 Hormones, mood and cognitive functioning in postmenopausal women. Obstetrics and Gynecology 87(2S): 20–26
2. Maggi A, Perez J 1985 Role of female gonadal hormones in the CNS: clinical and experimental aspects. Life Sciences 37: 893–906
3. Crowley WR 1982 Effects of ovarian hormones on norepinephrine and dopamine turnover in individual hypothalamic and extrahypothalamic nuclei. Neuroendocrinology 34: 381–386
4. Luine VN, McEwen BS 1977 Effect of estradiol on turnover of type A monoamine oxidase in brain. Journal of Neurochemistry 28: 1221–1227
5. Aylward M 1973 Plasma tryptophan levels and mental depression in postmenopausal subjects. Effects of oral piperazine oestrone sulphate. IRCS Medical Science 1: 30–34
6. McEwen BS 1993 Ovarian steroids have diverse effects on brain structure and function. In: Berg G, Hammar M (eds.) The modern management of the menopause. Parthenon Publishing Group, New York, pp 269–278
7. Zimmerman E, Parlee MB 1973 Behavioural changes associated with the menstrual cycle: an experimental investigation. Journal of Applied Social Psychology 3: 335–344

8. Broverman DM, Klaiber EL, Kobayashi Y, Vogel W 1968 Roles of activation and inhibition in sex differences in cognitive abilities. Psychology Reviews 75: 23–50
9. Fillit H 1994 Estrogens in the pathogenesis and treatment of Alzheimer's disease in postmenopausal women. Annals of the New York Academy of Sciences 743: 233–238
10. Magos AL, Studd JWW 1985 Effects of the menstrual cycle on medical disorders. British Journal of Hospital Medicine 33: 68–77
11. Montgomery JC, Brincat M, Studd JWW et al 1987 Effect of oestrogen and testosterone implants on psychological disorders in the climacteric. Lancet i: 297–299
12. Phillips S, Sherwin BB 1991 Effects of estrogen on memory function in surgically menopaused women. Psychoneuroendocrinology 17: 485–495
13. Barrett-Connor E, Kritz-Silverstein D 1993 Estrogen replacement therapy and cognitive function in older women. Journal of the American Medical Association 260: 2637–2641
14. Kampen DL, Sherwin BB 1994 Estrogen use and verbal memory in healthy postmenopausal women. Obstetrics and Gynecology 83: 979–983
15. Daly E, Gray A, Barlow D et al 1993 Measuring the impact of menopausal symptoms on quality of life. British Medical Journal 307: 836–840
16. Limouzin-Lamothe M, Mairon N, LeGal J et al 1991 Quality of life after the menopause: influence of hormone replacement therapy. American Journal of Obstetrics and Gynecology 78(Pt 6): 991–995
17. Ditkoff EC, Crary WG, Cristo M, Lobo RA 1991 Estrogen improves psychological functioning in asymptomatic postmenopausal women. Obstetrics and Gynecology 78: 991–995
18. Best N, Rees M, Barlow D et al 1992 Effect of estradiol implant on noradrenergic function and mood in menopausal patients. Psychoneurendocrinology 17(Pt 1): 87–93
19. Klaiber EL, Broverman DM, Vogel W et al 1979 Estrogen replacement therapy for severe persistent depression in women. Archives of General Psychiatry 36: 550–554
20. Coope J, Thomson J, Poller L 1975 Effect of 'natural estrogen' replacement therapy on menopausal symptoms and blood clotting. British Medical Journal 4: 139–143
21. Shapira B, Oppenheim G, Zohar J et al 1985 Lack of efficacy of estrogen supplementation to imipramine in resistant female depressives. Biology Psychiatry 20: 570–583
22. Funk JL, Mortel KF, Meyer JS 1991 Effects of estrogen replacement therapy on cerebral perfusion and cognition amongst postmenopausal women. Dementia 2: 268–272
23. Butler RN, Aronheim H, Fillet H, Rapoport S, Tatemichi TK 1993 Vascular dementia: stroke prevention takes on new urgency. Geriatrics 48: 32–34
24. Bueb LP, Hob PR, Bouras C, Delacourie A et al 1994 Pathological alterations of the cerebral microvasculature in Alzheimer's disease and related dementing disorders. Acta Neuropathol Berlin 87: 469–480
25. Fillit H, Weinreb H, Cholst I, Luine V, McEwen B, Amador R, Zabriskie J 1986 Observations in a preliminary open trial of estradiol therapy for senile dementia — Alzheimer's type. Psychoneuroendocrinology 11(3): 337–345
26. Honjo H, Ogino Y, Naithoh K et al 1989 In vivo effects by estrone sulphate on the central nervous system — senile dementia (Alzheimer's type). Journal of Steroid Biochemistry 34: 521–525
27. Slap GB 1981 Oral contraceptives and depression: impact, prevalence and cause. Journal of Adolescent Health Care 2(1): 53–64
28. Forrest ARW 1979 Cyclical variations in mood in normal women taking oral contraceptives. British Medical Journal 2(6202): 1403
29. Shaarawy M, Fayad M, Nagui AR, Abdel-Azim S 1982 Serotonin metabolism and depression in oral contraceptive users. Contraception 26(2): 193–204
30. Cullberg J 1972 Mood changes and menstrual symptoms with different gestagen/estrogen combinations. A double blind comparison with placebo. Acta Psychiatrica Scandinavica 236 (Suppl): 1–46
31. Backstrom T, Smith S, Lothian H, Baird DT 1985 Prolonged follicular phase and depressed gonadotrophins following hysterectomy and corpus luteectomy in women with premenstrual tension syndrome. Clinical Endocrinology 22: 723–732
32. Backstrom T, Lindhe B-A, Cavalli-Bjorkman B, Nordenstrom S, Hansson Y 1985 Effects of oral contraceptives on mood: a randomised comparison of three phasic and monphasic preparations. Contraception 46: 253–268
33. Fleming O, Seager CP 1978 Incidence of depressive symptoms in users of the oral contraceptive. British Journal of Psychiatry 132: 431–440
34. Warner P, Bancroft J 1988 Mood, sexuality, oral contraceptives and the menstrual cycle. Journal of Psychosomatic Research 32(4–5): 417–427
35. Kay CR 1984 The Royal College of General Practitioner's oral contraceptive study: some recent observations. Clinics in Obstetrics and Gynaecology 11(3): 759–786
36. Guillebaud J (ed) 1993 Oestrogen-free hormonal contraception. In: Contraception: your questions answered. Churchill Livingstone, Edinburgh, pp 225–292
37. McCann MS, Potter L 1994 Progestin-only oral contraception: a comprehensive review. Contraception 50(S): S1–S195
38. Fraser IS, Weisberg E 1981 A comprehensive review of injectable contraceptives, with special emphasis on depot medroxyprogesterone acetate. Medical Journal of Australia 1(Suppl): 1–19
39. Sihvo S, Ollila E, Hemminki E 1995 Perceptions and satisfaction among Norplant users in Finland. Acta Obstetrica Gynecologica Scandinavica 74(6): 441–445
40. Wagner KD, Berenson AB 1994 Norplant-associated major depression and panic disorder. Journal of Clinical Psychology 55(11): 478–480
41. Nilsson CG, Lahteenmaki PLA, Luukkainen T 1984 Ovarian function in amenorrhoeic and menstruating users of a levonorgestrel-releasing intrauterine device. Fertility and Sterility 41(1): 52–55
42. Nilsson CG, Lahteenmaki PLA, Luukkainen T et al 1986 Sustained intrauterine release of levonorgestrel over 5 years. Fertility and Sterility 45: 805–807
43. Luukkainen T, Allonen H, Haukkamaa M et al 1990 Five year's experience with levonorgestrel releasing IUD's. Contraception 33: 139–148

44. Luukkainen T, Lahteenmaki P, Toivonen J 1990 Levonorgestrel-releasing intrauterine device. Annals of Medicine 22: 85–90
45. Andersson K, Mattsson L-A, Rybo G et al 1992 Intrauterine release of levonorgestrel — a new way of adding progestogen in hormone replacement therapy. Obstetrics and Gynecology 79: 963–967
46. Suhonen SP, Holmstrom T, Allonen H O et al 1995 Intrauterine and subdermal progestin administration in postmenopausal hormone replacement therapy. Fertility and Sterility 63: 336–342
47. Studd JWW 1979 Premenstrual tension syndrome. British Medical Journal 1: 410
48. Magos AL, Studd JWW 1984 The premenstrual syndrome. In: Studd J (ed) Progress in obstetrics and Gynaecology, vol. 4. Churchill Livingstone, London, pp 334–350
49. Magos AL, Brincat M, Studd JWW 1986 Treatment of the premenstrual syndrome by subcutaneous oestradiol implants and cyclical oral norethisterone: placebo controlled study. British Medical Journal 292: 1629–1633
50. Studd JWW, Smith RNJ 1993 Oestradiol and testosterone implants. Ballière's Clinical Endocrinology and Metabolism 7: 203–223
51. Watson NR, Studd JWW, Riddle AF et al 1988 Suppression of ovulation by transdermal oestradiol patches. British Medical Journal 297: 900–901
52. Watson NR, Studd JWW, Savvas M et al 1989 Treatment of severe premenstrual syndrome with oestradiol patches and cyclical oral norethisterone. Lancet i: 730–734
53. Smith RNJ, Studd JWW, Zamblera D et al 1995 A randomised comparison over 8 months of 100 μg and 200 μg twice weekly doses of transdermal oestradiol in the treatment of severe premenstrual syndrome. British Journal of Obstetrics and Gynaecology 102: 475–484
54. Pitt B 1968 Atypical depression following childbirth. British Journal of Psychiatry 114: 1325–1335
55. Henderson A, Studd JWW 1995 Oestrogens and postnatal depression. Cont Reviews in Obstetrics and Gynaecology 7: 90–96
56. Wagner HR, Davis JN 1980 Decreased beta-adrenoceptor responses in female rats are eliminated by ovariectomy: correlation of 3H-dihydroalprenolol binding and catecholamine stimulated cAMP levels. Brain Research 201: 235–239
57. Harris B, Johns S, Fung H et al 1989 The hormonal environment of postnatal depression. British Journal of Psychiatry 154: 660–667
58. Harris B, Lovett L, Newcombe R et al 1994 Maternity blues and major endocrine changes: Cardiff puerperal mood and hormone study II. British Medical Journal 308: 49–53
59. Alder EM, Cox JL 1983 Breast feeding and postnatal depression. Journal of Psychosomatic Research 27(2): 139–144
60. Henderson A, Gregoire AJP, Kumar R, Studd JWW 1991 The treatment of severe postnatal depression with oestradiol skin patches. Lancet i: 816
61. Gregoire AJP, Kumar R, Everitt B, Henderson AF, Studd JWW 1996 Transdermal oestrogen is an effective treatment for severe postnatal depression. Lancet 347: 930–933
62. Holst J, Backstrom T, Hammarback S et al 1989 Progestogen addition during oestrogen replacement therapy — effects on vasomotor symptoms and mood. Maturitas 11: 13–20
63. Watson NR, Studd JWW, Savvas M et al 1990 The long term effects of oestradiol implant therapy for the treatment of premenstrual syndrome. Gynaecological Endocrinology 4: 99–107
64. De Cleyn K, Buytaert P, Delbeke L et al 1986 Equine estrogen-dydrogesterone therapy in the management of post-menopausal women. European Journal of Obstetrics, Gynaecology and Reproductive Biology 23: 201–209
65. Magos AL, Brewster E, Studd JWW et al 1986 The effects of norethisterone in postmenopausal women on oestrogen replacement therapy: a model for premenstrual syndrome. British Journal of Obstetrics and Gynaecology 93: 1290–1296
66. Barlow DH, Grosset KA, Hart H, Hart DM 1989 A study of the experience of Glasgow women in the climacteric years. British Journal of Obstetrics and Gynaecology 96: 1192–1197
67. Studd JWW 1995 Shifting indications for hysterectomy. Lancet 345: 388
68. Dalton K 1977 Premenstrual syndrome and progesterone therapy. Heinemann, London
69. Arafat ES, Hargrove JT, Maxson WS et al 1988 Sedative and hypnotic effects of oral administration of micronised progesterone may be mediated through its metabolites. American Journal of Obstetrics and Gynecology 159: 1203–1209
70. van de Mer YG, Bendek-Jaszmann LJ, van Loenan AC 1983 Effect of high dose progesterone on the premenstrual syndrome: a double blind cross-over trial. Journal of Psychosomatic Obstetrics and Gynaecology 2: 220–223
71. Dennerstein L, Spencer Gardner C, Gotts G et al 1985 Progesterone and the premenstrual syndrome: a double blind cross-over trial. British Medical Journal 290: 1617–1621
72. Magos AL, Studd JWW 1985 Progesterone and the premenstrual syndrome: a double blind cross-over trial. British Medical Journal 291: 213–214 (letter)
73. Hallbreich U 1990 Treatment of premenstrual syndromes with progesterone antagonists (e.g. RU486): political and methodological issues. Psychiatry 53: 407–409
74. Schmidt PJ, Neiman LK, Grover GN et al 1991 Lack of effect of induced menses on symptoms in women with premenstrual syndrome. New England Journal of Medicine 324: 1174–1179
75. Chan AF, Mortola JF, Wodd SH, Yen SSC 1994 Persistence of premenstrual syndrome during low-dose administration of the progesterone antagonist RU 486. Obstetrics and Gynecology 84: 1001–1005

65. Psychosexual effects

Lorraine Dennerstein

Introduction

Many women notice changes in their sexual functioning during phases of endogenous or exogenous hormonal variation. This chapter reviews the changes in sexuality reported during certain defined phases of endocrine change (menstrual cycle and menopause) and then evaluates the effects of added hormone therapies.

ASSESSMENT OF FEMALE SEXUALITY

In the clinical setting female sexuality is usually assessed by interview. Questioning relates to each component of sexuality and the various factors which may be having an effect. These include factors present in the past as well as those still current. Physical examination may be necessary to determine the role of physical factors.

Research into female sexuality may involve interviews with structured or open questions. Questionnaires are used in both clinical trials and surveys. Answers may be rated on a true/false, ordinal, analog or actual frequency basis. Most questionnaires for female sexuality detail the type and frequency of sexual activities/behaviors rather than assessing aspects of female libido or responsivity. This may reflect the effect of the AIDS epidemic on research about sexuality. Few of the questionnaries which purport to measure female libido or responsivity have provided adequate documentation of validity and reliability and are brief enough to use in surveys or in clinical trials. Two scales which look promising on data to date are the Brief Index of Sexual Functioning for Women[1] and the McCoy Female Sexuality Questionnaire.[2]

Faced with the paucity of adequately validated instruments, researchers have tended to develop their own measures for specific projects. Sources of methodological difficulty include whether the same meaning is ascribed to terms by the woman subject and the researcher, the problems and biases inherent in retrospective recall, particularly where long time periods are allowed, and biases which may reflect sampling method. Ethnic and other social differences such as education and occupation may influence how women interpret and express any changes in their sexual feelings or behavior.

Female sexual responsivity has also been measured physiologically in the laboratory setting. Such studies measure vaginal blood flow (and sometimes other extragenital changes) in response to fantasies, prose, audiotapes or erotic videotapes. This type of research may not reflect the woman's sexuality in the real life setting. Biases are likely as the sort of person who volunteers for such a study is likely to be very different from women in the community overall.

The menstrual cycle

Conflicting findings have been reported regarding the influence of the menstrual cycle on female sexuality. An earlier review[3] reported that different studies had found increases in sexual behavior to occur with ovulation, premenstrually, postmenstrually and during menstruation. The lack of consensus reflects the many methodological problems involved in assessing sexuality described above, compounded by the problems inherent in menstrual cycle research. A crucial problem has been the lack of daily endocrine measures so that menstrual cycle phases of each woman can be adequately delineated. Both Doty[4] and Udry and Morris[5] have demonstrated that without careful categorization of menstrual cycle phases determined endocrinologically, peaks and troughs in sexual behavior can erroneously be found at any time of the menstrual cycle. Even with endocrine markers there are manifold statistical problems in comparing changes between women as there will be differences in the length of cycles, time of ovulation, onset and duration of menses and in the baseline variable under study.[6]

Many studies have measured coital rates.[7,8] Hedricks et al[7] found a peak in coital rate at ovulation (determined endocrinologically). It is not quite clear whether this reflects an increase in female sexual interest, increased attractivity to the male and/or the intention of the couples studied to conceive. Sex may serve a number of functions in addition to reproduction and the provision of pleasure. These functions include those of enhancing the intimacy of interpersonal relationships, maintenance and bolstering of self-esteem and identity, exerting control, dominance and hostility and even those of material gain.[9] Women have not been encouraged to initiate sexual activity in many societies. Thus coital rate may reflect more about male sexual drive and social needs and expectations than it does about female sexual interest or drive. This type of study of female sexuality also assumes that all women are heterosexual in orientation and that sexual activity is necessarily penetrative.

Few studies have investigated menstrual cycle-related changes in female sexuality in settings in which the effect of male sexual desire is excluded. An early study by Stopes[10] involved women whose husbands were away at war. She found two peaks of sexual desire reported by these women, one just before menstruation, the other two weeks later. In a more recent investigation, Matteo and Rissman[11] analyzed daily records of sexual thoughts and activities from seven lesbian couples. Significant peaks in orgasms and self-initiated and total sexual encounters were found around the presumed midcycle portion of the menstrual cycle. It is unfortunate that hormonal measures were not utilized in order to accurately delineate cycle phase.

Investigation of physiological responses (such as vaginal blood flow) in a laboratory setting suggest that vaginal arousal or responsivity does not vary consistently across the menstrual cycle.[12,13]

Some research has tried to distinguish aspects of female sexuality from those that may be male initiated.[14,15] These researchers included a measure of female sexual desire or interest in their studies. A working definition of sexual desire is that of 'a subjective feeling state that may be triggered by both internal and external cues, and that may or may not result in overt sexual behavior'.[16]

Adams et al[14] identified female-initiated sexual behavior, including masturbation and the use of erotic fantasy and literature, and reported a peak of such behaviour around ovulation. Stanislaw and Rice[15] also found a periovulatory peak in female sexual desire. However, these researchers used the basal body temperature method to identify ovulation. This method is only able to identify the day of ovulation in 34% of cycles.[17] Some other studies attempted to correlate female sexual interest with hormonally determined cycle phases. Sanders et al[18] and Udry and Morris[5] found peak levels for sexual interest in the follicular phase followed by a luteal trough. However daily endocrine data were only available for a small subset of the Udry and Morris sample[5] and not available (on a daily basis) for the Sanders et al study.[18]

Many of these methodological difficulties were overcome in a study in which, for a whole menstrual cycle, 168 women recorded their sexual interest and moods daily and also collected daily 24 hour urinary samples so that total estrogens and pregnanediol could be measured.[6] This method allows the accurate identification of menstrual cycle hormonal phases. The statistical method described by Doty[4] was used so that data could be compared from cycles of different lengths and differing days of ovulation. A general pattern was found of a rise in sexual interest during menses, sustained higher levels of interest during the follicular phase, a small ovulatory peak and a sharp decrease following ovulation. This pattern was present independent of whether women suffered from premenstrual symptoms. Statistical analyses confirmed that sexual interest was significantly higher in the follicular and ovulatory phases (the potentially fertile parts of the cycle) than for other phases of the cycle. Knowledge that there is a pronounced change in female sexual interest with menstrual cycle phase may help women in understanding their sexual behavior and in reducing the unrealistic expectations present in many societies for women to maintain sexual interest across the menstrual cycle. The finding that female sexual interest peaks at the most fertile time of the cycle places women at risk for pregnancy and introduces some paradoxes for those contraceptive methods that instruct women to desist from sexual intercourse during the fertile phase of the menstrual cycle.

Although this study did find a strong pattern of change in sexual interest with menstrual cycle phase, correlation with actual hormonal levels of estrogens or pregnanediol were weak. It is unclear whether cyclical changes are dependent on ovulation, normal corpus luteum function,[19] or other substances varying across the menstrual cycle.

COMBINED ORAL CONTRACEPTIVE (COC) PILL

Bancroft and Sartorius[19] carried out an extensive methodological critique of the effects of oral contraceptives on well-being and sexuality. They concluded that a proportion of women who begin oral contraceptives do suffer adverse effects which may lead to discontinuation, reduction in the quality of life, or reduced efficacy of COC. Guichoux[20] noted the need to have baseline comparisons of users with nonusers with regard to sexual functioning. Because of the menstrual cycle variation described above, at least one month of daily observation is needed. Other concerns were the lack of documentation of drop-outs, and the influence of confounding factors such as that of mood, marital status, multiple partners, fear of sexually transmitted diseases, age, socioeconomic and educational status, desire for contraception, and willingness to answer questions on sexuality.

There are several different research methods with which to examine the effects of COC on sexuality.

Surveys — cross-sectional

Cross-sectional surveys have generally found those women who have taken up and continued to use COC to be more sexually active: they are more likely to have a sexual partner and less likely to be a virgin;[21] have a higher coital frequency;[22] have higher psychosexual interest;[2] have more enjoyment of sex;[21] have more liberal and less inhibited attitudes to sexuality.[19,21] Other attitudinal factors discriminating COC users from nonusers include perceived support for the method from those in authority and a greater need to avoid pregnancy.[23] Thus psychological factors including attitudes, personality, prior sexual adjustment and relationship phase may influence whether women elect to use oral contraceptives.

A major problem in sampling is whether to include only those women beginning COC use or to study those women who are established COC users. The high discontinuation rate (more than 25% during the first year of COC use) implies that the established COC users group have already excluded those who experienced sexual and other side effects and discontinued use.[19] Women with a tendency to premenstrual symptoms are more likely to discontinue COC,[24] as were those who suffer from depression premorbidly or postnatal depression.[19]

A number of surveys have also reported that COC users are less likely to report menstrual cycle-linked changes in their sexual behavior. A retrospective study of over 4000 women,[25] found that nonusers were more likely to report fluctuations in their levels of sexual desire across the cycle, with highest levels postmenstrually compared to premenstrually or menstrually. The least variation was shown by monophasic pill users, with triphasic pill users intermediate between monophasic and non-pill users. McCoy and Matyas[2] found triphasic users to be more sexually interested, sexually active and aroused and to enjoy sex more than monophasic users.

Cross-sectional studies are useful for providing an overview of women's experiences and for suggesting areas for further research, but have some inherent problems which limit the conclusions which can be drawn. First, this sort of study design is unable to sort out differences which may have been present before the study. As noted above women who *choose* to take COC as a contraceptive method differ from nonusers in their attitudes towards sexuality, previous sexual experience and satisfaction with current sexual relationships.[21] Further, the study sample of COC users are those women who have *continued* to take the pill. Longitudinal studies are needed, preferably in which women are studied before commencing the COC. These prospective studies should include both observational investigations and clinical trial interventions. Where possible, clinical trials should be blinded and include a placebo comparison in order to separate psychological from pharmacological effects.

Prospective — observational

As noted above, cross-sectional survey findings suggest that COC users may not show the cyclical changes in parameters of sexuality evident in nonusers. Prospective studies in which women have kept daily ratings of sexual interest and activities provide confirmatory evidence. For example Adams et al,[14] found a midcycle peak in the frequency of female initiated sexual behaviors for nonusers that was not apparent for COC users. Alexander et al[26] also found that COC users did not show the cyclical pattern for sexual desire evident for nonusers. In this study weekly levels of autosexual behaviors and sexual activities with partners did not vary across either COC or menstrual cycles.

Prospective — clinical trials

A major methodological issue at present unresolved relates to the way in which adverse side effects are sought, i.e. whether spontaneous or elicited methods are used. Most studies find higher rates when elicited reports are sought, but there is little information about which method is more valid.[19]

Adverse effects of COC on sexuality may reflect psychological effects. Some years ago Aznar-Ramos et al[27] carried out a study in which women who had recently suffered a spontaneous abortion and desired a pregnancy, were given a placebo but informed that they had been given a COC. A 'decrease in libido' was reported by 30%. There would be ethical concerns in initiating such a study today.

Cullberg[28] was able to introduce the difficult placebo-controlled double-blind condition by telling the 320 women studied they would receive weak female hormones to assess what effect they had on premenstrual symptoms. He found significant adverse effects on mood but not on sexual behavior when women who received COC were compared with the control group who received placebo. A different type of design (a cross-over design) was used by Leeton et al.[29] In this smaller study (n = 20) the researchers found a significant decrease in sexual response during COC use.

In a double-blind study of 45 women with prospectively confirmed premenstrual symptoms who had been allocated either a triphasic COC or placebo, Graham and Sherwin[30] also found that the women prescribed COC suffered decreased sexual interest after starting the pill independent of any effect on mood.

Other studies have compared COC types in terms of constituents, dosage or temporal pattern of use. Cullberg[28] found no association between loss of sexual interest and progestogen dosage. Warner and Bancroft[25] found that there was a relative lack of peaks of sexual interest in the monophasic group especially those who had been using the pill for four or more years.

There is very little evidence about the effect of progestogen-only pills, injectables or IUDs on sexuality.[19] Menstrual cycle studies suggest that progesterone may have a negative effect on some parameters including that of female sexual interest.[6] Synthetic progestogens may combine effects of natural progesterone with androgenic effects and even anti-androgenic effects. For example, medroxyprogesterone acetate may be antigonadotropic and hence antiandrogenic. Some progestogens show more binding to androgen receptors than others.[19]

Mechanisms

Oral contraceptives are known to suppress FSH and LH. This will result in lower levels of endogenous estrogens and progesterone. Reduced gonadotropin response occurs most convincingly with 50 µg estrogen-containing pills and may be much less with low-dose pills. Such central effects may influence the central control of mood and sexuality.[19]

There is general agreement that in combined pill users, ovulation is blocked in the majority of cycles but that with the low-dose estrogen pills, especially the triphasic pills, follicular development may occur in 20% or more cycles.[19] COC also suppress the midcycle ovarian increase in androgens, lower levels of total and free testosterone (T),[21] and raise sex hormone-binding globulen.[26] Differential effects of triphasic pills compared to monophasic pills on ovarian function may result in a different hormonal milieu and explain some of the differences observed.

The role of androgens is unclear. COC users have been found to have substantially lower free testosterone than nonusers but to have a higher level of sexuality.[31] Bancroft et al[32] compared 20 women complaining of sexual problems while using COC with 20 women using the same COC but without sexual problems and found androgen levels to be similarly low in both groups. When androstenedione was added in a double-blind placebo-controlled trial to the sexual problem group, there was no significant improvement in sexuality.

THE MENOPAUSE AND HORMONE THERAPIES (HRT)

Studies of menopause clinic populations report a high prevalence of sexual difficulties and marital problems.[33] A critical question for clinicians is the possible relationship of any deterioration in sexual functioning to changing endocrine status during the menopausal transition. A methodological critique[34] has pointed out that major biases in published menopause research reflect sampling from clinical populations, low measurement sensitivity and an assumption that all respondents are heterosexual. The authors called for more large scale, objective, methodologically sophisticated studies to explore changes in sexual functioning of women experiencing natural menopause as well as those who have undergone surgical menopause by hysterectomy and oophorectomy — a procedure reputed to be associated with significant sexual sequelae.[35]

In a more recent methodological review and meta-analysis of 33 empirical studies which have examined sexuality, hormone therapies and menopausal status between 1972–92, Myers[36] found that significantly higher effect sizes were found in those studies rated as having adequate measures of hormone status or adequate hormone manipulation, including appropriate controls, and had less confounding variables. Studies having adequate measures of sexuality also had a slightly higher effect size. Multiple regression analysis found that overall ratings of methodological adequacy accounted for 31% of the variance of effect sizes. Eighteen of the studies involved hormone therapy with either estrogen, progestogen, estrogen and progestogen, androgen, estrogen and androgen, or placebo. The meta-analysis did find a mean treatment effect size of 0.67, indicating that hormones (both endogenous and exogenous) have some importance in pre-postmenopausal sexuality. However, when the individual treatment effect sizes of studies were examined, the highest differences came from studies that compared surgically menopausal women to intact pre/menopausal women[37] with the next highest effect sizes coming from those studies which compared surgically menopausal women being treated with hormones to those who were not.

As the majority of women go through a natural menopause it is difficult to generalize from studies involving surgically menopausal women. When the amount of variance contributed by hormonal factors was examined this was often found to be small, indicating that other factors such as methodological issues and social and interpersonal factors may have larger effects on sexuality than do hormones. The largest amount of variance (still quite small — 7%) due to hormones occurred when surgically menopausal women were administered estrogen and androgen rather than estrogen alone. This suggests that androgens may have an incrementally greater positive effect on some parameters of female sexuality than estrogens alone for oophorectomized women, but reveals little about the role of androgens for those women with intact uterus and ovaries. A recent review by Campbell and Udry,[38] found that while the presence of some amount of androgens appears to be important in maintaining female sexual motivation, there is little evidence that variation in testosterones within the normal range is associated with variation in sexual motivation. Stimulatory effects of androgens occur in hyperandrogenized states as in the clinical trials of Sherwin and Gelfand.[39]

In summary, evidence from clinical trials is often limited by poor methodology and by a focus on surgically menopausal women. The results to date from double-blind trials suggest positive effects on female sexual interest/arousal of oophorectomized women for estrogen,[40] estrogen and androgen or androgen alone.[37] Most studies have not found any effect of hormone therapies on frequency of sexual intercourse. Studies involving naturally postmenopausal women have found positive effects of estrogen often confined to beneficial effects on vaginal dryness,[41,42] and less effectiveness of the addition of androgens.[43] A larger Swedish study,[44] involving 242 naturally postmenopausal women suffering from vasomotor symptoms in a double-blind placebo-controlled trial of transdermal estrogen did find significant improvement in frequency of sexual activity and fantasies, enjoyment, well-being and quality of life, as well as vaginal lubrication and dyspareunia.

There have been few studies of the effects of progestogen therapy on sexuality of postmenopausal women. A double-blind study of oophorectomized women,[40] found less favorable effects on sexual parameters when progestogen was given alone (norgestrel 250 μg/day) compared to the results for estrogen alone. A study of naturally postmenopausal women[45] found that the addition of progestogen (5 mg medroxyprogesterone acetate for 10 days) had no adverse effects on sexual functioning but did affect mood negatively.

Relatively few of the population studies of the menopausal transition in mid-aged women have inquired about sexual functioning. A cross-sectional study[46] of 800 Swedish women aged 38, 46, 50 and 54, randomly selected from the general population, found a decline in sexual interest, capacity for orgasm and coital frequency with menopausal status rather than with aging. Decline in sexual interest was also associated with low social class and psychiatric disorder.[47] Osborn et al[48] studied 436 women aged 35–59 years, registered with two Oxford general practices. Sexual dysfunction was significantly associated with increasing age, psychiatric disorder, neuroticism and marital disharmony. No association between sexual dysfunction and menopause appeared. A Danish postal questionnaire study[49] of 474 women also found that menopausal status did not predict decreased or infrequent sexual desire at age 51 years. The only significant predictor of decreased sexual desire at age 51 was women's prior anticipation of decreased sexuality as a result of menopause. This variable also significantly predicted infrequent sexual desire, as did low frequency of sex, single status, poor physical fitness, low social class and 'weak nerves'. However, the question regarding changed sexual desire covered a very long time frame (11 years) and may have been subject to recall bias. Other epidemiological studies[50] have also shown a significant association between social factors (such as social background, marital status and educational level) and sexual behavior.

A Melbourne study[51] reported the results of a cross-sectional telephone survey of 2001 randomly selected Australian-born women aged between 45–55 years. The major outcome variables were questions relating to changes in sexual interest over the prior 12 months, reasons for any changes, occurrence of sexual intercourse, and of unusual pain on intercourse. The natural menopausal transition was clearly associated with declining sexual interest, decreased likelihood of intercourse and increased likelihood of discomfort with intercourse. Logistic regression was used to identify explanatory variables for change in sexual interest. The majority of women (62%) reported no change in sexual interest, although 31% reported a decrease. Decline in sexual interest was significantly and adversely associated with natural menopause ($P < 0.01$) rather than age, decreased well-being ($P < 0.001$), decreasing employment ($P < 0.01$) and symptomatology (vasomotor $P < 0.05$, cardiopulmonary $P < 0.001$ and skeletal ($P < 0.01$). Eleven to twelve years of education was associated with a lowered risk of decreased sexual functioning ($P < 0.01$). Heterogenous results were reported by users of hormone replacement therapies. Most observational studies of population cohorts have not included hormone levels. Longitudinal studies or clinical trials may help establish the effects of hormone therapies on female sexuality.

Few longitudinal studies of the menopausal transition have assessed sexual functioning. McCoy and Davidson[52] followed 16 of 39 women through the transition. They found a significant decline in sexual functioning from pre- to postmenopause. Decline in a number of aspects of sexual functioning (sexual thoughts, dyspareunia, lack of vaginal lubrication, less satisfaction with partners as lovers or partner's level of interest in the woman) were associated with low serum E_2 levels.[53] Testosterone was the hormone most consistently related to coital frequency.[54]

For postmenopausal women, there have been a number of cross-sectional studies of clinical or convenience samples which have included assessments of sexual functioning and hormone levels. Bachmann and Leiblum[55] found that the sexagenarian women had significantly less genital atrophy, and significantly higher levels of desire and sexual satisfaction then younger postmenopausal women. From this cross-sectional study of older postmenopausal women it is not clear whether increased coital activity caused increased release of androgens and decreased genital atrophy, perhaps consequent on conversion of androgens to estrogen, or whether causation flows in other directions.

Conclusion

Estrogen and progestogens, whether administered for contraception, control of gynecological disorders or for therapy associated with menopause, should be subjected to rigorous study in order to determine side effects, including effects on sexuality. Most studies to date suggest a great deal of variance between individual women both in their experience of sexual cognitions and behaviors and in any effects (positive or negative) of hormones. Prospective studies of large and representative groups of women are needed. Greater attention to methodological issues including the use of valid and reliable measures of sexuality and adequate determination of hormonal status are also needed.

REFERENCES

1. Taylor JF, Rosen RC, Leblum SR 1994 Self report assessment of female sexual function. Psychometric evaluation of the brief index of sexual functioning for women. Archives of Sexual Behavior 23: 627–643
2. McCoy NL, Matyas JR 1996 Birth control pill use and sexuality in university women. Archives of Sexual Behaviour 25: 73–79
3. Schreiner-Engel P 1980 Female sexual arousability in relation to gonadal hormones and the menstrual cycle. Dissertation Abstracts International 41(02B): 730
4. Doty RL 1979 A procedure for combining menstrual cycle data. Journal of Clinical Endocrinology and Metabolism 48: 912–918
5. Udry JR, Morris NM 1977 The distribution of events in the human menstrual cycle. Journal of Reproduction and Fertility 51: 419–425
6. Dennerstein L, Gotts G, Brown JJ, Morse CA, Farley TM, Pinol A 1994 The relationship between the menstrual cycle and female sexual interest in women with PMS complaints and volunteers. Psychoneuroendocrinology 19: 293–304
7. Hedricks C, Piccinino LJ, Udry JR, Chimbira THK 1987 Peak coital rate coincides with onset of luteinising hormone surge. Fertility and Sterility 48: 234–238
8. Morris NM, Udry JR, Khan-Dawood F, Dawood MY 1987 Marital sex frequency and midcycle female testosterone. Archives of Sexual Behaviour 16: 27–37
9. Bancroft J 1980 Endocrinology of sexual function. Clinics In Obstetrics and Gynecology 7: 253–281
10. Stopes MC 1931 Married love. Putnams, London
11. Matteo S, Rissman EF 1984 Increased sexual activity during the midcycle portion of the human menstrual cycle. Hormones and Behaviour 18: 249–255
12. Meuwissen I, Over R 1992 Sexual arousal across phases of the human menstrual cycle. Archives of Sexual Behaviour 21: 101–119
13. Schreiner-Engel P, Schiavi RC, Smith H, White D 1981 Sexual arousability and the menstrual cycle. Psychosomatic Medicine 43: 199–214
14. Adams DB, Gold AR, Burt AD 1978 Rise in female initiated sexual activity at ovulation and its suppression by oral contraceptives. New England Journal of Medicine 299: 1145–1150

15. Stanislaw H, Rice FJ 1988 Correlation between sexual desire and menstrual cycle characteristics. Archives of Sexual Behaviour 17: 499–508
16. Leiblum SR, Rosen RC 1988 Introduction: changing perspectives on sexual desire. In: Leiblum SR, Rosen RC (eds) Sexual desire disorders. Guilford Press, New York, pp 1–17
17. Lenton EA, Weston GA, Cooke ID 1977 Problems in using basal body temperature recordings in an infertility clinic. British Medical Journal 1: 803–805
18. Sanders D, Warner GA, Cooke ID 1983 Mood, sexuality, hormones and the menstrual cycle 1. Changes in mood and physical state: description of subjects and method. Psychosomatic Medicine 45: 487–501
19. Bancroft J, Sartorius N 1990 The effects of oral contraceptives on well-being and sexuality. Oxford Review of Reproductive Biology 12: 57–92
20. Guichoux JY 1993 Methodological problems in the evaluation of drug induced sexual dysfunction for oral contraceptives. Therapie 48(5): 447–451
21. Bancroft J, Sherwin BB, Alexander GM, Davidson DW, Walker A 1991 Oral contraceptives, androgens and the sexuality of young women 1. A comparison of sexual experiences, sexual attitudes, and gender role in oral contraceptive users and non-users. Archives of Sexual Behaviour 20: 105–120
22. Westoff CF 1974 Coital frequency and contraception. Family Planning Perspective 6: 136–141
23. Condelli L 1986 Social and attitudinal determinants of contraceptive choice: using the Health Belief Model. Journal of Sex Research 22: 478–491
24. Dennerstein L, Spencer-Gardner C, Brown JB, Smith MA, Burrows GD 1984 Premenstrual tension hormonal profiles. Journal of Psychosomatic Obsterics and Gynecology 3: 37–51
25. Warner P, Bancroft J 1988 Mood, sexuality, oral contraceptives and menstrual cycle. Journal of Psychosomatic Research 32: 417–427
26. Alexander GM, Sherwin BB, Bancroft J, Davidson DW 1990 Testosterone and sexual behavior in oral contraceptive users and nonusers: a prospective study. Hormones and Behaviour 24: 388–402
27. Aznar-Ramos R, Giner-Vallazques J, Lara-Ricalde R et al 1969 Incidence of side effects with contraceptive placebo. American Journal of Obstetrics and Gynecology 105: 1144–1149
28. Cullberg J 1972 Mood changes and menstrual symptoms with different gestagen/estagen combinations. Acta Psychiatrica Scandinavica 236 (Suppl): 1–86
29. Leeton J, McMaster RR, Worsley A 1978 The effects on sexual response and mood after sterilisation of women taking long term oral contraceptives: results of a double blind crossover study. Australian and New Zealand Journal of Obstetrics and Gynaecology 18: 194–197
30. Graham CA, Sherwin BB 1992 A prospective treatment study of premenstrual symptoms using a triphasic oral contraceptive. Journal of Psychosomatic Research 36(3): 257–266
31. Bancroft J, Sherwin BB, Alexander GM, Davidson DW, Walker A 1991 Oral contraceptives, androgens and the sexuality of young women 2. The role of androgens. Archives of Sexual Behaviour 20: 121–135
32. Bancroft J, Davidson DW, Warner P, Tyrer G 1980 Androgens and sexual behavior in women using oral contraceptives. Clinical Endocrinology 12: 327–340
33. Sarrel PM, Whitehead MI 1985 Sex and menopause: defining the issues. Maturitas 7: 217–224
34. Cole E, Rothblum E 1990 Commentary on sexuality and the midlife woman. Psychology of Women Quarterly 14: 509–512
35. Dennerstein L, Wood C, Burrows GD 1977 Sexual response following hysterectomy and oophorectomy. Obstetrics and Gynecology 49: 92–96
36. Myers LS 1995 Methodological review and meta-analysis of sexuality and menopause research. Neuroscience and Biobehavioral Reviews 19: 331–341
37. Sherwin BB, Gelfand MM, Brender W 1985 Androgen enhances sexual motivation in females: a prospective, cross-over study of sex steroid administration in the surgical menopause. Psychosomatic Medicine 47: 339–351
38. Campbell BC, Udry JR 1994 Implications of hormonal influences on sexual behavior for demographic models of reproduction. Annals of the New York Academy of Science 709: 117–127
39. Sherwin BB, Gelfand MM 1987 The role of androgen in the maintenance of sexual functioning in oophorectomized women. Psychosomatic Medicine 49: 397–409
40. Dennerstein L, Burrows GD, Hyman GJ, Sharpe K 1980 Hormones and sexuality: effects of estrogen and progestogen. Obstetrics and Gynecology 56: 316–322
41. Campbell S 1976 Double blind psychometric studies on the effects of natural estrogens on post-menopausal women. In: Campbell S (ed) The management of the menopause and the post-menopausal years. MTP Press, Lancaster, pp 149–158
42. Myers LS, Morokoff PJ 1986 Physiological and subjective sexual arousal in pre- and postmenopausal women and postmenopausal women taking hormone replacement therapy. Psychophysiology 23: 283–292
43. Myers LS, Dixen J, Morrissette D, Carmichael M, Davidson JM 1990 Effects of estrogen, androgen, and progestin on sexual psychophysiology and behavior in postmenopausal women. Journal of Clinical Endocrinology and Metabolism 70(4): 1124–1131
44. Nathorst-Boos J, von Schoultz B, Carlstrom K 1993 Elective ovarian removal and estrogen replacement therapy — effects on sexual life, psychological well-being and androgen status. Journal of Psychosomatic Obstetrics and Gynaecology 14: 283–293
45. Sherwin BB 1991 The impact of different doses of estrogen and progestin on mood and sexual behavior in postmenopausal women. Journal of Clinical Endocrinology and Metabolism 72: 336–343
46. Hallstrom T 1977 Sexuality in the climacteric. Clinics in Obstetrics and Gynaecology 4: 227–239
47. Hallstrom T 1973 Mental disorder and sexuality in the climacteric: a study in psychiatric epidemiology. Scandinavian University Books, Goteborg, Sweden
48. Osborn M, Hawton K, Gath D 1988 Sexual dysfunction among middle aged women in the community. British Medical Journal 296: 959–962
49. Koster A, Garde K 1993 Sexual desire and menopausal development. A prospective study of Danish women born in 1936. Maturitas 16: 49–60
50. Van Keep PA, Kellerhals JM 1976 The ageing woman. Acta Obstetrica Gynecologica Scandinavica 51 (Suppl): 17–27

51. Dennerstein L, Smith AMA, Morse CA, Burger HG 1994 Sexuality and the menopause. Journal of Psychosomatic Obstetrics and Gynecology 15: 59–66
52. McCoy N, Davidson J 1985 A longitudinal study of the effects of menopause on sexuality. Maturitas 7: 203–210
53. McCoy N 1990 Estrogen levels in relation to self-reported symptoms and sexuality in perimenopausal women. In: Flint M, Utian W (eds) Multidisciplinary perspectives on menopause. New York Academy of Sciences, New York, pp 450–452
54. McCoy, N 1991 The menopause and sexuality. In: Sitruk-Ware R, Utian WH (eds). The menopause and hormone replacement therapy. Facts and controversies. Marcel Dekker Inc., New York, pp 73–100
55. Bachmann GA, Leiblum SR 1991 Sexuality in sexagenarian women. Maturitas 13: 43–50

66. Effects on other tissues

Joseph W. Goldzieher

Introduction

The estrogens and progestogens are generally regarded as 'sex hormones', and rightly so, for their discovery, biology, and applications have first occurred in that domain. Today, however, this narrow concept is obsolete. From brain to bone, from coronary artery to colon, from immune system to insulin these 'sex hormones' exert an enormous array of effects outside the reproductive system. A few of them are discussed below; future research will show how much wider our perspective really should be.

SKIN

The effect of estrogen deficiency on the skin is well known.[1] The beneficial effect of estrogens applied topically to senile skin was demonstrated years ago[2] and has recently been rediscovered. There is regeneration of the epidermis and collagen, but elastic fibers are not restored. The low exposure of skin to estrogens in the course of estrogen replacement therapy (ERT) is not likely to have cosmetically significant effects. Topically applied estrogens, depending on the vehicle, are well absorbed through the skin, as evidenced by transdermal delivery systems.

On the other hand higher estrogen exposures (for example, in pregnancy) lead in some women with susceptible skin and substantial exposure to sunlight to the well-known condition of melasma (Shakespeare's 'mask of pregnancy'). The high estrogen oral contraceptives used in the 1960s and 70s reproduced this condition in some women; however, as the estrogen dosage has been lowered, less and less of this condition is seen. It is easily prevented with the use of sun blocking agents.

Acne and seborrhea are manifestations of androgen activity on the skin. The effect is produced by the local conversion of testosterone to dihydrotestosterone and varies not only with this hormonal exposure but also with the (genetic) susceptibility of the skin. Many women who are advised to use ERT are afraid 'that they will grow a mustache'. This belief has two origins: it is common knowledge that some old women develop mustaches with age, hence there is concern that 'hormones' will aggravate this tendency. (Actually, the endocrinology of androgenic effects in aged women is underexplored.) Secondly, the use of androgens together with ERT in an effort to manage the diminished libido of some (about half) of postmenopausal women has resulted occasionally in hyperandrogenic manifestations, such as increase in facial hair. In fact, the choice of androgens for administration to women is very limited: oral androgens are not available in suitably low doses, and injectables and transdermal patches present an even worse problem. Implants of testosterone and estrogen have been used, but the formulations available so far have inconsistent delivery rates and tend to become encapsulated by fibrous tissue. There is no reason why modern delivery systems could not be delivered for specific applications, not just for total replacement. Dehydroepiandrosterone (DHEA), a secretory product of the adrenal, is converted endogenously into testosterone and androstenedione, and orally bioavailable DHEA may provide a physiological delivery system in the future.

Oral contraceptives have been reported to produce acne and/or hirsutism. For the most part, these are anecdotal observations, reinforced by the notion that some 19-norprogestogens (especially levonorgestrel) are more 'androgenic' and therefore less desirable than others. This has been used as a marketing ploy by some pharmaceutical manufacturers, even though such androgenicity has always been measured on the progestogen alone (never on the combination with estrogen) either in animal models of questionable relevance to human skin effects, or by using indirect parameters such as changes in plasma LDL or by measuring changes in certain hepatic protein levels, whose correlation with skin effects is equally problematic. While some progestogens such as cyproterone acetate are clearly antiandrogenic and have been used for therapy of acne and hirsutism, even the 'androgenic' progestogens in low-dose oral contraceptives produce relief of postpubertal acne.[3] This is due to several effects common to all combined oral contraceptives (COC): inhibition of ovarian function reduces androgen production from this source (the origin of most adolescent acne in women), suppression of adrenal androgen production, and an increase (due to the estrogen in the COC) of sex hormone-binding globulin (SHBG) levels, thus diminishing the concentration of unbound testosterone in the blood. Some formulations raise SHBG levels more than others; whether this difference is reflected clinically is uncertain. The relationship between testosterone/SHBG levels and clinical parameters such as acne and hirsutism is not at all straightforward.

Melanoma

In 1968 a physician (who deserves to be forgotten) published a report of a single case of melanoma occurring in a woman who used a variety of drugs including an oral contraceptive taken for 90 days. The COC was held responsible for this event. This triggered an avalanche of epidemiological studies on the association of oral contraceptives and this tumor, presumably because of the stimulatory effect of estrogens on melanocytes, as in melasma. Such studies are rendered ambiguous by biases due to ethnicity, sunlight exposure, etc. but a review of ten studies, some of them very substantial[4] has pretty well laid this issue to rest.

BONE

Estrogen-deficiency osteoporosis was clearly documented by Albright and his colleagues in Boston more than half a century ago.[5] The effect of estrogens in slowing bone loss and producing a small increase in trabecular and cortical bone mass is documented beyond any question;[6] only dose/response details and individual variability in response need to be further elucidated. It is clear that the osteoporotic process resumes promptly on estrogen withdrawal. Progesterone itself is a bone-trophic hormone.[7] Progestogens have osteoblast-stimulating activity *in vitro*.[8]

There are conflicting reports on the effect of COC on bone mass, some showing a significant positive effect,[9] others not.[10] The mechanism has not been elucidated but is presumably the same as that of estrogen alone. However, Gallagher et al[11] felt that 20 mg/day of medroxyprogesterone acetate (MPA) combined with conjugated equine estrogens (CEE) had a positive synergistic effect. A small study on contraceptors using DMPA[12] suggested that the 'relative degree of estrogen deficiency' induced by this agent had an adverse effect on bone density, which may be a matter for concern. Larger, more definitive studies which include parameters of bone turnover are being performed with DMPA as well as other progestogen-only contraceptives.

LIVER

The effects of estrogens on the liver, especially when delivered through the portal circulation, are protean.[13] Estrogens are known to increase the lithogenic properties of bile (c.f. the normal cholestasis of pregnancy).[14] Jaundice of pregnancy may have a genetic basis; it is said to be more prevalent in Scandinavian and Chilean women.

There may be a slight increase in the incidence of gallbladder disease in women on ERT,[13] but this is not well documented. Progestogens have far less effect on the liver, which has no progesterone receptors. Liver function tests have been carried out in oral contraceptive users in virtually every phase II and phase III trial ever conducted; these have proved uniformly negative. Similar results have been obtained with progestogen-only minipills (POP) and there are no data on which to base withholding steroid contraceptives, especially progestogen-only types, from women with past (or present) liver disease.[15] Estrogens have a cholestatic action[14] (c.f. pregnancy) and liver disease with jaundice or biliary tree involvement would not be a circumstance where estrogen administration would be appropriate. A meta-analysis of publications on gallbladder disease and COC use found only a slight increase in relative risk, which disappeared with time.[16] Considering the natural history of gallstones, this is highly improbable; it may suggest that COC use enhances the development of symptoms from pre-existing gallstones.

Interactions between COC and other drugs take place chiefly in the liver, largely at the level of the cytochrome P450 enzymes. This subject, heavily dependent on anecdotal information, has been reviewed by Back and Orme.[17] Of the antibiotics, rifampicin is the only one for which there is substantive evidence that it has reduced oral contraceptive bioavailability; griseofulvin is possibly implicated as well.

Anticonvulsants (except sodium valproate) may also reduce efficacy, and there is some suspicion that barbiturates may act similarly. On the other hand, COC may reduce the effectiveness of acetaminophen, aspirin, morphine, corticosteroids and possibly a number of other agents. Finally, the combination of troleandomycin or cyclosporine and COC may produce liver damage.

Liver tumors

In 1973, three cases of liver tumor in COC users were reported; by 1979 there were 109 publications describing 220 case reports of hepatoma (HCA) and carcinoma (HCC) associated with COC use. (During the same period, there were 136 case reports from 75 publications where no hormone use was implicated.) By 1991 four small and one sizable case-control studies of HCC reported an increased relative risk for ever-use or long-term use of COC. Most disturbing of all was a case-control study by Rooks et al[18] which estimated a relative risk for HCC of 104(!) with 5+ years of COC use. In all this work there were confounders: Yu[19] noted a doubling of risk from smoking and a tripling of risk with diabetes. Amazingly, the most important confounder of all — infection with hepatitis B virus (HBV) — was totally ignored in most studies or dismissed in passing as 'negative history for liver disease'. Yet evidence of HBV infection is found in 74–95% of HCC cases worldwide. A WHO multinational study[20] carried out in countries where HBV is endemic and the rates of HCC are relatively high showed no increase in risk with ever-use of COC. The contrast between this epidemiology and the large, long-term prospective studies is startling: *none* of the three major USA or two UK studies, carried out for more than two decades, observed a single case of HCC, and no liver tumors were reported in Europe with 13 million cycles of a cyproterone acetate COC. If anything, the issue of hepatomas and COC use underscores that caution that must be applied to anecdotal case reports and epidemiological calculations that yield relative (rather than attributable) risks.

OBESITY, BODY WEIGHT

While it is almost universally believed by women who are using or are planning to use ERT or COC that these modalities cause weight gain, there is nothing except anecdote to support this belief. Innumerable pre- and postmarketing studies of COC have shown that 'as many women lose weight as gain weight' over a specified period of time; however, there are simply no long-term studies with appropriate controls, because women who elect to use COC or ERT differ in important ways from women who do not. A careful metabolic balance study in women maintained on a constant diet and 801 µg mestranol daily and given 5 mg norethynodrel or 2 mg chlormadinone acetate for several weeks showed an increase in sodium retention and lean body mass and a decrease in body fat attributable to the progestogen.[21] As diet was constant, no change in total body weight was expected, or found. In contrast to uncontrolled WHO studies which reported a significant increase in body weight of DMPA users, a comparative one year study of COC, Depoprovera and Norplant failed to show any statistically significant weight gain or difference between any of these agents.[22]

GASTROINTESTINAL TRACT

The relationship of chronic inflammatory bowel disease and use of COC is confounded (as in the case of cardiovascular disease) by cigarette smoking. Even so, there have been several reports suggesting that both ulcerative colitis and Crohn's disease are more common in COC users. The most recent large epidemiologic study[23] found a doubling of the risk of either disorder. COC use for more than five years yielded a relative risk of 5.1 for Crohn's disease whereas duration of use was not a factor with ulcerative colitis. However, higher ulcerative colitis risk tended to occur more among high-estrogen COC users, while the relative risk of Crohn's disease was unaffected by estrogen dose. On the other hand, a meta-analysis by Godet et al[24] found only a weak, probably noncausal association between inflammatory bowel disease and COC use.

It has been suggested that COC use protects against colon cancer. An Australian study[25] found no effect on large bowel cancer, and a meta-analysis of 14 studies showed no impact.[26] However, a very large prospective cohort study enrolling 676 526 females found a decreased relative risk of colon cancer of 0.55 (95% confidence limits 0.40–0.76) in current ERT users and 0.71 (0.61–0.83) in ever-users.[27] Since colon cancer is the third most common malignancy in women, these and many similar epidemiologic findings are of great interest.

RENAL SYSTEM

While hypertension is less common in postmenopausal estrogen users than in nonusers, there are cases where ERT actually raises blood pressure. The mechanism for this event is believed to reside in the renin-angiotensin-aldosterone system. Under physiological conditions, renin substrate is the rate-limiting step of the renin reaction. Estrogen stimulates the hepatic synthesis of this protein, but only a small percentage of women with elevated renin substrate levels develop hypertension, and it has been speculated that a large molecular weight isoform of renin is involved.[28] Prorenin is affected by hormone levels even in the various phases of the menstrual cycle, and is significantly depressed by both monophasic and triphasic COC.[29]

Epidemiological studies with older high-dose COC reported an average increase of a few mm Hg in systolic and diastolic blood pressure, and an increased incidence (1–3%) of de novo hypertension, but this does not appear to be the case for the lower-dose COC in current use. Endogenous creatinine clearance is increased in COC users; the mechanism for this action is unknown.[30] In this study, sodium and/or potassium excretion rate was also increased, suggesting a renal tubular effect.

Renal disease is a common complication of diabetes, and it has been speculated on the basis of COC effects on blood pressure, cholesterol fractions and carbohydrate metabolism that an increase in nephropathy might occur. However, the use of COC in insulin-dependent diabetics had no effect on hemoglobin A_{1c}, albumin excretion rates or retinopathy scores.[31]

VITAMIN AND MINERAL METABOLISM

Nearly all of the research on the effect of sex hormones on these parameters has focussed on oral, injectable and implantable contraceptives, because of the importance of nutritional problems in underdeveloped countries and the concern that these agents might have adverse effects. This field has been reviewed recently by Amatayakul.[32] Studies under the auspices of the WHO[33] have been carried out in Thailand, India, Mexico, South Korea, Australia and Great Britain.

Although estrogens increase retinol-binding protein and therefore total plasma vitamin A levels, the storage and availability of vitamin A are unaffected. Thiamin nutritional status is either marginally or not at all affected by COC in Third World women. Riboflavin deficiency might be of particular importance in women with glucose-6-phosphate dehydrogenase deficiency, but studies with low-dose COC showed no effect on riboflavin status. The alteration in the tryptophane-niacin metabolic pathway seen in COC users has been linked to increased hepatic synthesis and release of tryptophane oxygenase, which shunts more of the available tryptophane into this pathway. Additionally, the metabolism of tryptophane is partially blocked by the metabolic products of estrogen, which interfere with the binding of pyridoxine coenzyme to the pyridoxine-dependent apoenzyme systems. Thus, the increased xanthurenic acid excretion in COC users is based on a different mechanism from that seen in pyridoxine-deficient individuals, and it took some time before the notion that COC cause pyridoxine deficiency was laid to rest. Some have reported a slight increase in both serum and red cell folate after a year of COC use; on the other hand cyanocobalamin levels are reduced, possibly due to a decrease of B_{12} binding capacity, but this reduction was still above the levels seen in B_{12} deficiency. Vitamin C levels may be slightly decreased, possibly due to estrogen-induced increases in serum ceruloplasmin, which has strong ascorbate-oxidase activity. Clinical consequences have not been observed. Limited studies of niacin or pantothenic acid have shown no changes.

Of the minerals, iron metabolism is most affected, by the reduction of menstrual hemoglobin loss in COC users. The observed increase in serum copper is due entirely to the increased levels of copper-binding ceruloplasmin. No effect of COC on zinc absorption and excretion has been observed, although in India decreased serum zinc levels were noted in users of Depoprovera and norethisterone enanthate.

Conclusion

This chapter is not intended to be a comprehensive summary of estrogen/progestogen effects outside the reproductive system. It does purport to show how scanty our knowledge in some of these areas really is, and suggests that there are many territories still to be explored, chiefly in terms of developing new, beneficial uses for these compounds. New molecules targeted at specific applications can be synthesized readily today; what needs to be done is to identify these targets.

REFERENCES

1. Kuhl H 1994 Ovarian failure and the skin. In: Berg G, Hammar M (eds) The modern management of the menopause. Parthenon Publishing Group, New York, pp 381–385
2. Goldzieher JW 1949 The direct effect of steroids on the senile human skin: a preliminary report. Journal of Gerontology 4: 104–112

3. Lemay A, Dewailly SD, Grenier R et al 1990 Attentuation of mild hyperandrogenic activity in postpubertal acne by a triphasic oral contraceptive containing low doses of ethynyl estradiol and d,l-norgestrel. Journal of Clinical Endocrinology and Metabolism 71: 8–14
4. Hannaford PC, Villard-Mackintosh L, Vessey MP et al 1991 Oral contraceptives and malignant melanoma. British Journal of Cancer 63: 430–433
5. Albright F, Smith PH, Richardson AM 1941 Postmenopausal osteoporosis; its clinical features. Journal of the American Medical Association 116: 2465–2497
6. Christiansen C 1994 Hormone replacement therapy — standardized or individually adapted doses? — effect on bone mass. In: Berg G, Hammar M (eds) The modern management of the menopause. Parthenon Publishing Group, New York, pp 337–342
7. Prior JC: 1990 Progesterone as a bone-trophic hormone. Endocrine Reviews 11: 386–398
8. Verhaar HJJ, Damen CA, Duursma SA et al 1994 Comparison of the effects of estrogen and the progestins progesterone, dydrogesterone and 20a-dihydroxydydrogesterone on proliferation and differentiation of normal adult human osteoblast-like cells. In: Berg G, Hammar M (eds) The modern management of the menopause. Parthenon Publishing Group, New York, pp 343–352
9. Lindsay R, Tohme J, Kanders B 1986 The effect of oral contraceptive use on vertebral bone mass in pre- and postmenopausal women. Contraception 34: 333–340
10. Mazess RB, Barden HS 1991 Bone density in premenopausal women: effects of age, dietary intake, physical activity, smoking and birth control pills. American Journal of Clinical Nutrition 53: 132–142
11. Gallagher JC, Kable WT, Goldgar D 1991 Effect of progestin therapy on cortical and trabecular bone: comparison with estrogen. American Journal of Medicine 90: 171–178
12. Cundy T, Evans M, Roberts H et al 1991 Bone density in women receiving depot medroxyprogesterone acetate for contraception. British Medical Journal 303: 13–16
13. Judd HL 1987 Effects of estrogen replacement on hepatic function. In: Mishell DR Jr (ed) Menopause: physiology and phramacology. Year Book Medical Publishers, Chicago, p 237
14. Sillem MH, Teichmann AT 1994 The liver. In: Goldzieher J, Fotherby K (eds) Pharmacology of the contraceptive steroids. Raven Press, New York, pp 247–258
15. McCann MF, Potter LS 1994 Progestin-only oral contraception: a comprehensive review. Contraception 50: S1
16. Thijs C, Knipschild P 1993 Oral contraceptives and the risk of gallbladder disease: a meta-analysis. American Journal of Public Health 83: 1113–1120
17. Back DJ, Orme M L'E 1994 Drug interactions. In: Goldzieher J, Fotherby K (eds) Pharmacology of the contraceptive steroids. Raven Press, New York, pp 407–425
18. Rooks JB, Ory HW, Ishak KG et al 1979 Epidemiology of hepatocellular adenoma. The role of oral contraceptive use. Journal of the American Medical Association 242: 644–648
19. Yu MC, Tong MJ, Govindarajan S et al 1991 Nonviral risk factors for hepatocellular carcinoma in a low-risk population: the non-Asians of Los Angeles County CA. Journal of the National Cancer Institute 83: 1820–1826
20. World Health Organization 1989 The WHO collaborative study of neoplasia and oral contraceptives: combined oral contraceptives and liver cancer. International Journal of Cancer 43: 254–259
21. Lecocq FR, Bradley EM, Goldzieher JW 1967 Metabolic balance studies with norethynodrel and chlormadinone acetate. American Journal of Obstetrics and Gynecology 99: 374–381
22. Moore LL, Valuck R, McDougall C et al 1995 A comparative study of one-year weight gain among users of medroxyprogesterone acetate, levonorgestrel implants, and oral contraceptives. Contraception 52: 215–219
23. Boyko EJ, Theis MK, Vaughan TL et al 1994 Increased risk of inflammatory bowel disease associated with oral contraceptive use. American Journal of Epidemiology 140: 268–278
24. Godet PG, May GR, Sutherland LR 1995 Meta-analysis of the role of oral contraceptive agents in inflammatory bowel disease. Gut 37: 668–673
25. Kune GA, Kune S, Watson LF 1990 Oral contraceptive use does not protect against large bowel cancer. Contraception 41: 19–25
26. MacLennan SC, MacLennan AH, Ryan P 1995 Colorectal cancer and oestrogen replacement therapy. A meta-analysis of epidemiological studies. Medical Journal of Australia 162: 491–493
27. Calle EE, Miracle-McMahill HL, Thun MJ et al 1995 Estrogen replacement therapy and risk of fatal colon cancer in a prospective cohort of postmenopausal women. Journal of the National Cancer Institute 87: 517–523
28. Shionoiri H, Eggena P, Barrett JD et al 1983 An increase in high-molecular-weight renin substrate associated with estrogenic hypertension. Biochemistry in Medicine 29: 14–22
29. Schumacher M, Nanninga A, Delfs T et al 1992 A direct immunoradiometric assay for human plasma prorenin: concentrations in cycling women and in women taking oral contraceptives. Journal of Clinical Endocrinology and Metabolism 75: 617–623
30. Brändle E, Gottwald E, Melzer H et al 1992 Influence of oral contraceptive agents on kidney function and protein metabolism. European Journal of Clinical Pharmacology 43: 643–646
31. Garg SK, Chase HP, Marshall G et al 1994 Oral contraceptives and renal and retinal complications in young women with insulin-dependent diabetes mellitus. Journal of the American Medical Association 271: 1099–1102
32. Amatayakul K 1994 Metabolism: vitamins and trace minerals. In: Goldzieher J, Fotherby K (eds) Pharmacology of the contraceptive steroids. Raven Press, New York, pp 363–377
33. World Health Organization 1985 WHO task force on oral contraceptives: impact of hormonal contraceptives vis-a-vis non-hormonal factors on the vitamin status of malnourished women in India and Thailand. Human Nutrition and Clinical Nutrition 40C: 205

67. The influence of steroids on gynecologic cancers

James J. Schlesselman John A. Collins

Introduction

Steroidal contraception first became available for general clinical use in June 1960 when GD Searle and Co. began marketing Enovid[R] in the United States after approval by the Food and Drug Administration (FDA). This combination type oral contraceptive contained 9.85 mg norethynodrel as the progestogen and 0.15 mg mestranol as the estrogen, a formulation that has been superseded by many alternatives over the past 35 years. Subsequent formulations were based on mestranol or ethinyl estradiol (EE) at dosages of 50 μg or more, and progestogens such as ethynodiol, lynoestrenol, norethisterone and norethisterone acetate. In the early 1970s products containing less than 50 μg of estrogen were introduced, and some of these were combined with progestogens such as norgestrel or levonorgestrel. Products marketed during the past 15 years in Europe and North America contain 20–35 μg of EE and one of three progestogens: gestodene, desogestrel or norgestimate.

At the time of the initial FDA approval, it was known from clinical studies in humans and experiments in animals that sex steroids play a role in the development of neoplasia.[1] While recent studies suggest that progestogens can be carcinogenic,[2] the initial concern was principally with estrogen.[3–5] As early as 1896, Beatson had reported that ovariectomy ameliorated the clinical course of breast cancer in women,[6] a finding later demonstrated experimentally in mice.[7] Animal studies in the 1920s and 1930s indicated that ovarian extracts were potent agents in producing tissue proliferation in the female genital tract, a common site of cancer in women.[1] There were also isolated case reports in which estrogen therapy was suspected of playing a role in the development of cancer of the breast and endometrium.[8–11] The possibility that steroidal contraception or hormone replacement therapy might have an effect on the development of cancer in humans, however, still lay within the realm of conjecture until the completion of epidemiologic studies over the past 20 years.

Before we begin our survey of this literature and comment on its relevance to clinical practice, we first present some of the pertinent epidemiology of cancer of the breast and reproductive tract. We next discuss the biologic plausibility for effects of exogenous hormones on cancer risk. This background should prove advantageous for placing in clinical perspective the results of the epidemiologic studies that follow.

EPIDEMIOLOGIC BACKGROUND

Age-specific rates of cancer occurrence

The two most striking and well known features of cancer occurrence are its dramatic variations by age and race. Figure 67.1 shows the age-specific incidence rates of invasive cancer of the breast, cervix uteri, corpus uteri and ovary in females in the United States.[12] Incidence refers here to the number of *newly* diagnosed cases of primary cancer within the five year period 1987–91. Incidence *rate* is the ratio of the number of these cases to the corresponding total *person-time at risk*, which is determined from the amount of follow-up time contributed by each person who is under observation either directly or conceptually.

Cancer incidence rates are often expressed in officially reported statistics as the number of cases 'per 100 000 persons per year'. Thus, if r denotes the annual incidence rate, $5 \times r$ would be the risk of developing cancer within a 5 year period. Likewise, if r_1 and r_2 denote the annual cancer incidence rates for women age 45–49 and 50–54, the risk of cancer within 10 years for a 45-year-old woman would be estimated as $5 \times (r_1 + r_2)$.

Figure 67.1 shows that as of 1987–91, invasive breast cancer was diagnosed among American women age 20–24 at the rate of 10 cases per million women per year. In women age 50–54, the corresponding rate

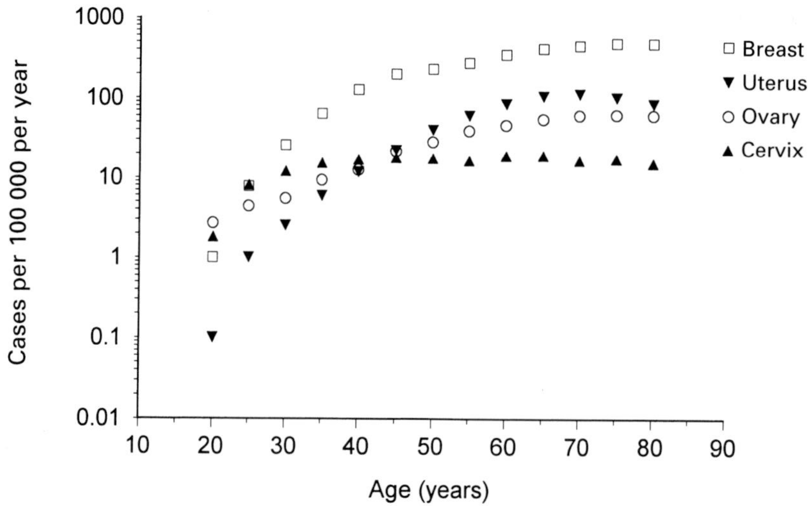

Fig. 67.1 Age specific rates of invasive cancer in United States females, 1987–91. (All races. Uterus = corpus uteri & NOS)

of diagnosis was 2.3 cases per thousand per year, and in women age 70–74, the rate was 4.5 per thousand per year, a 450-fold increase over the incidence rate in women age 20–24.

Figure 67.1 also shows that by age 35 the incidence rate of invasive cervical cancer began to plateau at 15–20 cases per 100 000 women per year, a result due to screening that detects and treats preinvasive lesions. The incidence rate of ovarian cancer continued to increase until age 75, however, at which point the rate of diagnosis was 62 cases per 100 000 women per year.

Epidemiologic studies of steroidal contraception in relation to cancer of the corpus uteri have focused on endometrial cancer. Although Figure 67.1 shows the incidence rates of cancer of the uterine corpus, including corpus sites not otherwise specified (NOS), these rates reflect primarily those of endometrial cancer because most cancers of the uterine corpus are endometrial carcinomas: adenocarcinomas, andenocanthomas, adenosquamous carcinomas and other histological subtypes. For example, in the United States about 93% of whites and 79% of blacks diagnosed with cancer of the uterine corpus have endometrial cancer.[13] The remaining cancers are predominantly leiomyosarcomas occurring within the myometrium and malignant lesions of mixed origin, such as carcinosarcoma and Mullerian mixed tumors.[14–16]

Adjustment of rates for population at risk

One shortcoming in the incidence rates of gynecologic cancer shown in Figure 67.1 is that they are based on the total number of women in the population, rather than the number of women actually at risk of gynecologic cancer. For example, women who have had a complete hysterectomy are no longer at risk of cancer of the uterine cervix or uterine corpus, and women who have had a bilateral oophorectomy are no longer at risk of ovarian cancer. As a consequence of these surgical procedures, the incidence rates in Figure 67.1 would be substantially higher at older ages if they were expressed as rates per 100 000 women who remain at risk of gynecologic cancer.

To be specific about this, Figure 67.2 shows estimates of the percentage of women in Finland and in the United States who have had a hysterectomy by the time they reach age 70. By 40 years of age, 3% of Finnish women and 11% of American women have had a hysterectomy. By age 70 the corresponding figures are 26% and 33%, respectively. The estimates for Finnish women are based on patient discharges from all Finnish hospitals over the three year period 1987–89.[17] The figures for Americans are based on our own calculations using reported age-specific rates of hysterectomy from the National Hospital Discharge Survey in 1988–90,[18] adjusted for the number of women who have already had a hysterectomy. The percentages shown in Figure 67.2 are similar to estimates of the age-specific prevalence of hysterectomy in South Australia as of 1991, where 31% of women age 65 or older had had a hysterectomy.[19] At younger ages, the corresponding figures from South Australia were 19% (40–44 yrs), 27% (45–54 yrs) and 31% (55–64 yrs).

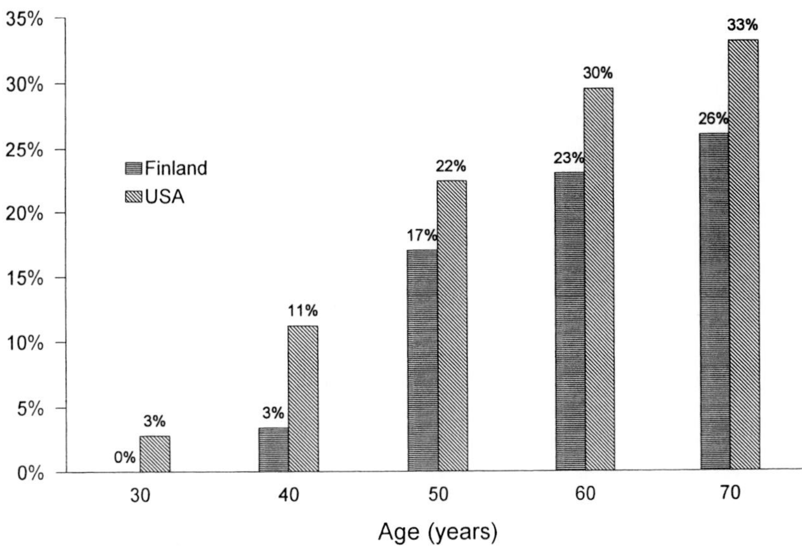

Fig. 67.2 Cumulative incidence (%) of hysterectomy.

If the rates of uterine cancer in US women shown in Figure 67.1 were expressed as rates per 100 000 actually at risk of this disease, then based on the data in Figure 67.2, the incidence rates would be about 3% higher in women age 30, about 12% higher in women age 40 and about 49% higher in women age 70. Obviously the need for such adjustment will vary not only by age but also by country. Since there are no systematic data that permit us to take account of this properly, we cite incidence rates per 100 000 women, recognizing that these rates *underestimate* gynecologic cancer risk, particularly at older ages.

Figure 67.3 shows that while Japanese women have a markedly lower overall risk of gynecologic cancer than Americans, they have similar age-specific patterns of cancer incidence.[20] One noteworthy difference, however, is that the incidence rate of breast cancer plateaus at age 50 for the Japanese, with an actual decline in the rate of the disease beyond age 75.

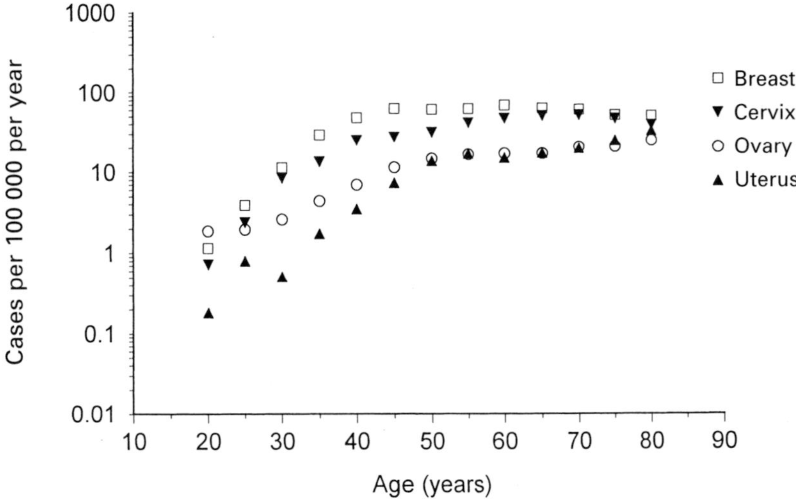

Fig. 67.3 Age specific rates of invasive cancer in Japanese females, 1983–87. (Osaka, Japan. Uterus = corpus uteri & NOS)

Risk of cancer within a range of age

Age-specific incidence rates show clearly how the risk of cancer varies throughout a woman's life, but they do not state directly the risk of cancer occurring at some time within a range of age. For example, Table 67.1 shows that as of 1989–91 a 20-year-old American woman had only a 0.04% chance of developing breast cancer within 10 years of life and a 2.0% chance of developing breast cancer within 30 years. The corresponding 10-year risk of breast cancer for a 50-year-old woman was 2.4% and her 30-year risk was 8.7%.

Despite the fact that a 20-year-old woman's risk of cancer within 10 or 30 years is lower than the risk for a 50-year-old woman, a 20-year-old's lifetime risk of cancer is *greater*, mainly because her life expectancy, and therefore her 'time at risk' for developing cancer, is greater.

The figures cited in Table 67.1 are estimates based on age-specific rates as of 1987–91. Thus, not only are these figures subject to change over time, but they will vary materially by factors that influence gynecologic cancer risk, such as a family history of cancer or a woman's reproductive history, points to which we shall return in later sections.

International variation in cancer risk

Age-specific incidence rates do not facilitate a discussion of how the risk of cancer varies among countries. We therefore consider the *cumulative risk* of cancer, by which we mean the probability (risk) that cancer will be diagnosed at some time within a specified range of age in women who do not have cancer at the outset and are subject to the risk of cancer either throughout the entire span of time under consideration, or until they develop clinically evident cancer at some point within it. The important point to note about the definition of cumulative risk is that its computation is based on a hypothetical condition — the assumption of no premature deaths over the period of time in question. This provides the very rationale, however, for the use of cumulative risk: it allows comparisons of cancer incidence across populations that are subject to markedly different forces of mortality.[21] For example, if a woman who is free of cancer dies at age 30 in an automobile accident or at age 50 from cardiovascular disease, she is obviously not at risk of developing cancer at older ages, the time at which the incidence rate is greatest.

Table 67.1 Risk of invasive cancer (%) within 10 years, 30 years and in remaining lifetime, given cancer-free at current age.*

	Current age (yrs)	Cancer risk within +10 yrs	+30 yrs	Lifetime
Breast	20	0.04	1.98	12.48
	50	2.36	8.67	11.05
Cervix	20	0.05	0.35	0.90
	50	0.17	0.46	0.56
Ovary	20	0.04	0.29	1.80
	50	0.33	1.24	1.57
Uterus**	20	0.01	0.21	2.68
	50	0.50	2.14	2.57

*USA SEER data, all races, 1989–91;[12] **Corpus uteri + NOS.

One further point to bear in mind is that cumulative risk continually increases with age, despite the fact that the age-specific incidence rates may be constant or even falling. This point is illustrated in Figure 67.4, which shows both the incidence rates[12] and the cumulative risk of invasive cancer of the uterine cervix in white women in the United States as of 1987–91.

Since 75 years of age approximates a woman's median lifespan, we consider the cumulative risk of cancer from 0–74 years of age, which is plotted in Figure 67.5 for 58 cancer registries throughout the world that cover populations of at least one-half million females.[20] The data for this figure are based on the cumulative rates of cancer published by the IARC.[20] The cumulative rate, which is defined as the sum over each year of age of the age-specific incidence rates, is an approximation to the cumulative risk.[21]

Figure 67.5 shows that the cumulative risk of developing invasive cancer at any anatomic site, excluding ICD-9 173 (squamous and basal cell cancer of the skin), ranges from a low of about 11% (in Qidong, China and Ahmedabad, India) to a high of about 27% (in white females in the United States). In other words, the cumulative risk of females developing cancer by 75 years of age varies among countries from a low of about 1 in 9 females to a high of about 3 in 11, a 2.7-fold difference.

Figure 67.5 also shows the corresponding figures for cancer of the breast and reproductive tract. These show three fold to ten fold differences in cumulative risk among countries. For example, the cumulative risk of invasive breast cancer ranges from a low of 1% (in Qidong, China and Khon Kaen, Thailand) to a high of 9.8% (in whites in the United States), almost a ten fold difference. The highest risk of cancer of the uterine cervix occurs in Madras, India and Goiania, Brazil, where the cumulative risk is 4.9%. The lowest

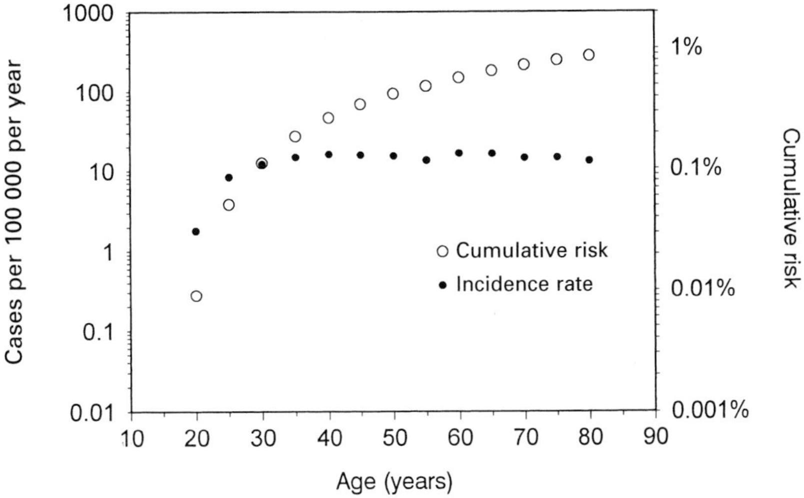

Fig. 67.4 Cervix cancer in United States white females. (All SEER centers, 1987–91)

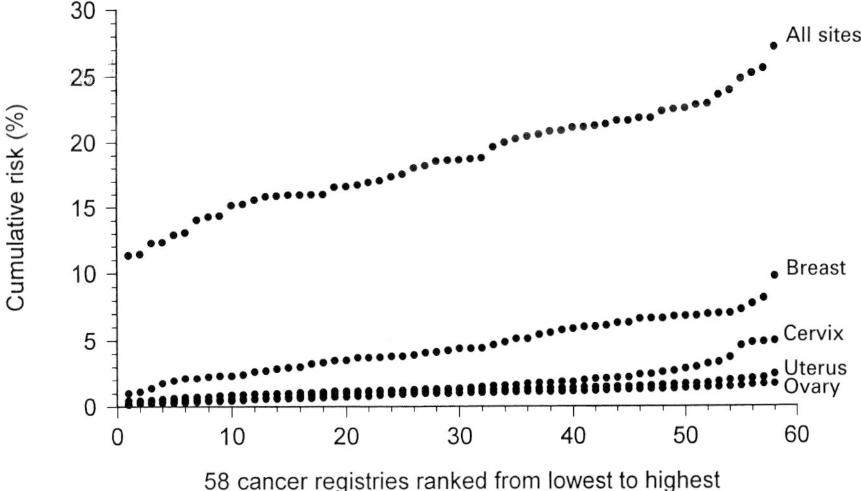

Fig. 67.5 International variation in the cumulative risk of invasive cancer from age 0–74 years. (Females, all anatomic sites except 173. Uterus = corpus uteri & NOS)

cumulative risk is found in Finland, in Qidong, China, and among Jews in Israel, where the cumulative risk is under 0.5%.

Cancer of the uterine corpus (+NOS) occurs most commonly among women in Canada (2.1%), Czechoslovakia (2.2%) and whites in the United States (2.5%), and least commonly among Asian women, where the cumulative risk is under 0.5% for India, China, Thailand and all but one cancer registry in Japan. The highest cumulative risk of ovarian cancer (1.7%) occurs in Denmark, Sweden and Norway. A number of cancer registries in Japan, India and China report some of the lowest values, 0.6% or less.

Table 67.2 gives a systematic overview of the cumulative risk of cancer for selected countries throughout the world. Since cumulative risk from age 0–74 years approximates the lifetime risk of cancer, one can think of lifetime risk when perusing the figures in Table 67.2, although a proper calculation of lifetime risk would be based on life-table methods[22] that account for both all-cause mortality throughout life and cancer incidence at age 75 years and beyond. With

Table 67.2 Cumulative risk (%) of females developing invasive cancer from age 0–74 years, by anatomic site and country.*

	Anatomic site				
	Breast	Cervix	Ovary	Uterus**	All sites+
Asia					
China, Shanghai	2.3	0.6	0.5	0.4	15.6
Japan, Osaka	2.4	1.5	0.6	0.5	15.9
Thailand, Chiang Mai	1.4	3.0	0.6	0.3	17.1
Europe					
Denmark	7.3	1.6	1.7	2.0	25.2
Finland	5.5	0.5	1.1	1.5	18.2
Italy, Florence	7.0	0.8	1.1	1.7	21.8
England & Wales	6.0	1.2	1.3	1.1	20.2
North America					
Canada	7.8	1.0	1.3	2.1	24.8
USA whites	9.8	0.7	1.5	2.5	27.2
USA blacks	7.0	1.2	0.9	1.3	22.8
South America					
Brazil, Goiania	4.7	4.9	0.5	0.9	21.1
Colombia, Cali	3.8	4.6	1.0	0.9	21.3
Paraguay, Asuncion	3.9	4.8	0.6	1.5	17.0

*Cumulative risk calculated from cumulative rates (age 0–74);[20] **Corpus uteri + NOS; +All anatomic sites, except ICD-9 173.

this caveat in mind, the cumulative risk of cancer (excluding ICD-9 173) occurring at any anatomic site is seen to be lowest among Asian women, ranging from 15.6% in Chinese to 17.1% in Thai. The highest cumulative risk is found among women in Europe and North America: 25% in Danes and Canadians, and 27% in American whites. Breast cancer is seen to be quite low in Asian women, ranging from 1.4% in Thai to 2.4% in Japanese. Women in Europe and North America have substantially greater risk of breast cancer, ranging from 5.5% in Finnish women to 9.8% in American whites.

Women in South America have an intermediate risk of breast cancer, on the order of 4–5%, but they have some of the highest risks of cervical cancer throughout the world, ranging from 4.6% in Cali, Columbia to 4.9% in Goiania, Brazil. A South American woman is as likely to develop invasive cancer of the uterine cervix as she is cancer of the breast.

Survival after cancer diagnosis

Table 67.3 shows that the prospect for survival after the diagnosis of breast cancer or gynecologic cancer can be very good, provided that detection has occurred when the disease is localized. The five year relative survival rates, which are 90% or greater for localized disease, fall to less than 30% for cancers whose stage at diagnosis is distant. The relative survival rate shown in Table 67.3 is the ratio of the five year survival rate observed among cancer patients to the five year survival rate expected on the basis of their age, race, sex, area of residence and calendar year.[12]

Table 67.3 also shows the relative survival rates by age at diagnosis. While the five year relative survival rate after the diagnosis of invasive breast cancer was

Table 67.3 Five year relative survival rates (%) by cancer stage at diagnosis and age.*

	Anatomic site			
	Breast	Cervix	Ovary	Uterus**
Stage				
Localized	94	90	90	94
Regional	73	51	41	67
Distant	18	12	21	27
All stages	80	67	42	83
Age (yrs)				
<45	76	79	74	92
45–	81	66	52	90
55–	80	63	38	86
65–	83	54	30	81
75–	81	40	20	71

*USA SEER data, all races, 1989–91;[12] **Corpus uteri + NOS.

Table 67.4 Cause of death (%) in females in 1990.[23]

	Europe*		Japan		USA	
	All ages	*35–69*	*All ages*	*35–69*	*All ages*	*35–69*
Vascular	47.9	28.2	41.7	27.0	45.9	30.3
Cancer	21.4	43.6	23.1	43.9	22.9	40.5
breast	4.0	11.1	1.6	5.1	4.2	9.3
cervix	0.4	1.3	0.5	1.3	0.4	1.1
uterus	0.7	1.5	0.7	1.4	0.6	0.9
ovary	1.2	3.2	0.9	2.5	1.2	2.4
Respiratory	11.0	5.2	11.0	5.2	8.9	6.8
Injuries	5.0	8.8	5.0	8.8	4.1	5.4
Infectious & parasitic	1.3	1.6	1.3	1.6	1.5	1.5
All other causes	17.9	13.5	17.9	13.5	16.7	15.5
All causes	100.0	100.0	100.0	100.0	100.0	100.0

*European Union (12 countries).

about 80% in American women regardless of their age, the relative survival rate after the diagnosis of ovarian cancer or invasive cervical cancer declined progressively and markedly with increasing age. For example, women who were under age 45 years at the time of the diagnosis of ovarian cancer had a relative survival rate of 74%; women age 65–74 years old at the time of diagnosis had a relative survival rate of 30%, and women who were age 75 years or older at the time of diagnosis had a relative survival rate of only 20%.

The age-related differences in survival shown in Table 67.3 reflect mainly differences in stage at diagnosis (data not shown). For example, 43% of women diagnosed with ovarian cancer under the age of 50 years had localized disease, but this was true of only 17% of the diagnoses in women age 50 or above, for whom distant disease was diagnosed in 57% of the cases. For cancer of the uterine cervix, 65% of cases under age 50 years had localized disease, whereas only 34% of cases age 50 or older had localized disease. By contrast, 52% of the cases of invasive cancer of the breast diagnosed under age 50 had localized disease, and 56% of cases age 50 or older had localized disease.[12]

Table 67.4 places deaths from cancer in perspective of other causes of mortality.[23] Among European females who died in 1990, 48% of deaths were from vascular disease and 21% were from cancer. However, among European women age 35–69 who died, deaths from cancer (43.6%) were far more common than deaths from vascular disease (28.2%), a reversal in cause of death that occurred also in Japan and in the USA. Cancer of the breast, cervix, uterine corpus and ovary accounted for 17.1% of deaths in European women age 35–69. Over the same range of age, these cancers represented 10.3% of deaths in Japanese women and 13.7% of deaths in Americans.

BIOLOGIC PLAUSIBILITY FOR EFFECTS OF EXOGENOUS HORMONES

Uterine cervix

Squamous cell cancer of the uterine cervix, which accounts for approximately 95% of invasive cervical neoplasms,[24] is considered to arise primarily from venereal transmission of the human papillomavirus (HPV).[24,25] A worldwide study in 22 countries detected HPV DNA in 93% of tumor specimens, the predominant subtypes being HPV 16, 18, 31 and 45, which were present in 50%, 14%, 5% and 8% of invasive cancers.[24] Although an HPV etiology does not rule out other causes, previously established risk factors for cervical cancer such as low social class, early age at first coitus, multiple sexual partners, multiparity and cigarette smoking, are now being re-evaluated to determine whether they are simply correlates of HPV infection, cofactors that operate only in the presence of HPV, or independent determinants of risk.[25]

Oral contraception could be associated with cervical cancer and not a cause of the disease simply because it may be a choice made by women with established risk factors, such as early age at first coitus or a habit of cigarette smoking. Alternatively, use of

COC could affect cervical cancer risk more directly by a variety of possible biologic mechanisms: through a promotional effect on tumor growth,[26–29] by the production of 'clear channel' mucus that facilitates the entry of mutagens,[30,31] by the alteration of immune response which might make women more susceptible to viral infection,[32] or by the production of a localized folate deficiency in the cervix that could alter the expression of steroid hormones[33] or facilitate the incorporation of HPV genomes at a fragile chromosomal site.[34] Similar mechanisms might also increase the risk of cervical cancer among users of hormone replacement therapy (HRT), but the peak incidence of squamous cell cancer of the uterine cervix occurs prior to the menopause, the time at which HRT is usually prescribed.

Ovary

Approximately 80–90% of ovarian cancers arise from tumors of the ovarian surface epithelium.[35–37] The other principal sites of origin are the follicles and germ cells,[38] the latter site predominating in cancers appearing in childhood and infancy.[37] Thus, most of what is known from epidemiologic studies of ovarian cancer in relation to use of steroid hormones is based on the epithelial tumors.

The etiology of epithelial ovarian cancer remains unknown, but two factors in addition to age have been consistently implicated with an increased risk: nulliparity[39,40] and a history of ovarian cancer in first or second degree relatives.[41–43] The risk of ovarian cancer declines with increasing numbers of live births, and data suggest that infertility may be an underlying cause of some ovarian cancers that are associated with nulliparity.[44,45] The familial aggregation is attributable in part to a gene or genes located on chromosome 17q12–21 that predispose women to both breast cancer and ovarian cancer.[46,47]

Two hypotheses concerning a hormonal etiology for ovarian cancer lead one to expect a protective effect from use of oral contraceptives. The ovulation hypothesis[48] is based on evidence that repeated ovulation fosters neoplastic growth, presumably a consequence of both minor trauma sustained by the ovarian surface epithelium with the release of an egg and the exposure of the epithelium to an estrogen-rich follicular fluid. By suppressing ovulation, COC would be expected to reduce the risk of epithelial tumors. The gonadotropin hypothesis[49] is based on experimental evidence linking elevated levels of gonadotropins to ovarian tumors in animals.[35] Since use of COC suppresses pituitary gonadotropins, one would expect their use to reduce the risk of ovarian neoplasms.

Results of epidemiologic studies provide both support for and exceptions to both hypotheses.[50] To give two examples of exceptions, a prospective population-based study[51] found that serum levels of FSH were 20% *lower* on average in women who developed ovarian cancer compared to normal controls. The risk of ovarian cancer, moreover, declined progressively with increasing serum levels of FSH and with increasing levels of serum LH. These findings are contrary to expectations from the gonadotropin hypothesis. With regard to the ovulation hypothesis, one would expect that each month of oral contraception or pregnancy would confer equal protection from ovarian cancer, since both conditions are equally effective in suppressing ovulation. Pregnancy, however, appears to be more effective in reducing ovarian cancer risk, particularly in young women.[44,52]

Presumably the ovulation hypothesis does not apply to any associations between HRT use and ovarian cancer. With respect to the gonadotropin hypothesis, the high levels of FSH and LH in postmenopausal women are reduced by HRT use, and it would follow that HRT might reduce ovarian cancer risk. It has also been suggested that HRT might increase risk by promoting the proliferation of ovarian epithelial cells.[53]

Uterine corpus (endometrium)

Endometrial cancer, long considered an estrogen-dependent neoplasm,[54] is now regarded as the consequence of an excess of estrogen accompanied by inadequate cyclic exposure to progestogen.[55–56] Biologic support for this mechanism is based on findings that estrogenic stimulation increases proliferation and induces nuclear estradiol receptors in the endometrium,[57] and that progestationally active compounds reduce endometrial DNA synthesis,[58–60] reverse hyperplasia,[61] and induce regression of endometrial carcinoma.[62]

Endometrial neoplasms probably originate with a single cell that has survived genetic damage; if the result impairs DNA synthesis regulation, the affected cell has the potential to develop into cancer. The initial damage may arise through spontaneous mutation, radiation or viral exposure. Chemical damage is also possible, but the estrogen molecule is not typical of chemical initiators of oncogenesis. Estradiol is a polycyclic aromatic hydrocarbon, but is more stable than known aromatic hydrocarbon carcinogens such as dibenzanthracene.[63] Although estrogen is an unlikely initiator of cancer growth, an effect of estrogen as a promoter of endometrial cancer development is accepted, and a role for estrogen at later stages of cancer development is also plausible.[50] Promotion occurs when endometrial cells that have undergone genetic damage are exposed to potent growth stimuli such as estrogen. The successive cell replications promote the cancer potential of the initiated cell or cells, presumably because attaining a larger cell mass increases the likelihood that the damaged cells will gain autonomy.

With respect to endometrial cancer, special conditions may influence the operation of these theoretical concepts. The typical premenopausal endometrium is unlikely to serve as a repository of cells with DNA damage because the majority of the endometrium is shed with each ovulatory menstrual cycle. Among women with anovulatory cycles, however, initiated cells are more likely to accumulate and undergo further development.[64,65] Initiation and promotion probably represent early stages in tumor development, and progression to clinical cancer most likely depends on additional influences, some of which may also be subject to steroid hormone modification.

To grow beyond a few cells in size, the nest of potential endometrial cancer cells must attain some degree of control over the body's immune defenses. Numerous studies have indicated that elevated levels of estrogen depress the cell-mediated immune response, possibly through a thymic mechanism.[66] A role for estrogen is therefore possible in thwarting the immune defenses against the nidus of tumor cells. Moreover, before the potential cancer can exceed a few millimeters in size it must co-opt angiogenesis functions to mobilize the necessary blood supply. Spiral arterioles grow exponentially during the proliferative phase of the menstrual cycle under the influence of estradiol.[67] Furthermore, estradiol enhances vasodilatation by stimulating nitric oxide synthesis and prostacyclin activity, and by attenuating the vasoconstrictor activity of endothelin on vascular smooth muscle.[68] These actions of estrogen are consistent with an effect on the dilation of capillaries and out-migration of endothelial cells that appears to precede angiogenesis.[69]

Thus, promotion of the growth of autonomous cells with genetic damage could be an estradiol effect early in tumor development. Early estrogen effects on tumor development would be consistent with a long subclinical phase, whereby tumor risk is seen to rise only after a relatively long period of exposure. Estradiol also may augment tumor growth late in the preclinical stage through immune or vascular mechanisms. Late stage estrogen effects would be consistent with a short subclinical phase and an association with current use.

While the exact molecular mechanisms still remain to be elucidated,[56,70] further evidence for a hormonal etiology of endometrial cancer comes from factors known to be associated with increased risk, all of which can be linked in one way or another to endogenous estrogenic stimulation: obesity, anovulatory menstrual cycles, polycystic ovaries, nulliparity, early age at menarche and late age at menopause.[50,71] Cigarette smoking appears to reduce the risk of endometrial cancer, possibly through its association with lower levels of circulating estrogen.[72] Clinical observations also indicate strong associations with Stein-Leventhal syndrome and theca cell and granulosa cell tumors of the ovary.[50]

ESTIMATED EFFECT OF ORAL CONTRACEPTIVES

This section begins with a presentation and discussion of estimates of the relative risk of gynecologic cancer in relation to use of oral contraceptives. Relative risk refers here to the risk of invasive cancer in women who have used COC for some specified duration ($Risk_{dur}$) divided by the corresponding risk of invasive cancer in women who have never used COC ($Risk_{nev}$). In other words:

$$RR_{dur} = Risk_{dur}/Risk_{nev}. \qquad [1]$$

A relative risk of 1, therefore, corresponds to no increase or decrease in the risk of invasive cancer among COC users; a relative risk of 1.4 corresponds to a 40% increase in risk, and a relative risk of 0.7 corresponds to a 30% reduction in risk. At the end of this section, our estimates of relative risk are placed in perspective of the absolute risk of gynecologic cancer arising from age 20–54 years in US women and in Japanese.

Uterine cervix (squamous cell cancer)

Figure 67.6 shows estimates of the relative risk of invasive squamous cell cancer of the uterine cervix by duration of oral contraceptive use. The data are from 11 epidemiologic studies reporting such information for 3118 women with invasive disease, 1080 of whom had used COC. The open circles in Figure 67.6 represent the reported estimates of relative risk from nine case-control studies;[73–81] the solid points correspond to the estimates of relative risk from two cohort studies.[82,83] Using methods published earlier,[84] the fitted curve represents relative risk by duration of

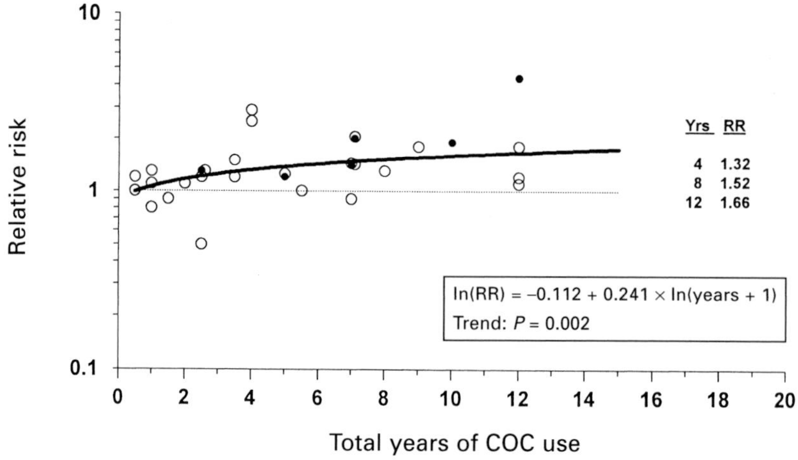

Fig. 67.6 Invasive cervix cancer: relative risk by duration of oral contraceptive use.

COC use (total years of oral contraception). It was estimated from our meta-analysis of the studies' data based on the regression equation below, where 'ln' denotes natural logarithm:

$$\ln(RR_{dur}) = b_0 + b_1 \times \ln\,(\text{duration} + 1). \quad [2]$$

Each reported estimate of relative risk shown in Figure 67.6 was weighted by its corresponding precision (inverse variance) in the analysis. The resulting estimates of b_0 and b_1 are given in Figure 67.6.

Figure 67.6 shows a trend of increasing risk with increasing duration of COC use. The risk of invasive cervical cancer is increased by an estimated 32% with four years of oral contraception, by 52% with eight years of use, and by 66% with 12 years of COC use (RR = 1.32, 1.52, 1.66; trend: $P = 0.002$, one-sided). Since most of the individual estimates of relative risk shown in Figure 67.6 have been adjusted for major risk factors for cervical cancer, these do not plausibly account for the increased risk just cited. Data from six studies[73–76,78,80] suggest there is no delay beyond that required to accumulate sufficient use of COC before an increased risk occurs. In other words, there appears to be no 'latent effect'. Two of these studies[73,74] specifically took into account duration of use in addressing this issue.

Sources of bias

Before one attributes risk associated with use of COC to oral contraception itself, one has to consider possibilities that might bias the results. For cervical cancer, there are substantial problems to avoid in this regard.[83,85,86] For example, women using COC for extended periods of time are less likely to use barrier methods of contraception. Since these protect against cervical cancer,[87,88] an apparently increased risk of this disease in COC users could be due simply to the reduced risk among the women using barrier methods. The resulting biased comparison of COC users versus nonusers might well show a dose response by duration of COC use, since cervical cancer risk associated with but not caused by use of COC ought to increase in proportion to the amount of time a woman is not using protective methods. The upshot is that a dose response by duration of use, which is often used to support an inference of cause-effect, could result simply from a biased comparison. One way to avoid this problem is to compare use of COC with use of nonbarrier contraceptive methods.[89,90] Another is to compare COC users and nonusers, but adjust the comparison for the total time during which barrier methods are used in the two groups.[73]

Assessment of COC use in relation to cervical cancer is further complicated by regular screening for the disease. Since dysplasia and pre-invasive lesions can be detected by Papanicolaou smear, one expects that women who use COC, who are typically under greater medical surveillance, will be diagnosed more frequently with dysplasia and carcinoma *in situ* even in the absence of an adverse effect of oral contraception. On the other hand, women who have frequent Papanicolaou tests are at substantially reduced risks of invasive cancer.[91–93] This occurs because pre-invasive lesions are found and treated before they progress to invasive disease. As a consequence, one expects that invasive cervical cancer will be diagnosed less frequently among COC users,[89] possibly even when

COC has an adverse effect. The preceding line of reasoning implies that opposing sources of bias are expected in these studies: some biases will act to spuriously increase cervical cancer risk in women using COC, others will act to spuriously reduce the risk.

A well designed study of invasive cervical cancer should ideally compare use of COC with use of methods that do not protect against cervical cancer. Furthermore, the comparison ought to be made under conditions of uniform screening for the disease in women at equal risk of exposure to HPV. None of the reported studies attains these ideals, and they vary in their attempts to approximate them by various maneuvers in their analyses.

Discontinued use

If the risk of cervical cancer is indeed elevated among women using COC, and if the effect is *due* to oral contraception, then one might expect an eventual decline in risk upon discontinuation. Relatively few studies have examined this in detail. Figure 67.7 shows the available data for recency of use (years since last use of COC) from six studies involving 2012 women with invasive disease, 606 of whom had used COC.[73–76,78,80] Relative risk by recency of use (RR_{rec}) was estimated from equation [2] above, except that years since last use of COC (recency) was the independent variable.

Figure 67.7 shows only a marginal trend of decreasing risk with increasing time since discontinuation: the relative risk of invasive cervical cancer is estimated at 1.28, 1.23 and 1.18 for 5,10 and 20 years after stopping use of COC (trend: $P = 0.31$, one-sided). It would be better to examine separately the effect of stopping COC use among long-term users, which is not addressed by Figure 67.7 and its accompanying analysis. Unfortunately, the reported data[73,74] are insufficient to address the issue well.

Other factors

Data relating to COC formulations have not been reported systematically, so there is no foundation upon which to build a strong case for or against any particular type or brand of COC having a different effect on cervical cancer risk. Likewise, the epidemiologic data reported to date reveals no 'susceptible subgroup' of women for whom use of COC *per se* should be avoided on the basis of cervical cancer risk. Obviously, however, since promiscuity is a major risk factor for contracting an HPV infection, women at risk should consider this in choosing their method of contraception. Barrier methods, such as the condom or diaphragm, offer some protection. Whether use of COC can promote HPV activity once infection has occurred[25,94] is an hypothesis that has yet to be established or refuted.

Adenocarcinoma

Data from several case-control studies indicate that women who use COC are at increased risk of adenocarcinoma of the cervix.[74,78,95] Evidence of a trend of increasing risk with increasing duration of use is not clear cut, however. The results of studies

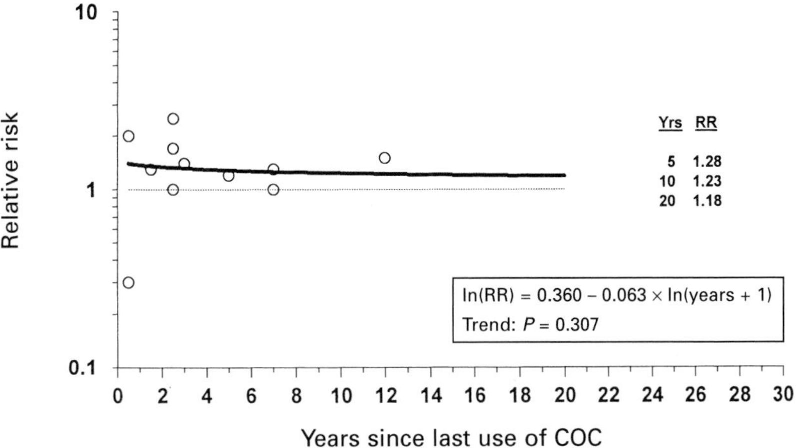

Fig. 67.7 Invasive cervix cancer: relative risk by time since last use of oral contraceptives.

comparing women with adenocarcinoma with those with squamous cell carcinoma,[96–100] however, indicate that women with these two disease entities are comparable with regard to their use of oral contraceptives. This suggests to us that there is an increased risk of adenocarcinoma of the cervix associated with use of COC. Whether the increased risk of invasive cervical cancer (adenocarcinoma and squamous cell) associated with COC is *due to* use of COC is still an open question. From a practical perspective, however, it seems prudent to act as if it is, by assuring that recommended screening guidelines for cervical cancer are followed by women using oral contraception.

Ovary (epithelial cancer)

Figure 67.8 shows estimates of the relative risk of epithelial cancer of the ovary by duration of use of oral contraceptives. The data are from 15 case-control studies[101–112] and two cohort studies[113,84] involving a total of 3785 women with invasive disease, 937 of whom had used COC. The open circles in Figure 67.8 correspond to the case-control studies and the solid points represent the estimates of relative risk from the cohort studies.

The risk of ovarian cancer declines with increasing duration of COC use. Risk is reduced by an estimated 41% in women using COC for 4 years, and by an estimated 54% and 61% in women using COC for 8 years and 12 years, respectively (RR = 0.59, 0.46, 0.39; trend: P <0.001, one-sided). Data from five studies suggest that the reduced risk of ovarian cancer begins to appear by five years after initiating use [104,105,44,108,82] a generalization supported by the results from the two studies that specifically analyzed latency in relation to duration of use.[105,108] One study from Shanghai, China, however, reported no reduction in ovarian cancer risk in women who had used COC.[106] The result is difficult to interpret since there was a very low prevalence of COC use in the population (only 7% of women had ever used oral contraceptives) and no details were given about the formulations.[106]

All of the estimates of relative risk shown in Figure 67.8 have been adjusted for age and most have been adjusted for nulliparity as well. These comprise two of three major risk factors for ovarian cancer. A family history of the disease, which is uncommon, is not a plausible explanation for the reduced risk in COC users: widespread avoidance of COC use on the basis of a family history of ovarian cancer would have had to occur to produce a spurious reduction in risk among users. This, moreover, would not account for a dose response by duration of use unless one were prepared to accept some convoluted reasoning. Although studies of COC and cervical cancer are susceptible to bias arising from more extensive screening for cancer in users of COC, this specific concern does not apply to ovarian cancer. Thus, in light of the biologic rationale reviewed earlier in this chapter we believe that the reduced risk of epithelial ovarian cancer associated with use of COC is in fact *due to* COC. Since studies to date pertain mainly to ovarian cancer in women under age 60 years, one cannot tell whether the reduction in risk represents only a postponement of cancer occurrence or the lifetime prevention of ovarian

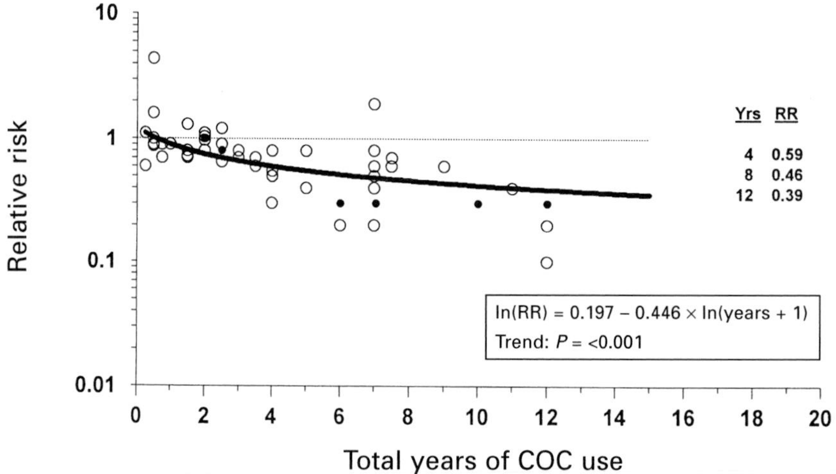

Fig. 67.8 Epithelial ovarian cancer: relative risk by duration of oral contraceptive use.

cancer in a fraction of women who would have developed the disease had they not used COC.

Discontinued use

Figure 67.9 shows that the protective effect associated with oral contraception continues unabated long after stopping use. Data from eight studies,[101,104,105,44,45,82,113,114] suggest that even 20 years after discontinuation the reduced risk of ovarian cancer in former COC users does not rise to the levels of risk observed in women who have never used COC. On the basis of the data shown in Figure 67.9, we estimate the relative risk of ovarian cancer at 5, 10 and 20 years after stopping use of COC to be 0.68, 0.65 and 0.61, respectively.

Formulation

Three studies have reported in some detail on risk in relation to formulation.[101,108,115] Most of the data relate to combination monophasic pills. Bearing in mind that analyses of specific formulations are limited by women's recall and by few women using any one preparation exclusively, the data are compatible with equal protection regardless of the type of progestogen or the amount of estrogen used. These findings are supported by earlier studies of the issue.[109,111] Limited data also suggest that progestogen-only COC is protective.[101] The risk of ovarian cancer has not yet been adequately characterized in relation either to the newer progestogens (desogestrel, gestodene, norgestimate) or to biphasic and triphasic pills. From the biologic background presented on page 838, however, we would expect that these would also protect against ovarian cancer.

Histology

The four major histologic types of epithelial tumors (serous, mucinous, endometrioid, clear cell) have been studied in limited fashion by examining their relation to 'ever use' of oral contraception.[105,108,109,111] With exception of mucinous tumors,[105,109] the risk of each subtype has been consistently reported to be reduced in women who have used COC. Since analyses did not take into account duration of use, the disparate results for mucinous tumors could be due to this factor or simply the result of chance.

Nonepithelial tumors

The limited data on nonepithelial ovarian tumors suggest that COC use may not protect against them.[106,108] A US population-based study estimated the relative risk of germ cell tumors at 1.6 (95% confidence interval: 0.5–4.7) for women who had used COC; the relative risk was 1.0 (0.2–4.0) among women whose use lasted five or more years, however.[108] That same study found the risk of sex chord-stromal tumors to be significantly reduced in women age 45–54 who had used COC (RR = 0.0, upper 95% confidence limit = 0.4), but non-significantly increased (RR = 1.4, 95% CI: 0.2–11.9) in women under age 45.[108] A second study, from Shanghai, China, reported a relative risk of 1.0 (0.3–4.3) for nonepithelial ovarian cancer in women who had used oral contraception.[106]

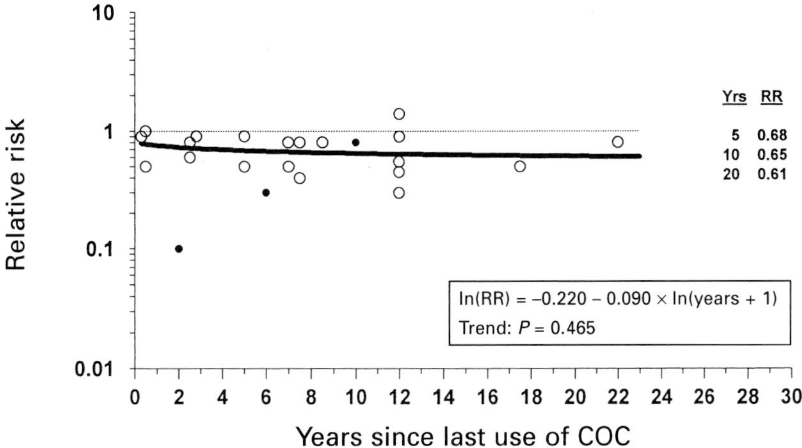

Fig. 67.9 Epithelial ovarian cancer: relative risk by time since last use of oral contraceptives.

Use of COC by women with a family history of ovarian cancer

An informed and judicious use of COC might offer the possibility of an effective means of primary prevention in women at high risk of a cancer that carries a very poor prognosis. For example, it has been estimated that 10 years of COC use by women with a positive family history of ovarian cancer might reduce their risk to a level below that for COC nonusers whose family history is negative.[116] Such a result, however, requires confirmation before it can be accepted as fact.

Corpus uteri (endometrium)

Figure 67.10 shows 33 estimates of the relative risk of endometrial cancer by duration of use of combined oral contraceptives. The results are from 11 studies involving 1660 women with invasive disease, 232 of whom had used combined COC.[117–125] All but two of the estimates were adjusted for age, and many have been further adjusted for endometrial cancer risk factors such as adiposity, parity and use of estrogen replacement therapy. There is a significant trend of decreasing risk with increasing duration of use: the risk of endometrial cancer is reduced by an estimated 56% with four years of use, by 67% with eight years of use, and by 72% with 12 years of use of combined COC (RR = 0.44, 0.33, 0.28; trend: $P < 0.0001$, one-sided).

Four other studies[113,127–129] report substantially reduced risks in relation to 'ever use' of combined COC (RRs range from 0.1 to 0.6), thereby supporting our estimates of relative risk in Figure 67.10. Two investigations,[130,131] however, did not find a protective effect of COC use, but these did not distinguish between use of combination type COC and sequential COC, the latter preparations being implicated in increasing the risk of endometrial cancer.[121,125,132]

Two studies[108,117] have estimated risk in relation to latency (time since first use), but only one explicitly took into account duration of use.[117] In view of the limited data, one cannot be precise, but the results suggest that the reduced risk of endometrial cancer occurs well within 10 years of initiating use of combined COC.[108]

In light of the consistency of findings for combination-type oral contraceptives, the duration-related effect of COC use and the biologic rationale reviewed on page 838, we believe that the reduced risk of endometrial cancer associated with combined COC is in fact *due to* its use.

Discontinued use

Figure 67.11 shows data for recency of use based on 19 estimates of relative risk from seven studies.[117,118,82,123,126] These involved 1340 women with endometrial cancer, 200 of whom had used combination-type oral contraceptives. The results suggest that after stopping COC use the risk of endometrial cancer begins to rise from its reduced levels associated with oral contraception (trend: $P = 0.01$, one-sided), although even 20 years later the risk in former users is still almost 50% below that in women who have never used oral contraception.

There is evidence to suggest that some residual protective effect from prior oral contraception will

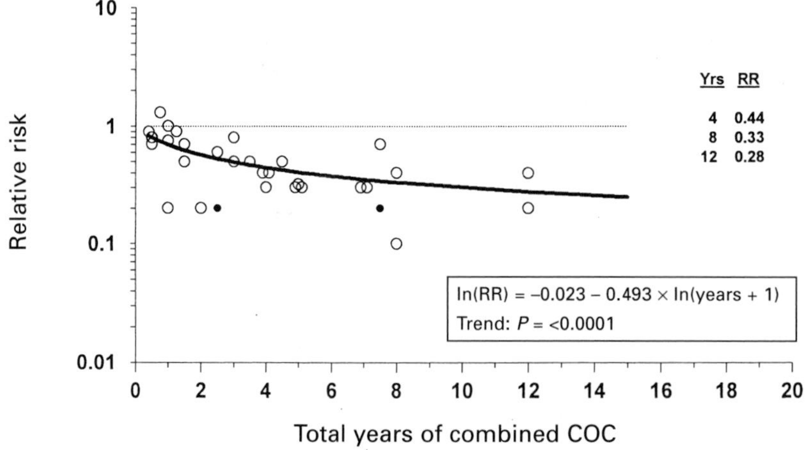

Fig. 67.10 Endometrial cancer: relative risk by duration of use of combined oral contraceptives.

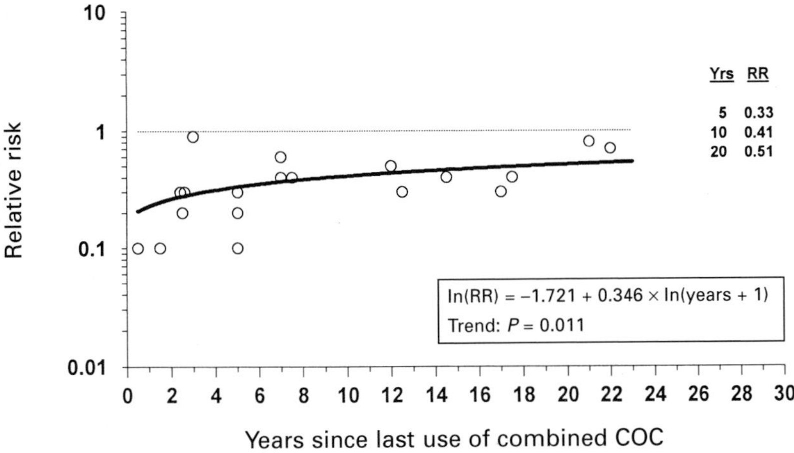

Fig. 67.11 Endometrial cancer: relative risk by time since last use of combined oral contraceptives.

continue throughout the menopause,[117] a time when the risk of endometrial cancer is greatest. In women age 55–64 years, the relative risk of invasive disease among former users of combined OC has been estimated at RR = 0.6 (95% CI: 0.3–1.1),[117] with an estimate of RR = 0.5 (95% CI: 0.1–1.7) in women age 65+. Such a result was anticipated by Key and Pike,[133] who predicted that five years of combined OC use beginning at age 28 years would produce a 60% reduction in lifetime risk. Their estimate was based on the assumption that use of combined OC suppresses endometrial mitotic activity to such an extent that five years of such use will delay the rise in the age-specific incidence rate of endometrial cancer by five years,[134] which in turn will produce lower rates of cancer at older ages.

Formulation

Two early reports examining effects of different formulations suggested on the basis of very small numbers that estrogen-predominant preparations may provide less protection against endometrial cancer.[123,125] This was not confirmed by two subsequent large studies which reported that the effect of combined OC did not differ materially among the major formulations then in use in the United States,[119] nor did the risk of endometrial cancer differ by estrogen:progestogen 'potency ratio,' defined[121] as:

$$\text{E:P} = \frac{\mu\text{g estrogen} \times \text{relative estrogen potency}}{\text{mg progestogen} \times \text{relative progestogen potency.}} \quad [3]$$

The two estrogens, mestranol and ethinyl estradiol, were assigned relative potencies of 1 and 2, and the progestogens were assigned relative potencies based on the delay of menses test.[135] Regardless of whether these assignments are correct, the risk of endometrial cancer was reduced by about 50% in women who had ever used combined OC, and the risk of early-onset (before age 45) endometrial cancer was found to decline with increasing duration of use of either high or low E:P-ratio oral contraceptives.[121]

Analyses of data from a WHO multinational study of endometrial cancer re-opened the issue.[136] Classifying the potency of progestogens on their capacity to induce subnuclear vacuolization in the human endometrium,[137,138] the investigators found that endometrial cancer risk was not reduced in women who had used high-dose estrogen:low-dose progestogen COC (RR = 1.1, 95% CI: 0.1–9.0). The risk of endometrial cancer was reduced, however, in women who had used high-dose progestogen COC, regardless of whether the estrogen dose was low (RR = 0.0, 95% CI: 0.0–1.1) or high (RR = 0.15, 95% CI: 0.0–0.5) and regardless of whether use of OC was short-term (less than two years) or longer. For women who had used COC that was low in both progestogen and estrogen, the relative risk of endometrial cancer was estimated at RR = 0.6 (95% CI: 0.3–1.3).

Since the findings from the WHO study depend critically on only 12 exposed cases, and since duration of use was not taken into account, the results are obviously in need of replication despite their appealing biologic rationale. Only partial confirmation has arisen thus far.[139] Using the same classification of progestogens, a study involving 20 exposed cases suggests that there is no reduction in endometrial cancer risk among women who use low progestogen COC short term (less than five years). Duration of use rather than progestogen potency seems to be the critical factor, because longer term use (five or more years) of both low progestogen and high progestogen COC was associated with a comparably reduced risk of endometrial cancer (RR ≈ 0.25).

Estrogen replacement therapy

The risk of endometrial cancer in postmenopausal women is increased by the administration of replacement estrogens without a cyclic opposing progestogen. The question therefore arises whether the protective effect of prior use of combined OC is diminished by estrogen replacement therapy (ERT). There is presently no consensus on the answer. Two studies[117,125] suggest that use of ERT for three or more years essentially eliminates the protective effect of prior oral contraception. Four other investigations,[118,123,124,140] however, do not lend support to this conclusion. These studies found that effect of COC use was not materially altered by whether or not ERT had been used, although only one study[140] considered the effect of duration of ERT. The remaining three studies simply examined prior COC use (duration unspecified) among women who had or had not used ERT.

Parity

Nulliparous women are at increased risk of endometrial cancer.[117,119,121] One would therefore hope that their use of combined OC would substantially diminish their risk. There are conflicting findings on this point. Data from a population-based study[119] suggest that the protective effect of COC use is indeed greatest in nulliparous women. Compared to never use, the relative risk of endometrial cancer from combined OC use of one or more years was estimated in women of parity 0, 1–2, 3–4 and 5+ at RR = 0.2, 0.3, 0.6 and 0.8 respectively. The decline in relative effectiveness of COC use with increasing parity is statistically significant, P = 0.01 (one-sided test of trend). However, since women of higher parity might have had shorter durations of use, this could have produced the result observed.

One study of early onset (before age 45) endometrial cancer implied that the effect of combined OC use was greatest in women of low parity. The study found that use of combined OC did not confer additional protection against endometrial cancer in women who had had more than three full term pregnancies.[121] Details of the results were not given, however, nor was there any mention of taking duration of use into account. Results from three other studies that considered parity-specific effects of combined OC use do not lend support to the aforementioned findings. A multinational study reported that ever-use of combined OC (compared to never use) was associated with a relative risk of endometrial cancer of 0.65 (95%, CI: 0.2–1.5) in women with four or fewer pregnancies and a relative risk of 0.3 (95%, CI: 0.1–1.5) in women with five or more pregnancies.[128] Another study reported that the corresponding relative risk was RR = 0.8 in women of parity 0 and RR = 0.3 in women of parity 1 or more.[118] Since the latter results were based on only 17 exposed cases, the difference in relative risk is compatible with chance. The one study that took duration of use into account when examining parity-specific effects of combined OC use reported that the protective effect was considerably diminished in nulliparous women:[117] compared to never users, the relative risk was 0.7 in nulliparous women who had used combined OC for less than three years and 0.9 in nulliparous women who had three or more years of such use. In women of parity 3–4, by contrast, the corresponding values of relative risk by duration of use were 0.6 and 0.3, respectively, and in women of parity 5 or more, the corresponding values of relative risk by duration of use were 0.4 and 0.3.

Body weight

Obese women are at substantially increased risk of endometrial cancer. For women whose body weight exceeds 200 pounds, endometrial cancer risk has been estimated to be approximately seven-fold[117] to nine-fold[121] higher than the risk for women whose body weight is 150 pounds or less. The risk for women whose body mass index (BMI) exceeds 27.4 kg/m^2 has been estimated to be about three-fold higher than the risk for women with a BMI lower than 22.5 kg/m^2.[114] Thus, one would like to know whether body weight has an influence on the protective effect of oral contraception.

There are discrepant results on this point. The first study to examine the issue reported that use of combined OC did not reduce the risk of early-occurring endometrial cancer in women whose body weight was 170 pounds or more.[121] For such women, even relatively long-term use (6+ years) was not associated with any reduction in risk. For women weighing less than 170 pounds, however, risk of endometrial cancer declined progressively with increasing duration of use of combined OC: RR = 0.6 (<2 yrs OC use), 0.7 (2–3 yrs), 0.2 (4–5 yrs) and 0.2 (6+ yrs); $P < 0.001$, one-sided test of trend. These findings were explained by hypothesizing that the amount of progestogen was insufficient to inhibit endometrial proliferation in obese women.[121] Although the explanation is attractive, three subsequent studies have not provided support for what remains an intriguing hypothesis. All three studies found that use of combined OC reduces the risk of endometrial cancer, regardless of women's adiposity.[117,118,119]

Histologic subtypes

Two studies[119,128] report details on histologic subtypes of endometrial cancer: adenocarcinoma, adenocanthoma and adenosquamous cancer. Both studies indicate that women who have used combined OC have reduced risks of similar magnitude for each histologic subtype.

Uterine sarcomas

Uterine sarcomas, which comprise about 3–5% of uterine malignancies in the United States,[16] have not been studied extensively in relation to oral contraceptive use. One investigation, however, suggests that women who have used COC may be at increased risk of leiomyosarcoma.[141] Based on a small number of cases ($n = 56$), the relative risk of this cancer was estimated at 1.7 (95%, CI: 0.7–4.1) in women who had used combination type COC. There was no clear relationship to duration use, and risk was not increased until at least 10 years after discontinuation. There was no mention of OC use affecting the risk of either mixed mullerian tumors ($n = 85$) or endometrial stromal sarcomas ($n = 26$). Thus, coincidence cannot be ruled out as a plausible explanation for the finding with respect to leiomyosarcoma.

Net effect of OC use on gynecologic cancers

To place the estimates of relative risk shown in Figures 67.6–67.11 in perspective of absolute risk, we estimated the cumulative incidence of invasive cancer of the cervix, ovary and uterus by duration of COC use and recency of use. This was based on our estimates of the age-specific incidence rate of each cancer in women using COC (I_{oc}) calculated as a function of women's age, duration of COC use and recency of use by means of equation [4] below.

$$I_{oc} = I_{age} \times RR_{dur} \times RR_{rec} \qquad [4]$$

For each cancer site, I_{age} denotes the age-specific rates of invasive cancer in nonusers of COC. The values were assumed to equal the incidence rates reported for the time period 1981–85 in either US white females or Japanese females in Osaka.[20]

Table 67.5 shows the results of calculating cumulative incidence by standard life-table methods[22] applied to the values of I_{oc} under the assumption that any duration-related effect of COC use appears immediately, that is, there is no latent effect, and that COC use begins at age 20 and continues without interruption for either 4, 8 or 12 years. For example, the first row of Table 67.5 estimates total number of women developing invasive cancer of the uterine cervix, ovary and uterine corpus from age 20–54 years in a cohort of 100 000 US white women who never use COC. Among 100 000 such women, 405 are estimated to develop invasive cancer of the uterine cervix over 35 years, 405 invasive ovarian cancer and 448 invasive cancer of the uterine corpus.

Rows 2–4 of Table 67.5 estimate the number of additional or fewer cancer cases in a cohort of 100 000 users of combination type OC. Thus, among 100 000 US white women who use COC for four years beginning at age 20, an *additional* 107 cases of invasive

Table 67.5 Cumulative incidence of cancer from age 20–54 in 100 000 women who never use COCs, and estimated number of added/fewer cases per 100 000 women using COCs for 4, 8 or 12 years.

	American Women (whites)		
OC use	Cervix	Ovary	Uterus
	Total cases		
Never	405	405	448
	Added/fewer cases		
4 years	107	–174	–165
8 years	176	–216	–206
12 years	219	–242	–234

	Japanese Women (Osaka)		
OC use	Cervix	Ovary	Uterus
	Total cases		
Never	542	219	136
	Added/fewer cases		
4 years	141	– 93	–50
8 years	233	–115	–63
12 years	296	–129	–71

cervical cancer are estimated to occur from age 20–54 years. The total number developing cervical cancer is estimated to be 512 (= 405 + 107). For women using COC for eight years or 12 years, the additional number of invasive cervical cancers among 100 000 users is 176 and 219, respectively. Taking ovarian cancer as a second example, a cohort of 100 000 US white women using COC for four years is estimated to incur 174 fewer cases from age 20–54, the total number of such cancers being estimated at 231 (= 405 – 174). The lower panel of Table 67.5 applies the preceding analysis to Japanese women in Osaka.

The results in Table 67.5 suggest that COC use prevents a proportionately large number of ovarian and uterine cancers and causes a proportionately large number of invasive cervical cancers. The absolute numbers are small, however. Thus, from a population perspective there are only small gynecologic cancer related risks and benefits associated with oral contraceptive use. On balance, the net effect is negligible, a conclusion that applies even when breast cancer is included in the analysis.[84]

Obviously, our analysis should not be applied uncritically in deciding whether or not an individual should use COC because other medical and personal considerations must weigh in the decision.[142,143] Furthermore, while many would agree that the reduced risks of ovarian and endometrial cancer associated with use of COC represent cause–effect, a consensus has yet to emerge about cervical cancer. Finally, none of the results is an 'individualized' estimate of risk that takes account of important personal characteristics such as a family history of early-onset cancer.

Other issues

Tumor stage and histologic grade

Tumor stage at diagnosis and histologic grade of invasive gynecologic cancers have not been studied systematically in relation to use of COC. Stage at diagnosis, which depends on tumor size, the presence or absence of nodal involvement and metastases can be affected by numerous extraneous factors. Among these are patients' decisions to seek or avoid medical attention when symptoms appear, the availability of medical and preventive care, the promotion and use of cancer screening and the sensitivity of diagnostic procedures.[144] Thus, tumor stage *per se* is not an intrinsic characteristic of cancer that use of COC can either cause or prevent, although in principle the use of COC could either mask or help reveal signs or symptoms of cancer, which in turn might affect tumor detection and therefore stage at diagnosis.

Survival after cancer diagnosis

Survival after the development of cancer depends heavily on tumor stage at diagnosis and the effectiveness of treatment(s) used. Since one cannot distinguish between tumors 'caused by' use of COC and those arising from other sources, one cannot compare survival on the basis of cancer cause. One can, however, compare survival after cancer diagnosis in patients who have and have not used COC. To our knowledge this has not been done for gynecologic cancers. However, in view of the results of studies concerning survival after the diagnosis of breast cancer, which indicate that COC users are at no greater risk of early death compared to nonusers,[145,146] we expect that little if any difference in survival would be found for gynecologic cancer.

Total mortality and morbidity

Oral contraception obviously has a very favorable health-benefit:risk ratio, otherwise COC would not be approved for use by drug regulatory authorities throughout the world. Recent studies have shown no significant evidence of any adverse effect of COC use on overall mortality.[147,148] Several attempts have been made to quantitate other health effects of COC use and place them in perspective of the health consequences of other contraceptive methods.[149–152] Much work remains to be done to achieve a comprehensive assessment that has clinical utility and can truly help patients make an informed choice when confronted with a wide range of contraceptive options.

Injectables

As of 1995, 12 million couples throughout the world were using injectable contraceptives. The majority contained only a progestogen, either depot-medroxy-progesterone acetate (DMPA), which is injected every three months, or norethisterone enanthate (NE), which is injected monthly.[153] There have been relatively few studies of gynecologic cancer risk in relation to use of these compounds.

Uterine cervix (squamous cell cancer)

Three case-control studies of invasive cervical cancer[154,155,156] suggest that its risk is not materially affected by the use of injectable contraceptives. One study from Costa Rica[154] estimated the relative risk at 1.4 (95% CI: 0.6–3.1) in women who had ever used DMPA. Use by most women was for less than one year, there was no indication of an increased risk with longer term use and the effect of chance or detection bias could not be ruled out as plausible explanations for the finding. A second study from Latin America reported a reduced risk of invasive cervical cancer associated with use of injectables for less than five years (RR = 0.5; 95% CI: 0.3–0.9) but an increased risk (RR = 2.4; 95% CI: 1.0–5.7) with longer term use.[155] Based on the reported frequency of injection, DMPA and NE were thought to comprise 45% and 55%, respectively, of the injectables used by women in this study. The relative risk of invasive cervical cancer was said to be particularly high in a subgroup of women who had long term use (≥ 5 years) and infrequent Pap smears (RR = 6.3, 95% CI: 2.1–18.7). There were only 11 cases who had used injectables for five years or more, however, and the biologically implausible findings with regard to duration of use made the authors advise caution about over interpreting the study's findings.

The largest study to date, a WHO multinational investigation involving 2009 women with invasive squamous cell cancer of the cervix and 9583 controls,[156] estimated the relative risk of invasive squamous cell cancer of the cervix at 1.1 (95% CI: 1.0–1.3) in women who had used DMPA. There were no trends in risk by duration of use or by time since initial or last use, nor was there evidence of an increased risk of cervical cancer even if DMPA had been used in excess of 10 years. The results of this study provide evidence against an adverse effect of DMPA on cervical cancer.

Ovary (epithelial cancer)

The one internally-controlled study of ovarian cancer incidence in relation to use of injectable contraceptives found no evidence of either a beneficial or adverse effect from use of DMPA.[157] Since depot-medroxy-progesterone acetate and oral contraceptives both suppress ovulation and reduce secretion of pituitary gonadotropins, the study's *a priori* hypothesis was that use of DMPA, like use of COC, would reduce the risk of epithelial ovarian cancer. For women who had used DMPA, their relative risk compared to never use was estimated at 1.1 (95% CI: 0.6–1.8). There was no evidence of a trend of either increasing or decreasing risk by duration of use, time since first use, recency of use or age at first use. Study bias was thought to be an unlikely explanation for the findings, but no alternative explanation apart from chance was apparent.

Corpus uteri (endometrium)

Only one internally-controlled study of endometrial cancer incidence in relation to use of injectable contraceptives has been reported to date.[158] Based on 122 histologically confirmed cases and 939 controls from Bangkok and Chiang Mai, Thailand, the relative risk for women who had used DMPA compared to never use was estimated at 0.2 (95% CI: 0.1–0.8). Although based on small numbers, the protective effect of DMPA appeared to continue after cessation of use, the relative risk being estimated at 0.2 (95% CI: 0.1–1.2) for women whose use had ceased at least eight years. Risk in relation to duration of use, recency of use, and time since first use could not be precisely estimated, however.

Implants

At the time of writing, gynecologic cancer risk has yet to be evaluated in relation to use of contraceptive implants containing progestogens such as levonorgestrel, 3-keto desogestrel and norethindrone.

ESTIMATED EFFECT OF HORMONE REPLACEMENT THERAPY

Estrogenic compounds first became available for the treatment of menopausal symptoms during the late 1930s. Shortly afterward there were calls for caution to prevent continuous stimulation of the endometrium.[159] Although most studies in the 1950s and 1960s found only small increased risks of endometrial cancer in women using estrogen,[160,161] the possibility of a significant increase in risk with estrogen use was suggested by others.[162] Unfortunately, since 1975 this latter possibility has been confirmed by numerous epidemiologic studies which have consistently found materially higher risks of endometrial cancer.[163–166]

Patterns of hormone replacement therapy have altered in response to physicians' perceptions of the attendant risks and benefits. In the United States, total prescriptions, mainly for unopposed estrogen, declined from 28 million per annum in 1975 to 14 million in 1980.[167] Use of estrogens and progestogens has returned to pre-1975 levels since 1980. Surveys indicate, however, that only one quarter of the HRT prescriptions include a progestogen.[168,170] For example, 32% of surveyed respondents in a California community were taking HRT in 1986–87, 81% of whom were using estrogen alone; only 19% of users took estrogen and a progestogen.[170] The proportion taking progestogen was only marginally higher in 1992.[168] Of course, some women who do not take a progestogen have had a hysterectomy and do not need endometrial protection. As shown in Figure 67.2, however, only 23–33% of postmenopausal US women have had a hysterectomy. Therefore, a substantial proportion of women are at risk for endometrial conditions that may arise as a consequence of using unopposed estrogen. Endometrial cancer thus continues to be a pertinent issue more than 20 years after the first of several major studies clearly established its association with estrogen use.

The HRT-associated conditions that are covered in this section include endometrial hyperplasia and endometrial cancer. A possible association between HRT use and epithelial ovarian cancer has been addressed by several studies, and the results of these will also be summarized.

Endometrial hyperplasia

The term endometrial hyperplasia (EH) identifies morphologic alterations of the endometrial glands and stroma ranging from a simple exaggerated physiologic response to carcinoma *in situ*.[171,172] EH is currently classified as simple, or complex with or without atypia.[173] Lesions in the complex category display alterations in the architecture of the glands: crowded glands, with irregular outlines and little stroma remaining between the glands. Atypical lesions manifest cellular changes such as nuclear enlargement, irregularities of shape and prominent nucleoli.[171]

Atypical lesions are more likely to progress to endometrial cancer. For example, among 170 women with endometrial hyperplasia, progression to cancer occurred in 1% (1/93) with simple EH, 3% (1/29) with complex EH, 8% (1/13) with simple atypical EH and 29% (10/35) with complex atypical EH.[173] Regression of endometrial hyperplasia is also a common outcome with long-term follow-up: the lesion regressed in 56 patients (33%), including 15 with atypia, who received no treatment.[173]

Hormone replacement therapy with unopposed estrogen is associated with a high risk of EH, which can be minimized by the addition of cyclic or continuous progestogen.[174] In a one year study that included 1385 patients with endometrial biopsies, EH developed in 20% of women using unopposed estrogen (conjugated estrogens, 0.625 mg daily) and in only 0.3% of women who received progestogen in one of four dose and administration protocols.[175] Endometrial cancer was found in a post-study biopsy in one patient using unopposed estrogen and in one patient in the high-dose progestogen treatment group. In the postmenopausal estrogen/progestogen interventions (PEPI) trial, 62% of women on unopposed estrogen developed EH during three years of follow-up, compared with 4% using progestogen and 2% on placebo.[176] In patients using unopposed estrogen, 14 (11.8%) developed atypical EH. The only adenocarcinoma in the study occurred in a woman taking placebo.

Accepting that endometrial hyperplasia and endometrial cancer may arise independently of steroid hormone treatment, and that the majority of the EH lesions may regress when unopposed estrogen is withdrawn, it is nevertheless prudent to make use of treatment protocols that will reduce the risk of developing EH. The key preventive element appears to be a sufficient duration of progestogen exposure rather than a higher dose.[174,177] In the two studies cited above, progestogens were administered for 14 days and 12 days, respectively.[175,176]

Endometrial cancer

Endometrial cancer arises within the glandular epithelium of the endometrium. It is the most common gynecologic malignancy, primarily found in women in the postmenopausal years. The peak incidence is in the late 50s and early 60s (see Figs 67.1 and 67.3). The endometrioid type of endometrial cancer develops in an estrogenic setting, and is frequently found in the presence of endometrial hyperplasia.[178] Serous or papillary serous varieties appear to occur more often in older women who have not received estrogens.

The evidence for an association with hormone replacement therapy is based mainly on studies in which unopposed estrogen, which is usually in the form of conjugated estrogens in North America, was the dominant therapy. The association with 'ever use' is addressed first in our discussion.

Ever use

Figure 67.12 shows estimates of endometrial cancer risk associated with ever use of HRT in 29 case-control studies and seven cohort studies:[150,160,161,163–165,166,178–207]. There were 7749 cases of endometrial cancer, 2442 of whom (32%) had used unopposed estrogen for HRT. On average, risk was increased 2.7-fold (95% CI: 2.5–2.9) in the case-control studies, 2.7-fold (2.3–3.3) in the cohort studies, and 2.7-fold (2.5–2.9) if all of the estimates are taken into account. Although characterizing use of HRT by ever or never use is of limited clinical value and potentially inaccurate, the funnel plot in Figure 67.12 shows that ever use is uniformly associated with increased risk, regardless of study design and study size.[208]

Duration of use

Figure 67.13 shows 95 estimates of the risk of endometrial cancer by duration of hormone replacement therapy using unopposed estrogen. The data are from 25 case-control studies and six cohort studies.[150,163–166,179,180,184,185,188–190,193–197,199–202,204–207,209–214]

Most of the estimates were adjusted for age, and many were also adjusted for obesity, diabetes, smoking and other possibly confounding variables. There is a significant trend of increasing risk with increasing duration of use. The estimated relative risk is 1.7 at one year of use, 3.6 at four years, 5.8 at eight years and 7.7 at 12 years (trend: $P < 0.001$). The increased risk with longer duration of use has been reported in at least three other reviews.[215–217]

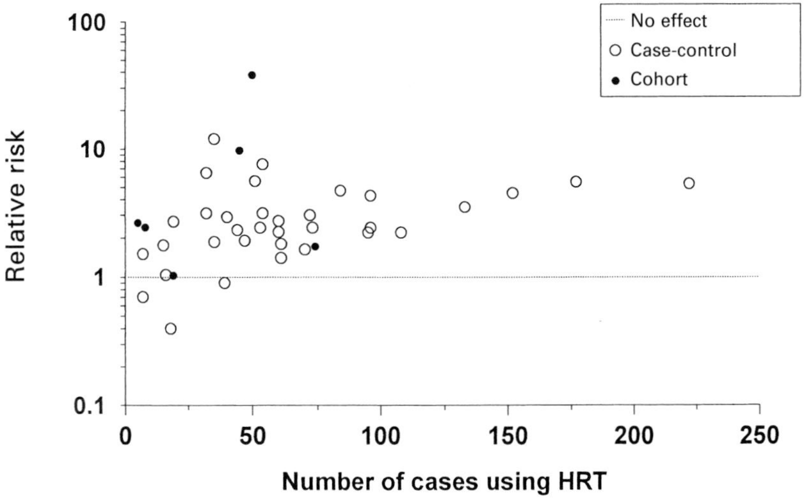

Fig. 67.12 Relative risk of endometrial cancer associated with ever use of HRT, by study size and design.

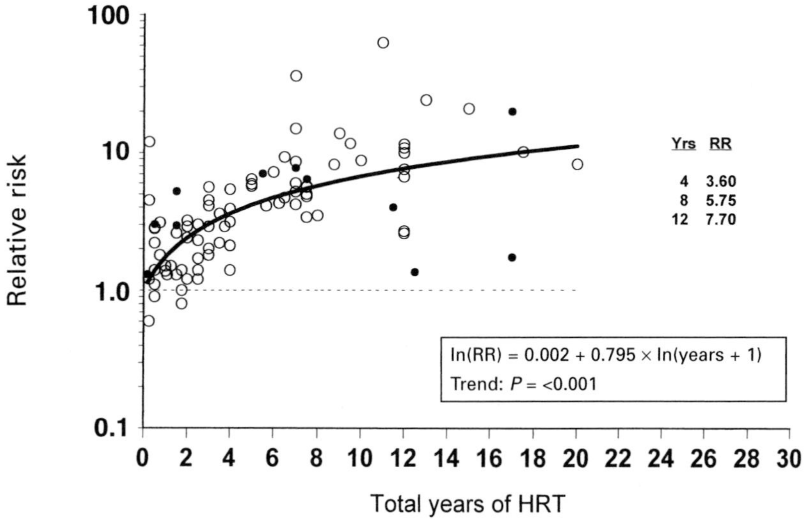

Fig. 67.13 Relative risk of endometrial cancer by total years of estrogen use.

Discontinued use

Figure 67.14 shows 35 estimates of endometrial cancer risk after discontinuing HRT consisting of unopposed estrogen. The estimates are drawn from 11 case-control studies and one cohort study[150,179,185,189,190,196,198,201,202,204,206,209] There appears to be a residual risk long after use is stopped. The estimated relative risk is 3.7 at one year after discontinuation; 10 years after stopping HRT, the risk of endometrial cancer is estimated to remain 2.2 times higher than the risk in nonusers.

Estrogen type and dose

Conjugated estrogen is the most frequently prescribed form of HRT in North America. Eleven studies reported estimates of endometrial cancer risk for users of conjugated estrogens compared with the risk in users of other types of estrogen.[165,166,184,186,189,194,196,199,202,204,218] Compared to nonuse, the adjusted relative risk of endometrial cancer is 2.6 for HRT consisting of other estrogens (95% CI: 2.0–3.4) and 3.0 (2.5–3.7) for HRT consisting of conjugated estrogen, a difference which is not significant ($P = 0.65$).

Fifteen studies reported estimates of endometrial cancer risk according to estrogen dose.[150,165,166,179,184,185,188–190,196,198,202,205,206,211] There is a trend of increasing risk with higher dose: the estimated relative risk is 2.5 for less than 0.625 mg, 3.6 for 0.625 mg and 5.0 for more than 0.625 mg (trend: $P = 0.035$).

Use of progestogens

Because use of progestogens is relatively recent and applies only to a minority of HRT users in North America, there are few published estimates of endometrial cancer risk associated with combined estrogen-progestogen therapy. Four studies, however, have reported adjusted estimates of relative risk associated with ever use of combined therapy (duration unspecified).[186,189,207,209] From this we derive an overall estimate of relative risk of 1.3 (95% CI: 0.9–2.0), a result compatible with only a small to moderate effect. There were insufficient data to confirm whether risk is diminished in proportion to the number of days in which progestogen is used in each cycle. There were also insufficient data to reliably estimate the risk of endometrial cancer by duration of use of combined HRT. Thus, although the data summarized here are sparse, they do suggest that use of progestogens lessens the adverse effect of unopposed estrogen on the risk of endometrial cancer.

Endometrial cancer prognosis

Estrogen use is associated with favorable tumor characteristics at diagnosis, including earlier clinical stage, decreased frequency of myometrial invasion and lower histologic grade.[166,188,190,197,202]

Eight studies reported estimates of endometrial cancer risk among estrogen users according to clinical stage at the time of diagnosis.[165,166,188,190,194,197,199,219] We estimate that estrogen use is associated with a

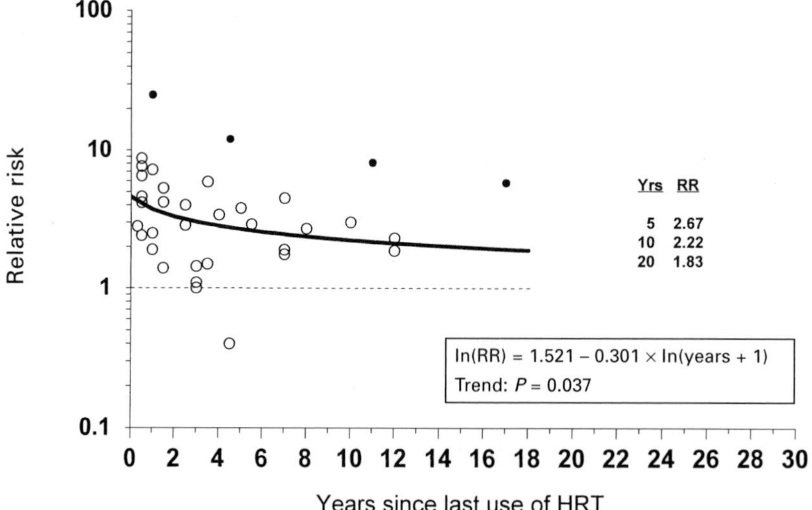

Fig. 67.14 Relative risk of endometrial cancer by time since last use of estrogens.

relative risk of 3.1 (95% CI: 2.3–4.1) for stage I disease, compared with a relative risk of 2.3 (1.7–3.1) for more advanced stages.

Seven studies reported estimates of endometrial cancer risk for estrogen users according to myometrial invasion.[166,179,188,190,197,202,219] Since the degree of invasion was not reported uniformly, and different methods exist for measurement,[178] we classified no myometrial invasion, superficial myometrial invasion and penetration of less than one-third depth or one-half depth under the heading of 'minimal invasion'. Our resulting estimate of the relative risk of minimal invasion associated with estrogen use is 5.9 (95% CI: 4.0–8.7) compared with a relative risk of 3.6 (2.0–6.6) for deeper degrees of myometrial invasion.

Nine studies reported estimates of endometrial cancer risk for estrogen users according to the histologic grade of the tumor.[165,166,188,190,194,197,199,202,219] Grade 1 tumors are well-differentiated and generally are associated with a good prognosis.[178] There is a significant trend of decreasing risk with increasing histologic grade: RR = 5.2, 3.9, 2.9 and 2.2 for grade 1, 2, 3 and 4 (trend: $P = 0.011$). Thus, it appears that the elevated risk of endometrial cancer which arises from estrogen use declines by approximately 25% for each higher level of histologic grade.

Clinical stage, myometrial invasion and histologic grade of endometrial cancer are all correlated with tendency to metastasize and with survival. Of these measurements, the most reproducible is histologic grade.[178] Estrogen use is significantly associated with well differentiated tumors at the time of diagnosis, a category associated with superior prognosis.

Better prognosis for estrogen users compared with nonusers is also supported by the results of follow-up of patients with endometrial cancer. Five studies involving 2198 cancer patients, 805 of whom (37%) were estrogen users, reported superior survival rates among estrogen users compared with nonusers.[185,197,220–222] In one study, the 10-year mortality of endometrial cancer patients who had been estrogen users was indistinguishable from the mortality in the female population of comparable age.[221]

The preceding studies address an important public health issue, but a pertinent question remains for women contemplating use of estrogen replacement therapy: given that the incidence of endometrial cancer is increased among users of HRT, is the risk of death from endometrial cancer also increased? Five epidemiologic studies involving 22 endometrial cancer deaths, 17 of which (77%) were among users of HRT, provide data on this question.[185,187,210,212,213] On average, the risk of endometrial cancer death is estimated to be 2.1-fold higher (95% CI: 0.8–5.9) among ever users. Overall mortality from endometrial cancer is relatively low, however, and none of the studies reports on the use of estrogen with progestogen. Therefore, there are insufficient data to determine whether use of an opposing progestogen reduces endometrial cancer mortality below that in women using unopposed estrogen.

Interpretation of the endometrial cancer HRT association

The findings of increased endometrial cancer risk with use of HRT are consistent among the reported studies, and the known sources of bias and confounding have been taken into account. The increasing risk with increasing duration of use, the trend to increased risk with higher dosage, the residual increased risk from prior use of HRT and the biologic rationale reviewed on earlier, indicate that the increased risk of endometrial cancer associated with use of HRT is in fact *due to* use of HRT.

The increased risk that appears shortly after initial use of HRT suggests there is no latent period, and the partial decline after discontinuation suggests that a residual effect remains. This would be consistent with a dual effect of estrogenic hormones on endometrial cancer risk: a short term effect, possibly related to enhancement of the growth of existing preclinical cancers, and a long-term effect, possibly related to the promotion of initiated cells that would not otherwise have had the potential to develop into cancers.

Thus, for HRT users the risk of endometrial cancer appears to consist of three components: a baseline risk, a risk due to hormonal enhancement of the growth of preclinical cancers and an added risk due to promotion. Progesterone appears to ameliorate the estrogen-related components of the HRT risk.

Epithelial ovarian cancer

Epithelial ovarian cancer shares certain reproductive and hormonal risk factors with endometrial cancer: the tumor is less common in parous women and in those who have used oral contraceptives or had an early menopause.[223–225] Thus, a potential association with HRT therapy was considered to be worthy of study. The issue is important because HRT is a common treatment among postmenopausal women, and ovarian cancer is associated with high mortality rates in this age group. There are, however, only a few controlled studies of hormone replacement therapy in relation to ovarian cancer.

Ever use of HRT

Figure 67.15 shows ten estimates of the relative risk of invasive epithelial ovarian cancer associated with ever use of HRT. The results are based on 2486 women with ovarian cancer, 396 of whom (16%) had used HRT.[223-232] On average the risk of invasive cancer is estimated to be only 10% higher in ever users (RR = 1.1, 95% CI: 1.0–1.3).

Duration of HRT use

The risk of ovarian cancer appears to increase very slightly with increasing duration of HRT use (Fig. 67.16). Based on data from five studies,[224,226,227,228,230] we estimate the relative risk of ovarian cancer at 1.19, 1.28 and 1.34 in women using HRT for 4, 8 and 12 years, respectively. The trend is not significant statistically (trend: $P = 0.205$).

Discontinued use

Two studies[228,230] have attempted to answer the question whether the small increased risk of ovarian cancer associated with use of HRT persists after discontinuation. Relative risk has been estimated at 1.4 (95% CI: 0.8–2.4) and 1.1 (95% CI: 0.8–1.6) 10 or more years after stopping HRT.

Interpretation

Ovarian cancer incidence is higher among well-educated women and those in the highest social class.[223] These women are also most able to pay for HRT, possibly giving rise in part to its small observed association with ovarian cancer. Of the estimates shown in Figure 67.16, one was adjusted for social class[223] and two were adjusted for education.[228,230] The average relative risk estimated from the studies which adjusted for socio-economic factors is 1.3 (95% CI: 1.1–1.5), a result which indicates that socio-economic status is unlikely to account for the observed association.

Use of HRT could also be linked to epithelial ovarian cancer through an association with the histologic subtype of endometrioid lesions. Such an association would be plausible if endometrioid ovarian cancer, which is similar in appearance to endometrioid tumors of the uterus, responded to estrogen in a parallel manner. A higher proportion of estrogen users has been reported among women with endometrioid and clear cell cancers as compared to women with serous or mucinous cancers.[224] The difference was not significant, however, and the data were not given. Other studies report contradictory estimates of the HRT-associated risk of endometrioid cancer: one estimate,[226] based on 18 HRT-exposed cases, suggests a reduced risk (RR = 0.5, 95% CI: 0.3–1.0) and

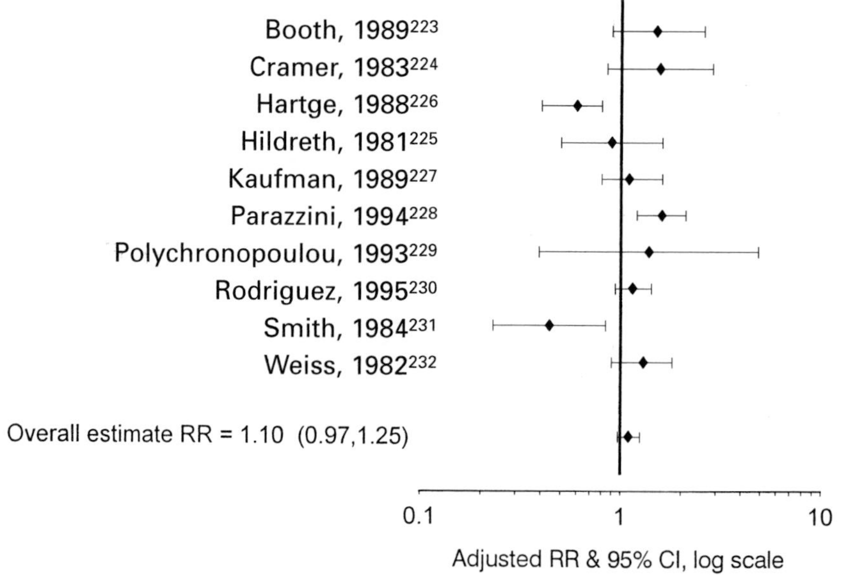

Fig. 67.15 HRT-associated risk of invasive epithelial ovarian cancer. (Homogeneity chi square = 25.7, $P = 0.002$ (9 df))

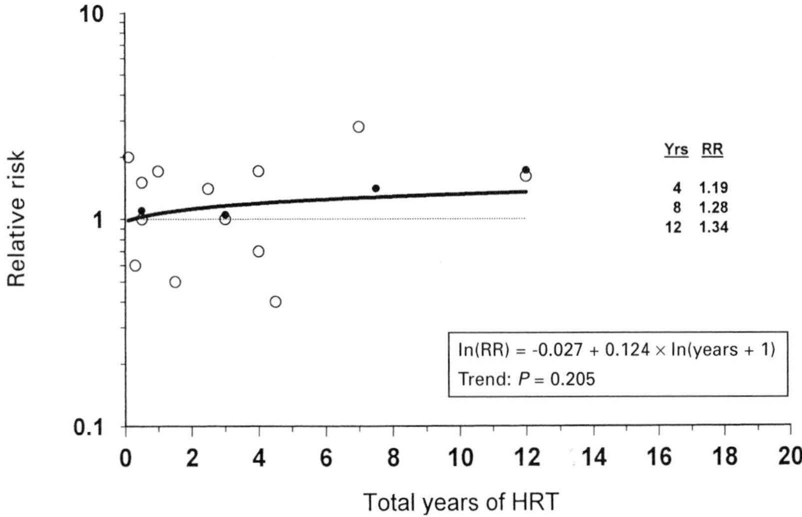

Fig. 67.16 Relative risk of epithelial ovarian cancer by total years of estrogen use.

another, involving 12 exposed cases, suggests an increased risk (RR = 3.1, 95% CI: 1.0–9.8).[232] On the basis of available publications, insufficient evidence exists to confirm or refute any distinct link between HRT use and endometrioid cancers of the ovary.

Comment

Studies of HRT use in relation to epithelial ovarian cancer are limited by what appears to be an association of small magnitude, if in truth an association exists at all. A further limitation is the relative paucity of data from controlled studies, which to date comprise only 396 HRT-exposed ovarian cancer cases; this contrasts with 2442 HRT-exposed cases in the studies of HRT use and endometrial cancer.

Given the serious nature of ovarian cancer and the frequency of HRT use among postmenopausal women, the possibility of an association between the two is a legitimate concern and warrants further study. Nonetheless, the results of epidemiologic studies at this time do not suggest that epithelial ovarian cancer should be listed among the risks associated with use of HRT.

Net effect of HRT use on gynecologic cancers

To place our estimates of relative risk shown in Figures 67.13 and 67.14 in perspective of absolute risk, we estimated the cumulative incidence of endometrial cancer by duration and recency of HRT use. The analysis was carried out solely for endometrial cancer because of the uncertainties associated with the results of studies of HRT and ovarian cancer. The calculation was based on our estimates of the age-specific incidence rate of endometrial cancer in women using HRT (I_{HRT}) calculated as a function of women's age, duration of HRT use and recency of use by means of equation[5] below.

$$I_{HRT} = I_{age} \times RR_{dur} \times RR_{rec} \quad [5]$$

For each cancer site, I_{age} denotes the age-specific rates of invasive cancer of the uterine corpus (+ NOS) in *nonusers* of HRT. The values were assumed to equal the population incidence rates reported for the time period 1981–85 in either US white females or Japanese females in Osaka.[20] We did not attempt to estimate the incidence rate of endometrial cancer specifically, because cancer rates are changing with time and enough assumptions are already involved in the analysis to make the estimates subject to some uncertainty.

Table 67.6 shows the results of calculating cumulative incidence by standard life-table methods[22] applied to the values of I_{HRT}, which were estimated under the assumptions that:

1. Any duration-related effect of HRT use appears immediately, that is, there is no latent effect
2. HRT use begins at age 50 and continues without interruption for either four, eight or 12 years
3. Women have an intact uterus.

For example, the first column in the upper panel of Table 67.6 shows estimates of the total number of US white women developing invasive cancer of the uterine

Table 67.6 Estimated cumulative number of cancer cases (uterine corpus + NOS) by age 75 and 80 years in 100 000 women, by duration of HRT.

	Use of HRT (years)			
	0	4	8	12
USA: white women				
Age 75	2219	5017	7710	9847
Age 80	2712	5973	9068	10557
Japan: Osaka				
Age 75	410	954	1458	1816
Age 80	483	1099	1669	1928

corpus from age 50 up to age 75 years or 80 years in a cohort of 100 000 women who never use HRT. Among 100 000 such women, 2219 are estimated to develop invasive cancer of the uterine corpus up to the end of their 74th year and 2712 up to the end of their 79th year.

Columns 2–4 of Table 67.6 estimate the number of cancer cases in a cohort of 100 000 users of HRT. Thus in column 2, among 100 000 US white women who use HRT for four years beginning at age 50, a total of 5017 cases, or an *additional* 2798 cases of invasive cancer of the uterine corpus, are estimated to occur from age 50 to 75 years. For women using HRT for eight years or 12 years, the additional number of invasive cancers among 100 000 users is 5491 and 7628, respectively. Taking follow-up to age 80 as another example, a cohort of 100 000 US white women using HRT for 12 years is estimated to incur 10 557 cancers, or 7845 additional cases from age 50 to age 80. The lower panel of Table 67.6 applies the preceding analysis to Japanese women in Osaka.

Table 67.6 indicates that use of unopposed estrogens can lead to a large number of uterine cancers. While the consequences of oral contraceptive use on gynecologic malignancies are small in terms of absolute numbers of women affected, this is not true for use of unopposed estrogen replacement therapy, for which a high multiple of risk applies to a relatively high cancer incidence rate. The potential number of incident cases in HRT users is of concern, particularly if one considers that two-thirds of the 26% of postmenopausal women using unopposed estrogen have a uterus and are at risk.[170] It matters very little that there may be no surplus mortality associated with endometrial cancer for HRT users. The diagnosis of cancer leads to significant morbidity and cost, not to speak of attendant anxiety.

HRT use offers symptomatic relief and potentially is associated with important benefits, including a reduced likelihood of osteoporotic fractures and myocardial infarction.[233–235] Although the cardiovascular benefits may be attenuated by the use of progestogen,[236] this has to be viewed in context of a substantial risk of endometrial cancer in the absence of progestogen. The estimates shown in Table 67.6 indicate that 10% of a cohort of American women who use unopposed estrogen for 12 years would develop endometrial cancer before reaching 80 years of age. The baseline risk is much lower among Japanese women, and the corresponding number would be less than 2%. From a North American perspective, the cardiovascular benefits of unopposed estrogen versus the combination with progestogen would have to be very well-proven to warrant a policy of prescribing unopposed estrogen for a long period of time.

SUMMARY AND CONCLUSIONS

Oral contraceptives

Oral contraception with products containing both estrogen and progestogen is associated with a reduced risk of endometrial cancer, a reduced risk of ovarian epithelial cancer and an increased risk of invasive squamous cell cancer of the uterine cervix. In all three instances the magnitude of the effect depends on duration of COC use, not on formulation. There appears to be a residual effect of reduced or increased risk for each of these three target organs long after use of COC is discontinued.

If one estimates the cumulative number of gynecologic cancers arising from age 20–54 years in four cohorts of women, COC never users and COC users of four, eight or 12 years duration, one finds that COC use prevents a proportionately large number of ovarian and uterine cancers and 'causes' a proportionately large number of invasive cervical cancers. The absolute numbers are small, however, so that from a population perspective there are only small gynecologic-cancer related risks and benefits associated with oral contraceptive use, and on balance the net effect is negligible.

Hormone replacement therapy

Hormone replacement therapy offers relief of menopausal symptoms and is potentially associated with other important benefits, including a reduced likelihood of osteoporotic fractures and myocardial infarction. Use of unopposed estrogens (ERT), however, is associated with a high risk of endometrial hyperplasia. This risk is minimized by the addition of cyclic or continuous progestogen, the key preventive element of which appears to be a sufficient duration of progestogen exposure rather than a high dose.

There is a significant trend of increasing risk of endometrial cancer associated with increasing duration of use of unopposed estrogens. There is also a trend of increasing risk with higher dosage preparations. The elevated risk among users of ERT appears to remain long after discontinuation.

We estimate that the risk of endometrial cancer in users of ERT is increased, compared to the risk in never users, 1.7-fold with one year of use, 3.6-fold with four years of use, 5.8-fold with eight years of use, and 7.7-fold with 12 years' use of ERT. If cancer occurs, use of unopposed estrogens is associated with favorable tumor characteristics at diagnosis and better survival. Nevertheless, a diagnosis of cancer leads to significant morbidity and cost, not to speak of attendant anxiety.

Presently only limited data are available to establish that use of progestogens materially lessens the adverse effect of unopposed estrogens on the overall risk of endometrial cancer. There are few controlled studies investigating what effect HRT might have on the risk of ovarian epithelial cancer. The results presently available, however, suggest that use of HRT does not have any adverse effect in this regard.

REFERENCES

1. Hertz R 1977 Evaluation of current information concerning the relationship between hormonal usage and cancer. Clinics in Obstetrics and Gynecology 20: 165–175
2. IARC Working Group on the Evaluation of Carcinogenic Risks to Humans 1987 Overall evaluations of carcinogenicity: an updating of IARC monographs volumes 1 to 42. International Agency for Research on Cancer, Lyon, pp 289–296
3. Hertz R, Bailar JC III 1966 Estrogen-progestogen combinations for contraception. Journal of the American Medical Association 198: 136–142
4. Hertz R 1967 The role of steroid hormones in the etiology and pathogenesis of cancer. American Journal of Obstetrics and Gynecology 98: 1013–1019
5. Hertz R 1969 The problem of possible effects of oral contraceptives on cancer of the breast. Cancer 24: 1140–1145
6. Beatson GT 1896 On the treatment of inoperable cases of carcinoma of the mammae. Lancet 2: 104–107
7. Loeb L 1919 Further investigations on the origin of tumors in mice VI. Internal secretions as a factor in the origin of tumors. Journal of Medical Research 40: 477–496
8. Allaben GR, Owens SE 1939 Adenocarcinoma of the breast coincidental with strenuous estrogen therapy. Journal of the American Medical Association 112: 1933–1934
9. Auchincloss H, Haagemen CD 1940 Cancer of the breast possibly induced by estrogenic substance. Journal of the American Medical Association 114: 1517–1523
10. Parsons WH, McCall EF 1941 The role of estrogenic substances in the production of malignant mammary lesions with report of a case of adenocarcinoma of the breast. Surgery 9: 780–786
11. Fremont-Smith M, Meigs JV, Graham RM, Gilbert HH 1946 Cancer of the endometrium and prolonged estrogen therapy. Journal of the American Medical Association 131: 805–808
12. Ries LAG, Miller BA, Hankey BF, Kosary CL, Harras A, Edwards BK (eds) 1994 SEER cancer statistics review, 1973–1991: tables and graphs. NIH Pub. No. 94–2789, National Cancer Institute, Bethesda, MD
13. Young JL, Percy CL, Asire AJ (eds) 1981 Surveillance epidemiology end results. Incidence and mortality data: 1973–1977. National Institutes of Health, Bethesda, p 152
14. Hoskins WJ, Perez C, Young RC 1989 Gynecologic tumors. In: DeVita VT Jr, Hellman S, Rosenberg SA (eds) Cancer: principles and practice of oncology, vol 1, 3rd edn. JB Lippincott, Philadelphia, pp 1144–1146
15. Hannigan EV 1993 Uterine sarcomas. In: Copeland LJ, Farrell JF, McGregor JA (eds) Textbook of gynecology. WB Saunders, Philadelphia, pp 1034–1045
16. Creasman WT 1994 Malignant lesions of the uterine corpus. In: Scott JR, DiSaia PJ, Hammond CB, Spellacy WN (eds) Danforth's obstetrics and gynecology, 7th edn. Lippincott, Philadelphia, pp 941–956
17. Luoto R, Kaprio J, Keskimaki I, Pohjanlahti JP, Rutanen EM 1994 Incidence, causes and surgical methods for hysterectomy in Finland, 1987–1989. International Journal of Epidemiology 23: 348–358
18. Wilcox LS, Koonin LM, Pokras R, Strauss LT, Xia Z, Peterson HB 1994 Hysterectomy in the United States, 1988–1990. Obstetrics and Gynecology 83: 549–555
19. MacLennan AH, MacLennan A, Wilson D 1993 The prevalence of hysterectomy in South Australia. Medical Journal of Australia 158: 807–809

20. Parkin DM, Muir CS, Whelan SL, Gao YT, Ferlay J, Powell J (eds) 1992 Cancer incidence in five continents, vol. VI. IARC, Lyon
21. Day N 1992 Cumulative rate and cumulative risk. In: Parkin DM, Muir CS, Whelan SL, Gao YT, Ferlay J, Powell J (eds) Cancer incidence in five continents, vol. VI. IARC, Lyon, pp 862–864
22. Selvin S 1996 Statistical analysis of epidemiologic data, 2nd edn. Oxford University Press, New York, pp 311–355
23. Peto R, Lopez AD, Boreham J, Thun M, Health C Jr 1994 Mortality from smoking in developed countries 1950–2000. Oxford University Press, Oxford, pp 248–249; 392–393; 530–531
24. Bosch FX, Manos MM, Munoz N, Sherman M, Jansen AM, Peto J, Schiffman MH, Moreno V, Kurman R, Shah KV 1995 Prevalence of human papillomavirus in cervical cancer: a worldwide perspective. Journal of the National Cancer Institute 87: 796–802
25. Schiffman MH, Brinton LA 1995 The epidemiology of cervical carcinogenesis. Cancer 76: 1888–1901
26. Allen E, Gardner WU 1941 Cancer of the cervix of the uterus in hybrid mice following long continued administration of estrogen. Cancer Research 1: 359–366
27. Murphy ED 1961 Carcinogenesis of the uterine cervix in mice: effect of diethylstilbestrol after limited application of 3-methylcholanthrene. Journal of the National Cancer Institute 27: 611–653
28. Kaminetzky HA 1966 Methylcholanthrene induced cervical dysplasia and the sex steroids. Obstetrics and Gynecology 27: 489–493
29. Dunn TB 1969 Cancer of the uterine cervix in mice fed a liquid diet containing an antifertility drug. Journal of the National Cancer Institute 43: 681–692
30. Jordan JA, Singer A 1976 The cervix. WB Saunders, Philadelphia
31. Cramer DW 1982 Uterine cervix. In: Schottenfeld D, Fraumeni JF (eds) Cancer epidemiology and prevention. WB Saunders, Philadelphia, pp 881–900
32. Mentlein R, Staves R, Rix-Matzen H, Tinneberg HR 1991 Influence of pregnancy on dipeptidyl peptidase IV activity (CD 26 leukocyte differentiation antigen) of circulating lymphocytes. European Journal of Clinical Chemistry and Clinical Biochemistry 29: 477–480
33. Butterworth CE Jr, Hatch KD, Gore H et al 1982 Improvement in cervical dysplasia associated with folic acid therapy in users of oral contraceptives. American Journal of Clinical Nutrition 35: 73–82
34. Butterworth CE Jr 1992 Effect of folate on cervical cancer. Synergism among risk factors. Annals of the New York Academy of Science 669: 293–299
35. Godwin AK, Perez RP, Johnson SW, Hamaguchi K, Hamilton TC 1992 Growth regulation of ovarian cancer. Hematology and Oncology Clinics of North America 6: 829–841
36. Dietl J, Marzusch K 1993 Ovarian surface epithelium and human ovarian cancer. Gynecologic and Obstetric Investigation 35: 129–135
37. Merino MJ, Jaffe G 1993 Age contrast in ovarian pathology. Cancer 71: 537–544
38. Weiss NS 1982 Ovary. In: Schottenfeld D, Fraumeni JF (eds) Cancer epidemiology and prevention. WB Saunders, Philadelphia, pp 871–880
39. Sanford JL 1991 Oral contraceptives and neoplasia of the ovary. Contraception 43: 543–556
40. Whittemore AS, Harris R, Itnyre J, and the Collaborative Ovarian Cancer Group 1992 Characteristics relating to ovarian cancer risk: collaborative analysis of 12 US case-control studies II. Invasive epithelial ovarian cancers in white women. American Journal of Epidemiology 136: 1184–1203
41. Amos CI, Shaw GL, Tucker MA, Hartge P 1992 Age at onset for familial epithelial ovarian cancer. Journal of the American Medical Association 268: 1896–1899
42. Kerlikowske K, Brown JS, Grady DG 1992 Should women with familial ovarian cancer undergo prophylactic oophorectomy? Obstetrics and Gynecology 80: 700–707
43. Hankinson SE, Colditz GA, Hunter DJ, Spencer TL, Rosner B, Stampfer MJ 1992 A quantitative assessment of oral contraceptive use and risk of ovarian cancer. Obstetrics and Gynecology 80: 708–714
44. Hartge P, Schiffman MH, Hoover R, McGowan L, Lesher L, Norris HJ 1989 A case-control study of epithelial ovarian cancer. American Journal of Obstetrics and Gynecology 161: 10–16
45. Booth M, Beral V, Smith P 1989 Risk factors for ovarian cancer: a case-control study. British Journal of Cancer 60: 592–598
46. Weber BL, Abel KJ, Couch FJ, Merajver S, Castilla L, Brody LC, Collins FS 1995 Transcript identification in the BRCA1 candidate region. Breast Cancer Research and Treatment 33: 115–124
47. Narod SA 1994 Genetics of breast and ovarian cancer. British Medical Bulletin 50: 656–676
48. Fathalla MF 1971 Incessant ovulation — a factor in ovarian neoplasia? Lancet ii: 163
49. Stadel BV 1975 The etiology and prevention of ovarian cancer. American Journal of Obstetrics and Gynecology 123: 772–773
50. Kelsey JL, Whittemore AS 1994 Epidemiology and primary prevention of cancers of the breast, endometrium, and ovary. A brief overview. Annals of Epidemiology 4: 89–95
51. Helzlsouer KJ, Alberg AJ, Gordon GB, Longcope C, Bush TL, Hoffman SC, Comstock GW 1995 Serum gonadotropins and steroid hormones and the development of ovarian cancer. Journal of the American Medical Association 274: 1926–1930
52. Gwinn ML, Lee NC, Rhodes PH, Layde PM, Rubin GL 1990 Pregnancy, breast feeding, and oral contraceptives and the risk of epithelial ovarian cancer. Journal of Clinical Epidemiology 43: 559–568
53. Cramer DW, Welch WR 1983 Determinants of ovarian cancer risk. II Inferences regarding pathogenesis. Journal of the National Cancer Institute 71: 717–721
54. Novak E, Yui E 1936 Relation of endometrial hyperplasia to adenocarcinoma of the uterus. American Journal of Obstetrics and Gynecology 32: 674–698
55. Henderson BE, Ross R, Bernstein L 1988 Estrogens as a cause of human cancer: The Richard and Hinda Rosenthal Foundation Award Lecture. Cancer Research 48: 246–253
56. King RJB 1991 Biology of female sex hormone action in relation to contraceptive agents and neoplasia. Contraception 43: 527–542

57. Whitehead MI, Townsend PT, Pryse-Davies J, Ryder TA, King RJB 1981 Effects of estrogens and progestins on the biochemistry and morphology of the postmenopausal endometrium. New England Journal of Medicine 305: 1599–1605
58. Martin I, Finn CA 1971 Oestrogen-gestagen interactions on mitosis in target tissues. In: Hubinont PO, LeRoy F, Galand P (eds) Basic actions of sex steroids on target organs. Karger, Basel, pp 172–188
59. Lane G, Siddle NC, Ryder TA, Pryse-Davies J, King RJB, Whitehead MI 1983 Dose dependent effects of oral progesterone on the oestrogenised postmenopausal endometrium. British Medical Journal 287: 1241–1245
60. Kim S, Korhonen M, Wilborn W, Foldesy R, Snipes W, Hodgen GD, Anderson FD 1996 Antiproliferative effects of low-dose micronized progesterone. Fertility and Sterility 65: 323–331
61. Gambrell RD 1986 The role of hormones in the etiology and prevention of endometrial cancer. Clinics in Obstetrics and Gynecology 13: 695–723
62. Kneale BLG 1986 Adjunctive and therapeutic progestins in endometrial cancer. Clinics in Obstetrics and Gynecology 13: 789–809
63. Hoffman D, Hecht S, Schmeltz I, Wynder E 1978 Polynuclear aromatic hydrocarbons: occurence, formation, and carcinogenicity. In: Asher IM, Zervos C (eds) Structural correlates of carcinogenesis and mutagenesis: a guide to testing priorities? Department of Health, Education and Welfare, Public Health Service, Food and Drug Administration, Scientific Liaison Staff, Office of Science, Rockville, Maryland, pp 120–127
64. McDonald T, Malkasian G, Gaffey T 1977 Endometrial cancer associated with feminizing ovarian tumor and polycystic ovarian disease. Obstetrics and Gynecology 49: 654–658
65. Wynder EL, Escher GC, Mantel N 1966 An epidemiologic investigation of cancer of the endometrium. Cancer 10: 489–520
66. Grossman C 1984 Regulation of the immune system by sex steroids. Endocrine Reviews 5: 435–455
67. Giudice LC, Ferenczy A 1996 The endometrial cycle. In: Adashi EY, Rock JA, Rosenwaks Z (eds) Reproductive endocrinology, surgery and technology. Lippincott-Raven, Philadelphia, pp 271–300
68. White MM, Zamudio S, Stevens T, Tyler R, Lindenfeld J, Leslie K et al 1995 Estrogen, progesterone, and vascular reactivity: Potential cellular mechanisms. Endocrine Reviews 16: 739–751
69. Folkman J 1995 Clinical applications of research on angiogenesis. New England Journal of Medicine 333: 1757–1763
70. Murphy LJ 1994 Growth factors and steroid hormone action in endometrial cancer. The Journal of Steroid Biochemistry and Molecular Biology 48: 419–423
71. Kelsey JL, Hildreth NG 1983 Breast and gynecologic cancer epidemiology. CRC Press, Boca Raton
72. Key TJ, Pike MC 1988 The dose-effect relationship between 'unopposed' oestrogens and endometrial mitotic rate: its central role in explaining and predicting endometrial cancer risk. British Journal of Cancer 57: 205–212
73. Kjaer SK, Engholm G, Dahl C, Bock JE, Lynge E, Jensen OM 1993 Case-control study of risk factors for cervical squamous-cell neoplasia in Denmark III. Role of oral contraceptive use. Cancer Causes and Control 4: 513–519
74. Brinton LA, Reeves WC, Brenes MM et al 1990 Oral contraceptive use and risk of invasive cervical cancer. International Journal of Epidemiology 19: 4–11
75. Parazzini F, La Vecchia C, Negri E, Maggi R 1990 Oral contraceptive use and invasive cervical cancer. International Journal of Epidemiology 19: 259–263
76. Irwin KL, Rosero-Bixby L, Oberle MW et al 1988 Oral contraceptives and cervical cancer risk in Costa Rica: detection bias or causal association? Journal of the American Medical Association 259: 59–64
77. Ebeling K, Nischan P, Schindler C 1987 Use of oral contraceptives and risk of invasive cervical cancer in previously screened women. International Journal of Epidemiology 39: 427–430
78. Brinton LA, Huggins GR, Lehman HF et al 1986 Long-term use of oral contraceptives and risk of invasive cervical cancer. International Journal of Cancer 38: 339–344
79. Peters RK, Thomas D, Hagan DG, Mack TM, Henderson BE 1986 Risk factors for invasive cervical cancer among Latinas and non-Latinas in Los Angeles County. Journal of the National Cancer Institute 77: 1063–1077
80. La Vecchia C, Decarli A, Fasoli M et al 1986 Oral contraceptives and cancers of the breast and of the female genital tract. Interim results from a case-control study. British Journal of Cancer 54: 311–317
81. World Health Organization 1985 Collaborative study of neoplasia and steroid contraceptives. Invasive cervical cancer and combined oral contraceptives. British Medical Journal 290: 961–965
82. Beral V, Hannaford P, Kay C 1988 Oral contraceptive use and malignancies of the genital tract. Results from the Royal College of General Practitioners' Oral Contraception Study. Lancet ii: 1331–1335
83. Vessey MP, Lawless M, McPherson K, Yeates D 1983 Neoplasia of the cervix uteri and contraception: a possible adverse effect of the pill. Lancet ii: 930–934
84. Schlesselman JJ 1995 Net effect of oral contraceptive use on the risk of cancer in women in the United States. Obstetrics and Gynecology 85: 793–801
85. Swan SH, Petitti DB 1982 A review of problems of bias and confounding in epidemiologic studies of cervical neoplasia and oral contraceptive use. American Journal of Epidemiology 50: 10–18
86. Schlesselman JJ 1989 Cancer of the breast and reproductive tract in relation to use of oral contraceptives. Contraception 40: 1–38
87. Boyce JG, Lu T, Nelson JH, Fruchter RG 1977 Oral contraceptives and cervical carcinoma. American Journal of Obstetrics and Gynecology 128: 761–766
88. Wright NH, Vessey MP, Kenward B, McPherson K, Doll R 1978 Neoplasia and dysplasia of the cervix uteri and contraception: a possible protective effect of the diaphragm. British Journal of Cancer 38: 273–279
89. Vessey MP, Lawless M, McPherson K, Yeates D 1983 Oral contraceptives and cervical cancer. Lancet ii: 1358–1359
90. Peritz E, Ramcharan S, Frank J, Brown WL, Huang S, Ray R 1977 The incidence of cervical cancer and duration of oral contraceptive use. American Journal of Epidemiology 106: 462–469

91. Brinton LA, Tashima KT, Lehman HF et al 1987 Epidemiology of cervical cancer by cell type. Cancer Research 47: 1706–1711
92. Ebeling K, Nischan P, Schindler C 1987 Use of oral contraceptives and risk of invasive cervical cancer in previously screened women. International Journal of Cancer 39: 427–430
93. Irwin KL, Rosero-Bixby L, Oberle MW et al 1988 Oral contraceptives and cervical cancer risk in Costa Rica. Journal of the American Medical Association 259: 59–64
94. Eluf-Neto J, Booth M, Munoz N et al 1994 Human papillomavirus and invasive cancer in Brazil. Brazilian Journal of Cancer 69: 114–119
95. Ursin G, Peters RK, Henderson BE, d'Ablaing G, III Monroe KR, Pike MC 1994 Oral contraceptive use and adenocarcinoma of cervix. Lancet 344: 1390–1394
96. Persson E, Einhorn N, Pettersson F 1987 A case-control study of oral contraceptive use in women with adenocarcinoma of the uterine cervix. European Journal of Obstetrics, Gynaecology and Reproductive Biology 26: 85–90
97. Silcocks PBS, Thornton-Jones JH, Murphy M 1987 Squamous and adenocarcinoma of the uterine cervix: a comparison using routine data. British Journal of Cancer 55: 321–325
98. Horowitz IR, Jacobson LP, Zucker PK, Currie JL, Rosenshein NB 1988 Epidemiology of adenocarcinoma of the cervix. Gynecological Oncology 31: 25–31
99. Jones MW, Silverberg SG 1989 Cervical adenocarcinoma in young women: possible relationship to microglandular hyperplasia and use of oral contraceptives. Obstetrics and Gynecology 73: 984–989
100. Honore LH, Koch M, Brown LB 1989 Comparison of oral contraceptive use in women with adenocarcinoma and squamous cell carcinoma of the uterine cervix. Gynecological and Obstetrical Investigation 32: 98–101
101. Rosenberg L, Palmer JR, Zauber AG, Warshauer ME, Lewis JL Jr, Strom BL, Harlap S, Shapiro S 1994 A case-control study of oral contraceptive use and invasive epithelial ovarian cancer. American Journal of Epidemiology 139: 654–661
102. Badawy YA, Bayoumi DM 1992 An epidemiologic study of ovarian cancer. Part II: Oral contraceptive use and menstrual events. Journal of the Egyptian Public Health Association 67: 579–591
103. Harlow BL, Cramer DW, Geller J, Willett WC, Bell DA, Welch WR 1991 The influence of lactose consumption on the association of oral contraceptive use and ovarian cancer risk. American Journal of Epidemiology 134: 445–453
104. Parazzini F, La Vecchia C, Negri E et al 1991 Oral contraceptive use and the risk of ovarian cancer: an Italian case-control study. European Journal of Cancer 27: 594–598
105. World Health Organization 1989 Collaborative Study of Neoplasia and Steroid Contraceptives. Epithelial ovarian cancer and combined oral contraceptives. International Journal of Epidemiology 18: 538–545
106. Shu XO, Brinton LA, Gao YT, Yuan JM 1989 Population-based case-control study of ovarian cancer in Shanghai. Cancer Research 49: 3670–3674
107. Wu ML, Whittemore AS, Paffenbarger RS et al 1988 Personal and environmental characteristics related to epithelial ovarian cancer I. Reproductive and menstrual events and oral contraceptive use. American Journal of Epidemiology 128: 1216–1227
108. The Cancer and Steroid Hormone Study of the Centers for Disease Control and the National Institute of Child Health and Human Development 1987 The reduction in risk of ovarian cancer associated with oral contraceptive use. New England Journal of Medicine 316: 650–655
109. Cramer DW, Hutchinson GB, Welch WR, Scully RE, Knapp RC 1982 Factors affecting the association of oral contraceptives and ovarian cancer. New England Journal of Medicine 307: 1047–1051
110. Willett WC, Bain C, Hennekens CH, Rosner B, Speizer F 1981 Oral contraceptives and risk of ovarian cancer. Cancer 48: 1684–1687
111. Weiss NS, Lyon JL, Liff JM, Vollmer WM, Daling JR 1981 Incidence of ovarian cancer in relation to the use of oral contraceptives. International Journal of Cancer 28: 669–671
112. Casagrande JT, Louie EW, Pike MC, Roy S, Ross RK, Henderson BE 1979 'Incessant ovulation' and ovarian cancer. Lancet ii: 170–173
113. Vessey MP, Painter R 1995 Endometrial and ovarian cancer and oral contraceptives — findings in a large cohort study. British Journal of Cancer 71: 1340–1342
114. The Centers for Disease Control Cancer and Steroid Hormone Study 1983 Oral contraceptive use and the risk of ovarian cancer. Journal of the American Medical Association 249: 1596–1599
115. Rosenblatt KA, Thomas DB, Noonan EA, WHO Collaborative Study 1992 High-dose and low-dose combined oral contraceptives: protection against epithelial ovarian cancer and the length of the protective effect. European Journal of Cancer 28A: 1872–1876
116. Gross TP, Schlesselman JJ 1994 The estimated effect of oral contraceptive use on the cumulative risk of epithelial ovarian cancer. Obstetrics and Gynecology 83: 419–424
117. Stanford JL, Brinton LA, Berman ML, Mortel R, Twiggs LB, Barrett RJ, Wilbanks GD, Hoover RN 1993 Oral contraceptives and endometrial cancer: do other risk factors modify the association? International Journal of Cancer 54: 243–248
118. Levi F, La Vecchia C, Gulie C, Negri E, Monnier V, Franceschi S, Delaloye JF, De Grandi P 1991 Oral contraceptives and the risk of endometrial cancer. Cancer Causes and Control 2: 99–103
119. The Cancer and Steroid Hormone Study of the Centers for Disease Control and the National Institute of Child Health and Human Development 1987 Combination oral contraceptive use and the risk of endometrial cancer. Journal of the American Medical Association 257: 796–800
120. Pettersson B, Adami HO, Bergstrom R, Johansson EDB 1986 Menstruation span — a time-limited risk factor for endometrial cancer. Acta Obstetrica Gynecologica Scandinavica 65: 247–255
121. Henderson BE, Casagrande JT, Pike MC, Mack T, Rosario I, Duke A 1983 The epidemiology of endometrial cancer in young women. British Journal of Cancer 47: 749–756

122. Kelsey JL, LiVolsi VA, Holford TR et al 1982 A case-control study of cancer of the endometrium. American Journal of Epidemiology 116: 333–342
123. Hulka BS, Chambless LE, Kaufman DG, Fowler WC, Grenberg BG 1982 Protection against endometrial carcinoma by combination-product oral contraceptives. Journal of the American Medical Association 247: 475–477
124. Kaufman DW, Shapiro S, Slone D et al 1980 Decreased risk of endometrial cancer among oral contraceptive users. New England Journal of Medicine 303: 1045–1047
125. Weiss NS, Sayvetz TA 1980 Incidence of endometrial cancer in relation to the use of oral contraceptives. New England Journal of Medicine 302: 551–554
126. The Centers for Disease Control Cancer and Steroid Hormone Study 1983 Oral contraceptive use and the risk of endometrial cancer. Journal of the American Medical Association 249: 1600–1604
127. Koumantaki Y, Tzonou A, Koumantakis E, Kaklamani E, Aravantinos D, Trichopoulos D 1989 A case-control study of cancer of the endometrium in Athens. International Journal of Cancer 43: 795–799
128. World Health Organization 1988 Study of neoplasia and steroid contraceptives. Endometrial cancer and combined oral contraceptives. International Journal of Epidemiology 17: 263–269
129. Ramcharan S, Pellegrin FA, Ray R, Hsu JP 1981 The Walnut Creek Contraceptive Drug Study: A prospective study of the side effects of oral contraceptives, vol 3. National Institute of Child Health and Human Development, Bethesda, p 62
130. Trapido EJ 1983 A prospective cohort study of oral contraceptives and cancer of the endometrium. International Journal of Epidemiology 12: 297–300
131. Horwitz RI, Feinstein AR 1979 Case-control study of oral contraceptive pills and endometrial cancer. Annals of Internal Medicine 91: 226–227
132. Cole P 1980 Oral contraceptives and endometrial cancer. New England Journal of Medicine 302: 575–576
133. Key TJ, Pike MC 1988 The dose-effect relationship between 'unopposed' oestrogens and endometrial mitotic rate: its central role in explaining and predicting endometrial cancer risk. British Journal of Cancer 57: 205–212
134. Pike MC 1987 Age-related factors in cancers of the breast, ovary and endometrium. Journal of Chronic Diseases 40(Suppl 2): 59s–69s
135. Greenblatt RB 1967 Progestational agents in clinical practice. Medical Science 18: 37–49
136. Rosenblatt KA, Thomas DB, WHO Collaborative Study 1991 Hormonal content of combined oral contraceptives in relation to the reduced risk of endometrial carcinoma. International Journal of Cancer 49: 870–874
137. Dickey RP, Stone SC 1976 Progestational potency of oral contraceptives. Obstetrics and Gynecology 47: 106–112
138. Dickey RP 1984 Managing contraceptive pill patients, 3rd edn. Creative Informatics, Durant, OK
139. Voigt LF, Deng Q, Weiss NS 1994 Recency, duration, and progestin content of oral contraceptives in relation to the incidence of endometrial cancer (Washington, USA). Cancer Causes and Control 5: 227–233
140. Rubin GI, Peterson HB, Lee NC, Maes EF, Wingo PA, Becker S 1990 Estrogen-replacement therapy and the risk of endometrial cancer: remaining controversies. American Journal of Obstetrics and Gynecology 162: 148–154
141. Schwartz SM, Weiss NS, Daling JR, Gammon MD et al 1996 Exogenous sex hormone use, correlates of endogenous hormone levels, and the incidence of histologic types of sarcomas of the uterus. Cancer 77: 717–724
142. Speroff L, Glass RH, Kase NG 1994 Clinical gynecologic endocrinology and infertility, 5th edn. Williams and Wilkins, Baltimore, pp 715–755
143. Hatcher RA, Trussell J, Stewart F et al 1994 Contraceptive technology, 16th revised edn. Irvington, New York, pp 228–279
144. Schlesselman JJ, Stadel BV, Korper M, Yu W, Wingo PA 1992 Breast cancer detection in relation to oral contraception. Journal of Clinical Epidemiology 45: 449–459
145. Rosner D, Joy J, Lane WW 1985 Oral contraceptives and prognosis of breast cancer in women aged 35 to 50. Journal of Surgical Oncology 30: 52–59
146. Millard FC, Bliss JM, Chilvers CED, Gazet JC 1987 Oral contraceptives and survival in breast cancer. British Journal of Cancer 56: 377–378
147. Colditz GA 1994 Oral contraceptive use and mortality during 12 years of follow-up: the Nurses' Health Study. Annals of Internal Medicine 120: 821–826
148. Vessey MP, Villard-Mackintosh L, McPherson K, Yeates D 1989 Mortality among oral contraceptive users: 20 year follow up of women in a cohort study. British Medical Journal 299: 1487–1491
149. Ory HW, Forrest JD, Lincoln R 1983 Making choices: evaluating the health risks and benefits of birth control methods. Alan Guttmacher Institute, New York
150. Fortney JA, Harper JM, Potts M 1986 Oral contraceptives and life expectancy. Studies in Family Planning 17: 117–125
151. Vessey MP 1989 The Jephcott Lecture, 1989: an overview of the benefits and risks of combined oral contraceptives. In: Mann RD (ed) Oral contraceptives and breast cancer. Parthenon, Park Ridge, New Jersey, pp 121–135
152. Harlap S, Kost K, Forrest JD 1991 Preventing pregnancy, protecting health: a new look at birth control choices in the United States. Alan Guttmacher Institute, New York, pp 57–60
153. Lande RE 1995 New era for injectables. Population Reports, Series K, No.5. Johns Hopkins School of Public Health, Population Information Program, Baltimore (August)
154. Oberle MW et al 1988 Cervical cancer risk and use of depot-medroxyprogesterone acetate in Costa Rica. International Journal of Epidemiology 17: 718–723
155. Herrero R, Brinton LA, Reeves WC, Brenes MM, De Britton RC, Tenorio F, Gaitan E 1990 Injectable contraceptives and risk of invasive cervical cancer: evidence of an association. International Journal of Cancer 46: 5–7
156. Thomas DB, Ray RM 1992 Depot-medroxyprogesterone acetate (DMPA) and risk of invasive squamous cell cancer. Contraception 45: 299–312

157. Stanford JL, Thomas DB 1991 Depot-medroxyprogesterone acetate (DMPA) and risk of epithelial ovarian cancer. International Journal of Cancer 49: 191–195
158. Thomas DB, Ray RM 1991 Depot-medroxyprogesterone acetate (DMPA) and risk of endometrial cancer. International Journal of Cancer 49: 186–190
159. Henry JS 1945 The avoidance of untoward effects of estrogenic therapy in the menopause. Canadian Medical Association Journal 53: 31–37
160. Jensen EI, Ostergaard E 1954 Clinical studies concerning the relationship of estrogens to the development of cancer of the corpus uteri. American Journal of Obstetrics and Gynecology 67: 1094–1102
161. Dunn LJ, Bradbury JT 1967 Endocrine factors in endometrial carcinoma. American Journal of Obstetrics and Gynecology 97: 465–471
162. Quint BC 1975 Changing patterns in endometrial adenocarcinoma. American Journal of Obstetrics and Gynecology 122: 498–501
163. Smith DC, Prentice R, Thompson DJ, Hermann WL 1975 Association of exogenous estrogen and endometrial carcinoma. New England Journal of Medicine 293: 1164–1166
164. Ziel HK, Finkle WD 1975 Increased risk of endometrial carcinoma among users of conjugated estrogens. New England Journal of Medicine 293: 1167–1170
165. Gray LA, Christopherson WM, Hoover RN 1977 Estrogens and endometrial carcinoma. Obstetrics and Gynecology 49: 385–391
166. McDonald TW, Annegers JF, O'Fallon WM, Dockkerty MB, Malkasian GD, Kurland LT 1977 Exogenous estrogen and endometrial carcinoma: case-control and incidence study. American Journal of Obstetrics and Gynecology 127: 572–579
167. Kennedy DL, Baum C, Forbes MB 1985 Noncontraceptive estrogens and progestins: use patterns over time. Obstetrics and Gynecology 65: 441–446
168. Wysowski DK, Golden L, Burke L 1995 Use of menopausal estrogens and medroxyprogesterone in the United States, 1982–1992. Obstetrics and Gynecology 85: 6–10
169. Ross RK, Paganini-Hill A, Roy S, Chao A, Henderson BE 1988 Past and present preferred prescribing practices of hormone replacement therapy among Los Angeles gynecologists: possible implications for public health. American Journal of Public Health 78: 516–519
170. Harris RB, Laws A, Reddy VM, King A, Haskell WL 1990 Are women using postmenopausal estrogens? A community survey. American Journal of Public Health 80: 1266–1268
171. Kurman RJ, Norris HJ 1994 Endometrial hyperplasia and related cellular changes. In: Kurman RJ (ed) Blaustein's pathology of the female genital tract, 4th edn. Springer-Verlag, New York, pp 411–437
172. Christopherson WM, Gray LA 1992 Premalignant lesions of the endometrium: endometrial hyperplasia and adenocarcinoma in situ. In: Coppleson M, Monaghan JM, Morrow CP, Tattersall MHN (eds.) Gynecologic oncology, 2nd edn. Churchill Livingstone, Edinburgh, pp 731–745
173. Kurman R, Kaminski P, Norris H 1985 The behavior of endometrial hyperplasia: a long-term study of 'untreated' hyperplasia in 170 patients. Cancer 56: 403–412
174. Varma T 1985 Effect of long-term therapy with estrogen and progesterone on the endometrium of post-menopausal women. Acta Obstetrica Gynecologica Scandinavica 64: 41–46
175. Woodruff JD, Pickar JH 1994 Incidence of endometrial hyperplasia in postmenopausal women taking conjugated estrogens (Premarin) with medroxyprogesterone acetate or conjugated estrogens alone. American Journal of Obstetrics and Gynecology 170: 1213–1223
176. PEPI Trial Writing Group 1996 Effects of hormone replacement therapy on endometrial histology in postmenopausal women. Journal of the American Medical Association 275: 370–375
177. Whitehead M 1986 Prevention of endometrial abnormalities. Acta Obstetrica Gynecologica Scandinavica 134(Suppl) 81–91
178. Kurman RJ, Zaino RJ, Norris HJ 1994 Endometrial carcinoma. In: Kurman RJ (ed) Blaustein's pathology of the female genital tract, 4th edn. Springer-Verlag, New York, pp 439–486
179. Weiss NS, Szekely DR, English DR, Schweid AI 1979 Endometrial cancer in relation to patterns of menopausal estrogen use. Journal of the American Medical Association 242: 261–264
180. Wigle DT, Grace M, Smith ESO 1978 Estrogen use and cancer of the uterine corpus in Alberta. Canadian Medical Association Journal 118: 1276–1278
181. Gambrell RD, Massey F, Castaneda TA, Ugenas A, Ricci C, Wright J 1980 Use of the progestogen challenge test to reduce the risk of endometrial cancer. Obstetrics and Gynecology 55: 732–738
182. Folsom AR, Mink PJ, Sellers TA, Hong C, Zheng W, Potter JD 1995 Hormonal replacement therapy and morbidity and mortality in a prospective study of postmenopausal women. American Journal of Public Health 85: 1128–1132
183. Hoover R, Fraumeni JF, Everson R, Myers MH 1976 Cancer of the uterine corpus after hormonal treatment for breast cancer. Lancet 1: 885–887
184. Jick H, Watkins RN, Hunter JR, Dinan BJ, Madsen S, Rothman KJ et al 1979 Replacement estrogens and endometrial cancer. New England Journal of Medicine 300: 218–222
185. Paganini-Hill A, Ross RK, Henderson BE 1989 Endometrial cancer and patterns of use of oestrogen replacement therapy: a cohort study. British Journal of Cancer 59: 445–447
186. Persson I, Adami H, Bergkvist L, Lindgren A, Pettersson B, Hoover R et al 1989 Risk of endometrial cancer after treatment with oestrogens alone or in conjunction with progestogens: results of a prospective study. British Medical Journal 298: 147–151
187. Petitti D, Perlman J, Sidney S 1987 Noncontraceptive estrogens and mortality: long-term follow-up of women in the Walnut Creek study. Obstetrics and Gynecology 70: 289–293
188. Antunes C, Stolley P, Rosenshein N, Davies JW, Tonascia J, Brown C et al 1979 Endometrial cancer and estrogen use: report of a large case-control study. New England Journal of Medicine 300: 9–13

189. Brinton LA, Hoover RN, Endometrial Cancer Collaborative Group 1993 Estrogen replacement therapy and endometrial cancer risk: unresolved issues. Obstetrics and Gynecology 81: 265–271
190. Buring JE, Bain CJ, Ehrmann RL 1986 Conjugated estrogen use and risk of endometrial cancer. American Journal of Epidemiology 124: 434–441
191. Ewertz M, Schou G, Boice JD 1988 The joint effect of risk factors on endometrial cancer. European Journal of Cancer and Clinical Oncology 24: 189–194
192. Franks AL, Kendrick J, Tyler C, The Cancer and Steroid Hormone Study Group 1987 Postmenopausal smoking, estrogen replacement therapy, and the risk of endometrial cancer. American Journal of Obstetrics and Gynecology 156: 20–23
193. Henderson BE, Casagrande JT, Pike MC, Mack T, Rosario I, Duke A 1983 The epidemiology of endometrial cancer in young women. British Journal of Cancer 47: 749–756
194. Hoogerland DL, Buchler DA, Crowley JJ, Carr WA 1978 Estrogen use — risk of endometrial carcinoma. Gynecological Oncology 6: 451–458
195. Horwitz R, Feinstein AR 1978 Alternative analytic methods for case-control studies of estrogens and endometrial cancer. New England Journal of Medicine 299: 1089–1094
196. Hulka B, Fowler W, Kaufman D, Grimson R, Greenberg B, Hogue C et al 1980 Estrogen and endometrial cancer: cases and two control groups from North Carolina. American Journal of Obstetrics and Gynecology 137: 92–101
197. Jelovsek F, Hammond C, Woodard B, Draffin R, Lee K, Creasman WT et al 1980 Risk of exogenous estrogen therapy and endometrial cancer. American Journal of Obstetrics and Gynecology 137: 85–91
198. Jick SS, Walker AM, Jick H 1993 Estrogens, progesterone, and endometrial cancer. Epidemiology 4: 20–24
199. Kelsey JL, Livolsi VA, Holford TR, Fischer DB, Mostow ED, Schwartz PE et al 1982 A case-control study of cancer of the endometrium. American Journal of Epidemiology 116: 333–342
200. La Vecchia C, Franceschi S, Decarli A, Gallus G, Tognoni G 1984 Risk factors for endometrial cancer at different ages. Journal of the National Cancer Institute 73: 667–671
201. Levi F, La Vecchia C, Gulie C, Franceschi S, Negri E 1993 Oestrogen replacement treatment and the risk of endometrial cancer: an assessment of the role of co-variates. European Journal of Cancer 29A: 1445–1449
202. Mack TM, Pike MC, Henderson BE, Pfeffer RI, Gerkins VR, Arthur M et al 1976 Association of exogenous estrogen and endometrial cancer. New England Journal of Medicine 294: 1262–1267
203. Salmi T 1980 Endometrial carcinoma risk factors, with special reference to the use of oestrogens. Acta Endocrinologica 233(Suppl): 37–43
204. Shapiro S, Kelly J, Rosenberg L, Kaufman D, Helmrich S, Rosenshein N et al 1985 Risk of localized and widespread endometrial cancer in relation to recent and discontinued use of conjugated estrogens. New England Journal of Medicine 313: 969–972
205. Spengler R, Clarke E, Woolever C, Newman A, Osborn R 1981 Exogenous estrogens and endometrial cancer: a case-control study and assessment of potential biases. American Journal of Epidemiology 114: 497–506
206. Stavraky K, Collins JA, Donner A, Wells G 1981 A comparison of estrogen use by women with endometrial cancer, gynecologic disorders, and other illnesses. American Journal of Obstetrics and Gynecology 141: 547–555
207. Voigt LF, Weiss NS, Chu J, Daling JR, McKnight B, Van Belle G 1991 Progestagen supplementation of exogenous oestrogens and risk of endometrial cancer. Lancet 338: 274–277
208. Light RJ, Pillemer DB 1984 Summing Up: the science of reviewing research. Harvard University Press, Boston
209. Jick SS 1993 Combined estrogen and progesterone use and endometrial cancer. Epidemiology 4: 384
210. Ettinger B, Golditch IM, Friedman G 1988 Gynecologic consequences of long-term, unopposed estrogen replacement therapy. Maturitas 10: 271–282
211. Hammond CB, Jelovsek FR, Lee KL, Creasman WT, Parker RT 1979 Effects of long-term estrogen replacement therapy II. Neoplasia. American Journal of Obstetrics and Gynecology 133: 537–547
212. Hunt K, Vessey M, McPherson K, Coleman M 1987 Long-term surveillance of mortality and cancer incidence in women receiving hormone replacement therapy. British Journal of Obstetrics and Gynaecology 94: 620–635
213. Lafferty FW, Helmuth DO 1985 Post-menopausal estrogen replacement: the prevention of osteoporosis and systemic benefits. Maturitas 7: 147–159
214. Vakil D, Morgan R, Halliday M 1983 Exogenous estrogens and development of breast and endometrial cancer. Cancer Detection and Prevention 6: 415–424
215. Persson I 1985 The risk of endometrial and breast cancer after estrogen treatment: a review of epidemiological studies. Acta Obstetrica Gynecologica Scandinavica 130: 59–66
216. Grady D, Gebretsadik T, Kerlikowske K, Ernster V, Petitti D 1995 Hormone replacement therapy and endometrial cancer risk: a meta-analysis. Obstetrics and Gynecology 85: 304–313
217. Herrinton LJ, Weiss NS 1993 Postmenopausal unopposed estrogens. Annals of Epidemiology 3: 308–318
218. Shapiro S, Kaufman D, Slone D, Rosenberg L, Miettinen O, Stolley P et al 1980 Recent and past use of conjugated estrogens in relation to adenocarcinoma of the endometrium. New England Journal of Medicine 303: 485–489
219. Hulka B, Kaufman D, Fowler W, Jr, Grimson R, Greenberg B 1980 Predominance of early endometrial cancers after long-term estrogen use. Journal of the American Medical Association 244: 2419–2422
220. Chu J, Schweid A, Weiss N 1982 Survival among women with endometrial cancer: a comparison of estrogen users and nonusers. American Journal of Obstetrics and Gynecology 143: 569–573
221. Collins JA, Allen L, Donner A, Adams O 1980 Oestrogen use and survival in endometrial cancer. Lancet 2: 961–964
222. Elwood JM, Boyes D 1980 Clinical and pathological features and survival of endometrial cancer patients in relation to prior use of estrogens. Gynecological Oncology 10: 173–187

223. Booth M, Beral V, Smith P 1989 Risk factors for ovarian cancer: a case-control study. British Journal of Cancer 60: 592–598
224. Cramer DW, Hutchison GB, Welch WR, Scully RE, Ryan KJ 1983 Determinants of ovarian cancer risk 1. Reproductive experiences and family history. Journal of the National Cancer Institute 71: 711–716
225. Hildreth NG, Kelsey JL, LaVolsi VA, Fischer DB, Holford TR, Mostow ED et al 1981 An epidemiologic study of epithelial carcinoma of the ovary. American Journal of Epidemiology 114: 398–405
226. Hartge P, Hoover R, McGowan L, Lesher L, Norris HJ 1988 Menopause and ovarian cancer. American Journal of Epidemiology 127: 990–998
227. Kaufman DW, Kelly JP, Welch WR, Rosenberg L, Stolley PD, Warshauer ME et al 1989 Noncontraceptive estrogen use and epithelial ovarian cancer. American Journal of Epidemiology 130: 1142–1151
228. Parazzini F, La Vecchia C, Negri E, Villa A 1994 Estrogen replacement therapy and ovarian cancer risk. International Journal of Cancer 57: 135–136
229. Polychronopoulou A, Tzonou A, Hsieh C-C, Kaprinis G, Rebelakos A, Toupadaki N et al 1993 Reproductive variables, tobacco, ethanol, coffee and somatometry as risk factors for ovarian cancer. International Journal of Cancer 55: 402–407
230. Rodriguez C, Calle EE, Coates RJ, Miracle-McMahill HL, Thun MJ, Heath CWJ 1995 Estrogen replacement therapy and fatal ovarian cancer. American Journal of Epidemiology 141: 828–835
231. Smith EM, Sowers MF, Burns TL 1984 Effects of smoking on the development of female reproductive cancers. Journal of the National Cancer Institute 73: 371–376
232. Weiss NS, Lyon JL, Krishnamurthy S, Dietert SE, Liff JM, Daling JR 1982 Noncontraceptive estrogen use and the occurrence of ovarian cancer. Journal of the National Cancer Institute 68: 95–98
233. Naessen T, Persson I, Adami H, Bergstrom R, Bergkvist L 1990 Hormone replacement therapy and the risk of first hip fracture: a prospective, population-based cohort study. Annals of Internal Medicine 113: 95–103
234. Falkeborn M, Persson I, Adami HO, Bergstrom R, Eaker E, Lithell H et al 1992 The risk of acute myocardial infarction after oestrogen and oestrogen-progestogen replacement. British Journal of Obstetrics and Gynaecology 99: 821–828
235. Stampfer MJ, Willett W, Colditz GA, Rosner B, Speizer F, Hennekens C 1985 A prospective study of postmenopausal estrogen therapy and coronary heart disease. New England Journal of Medicine 313: 1044–1049
236. Grady D, Rubin SM, Petitti DB, Fox CS, Black D, Ettinger B et al 1992 Hormone therapy to prevent disease and prolong life in postmenopausal women. Annals of Internal Medicine 117: 1016–1037

68. Influence of therapeutic steroids on the incidence and severity of breast cancer

Susan E. Hankinson M. Stampfer

Introduction: breast cancer incidence rates

Breast cancer incidence rates vary approximately fivefold worldwide, with the highest rates in North America and Northern Europe and the lowest rates in Asia and Africa.[1] In the United States, breast cancer is the most frequently diagnosed malignancy in women, with over 180 000 new cases diagnosed annually. Please refer to chapter 67 for further details of the methodology and descriptive epidemiology of reproductive cancers. Because of these high breast cancer incidence rates, coupled with a high prevalence of exogenous hormone use, the relationship between hormones and breast cancer risk has received intensive study.

PREVALENCE OF HORMONE USE

Oral contraceptives

Since oral contraceptives were first introduced in the 1960s, they have been used by millions of women. In 1988, over 10.7 million US women were currently using oral contraceptives.[2] Most combined oral contraceptives (COC) contain ethinyl estradiol (or mestranol which is metabolized to ethinyl estradiol) and a progestogen. The estrogen dose in COC has ranged from more than 80 µg in 1960 to 30 µg, the dose most commonly used today; during this same time period at least nine different progestogens have been used.[3,4] Patterns of use also have changed considerably over time with both increasing durations of use and a trend towards earlier ages at first use.

Postmenopausal hormones

Postmenopausal estrogens have been used for over half a century. By the mid 1970s almost 30 million prescriptions were being filled annually in the US.[5] Both the formulations prescribed (e.g. estrogen vs. estrogen plus progestogen), patterns of use (e.g. use over several years vs. a trend to long-term use today), and delivery systems (e.g. patch estrogen) have changed substantially over time.

One challenge in studying the relationships between exogenous hormones, either oral contraceptives or postmenopausal hormones, and breast cancer is the substantial variation in formulations and patterns of use over time. By the time sufficient use of one type of hormone has occurred to allow a detailed epidemiologic evaluation, new formulations are already being introduced.

BIOLOGIC PLAUSIBILITY OF AN ASSOCIATION WITH BREAST CANCER RISK

Several different lines of evidence support the hypothesis that exogenous estrogens play an important role in the etiology of breast cancer. Population studies from a variety of locations have shown that rates of breast cancer increase rapidly in the premenopausal years, but the rate of increase slows sharply at the time of menopause, when endogenous estrogens decline rapidly (Fig. 68.1). In addition, several reproductive variables that alter estrogen status affect risk of breast cancer (Table 68.1). For example, early age at menarche[6] and late age at menopause (reflecting prolonged ovarian function and estrogen production) are associated with increased risk of breast cancer.[7,8] During pregnancy, estrogen levels are markedly elevated, and this is associated with a temporary increase in breast cancer risk. The number of full-term pregnancies, and their timing, also affect the risk.[9,10] Estrogens and progesterone promote mammary tumors in animals, and hormonal manipulations such as anti-estrogens (e.g. tamoxifen) have been useful in the treatment of breast cancer.

Age at menopause also is a strong risk factor for breast cancer. Women who have menopause before age 45 have approximately half the risk of breast

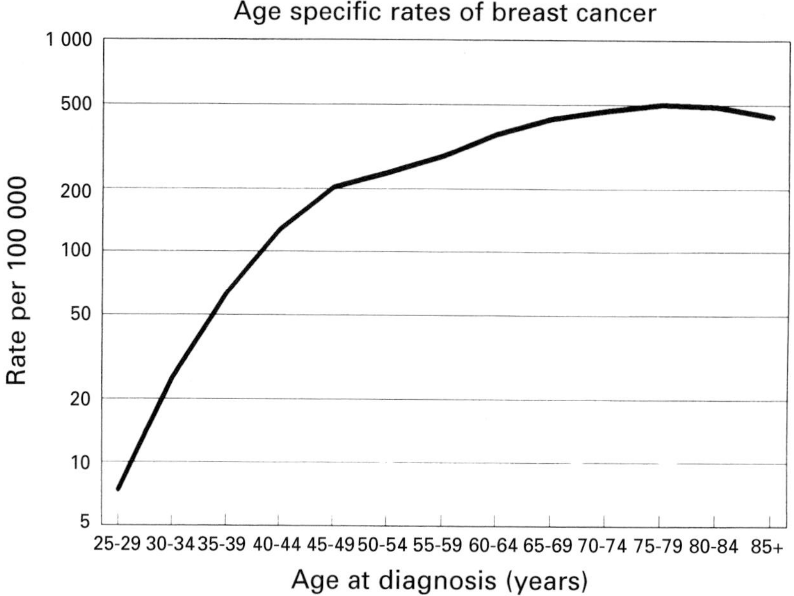

Fig. 68.1 Age-specific breast cancer incidence rates for US white women 1987–91. Surveillance, Epidemiology and End Results (SEER) Program, National Cancer Institute, National Institutes of Health, US Department of Health and Human Services

Table 68.1 Established hormonally-related risk factors for breast cancer.

Risk factor	Comparison category	Risk category	Typical relative risk	Study
Age at menarche	<12 years	12 years	0.9	Brinton et al 1988[6]
		13 years	0.8	
		14 years	0.9	
		≥15 years	0.8	
Age at birth of 1st child	Before 20 years	20–24 years	1.3	White 1987[9]
		25–29 years	1.6	
		≥30 years	1.9	
		Nulliparous	1.9	
Age at menopause	45–54 years	After 55 years	1.5	Trichopoulos et al 1972[11]
		Before 45 years	0.7	
		Oophorectomy before 35 years	0.4	
Obesity	BMI≤21*	BMI≥28	1.6	Huang et al 1997[12]

* BMI = kg/m²; relative risks given are among never users of postmenopausal hormones.

cancer compared to women who become menopausal after age 55 years.[11] In addition, after menopause, adipose tissue is the major source of estrogen and obese postmenopausal women have both higher levels of endogenous estrogen and a higher risk of breast cancer.[12,13,14] These observations suggest that altering the postmenopausal hormonal milieu to approach that of premenopausal women may lead to a continued acceleration rate of the breast cancer, as is observed in premenopausal women.

Epidemiologic study designs

Several different study designs have been used to address the relationship of exogenous estrogens and breast cancer risk. Each study design has unique strengths and limitations.

Case-control studies

In a case-control study, cases with and controls without the disease are queried about their past exposures. In the statistical analysis, the exposure experience in these two groups is compared. There are two primary types of case-control studies: hospital-based and population-based. In hospital-based studies, control subjects are patients hospitalized for conditions other than breast cancer. In a population-based study, controls are chosen from the general population.

The advantages of case-control studies are that they can be conducted relatively quickly and at a low cost. Thus, in general, case-control studies are quite helpful in evaluating exposures that are new or have changed recently. In addition, rare diseases can be evaluated quickly. Disadvantages are that these studies are more susceptible to selection and recall bias than are cohort studies. Selection bias occurs when selection of study subjects is related to both the exposure of interest and their case or control status. For example, in a hospital-based case-control study of postmenopausal hormones and heart disease, if enrolled controls have diagnoses related to estrogen use (e.g. patients with osteoporotic fractures) then the expected inverse association will be biased away from observing a benefit. The possibility of selection bias is a particular concern when participation rates among eligible subjects are low. Recall bias will occur if study subjects differentially report past exposures because of their current disease status.

Cohort studies

In a cohort study, healthy subjects are enrolled and then queried as to their current or past exposure history. These participants are followed over time and their disease status tracked. Disease rates in the exposed and nonexposed are then compared.

A major advantage of cohort studies is that, because the disease has not yet occurred at study entry, neither participation nor exposure information collected will depend on disease status, thus avoiding selection and recall biases. The main disadvantage of cohort studies is that they are either expensive (to accrue a sufficient number of cases in a reasonable period of time, thousands of subjects must be enrolled) or, if only a small cohort is established, few cases of disease will occur and thus statistical power will be limited. Thus, although this design is generally less subject to potential biases than case-control studies, few large cohort studies have been or are being conducted. Biases also can occur in a cohort study. If the completeness of follow-up varies by exposure and disease status, biased relative risks may be obtained. This type of bias can occur when medical surveillance is heightened in one of the exposure groups such that disease is detected earlier or more often, or if there is differential loss to follow-up in the different exposure groups.

In any observational study, either case-control or cohort, an additional type of bias, confounding, can occur and must be carefully evaluated. If a third factor, which is both correlated with the exposure of interest and an independent risk factor for disease, is unaccounted for in the analysis, biased relative risks may result. For example, in an evaluation of postmenopausal hormone use and breast cancer risk, it is important that body mass index (a measure of obesity) be accounted for in the analysis. Obesity is positively associated with breast cancer risk, and, as obese women are less likely to experience menopausal symptoms, tends to be inversely correlated with hormone use. Thus, if a true positive association exists between hormone use and breast cancer, failure to account for obesity may bias the relative risk towards no effect.

Randomized intervention trials

In a randomized trial, study subjects are randomly assigned use of an active agent (e.g. postmenopausal hormones) or a placebo. Ideally, to minimize the chance of bias, neither the study subjects nor the investigators interacting with the subjects know who is on active agent or placebo (i.e. a double-blind system). The study subjects are followed over time to assess their risk of disease. The randomization process is a major strength of these studies. Providing the study is large, randomization provides considerable reassurance that any observed study effects are not due to bias (including confounding). Although in theory the randomized trial is the best way to assess the relationship between exposure and disease, because of the high cost of these studies, the small number of formulations that can be addressed in any one study and the long study duration required, in practice much of what we know about exogenous estrogens and breast cancer will continue to be provided by observational studies.

ORAL CONTRACEPTIVES: EPIDEMIOLOGIC FINDINGS

Over 50 epidemiologic studies have evaluated the relationship between oral contraceptive use and breast cancer risk. Generally, the results have been quite reassuring in showing little if any increase in risk overall among ever users or users for extended durations. Several aspects of COC use, particularly long durations of use in young women or prior to a first pregnancy, have remained of concern. These findings are summarized below.

Any use of oral contraceptives

In several recent meta-analyses[15,16] and reviews[17] ever use of COC was unassociated with breast cancer risk with summary relative risks all being about 1.0 (e.g. RR = 1.1; 95% confidence interval (CI) = 0.9–1.4[16]). Although this finding is reassuring, defining COC use this way is misleading because women in the 'ever' use category will be a mix of women with long and short-term use, so that any true relationship with one particular aspect of COC use may be missed.

Duration of use

Overall

Most studies have observed no significant increase in breast cancer risk with long durations of use (≥5 years). In one meta-analysis where results from 10 studies were combined, the relative risk associated with 10 or more years of use was 1.14 (95% CI = 0.90–1.42).[16] In a second meta-analysis, the relative risk was 1.1 for greater than five years of use when results were combined for either nine case-control studies (95% CI = 0.9–1.2) or four cohort studies (95% CI = 0.9–1.4).[15] These results were from analyses where women of all ages were combined and provide considerable evidence against any material adverse effect of long-term COC use overall. Similar findings have generally been observed when long-term use was evaluated among either postmenopausal women or women over the age of 45 years. However, findings have not been quite as consistent or reassuring in analyses of long-term use in young women.

Duration of use among young women

In several studies[18–21] an elevated relative risk was observed among young women (generally less than 45 years) who used COC for extended durations. In two meta-analyses, summary relative risks for long durations of use in young women were 1.5[16] and 1.4 (95% CI = 1.3–1.6).[15] The greatest increase tended to be observed in the youngest women, generally women less than 35 years of age;[20,21,22] this observation also was noted in several more recent case-control studies.[23,24,25]

Recently, a large case-control study was conducted to specifically address this issue.[24] COC use data and information on standard breast cancer risk factors was collected from over 2000 breast cancer cases and a similar number of age-matched population-based controls, all of whom were less than 45 years of age. Participation rates were 86% among cases and 71% among controls.

Although women using COC for more than six months had an elevated risk of breast cancer (OR = 1.3; 95% CI = 1.1–1.5), when this association was examined in finer (five year) age strata, the increased risk was noted primarily among the youngest women. Among women <35 years, the relative risk associated with using COC for ≥10 years, compared to never use, was 2.3 (95% CI = 1.2–4.1). In contrast, among women 35–39 years of age, COC users had a small nonsignificant increased disease risk (≥10 years of use relative to never use: OR = 1.2; 95% CI = 0.8–1.9) and, among women 40–44 years of age, essentially no increase in risk was noted (≥10 years relative to never use: OR = 1.1; 95% CI = 0.8–1.6). The increased risk in the youngest women did not appear to be due to increased screening for breast cancer among the cases.

The primary limitation of the study was the 29% refusal rate among potential controls. However, the investigators collected some limited data from a proportion of the nonparticipants; including these data resulted in participation rates of 88.4% among cases and 84.8% among controls. Analyses using these additional data apparently yielded very similar findings. Thus, overall, results from this large and carefully conducted case-control study suggest that COC use among young women (predominantly those <35 years of age) may increase their breast cancer risk.

Several cohort studies also have evaluated these relationships.[26,27,28] In the Oxford Family Planning Association study, over 17 000 women aged 25–39 years were recruited in 1968–74 and followed until 1987, by which time 189 breast cancer cases had occurred.[26] No association was observed with increasing duration of use among women 25–44 years (relative risks varied from 0.8–1.1 for categories up to 10 or more years of use); only 14 cases were <35 years of age. In the Royal College of General Practitioners' cohort, 23 000 women who used COC and 23 000 nonusers were enrolled in 1968 and followed to 1985.[27] Although little if any increase in risk was noted with increasing duration of use overall, a substantial increased risk was observed among women ages 30–34 years (relative risks of 4.1, 2.2, 2.5 and 10.2 for COC use of 4–5, 6–7, 8–9, and 10+ years — all relative to never users). However, these results must be interpreted cautiously for several reasons. Only 24 cases of breast cancer occurred among women 30–34 years so the relative risk estimates were unstable, the follow-up rate in this cohort was low (as of 1985, the investigators had accounted for less than 60% of the total possible number of person-years of follow-up) and the incidence rate among the 30–34 year old women who did not use COC was considerably lower than the age-specific national breast cancer rates (especially in the youngest women).

The largest prospective study of this association was the Nurses' Health Study cohort. 121 700 women were enrolled in 1976 and have been followed every two years since that time. The follow-up rate in this cohort has been consistently 90% or higher. From 1976–86 (during which time 1799 breast cancers were reported and confirmed), no significant association was noted between duration of use and breast cancer risk among premenopausal women (relative risks of 1.05 and 0.59 for 10–15 and >15 years of use, relative to never use).[28] In a recent reanalysis of these data, with follow-up up to 1992, again no positive association was noted either among premenopasual women or among women over 35 years of age.[29] Both the Oxford and the Nurses' Health Study cohorts have provided considerable reassurance that no substantial increase in risk occurs among women over 35 years who used COC for extended durations. However, neither of these cohorts had a sufficient number of women under 35 years of age enrolled to evaluate the risk in this specific group. This issue will be addressed in detail within the next several years in a second Nurses' Health Study cohort which was started in the US in 1989 among 116 000 women who were 25–42 years of age in 1989.

Use before a first full-term pregnancy

Because any influence of COC on the breast was hypothesized to be greatest prior to the cellular differentiation that occurs with a full-term pregnancy,[30] a number of investigators have evaluated the effect of COC use prior to a first full-term pregnancy. In both meta-analyses, the summary relative risk indicated a modest increase in risk with long-term use (RR = 1.7;[16] RR = 1.4[15]). However, although the summarized relative risk was indeed elevated, results of individual studies tended to vary substantially and in few of the studies was a dose-response relationship noted between duration of use and disease risk.

Additionally, in several recent studies not included in these meta-analyses,[23,24,31] and in the large Nurses' Health Study cohort,[28,29] no increase in risk was observed specifically in relation to use prior to a first pregnancy.

Recency of use

Only a handful of studies have specifically evaluated the relationship between current or very recent use of COC and breast cancer risk, but in most that have at least a modest increased risk has been noted[21,24,28] relative to never users. These data suggest that COC may act as late stage promoters. In the Nurses' Health Study cohort, current users had a 50% higher risk than never users.[28] This increased risk did not appear attributable to increased disease detection among current COC users as these women tended to have larger tumors that were more likely to be metastatic at diagnosis.

Recently, individual data from 54 epidemiologic studies were collected and analyzed centrally to try to best summarize almost all the available data on oral contraceptive use and breast cancer risk.[32] In this large pooled analysis, data from 53 297 women with breast cancer and 100 239 women without breast cancer were evaluated. Overall, current and recent users of oral contraceptives were observed to have an increased risk of breast cancer (RR for current vs never users = 1.24; 95% CI = 1.15–1.33) (Table 68.2).

This increased risk subsided within 10 years of stopping COC use (RR by years since stopping use vs never use: 1–4 years 1.16, 5–9 years 1.07, 10–14 years 0.98, ≥15 years 1.03). Importantly, the authors observed a modest increased risk of breast cancer only among current and recent COC users, and did not observe any independent effect of long durations of use on risk of breast cancer even among very young women. Thus, based on this large pooled analysis, it would appear that the increased risk of breast cancer observed among young (<35 yrs), long-term COC users in past individual studies was due to recency of COC use rather than duration of use.

Type and dose of COC

The specific formulation of the COC might be important in determining cancer risk, but studies of this issue are difficult because study participants may not be able to remember specific formulations, very large studies are needed to have enough statistical power to examine individual brands and, finally, no satisfactory classification system exists to categorize specific COC

Table 68.2 Collaborative group on hormonal factors in breast cancer: duration of oral contraceptive use and recency of use in relation to breast cancer risk.

Duration of use and time since use	Relative risk* (standard deviation)
Never user	1.00 (0.01)
Current user	
Duration of use: ≤12 months	1.18 (0.12)
1–4 years	1.27 (0.08)
5–9 years	1.21 (0.06)
≥10 years	1.29 (0.06)
Last use 1–4 years ago	
Duration of use: ≤12 months	1.05 (0.08)
1–4 years	1.12 (0.06)
5–9 years	1.26 (0.06)
≥10 years	1.14 (0.06)
Last use 5–9 years ago	
Duration of use: ≤12 months	1.05 (0.06)
1–4 years	1.05 (0.04)
5–9 years	1.13 (0.04)
≥10 years	1.14 (0.06)
Last use 10–14 years ago	
Duration of use: ≤12 months	1.00 (0.04)
1–4 years	0.97 (0.04)
5–9 years	0.99 (0.05)
≥10 years	1.01 (0.08)
Last use ≥15 years ago	
Duration of use: ≤12 months	1.05 (0.04)
1–4 years	1.04 (0.04)
5–9 years	0.87 (0.06)
≥10 years	0.90 (0.15)

Collaborative Group on Hormonal Factors in Breast Cancer 1996 Lancet 347: 1713–1727
* Relative to never users, stratified by study, age at diagnosis, parity, age at first birth and age at which risk of conception ceased.

formulations by their effect on breast tissue. For these reasons, few studies have evaluated specific COC formulations in relation to breast cancer risk.

Most studies observed no apparent difference between formulations.[19,26,33,34] Other studies observed a modest increased risk[20,35] or decreased risk[23] among women who used pills with a higher estrogen dose (generally >50 µg). In one study, women using ethinyl estradiol versus mestranol (which is converted into ethinyl estradiol) appeared to have a slightly higher breast cancer risk[36] however this finding was not replicated in other studies. Thus, overall, there is little evidence overall of a differential effect according to type or dose of either estrogen or progestogen.

In the Nurses' Health Study II cohort, described above, data on the specific formulations used was collected and the validity of these self-reported data has been confirmed.[37] Therefore within the next five years additional data on effects of specific, contemporary COC formulations will be available from a large prospective cohort.

Interactions with other breast cancer risk factors

The possible interaction of COC use with other breast cancer risk factors has been evaluated in a substantial number of studies. However, limited statistical power in these subgroup analyses resulted in wide confidence limits (thus a limited ability to detect true differences) and the categorization of COC as ever versus never use – a crude and generally uninformative exposure definition. In the largest studies where any true differences are most likely to be detected (and defined here as those with over 1000 cases and a high prevalence of COC use), the relationship between COC use did not vary appreciably by family history of breast cancer,[15,21,24,25,38] history of benign breast disease,[21,39] or postmenopausal hormone use.[25] The relation between COC use and breast cancer within categories of age at menarche, body mass index and alcohol use also has been examined in a number of smaller studies, and overall no substantial differences have emerged.

Progestogen-only contraceptives

These contraceptives include progestogen-only pills ('mini-pill'), depot medroxyprogesterone acetate (DMPA) and implantable levonorgestrel (Norplant®). Although the progestogen-only pill has been evaluated in few studies, to date no increase in breast cancer risk has been observed for ever users[20,33,35,40,41] and, in the two studies where duration of use was evaluated[20,35] longer term users were observed to have either a similar or lower risk of breast cancer compared to never users. DMPA, an injectable contraceptive, also has had limited study in relation to breast cancer risk. In the most comprehensive study[42] of this relationship, no significant increase in risk was observed with increasing duration of use (RR for >3 years of use vs never use = 0.9, 95% CI = 0.6–1.4), although both long-term users who began use before age 25 and users under age 35 overall were observed to have a modest increase in breast cancer risk. Norplant, a long-acting contraceptive which is implanted subdermally, was introduced in the United States in 1990. No epidemiologic data have been published on Norplant's influence, if any, on breast cancer risk. Further epidemiologic research is needed for each of these drugs, particularly DMPA and Norplant.

Summary

Whether use of COC increases risk of breast cancer has been a long-standing concern and, as such, this relationship has been evaluated in over 50 epidemiologic studies. Results of these studies have provided considerable reassurance that there is little, if any, increase in risk with COC use in general, even among women who used COC for 10 or more years. Although there has been concern that long-term use prior to a first term pregnancy might increase breast cancer risk, accumulating data suggest that this aspect of COC use does not appreciably increase risk.

A relatively consistent finding among previous case-control studies, however, is an increase in risk among young women who used COC for extended durations. This observation has not been confirmed by the larger prospective studies, although these studies had few very young women (<35 years of age), the group most consistently observed to be at increased risk. In a recent pooled analysis on this topic (where original data from almost all of the individual studies was combined), long-term use among young women was not independently associated with an increase in breast cancer risk. Rather, current users and recent users (<10 years since last use) were observed to have a modest elevation in risk compared to never users. This relationship most likely could not be discerned from the individual studies, as duration of use, rather than recency of use, was often reported. Among young women, the long-term users are more likely to be recent users; large data sets (such as the pooled analysis) were needed to determine the independent effect of these variables.

It is important to note that current and recent users, the group that appears to have a modest increase in risk, are generally young (<45 years) and thus have a low absolute risk of breast cancer. Hence, a modest increase in their risk will result in few additional cases of breast cancer. Nevertheless, this apparent increased risk among current and recent users should be factored into the overall decision on whether or not to use COC.

POSTMENOPAUSAL HORMONE USE: EPIDEMIOLOGIC FINDINGS

Estrogen only

The possible relation between postmenopausal estrogen use (hormone replacement therapy, HRT) and risk of breast cancer has been investigated in over three dozen epidemiologic studies over the past 20 years.[43–47] Most of these studies have been summarized in six meta-analyses[42,48–52] and a recent large pooled analysis.[53] A summary of these findings, plus a more detailed discussion of several of the most important and most recent studies, is provided below.

Any use

All the meta-analyses have concluded that overall, ever users of postmenopausal estrogens have little or no increase in risk of breast cancer compared with women who have never used this therapy. Depending upon the inclusion criteria for the meta-analyses, the relative risk estimates across studies range from 1.01–1.07. Moreover, the 95% confidence limits around these summary estimates are narrow, and the highest upper bound observed in these analyses was 1.12.

Duration of use

Although the overall results comparing risk estimates in ever to never users provide a useful first step, these findings have the potential to underestimate the true effect. The group of all 'ever users' will, in many populations, include a large number of women with relatively short durations of use, perhaps many with just a few months of use. Moreover, the broad 'ever use' category will include a mix of both women who are currently using estrogen and those whose only exposure was in the distant past. Recognizing these limitations, several investigators have provided summary findings from studies that have examined risk of breast cancer by duration of postmenopausal hormone use (Table 68.3). In a meta-analysis limited to case-control studies, Steinberg et al[49] used a statistical model to evaluate the relation between duration of use and risk; they reported a significant increase in risk with longer duration of use, estimating a 30% increase in risk with more than five years of use. In a subsequent analysis, Steinberg et al found a 45% increase in risk after 10 years of use when combining results from the follow-up studies.[49] In another meta-analysis, Colditz et al[51] calculated a summary relative risk of 1.23 (95% CI: 1.08–1.40) for 10 or more years of hormone use. Sillero-Arenas[50] found the same overall estimate, but when stratified by menopause type, the relative risks were somewhat higher: for more than 12 years of use, among women with a natural menopause, the relative risk was 1.32 (1.08–1.40), and for those with a surgical menopause, 1.63 (95% CI: 1.26–2.12). Grady et al also calculated a significant increase in risk with eight or more years of use, with a relative risk of 1.25 (95% CI: 1.04–1.51).[43]

Table 68.3 Summary of epidemiologic studies of the relationship between duration of postmenopausal hormone use and breast cancer risk.

Hormone use Meta-analysis	Number of studies in meta-analysis		Duration of relative risk (95% CI)		
Steinberg et al 1991[49]	18 case-control		Never	1.0	
	6 cohort		≥15 years	1.3	(1.2–1.6)
Sillero-Arenas et al 1992[50]	23 case-control		Never	1.0	
	13 cohort		≤1 year	1.1	(0.9–1.2)
	1 clinical trial		1–3 years	1.0	(0.9–1.1)
			4–7 years	1.2	(1.1–1.3)
			8–11 years	0.9	(0.7–1.2)
			≥12 years	1.2	(1.1–1.4)
Grady et al 1992[43]	24 case-control				
	10 cohort		Never	1.0	
	1 clinical trial		≥8 years	1.3	(1.0–1.5)
Colditz et al 1993[51]	25 case-control		Never	1.0	
	6 cohort		≥10 years	1.2	(1.0–1.4)
Recent studies	**Type**	**Size***	**Duration of hormone use**		
Schairer et al 1994[56]	Cohort	640/313 902	None	1.0	
			<5 years***	1.4	(1.1–1.9)
			5–9 years	1.2	(0.9–1.7)
			10–14 years	1.0	(0.7–1.5)
			≥15 years	1.3	(1.0–1.7)
Colditz et al 1995[46]	Cohort	1935/725 550	Never	1.0	
			<2 years***	1.1	(0.9–1.4)
			2–4 years	1.1	(0.9–1.4)
			5–9 years	1.4	(1.2–1.6)
			≥10 years	1.5	(1.2–1.8)
Stanford et al 1995[54]	Case-control	537/492	Never	1.0	
			1–3 months	1.1	(0.5–2.0)
			4–35 months	1.0	(0.6–1.6)
			3–4 years	0.9	(0.4–1.8)
			5–7 years	1.2	(0.7–2.2)
			8–11 years	0.5	(0.3–0.9)
			12–14 years	1.0	(0.5–2.0)
			15–19 years	0.5	(0.3–1.0)
			20+ years	1.0	(0.5–2.0)
Schuurman et al 1995[45]	Cohort	471/5446**	Never	1.0	
			≤1 year	0.8	(0.5–1.5)
			2–4 years	1.4	(0.7–2.7)
			≥5 years	0.9	(0.4–2.1)
Newcomb et al 1995[44]	Case-control	3130/3698	Never	1.0	
			<2 years	0.9	(0.7–1.1)
			2–4 years	1.1	(0.9–1.4)
			5–9 years	0.9	(0.7–1.2)
			10–14 years	0.9	(0.7–1.3)
			≥15 years	1.0	(0.8–1.3)

* Number of cases and controls (case-control studies) or cases/person-years (cohort studies);
** Overall cohort consisted of 62 573 members. A case-cohort design was used in the data analysis;
*** Duration among *current* hormone users only for each exposure category.

Results of several large studies have become available since the publication of these meta-analyses. The largest of these, in terms of number of cases, was a population-based case-control study of 3130 cases and 3698 controls conducted in Wisconsin, Massachusetts, Maine and New Hampshire.[44] Study subjects were all less than 75 years of age and participation rates were 81% among cases and 84% among controls. The investigators did not observe a significant positive association between postmenopausal hormone use and breast cancer risk, even among long-term users. The risk associated with ≥15 years of estrogen use, relative to never use, was 1.11 (95% CI: 0.87–1.43).

In another recent case-control study, Stanford et al[54] enrolled 537 women with breast cancer and 492 randomly selected control women, all 50–64 years of age. Cases were ascertained through a population-based cancer surveillance system (SEER program). In this study, no significant associations between postmenopausal hormone use and breast cancer risk were noted, regardless of duration of use. Compared to never users, women using HRT for 12–14, 15–19 and ≥20 years had a breast cancer risk of 1.0 (95% CI = 0.5–2.0), 0.5 (95% CI = 0.3–1.0) and 1.0 (95% CI = 0.5–2.0) respectively. However, as with the study by Newcomb et al the 95% confidence intervals were broad enough to encompass the elevated relative risks observed in the meta-analyses.

One potential difficulty in interpreting the results of case-control studies is the impact of nonparticipation, particularly among the controls. For example, in the Stanford study, the response rate among controls was approximately 70%. In the general population, estrogen users tend to have a somewhat higher socio-economic status on average[55] and, typically, better educated individuals are more likely to participate as controls in health-related research studies. Thus, if the responding controls were more likely to be estrogen users than the nonresponding controls, the observed relative risk may have been biased towards 1.0 (no effect). As any true increase in risk is likely to be small, even a modest bias in control participation could obscure the results.

Data from several recent cohort studies, not included in the meta-analyses, are available. Initial results from the prospective Netherlands Cohort study of 62 573 women (including 471 cases) were recently reported.[45] However, long-term use was uncommon, with only 14 cases in the category of five or more years of use. The relative risk in this category was 0.9 (95% CI = 0.4–2.1); these broad confidence intervals are clearly compatible with a wide range of true effects. Similar null findings with broad confidence intervals were observed among the small number of recent users.

Colditz et al recently reported updated results from the Nurses' Health Study.[46] This is the largest prospective study conducted to date on this topic, with 725 550 person-years of follow-up among postmenopausal women, and 1935 cases of newly diagnosed invasive breast cancer. In this analysis, because of the similar findings for estrogen and estrogen plus progestogen use, results were presented for all hormone use combined. An excess risk of breast cancer was limited to women with current or very recent use of postmenopausal hormones. The risk increased with increasing duration of use, and was statistically significant among current users of five or more years duration (compared to never users of HRT: RR for 5–9 years of use = 1.36, 95% CI = 1.15–1.61; RR for ≥10 years of use = 1.47, 95% CI = 1.22–1.76).

Recency of use

Data on recency of use have been sparse because many studies did not distinguish current from past users. The Sillero-Arenas meta-analysis calculated a relative risk for current use of 1.63 for women with natural menopause and 1.48 for women with surgical menopause. Colditz et al estimated a summary relative risk of 1.40 (95% CI = 1.20–1.63) comparing current to never users.

In the recently published multi-center case-control study,[44] recent long-term use (at least five years use within two years of the cases' date of diagnosis) was not associated with an increased risk, with a relative risk of 0.91 (0.72–1.14), based on 174 cases. Similarly, in the case-control study by Stanford et al[53] no significant associations between postmenopausal hormone use and breast cancer risk were noted regardless of recency of use (RR for current use vs never use = 0.9; 95% CI = 0.7–1.3). In this study, the 95% confidence intervals were broad enough to encompass the modestly elevated relative risks observed in the meta-analyses and the duration of use was not distinguished in the current use group.

In the recent report from the large Nurses' Health Study cohort,[46] an excess risk of breast cancer was limited to women with current or very recent use of postmenopausal hormones. In contrast, past users did not appear to be at increased risk regardless of duration of use. Specifically, among current users, only women with five or more years of use had a significantly increased risk of breast cancer (RR for 5–9 years of use = 1.36, 95% CI = 1.15–1.61; RR for ≥10 years of use = 1.47; 95% CI = 1.22–1.76, all compared to never users). The effect appeared to be slightly greater among older women, although these differences were not statistically significant. Women currently using HRT who had used it for less than five years were not observed to have an increased risk of breast cancer (compared to never use: use for <2 years RR= 1.09, 95% CI = 0.87–1.37; use for 2–4 years RR= 1.13, 95% CI = 0.94–1.35). In the Breast Cancer Detection Demonstration project cohort a positive association with invasive breast cancer was noted among current users of 5–≥15 years duration that varied little by duration of use (relative risks ranged from 1.0 to 1.4).[56]

This relationship was evaluated in considerable detail in the recently published pooled analysis, which combined results of 51 epidemiologic studies.[53] The investigators observed a statistically significant association between current or recent use of HRT and risk of breast cancer; the positive association was strongest among those with the longest duration of use. For example, among women who used HRT within the previous five years (compared to never HRT users), the relative risks for duration of use were 1.08 for 1–4 years of use, 1.31 for 5–9 years, 1.24 for 10–14 years and 1.56 for ≥15 years of use. No significant increase in breast cancer risk was noted for women who had quit using HRT five or more years in the past, regardless of their duration of use.

Some investigators have suggested that the increased risk observed in many of the studies may be an artifact of increased surveillance for breast cancer among women taking hormones. Consistent with such a possibility, both Colditz et al and Schairer et al[55] reported a higher relative risk associated with *in situ* disease than invasive disease. However, in both of these studies a significant positive (although weaker) association was noted when only invasive breast cancer cases were considered. Colditz et al also evaluated the potential for this bias in several other ways. In this population of nurses, mammography rates were uniformly high, exceeding 90% even among women who never used hormones. Moreover, past users and current users of short duration were not observed to have an elevated risk, despite higher mammography rates than the never users of HRT. Finally, a higher death rate from breast cancer was observed among current users of 10 or more years duration at the time of diagnosis. This latter analysis indicates that the breast cancers detected among the long-term hormone users were not being detected at an earlier stage (and would result in a better prognosis), thus providing further evidence that the association cannot be explained as an artifact of screening. It should be noted that two large studies have reported a lower mortality rate from breast cancer in women whose cancers were detected while they were taking HRT compared with the group whose cancers were detected when they were not using HRT.[57,58] This issue of death rates from breast cancer in users and nonusers of HRT requires further study.

Type, dose and mode of delivery of estrogen

Limited data are available regarding the effects of dose or type of estrogen on breast cancer risk. In most studies where the issue was examined, typically the analysis was limited to a comparison of ever versus never use.

In the US, approximately three quarters of the hormone use has been conjugated equine estrogens, thus findings from most US studies represent use of conjugated estrogens only. Colditz et al[46] observed similar increases in breast cancer risk among current users of conjugated estrogen alone (RR = 1.32; 95% CI = 1.14–1.54) and other estrogen formulations (RR = 1.28; 95% CI = 0.97–1.71), all compared to never users. In the Swedish cohort, the relative risk of breast cancer appeared slightly higher among users of estradiol formulations (relative risks of 2.3 and 1.8 for 6–9 and >9 years respectively) than among women using conjugated estrogens (RR 1.3 for ≥6 years of use) although relatively few women used conjugated estrogens and thus the estimates were imprecise.[59] In addition, approximately one third of these women also used a progestogen. In a meta-analysis where published results from European (n=3) and US studies (n=9) were separately pooled,[51] the relative risk for ever use was higher in Europe (1.31) than in the US (1.05), again suggesting that synthetic estrogens may confer a slightly higher breast cancer risk than use of conjugated estrogens.

The most commonly prescribed dosages of conjugated estrogen have been 0.625 and 1.25 mg/day, although both lower and higher doses have been available. In several meta-analyses that examined the influence of dose on breast cancer risk (generally <1.25 mg/day vs ≥1.25 mg/day), no substantial variation in effect was observed[48,51] although the relative risks observed for higher doses tended to vary from study to study. Colditz et al,[60] in the Nurses' Health Study data, observed similar associations for all doses up to 1.25 mg/day (for current vs never use: 0.3 mg/day RR = 1.55, 95% CI = 1.0–2.5; 0.625 mg/day RR = 1.42, 95% CI = 1.0–1.9; 1.25 mg/day RR = 1.48, 95% CI = 1.0–2.2) and a somewhat higher relative risk among women who used >1.25 mg/day (RR = 2.27; 95% CI = 1.0–5.3). Because of the small number of women using these higher doses, this estimate is imprecise and not significantly different from the RRs associated with the lower dose formulations. Stanford et al recently observed no difference in risk according to dose of conjugated estrogen (≤0.625 mg vs >0.625 mg) or by type of estrogen formulation (conjugated estrogen vs other estrogens).[53]

Although the effect of estrogen use on breast cancer risk could be reasonably hypothesized to vary by mode of estrogen delivery (e.g. patch estrogen, by avoiding the first pass effect in the liver, does not increase SHBG to the extent that oral preparations do), insufficient data are currently available to evaluate these potential differences.

Risk according to breast cancer risk factor profile

Several studies have evaluated the association between estrogen use and breast cancer risk within strata of other breast cancer risk factors, such as age, family history of breast cancer, adiposity, previous oral contraceptive use and alcohol intake. However, to date these analyses have generally been limited by the small number of participants in any one subgroup, thus leading to the examination of ever versus never hormone use (instead of the preferred duration and recency of use) and to imprecise estimates of relative risk.

In a meta-analysis, Colditz et al observed that the estrogen/breast cancer relationship did not vary substantially by family history of breast cancer (evaluated in 10 studies), benign breast disease (12 studies), and type of menopause or number of ovaries. In some[49,61,62,63] but not all studies, a slightly higher relative risk has been observed among older women.

Although the findings have not been entirely consistent, at least six studies have reported a modestly stronger association between estrogen use and breast cancer among leaner women.[46,62,64,65] Additional support for this relation was provided by the recent pooled analysis.[53] In two prospective studies,[59,66] this association was stronger among women who reported alcohol use.

Estrogen plus progestogen use

The addition of a progestogen to estrogen regimens has become increasingly common as it minimizes or eliminates the increased risk of endometrial hyperplasia and cancer associated with using unopposed estrogens. In the US, by the mid-1980s, almost 30% of postmenopausal hormone prescriptions included a prescription for progestogen.[67] The impact, if any, of an added progestogen to the risk of breast cancer has been evaluated only in the last few years and remains controversial.

Two of the first studies to assess this relationship suggested that the addition of a progestogen could decrease breast cancer risk.[68,69] However, these studies were small and potentially important confounders (e.g. age, parity) were not accounted for in the analysis. Since this time, several additional studies have assessed this relationship and together these studies indicate that a substantial protective effect of typical doses used in postmenopausal hormone therapy can be ruled out.[46]

Findings from these latter studies have not been consistent however. In several case-control studies[70,71] but not others[62,72] an increased risk with use of estrogen plus progestogen was suggested. Neither of the two most recent case-control studies has observed a significant increase in risk with estrogen plus progestogen use.[44,53] Stanford et al reported relative risks of 1.0 (95% CI = 0.4–2.2) and 0.4 (95% CI = 0.2–1.0) for 5–<8 and ≥8 years of use, respectively. Newcomb et al observed a relative risk of 1.1 (95% CI = 0.5–2.3) among users for ≥15 years. In both of these studies, medroxyprogesterone acetate was the progestogen used most commonly.

Only two prospective studies have reported on this relationship and their findings were similar. Bergkvist et al observed a relative risk of 4.4 (95% CI = 0.9–22.4) among women who used estrogen plus progestogen for ≥6 years compared to never users.[56] Women using hormones for shorter duration did not appear at an increased risk (relative risks varied from 0.5–0.9) but confidence intervals again were wide and did not exclude either a modest increase or decrease in risk. The type of progestogen used among these women was not specified. Colditz et al recently reported findings from the Nurses' Health Study where, among women using progestogens, about two-thirds used 10 mg of medroxyprogesterone for 14 or fewer days per month.[46] The relative risk associated with current estrogen plus progestogen use versus never use was 1.4 (95% CI = 1.2–1.7), very similar to that reported for estrogen use alone. Thus, overall, although the recently published papèrs differed in their findings, within each study no material difference in risk was observed comparing those who used estrogen alone and those using estrogen plus progestogen. To date, the weight of the evidence suggests that a modest increase in breast cancer risk also is observed among women using estrogen plus progestogens for extended durations.

Widespread use of estrogen plus progestogen is so recent that few data are available to evaluate the effect of different formulations, doses or schedules of use on risk of breast cancer.

Summary of data on postmenopausal hormone use and breast cancer risk

Although aspects of the relationship between HRT and breast cancer risk remain unresolved, several areas of agreement have emerged. The finding of no increase in risk comparing ever to never users is consistent and reassuring. Much of that observation reflects the experience among short-term users, and hormone use in the past. Among these groups, most studies are in agreement that little if any excess risk is present.

Although not entirely consistent, overall, the findings also suggest an increased risk in two important subgroups of users: users of long duration and current users. In general, users of long duration are more likely to be current users, so in many studies these two groups overlap substantially. Part of the inconsistency in findings between studies likely stems from the limited number of cases in any given study in these two groups. From a biological perspective, these are the groups one would most expect to demonstrate a relation with breast cancer risk. If one applies the model of postmenopausal hormone use as mimicking delayed menopause, one might expect increases in the relative risk of the approximate magnitude observed for an increase of five years of premenopausal status. In addition, exogenous estrogens are well known to increase progression of mammary tumors in animal models, and appear to act in a very late stage, perhaps stimulating growth in tumors which are already present but undiagnosed.

Although better and more complete information will be forthcoming in the future, as a number of additional studies are being conducted, it is unlikely that the current controversies will be fully settled in the foreseeable future. For now, the weight of the evidence suggests little or no increase in risk among users of short duration, or of use in the past. However, current longer term use does appear to be associated with an increased risk of breast cancer. This increase in risk is small in relative terms but is large enough, and well enough supported, to be considered as part of a balanced perspective along with the other risks and benefits of postmenopausal hormone therapy.

REFERENCES

1. Kelsey JL, Ross-Horn PL 1993 Breast cancer: magnitude of the problem and descriptive epidemiology. Epidemiology Reviews 15: 7–16
2. Committee on the Relationship Between Oral Contraceptives and Breast Cancer, Institute of Medicine 1991 Oral contraceptives and breast cancer. National Academy Press, Washington, DC
3. Piper JM, Kennedy DL 1987 Oral contraceptives in the United States: trends in content and potency. International Journal of Epidemiology 16: 215–221
4. Annegers JF 1989 Patterns of oral contraceptive use in the United States. British Journal of Rheumatology 28 (Suppl 1): 48–50
5. Kennedy DL, Baum C 1985 Noncontraceptive estrogens and progestins: use patterns over time. Obstetrics and Gynecology 65: 441–446
6. Brinton LA, Schairer C, Hoover RN et al 1988 Menstrual factors and risk of breast cancer. Cancer Investigation 6: 245–254
7. Lilienfeld AM 1956 The relationship of cancer of the female breast to artificial menopause and marital status. Cancer 9: 927–934
8. Feinleib M 1968 Breast cancer and artificial menopause: a cohort study. Journal of the National Cancer Institute 41: 315–329
9. White E 1987 Projected changes in breast cancer incidence due to the trend toward delayed childbearing. American Journal of Public Health 77: 495–497
10. Rosner B, Colditz GA, Willett WC 1994 Reproductive risk factors in a prospective study of breast cancer: The Nurses' Health Study. American Journal of Epidemiology 139: 819–835
11. Trichopoulos D, MacMahon B, Cole P 1972 Menopause and breast cancer risk. Journal of the National Cancer Institute 48: 605–613
12. Huang Z, Hankinson SE, Colditz GA, Stampfer MJ, Hunter DJ, Manson JE et al 1997 Dual effects of weight and weight gain on breast cancer risk. Journal of the American Medical Association 278: 1407–1411
13. Tretli S 1989 Height and weight in relation to breast cancer morbidity and mortality: a prospective study of 570,000 women in Norway. International Journal of Cancer 129: 22–30
14. Lew EA, Garfinkel L 1979 Variations in mortality by weight among 750,000 men and women. Journal of Chronic Disease 32: 563–576
15. Thomas DB 1991 Oral contraceptives and breast cancer: review of the epidemiologic literature. Contraception 43: 597–642
16. Romieu I, Berlin JA, Colditz GA 1990 Oral contraceptives and breast cancer: review and meta-analysis. Cancer 66: 2253–2263
17. Malone KE, Daling JR, Weiss NS 1993 Oral contraceptives in relation to breast cancer. Epidemiology Reviews 15: 80–97
18. Meirik O, Farley TMM, Lund E, Adami H-O, Christoffersen T, Bergsjö P 1989 Breast cancer and oral contraceptives: patterns of risk among parous and nulliparous women — further analysis of the Swedish-Norwegian material. Contraception 39: 471–475
19. Miller DR, Rosenberg L, Kaufman DW, Stolley P, Warshauer ME, Shapiro S 1989 Breast cancer before age 45 and oral contraceptive use: new findings. American Journal of Epidemiology 129: 269–280
20. UK National Case-Control Study Group 1989 Oral contraceptive use and breast cancer risk in young women. Lancet i: 973–982

21. The WHO Collaborative Study of Neoplasia and Steroid Contraceptives 1990 Breast cancer and combined oral contraceptives: results from a multinational study. British Journal of Cancer 61: 110–119
22. Wingo PA, Lee NC, Ory HW, Beral V, Peterson HB, Rhodes P 1991 Age-specific differences in the relationship between oral contraceptive use and breast cancer. Obstetrics and Gynecology 78: 161–170
23. Rookus MA, Leeuwen FE, for the Netherlands Oral Contraceptives and Breast Cancer Study Group 1994 Oral contraceptives and risk of breast cancer in women aged 20–54 years. Lancet 344: 844–851
24. Brinton LA, Daling JR, Liff JM, Schoenberg JB, Malone KE, Stanford JL et al 1995 Oral contraceptives and breast cancer risk among younger women. Journal of National Cancer Institute 87: 827–835
25. Rosenberg L, Palmer JR, Rao S, Zauber AG, Strom BL, Warshauer ME, Harlap S, Shapiro S 1996 Case-control study of oral contraceptive use and risk of breast cancer. American Journal of Epidemiology 143: 25–37
26. Vessey MP, McPherson K, Villard-Mackintosh L, Yeates D 1989 Oral contraceptives and breast cancer: latest findings in a large cohort study. British Journal of Cancer 59: 613–617
27. Kay CR, Hannaford PC 1988 Breast Cancer and the pill — a further report from the Royal College of General Practitioners' oral contraception study. British Journal of Cancer 58: 675–680
28. Romieu I, Willett WC, Colditz GA, Stampfer MJ, Rosner B, Hennekens CH, Speizer FE 1989 Prospective study of oral contraceptive use and risk of breast cancer in women. Journal of National Cancer Institute 81: 1313–1321
29. Hankinson SE, Colditz GA, Manson JE, Willett WC, Hunter DJ, Stampfer MJ, Speizer FE 1997 A prospective study of oral contraceptive use and risk of breast cancer (Nurses' Health Study, United States). Cancer Causes and Control 8: 65–72
30. Russo J, Gusterson BA, Rogers AE, Russo IH, Wellings SR, van Zwieten MJ 1990 Biology of disease: comparative study of human and rat mammary tumorigenesis. Laboratory Investigation 62: 244–278
31. White E, Malone KE, Weiss NS et al 1994 Breast cancer among young US women in relation to oral contraceptive use. Journal National Cancer of Institute 86: 505–514
32. Collaborative Group on Hormonal Factors in Breast Cancer 1996 Breast cancer and hormonal contraceptives. Lancet 347: 1713–1727
33. Clavel F, Andrieu N, Gairard B, Bremond A, Piana L, Lansac J et al 1991 Oral contraceptives and breast cancer: a French case-control study. International Journal of Epidemiology 20: 32–38
34. Thomas DB, Noonan EA, and the WHO Collaborative Study of Neoplasia and Steroid Contraceptives 1992 Breast cancer and specific types of combined oral contraceptives. British Journal of Cancer 65: 108–113
35. Ewertz M 1992 Oral contraceptives and breast cancer risk in Denmark. European Journal of Cancer 28A: 1176–1181
36. McPherson K, Vessey MP, Neil A, Doll R, Jones L, Roberts M 1987 Early oral contraceptive use and breast cancer: results of another case-control study. British Journal of Cancer 56: 653–660
37. Hunter D, Colditz G, Manson J, Stampfer M, Speizer F, Willett WC 1993. Prospective study of oral contraceptive use before first pregnancy and breast cancer risk among younger women. American Journal of Epidemiology 138: 643 (abstract)
38. Murray PP, Stadel BV, Schlesslman JJ 1989 Oral contraceptive use in women with a family history of breast cancer. Obstetrics and Gynecology 73: 977–983
39. Sattin RW, Wingo PA, Lee NC 1987 Oral-contraceptive use the risk of breast cancer. New England Journal of Medicine 316: 163–164
40. Vessey M, Baron J, Doll R et al 1983 Oral contraceptives and breast cancer: final report of an epidemiological study. British Journal of Cancer 47: 455–462
41. The Cancer and Steroid Hormone Study of the Centers for Disease Control and the National Institute of Child Health and Human Development 1986 Oral contraceptive use and the risk of breast cancer. New England Journal of Medicine 315: 405–411
42. WHO Collaborative Study of Neoplasia and Steroid Contraceptives 1991 Breast cancer and depot-medroxyprogesterone acetate: a multinational study. Lancet 338: 833–838
43. Grady D, Rubin SM, Petitti DB, Fox CS, Black D, Ettinger B, Ernster VL, Cummings SR 1992 Hormone therapy to prevent disease and prolong life in postmenopausal women. Annals of Internal Medicine 117: 1016–1036
44. Newcomb PA, Longnecker MP, Storer BE, Mittendorf R, Baron J, Clapp RW, Bogdan G, Willett WC 1995 Long-term hormone replacement therapy and risk of breast cancer in postmenopausal women. American Journal of Epidemiology 142: 788–795
45. Schuurman AG, van den Brandt PA, Goldbohm RA 1995 Exogenous hormone use and the risk of postmenopausal breast cancer: results from the Netherlands Cohort Study. Cancer Causes and Control 6: 416–424
46. Colditz GA, Hankinson SE, Hunter DJ, Willett WC, Manson JE, Stampfer MJ et al 1995 The use of estrogens and progestins and the risk of breast cancer in postmenopausal women. New England Journal of Medicine 332: 1589–1593
47. Stanford JL, Thomas DB 1993 Exogenous progestins and breast cancer. Epidemiology Reviews 15: 98–107
48. Dupont WD, Page DL 1991 Menopausal estrogen replacement therapy and breast cancer. Archives of International Medicine 151: 67–72
49. Steinberg KK, Thacker SB, Smith SJ, Stroup DF, Zack MM, Flanders WD, Berkelman RL 1991 A meta-analysis of the effect of estrogen replacement therapy on the risk of breast cancer. Journal American of Medicine Association 265: 1985–1990
50. Sillero-Arenas M, Delgado-Rodriquez M, Rodigues-Canteras R, Bueno-Cavanillas A, Galvez-Vargas R 1992 Menopausal hormone replacement therapy and breast cancer: a meta-analysis. Obstetrics and Gynecology 79: 286–294
51. Colditz GA, Egan KM, Stampfer MJ 1993 Hormone replacement therapy and risk of breast cancer: results from epidemiologic studies. American Journal of Obstetrics and Gynecology 168: 1473–1480
52. Steinberg KK, Smith SJ, Thacker SB, Stroup DF 1994 Breast cancer risk and duration of estrogen use: the role of study design in meta-analysis. Epidemiology 5: 415–421

53. Collaborative Group on Hormonal Factors in Breast Cancer 1997 Breast cancer and hormone replacement therapy: collaborative reanalysis of data from 51 epidemiologic studies of 52 705 women with breast cancer and 108 411 women without breast cancer. Lancet 350: 1047–1059
54. Stanford JL, Weiss NS, Voigt LF, Daling JR, Habel LA, Rossing MA 1995 Combined estrogen and progestin hormone replacement therapy in relation to risk of breast cancer in middle-aged women. Journal of the American Medicine Association 274: 137–142
55. Egeland GM, Matthews KA, Kuller LH, Kelsey SF 1988 Characteristics of noncontraceptive hormone users. Preventive Medicine 17: 403–411
56. Schairer C, Byrne C, Keyl PM, Brinton LA, Sturgeon SR, Hoover RN 1994 Menopausal estrogen and estrogen-progestin replacement therapy and risk of breast cancer (United States). Cancer Causes and Control 5: 491–500
57. Willis DB, Calee EE, Miracle-McMahill H, Heath C 1996 Estrogen replacement therapy and risk of fatal breast cancer in a prospective cohort of postmenopausal women in the United States. Cancer Causes and Control 7: 449–457
58. Holli K, Isola J, Cusick J 1998 Hormone replacement therapy and biological ?????? 350: 1704–1705???
59. Bergkvist L, Adami H-O, Persson I, Hoover R, Schairer C 1989 The risk of breast cancer after estrogen and estrogen-progestin replacement. New England Journal of Medicine 321: 293–297
60. Colditz GA, Stampfer MJ, Willett WC, Hennekens CH, Rosner B, Speizer FE 1990 Prospective study of estrogen replacement therapy and risk of breast cancer in postmenopausal women. Journal of the American Medical Association 264: 2648–2653
61. Brinton LA, Hoover R, Fraumeni JR Jr 1986 Menopausal oestrogens and breast cancer risk: an expanded case-control study. British Journal of Cancer 54: 825–832
62. Wingo PA, Layde PM, Lee NC et al 1987 The risk of breast cancer in postmenopausal women who have used estrogen replacement therapy. Journal of the American Medical Association 257: 209–215
63. Palmer JR, Rosenberg L, Clarke EA et al 1991 Breast Cancer risk after estrogen replacement therapy: results from the Toronto Breast Cancer Study. American Journal of Epidemiology 134: 1386–1395
64. Mills PK, Beeson L, Phillips RL et al 1989 Prospective study of exogenous hormone use and breast cancer in Seventh-day Adventists. Cancer 64: 591–597
65. Harris RE, Namboodiri KK, Wynder EL 1992 Breast cancer risk: effects of estrogen replacement therapy and body mass. Journal of National Cancer Institute 84: 1575–1582
66. Gapstur SM, Potter JD, Sellers TA et al 1992 Increased risk of breast cancer with alcohol consumption in postmenopausal women. American Journal of Epidemiology 136: 1221–1231
67. Hemminki E, Kennedy DL, Baum C, McKinlay SM 1988 Prescribing of noncontraceptive estrogens and progestins in the United States, 1974–1986. American Journal of Public Health 78: 1479–1481
68. Nachtigall LE, Nachtigall RH, Nachtigall RD, Beckman EM 1979 Estrogen replacement therapy II: a prospective study in the relationship to carcinoma and cardiovascular and metabolic problems. Obstetrics and Gynecology 54: 74–79
69. Gambrell RD, Maier RC, Sanders BI 1983 Decreased incidence of breast cancer in postmenopausal estrogen-progestogen users. Obstetrics and Gyencology 62: 435–445
70. Ewertz M 1988 Influence of non-contraceptive exogenous and endogenous sex hormones on breast cancer risk in Denmark. International Journal of Cancer 42: 832–838
71. Kaufman DW, Miller DR, Rosenberg L et al 1984 Noncontraceptive estrogen use and the risk of breast cancer. Journal of the American Medical Association 252: 63–67
72. Yang CP, Daling JR, Band PR et al 1992 Noncontraceptive hormone use and risk of breast cancer. Cancer Causes and Control 3: 475–479

Index